Pathophysiology of Shock, Anoxia, and Ischemia

Editors

R Adams Cowley, M.D.

Director, Maryland Institute for Emergency
Medical Services Systems
Baltimore, Maryland

Benjamin F. Trump, M.D.

Chairman, Department of Pathology
University of Maryland School of Medicine
Baltimore, Maryland

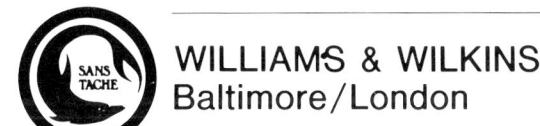

WILLIAMS & WILKINS
Baltimore/London

The Publishers have made every effort to trace the copyright holders for borrowed material. If they have inadvertantly overlooked any, they will be pleased to make the necessary arrangements at the first opportunity.

This monograph on cell injury in shock, anoxia, and ischemia was supported by a grant from The UpJohn Company, Kalamazoo, Michigan 49001.

Copyright ©, 1982
Williams & Wilkins
428 East Preston Street
Baltimore, MD 21202, U.S.A.

All rights reserved. This book is protected by copyright. No part of this book may be reproduced in any form or by any means, including photocopying, or utilized by any information storage and retrieval system without written permission from the copyright owner.

Made in the United States of America

Library of Congress Cataloging in Publication Data

Main entry under title:

Pathophysiology of shock, anoxia, and ischemia.

Includes index.
1. Shock. 2. Hypoxia. 3. Ischemia. 4. Physiology, Pathological. I. Cowley, R Adams, 1917- II. Trump, Benjamin F. [DNLM: 1. Shock—Physiopathology. 2. Anoxia—Physiopathology. 3. Ischemia—Physiopathology. QZ140 P296]
RB150.S5P37   616'.047   80-20637
ISBN 0-683-02149-4

Composed and printed at the
Waverly Press, Inc.
Mt. Royal and Guilford Aves.
Baltimore, MD 21202, U.S.A.

Dedication

This book is dedicated to three of the authors, Dr. Walter Sandritter, Dr. Lars-Erik Gelin, and Dr. Richard C. Lillehei, who died during the preparation of this book. These distinguished scientists will be remembered for their many contributions to this field.

The authors especially want to acknowledge the editorial assistance of Mrs. Cecily Orlando, Mrs. Elaine Adelberg, Mrs. Gloria Taylor, and Mrs. Sandra Minton.

Preface

This book represents one outcome of a long-term research and clinical collaboration between the editors. We came together about 10 years ago with similar goals but different approaches. One of us was focussing on the pathophysiology and treatment of shock, ischemia, and anoxia in patients while the other was primarily concerned with the effects of injury on cells and subcellular systems. This blend, between the cardiac surgeon and the cellular pathologist, has been an immense source of intellectual satisfaction to both of us and, we hope, a synergism that will advance the understanding of human disease. Clearly, the time is ripe for interdisciplinary collaboration of this kind. Our philosophy of shock is that if it can be anticipated, controlled, prevented, and treated, many human deaths can be prevented within the limits of current medical and surgical technology.

The primary goal of all biomedical research is the understanding and prevention of disease in man. The vast knowledge gained in the past few decades has been accomplished through comparison of human and animal data; evidence clearly indicates that even though cellular organization is basically the same throughout all living systems, important differences probably do exist. Although we need to study both experimental model systems and humans, it is often difficult or impossible to extrapolate data from the one to the other. Without model systems, however, it is impossible to know the relevance to human disease while, on the other hand, without studies of human diseases, it is impossible to achieve any progress concerning their prevention or modification. On this basis, we have recently stressed the need for much more experimentation using human tissues in culture (Trump and Harris, 1979) and at immediate autopsy (Cowley et al., 1979; Trump et al., 1973). Recent developments in the collection, transport, storage, culture, and xenotransplantation of human tissues have made the direct testing of important hypotheses in human tissues in vivo and in vitro quite possible by performing comparative studies on tissues from animals and transplantation into immunocompatible animals. This method of approach will not only be extremely helpful in the field of ischemia and anoxia but also in the areas of infectious disease, neoplasia, myocardial infarction, atherosclerosis, stroke, and environmental disease (Harris et al., 1980a and b).

Little information on humans in shock has been available except in time of war (Beecher, 1949). In 1960, under the auspices of the R & D Command of the Surgeon General and later the National Institutes of Health, a systemized effort to examine and observe the effects of shock and injury on man in a specialized facility was initiated, resulting in the establishment of a large physiological and biochemical data bank. This bank has been used by the authors and others to gain further insight and knowledge of the shock process and how this phenomena can be better diagnosed, managed, and treated in man.

While during the years many studies had, through animal experimentation, shed light on the shock process, it became apparent in our studies that shock, ischemia and anoxia represent multidisciplinary problems which required for solution not only the knowledgeable physician but also the basic scientist. As a result, the cell biologist, biochemist, engineer, mathematician, and others were assigned to the project. Many of the research efforts of this group soon became the standard for management and therapy, while at the same time, posed those questions which could not be obtained through the study of man alone, again necessitating our falling back to controlled animal experimentation either for verification or searching for newer techniques to treat the shock process. For example, the origin of the immediate autopsy to study fresh tissues and fluids required a public law, making a trauma victim the property of the State Medical Examiner's system and thereby relieving the physician of obtaining consent for autopsy. Thus, at the time of death, tissues are gathered and prepared for electron microscopic study. The use of this tool in our program is producing a quantum leap in the better understanding of the shock process not unlike when Virchow (1858) first applied the light microscope to a better understanding of cellular pathology in disease. As a result we are now able to apply this and a variety of related techniques to the study of the injured cell and to compare these findings with the biochemical and physiological studies found in life. It also offered comparison of surgical tissues obtained at biopsy with those found at death.

The purpose of this book is to present a comprehensive picture of the pathophysiology and treatment of shock, ischemia, and anoxia. We hope to cover the developments since the monograph edited by Mills and Moyer in 1965. It is hoped that this presentation will not only stimulate work in this field but will also serve as a background for practitioners, researchers, and students working in the area.

The book is organized into several sections which correspond to our concepts of the major problems in shock, ischemia, and anoxia. It is our philosophy that each section should have a summary that explains the relevance of the area. In the future, much or all of the research in this area should correlate human observations with animal models.

References

Beecher, H.K.: *Resuscitation and Anesthesia for Wounded Men; The Management of Traumatic Shock.* Charles C Thomas, Springfield, IL, 1949.

Cowley, R.A., Mergner, W.J., Fisher, R.S., Jones, R.T., and Trump, B.F.: The subcellular pathology of shock in trauma patients: Studies using the immediate autopsy. Am. Surg. 45: 255–269, 1979.

Harris, C.C., Trump, B.F., and Stoner, G.D. (Eds): Normal human tissue and cell culture. Respiratory, cardiovascular, and integumentary systems. In *Methods in Cell Biology*, vol. 21A. Academic Press, New York, 1980a.

Harris, C.C., Trump, B.F., and Stoner, G.D. (Eds.): Normal human and cell culture. Endocrine, urogenital, and gastrointestinal systems. In *Methods in Cell Biology*, vol. 21B, Academic Press, New York, 1980b.

Mills, L.C., and Moyer, J.H. (Eds.): *Shock and Hypotension: Pathogenesis and Treatment.* Grune & Stratton, New York, 1965.

Trump, B.F., and Harris, C.C.: Human tissues in biomedical research (editorial). Hum. Pathol. 10:245–248, 1979.

Trump, B.F., Valigorsky, J.M., Dees, J.H., Mergner, W.J., Kim, K.M., Jones, R.T., Pendergrass, R.E., Garbus, J., and Cowley, R.A.: Cellular change in human disease. A new method of pathological analysis. Hum. Pathol. 4: 89–109, 1973.

Virchow, R.: Die Cellularpathologie in ihrer Begrundung of physiologische und pathologische Gewebelehre. A Hirschwald, Berlin, 1858.

Contributors

Stephen M. Ayres, M.D.
Professor and Chairman
Department of Internal Medicine
St. Louis University School of Medicine
St. Louis Missouri

Jeffrey L. Barnes, Ph.D.
Department of Pathology
The University of Texas Health Sciences Center at San Antonio
San Antonio, Texas

Arthur E. Baue, M.D.
Professor and Chairman
Department of Surgery
Yale University School of Medicine
New Haven, Connecticut

Donald P. Becker, M.D.
Professor and Chairman
Division of Neurosurgery
Virginia Commonwealth University
Medical College of Virginia
Richmond, Virginia

Irene K. Berezesky, B.A.
Department of Pathology
University of Maryland School of Medicine
Baltimore, Maryland

Samuel P. Bessman, M.D.
Department of Pharmacology and Nutrition
University of Southern California School of Medicine
Los Angeles, California

John R. Border, M.D.
Department of Surgery
Erie County Comprehensive Health Care Center
The State University of New York at Buffalo
Buffalo, New York

Captain Mark E. Bradley, M.D., F.A.C.P.
Director, Hyperbaric Medicine Program Center
Naval Medical Research Institute
National Naval Medical Center
Bethesda, Maryland

Richard A. Brunswick, M.D.
Department of Surgery, Tulane University School of Medicine,
New Orleans, Louisiana

Yale H. Caplan, Ph.D.
Chief Toxicologist
Office of the Chief Medical Examiner
Baltimore, Maryland

Ernesto Carafoli, M.D.
Laboratorium für Biochemie
Eidgenössische Technische Hochschule Zürich
Zurich, Switzerland

Frank B. Cerra, M.D.
Department of Surgery
State University of New York at Buffalo
and The Buffalo General Hospital
Buffalo, New York

Irshad H. Chaudry, Ph.D.
Department of Surgery
Yale University School of Medicine
New Haven, Connecticut

Leland C. Clark, Jr., Ph.D.
Division of Neurophysiology,
Children's Hospital Research Foundation
Cincinnati, Ohio

Bill Coleman
Surgical Research Computer Facility
The Buffalo General Hospital
Buffalo New York

Karl A. Conger, Ph.D.
Department of Pathology
University of Alabama in Birmingham
Birmingham, Alabama

R Adams Cowley, M.D.
Director, Maryland Institute for Emergency Medical Services Systems
Baltimore, Maryland

Ingemar Dawidson, M.D., Ph.D.
Department of Surgery I, Sahlgrenska Sjukhuset
University of Goteborg
Goteborg, Sweden

R. Ben Dawson, M.D.
Director, Blood Bank and Transfusion Services
Division of Clinical Pathology
University of Maryland Hospital
Baltimore, Maryland

Nicholas DeClaris, Sc.D.
Maryland Institute for Emergency Medical
 Services Systems
Baltimore, Maryland

Robert H. Demling, M.D.
Department of Surgery
School of Medicine
University of California, Davis
Sacramento, California

A. A. Driedger, M.D., F.R.C.P.(C), F.A.C.P.
Department of Medicine
Victoria Hospital
London, Ontario, Canada

Thomas B. Ducker, M.D., F.A.C.S.
Professor and Head
Department of Neurosurgery
University of Maryland Hospital
Baltimore, Maryland

Walter Flamenbaum, M.D.
Chief, Renal Section
Boston Veterans Administration Center
Boston, Massachusetts

John T. Flynn, Ph.D.
Department of Physiology
Jefferson Medical College
Thomas Jefferson University
Philadelphia, Pennsylvania

Julio H. Garcia, M.D.
Departments of Pathology and Neurology
University of Alabama in Birmingham
The Medical Center
Birmingham, Alabama

Marc Gehr, M.D.
Renal Section
Boston Veterans Administration Center
Boston, Massachusetts

Lars-Erik Gelin, M.D., Ph.D., F.A.C.S., D.Sc.
Chairman, Department of Surgery I
University of Goteborg, Sahlgrenska Sjukhuset
Goteborg, Sweden

Michael Gross, M.D.
Renal Section
Boston Veterans Administration Center
Boston, Massachusetts

John R. Hankins, M.D.
Maryland Institute for Emergency Medical
 Systems Services
Baltimore, Maryland

Robert M. Hardaway, M.D.
Department of Surgery
Texas Tech University School of Medicine
El Paso, Texas

Lerner B. Hinshaw, Ph.D.
Veterans Administration Hospital
Oklahoma City, Oklahoma

R. Horn, M.D.
University of Freiburg
Freiburg, West Germany

Richard B. Hornick, M.D.
Chairman, Department of Medicine
Infectious Diseases Unit
University of Rochester School of Medicine
 and Dentistry
Rochester, New York

Jerome F. Hruska, M.D., Ph.D.
Department of Medicine
Infectious Diseases Unit
University of Rochester School of Medicine
Rochester, New York

John A. Jane, M.D., Ph.D.
Department of Neurosurgery
University of Virginia Hospital
Charlottesville, Virginia

Robert B. Jennings, M.D.
Professor and Chairman
Department of Pathology
Duke University Medical Center
Durham, North Caroline

Raymond T. Jones, Ph.D.
Department of Pathology
University of Maryland School of Medicine
Baltimore, Maryland

Myong Won Kahng, Ph.D.
Department of Pathology
University of Maryland School of Medicine
Baltimore, Maryland

Contributors

Allan M. Lefer, Ph.D.
Professor and Chairman
Department of Physiology
Jefferson Medical College
Thomas Jefferson University
Philadelphia, Pennsylvania

Richard C. Lillehei, M.D., P.A.
Department of Surgery
University Hospitals
Minneapolis, Minnesota

Richard Lindenberg, M.D.
Towson, Maryland

George E. Linhardt, Jr., M.D.
Department of Surgery
University of Maryland School of Medicine
Baltimore, Maryland

Česlovas Masaitis, Ph.D.
U.S. Army Ballistics Research Laboratory
Aberdeen Proving Ground, Maryland

Robert S. McCuskey, Ph.D.
Professor and Chairman
Department of Anatomy
School of Medicine
West Virginia University
Morgantown, West Virginia

Elizabeth M. McDowell, B. Vet. Med., Ph.D.
Department of Pathology
University of Maryland School of Medicine
Baltimore, Maryland

Rapier H. McMenamy, Ph.D.
Department of Biochemistry
The State University of New York at Buffalo
Buffalo, New York

Leena M. Mela, M.D.
Department of Physiology
Michigan State University
East Lansing, Michigan

Wolfgang J. Mergner, M.D., Ph.D.
Department of Pathology
University of Maryland School of Medicine
Baltimore, Maryland

Arthur V. Milholland, M.D., Ph.D.
Maryland Institute for Emergency Medical Services
    Systems
Baltimore, Maryland

Christian Mittermayer, M.D.
Head, Department of Pathology
Aachen Technical University
D-5100-Aachen, West Germany

James E. Muller, M.D.
Harvard Medical School
Boston, Massachusetts

Ferid Murad, M.D., Ph.D.
Department of Internal Medicine
School of Medicine
University of Virginia
Charlottesville, Virginia

Kazue Ozawa, M.D.
First Department of Surgery
Kyoto University Medical School
Kyoto, Japan

Joseph Ransohoff, M.D.
Professor and Chairman, Department of Neurosurgery
School of Medicine
New York University-Bellevue Medical Center
New York, New York

Keith A. Reimer, M.D., Ph.D.
Department of Pathology
Duke University Medical Center
Durham, North Carolina

V. Jayne Renner
Department of Pharmacology and Nutrition
University of Southern California
    School of Medicine
Los Angeles, California

Urs N. Riede, M.D.
Department of Pathology
University of Freiburg
Freiburg, West Germany

William C. Roberts, M.D.
Chief, Pathology Branch
National Heart, Lung, and Blood Institute
National Institutes of Health
Bethesda, Maryland

Peter Safar, M.D.
Resuscitation Research Institute
University of Pittsburgh
Pittsburgh, Pennsylvania

Walter Sandritter, M.D.
Director, Department of Pathology
University of Freiburg
Freiburg, West Germany

Thomas G. Saul, M.D.
Department of Neurosurgery
University of Maryland Hospital
Baltimore, Maryland

Mohammed M. Sayeed, Ph.D.
Department of Physiology
Loyola University Medical Center
2160 South First Avenue
Maywood, Illinois

Jutta Schaper, M.D.
Max-Planck-Institut für Physiol Klinische Forschung
Abterlung Experimentalische Kardiologie
Bad Nauheim
West Germany

Gunther Schmitt, M.D.
Renal Section
Boston Veterans Administration Center
Boston, Massachusetts

William Schumer, M.D.
Professor and Chairman, Department of Surgery
University of Health Sciences
The Chicago Medical School at Veterans Administration
    Hospital
North Chicago, Illinois

Clayton H. Shatney, M.D.
Director of Traumatology
Maryland Institute for Emergency Medical Services
    Systems
Baltimore, Maryland

William C. Shoemaker, M.D.
Department of Surgery, Harbor Medical Center
University of California at Los Angeles
Torrance, California

William J. Sibbald, M.D., F.R.C.P.(C)
Department of Medicine
Victoria Hospital
London, Ontario,
Canada

John H. Siegel, M.D.
Department of Surgery
The State University of New York at Buffalo
    and The Buffalo General Hospital
Buffalo, New York

Paul R. Sohmer, M.D.
Division of Blood Research, Department of the Army
Letterman Army Institute of Research
Presidio, California

Benjamin F. Trump, M.D.
Professor and Chairman
Department of Pathology
University of Maryland School of Medicine
Baltimore, Maryland

George W. Tyson, M.D.
Division of Neurosurgery
School of Medicine
University of North Carolina at Chapel Hill
Chapel Hill, North Carolina

Watts R. Webb, M.D.
Professor and Chairman
Department of Surgery
Tulane University School of Medicine
New Orleans, Louisiana

Robert F. Wilson, M.D., F.A.C.S.
Department of Thoracic Surgery
Harper Hospital
Detroit, Michigan

Harold F. Young, M.D.
Co-Director, Division of Neurosurgery
Medical College of Virginia
Virginia Commonwealth University
Richmond, Virginia

Contents

Preface vii
Contributors ix

Section 1. Basic Pathophysiology 1

Part 1. Cellular Injury and Metabolic Responses 3
Editors' Summary 3

Chapter 1. The Cellular and Subcellular Characteristics of Acute and Chronic Injury with Emphasis on the Role of Calcium
Benjamin F. Trump, Irene K. Berezesky, and R Adams Cowley 6

Chapter 2. On the Qualitative Dynamics of Cell Response to Injury
Nicholas DeClaris 47

Chapter 3. The Biphasic Hormonal Nature of Stress
Samuel P. Bessman and V. Jayne Renner 60

Chapter 4. Intermediary Metabolism
Myong Won Kahng 66

Chapter 5. Energy Metabolism
Kazue Ozawa 74

Chapter 6. Mitochondrial Function in Shock, Ischemia, and Hypoxia
Leena Mela 84

Chapter 7. Membrane Transport and the Regulation of the Cell Calcium Levels
Ernesto Carafoli 95

Chapter 8. Membrane Na^+-K^+ Transport and Ancillary Phenomena in Circulatory Shock
Mohammed M. Sayeed 112

Chapter 9. Ion and Water Shifts, Cellular
Keith A. Reimer and Robert B. Jennings 132

Chapter 10. Regulation and Roles of Cyclic Nucleotides
Ferid Murad 147

Part 2. Alterations in the Microcirculation 155
Editors' Summary 155

Chapter 11. Microcirculation—Basic Considerations
Robert S. McCuskey 156

Chapter 12. Vascular Mediators in Ischemia and Shock
Allan M. Lefer 165

Chapter 13. Microcirculation in Shock—Clinical Review
Watts R. Webb and Richard A. Brunswick 181

Chapter 14. Pathology and Pathophysiology of Disseminated Intravascular Coagulation Robert M. Hardaway	186

Section 2. Shock and Related Phenomena ... 199

Part 1. General Considerations ... 201
Editors' Summary ... 201

Chapter 15. Overview of Hemorrhagic Shock Irshad H. Chaudry and Arthur E. Baue	203
Chapter 16. Overview of Endotoxin Shock Lerner B. Hinshaw	219
Chapter 17. Human Response to Sepsis. A Physiologic Manifestation of Disordered Metabolic Control John H. Siegel, Frank B. Cerra, John R. Border, Bill Coleman, and Rapier H. McMenamy	235
Chapter 18. Multiple Systems Organ Failure Frank B. Cerra, John R. Border, Rapier H. McMenamy, and John H. Siegel	254
Chapter 19. Pathology and Pathophysiology of the Systemic Toxicants Carbon Monoxide and Cyanide Yale H. Caplan	270

Part 2. Organ Dysfunction in Shock ... 281
Editors' Summary ... 281

Chapter 20. Pathology and Pathophysiology of the Liver R Adams Cowley, John R. Hankins, Raymond T. Jones, and Benjamin F. Trump	285
Chapter 21. Human Pathology of the Gastrointestinal Tract in Shock, Ischemia, and Hypoxemia Christian Mittermayer and Urs N. Riede	301
Chapter 22. Pathology and Pathophysiology of the Exocrine Pancreas in Shock Raymond T. Jones and George E. Linhardt, Jr.	309
Chapter 23. Pathology and Pathophysiology of Acute Renal Failure—A Review Jeffrey L. Barnes and Elizabeth M. McDowell	324
Chapter 24. Treatment of Acute Renal Failure Marc Gehr, Michael Gross, Gunther Schmitt, and Walter Flamenbaum	341
Chapter 25. Pathobiology at the Alveolar Wall in Human Shock Lung Urs N. Riede, Christian Mittermayer, R. Horn, and Walter Sandritter	358
Chapter 26. Pulmonary Alveolarcapillary Permeability in Human Septic Respiratory Distress Syndrome William J. Sibbald and A. A. Driedger	372
Chapter 27. Treatment of the Adult Respiratory Distress Syndrome Stephen M. Ayres	387
Chapter 28. Humoral Factors and Lung Injury During Shock, Trauma, and Sepsis Robert H. Demling and John T. Flynn	395

Contents xv

Part 3. Current Therapy of Shock 409
Editors' Summary 409

Chapter 29. Resuscitation in Hemorrhagic Shock, Coma, and Cardiac Arrest
Peter Safar 411

Chapter 30. Pathophysiology and Therapy of Hemorrhage and Trauma States
William C. Shoemaker 439

Chapter 31. Transfusion Therapy in Hemorrhagic Shock
Paul R. Sohmer and R. Ben Dawson 447

Chapter 32. Plasma Expanders and Hemodilution in the Treatment of Hypovolemic Shock
Lars-Erik Gelin and Ingemar Dawidson 454

Chapter 33. The Use of Corticosteroids in the Therapy of Hemorrhagic Shock
Clayton H. Shatney 465

Chapter 34. General Treatment of Septic Shock
William Schumer 479

Chapter 35. Treatment of Infection in Septic Shock
Jerome F. Hruska and Richard B. Hornick 482

Part 4. Strategies for Future Diagnosis and Therapy 499
Editors' Summary 499

Chapter 36. Future Treatment of Shock
Robert F. Wilson 500

Chapter 37. Theoretical and Practical Considerations of Fluorocarbon Emulsions in the Treatment of Shock
Leland C. Clark, Jr. 507

Chapter 38. Hyperbaric Oxygen Therapy
Mark E. Bradley 522

Chapter 39. Mathematical Models
Česlovas Masaitis 528

Chapter 40. Design Principles and Objectives for Medical Registries and Other Computer Systems
Arthur V. Milholland 545

Section 3. **Injury of the Central Nervous System** 553

Editors' Summary 555

Chapter 41. Pathology of Head Injury
Richard Lindenberg 558

Chapter 42. Pathophysiology of Head Injury
George W. Tyson and John A. Jane 570

Chapter 43.	Treatment of Head Injury **Joseph Ransohoff**	601
Chapter 44.	Spinal Cord Injury **Harold F. Young and Donald P. Becker**	613
Chapter 45.	Treatment of Spinal Cord Injury **Thomas G. Saul and Thomas B. Ducker**	624

Section 4. Vascular Insufficiency ... 641
Editors' Summary ... 643

Chapter 46.	Pathology and Pathophysiology of Cerebral Ischemia **Julio H. Garcia and Karl A. Conger**	645
Chapter 47.	Cellular and Subcellular Changes in Myocardial Infarction **Wolfgang J. Mergner and Jutta Schaper**	658
Chapter 48.	Fatal Acute Myocardial Ischemia. An Analysis of the Extent of Coronary Narrowing at Necropsy **William C. Roberts**	681
Chapter 49.	Treatment of Myocardial Infarction **James E. Muller**	684
Epilogue.	Cultivating a Climate of Research. The Wangensteen System, 1930–1967 **Richard C. Lillehei**	701
Index		705

Section 1

Basic Pathophysiology

PART 1

CELLULAR INJURY AND METABOLIC RESPONSES

EDITORS' SUMMARY

The purpose of this portion of the book is to introduce the reader to some basic concepts of cellular and subcellular changes in ischemia, anoxia, and shock.

This section begins with a chapter by Trump et al. on cellular and subcellular injury, which presents an overview of cell and organelle reactions to injury as they occur in various human disease and experimental processes. The emphasis of the chapter is on the relationship between altered ion movements, especially calcium, and reversible or irreversible cell injury. Following either type of injury, the cell enters a series of stages which can be characterized morphologically, biochemically, and functionally. These stages have been compared in both human studies and experimental animal models. It is now possible to characterize both reversible and irreversible cell injury at the ultrastructural level. Future studies on metabolic and pharmacologic interventions will need to take this information into account, and hopefully it will be possible to find agents or conditions to modify and improve the cell response.

In his chapter on the dynamics of cell response to injury, DeClaris utilizes a systems approach to present the elements of his theory, which is distinctly different from traditional medical viewpoints. Utilization of this type of analysis may be extremely helpful in designing new experiments or in helping to analyze data from old ones. He suggests that the behavior of cells or physiological systems following injury can be described in terms of state variables and control variables and that improved methods of plotting or otherwise utilizing the data may be extremely important in understanding the processes involved. This approach promises to be more widely used in the future.

In their chapter on the biphasic hormonal nature of stress, Bessman and Renner have developed a fundamental hypothesis that there are two hormonal phases of stress: phase I, the catecholamine phase, and phase II, the peptide-steroid phase. Both are under the regulatory control of the CNS. Although the first phase is short and immediate, the second is more prolonged, with metabolic consequences lasting for several days. It is of interest to correlate these results with those in Chapter 1 by Trump et al., in which the massive autophagocytosis characterizing the chronic phase of shock in several organ systems is probably the proximate cell mechanism involved in much of this increased catabolism. Bessman also suggests that, in the future, attempts be made to design therapeutic interventions which modify the hormone response, since therapeutic efforts with insulin, anabolic steroids, and parenteral nutrition have little effect once the body is in this new steady state.

In the next series of chapters by Kahng, Ozawa, and Mela, various aspects of intermediary and energy metabolism are discussed. The central theme of these chapters is the basic importance of energy metabolism in the pathophysiology of hemorrhagic and septic shock as well as in the cellular consequences of vascular occlusion. The details of current knowledge concerning this metabolism are extensively reviewed. One central problem brought out in the chapter by Kahng is that, in contrast to many other animals, terrestrial vertebrates have a very limited capacity for anaerobiosis, especially in the CNS. Since very limited stores of available substrates such as glycogen are available, glucose is the principal substrate for the brain; even in other organs, however, glycogen stores often cannot be utilized effectively. In contrast to some other animals, only mammals have the pyruvate-lactate mechanism to lower reducing equivalents and to synthesize ATP anaerobically. Another peculiar aspect is the reduction of total nucleotides, especially the hydrolysis of AMP resulting from conversions of ATP and ADP. In fact, in some organ systems the destruction of AMP has the possibility of being a correlate of loss of reversibility. Rapid reconstitution of AMP for conversion to ADP and ATP during reflow or oxygenation is a complex process which may not always be completed properly. In this context, evidence is also presented in Chapter 1 that irreversible irreparable damage to mitochondria, especially their inner membrane, may be a limiting factor in whether or not the cells can recover. Most available evidence indicates that mitochondria are the site of alterations which render the cell irreversible.

Different tissues differ considerably in the rate at which these irreversible changes take place. The reasons for this are poorly understood but based on the information in these chapters they may well include differences in calcium metabolism, activity of phospholipases, availability of alternate substrate sources, and availability of alternate substrates. The brain, for example, is in a precarious position even during reflow since fatty acids cannot be utilized and glycogen is sparse. On the other hand, bronchial and pancreatic epithelium can survive up to 3 hr of total ischemia, even at body temperature. Obviously, the duration of survival is greatly modified by temperature; reduction of temperature to 0–4°C or even to room temperature is associated with markedly prolonged survival. Kahng also reviews some possible therapeutic interventions including modified substrates, membrane stabilizing compounds, inhibitors of total nucleotide breakdown, and modification of temperature, all of which deserve further consideration in this extremely difficult therapeutic area.

Ozawa's chapter also considers energy metabolism in hemorrhagic and septic shock. Interestingly, each is basically similar in terms of changing energy-producing pathways. This again re-emphasizes the probable role of mitochondria as limiting factors in cell survival. Moreover, septic shock, at least in experimental animals, has two distinct stages. These include an early stage in which oxidative phosphorylation is increased and a later stage in which it is markedly depressed. The later stage is similar to that seen in hemorrhagic shock and immediately precedes irreversible damage. This correlates very well with studies in our laboratory on human patients, which indicate similar changes in mitochondria and other organelles in the late stages. Ozawa also discusses the close correlation between hepatic energy charge and mortality rate in acute hemorrhagic shock and a strong negative correlation between volume of shed blood and energy charge. In Chapter 21, by Cowley et al., the possible central role of the liver is also discussed in the sense that animals with impaired liver function are much more susceptible to the effects of hemorrhagic shock.

In Chapter 6, Mela reviews the current literature on specific mitochondrial functional consequences of hypoxia, ischemia, and other circulatory deficits. Special emphasis is paid in the chapter to the relationship between the cause and effect, which is not always readily discernible in the case of mitochondrial changes. As discussed in Chapter 1, however, irreparable damage to the mitochondria during the ischemic phase probably explains the inability of tissues to recover even following reflow. Initially, mitochondrial membrane changes are reversible and this can even occur with membrane phospholipid modification. These changes may also imply alterations in membrane fluidity, intermembrane adhesions and fusions, and changes in the ability to maintain a proton gradient. It is also associated with defective ability to regulate cytosol calcium, which can be of great importance in many other calcium-mediated interactions (see Chs. 1 and 7). Initially, these changes are reversible in various organ systems, and it is interesting that incomplete ischemia followed by reflow can be even more damaging, possibly due to excessive formation of oxygen free radicals during the recirculation phase (see also Ch. 29). This has been related by some investigators to possible protective effects of barbiturate anesthesia. In a somewhat similar vein, mitochondrial functional impairment in septic shock occurs earliest in the brain, followed by liver, kidney, and very late in cardiac and skeletal muscle. This may again be due to alterations of blood flow though, at least in vitro, endotoxin is also directly damaging to mitochondrial membrane function. Both endotoxemia and anoxia affect regulation of intracellular calcium and the possible importance of a rise in intracellular ionized calcium is discussed here and in other chapters. The possible role of glucocorticoids in improving survival is also discussed. This may modify the microcirculation and may also more directly modify mitochondrial membrane function in septic shock. Whether or not direct effects of glucocorticoids can be observed in mitochondrial membranes is a significant question that needs further study.

Somewhat different mitochondrial changes in hypoxia or partial anoxia can occur, including partial adaptation. With partial acute hypoxia, the mitochondria increase their capacity to respire and synthesize ATP and with chronic hypoxia there are decrements in cytochrome oxidase and cytochrome b. In spite of this, mitochondrial respiratory capacities are very high. Indirect evidence suggests that the dehydrogenases are responsible for oxygen-induced control of respiratory activity and, through some unknown mechanism, activation of latent dehydrogenases may occur.

The chapter by Carafoli is a detailed review of the current state-of-the-art of regulation of cell calcium. Today there is increasing knowledge and concern about the probable role of ionized intracellular calcium regulation in a number of very important physiological and pathological phenomena. Many of these seem to be mediated through a recently discovered protein known as calmodulin, which has a rapidly increasing literature. In shock, ischemia, and anoxia, failure to regulate calcium by cell membranes, mitochondria, and endoplasmic reticulum may mediate many of the ultimately deleterious functions including damage to cell membranes through activation of phospholipases, modification of membrane fluidity, alteration of cytoskeleton with altered cell shape, contractility, cell division, formation and modification of prostaglandins, and modification of cell secretion. Thus, calcium regulation becomes an important focal point in these chapters and one which may be of increasing importance in the future in terms of therapeutic modification. Calcium levels are regulated by cell membrane extrusion systems, including sodium-calcium exchange at the cell surface, mitochondrial inner membrane transport and active transport systems in the endoplasmic reticulum. These work in concert with calcium-binding proteins in the cytosol and elsewhere of which calmodulin may be the most important (Means and Dedman, 1980).

In his chapter, Sayeed reviews the central role of membrane sodium-potassium transport in shock, ischemia, and anoxia. The plasmalemma sodium-potassium ATPase, which is inhibited by ouabain and other related cardiac glycosides in most cells, plays a key role in the maintenance of the intracellular environment. This transport system, which is energy-dependent, not only regulates sodium and potassium and, therefore, cell volume but, because of mechanisms such as the sodium-calcium exchange and other related exchange phenomena, also regulates intracellular calcium and a variety of other membrane transport systems. It is not surprising, therefore, that irreversible inhibition of this transport system, e.g., with ouabain or energy depletion, results in cell death (Ginn et al., 1968). Therefore, the effects of a variety of injuries either on the energy-generating systems of the cell or by toxic agents which interfere directly with the sodium-potassium pump can result in both reversible and irreversible cell injury. The pertinent literature relevant to this system is considered in detail in this chapter. So far there have been no therapeutic interventions designed to protect this pump or to modify its affinity for ATP. On the other hand, it is possible to develop ouabain-resistant mutants of mammalian cells with appropriate mutagens which would then make them much less susceptible to this particular toxin.

The chapter by Reimer and Jennings continues in the same context and stresses the pathophysiologic consequences of altered cell volume regulation. This involves not only parenchymal cells but also endothelium (see Chs. 26 and 27). Cell swelling of both can lead not only to altered intracellular metabolism but also to changes in the microcirculatory system (see Chs. 11–13). There is evidence that cell membrane regulation becomes limiting at the time of cell death, so "cause and effect" relationships between cell membrane function and irreversible changes in mitochondrial ATP generation remain moot. Membrane disruption actually occurs at or about the time of the "point-of-no-return"; the point-of-no-return may be induced by calcium-activated phospholipases. Membrane damage can also occur as a primary effect; for example, it occurs through the results of endotoxin and complement activation or as a result of direct acting toxins which affect membrane permeability. Such agents include mercury and other heavy metals. In this event, the sodium-potassium ATPase, even if an energy source is present, is unable to continue its regulation of cell ion composition and cell volume. There is also the possibility that membrane peroxidation during reflow could further accentuate weaknesses in the cell membrane, causing a harmful chain reaction (see Ch. 6). The disruption of the cell membrane at or about the time of cell death is presumed to be the basis of commonly used tests for cell viability such as staining with nigrosin or trypan blue.

The role of lysosomes in acute lethal cell injury requires more investigation. Wildenthal (1978) has recently reviewed the scientific and philosophical situation. Lysosomal enzymes may play a harmful role during the initiation phase and a beneficial function during the recovery or repair phases. The available evidence shows that the time course of lysosomal alterations parallels the evolution of irreversible ischemic damage as monitored by electron microscopy but, at the present time, does not permit a cause-and-effect relation to be established. Hawkins (1980) has also reviewed this entire subject recently.

The role of cyclic nucleotides is reviewed by Murad. Subsequent to their original discovery by Sutherland and Rall, it has become apparent that the cyclic nucleotides mediate a variety of hormone, toxin, and drug-induced responses in numerous tissues, the modification of which may be extremely important in cell injury. The details of these relationships are under continual study. More recently, cyclic GMP and cyclic AMP interactions have been related to a number of important cell changes, including regulation of calcium and cell division. Calcium, for example, is essential to cyclic GMP formation. An important additional site of regulation is control of the phosphodiesterase activity. Insulin, for example, increases the activity of this enzyme in liver. The role of increased cyclic AMP in the formation of numerous lysosomes in acute shock or following the administration of glucagon is discussed in Chapter 1. Similar increases in the same ratio occur with both human and experimental diabetes. The end result of autophagocytosis is increased lysosome formation with numerous residual bodies (see Ch. 3).

References

Ginn, F.L., Shelburne, J.D., and Trump, B.F.: Disorders of cell volume regulation. I. Effects of inhibition of plasma membrane adenosine triphosphatase with ouabain. Am. J. Pathol. *53*:1041–1071, 1968.

Hawkins, H.: In *Pathobiology of Cell Membranes*, vol. II, pp. 252–280. Academic Press, New York, 1980.

Means, A.R., and Dedman, J.R.: Calmodulin—an intracellular calcium receptor. Nature *285*:73–77, 1980.

Wildenthal, K.: Lysosomal alterations in ischemic myocardium: Result or cause of myocellular damage. J. Mol. Cell Cardiol. *10*:595–603, 1978.

CHAPTER 1

The Cellular and Subcellular Characteristics of Acute and Chronic Injury With Emphasis on the Role of Calcium

BENJAMIN F. TRUMP
IRENE K. BEREZESKY
R ADAMS COWLEY

The purpose of this chapter is to review current concepts on cell injury as they apply particularly to shock, ischemia, and anoxia. As will become evident during the development of this volume, all of these disease states are most meaningfully expressed at the cellular and subcellular levels, and these changes form the basis of the physiologic and morphologic changes that are observed. An analysis of the published investigations of the past 10 years reveals a unifying set of principles at the subcellular level which have begun to explain the fundamental basis of seemingly diverse disease states. In this initial chapter, we will consider how disease originates at the cell level as expressed by reactions of the cell to injury. For the most part, we will be considering injury to normally nondividing cells, but in some instances we will include cells that are capable of re-entry into the mitotic cycle following death or removal of adjacent cells. Many of the principles discussed apply to both populations; however, some additional types of damage involving cytoskeleton and macromolecular synthesis can have differential effects, especially on cells which are in the mitotic cycle. The latter is especially important in organs where continual cell replacement is occurring, such as in the epithelium of the gastrointestinal tract or in situations where regeneration is required to restore normal organ function, as in necrosis followed by regeneration of kidney tubules or hepatic parenchymal cells.

An injury applied to the cell, depending on the type, duration, and severity, may result in an acute, rapidly lethal injury followed by cell and tissue necrosis. With this type of injury, for example, after occlusion of a main vessel, the initial changes are not lethal but rather reversible. However, soon the cell passes the "point-of-no-return" or the point-of-cell-death, whereupon the degradative processes are collectively termed "necrosis" and the cell is converted to debris which ultimately reaches equilibrium with its environment. Such is the case in the central region of an acute myocardial infarction. On the other hand, a less severe injury such as partial ischemia or hypoxia results only in a reversible type of injury which sometimes leads to the cell acquiring a new steady state if the injury is prolonged. In the latter injury, the cell differs markedly from normal yet is able to continue its survival. Many examples of this type of injury occur in circulatory shock of various types. Either type of injury can cause death of the patient if not death of the cells involved depending on the significance of the site. For example, injuries to the myocardium which result in altered steady states cause loss of contractility. This can lead to death of the patient long before all of the myocardial cells die. Also, small areas of necrosis in critical parts of the brain can bring about brain death.

ACUTE LETHAL INJURY

Following an injury which will ultimately prove lethal, the reaction of the cell can be classified into two phases: a reversible phase which precedes the time of death (the point-of-no-return), and an irreversible phase consisting of those changes occurring after the death of the cell (Fig. 1.1). Therefore, the term acute lethal injury means that the injury will prove lethal in all cases if it is not removed prior to the point-of-no-return, a point beyond which the changes are irreversible.

Ischemia

One of the best examples of acute lethal injury in human disease as well as one of the best experimental

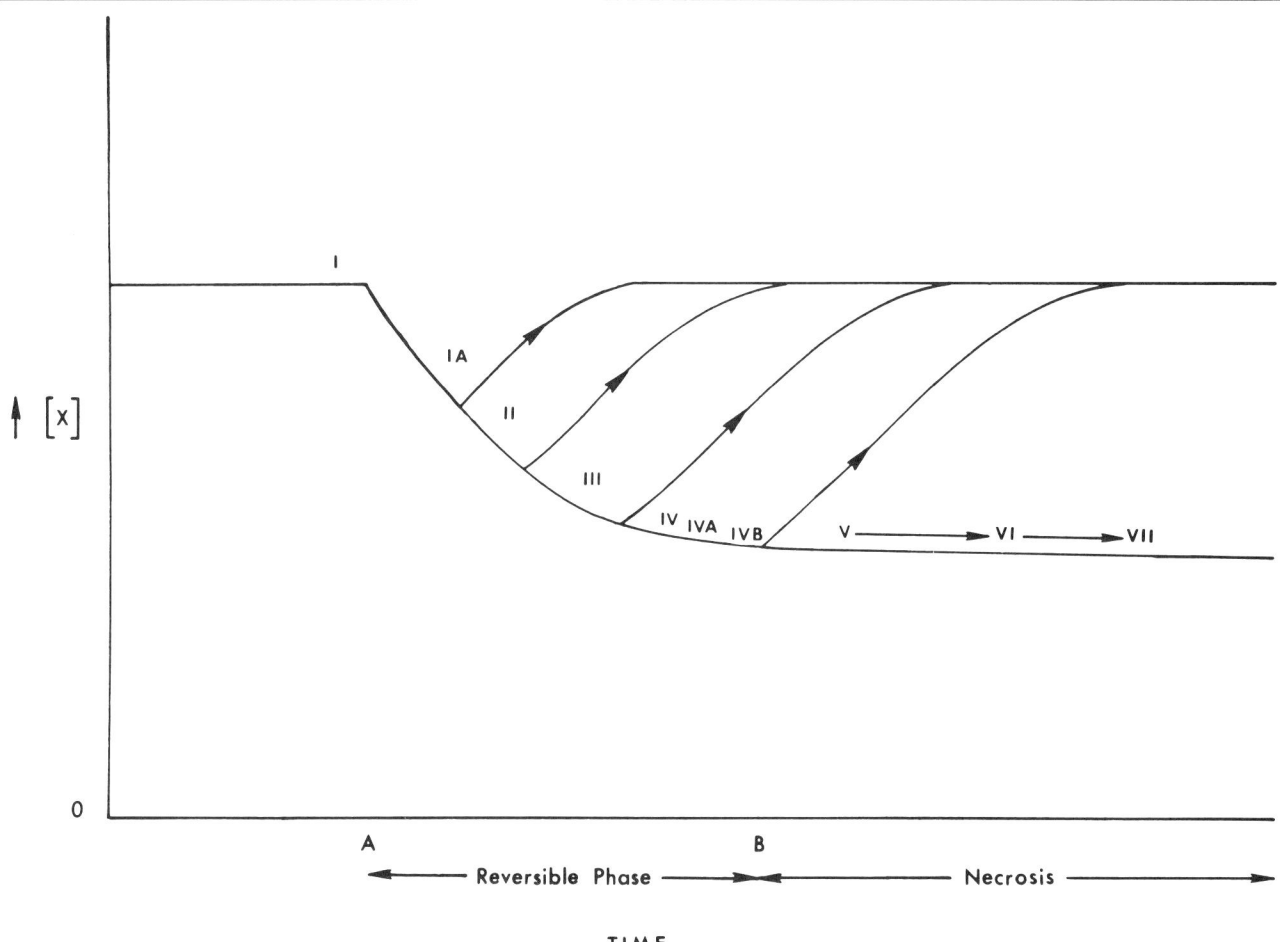

Figure 1.1. A diagram representing a conception of the effects of ischemic or anoxic injury on a cell. Plotted along the abscissa is time and along the ordinate, the level of homeostasis (X). The cell is injured at point A and becomes irreversible at point B. Roman numerals along the curve refer to the progression of stages during the reversible and irreversible phases. It should be noted that other types of injury such as direct membrane damage with complement or heavy metals results in mitochondrial calcifications in addition to the changes represented here (see text) and that the period of time from point A to point B varies depending upon the type of injury, temperature, etc.

models is acute total ischemia. Ischemia is produced by cessation of blood flow resulting in the combined effects of anoxia, lack of substrate, and absence of tissue perfusion. If complete, ischemia results in death of 100% of the cells in the affected region in a length of time varying from minutes to hours depending on such factors as temperature, magnitude of anaerobic glycolysis, availability of stored substrate (usually in the form of glycogen), and other undetermined factors. In the kidney proximal tubule, at 37°C, the time to the point-of-no-return is between 1 and 2 hr (Kahng et al., 1978); in the liver, it is approximately the same; in the bronchial epithelium and pancreas (Jones et al., 1975), it approximates 3 hr. In contrast, at 0–4°C, it approximates 24–48 hr in the kidney (Kahng et al.), 1 week in the bronchial epithelium, and perhaps 2 weeks in the mammary epithelium (Barrett et al., 1977).

These same interactions can be simulated in model cell systems by utilizing conditions which interfere with respiration and glycolysis or with respiration in the absence of substrate. Detailed studies from our laboratory on the effects of inhibitors such as cyanide or antimycin A and the effects of anoxia in the presence of glycolytic inhibitors or in the absence of glucose in the medium have been performed on in vitro isolated toad bladders (Saladino and Trump, 1968; Saladino et al., 1969; Croker et al., 1970), isolated flounder kidney tubules (Trump and Bulger, 1968a and b), Ehrlich ascites tumor cells (EATC) (Laiho and Trump, 1974a and b, 1975a and b; Trump and Laiho, 1975), and Hela cells (Arstila et al., 1971).

What is the sequence of changes during the reversible phase prior to the point-of-no-return? What happens at the point-of-no-return and what are the changes during the phase of necrosis? Moreover, is it possible to devise therapeutic interventions that would modify this progression in a favorable direction, and, if so, would such modifications affect clinical injury at the patient level?

STAGES OF CELL INJURY

In our laboratory, based on an extensive series of studies in a variety of cell types and species, it appears that a sequence of changes at the subcellular level following injury progress through a series of stages, beginning with the normal cell and ending with the necrotic cell. Although the rate of progression varies in many different cell types and with many different types of injury, the end point (namely stage V or Vc) remains the same. Therefore, for the purpose of convenience of notation, these stages have been documented in several previous publications (Trump and Ginn, 1969; Trump and Arstila, 1975; Trump and Mergner, 1974; Trump et al., 1974a). Additional data have necessitated some modifications and although these have been recently described in detail elsewhere (Trump et al., 1980a), we will again review them here in order to provide the reader with sufficient detail to facilitate easy comprehension of our concepts concerning cell injury.

Stage I is a normal cell with normal appearance and relationships of organelles (Fig. 1.2). Following lethal injury, progression through stages II-VII occurs. In the first stage, an injury such as ischemia results in a sudden decrease in the oxygen tension within the extracellular fluid and the cell. Because of the rapid fall in oxygen tension, the cell seems to attempt to maintain its homeostasis by using very rapid feedback control mechanisms. Such control mechanisms involve changes in ion concentrations as well as in various coenzymes and regulation of enzyme activities. As the oxygen concentration falls, mitochondrial phosphorylation decreases rapidly and contraction of the inner mitochondrial compartment begins. The drop in cellular ATP is believed to stimulate the activity of phosphofructokinase (PFK) in many cells which results in an increased rate of anaerobic glycolysis, assuming an ample supply of glycogen is present. This accelerated glycolysis leads to the accumulation of lactate which, together with the increased inorganic phosphate from ATP hydrolysis, soon reduces the intracellular pH. Since the circulation has ceased, metabolites such as lactate and hydrogen ions also tend to accumulate as well in the extracellular microenvironment, depressing the extra- as well as the intracellular pH. This decreased pH appears to be protective in that it has a stabilizing affect on the cell membrane (Penttila and Trump, 1974, 1975a–c; Penttila et al., 1976). The change in intracellular pH is probably reflected by the rapid clumping of nuclear chromatin (*stage IA*) which occurs very rapidly but which is clearly reversible. This change could also result from loss of bound K, which also occurs very quickly. Clumping of nuclear chromatin is known to be associated with decreased nuclear RNA synthesis. However, this is of no immediate consequence to the cell since, if circulation is not restored, the cell will die and undergo necrosis long before the decreased RNA synthesis has any significant effect. In addition to nuclear chromatin clumping and reduction in glycogen, cells in stage IA also show the disappearance of mitochondrial matrical granules as seen after glutaraldehyde-osmium fixation and Epon embedment. Meanwhile, the cell also begins to show the effects of the reduced ATP concentration. Among the consequences of the fall in ATP concentration is a decrease in the activity of the ion pumps at the cell membrane that leads to movements of sodium, potassium, calcium, and magnesium down their concentration gradients. Using x-ray microanalysis, such ion shifts are seen as early as 10 min following ischemia (Osornio et al., 1980) and probably occur even prior to that.

One of the earliest ultrastructural changes which can be seen in cells after a variety of acute lethal injuries is enlargement in the volume of the endoplasmic reticulum (ER) that is reflected in electron micrographs as dilatation of the cisternae (*stage II*) (Fig. 1.3). This initial change can be correlated with increased Na and decreased potassium content of the cell and often with increased water content, although studies by Laiho and Trump (1974a and b) indicate that significant dilatation of the ER can sometimes occur even with decreased total cell volume. The implied mechanism is intracellular redistribution of ions and water. This stage is clearly reversible and occurs before the point-of-no-return. Also in stage II, cell surface changes in the form of protrusions or "blebs" commonly begin to appear. These alterations in cell shape appear to reflect acute changes in the microtubules and microfilaments whose normal function is to maintain cell shape. Recent data have implied that lack of control of cell calcium levels during this phase, probably through effects on the cytoskeleton, may result in these changes (Trump et al., 1978c, 1979e). In addition, alterations in the inner membrane-associated magnesium-dependent ATPase can be seen (Mergner et al., 1972, 1977b and c, 1979). As the pH continues to drop in the cytosol, it is probable that inhibition of PFK occurs, with a gradual decrease in the rate of glycolysis, tending to stabilize the glycogen levels at low but significantly greater than zero values. The fall in cellular ATP concentration continues and ADP rises. This decreased ATP concentration begins to be reflected by decreased functions of the various energy-requiring systems such as protein synthesis, ion pumps at the cell surface, and most probably ion accumulation by mitochondria which begin to undergo shrinkage of the inner compartment.

In *stage III*, which can occur very rapidly, the mitochondria appear dense, showing marked condensation of the inner compartment and enlargement of the space between the inner and outer membranes of the envelope and the intracristal space (Fig. 1.4). This is associated with dilatation of the ER and the cell sap, both of which correlate with the gradual increases in Na and water contents as well as with decreases in potassium and magnesium. Loss of potassium and calcium from mitochondria inner compartments could result in shrinkage of that structure, while movements into the ER could explain the dilatation of such cisternae. Decreased po-

Cellular and Subcellular Characteristics

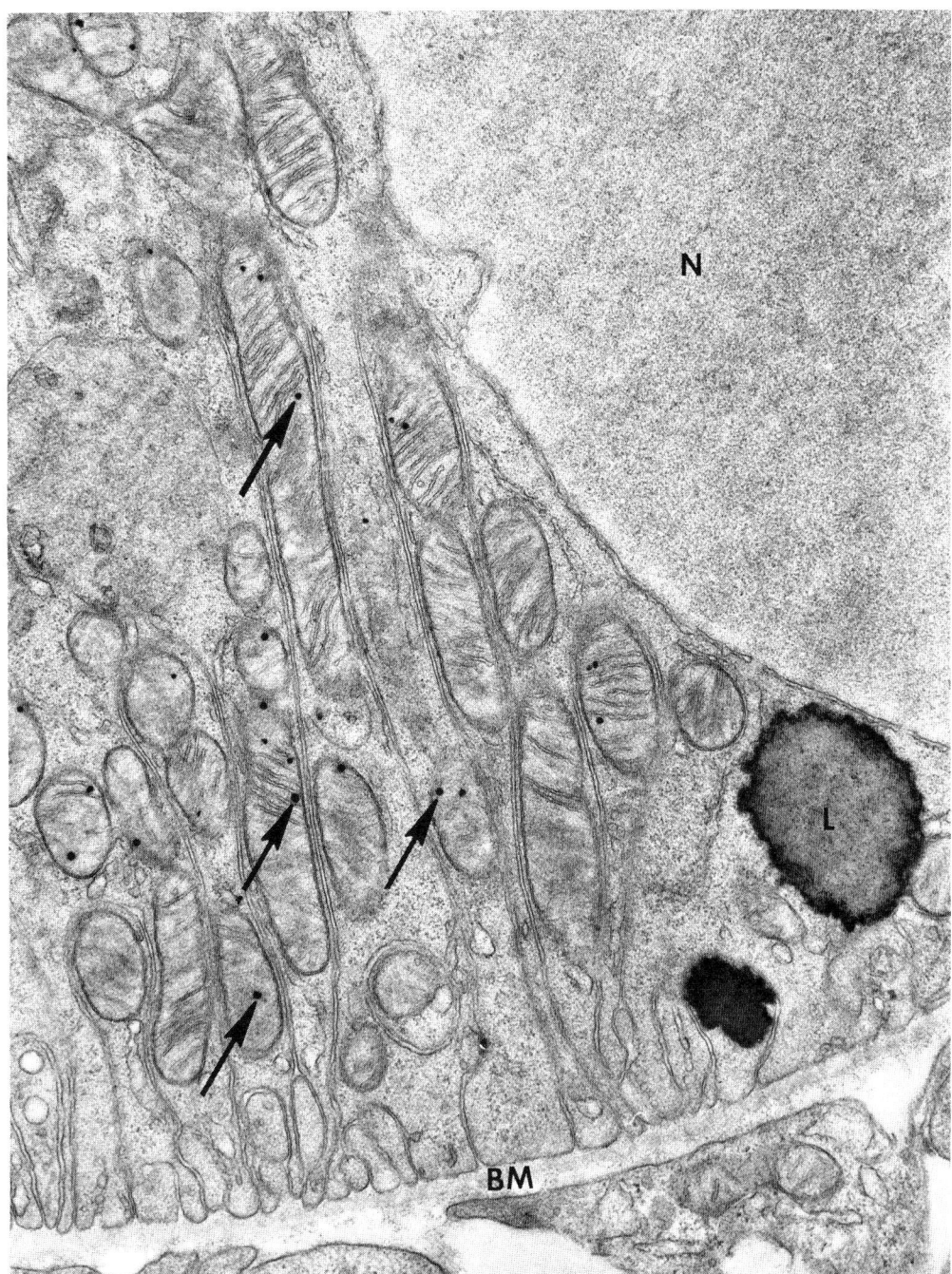

Figure 1.2. *Stage I.* Control rat proximal convoluted tubule cell fixed with 1% OsO$_4$ in Millonig's phosphate buffer. The elongated mitochondria are in orthodox conformation and most contain several prominent matrix granules (*arrows*). The nucleus (*N*) appears homogeneous with even distribution of chromatin. *L*, lipid droplet; *BM*, basement membrane. ×23,000. (Reprinted with permission from B. F. Trump and J. L. E. Ericksson: Laboratory Investigation *14:*1245–1323, 1965.)

tassium content is also a factor which is associated with inhibited protein synthesis, although at this stage the membrane-bound polysomes usually appear unaltered and maintain both their ordered arrangements and their membrane attachments (see Ch. 8 for early changes in acute renal failure). The increased water content at this stage is often reflected by the presence of blebs at the cell surface, although the latter may also involve modulations of the cytoskeleton. Mitochondrial function is inhibited because of the continued lack of oxygen and, as a consequence, ATP and now ADP levels are low (Kahng et al., 1978). If cells in this stage are restored to

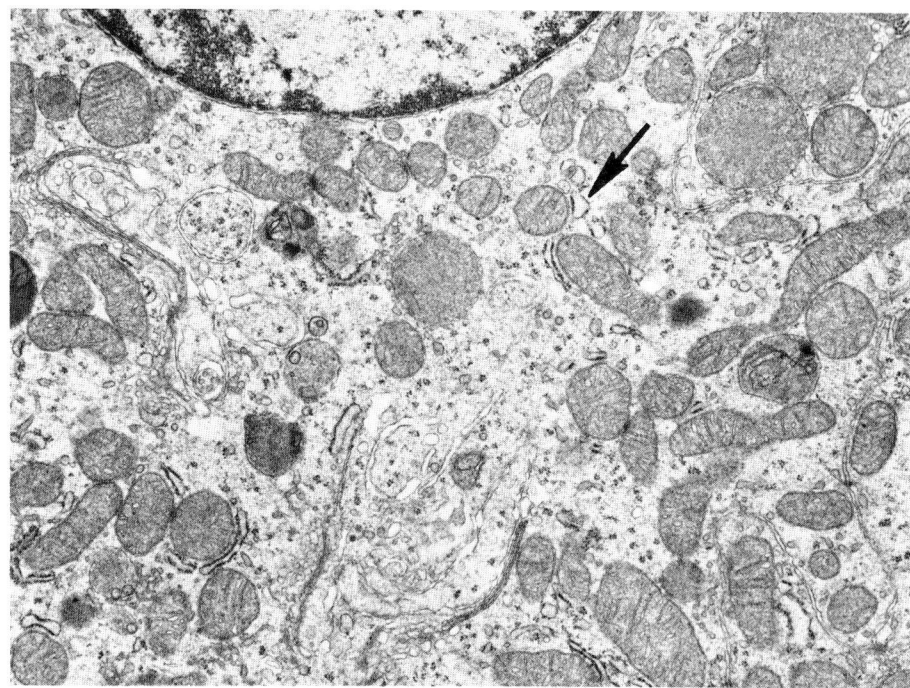

Figure 1.3. *Stage II.* Rat proximal pars recta tubule cell following 15 min of in vivo ischemia. Mitochondrial matrices are slightly condensed, the rough ER is beginning to show slight dilatation (*arrow*), and there is some clumping of the nuclear chromatin. ×10,000.

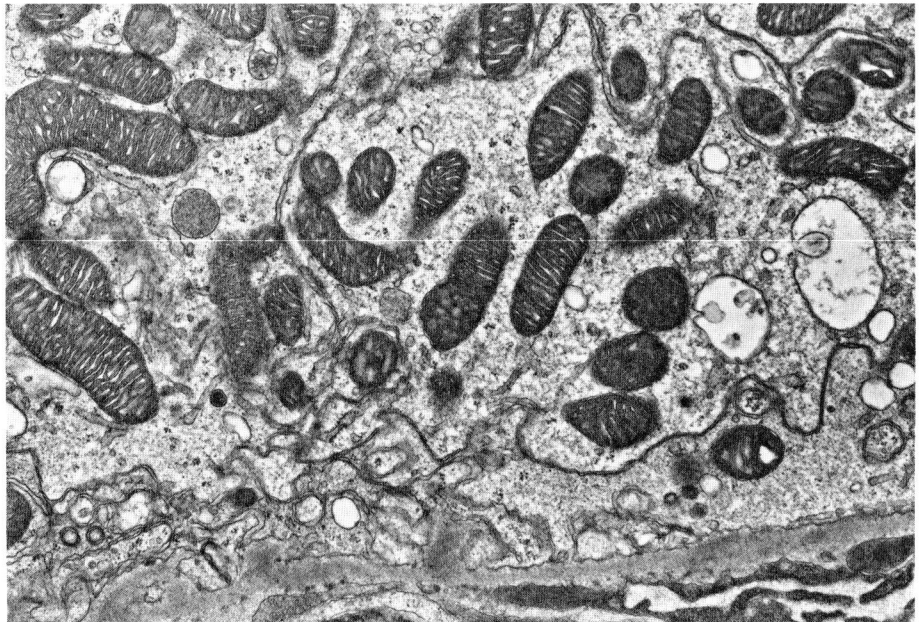

Figure 1.4. *Stage III.* Rat proximal convoluted tubule cell following 15 min of in vivo ischemia. The mitochondria show condensation of their inner compartments with increased density of the matrices and expansion of intracristal spaces. ×10,000.

normal conditions, the mitochondrial inner compartments re-expand, the ER cisternae contract, and the cells extrude sodium and calcium along with water and chloride. Therefore, although the mitochondria are temporarily although dramatically changed in form, they retain their ability to respire and phosphorylate as well as the ability to regain their normal internal compartment volume following restitution of a normal microenvironment both in vivo and in vitro. At this stage, protein synthesis remains severely inhibited and both free and bound polysomes are present as monosomes, some of which maintain their membrane attachments. The cell sap is swollen because of the increased water content. The lysosomes have a clear matrix and are often swollen, although significant macromolecular sized leaks in the lysosomal membranes apparently do not occur. At present, it is not clear whether the release of lysosomal hydrolases to the cytosol plays a significant role in this or later stages.

In *stage IV*, the transition across the point-of-no-return appears to begin. Here, some mitochondria begin to show high amplitude swelling, which seems to indicate initially reversible and later irreversible loss of the inner membrane function. As a result, some mitochondrial profiles show high amplitude inner compartment swelling while others remain condensed (Fig. 1.5). In some cells, such as renal tubular epithelium where two or more inner compartments are present in a given mitochondrion, one compartment may be condensed while others are swollen (Glaumann and Trump, 1975; Glaumann et al., 1975; Trump et al., 1974b; Kahng et al., 1978). The remaining organelles resemble those seen in stage III. This series of membrane permeability changes involving both the mitochondria and the cell membrane probably reflects basic chemical as well as structural modifications in the molecular architecture. The mitochondrial swelling is probably associated with the increased content of sodium and calcium in the inner compartments, although the precise ionic composition of the mitochondria probably depends upon that of the cytoplasm. Among the factors which may result in this structural damage to the mitochondrial inner membrane is the continued magnesium deficiency and the destruction of phospholipids and release of fatty acids. The role of changes in membrane fluidity is not known but may be important. Mitochondrial membranes possess endogenous phospholipases which can be activated by factors such as increased levels of calcium known to be present at this time (Goracci et al., 1978).

In *stage IVA*, in addition to the alterations mentioned above, all mitochondria are swollen with inner compartments expanded (Fig. 1.6). In *stage IVB*, not only are all mitochondria swollen but some also contain tiny dense aggregates (Fig. 1.7). These may represent early, reversible protein denaturation (Lehninger, 1970). This stage was recently described by Glaumann et al. (1977a and b) in proximal tubules from the pars convoluta of rat kidney following 30 and 60 min of ischemia. Both of these stages, however, are still capable of being resuscitated. Also, some membrane fusions or adhesions may be seen (see below). We still do not know whether all mitochondria are reversible or only the ones that do not have the tiny dense aggregates. In any case, the cells do survive.

In *stage V*, all mitochondria exhibit massive swelling and show marked increases in inner membrane permeability associated with loss of proteins, including matrical enzymes and cofactors to the cell sap, and ultimately through the cell membrane to the extracellular space. Cell sap enzymes are probably lost before mitochondrial or other organelle enzymes and the sum of adenosine nucleotides is only a small fraction of normal (Kahng et al., 1978). Also at this stage, prominent, large flocculent densities appear in the inner compartment, presumably the result of denaturation of matrix proteins (Fig. 1.8). Cells are swollen and the membranes of the cytocavitary

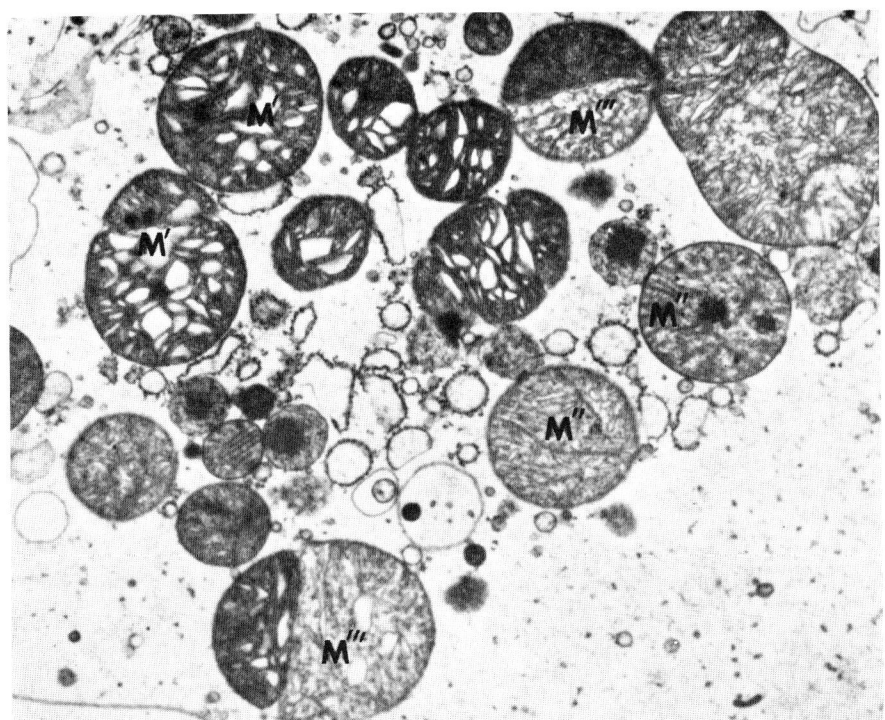

Figure 1.5. Rat proximal convoluted tubule cell from a slice incubated in Robinson's buffer at 4°C for 48 hr showing three types of mitochondria. In the first type (M'), the matrix is markedly condensed with expansion of intracristal spaces and flocculent densities. In the second type (M''), the inner compartments are expanded and contain flocculent densities. In the third type (M'''), both types of changes are present in the same mitochondrion, indicative of *Stage IV*, although those with flocculent densities may not be reversible. ×13,000. (Reprinted with permission from B. F. Trump, J. M. Strum, and R. E. Bulger: Virchows Archiv. B. Cell Pathology *16*:1–39, 1974b.)

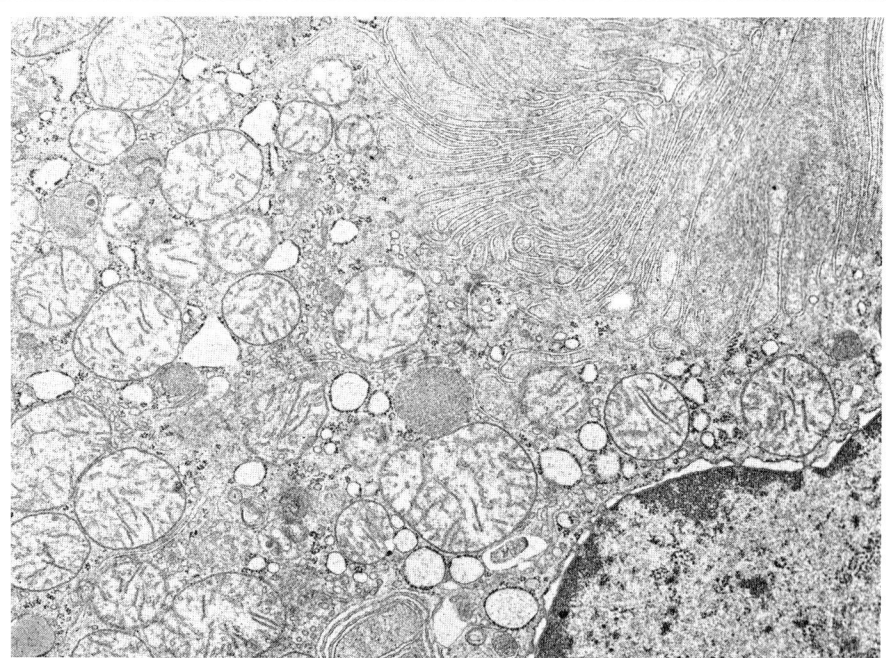

Figure 1.6. *Stage IVA.* Rat proximal pars recta tubule cell following 30 min of in vivo ischemia. Mitochondria show high amplitude swelling of their inner compartments. The rough ER is dilated, the nucleus shows chromatin clumping, and the microvilli are swollen and closely packed together. ×13,000. (Reprinted with permission from B. Glaumann and B. F. Trump: Virchows Archiv. B. Cell Pathology *19:*303–323, 1975.)

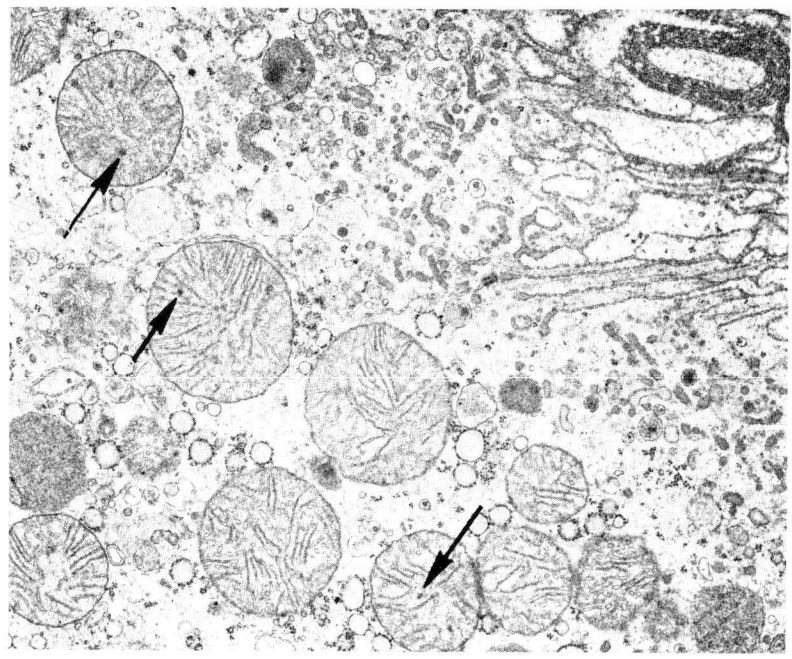

Figure 1.7. *Stage IVB.* Rat proximal convoluted tubule cell following 60 min of in vivo ischemia. The mitochondria are rounded with swollen inner compartments and some contain tiny dense aggregates (*arrows*). ×16,800. (Reprinted with permission from B. Glaumann, H. Glaumann, I. K. Berezesky, and B. F. Trump: Virchows Archiv. B. Cell Pathology *19:*281–302, 1975.)

network are fragmented. Distortion of intracellular membrane systems with whorl-like configurations often can be seen at the cell surfaces. Chromatin begins to undergo enzymatic attack and in later stages is completely dissolved (karyolysis), presumably by the combined action of proteolytic enzymes and DNase. Lysosomes continue to swell, as evidenced by increased size, clarification of the matrix, and condensation of the contents. The lysosomal swelling may result in hydrolase leak. In some cells, calcifications of the inner mitochondrial compartments can be seen consisting of amorphous calcium phosphate or crystalline deposits of hydroxyapatite along the inner membrane (Fig. 1.9).

In *stage VI*, the changes are mainly characterized by a rapid acceleration in the rate of digestion of intracellular constituents as measured by marked increases in free fatty acids, free amino acids, inorganic phosphorous, and decreases in phospholipids, triglycerides, protein, DNA, and RNA. This is reflected morphologically by continuing karyolysis and changes in the staining pattern of the cytoplasm. There is evidence that, at this stage, the lysosomal contents can escape into the cytosol and,

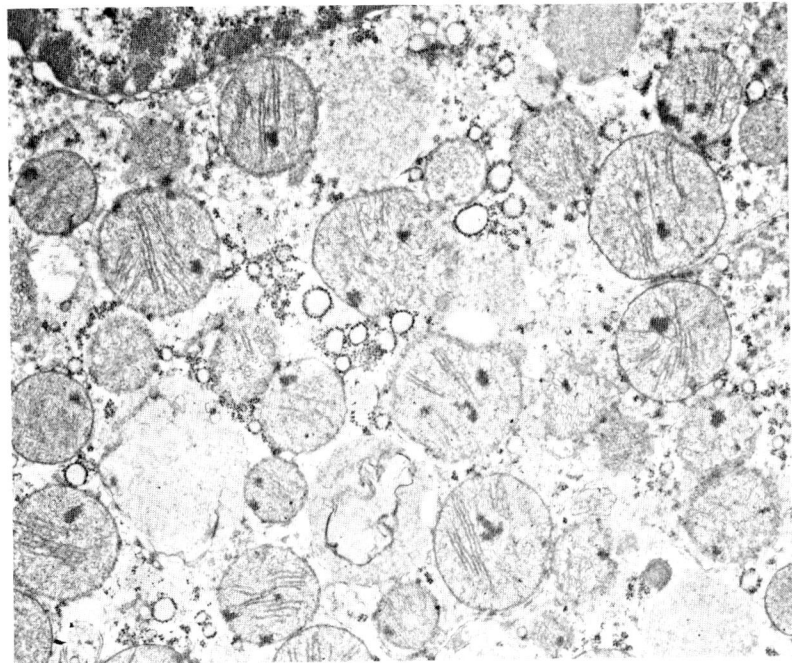

Figure 1.8. *Stage V.* Rat proximal convoluted tubule cell following 60 min of in vivo ischemia. All mitochondria are swollen and contain large flocculent densities, the hallmark of irreversibility. ×15,000.

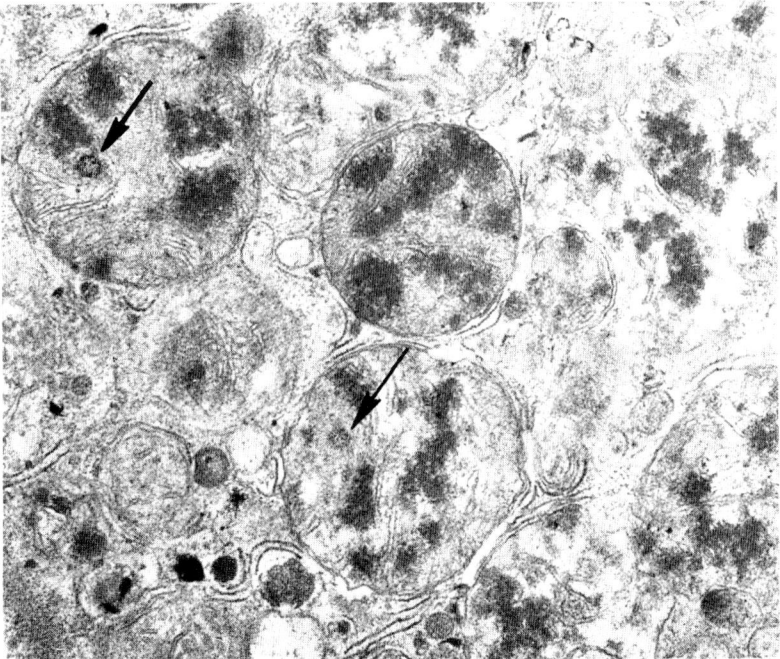

Figure 1.9. *Stage Vc.* Rat proximal convoluted tubule cell after 120 min of in vivo ischemia followed by 24 hr of reflow. Mitochondria are swollen and contain large flocculent densities and occasional calcifications (*arrows*). ×22,000. (Reprinted with permission from B. F. Trump, I. K. Berezesky, K. U. Laiho, A. R. Osornio, W. J. Mergner, and M. W. Smith: Scanning Electron Microscopy 2:437–462, 1980a.)

indeed, the disappearance of the macromolecular components of the cell as well as the persistence of lysosomal hydrolases as compared with the many other enzymes strongly indicates that lysosomal leakage is followed by digestion. Other membrane systems show dramatic rearrangements including vesiculation, wrappings, formation of tubular forms in the inner compartment of the mitochondria, disappearance of ribosomes from the ER membrane surface, alterations in the nucleolus, disappearance of microbody matrices, and frequent visualization of breaks in the plasma membrane contour (Fig. 1.10).

In stage VII, in spite of the fact that the cell is virtually completely degraded, new structures in the cytoplasm occur as large dense inclusions composed of dense, homogeneous, osmiophilic material with lamellar regions in lacunae within bodies or at the margins of the bodies. These periodic regions resemble stacks of membranes, although the fine structure within the bodies has not been discerned. However, they probably correspond to the myelin of Virchow, so named because of the resemblance to the bodies which Virchow described following autolysis in various cell types, especially the CNS. In

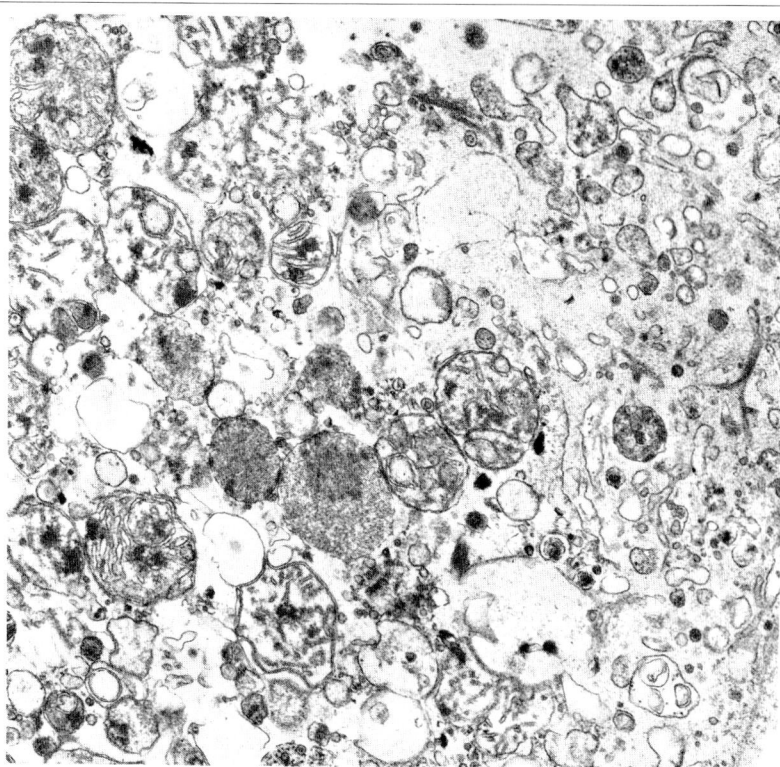

Figure 1.10. Rat proximal pars recta tubule cell after 60 min in vivo ischemia followed by 24 hr of reflow. Disrupted organelles are seen with swollen mitochondria containing large flocculent densities. Note that there are no epithelial cells lining the basement membrane. ×21,000. (Reprinted with permission from B. Glaumann and B. F. Trump: Virchows Archiv. B. Cell Pathology *19*:303–323, 1975.)

general, at this stage, most enzymatic activity has approached zero activity. Unless other sources of enzymes such as those produced by microorganisms are present, the cells are stabilized for long periods of time in this stage. However, equilibration once again occurs during this phase when the extracellular fluid pH approaches physiological levels. Greater and greater calcium binding by these cells is observed, possibly related to the change in pH as well as to changes in relative protein sites. How much of the calcium binding is mitochondrial is not known. At this stage, this type of calcification is often, however, extensive (dystrophic calcification) and it is almost certainly not energy-dependent.

COMMENTS ON THE STAGES

As mentioned above, the rate of progression through these stages varies dramatically in different cell types and with different types of injury. We do not yet know all of the reasons for this variation. For example, stage III is extremely variable. In hypoxic EATC (Trump and Laiho, 1975) or renal cortical slices at 0–4°C (Kahng et al., 1978; Trump et al., 1974b), stage III is prominent, as it also is with acute cell membrane damage by organic mercurials (Penttila and Trump, 1975a and c) or complement (Hawkins et al., 1972). On the other hand, this stage is absent or very transient in acute total ischemia of rat kidney (Glaumann and Trump, 1975; Glaumann et al., 1975), dog (Trump et al., 1976b and d) or rat myocardium (Osornio et al., 1980), human or rat pancreas (Jones et al., 1975), and human or hamster bronchus (Barrett et al., 1977). Both smooth and skeletal muscle also represent special cases, possibly based on their remarkable capacity for anaerobic glycolysis (Paul et al., 1979). We are currently investigating the former for its possible relationship to hypertension and atherosclerosis. Hochachka (1980) has recently re-examined some remarkable adaptations to anoxia in lower forms. In some situations, flocculent densities and presumably irreversibility can occur in this stage.

In addition, recent studies in our laboratories have necessitated modifications of stages IV and V. In proximal tubules from the pars convoluta of rat kidney following 30 and 60 min of ischemia, all mitochondria not only appear swollen (indicative of stage IVA) but some contain tiny dense aggregates (Glaumann et al., 1977a). These alterations were classified into stage IVB. Since these changes were compatible with the apparently complete recovery seen in the cortex, it was inferred that this stage was also a reversible one. The tiny dense aggregates are believed to represent reversible denaturation of matrix proteins in the mitochondria; it is well known that protein denaturation is initially reversible (Lehninger, 1970). Moreover, Majno et al. (1960) reported reversibility of protein denaturation prior to the point-of-no-return in light scattering studies of tissue slices following ischemic injury.

In stages III, IV, and V, under certain conditions, altered cells do occur in which there is calcification of mitochondria in addition to the other changes mentioned. These have been classified as stages IIIc, IVc, and Vc. This modification does not occur with total ischemia or chemicals which inhibit respiration or oxidative phosphorylation but does appear after ischemia followed by reflow (Glaumann et al., 1977a and b) or after lethal injury with membrane-damaging agents such as complement and antibody (Hawkins et al., 1972), amphotericin B (Saladino et al., 1969), penetrating or nonpenetrating mercurials (Gritzka and Trump, 1968; Sahaphong and Trump, 1971), inhibition of the sodium-potassium ATPase with ouabain (Ginn et al., 1968), and direct mechanical damage (Trump et al., 1974b).

Different cell types do not reach the irreversible stage V at the same time interval. For example, totally ischemic rat renal proximal tubule cells require approximately 1–2 hr (Glaumann and Trump, 1975; Glaumann et al., 1975), while hamster and human bronchial epithelia require over 3 hr (Barrett et al., 1977; Trump and Harris, 1979). The ambient temperature of the cells during the injurious process also has obvious relevance to the rate of change through these stages. Kidney cells at 37°C progress to stage V in 1–1.5 hr, while at 4°C, this same progression requires over 48 hr (Kahng et al., 1978). Similarly, at 0–4°C, human bronchus and mammary epithelia survive for over 1 week (Barrett et al., 1977).

Another stage modification is that of mitochondrial membrane fusions and adhesions. In acute myocardial infarction in the rat, and to some extent also in acute ischemia of the rat kidney, the mitochondrial inner membranes exhibit early fusions and adhesions, resulting in the formation of intracristal or intermembrane helical arrays with a periodicity of 15 nm (Osornio et al., 1980). These fusions typically appear in large numbers during early time intervals following occlusion and tend to decline and disappear in the later intervals (Fig. 1.11). Although the nature of these inner membrane fusions is not presently known, we speculate that they represent the effect of a calcium-induced phospholipase action with the release of membrane-fusing agents such as fatty acids or lysophosphatides or some direct action of calcium itself. In the same context, Sun et al. (1978) noted that the calcium-induced fusion of phosphatidylserine vesicles was temperature dependent with a peak in the region of 11°C. As the time after injury increased, the inner membrane fusions decreased in frequency. This could mean that completion of the fusion, as in fusion of secretory vesicles with the cell membrane, causes a return to a trilaminar membrane. It is essential to distinguish between membrane fusion and membrane adhesion. The word fusion implies a melting together, blending, or coalescence. This term is therefore used when two membranes (here the inner membranes) come together, usually on the outer side to produce a new membranous structure that is less than twice the thickness of the original membranes added together. The unusual result is a pentalaminar structure. The word adhesion means adhering or sticking together. Thus, this term is used when two membranes come into proximity, often with a thin intervening macromolecular layer. In the mitochondria, this change seems most often to occur between the inner membranes on the matrical sides, apparently representing an extreme form of inner compartment condensation. Such a phenomenon was described by Wakabayashi and Green (1977) in mitochondria in vitro.

In muscle, intermembrane mitochondrial inclusions have been observed in several diverse conditions such as ischemia (Hanzlikova and Schiaffino, 1977; Karpati et al., 1974), postmortem ageing (Cheah and Cheah, 1977; Saito et al., 1974), and anoxia (Schiaffino et al., 1979). However, the exact nature of these inclusions and the factors responsible for their formation remain to be determined. Recently, Hanzlikova and Schiaffino reported that the inclusions were protein in nature as

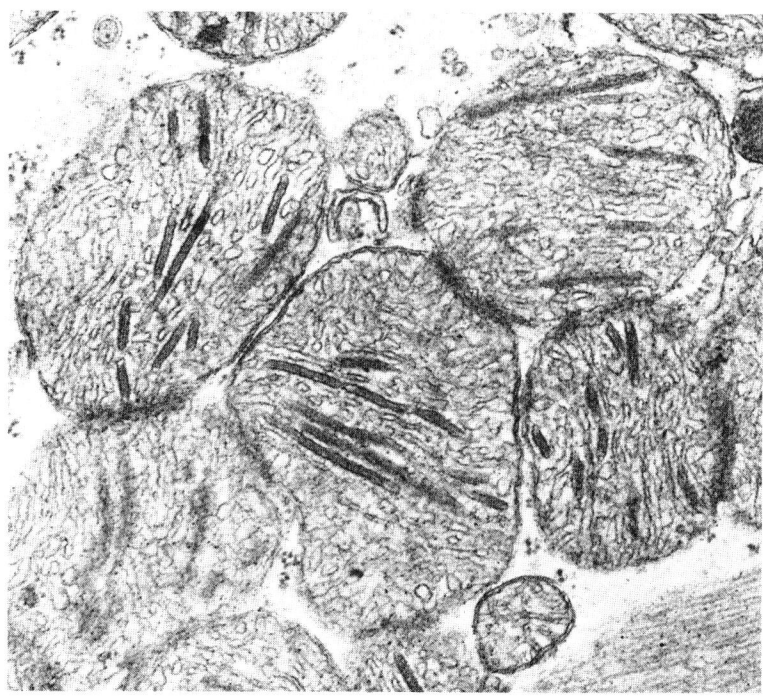

Figure 1.11. Mitochondria from a rat myocardial cell following a 60 min infarct illustrating abundant fusions of the cristae. ×50,000. (Reprinted with permission from B. F. Trump, I. K. Berezesky, K. U. Laiho, A. R. Osornio, W. J. Mergner, and M. W. Smith: Scanning Electron Microscopy 2:437–462, 1980a.)

shown by enzyme digestion experiments and suggested that they may result from the polymerization of enzymes such as creatine kinase present in the mitochondrial intermembrane space.

Stage V, which can only be recognized by electron microscopy, seems to be the hallmark of irreversible injury. Its definition has meant the difference between recognizing significant lesions in patients and animals using modern methods and failure to recognize such irreversible injury using the methods of the past. This, therefore, represents a hallmark in the progression of knowledge concerning the nature of cell injury. The problem is especially acute in humans because following somatic death all organs become acutely ischemic and progress over a period of minutes and hours to stage V. Therefore, unless an autopsy is performed virtually immediately following death (Trump et al., 1975), recognition of the reversible or the irreversible nature of cell injury becomes impossible. The same obviously applies to experimental animals; however, in these cases, it is ordinarily possible to control the initiation of studies.

Injury by Direct Attack on the Cell Membrane

Direct injury to the cell membrane often results in acute cell injury and cell death. This can be caused by various agents including specific antibodies to membrane antigens usually in the presence of complement (Hawkins et al., 1972), nonpenetrating mercurials such as *p*-chloromercuribenzene sulfonic acid (PCMBS) which act directly with membrane sulfhydryl groups causing rapid increase in permeability (Laiho et al., 1971), ultraviolet radiation (Ginn and Trump, 1970), direct mechanical damage (Trump and Bulger, 1968a and b), and antibiotics such as amphotericin B (Saladino et al., 1969) or gramicidin (Myers and Haydon, 1972), some of which may form membrane channels. All of these injuries have one fact in common, namely, they interact primarily with the cell surface and modify membrane permeability and/or transport systems. This interaction causes rapid ion movement down their concentration gradients and rapid cell swelling and lysis. Although the cells progress through the same stages as mentioned above, the rate of response and the magnitude of the cell volume alteration are different, causing the cells to pass quite rapidly to stage V. Following such a direct injury to the cell membrane, this stage contains mitochondria which not only exhibit high amplitude swelling and flocculent densities but also calcifications along their inner membranes (Fig. 1.12). Since the damage is to the cell membrane and not to the mitochondria, the rapid influx of calcium into the cell, accompanied by phosphate, results in mitochondrial accumulation of these elements.

RECOVERY OF CELLS FROM INJURY

As yet, there are relatively few studies on the progressive recovery of injured cells. We have, however, studied the recovery of temporarily ischemic proximal convoluted tubules in the rat kidney (Glaumann et al., 1977a and b). These studies revealed that recovery of many cells in the tubule can be remarkably rapid after periods of ischemia of up to 1 hr. Within a few hours after restoration of blood flow, the tubules regain a normal appearance, reflecting reversal of stages IV–IVB (Fig. 1.13). Somewhat similar studies have also been performed on anoxic EATC and in hamster trachea and human bronchus in explant culture (Barrett et al., 1977) (Fig. 1.14).

One interesting mechanism involved in the repair is apparently the loss of much of the plasmalemmal surface material caused by a pinching off of the blebs and

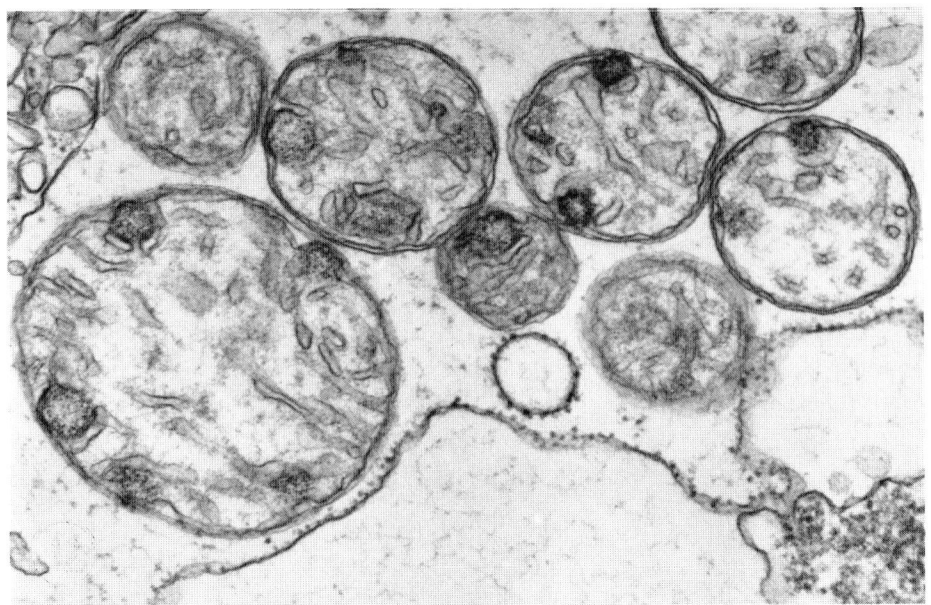

Figure 1.12. Portion of a tubule cell from an isolated flounder nephron treated with 10^{-5} M ouabain for 4 hr. Mitochondria are swollen and contain calcifications. ×50,000. (Reprinted with permission from F. L. Ginn, J. D. Shelburne, and B. F. Trump: American Journal of Pathology 53:1041–1071, 1968.)

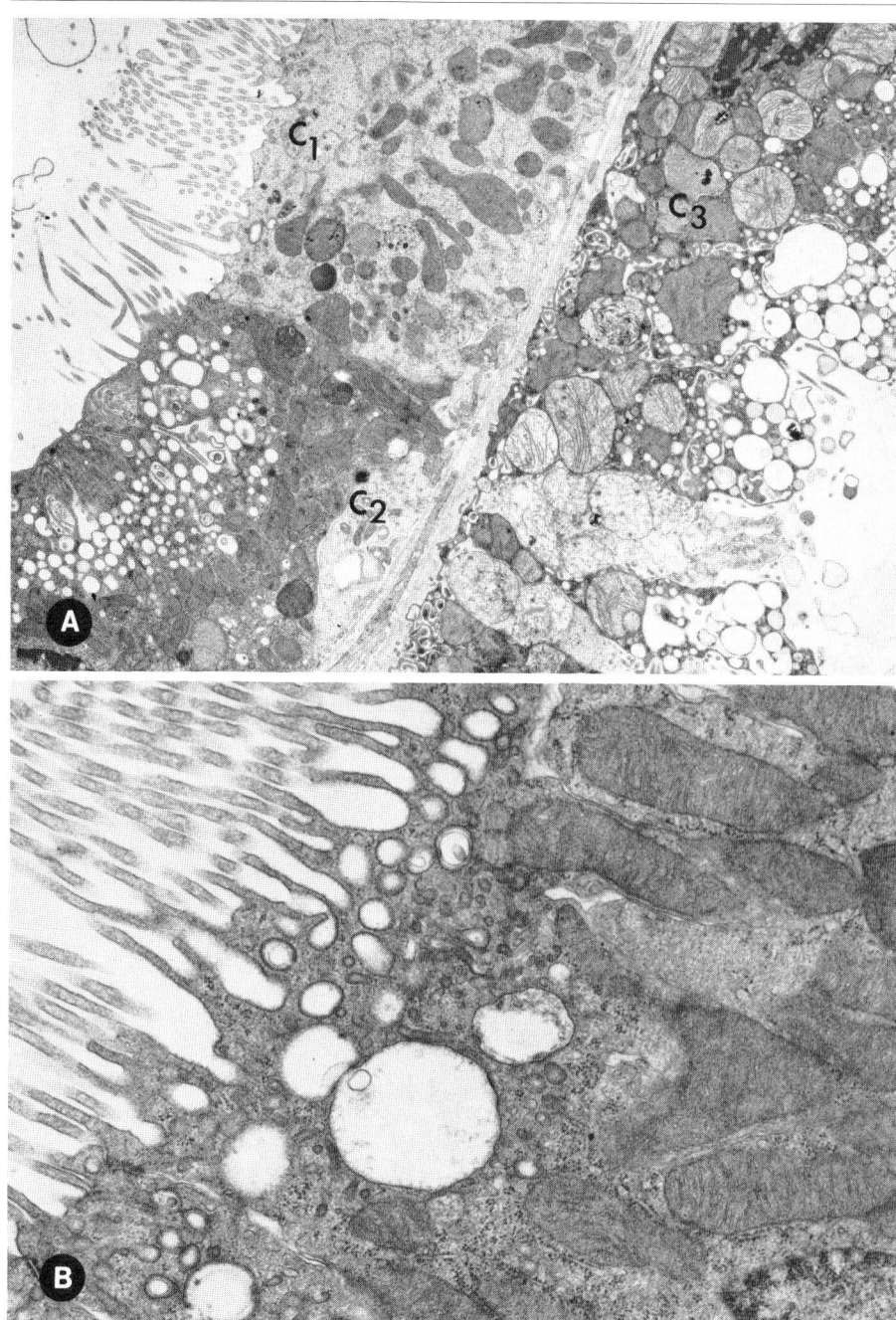

Figure 1.13. A, portions of three proximal pars recta tubule cells after 30 min in vivo ischemia followed by 3 hr of reflow showing different phases of viability. The C_1 cell contains well preserved mitochondria and has recovered from the injury. The C_2 cell shows autophagocytosis with interiorization of the microvilli, a dense cytoplasm, numerous clear vesicles and slightly swollen mitochondria. The C_3 cell contains many swollen mitochondria with flocculent densities and missing microvilli. ×9,000. (Reprinted with permission from B. Glaumann and B. F. Trump; Virchows Archiv. B. Cell Pathology 19:303–323, 1975.) B, rat proximal pars recta tubule cell after 60 min in vivo ischemia followed by 24 hr of reflow. The mitochondria, rough ER, nucleus, and microvilli have regained an almost normal appearance. ×18,500. (Reprinted with permission from B. Glaumann, H. Glaumann, I. K. Berezesky, and B. F. Trump: Virchows Archiv. B. Cell Pathology 19:281–302, 1975.)

distorted membrane contours at the cell surface. The cell membrane apparently seals off, and in the case of the ischemic proximal tubules these membrane fragments may pass down the nephron, while in EATC, they float away into the suspending medium. Some of this material may be phagocytized by the recovering cells and may contribute to the increased amount of lysosomal debris found during the recovery phase. In addition, some of this lysosomal debris may result from autophagocytosis of damage organelles within the cytoplasm, which cannot be repaired.

CHRONIC CELL INJURY

In chronic cell injury, we refer to sublethal changes resulting in structural and functional alterations of the cell that are existent for relatively long periods of time without loss of cell survival. By changing its physiologic state in such a way as to adapt to the presence of even a continuous injurious stimulus, the cell is able to continue its existence although in a new steady state. Such sublethal changes are quite common in many pathologic states including shock, ischemia, and anoxia. Examples of such adaptations include fatty changes, increased lysosome formation (especially by autophagy), hypertrophy, atrophy, neoplastic transformation, ageing, etc. In the present review, only brief summaries to emphasize the principal changes in this category will be presented.

Fatty Changes (Fatty Metamorphosis)

This is a very common reaction of cells to injury

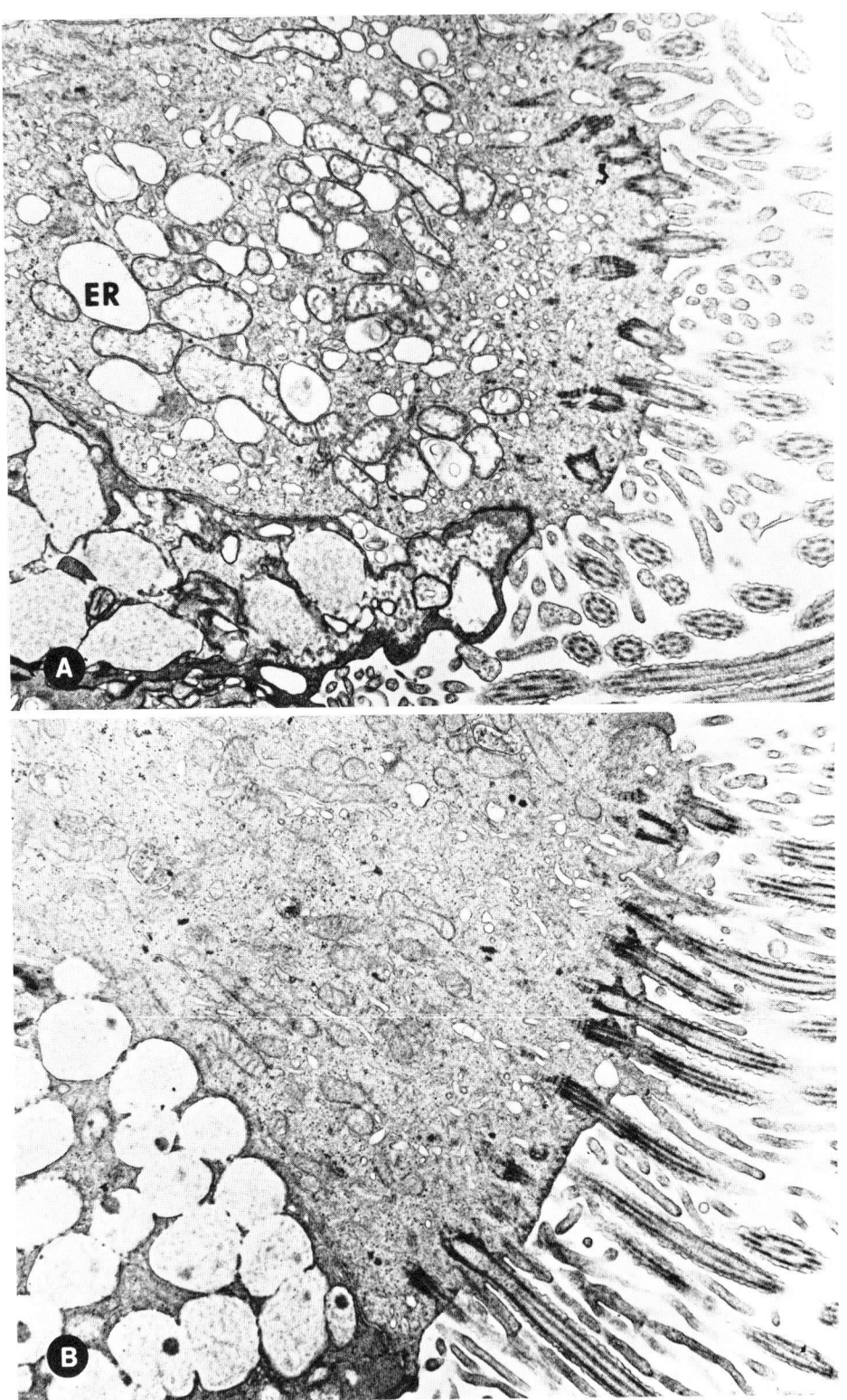

Figure 1.14. *A*, epithelial cells from human bronchus obtained at immediate autopsy and fixed after being stored in L-15 medium for 30 min at 4°C. The ER is dilated and the mitochondria are swollen. The ciliated cell is pale, indicating loss of volume regulation, and the mucous cell is dark due to shrinkage of the cytoplasm. ×11,000. *B*, epithelial cell from the same case as in Figure 1.14*A* after 24 hr in organ culture. The ER is no longer swollen and the matrical density and cristae of the mitochondria appear normal. The luminal surface of the central cell contains numerous cilia and microvilli. The mucous cell contains large mucous droplets. ×11,000. (Reprinted with permission from L. A. Barrett, E. M. McDowell, C. C. Harris, and B. F. Trump: Beitraege zur Pathologie *161:*109–121, 1977.)

known to pathologists for many decades. It is characterized by the accumulation of stainable lipid in cells, which mainly represents accumulations of triglyceride in the cytosol. The liver, heart, and kidney are especially susceptible to this type of change. The lipid appears as medium, electron-dense deposits in the cytosol which are not confined within any major membrane compartment. The usual explanation for such triglyceride accumulations is an imbalance between uptake, utilization, and secretion. For example, in the liver cell, inhibitors of protein synthesis which interfere with the formation of secretory lipoproteins result in triglyceride accumulations (Lombardi, 1966). Similarly, interference with microtubule function, for example, treatment of animals with vinblastine, also results in a similar lipid accumulation, presumably through interference with the normal role of microtubules on the secretion of lipoprotein-filled vesicles with the plasma membrane. Similar toxic factors may be operational in shock, ischemia, and anoxia but studies on mitochondrial oxidation of fatty acids, reduced or blocked in anoxic or hypoxic states, suggest that this may be a much more important cause, especially in the heart.

Accumulation of large amounts of lipid in cells does not seem to markedly interfere with cell function. Since many traumatized patients are affected by acute alcohol intoxication, it is difficult in clinical research to differentiate between other causes and an alcohol-induced fatty liver. Considerable data suggest that an alcohol-induced fatty liver also involves a defect in fatty acid oxidation.

Lysosome Formation

Embedded in the literature on shock, ischemia, and anoxia is the theory that activation or cell destruction by lysosomes plays an important role. This is no doubt the case; however, it has been difficult to dissect from the numerous experiments that have been performed precisely what this role may be (discussed under Acute Lethal Injury). In this section, we will review, in part, the increased formation of lysosomes which occurs in sublethal injury from these etiologic agents.

Predominantly, it appears through the mechanism known as autophagocytosis, which refers to the sequestration and ultimate digestion of portions of the cell, including most organelles. This is an active, energy-requiring process which appears to involve exotropic budding of portions of the cytoplasm and possibly portions of the nucleus into the cavities of the cytocavitary network including phagosomes and the ER (Arstila and Trump, 1968; Arstila et al., 1972). The process can be triggered by a variety of factors which may have in common modification of microtubule and microfilament functions and which probably includes activation of cyclic nucleotides, especially cyclic AMP. The process is shown in Figure 1.15 and involves an initial bud into a cavity (e.g., the ER) followed by total sequestration and subsequent fusion of the membranes, resulting in a double walled sac with ultimate dissolution of the inner membrane of the sac and fusion with pre-existing primary and/or secondary lysosomes, causing conversion to a residual body. It appears that such autophagosomes and autolysosomes can readily fuse with other heterophagosomes containing material taken in from the extracellular space.

The fundamental movements in various parts of the cytocavitary network and between the cell sap space and the extracellular space can be considered as forward or reverse movements of two geometrically opposite processes. Esotropy refers to a turning in of a membrane toward the cell sap followed by fission to form a new membrane-bound cavity. When this occurs in the opposite direction (reverse esotropy), the vesicle fuses with the membrane causing the contents of the vesicle to become continuous with the space within the cytocavitary network or extracellular space. Exotropy refers to the turning out of the membrane toward the extracellular space or toward the space of the cytocavity network. This is followed by fusion and formation of a new membrane-bound structure containing cell sap and organelles within it. It can also occur in the opposite direction (reverse exotropy) and results in the cell sap of the two compartments being brought together into continuity following fusion. Examples of esotropy include pinocytosis, the movement of transport vesicles from the ER to the forming side of the Golgi apparatus, and the formation of microbodies. Examples of reverse esotropy include fusion of secretory granules with the cell membrane, fusion of Golgi vesicles with phagosomes, and fusion between various granules. Exotropy results in eliminating a portion of the cell substance into the cytocavitary network or the extracellular space. Examples of this phenomenon include the formation of vesicles in multivesicular bodies (Arstila et al., 1971), autophagy in which portions of cytoplasm-containing organelles bud into the cavities of the ER (Arstila and Trump, 1968), cell division, lipid secretion in the mammary gland, and the budding of many viruses such as herpes, influenza, and mammary tumor viruses. Reverse exotropy occurs when a membrane-bound body fuses with another one, bringing the two portions of the cell sap into continuity. This is observed in intercellular fusions such as is seen in the formation of multinucleated giant cells in various virus infections or in the various fusions which occur during embryonic development. A diagramatic summary of esotropy and exotropy is shown in Figure 1.16.

Increased numbers of autophagic vacuoles are clearly a feature of several organ systems in both hemorrhagic and septic shock (Fig. 1.17) and probably contribute, possibly in a major way, to the increased protein catabolism and gluconeogenesis that are well known to accompany these states. The trigger or initiating mechanism involved in the formation of such autophagic vacuoles is still incompletely understood but may involve cyclic AMP. Our studies have suggested that changes in amino acid levels, possibly induced by glucagon, may initiate this response (Shelburne et al., 1973). Studies in our laboratory indicate that changes in the regulation of ionized intracellular calcium may constitute a final common pathway in the formation of autophagic vacu-

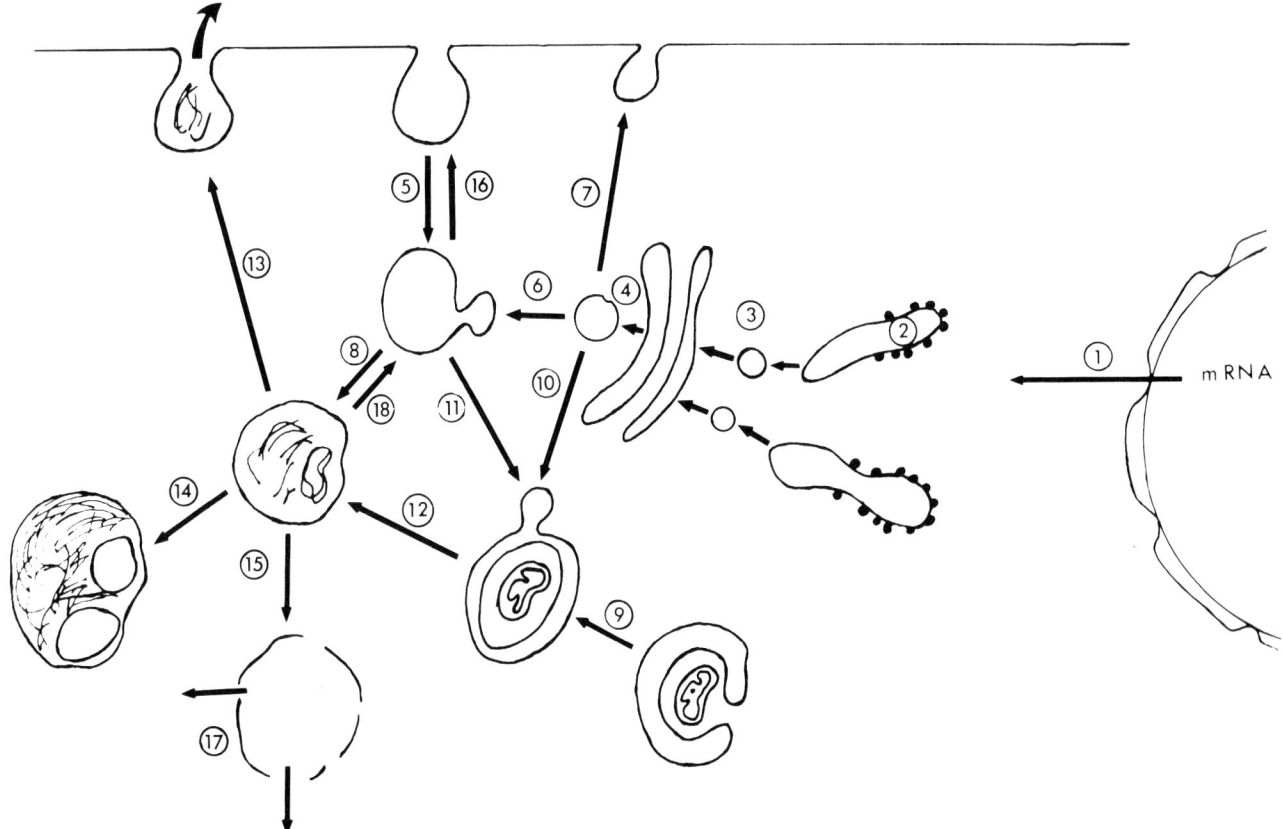

Figure 1.15. Diagram illustrating the basic reactions of the lysosome system to cell injury. *1*, messenger RNA for synthesis of acid hydrolases moves from the nucleus to the cytoplasm. If genetic defects exist, enzyme deficiencies will occur. *2*, acid hydrolases, presumably synthesized on membrane-bound ribosomes, are injected into the lumen of the ER and transported to the Golgi region. An obstacle to release from the ER, as in ATP-deficient states, may result in accumulation within the ER. *3*, transitional vesicles carry acid hydrolases and other materials from the ER to the forming face of the Golgi apparatus. This step has been shown to be ATP-dependent. In the Golgi apparatus, formation of secretion products occurs including addition of glycosyl moieties to form glycoproteins. *4*, hydrolases are released at the maturing face to form primary lysosomes. Primary lysosomes may exist not as vesicles but as tube-like extensions from the maturing face. 5, phagocytic vacuoles or phagosomes pinch from the cell surface and enter the cytoplasm, fusing with either primary lysosomes (*6*) or secretory lysosomes (*8, 18*). *7*, in some cases, primary lysosomes are discharged directly to the surface. This same process occurs in secretion of hormones. *9*, autophagic vacuoles are formed by exotropy, creating a double walled sac, the outer membrane of which may fuse with either primary (*10*) or secondary (*11*) lysosomes. *12*, conversion of the double walled stage to a residual body, or secondary lysosome occurs. *13*, in some cells, there is defecation of residual body contents to the cell surface. *14*, formation of increased amounts of residual bodies appears to be an event occurring in ageing, especially in neurons and muscle cells. It can also result from increased autophagic and/or heterophagic events in many cell types after injury. *15*, lysosomes in necrotic cells deteriorate, the membrane leaks, and enzymes escape to the cell sap (*17*). *16*, secondary lysosomes or enzyme-containing phagosomes may fuse with the cell surface, leaking enzymes into the extracellular space. (Reprinted with permission from B. F. Trump, E. M. McDowell, and A. U. Arstila: *Principles of Pathobiology*, edited by R. B. Hill, Jr. and M. F. La Via, pp. 20–111. Oxford University Press, New York, 1980b.)

oles, possibly through the effects of calcium on the cytoskeleton. Among the amino acids, a deficiency of glutamine may be important in the induction. Autophagic vacuole formation occurs in many organs including skeletal and cardiac muscle, the liver, the pancreas, the kidney, and the CNS. Such vacuoles probably play a significant role in organelle turnover and protein degradation in all of these organs and, as the process proceeds, release of sequestered hydrolases by secretion at the surface may result in increased circulating levels of

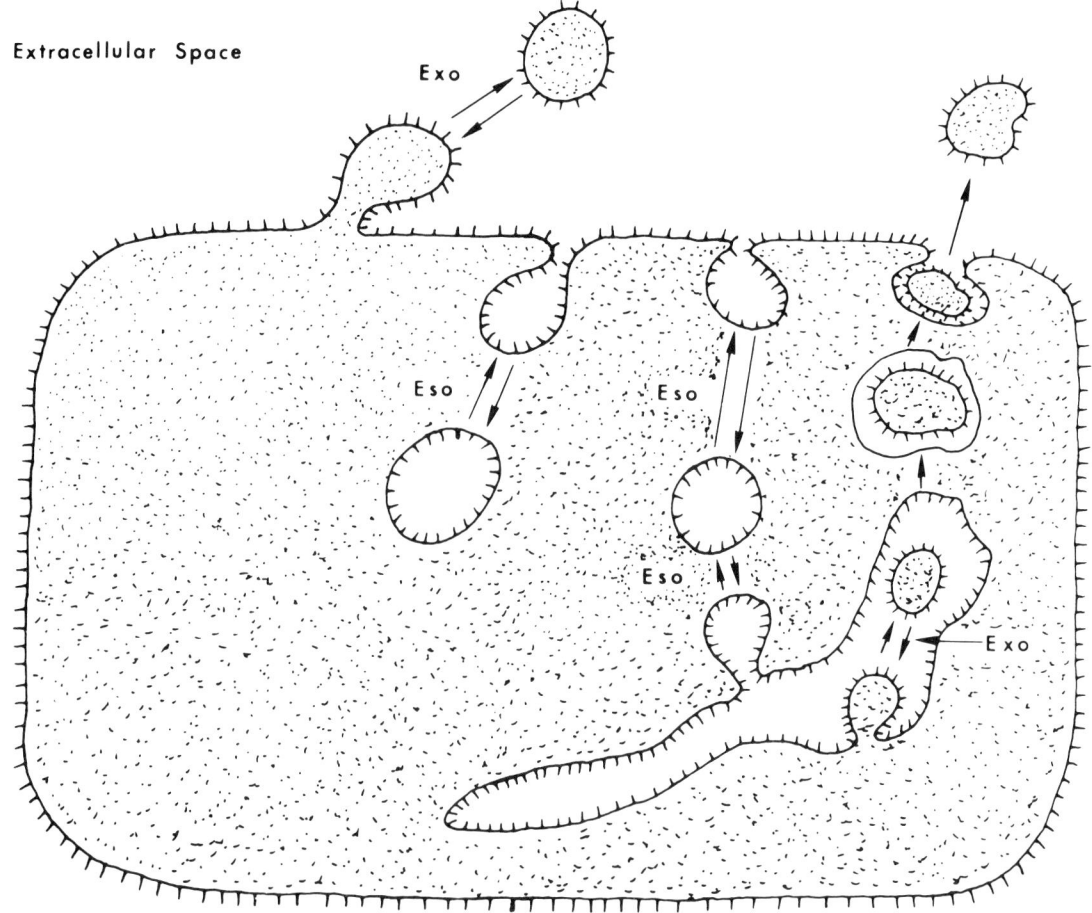

Figure 1.16. Diagram illustrating the principles of esotropy and exotropy. Esotropy results in the formation of a membrane-bound structure in which the membrane is turned inside out. The contents of the structure are topologically equivalent to extracellular space. Exotropy results in a structure that contains cell sap. Esotropic processes include phagocytosis, elaboration of vesicles from either face of the Golgi apparatus, fusions among lysosomes and phagosomes, and secretion of secretory granules. Exotropic processes include autophagocytosis, entry and release of viruses from cells, and fusion of one cell with another. (Reprinted with permission from B. F. Trump, E. M. McDowell, and A. U. Arstila: *Principles of Pathobiology*, edited by R. B. Hill, Jr. and M. F. La Via, pp. 20–111. Oxford University Press, New York, 1980b.)

lysosomal hydrolases (see Ch. 12). Increased secretion of lysosomal enzymes is an important facet of the inflammatory response with polymorphonuclear leukocytes and, later, of macrophages releasing such enzymes. Measurements of lysosomal enzymes in the urine may mirror tubular cell damage either lethal or sublethal. It is very important to realize that release of lysosomal enzymes to the extracellular space does not imply cell death, although when cells do die, enzyme release from the necrotic debris may also occur. The role of released lysosomal enzymes in causing local and even systemic damage needs further investigation. In our laboratories, the increased lysosome formation which we have observed in the hepatic parenchymal cells in shock may represent an important facet of liver cell damage (Trump et al., 1975; Jones et al., 1975). This is especially prominent in septic shock.

Hypertrophy

Hypertrophy clearly implies an increase in the dry mass of cells, usually resulting from increased synthesis of macromolecules. It is reflected by an increase in size and/or number of organelles and other subcellular components. Hypertrophy results from cellular adaptation to an increased workload, either chemical or mechanical, and is well known in both skeletal muscle cells and cardiac muscle. It also occurs in parenchymal organs such as the liver in response to chemical stimulation such as that following chronic administration of a number of organic lipid soluble compounds, including phenobarbital, polychlorinated biphenyls, and many polyaromatic hydrocarbon carcinogens. In a sense, therefore, hypertrophy is not a usual response to anoxia, ischemia, or shock, although some of the compounds implicated in hypertrophy and also under certain hypoxic conditions can alter

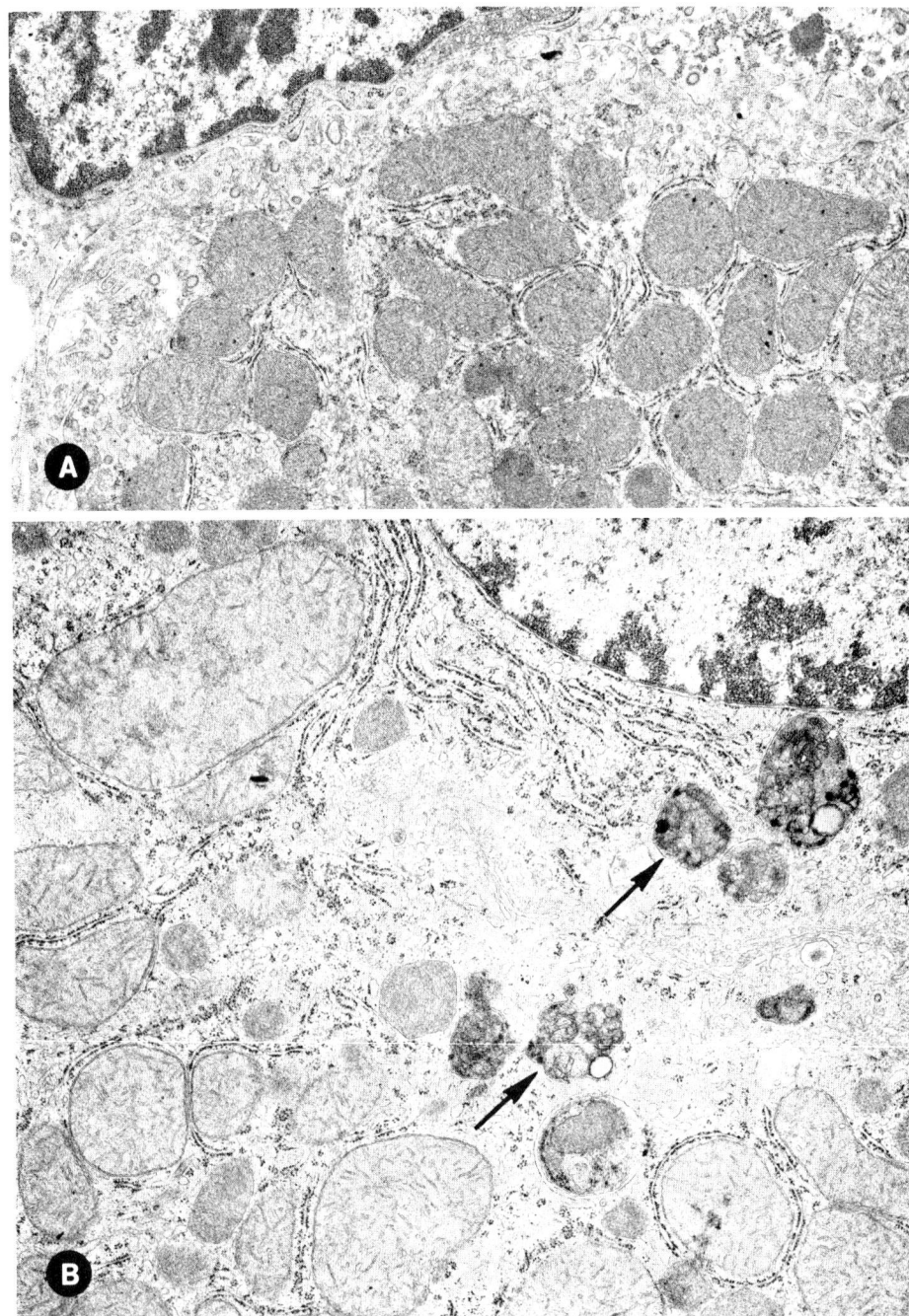

Figure 1.17. A, control rat liver illustrating a portion of a normal appearing parenchymal cell. ×12,000. B, rat liver following 21 hr treatment with an intravenous injection of live *Escherichia coli* (2.5–4.0 × 10^9 organisms per 200 g body wt) illustrating swollen mitochondria and numerous autophagic vacuoles (*arrows*). ×15,000. (Courtesy of T. Sato.)

mitochondria (see Ch. 6). Also, as mentioned above, hypertrophy of certain other organelles clearly does occur in shock and related states, notably the hypertrophy of the secondary lysosomes that results from stimulation in both hemorrhagic and septic shock.

Atrophy

Atrophy is the opposite of hypertrophy in the sense that it refers to a decrease in the dry mass of cells and their components resulting from decreased stimulation, nutrition, or oxygen. Although not occurring in acute ischemia or anoxia, chronic hypoxia definitely leads to atrophy of parenchymal cells and has been studied both in the CNS and in the heart. The atrophic cells are obviously not only smaller but, in addition, contain increased numbers of secondary lysosomes and residual bodies presumably derived from autophagic vacuoles. The residual bodies accumulate debris which often becomes auto-oxidized and form pigmented autofluorescent materials called lipofuscin or ageing pigment. This accumulation is especially prominent in the CNS.

Neoplastic Transformation

The transformation of one fully differentiated cell population into a differentiated population of another type occurs in response to abnormal stimuli. Such metaplastic cells are believed to have arisen from a new type of differentiation of undifferentiated basal or reserve cells rather than from division of pre-existing differentiated cells. However, recent studies in our laboratory of tracheal regeneration (McDowell et al., 1979) have shown that metaplasia may occur in the latter manner. Similar metaplasia may occur in epithelia injured by chemicals or there may be simple hyperplasia of mucous cells which replace the ciliated cells that are normally present. These lesions are usually reversible but when an injury is repeated and a carcinogen is present (such as benzo(a)pyrene), squamous metaplasia occurs followed by cytologic atypia characteristic of carcinoma in situ. Such foci are likely to progress to focally developed carcinoma. Therefore, regeneration, mucous cell hyperplasia, epidermoid metaplasia, and carcinoma in situ may arise as direct consequences of alteration in the structure and function of mucous cells in mucous-secreting epithelia.

Recently, much interest has evolved in the possibility that changes in various intracellular ion concentrations may act as intracellular messengers involved in modulations of growth regulation, cell adhesion, cell membrane properties, and cell-cell communication in neoplastically transformed cells (Rasmussen and Goodman, 1977). We recently initiated studies to investigate this phenomenon using a model of hepatocellular carcinoma produced in mice by safrole (Lipsky et al., 1979). Our x-ray data obtained from measurements of liver from control and tumor freeze-dried sections revealed marked increases in sodium and calcium and decreases in potassium and phosphate in the tumor versus the control (Trump et al., 1979a), suggesting that malignant transformation, at least in the liver, is indeed associated with marked changes in intracellular ion concentrations (Fig. 1.18). Cameron et al. (1980) have also been investigating this hypothesis and have found statistically higher concentrations of sodium and calcium in tumor cells than in any other cell population studied. Their x-ray data not only supports the theory that such high levels are associated with mitogenesis but also that even higher concentrations are associated with oncogenesis. They also reported that elevated intracellular concentrations of potassium and magnesium are associated with the maintenance of a high rate of mitotic activity in the nontumor cells but is not necessary for the maintenance of a high rate of mitotic activity in the tumor cells.

No doubt this phenomenon is much more complex than as visualized above. Because of the known importance of the sodium-calcium exchange mechanism at the plasmalemma, increased levels of cell sodium will be accompanied by increased levels of calcium. Calcium is

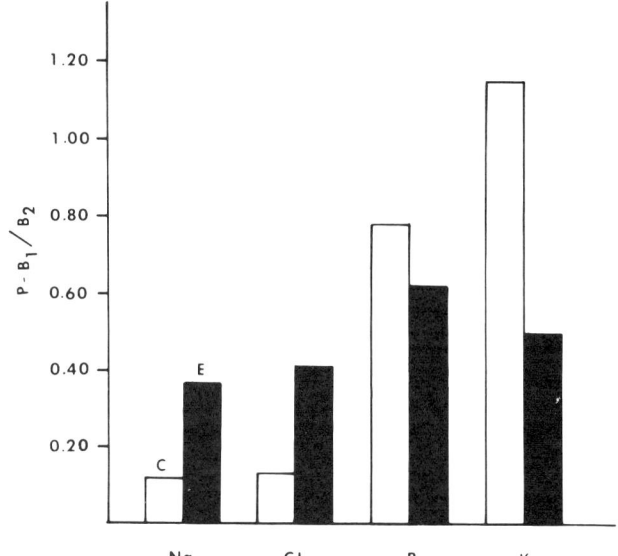

Figure 1.18. Bar graph illustrating peak to background ratios for Na, Cl, P, and K from microprobe measurements obtained over 10 μm freeze-dried cryosections of control hepatocytes (C) and tumor hepatocytes (E) induced in mice by safrole. (Reprinted with permission from B. F. Trump, I. K. Berezesky, S. H. Chang, et al.: Scanning Electron Microscopy 3:1–14, 1979a.)

known to have a controlling influence on cell division, to tend to separate intracellular functions, and to alter cell shape. All of these are known characteristics of regenerating and neoplastic cells; indeed, we suggest that this may be the stimulus for regeneration after ischemia and shock.

Ageing

Although no specific cellular features of ageing have been identified, many cells do exhibit alterations with time. One example of this is the accumulation of lipofuscin pigment in neurons which appear to increase in a linear fashion with age. Many theories of ageing have been proposed, including defective or altered immune recognition, thermal denaturation of cell proteins, free radical damage as by long-term action of cosmic irradiation, and accumulation of genetic errors; however, conclusive data have been difficult to obtain.

THE ROLE OF ION SHIFTS IN CELL INJURY

Since diffusible ions such as sodium, magnesium, phosphate, chlorine, potassium, and calcium, all of which are very important in the fine tuning of metabolic processes, are controlled within very fine limits in various intracellular compartments and between the cell and the extracellular space, numerous studies over the past decade have strongly indicated an extremely important if not a key role for their movements and redistributions in the pathophysiology of diverse types of cell injury (Arango et al., 1976; Campion et al., 1969; Chien et al., 1978; Cone, 1971, 1974; Farber et al., 1978; Haljamae et al., 1977; Cunningham et al., 1971; Polimeni and Al-Sadir, 1975; Jennische et al., 1978; Laiho and Trump, 1974a and b; Trump et al., 1976a and b, 1978a, 1979a, 1980a). The critical control of such ion concentrations is responsible not only for normal cell functions including cell shape maintenance, cell transport, cell junctions, cell-cell communication, energy production, protein and nucleic acid synthesis, and control of the cell cycle but also for any modifications of these concentrations, which are very important in many disease states including shock, trauma, myocardial infarction, stroke, acute renal failure, metaplasia, regeneration, and malignant transformation. At the same time, it is also well documented that many of these major ion shifts, although symptomatic of cell injury, by no means result in the death of the cell. The behavior of water is even more complex, as in some injurious situations cell water decreases and is associated with cell shrinkage, while in others, it increases in parallel with cell volume expansion. All of these modulations are reversible in the initial stages.

The recent development of x-ray microanalysis and other types of analytical microscopy has now made possible the measurement and quantitation of diffusible ions, not only extra- and intracellularly but also in specific intracellular compartments such as mitochondria, lysosomes, ER, nuclei, and cytosol. Space precludes any discussion of the theory and techniques involved; therefore, the interested reader is referred to two recently available reference books which outline these in detail (Chandler, 1977; Russ, 1978). Since it is impossible to use chemical fixatives for analyzing diffusible ions because of losses during tissue processing, the current preparative method of choice is direct, rapid quench-freezing of tissues by immersion in liquid propane or freon slush cooled by liquid nitrogen or the freezing and excision of small pieces of tissue in situ using a device such as the cryogun which was recently developed in our laboratory (Chang et al., 1980). This is followed by cutting thick (4 μm) sections in a conventional cryostat at $-20°C$ (Trump et al., 1979a) or by cutting ultrathin (100–150 nm) sections in an ultracryomicrotome at -70 to $-110°C$ (Appleton, 1974; Christensen, 1971). The sections are then completely dried under a dry nitrogen gas atmosphere of liquid nitrogen and brought to room temperature. Sections are analyzed in a scanning or transmission electron microscope equipped with a SiLi detector and interfaced with a multichannel analyzer. Bovine serum albumin (20%) standards of known electrolyte concentrations are frozen, cryosectioned, freeze-dried, and analyzed in the same manner. Peak to background ratios (P-B/B) for tissues and standards are then calculated and compared to standard curves giving the concentrations of each element of interest in millimole per kilogram dry weight (mmole/kg dry wt). Although technical problems still remain using this new analytical method, the correlation of ion shifts with altered cell function and structure will allow a better understanding of the pathophysiology of many diseases including shock, trauma, myocardial infarction, acute renal failure, and carcinogenesis.

Many theories have been proposed to explain the sequence of events which leads to irreversible shock and to account for the severe changes in multiple organ systems which occur during each of these phases. Such theories have included lysosomal disruption, deficits in energy metabolism, and damage to the cell membrane, among others (Baue, 1975). It has not been clear which, if any, of these events is primary and which secondary. In addition, several studies have suggested that one important alteration involved in cell function is manifested by decreased plasma membrane potential and ion and water shifts between extra- and intracellular compartments (Baue, 1974; Trump, 1974). Therefore, as part of our continuing series of studies on shock, we recently employed x-ray microanalysis to investigate the pattern of occurrence of ion shifts following 15 min of hemorrhagic shock in adult Sprague-Dawley rats. Preliminary results of measurements over liver hepatocytes and quadriceps femoris muscle revealed the patterns shown in Figure 1.19. Increases in sodium and calcium and decreases in phosphate and potassium were found in both tissues following shock although those quantitated over liver were more striking. Such early changes in liver cell function are commonly observed in human hemorrhagic shock (Champion et al., 1976; Cowley et al., 1969). Our x-ray probe data are consistent with the concept that deficiency in energy metabolism occurs at early intervals following hemorrhagic shock and leads to cessation or diminution of ion transport systems in the cell membrane, resulting in an influx of sodium and calcium and an efflux of potassium. By transmission electron microscopy (TEM), cells having such an acute energy deficit commonly show swelling of mitochondria and dilatation of the ER. These very early changes are doubtlessly reversible, since if blood is isotonic saline are reinfused within 15 min, the animals survive indefinitely.

Also of interest is the case of the hydrogen ion. Cellular as well as extracellular pH levels begin to decrease rapidly after cell and tissue ischemia. For many years this intra- and extracellular acidosis was considered to be a possible cause of irreversible cell injury (Katz and Hecht, 1969; Williamson et al., 1976). Recently, however, we have found that this factor may be a protective feedback mechanism. Anoxic incubation of cells at reduced pH results in a major prolongation of survival (Fig. 1.20). Indeed, anoxia at pH 6.5 or even lower doubles or triples the survival time of cells from the heart, liver (Penttila et al., 1976), kidney (Penttila and Trump, 1974), and EATC (Penttila and Trump, 1975a–c). The mechanism of this effect is not presently known; however, it is seemingly against the lysosomal theory of cell death since lysosomal hydrolases have an acid pH optimum. Currently, our hypothesis of the protection is that hydrogen ions can effectively compete with calcium ions for occupation of calmodulin-binding sites (see below). Another and clinical implication of this finding is

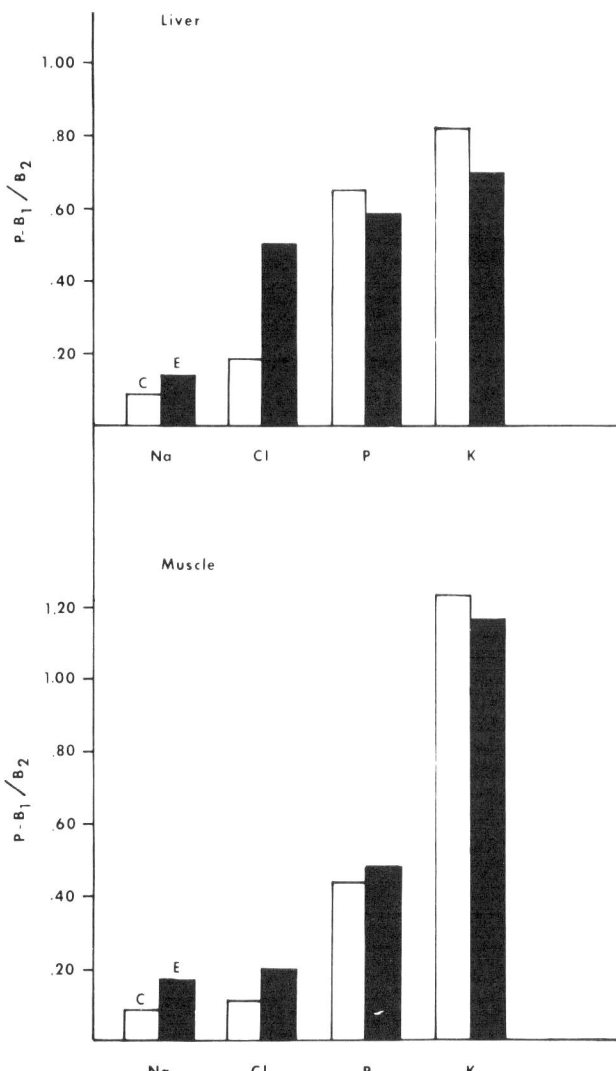

Figure 1.19. Bar graphs illustrating peak to background ratios for Na, Cl, P, and K from microprobe measurements obtained over 10 μm freeze-dried cryosections of liver and muscle. C, control; E, experimental following 15 min hemorrhagic shock. (Reprinted with permission from B. F. Trump, I. K. Berezesky, S. H. Chang, et al.: Scanning Electron Microscopy 3:1–14, 1979a.)

that overcorrection of metabolic acidosis may be extremely harmful to the cell.

THE ROLE OF CALCIUM IN CELL INJURY

Calcium is an extremely important intracellular electrolyte which plays a fundamental role in the regulation of many aspects of cell metabolism and activity (Table 1.1). Disturbances in cytosolic levels can, for example, alter the flux of glycogenolysis and glycolysis (Elbrink and Bihle, 1975) and increased calcium can activate membrane-bound phospholipases leading to alterations of the plasma membrane (Chien et al., 1979) as well as to interference with mitochondrial function (Mergner and McDonnell, 1978; French et al., 1971), thereby interfering with energy conservation.

The distribution of calcium across the cell membrane is far from equilibrium, with the concentration of free intracellular calcium being normally 10^{-7} M while extracellular calcium is 10^{-3} M (Baker, 1972; Blaustein, 1974; Kretsinger, 1976). Because of this distribution, specific processes exist both for the entry and removal of calcium. Control of calcium concentrations, especially that portion which is ionized and which exists extracellularly in only a small fraction of the total, has recently received a great deal of attention. However, total cell calcium may have little relationship to that which is physiologically active. It has been reported in the squid axon that of 50 μmole/kg calcium, only 0.06% is in the ionized form, although ionized calcium is higher in concentration in the extracellular compartment. The distribution of intracellular calcium is uneven, as has been shown by Brinley (1978), with almost 90% being localized in mitochondria. However, knowledge is still incomplete concerning calcium levels in various intracellular compartments. Using x-ray microanalysis, both we (Trump et al., 1979a) and Somlyo et al. (1979) have failed to find very great differences in total calcium concentrations between mitochondria and cytosol in normal cells. This does not necessarily indicate that large gradients could not exist for ionized calcium but rather that adequate methods for measuring ionized calcium at the subcellular level have not been developed. The estimation of calcium levels in various intracellular compartments is difficult in normal cells, and if one wishes to compare ionized and total calcium following injury, it is difficult in the extreme. However, as should be evident from the foregoing, it is of great interest to determine the common thread that could explain the progression of cells through the reversible and irreversible stages of cell injury. Especially, it would be of great importance to understand the factor or factors that result in the cell passing the point-of-no-return and, therefore, to be able to initiate interventions that could modify or delay this transition. Knowledge of the activities of calcium may well be pivotal in the understanding of these events.

It has long been well known to the anatomic pathologist that calcification of tissues is associated with cell death. Indeed, calcium phosphate precipitates act in histopathological sections as the gravestones of cells that were killed by a variety of injurious stimuli. This still remains an important characteristics of lethally injured cells; indeed, the process has recently been identified as the active accumulation of calcium by mitochondria, followed by precipitation with phosphate and subsequent conversion of the precipitates to hydroxyapatites (Fig. 1.21). Because of the active, energy-dependent accumulation of calcium, this process of dystrophic calcification occurs only at the edge of totally ischemic areas but is common in all areas of cell or tissue regions in which killing is the result of toxic, microbiological, or immunological stimuli.

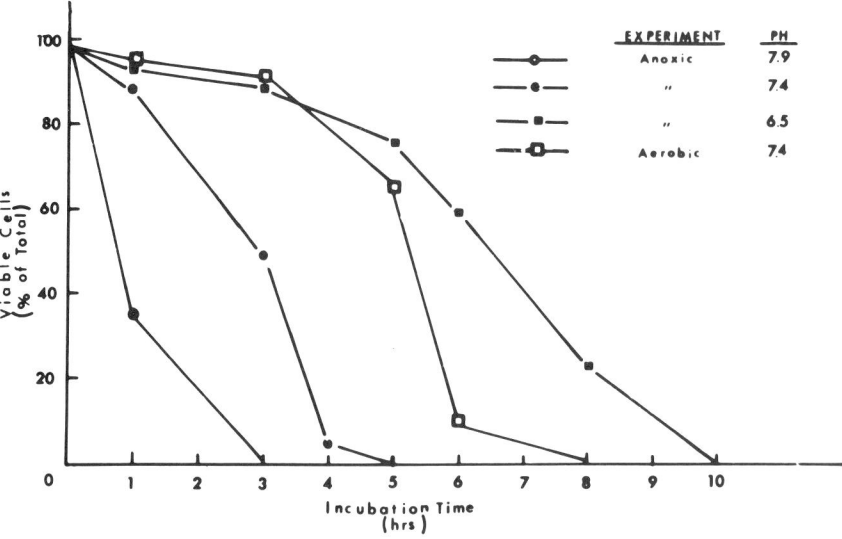

Figure 1.20. Viability of EATC incubated aerobically and anaerobically at various pH values. (Reprinted with permission from A. Penttila and B. F. Trump: Virchows Archiv. B. Cell Pathology 18:1–16, 1975b.)

Table 1.1
Calcium-Mediated Processes[a]

Activation of enzyme systems
    Glycogenolysis (phosphorylase b kinase)
    Lipases and phospholipases
    α-Glycerophosphate oxidation
    Pyruvate oxidation
    Succinate oxidation
Inhibition of enzyme systems
    Inhibition of pyruvate kinase
    Inhibition of phospholipid synthesis
Activation of contractile and motile systems
    Muscle myofibrils
    Cilia and flagella
    Microtubules and microfilaments
    Cytoplasmic streaming
    Pseudopod formation
Hormonal regulation
    Formation and/or function of cyclic AMP
    Release of insulin, steroids, vasopressin, catecholamines, thyroxine, and progesterone
Membrane-linked functions
    Excitation secretion coupling at nerve endings
    Excitation contraction coupling in muscles
    Exocrine secretion (pancreas, salivary glands and HCl in the stomach)
    Aggregation of platelets
    Action potential (nerve and muscle cells)
    ($Na^+ + K^+$)-activated adenosine triphosphatase of several membranes
    Tight junctions
    Cell contact
    Binding of prostaglandins to membranes

[a] From Carafoli, 1974.

Although the possibility that calcium might not act in its free ionic form but rather in the presence of a binding protein has been known for some time (Meyer et al., 1964; Cheung, 1970; Kakiuchi et al., 1970; Wolff and Siegel, 1972), it has not been until recently that this same calcium-binding protein was found to act as a calcium regulator in a variety of cellular enzyme systems and in most types of cell motility (Rasmussen and Goodman, 1977; Rubin, 1974; Dedman et al., 1979; Cheung, 1980). As a result, this recent discovery of calmodulin has excited a major stir in the biomedical community. This protein, apparently found in all nucleated cells, appears to play a major role in normal and abnormal cellular regulation because of its role as an intracellular intermediary for calcium (Table 1.2). Some time ago, Rasmussen (1974) suggested the possibility that calcium may act as a second messenger in cellular responses to many stimuli in a fashion somewhat analogous to the "second messenger" role of cyclic AMP in the action of hormones including glucagon and epinephrine (actually calcium regulation through calmodulin is evidently important as well in the actions of those hormones). The regulatory role of calcium in the overall cell economy involves a diversity of cell functions ranging from fertilization through muscle contraction and other cell movements to the events involved in both normal and frustrated phagocytosis, all of which have been recently reviewed by Means and Dedman (1980). Apart from these more or less productive activities, calcium, through calmodulin, is apparently involved in destructive cell processes as well since calcium can activate the seriously destructive cellular phospholipases. Until relatively recently, however, the manner in which calcium could modify or control such seemingly diverse functions defied analysis. With the discovery of calmodulin, we have, for the first time, possible insight into the mechanisms.

One such study is that of Welsh et al. (1979) who compared the immunofluorescent localization of calmodulin and tubulin in mitotic cells in culture and showed that the pattern of distribution of calmodulin was distinctly different from that of tubulin (Fig. 1.22). Calmodulin first appeared in association with the forming mitotic apparatus during midprophase and was also seen in metaphase and anaphase between the spindle poles and chromosomes. Tubulin was seen in the interzonal region throughout anaphase while calmodulin appeared

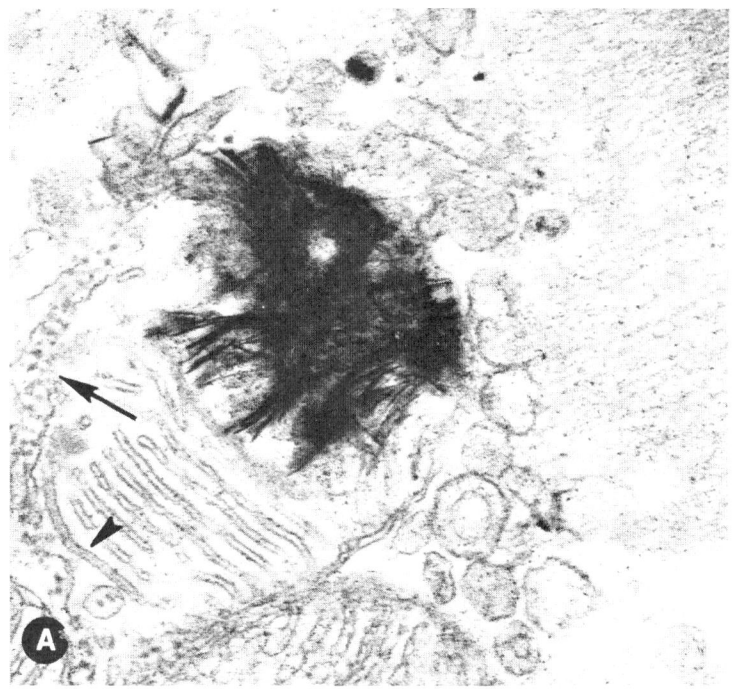
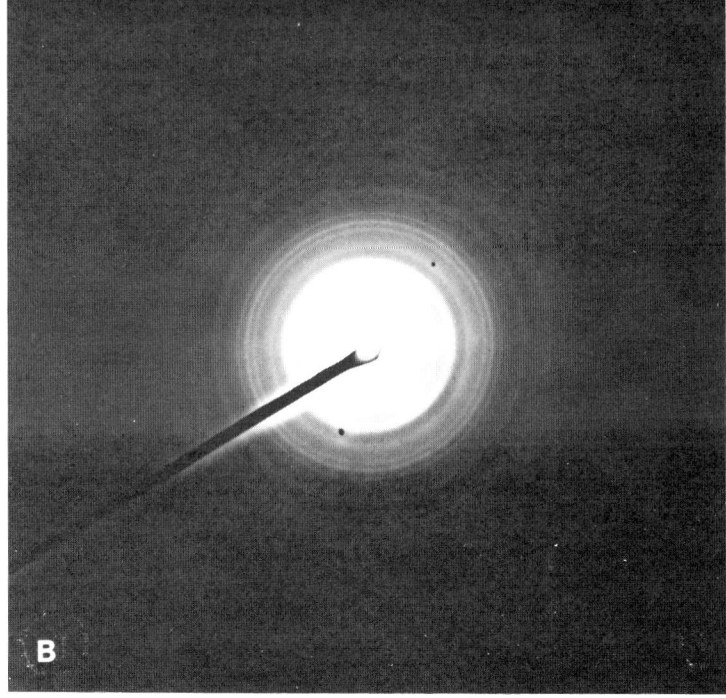

Figure 1.21. *A, Stage Vc.* A mitochondrion in a rat myocardial cell following a 60 min infarct. Needle-shaped inclusions are seen which reveal significant Ca and P peaks when analyzed with the electron probe. Note also the mitochondrial outer membrane disruption (*arrow*) and the intermembrane fusion (*arrowhead*). ×55,000. (Reprinted with permission from B. F. Trump, I. K. Berezesky, K. U. Laiho, A. R. Osornio, W. J. Mergner, and M. W. Smith: Scanning Electron Microscopy 2:437–462, 1980a.) *B*, electron diffraction pattern obtained over the needle-shaped inclusions illustrated in Figure 1.21A revealing a pattern characteristic of hydroxyapatite.

in the interzone region only at late anaphase. Also, calmodulin was not seen in the cleavage furrow. The localization of calmodulin during mitosis suggested that this calcium-binding protein may be interacting with some of the microtubules or microtubule-associated proteins of the mitotic apparatus.

Studies from our laboratory over the last 20 years have shown that there is, indeed, a close relationship between the total amount of cell calcium and cell death (Gritzka and Trump, 1968; Croker et al., 1970; Saladino et al., 1969; Sahaphong and Trump, 1971; Laiho and Trump, 1974a and b), but it has only been recently that the concept that calcium accumulation might be primary to cell death as well as a late and, therefore, secondary phenomenon has been added (Hearse, 1978; Trump et al., 1976c, 1978c). Recent studies which have added further support to this hypothesis include those from our laboratory (Trump et al., 1976d) as well as those of Shen and Jennings (1972) on reflow studies in dog myocardium. Kloner et al. (1974), in the transient ischemic

Table 1.2
Calmodulin-Mediated Processes[a]

Cyclic nucleotide metabolism
  Phosphodiesterase
  Adenylcyclase
Protein phosphorylation
  Membrane proteins
  Cytoplasmic proteins
Myosin light chain kinase
  Skeletal muscle
  Smooth muscle
  Nonmuscle
  Stress fiber localization
Microtubule assembly/disassembly
Glycogen metabolism
  Phosphorylase kinase
Calcium flux
  Ca^{2+}-Mg^{2+}-ATPase
  Ca^{2+} transport
Secretion
  Intestinal ion secretion
  Neurotransmitter release
Other enzyme systems
  NAD^+ kinase
  Tryptophan 5'-monooxygenase
  Phospholipase A_2

[a] From Means and Dedman, 1980.

model, and Goring and Spieckermann (1978), during reduced perfusion, all of which show dramatic increases in calcium. In addition, excellent correlation between total cell calcium and loss of viability has been found in EATC injured by agents which inhibit energy metabolism and inflict direct cell membrane damage (Laiho et al., 1971).

Since modifications of cytosolic ionized calcium take place within relatively narrow limits (Carafoli, 1979), any deviations from these limits can be expected to exert a number of dramatic and even disastrous effects on the structure and function of cells. Following cell injury of diverse types, not only is the regulation of calcium modified but also the regulation of many other cellular metabolic processes. It has been our experience that failure of intracellular calcium regulation, if it persists, shows a direct correlation with cell death (Laiho and Trump, 1974b) (Fig. 1.23). The same is not true for sodium, potassium, and chlorine which show early modulations prior to the point-of-no-return or for magnesium, which changes only after the loss of reversibility. In view of this, therefore, the answer to the question of exactly how calcium levels are modified following cell injury becomes the key. Although we do not yet know if the critical point is ionized or total calcium, three possibilities of primary modification exist. These include: 1) increased permeability or decreased extrusion at the plasma membrane; 2) increased efflux or decreased accumulation by mitochondria; 3) increased efflux or decreased accumulation by the ER. The second possibility may involve up to 90% of the control of calcium in many cells, and, therefore, particular attention must be directed to it. Following ischemic or anoxic injury, for example, mitochondrial uptake of calcium is arrested very rapidly. In addition, the lack of ATP results in the arrest of the plasma membrane calcium extrusion mechanism along with cessation of the sodium-potassium pump, causing the resultant increase in sodium to further interfere with mitochondrial calcium accumulation (Crompton et al., 1978). We have previously reported, for example, that in toad bladders following amphotericin treatment, Ringer's sucrose buffer promoted much more mitochondrial calcification than did Ringer's sodium buffer (Saladino et al., 1968). As a consequence of the loss of volume control which results from the cessation of the sodium-potassium pump, cellular swelling may accentuate the calcium control problem by cell membrane "stretching" with increased permeability and increased calcium influx. Further deleterious changes continue to occur as the injury progresses in time. For example, such changes in the mitochondrial inner membrane progressively lead to impaired calcium-accumulating ability (Trump et al., 1971; Mergner et al., 1977a). Although these alterations cannot presently be defined at the molecular level, our recent experiments indicate that they may correlate with modification of mitochondrial phospholipids, in particular, cardiolipin (Smith et al., 1980).

Using the calcium ionophore A23187 has also aided in our understanding of the role of calcium in cell injury. We recently reported on the synergistic effect of this compound on the progression of cell death following anoxic injury in EATC (Trump et al., 1979b; Laiho et al., 1980) (Fig. 1.24). Schanne et al. (1979) have also recently published similar data on rat hepatocytes using several membrane-active toxins and showing that the cells were killed much more rapidly in the presence of calcium than in its absence. Publicover et al. (1978) reported on the major ultrastructural damage in mammalian muscle following treatment with the ionophore A23187 and postulated that it resulted in release of calcium from the ER followed by calcium uptake in mitochondria which, after 40 min, then released the calcium. These results suggest that the cellular necrosis observed in various muscle diseases may be the result of an increased net influx of calcium into the cells, which in turn causes calcium overloading of the muscle mitochondria (Wrogemann and Pena, 1976). Borle and Studer (1978), in their study using kidney and liver slices, speculated that the ionophore may promote intracellular redistribution of calcium rather than influx of calcium from the extracellular fluid.

In addition to the above, evidence for the damaging effect of calcium has been further advanced by the "calcium paradox." Recently, Hearse et al. (1977) exposed myocytes to short periods of calcium-free perfusion at 37°C with energy metabolism uninhibited and found that under these conditions, if calcium-free perfusion is followed by calcium-containing solutions, unlimited influx of calcium occurs. Cell functions subsequently decline due to excessive accumulation of calcium by the mitochondria accompanied by a decline in creatine phosphate and ATP and by explosive cell swelling (Bulkley et al., 1978). Similarly, Ashraf et al. (1978)

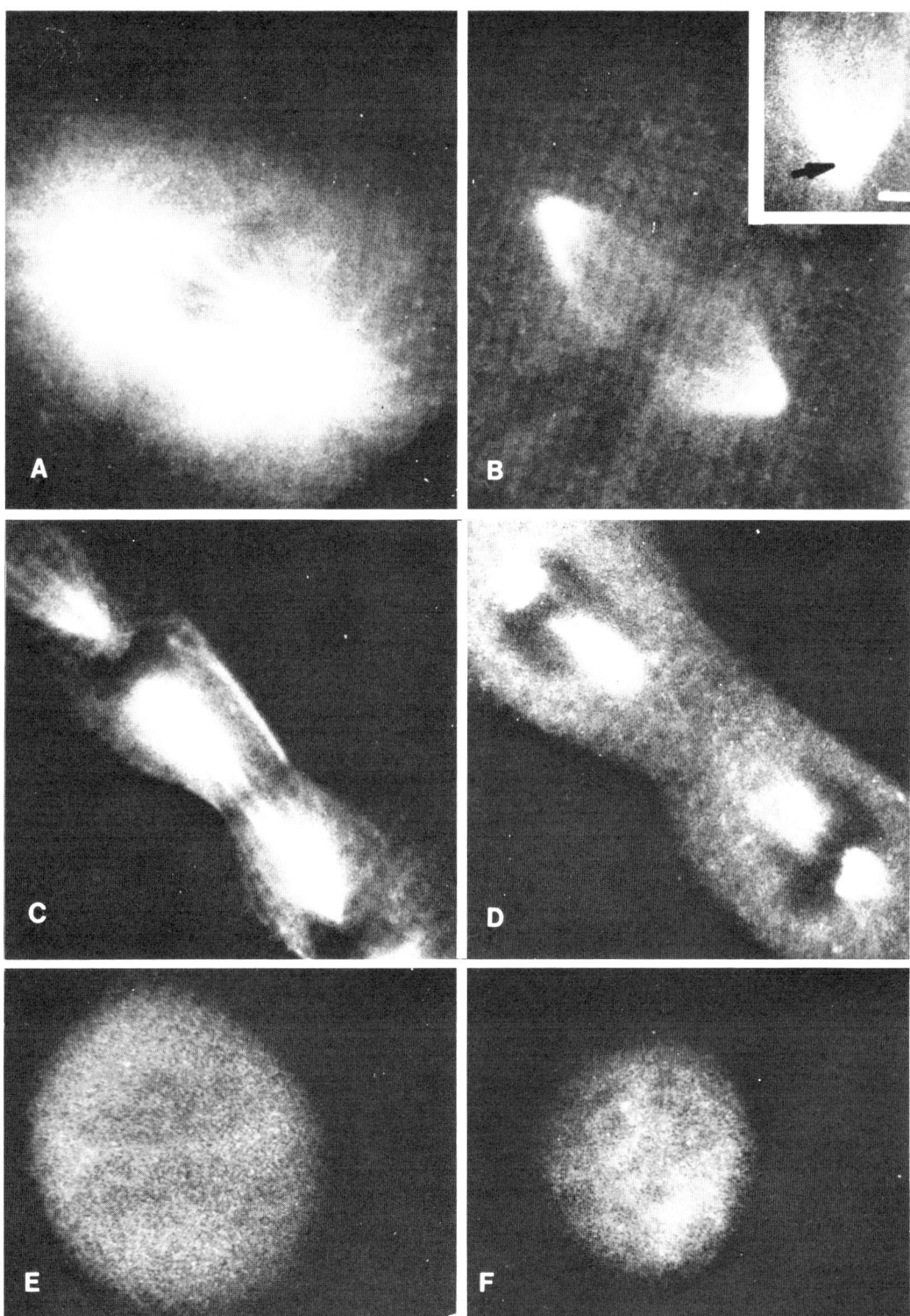

Figure 1.22. Indirect immunofluorescence localization of tubulin and calmodulin in rat kangaroo cells (PtK$_2$) at similar stages or mitosis. *A*, tubulin at metaphase illustrating a complete spindle with microtubule bundles passing from the spindle poles to the chromosomes and also microtubules traversing the metaphase plate. *B*, calmodulin at metaphase showing concentration near the poles. The inset illustrates that the concentration in the pericentriolar region is reduced at the centrioles (*arrow*) and in their immediate vicinity. ×2,200. *C*, tubulin at late anaphase continues to be localized both in the half spindle and interzone region. *D*, calmodulin at late anaphase appears in the interzone region but is absent from the developing cleavage furrow. *E*, tubulin immunofluorescence in a cell treated with 0.06 µg/ml colcemid for 1 hr at 37°C. All spindle fluorescence is abolished. *F*, calmodulin in a cell treated with colcemid. All spindle fluorescence is abolished. *A, C–F* ×900. (Reprinted with permission from M. J. Welsh, J. R. Dedman, B. R. Brinkley, and A. R. Means: Journal of Cell Biology *81:* 624–634, 1979.)

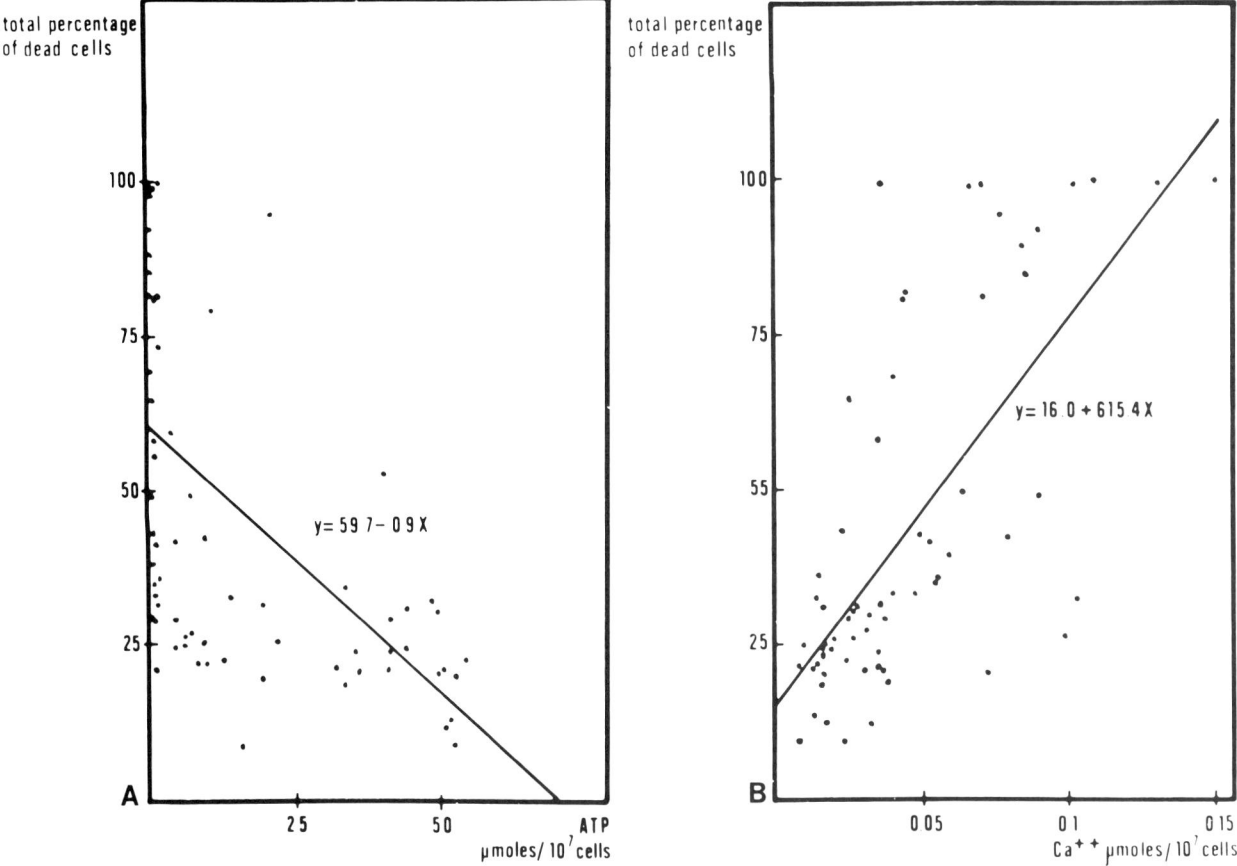

Figure 1.23. A, scatter plot with regression line showing a good positive correlation between Ca^{2+} content of cells and the total percentage of dead cells. Cellular injury was produced by an inhibitor of function of the plasma membrane (p-chloromercuribenzene sulfonic acid), by inhibitors of respiration (antimycin A), glycolysis (iodoacetic acid), or oxidative phosphorylation (2,4-dinitrophenol), or by combinations of inhibitors of respiration, glycolysis or oxidative phosphorylation ($r = 0.68$, $p < 0.001$, $n = 62$). B, scatter plot with regression line showing a moderate correlation between ATP content of the cells and the total percentage of dead cells. Cellular injury was produced as in Figure 1.23A ($r = 0.58$, $p < 0.001$, $n = 72$). (Reprinted with permission from K. U. Laiho and B. F. Trump: Virchows Archiv. B. Cell Pathology 15: 267–277, 1974b.)

reported that reperfusion of ischemic dog myocardium with calcium-free blood delayed the onset of ultrastructural alterations.

In summarizing the relationships of cell calcium to acute injury, it is important to distinguish between those effects which result from inhibition of energy metabolism such as in acute ischemia from those which result from primary attack on the plasma membrane. Both, of course, can be acting in concert such as occurs in many cases of shock, particularly when hemorrhagic shock is combined with the effects of sepsis, and in myocardial infarction.

CHANGES IN ORGANELLES

It is extremely difficult to put forward a general hypothesis that explains the cellular alterations following injury without first explaining our concepts of the pathophysiology of organelle changes. To this end, the following section is devoted.

Cell Membranes

Shortly after anoxic or ischemic injury, major changes involve redistribution of intramembrane particles (IMP) which, at least in the kidney, are more or less randomly distributed. These particles, presumably membrane proteins, become rapidly aggregated even during the reversible phase, having large irregular IMP fine particles. We believe that this redistribution is related to alterations in the cytoskeleton and in the attachments of the cytoskeleton to intra and transmembrane proteins. The significance of this reversible change is not known; however, available evidence indicates that it probably affects membrane permeability as well as membrane receptor sites. Although many more studies are needed, direct membrane damage may result in membrane channels allowing free exchange of sodium, potassium, and calcium. Entry of calcium into the cytosol seems to be of especial importance as calcium-binding to calmodulin

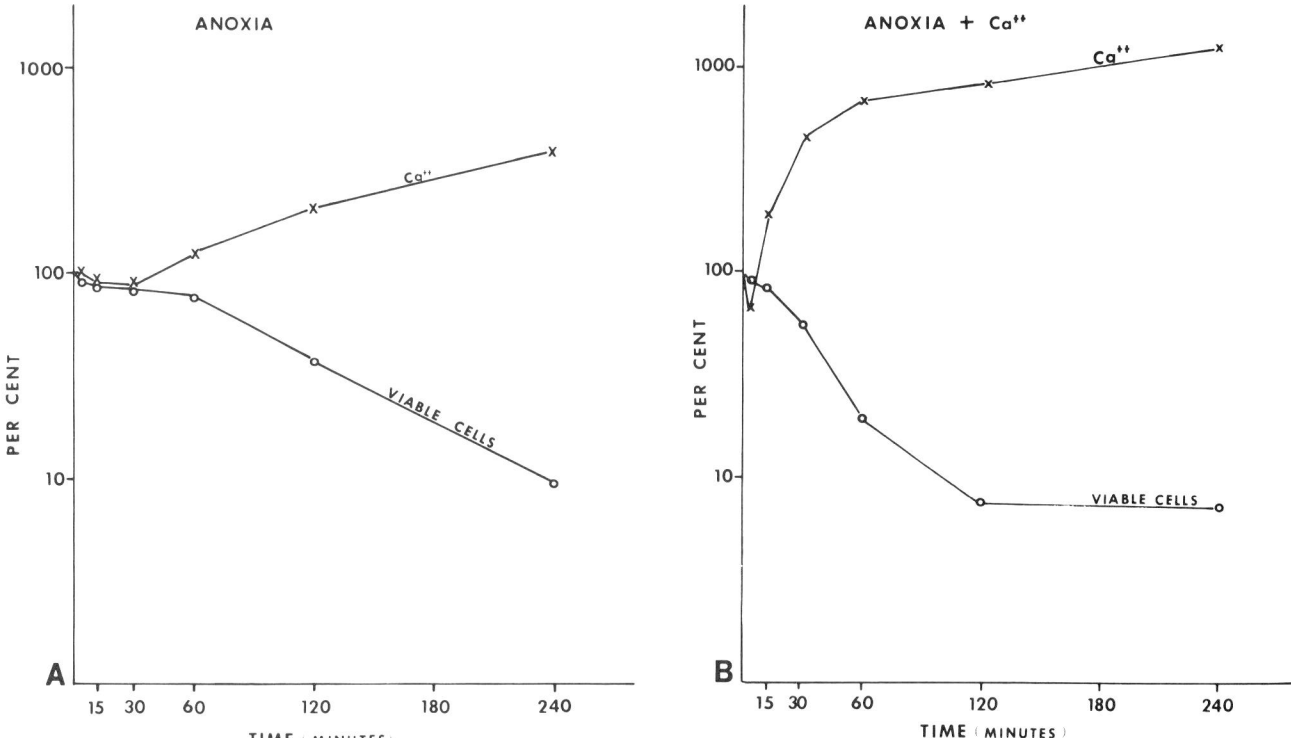

Figure 1.24. Graph illustrating percentage of viable cells and Ca^{2+} uptake in EATC following 0–240 min of anoxia. Cells were preincubated in Krebs-Ringer phosphate buffer (pH 7.4) for 10 min prior to the experiments, and at 0 time, the gassing phase was changed to purified nitrogen. Cell viability was determined by nigrosin staining. B, graph illustrating percentage of viable cells and Ca^{2+} uptake in anoxic EATC following 0–240 min treatment with 10 μm ionophore A23187. Experimentation was performed as in Figure 1.23A. Cell Ca^{2+} levels were determined by atomic absorption spectrophotometry using ^{14}C inulin to estimate extracellular space. (Reprinted with permission from B. F. Trump, I. K. Berezesky, K. U. Laiho, A. R. Osornio, W. J. Mergner, and M. W. Smith: Scanning Electron Microscopy 2:437–462, 1980a.)

can activate a number of important processes in the cell and may contribute, at least in part, to a final common pathway of cell injury.

Changes in the configuration of the cell membrane are dramatic after acute cell injury (Fig. 1.25). In addition, as is now recognized, the cell surface is involved in many important aspects of neoplasia including uncontrolled cell growth, invasion of normal tissues, and metastasis to secondary sites. Although the above are complex cell surface problems, knowledge of the normal cell membrane gained in the past few years has led us to a better understanding of the mechanisms involved. The dynamics of cell membrane organization and the hypothetical interactions involved between the various components are illustrated in Figure 1.26. Figure 1.27 illustrates microtubule arrangements as observed following peroxidase-antiperoxidase (PAP) staining of an epithelial cell outgrowth from a human lung tumor.

A typical example of the many cell membrane changes which occur following injury are the exotropic blebs of the acutely ischemic proximal convoluted tubule (PCT) cells of the kidney. Following acute ischemia, the apical surfaces of the PCT bulge out toward the tubule lumen (Glaumann et al., 1977a) (Fig. 1.28). In our view, it is because this is a "free" surface as compared with the lateral membranes and those toward the basal lamina. In contrast, anoxic cells in suspension, such as EATC, show similar blebs at random along their spherical periphery (Trump et al., 1979c and d) (Fig. 1.29). These blebs are free of the usual microvilli and, on section, contain a relatively clear cytosol (Fig. 1.30). In such areas, both contractile filaments and microtubules are inconspicuous. It is probably significant that this same type of effect can be readily produced in EATC by the addition of cytochalasin B, which modifies the contractile filaments (Fig. 1.31); vinblastine, which modifies microtubules; or the calcium ionophore A23187, which modifies both (Fig. 1.32). We believe that such experiments support the concept that lack of control of cytosol calcium results in analogous changes in the cytoskeleton bringing about similar changes after cell injury.

Detachment and/or depolymerization of microtubules may, therefore, result in these protrusions, possibly through release of attachment sites to the membrane followed by cytoplasmic pressure from contraction of microfilaments. The system also behaves as if the con-

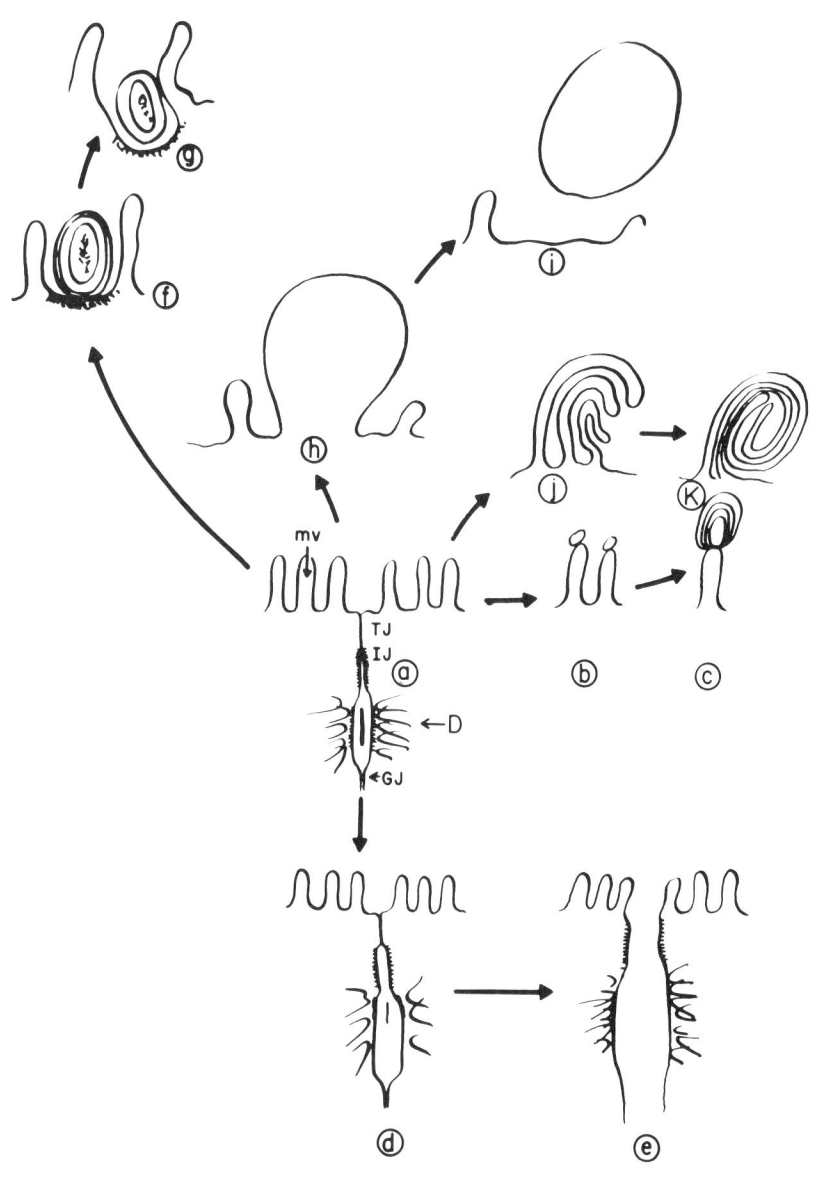

Figure 1.25 Conformational changes in the cell membrane following cell injury. a, a typical normal membrane with microvilli (mv) and components of junctional complex including tight junction (TJ), intermediate junction (IJ), desmosome (D), and gap junction (GJ). b, c, myelin forms produced and elaboration of bimolecular leaflets representing extracted phospholipid. d, e, stages of separation of junctional complexes occurring as a result of removal of calcium or treatment with chelating agents such as EDTA. f, g, stages in phagocytosis of bacteria in small intestine showing induced formation of spine-like coatings on the cytoplasmic surface of the membrane adjacent to the ingested organism. h, i, stages in elaboration of an exotropic bleb from the membrane surface. j, k, elaboration of tubular forms with formation of concentric arrangements when these protrude into a constrained space such as a kidney tubule or a bile canaliculus. l, stages of budding virus. (Reprinted with permission from B. F. Trump, E. M. McDowell, and A. U. Arstila: *Principles of Pathobiology*, edited by R. B. Hill, Jr. and M. F. La Via, pp. 20–111. Oxford University Press, New York, 1980b.

verse works as well; i.e., depolymerization of microfilaments leads to essentially the same effect, possibly in this case resulting from loss of contractile filaments and reciprocal action of microtubules.

These changes at the cell surface are clearly reversible. However, the protruding blebs can apparently detach, with subsequent sealing of the cell membrane. In some situations, however, this may produce secondary effects. In the kidney tubule, for example, the detached blebs float down the nephron and form casts in the distal tubules. This can result in tubular obstruction and may be one factor that contributes to the pathogenesis of ischemically-induced acute renal failure (Donohoe et al., 1978). In capillary and venular endothelium, the same type of change may result in decreased flow and contribute to tissue ischemia and later the "no-reflow" phenomena.

Somewhat the opposite effect causes formation of hypoxic vacuoles, at least in the hepatic parenchymal cells (Trump et al., 1976c). These consist of huge invaginations of the cell membrane along both the canalicular and the sinusoid margins and range in diameter up to that of the nucleus. These vacuoles are surrounded by bundles of contractile filaments in the subjacent cytoplasm and are aligned along the periphery of the vacuole, presumably to function in pulling in the invaginations.

Changes in Membrane Constituents

As yet, we know relatively little about membrane components in cell injury. As mentioned above, changes

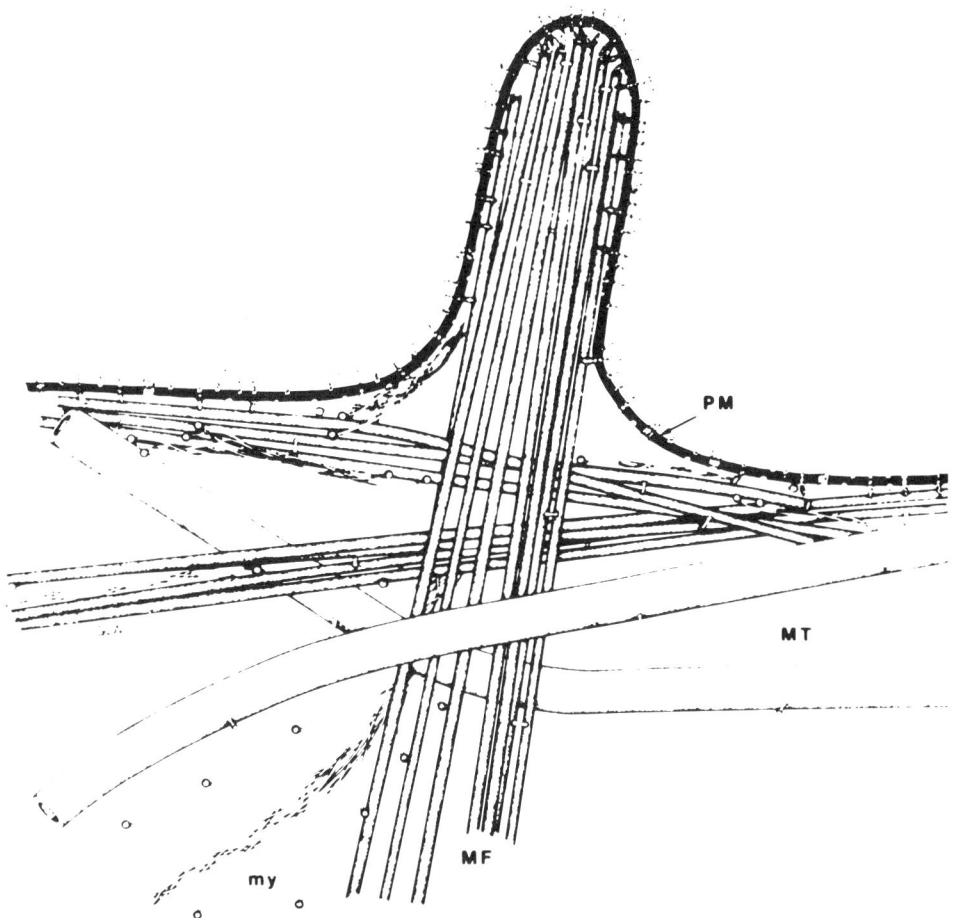

Figure 1.26. Model illustrating the relationship of cytoskeletal components and the cell membrane. The model demonstrates hypothetical interactions between membrane-associated microtubule (*MT*) and microfilament (*MF*) systems involved in transmembrane control over cell surface receptor mobility and distribution. This model envisages opposite but coordinated roles for microfilaments (contractile) and microtubules (skeletal) and suggests that they are linked to one another or to the same plasma membrane (*PM*) inner surface components. This linkage may occur through myosin molecules either in small bundles or the larger filaments (*my*) or through cross-bridging molecules such as α-actin. In addition, peripheral membrane components linked at the inner or outer plasma membrane surface may extend this control over specific membrane domains. (Reprinted with permission from G. L. Nicolson, et al.: *International Cell Biology,* edited by B. R. Brinkley and K. R. Porter, pp. 138–148. Rockefeller University Press, New York, 1977.

in phospholipid content may occur as a result of phospholipase activities even during the reversible phase. This is correlated with increased membrane permeability and potentially with membrane protein conformational damage because of altered lipid-protein interactions. Indeed, freeze-fractured studies of ischemic kidney proximal tubules reveal that the normally random even distribution of IMPs changes to aggregates with large particle-free zones or particles (Coleman et al., 1975). Similarly, Frank (1980) recently observed that in rabbit myocardium, anoxia caused a significant decrease in redistribution of IMPs. Somewhat analogous aggregations of IMPs may appear in the region of cap junctions yielding regular hexagonal arrays. Both of these changes not only indicate a severe alteration in membrane lipoprotein structure but may also relate to alterations in the cytoskeletal attachments to cell membrane proteins.

Functional changes that could relate to the altered IMPs include variations in permeability and transport proteins. Although gross defects in cell membrane continuity at the electron microscopic level have been reported, we doubt that they actually occur until after death (stage V) and, even then, may be the result of artifactual breakage that is perhaps related to increased membrane fragility.

Changes in Cell Junctions

The loosening and detachment of cell junctions that occur following injury often appear to have severe physiologic consequences. Since epithelia are frequently

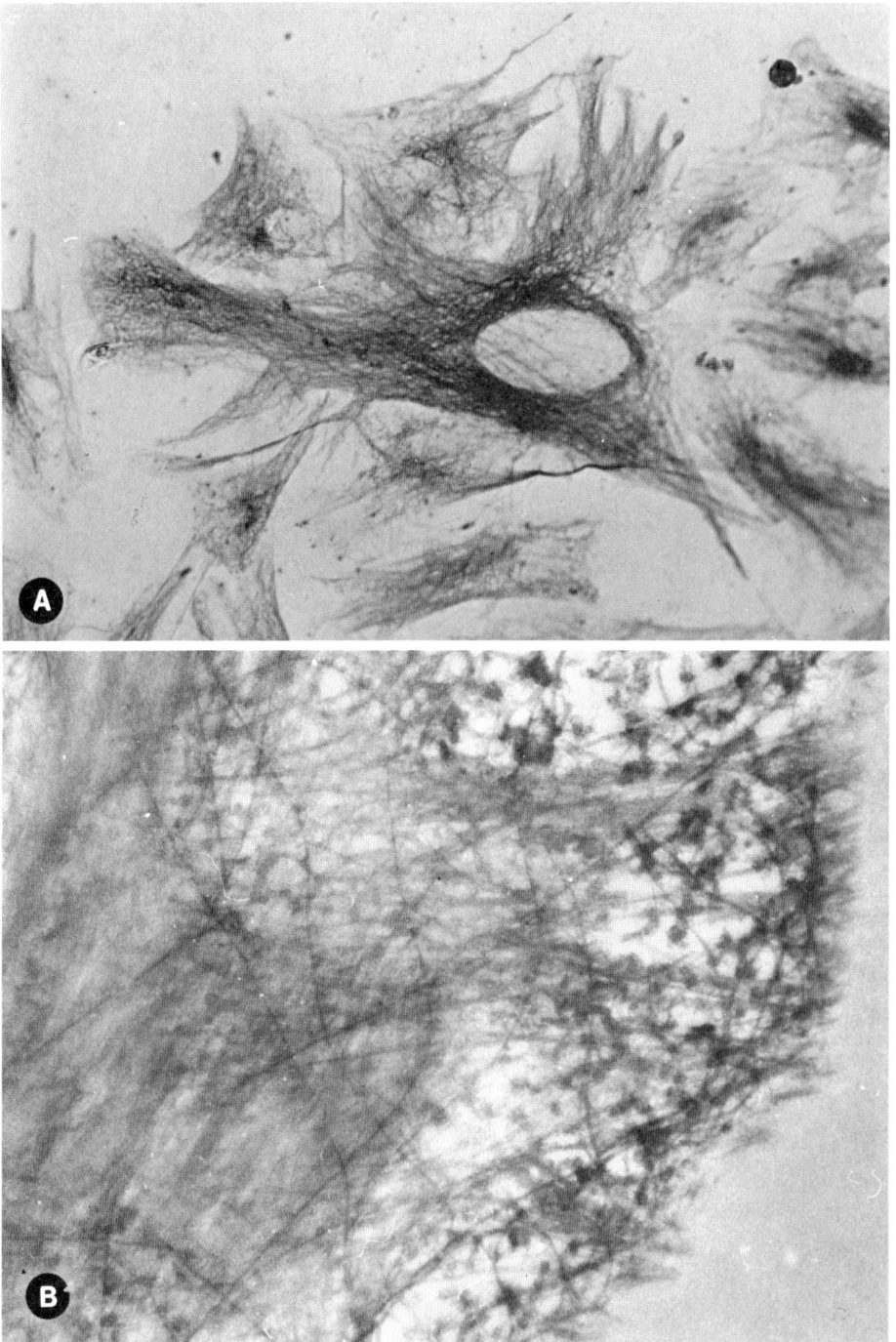

Figure 1.27. *A*, light micrograph of epithelial cell outgrowths from a human lung tumor grown in organ culture on plastic coverslips. The cells were fixed, treated with Triton-X100, and then stained by the Sternberger PAP immunohistochemical technique for microtubules. ×1,000. (Courtesy of P.C. Phelps.) *B*, TEM of the same central cell as in Figure 1.27*A* showing two specific PAP stainings of flat microtubules. The specimen was postfixed in OsO_4 and flat embedded, and 0.5 μm sections were viewed at 100 kv. ×15,000. (Courtesy of P. C. Phelps.)

communicating as a syncytium by means of gap junctions, loss of such junctions can be expected to alter cell physiology. Among such consequences in many epithelia is the cell entering the mitotic cycle, which may even occur in cells some distance away from the cells that disappeared as a result of the injury. Such mitotic activity is one of the first steps leading to the ultimate repair of the epithelial defects. The factors responsible for the detachment of cells are not well worked out. Loewenstein and Rose (1978), however, have presented evidence that

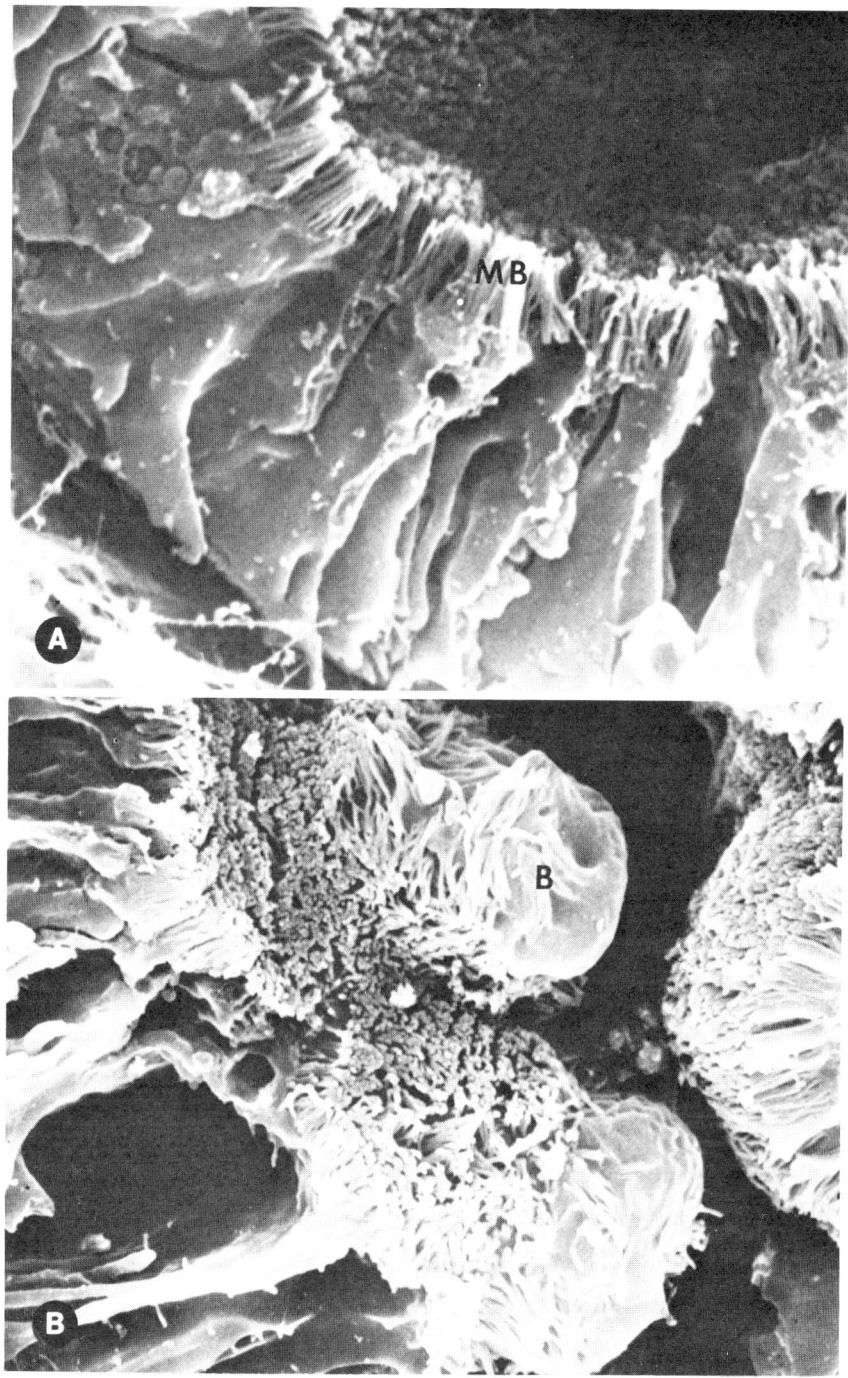

Figure 1.28. *A*, SEM of a portion of control kidney proximal tubule. The microvillous border (*MB*) is seen projecting into a patent lumen. Lateral membrane folds of the tubule cell are seen. ×5,000. *B*, SEM of a portion of a kidney proximal tubule following 15 min of in vivo ischemia. Note the distortion of the microvillous border forming large apical blebs (*B*) which protrude into the lumen. Some lateral membrane folds of the tubular cells appear greatly swollen. ×5,000. (Reprinted with permission from B. F. Trump, I. K. Berezesky, Y. Collan, M. W. Kahng, and W. J. Mergner: Beitraege zur Pathologie *158*:363–368, 1976b.)

increased levels of intracellular ionized Ca can result in this cell separation. Again, the cytoskeleton may be involved (Brinkley et al., 1979). He postulated that this may be a protective feedback in the sense that detachment of an injured cell from its neighbors may prevent or limit the spread of deleterious changes of the internal miliem to its neighbors.

In the case of epithelia with barrier functions, e.g., vascular endothelium, cell junctional separation may be quite harmful. In the case of "shock lung," for example, there is evidence that such separation of cell junctions is responsible for the abrupt increase in vascular permeability that occurs, especially in the presence of endotoxin. Also, in secretory or resorptive cells, e.g., kidney tubular epithelium, loss of leak-proof seals will result in dissipation of concentration gradients and thus loss of these functions. This may trigger acute renal failure (see below).

Endoplasmic Reticulum—Golgi Apparatus

The early dilation of ER cisternae is believed to reflect loss of cell and compartmental volume control and loss

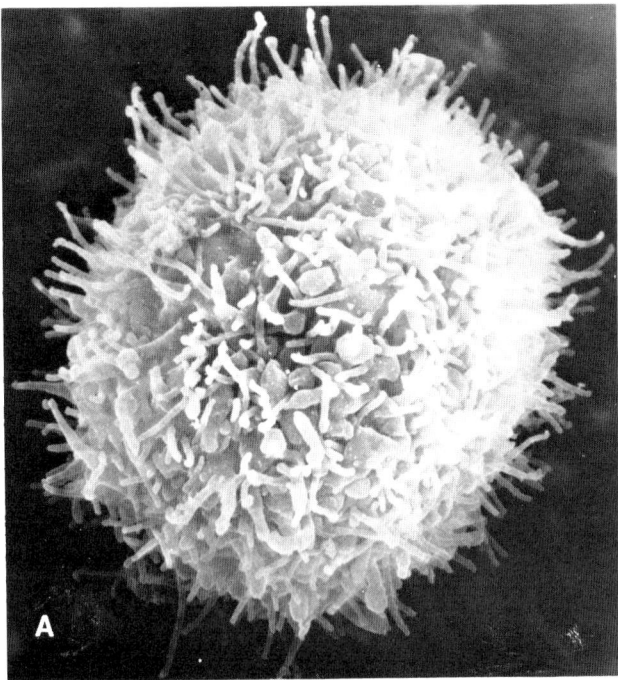

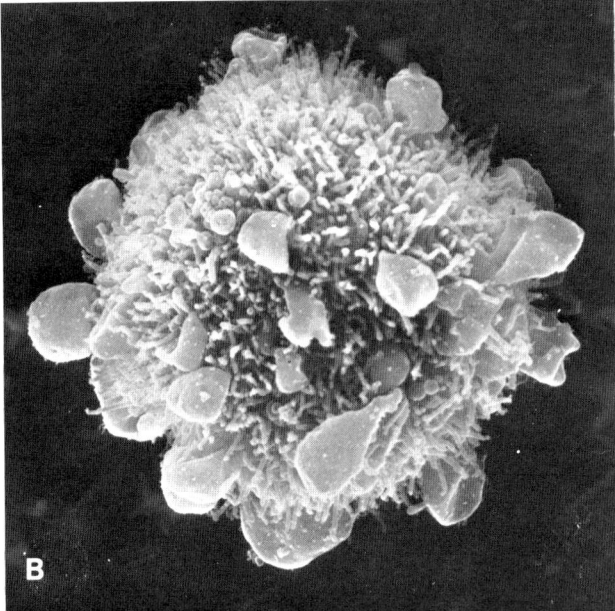

Figure 1.29. *A*, SEM of a control EATC. Note the many delicate, closely packed microvilli. ×5,000. (Reprinted with permission from B. F. Trump, A. Penttila, and I. K. Berezesky: Virchows Archiv. B. Cell Pathology 29:281–296, 1979c.) *B*, SEM of an EATC following 1 hr of anoxia. Although numerous microvilli remain, some areas of the cell surface contain large blebs. ×5,000.

of ion regulation attendant upon deenergization of plasmalemmal sodium-potassium ATPase. It always seems to correlate with reversal of the normal intracellular sodium/potassium ratio.

The energy deficit also presumably stops intracellular transport of secretory proteins within ER lumens, especially at the junction between the ER and Golgi. This may, in some cells, be associated with accumulation of "clouds" of the protein clathrin around elements of the Golgi apparatus. At about this same time, the Golgi complex loses its polarity and orientation and begins to curl in upon itself. We presume again that this is related to cytoskeletal changes (see above). Many other consequences of this Golgi change would doubtedly result if it were kept in this state, including changes in formation of membrane and secretory glycoproteins.

The rough ER shows early changes in the attached ribosomes including loss of polysome arrangements, although early membrane detachment does not occur. We have previously reported that detachment occurs only following irreversible injury (Smuckler and Trump, 1968).This early polysome dissociation may relate to potassium depletion and/or energy deficits which affect messenger-ribosome interactions, deficit of messenger itself, and conceivably changes in membrane fluidity with randomization of attached ribosomes.

Additional changes in the ER involve progressive vesiculation of the cisternae, the mechanism of which is unknown. It probably, however, reflects increased membrane fragility and passage from parallel cisternal systems to a lower energy state.

Lysosomes and Secretory Granules

These related, single membrane-bound granules exhibit somewhat similar reactions after injury. Some of these putative changes have been controversial for over 20 years and still are at the present time.

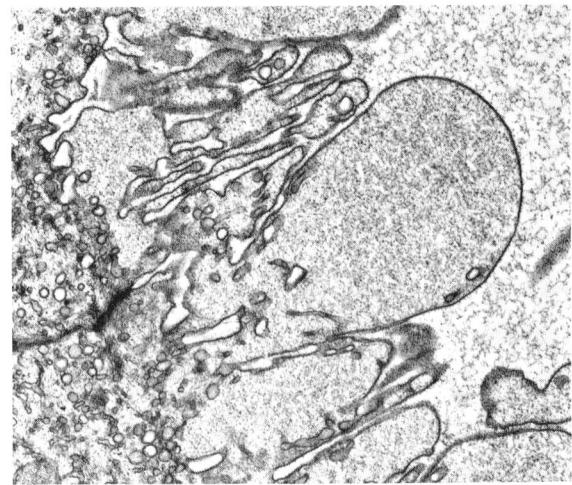

Figure 1.30. An apical bleb of the plasma membrane protruding into a flounder kidney tubule after exposure to 3×10^{-3} M potassium cyanide for 5 min. ×10,000. (Reprinted with permission from B. F. Trump, E. M. McDowell, and A. U. Arstila: *Principles of Pathobiology*, edited by R. B. Hill, Jr. and M. F. La Via, pp. 20–111. Oxford University Press, New York, 1980b.)

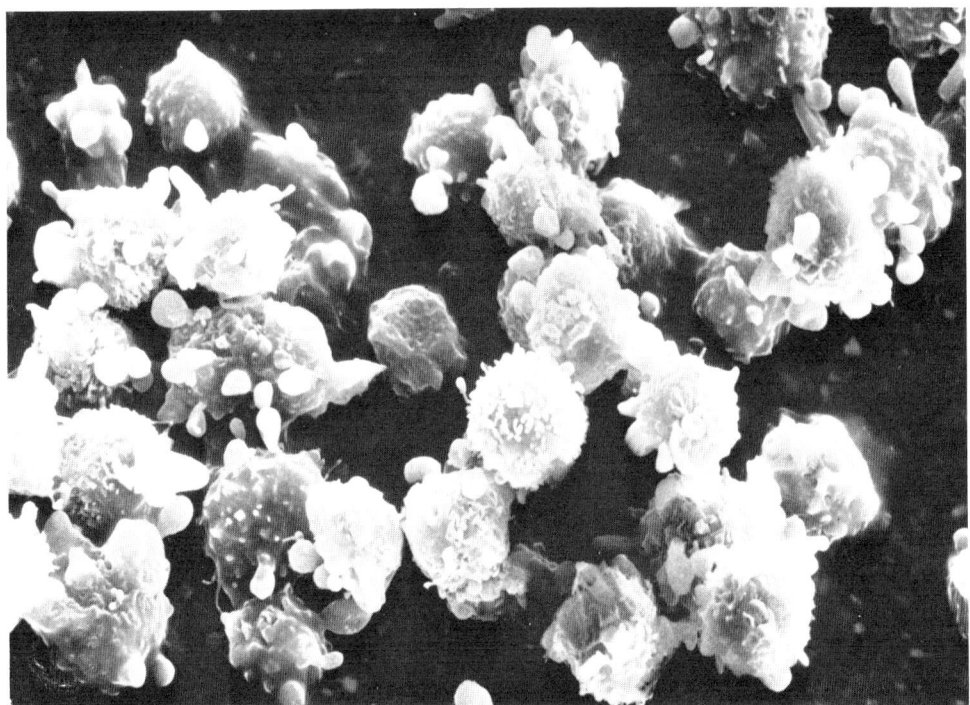

Figure 1.31. SEM of EATC following 30 min incubation with 10 µg/ml cytochalasin. Note the multiple medium sized blebs on the cell surfaces. ×2,000. (Courtesy of P. C. Phelps.)

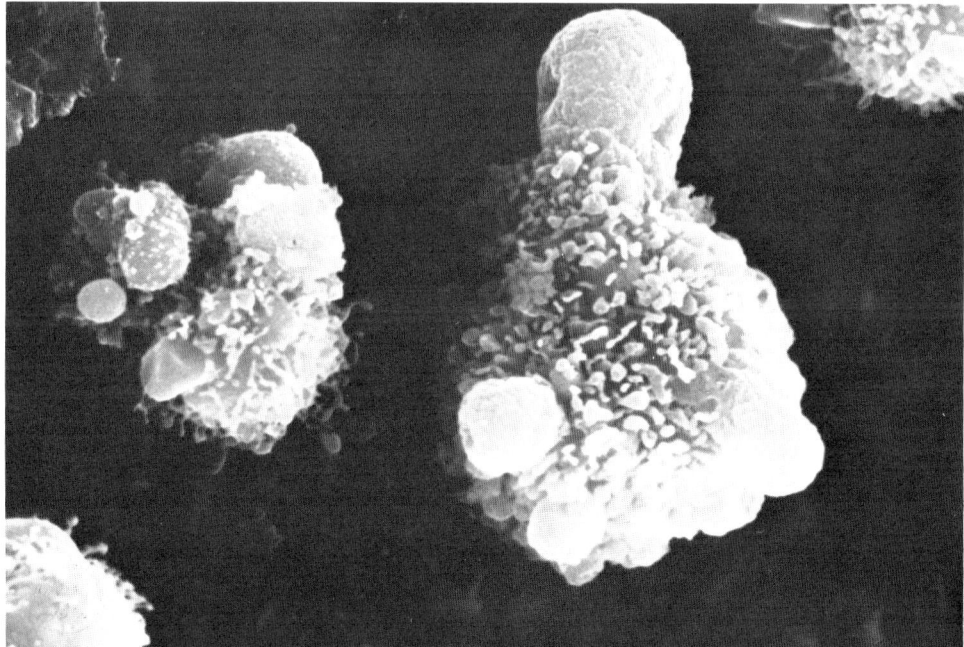

Figure 1.32. SEM of EATC following 60 min incubation with 10^{-3} M ionophore A23187. Note the large surface blebs. ×4,000. (Courtesy of P. C. Phelps.)

SUICIDE BAG HYPOTHESIS

It has been hypothesized for a number of years that the event which causes the cell to pass beyond the point-of-no-return is the leakage of lysosomes and the consequent destructive release of enzymes. Digestive vacuoles do, indeed, rupture during necrosis and release hydrolases into the cytosol but it appears to be the result of cell death rather than the cause. In fact, regions of the cell rich in acid hydrolase-containing structures have been observed well along into the necrotic phase (Trump and Ginn, 1969).

Much work, particularly on myocardial ischemia, has centered around the question of whether or not early damage to lysosomes and release of lysosomal degradative enzymes contributes to potentially reversible ischemic damage progressing to irreversible damage (Wildenthal, 1978). However, the assays commonly used to study lysosomes such as cell fractionation, biochemical enzyme assays, and histochemical tests are characterized by the difficulty that they cannot discriminate between changes due only to the injurious stimulus and those acquired during preparation. It is obvious that isolation procedures cause increased membrane fragility, thereby confusing outcomes. Recently, however, a method for indirect immunohistochemical localization of one major lysosomal enzyme, cathepsin D, has been refined (Decker et al., 1980), allowing for detection of early, subtle changes in ischemic myocyte lysosomes. Other studies concerning the effects of leakage of lytic enzymes from lysosomes have shown that these are released not in toto but slowy (Decker and Wildenthal, 1978). It might well be that smaller sized enzymes are released first; however, activation has to be proven for each lysosomal enzyme as it is leaked from the cytocavitary network during the early stages of cell injury before the situation can be thoroughly evaluated.

INCREASED LYSOSOME FORMATION, ORGANELLE TURNOVER AND CELLULAR AUTOPHAGY

This seemingly important phenomena was discussed above and will not be repeated here.

INCREASED EXTRACELLULAR RELEASE OF LYSOSOMAL ENZYMES

Another way in which the activities of the lysosome system can be harmful to cells is for one cell to secrete its contents, then deleteriously affect neighboring cells. Although this may occur with parenchymal cells, it is much more characteristic of inflammatory cells, e.g., polymorphonuclear cells and macrophages. Some regurgitation always seems to accompany phagocytosis and even more accompanies autophagocytosis. Stimulation of polymorphonuclear cell-lysosomal enzyme secretion can be induced by ionophore A23187.

FUSION OF SECRETORY GRANULES

As mentioned in Chapter 22, extensive fusions of secretory vacuoles may occur, resulting in confluent masses of zymogen granules. Eventually the limiting membranes themselves disappear and the contents appear to blend with the cytosol. This appears, however, to occur only after cell death. It is, nevertheless, the apparent reason for the rapid dissolution of pancreatic cells during the phase of autolysis. In vivo, such autolysis could, however, result particularly in the release of many products including toxic and vasoactive peptides.

Peroxisomes

These organelles are currently attracting increasing attention as more is learned about their structure and function. Their most important function may be in β-oxidation of fatty acids, the products of which enter the Krebs cycle. Failure of this oxidation in hypoxic or ischemic states may lead to the accumulation of triglycerides in organs, e.g., the heart and liver. In the heart, peroxisomes are in close proximity to the mitochondria. Of course, with complete ischemia, they cannot accumulate for long since the cells die and undergo necrosis. In partial ischemia or hypoxia, however, continued accumulation can occur.

Nucleus

The earliest change in the nucleus is chromatin clumping, which is initially quite reversible. It is probably produced by the decreased pH which rapidly develops in the cell and is exemplified by the condensation of the normally expanded chromosomes. In this condensed state, the DNA is inactive in RNA synthesis and the nuclear envelope remains intact, although dilatation of it may occur producing perinuclear vacuoles.

Later, especially after the point-of-no-return, progressive loss of chromatin occurs, presumably through the action of lysosomal DNAase and proteases, and gradually results in total disappearance of stainable DNA—the process known as karyolysis.

With the use of synchronized cell cultures, it is now possible to study variations in sensitivity to toxic agents throughout the division cycle. Following injury by ionizing irradiation or radiomimetic agents such as nitrogen mustards, cells in early G_1 and G_2 phases are the least sensitive, while cells in M, late G_1, or early phases are the most sensitive. Such treatments appear to prolong the interphase period and to delay the entry of cells into mitosis by prolonging the time in G_2; characteristic cytological changes observed in the nucleus during cell division include chromosome breaks, bridge formation between chromosomes at anaphase, and chromosomal fragmentation. In contrast, some cells such as lymphocytes and spermatogonia appear to undergo an immediate cytologic type of death after irradiation. The so called spindle poisons (colchicine, vinblastine, etc.) which exhibit differential effects during the cell cycle are in another category. These agents interfere with the formation of the mitotic spindle and stabilize or block the process of mitosis in metaphase. Of interest is the fact that some features of the M phase are quite similar to the phase of altered homeostasis following cell injury. During mitosis, the cells round up and show marked alterations in cell membrane permeability. Existing supplies of high energy compounds are used up and little or no further synthesis occurs. As a result, the stress of the M phase often proves lethal to the cell since the continuation through S and G_2 has been interfered with.

Mitochondria

Many details of mitochondrial changes were given above. This section will, therefore, only describe our current conception of their histogenesis, as shown in Figure 1.33.

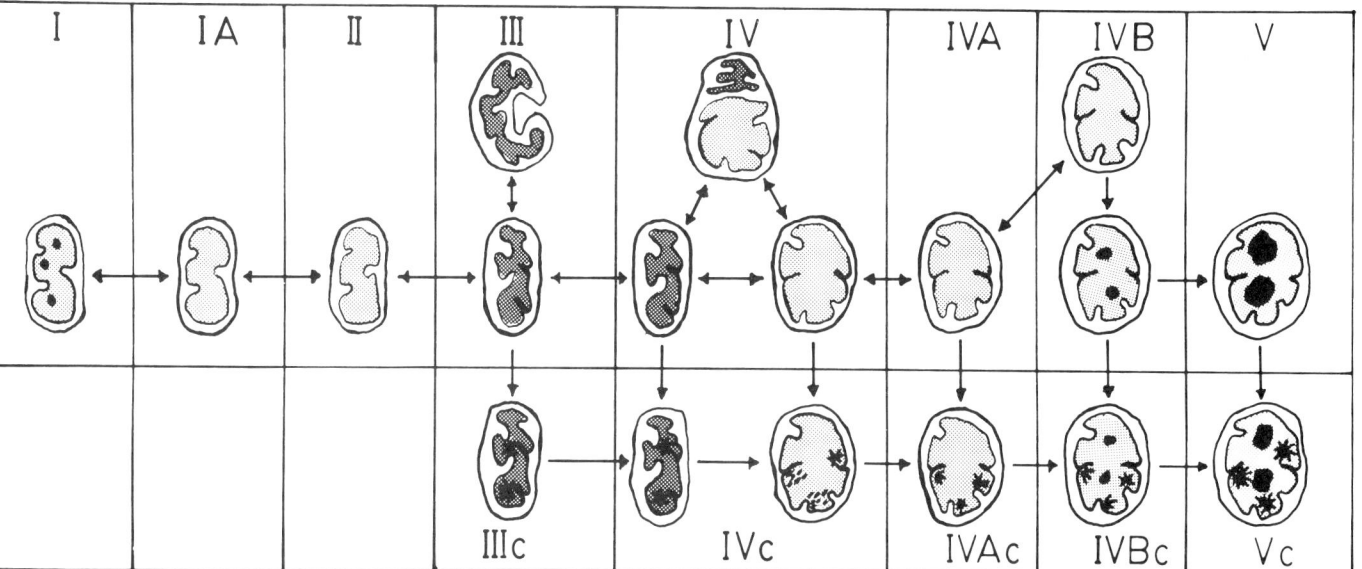

Figure 1.33. A diagrammatic representation of mitochondrial profiles following cell injury. This figure shows the configuration of mitochondria in each of the various stages of cell injury. The numbering on the stages is as defined in the text. In stage I, the mitochondria are in orthodox conformation with normal, electron-dense matrical granules. In stage IA, the mitochondria are unaltered except for the disappearance of the normal matrical granules; the same occurs in stage II. In stage III, the mitochondria assume a condensed configuration with increased density of the matrix and the beginning of fusions and adhesions of the inner membrane. When this is severe, the mitochondria can assume curved donut configurations, and when the matrix condensations is extremely severe, adhesion of cristae on the matrical side develops. Calcifications can also occur in this phase under some conditions (IIIc); also in some conditions, flocculent densities may develop. In stage IV, some mitochondria remain in the condensed configuration while others show inner compartment swelling. Still other mitochondria, in some cells where there are several inner compartments, may show one compartment condensed and the other swollen. This stage may also have each of the conformations also showing calcifications (IVc). In the next stage, IVA, all the mitochondria have swollen inner compartments. The matrical space is pale, presumably because of increased water content. In IVAc, calcific deposits occur especially in proximity to cristae. In IVB, some mitochondria retain the appearance of IVA, whereas others show the appearance of tiny dense aggregates. In IVBc, in addition to the tiny dense aggregates, small calcific deposits occur. In stage V, large flocculent densities appear within the matrical compartment, whereas in Vc, they occur together with large calcific deposits. It is to be emphasized that the progression of stages I through V is characteristic of certain types of injury, specifically, anoxia and ischemia. With reflow into ischemic areas, stages IIIc, IVc, IVAc, IVBc, and Vc may also occur. The c series can also occur with direct membrane injury. Flocculent densities can occur not only in stage V but in stages III and IV as well. This is a rare occurrence and may indicate irreversibility when it occurs. We do not presently know the factors responsible for it.

The earliest mitochondrial change may be loss of or modification of the normal matrix granules. Although these may, in part, be formed of phospholipid, the change correlates with loss of calcium due to the energy-depleted state and in part due to sodium-stimulated calcium loss, at least in some cells.

Mitochondrial condensation also occurs very rapidly. This may be correlated with increased ADP levels, although its mechanism is still not known. It is clearly reversible and also correlates with potassium loss. Part of the contraction may thus be part of a water loss accompanying the K efflux; another part could perhaps relate to mitochondrial matrix contraction, although little is known as yet concerning cytoskeletal elements in the mitochondria. This change also occurs readily in vitro after adding ADP to respiring mitochondria or after inhibiting respiration. Mitochondria are also in this state when freshly isolated in sucrose. In fact, they behave as if this state occurs when they are at a resting stage or when $[H^+]$ influx occurs in an abrupt fashion. Much more needs to be known about it.

Another early change, especially in some tissues, is the apparent fusion of the inner and outer membranes to form pentalaminar structures with thick, dense, rod-like central layers. This change occurs very early after ischemia, especially in the heart (Osornio-Vargas et al., 1980) and is probably associated with defective inner membrane functions. Although we do not know the precise mechanisms at present, we hypothesize that it is related to release of a membrane-fusing agent(s), e.g., fatty acid or lysophosphatides as a result of phospholipase activation. Apparently simultaneously with this state is the development of so called "adhesions" between the inner membranes on their matrical side (see above). Both fusions and adhesions are probably associated with decreased or absent inner membrane function. Both are apparently prior to the point-of-no-return.

The next change in the mitochondria involves a swelling of the inner compartment which occurs over a relatively short period of time and in some instances explosively. The cristae gradually unfold and the surface area increases. Ultimately the outer membrane breaks. As this occurs, the inner compartment is diluted due to the influx of water. Initially, this change is totally reversible, and following restoration of blood flow, the mitochondria quickly return to normal. Initially, therefore, the respiratory proteins and coupling factors are either intact or else can be repaired quickly during the recovery process. Respiration in mitochondria isolated during this stage is intact but coupling is loose (see Ch. 47). Total mitochondrial calcium is reduced.

The cell is now poised on an edge between life and death. In a short time, depending on the cell, the temperature, and other conditions, irreversible change takes place. Before the change occurs, however, the previously sparse and diluted marcomolecules in the matrix begin to aggregate forming tiny, fluffy aggregates which evidently represent reversible denaturation of matrical proteins. These initial loose aggregates quickly reverse if circulation is restored.

Soon, however, the time of cell death is heralded by the appearance of much larger and more compact aggregates of denatured protein in the matrix-flocculent densities. These denatured proteins may include those of both the matrix and the inner membrane and are the earliest signs of irreparable damage to mitochondria and thus of cell death. Cells showing these changes may be indistinguishable from normal cells by routine light microscopy of paraffin sections; by electron microscopy, however, they are easily evident.

HYPOTHESIS

It is apparent that the subcellular structural and functional changes that occur following ischemia are both diverse and complex. Our studies over the past 20 years have revealed a variety of effects—some of which seem critical and others which do not. Admittedly, most of the information is phenomenological. It is, however, the purpose of this chapter to leave the reader with our interpretation of all available observations on this process and to produce a new theory of the mechanisms of progression. Hopefully, this will lead not only to a better understanding of the processes but also to the development of improved therapeutic interventions.

As mentioned above, the organelles and other subcellular systems undergo a series of relatively reproducible changes following injury. The type of changes as well as the sequence and the rate of progression vary with the injury and probably with the genetic background of the host recipient. Nevertheless, we deem it of great importance to synthesize all of this information into a general theory of cell injury.

Our current working hypothesis of the progression of changes following acute ischemic injury is shown in Figure 1.34. Following acute ischemia, acute oxygen and substrate deficiencies occur within the cell rapidly, resulting in cessation of oxydative phosphorylation and rapid decreases of ATP concentration. These consequences have a number of important effects on the cell, as indicted in the diagram (see also Chs. 4–6), including stimulation of anaerobic glycolysis, inhibition of ATP-dependent reactions such as the sodium-potassium ATPase, and feedback on the control of other organelles. Also shown in the diagram is the possibility of peroxisomal hyperplasia as suggested by the work of Riede and colleagues (1980).

The cessation of sodium-potassium ATPase activity results in gradual increases of sodium and decreases of potassium in the cell. The increased concentration of sodium affects sodium entry and interferes with sodium-calcium exchange at the cell surface membrane. In some cells, this increased sodium concentration tends to displace calcium from the mitochondria. All of these changes result in increased phorbols of ionized calcium in the cytosol which increase binding to calmodulin. The increased level of calcium-calmodulin complexes are believed to activate a number of phenomena, including separation of cell junctions, uptake of calcium by mitochondria in certain states such as reflow and when substrate is available, alteration of microtubules and microfilaments, and activation of phospholipases. It is also possible that through affects on cyclic AMP formation this acts as a stimulus to cell division. At about the same time, the decreased potassium levels lead to mitochondrial contraction and condensation with loss of mitochondrial granules. Simultaneously, the ER accumulates water presumably with one or more ions and also dilates. The exact nature of the ions within the dilated ER awaits elucidation. Also simultaneously, increased glycolysis depletes cell glycogen, increases levels of lactate, and results in decreased cell pH. This is associated with chromatin clumping and decreased RNA synthesis but is a reversible change.

Many of the inital effects on cell shape, autophagic vacuole formation, and altered intermembraneous particles may relate to alterations of the cytoskeleton, including microtubules and microfilaments. These can be seen in cells both in vitro and in vivo as mentioned above.

The critical points in irreversibility are possibly related to membrane hydrolysis, especially membrane lipids, perhaps through the effects of phospholipase. This includes damage to the plasmalemma and the mitochondria and leads to changes in permeability including mitochondrial swelling. The released fatty acids may have a number of effects including membrane fusions which can be seen in mitochondria as well as in other

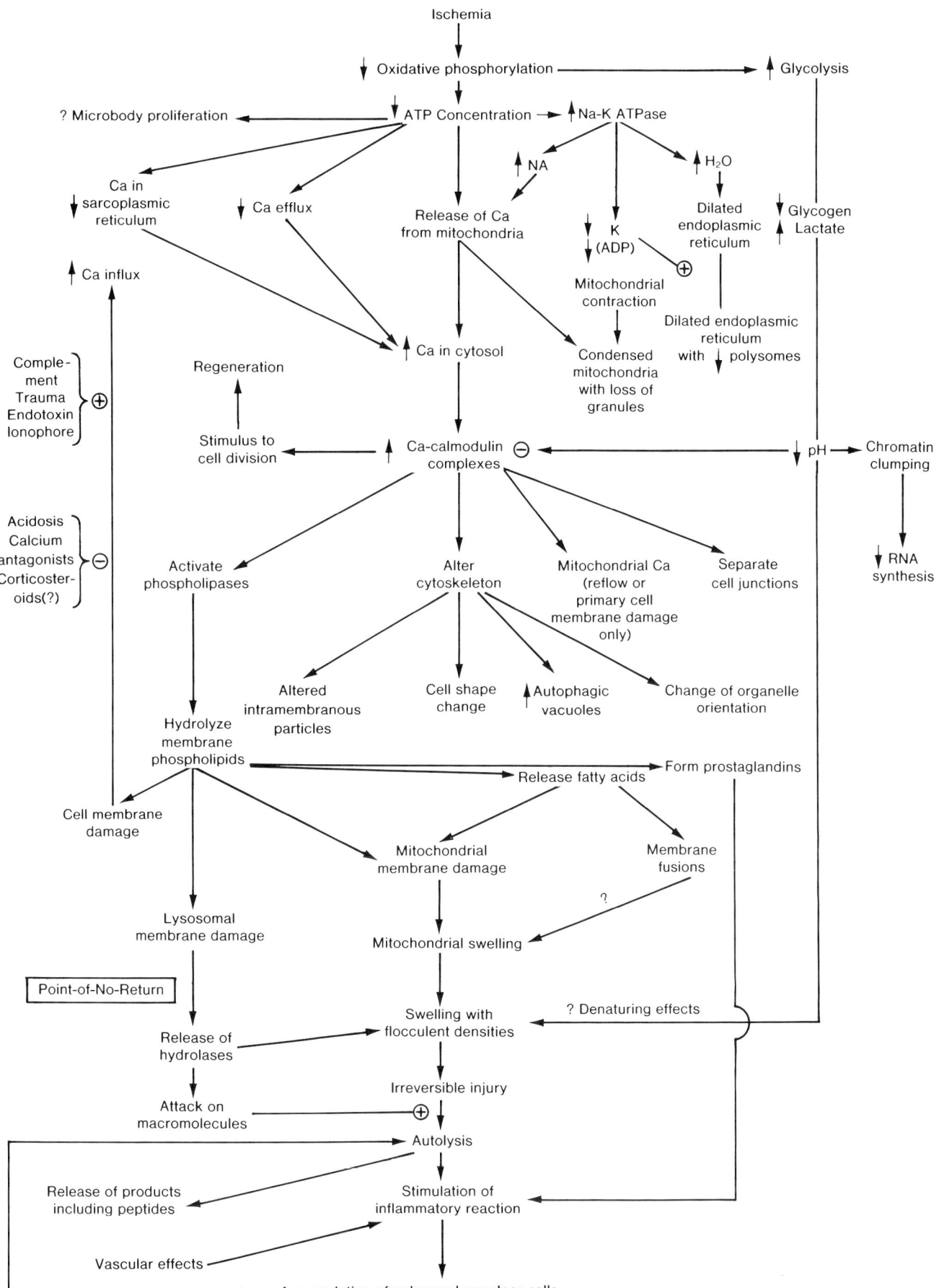

Figure 1.34. A diagram illustrating a conceptualization of the effects of ischemic injury on ion distributions and the cellular events which are triggered (see text for discussion).

organelles. Also, phospholipase activity could relate to prostaglandin formation. Irreversibility is indicated by the appearance of flocculent densities in the mitochondria and seems to occur in all systems studied. Lysosomal membrane damage with release of hydrolases is still somewhat controversial but, in our data, does not seem to occur until after the point-of-no-return. Among the effects of products resulting from proteolytic and phospholipase attack are products with vascular effects, including peptides and prostaglandins, which stimulate in inflammatory reaction.

Shown at the left side of Figure 1.34 are the effects of potentiating or inhibitory conditions or compounds which are visualized in the diagram to modify cell membrane damage and calcium influx.

In direct contrast to ischemic injury, other types of lethal injury which primarily attack the cell membrane can be produced by Hg and other heavy metals, complement, endotoxin, and chemical ionophores. These result in an increase in calcium entry into the cell either through specific diffusion sites or by nonspecific increases in membrane permeability caused by protein and/or lipid alterations. The increased calcium entry rapidly exceeds the buffering capacity of the ER, mitochondria, and cytosol proteins such as calmodulin and results in increased ionized calcium in the cytosol which, we believe, eventually triggers the phospholipase-induced cell membrane damage. The effects of this can be virtually explosive, with rapid cell volume changes, cell shape modifications due to alterations of the cytoskelton, and early cell lysis. Progression from normal to stage V or the necrotic cell is much more rapid with these plasma membrane damaging agents than that following ischemia. Mitochondrial calcium-loading almost always occurs because, we believe, the primary attack is directed against the cell membrane, with the mitochondrial membrane not being involved, at least not initially. Calcium is then translocated into the mitochondria and, since phosphate is present and increased as ATP hydrolysis occurs, is precipitated as calcium phosphate. Initially, this begins as annular deposits which do not resemble normal matrix granules or flocculent densities. At later stages, needle-like crystals occur which, in some cases, represent calcium hydroxyapatite. The mitochondria continue to progress through the stages, and stage VA is reached in which flocculent densities are associated with the mitochondrial calcifications. Calcium precipitates also occur in condensed mitochondria (stage IIIc). Agents such as mannitol, which reduce cell swelling, or those which modify calcium permeability such as Verapamil and methyl prednisolone modify this process. However, extracellular acidosis delays the response and modifies cell killing.

SUMMARY

As was stated earlier in this chapter, the understanding of the events following various types of cell injury is crucial to the development of our knowledge concerning the pathogenesis, treatment, and prevention of human diseases. We have been involved in such studies for many years, as have other investigators, and, as a result, believe that many of the cellular changes leading from the normal to the irreversibly injured cell are initiated and modified by primary and secondary effects of ion redistributions. In particular, we have been concerned with the role of calcium, both ionized and total, since considerable evidence has been accumulated which indicates that abnormal levels and distributions of this ion in the cytosol initiate catabolic processes, directly lead the cell beyond the point-of-no-return, or cell death. Regardless of the type of injury, the cell undergoes Ca accumulation either by impaired energy metabolism or plasma membrane alterations. This elevated intracellular calcium concentration is responsible for cytoskeletal modifications which alter cell shape, the activation of phospholipases which causes perpetuation of membrane damage, and, finally, mitochondrial calcification. Although these alterations have been somewhat characterized biochemically and morphologically, certain points continue to need clarification. New techniques such as x-ray microanalysis for measuring total cell calcium and organelle-localized calcium as well as methods for the estimation of ionized calcium should provide a much better understanding of the role of this important cation. Since the importance of determining the event(s) responsible for cell death is directly related to the potential capability of their manipulation, knowledge of this event could result in the development and/or modification of pharmacologic interventions for the control and prevention of many human diseases including shock.

References

Appleton, T.C.: Dry ultrathin frozen sections for electron microscopy and x-ray microanalysis: The cryostat approach. Micron 3:101–105, 1972.

Arango, A., Illner, H., and Shires, G.T.: Role of ischemia in the incubation of changes in cell membrane during hemorrhagic shock. J. Surg. Res. 20:473–476, 1976.

Arstila, A.U., and Trump, B.F.: Studies on cellular autophagocytosis. The formation of autophagic vacuoles in the liver after glucagon administration. Am. J. Pathol. 53:687–733, 1968.

Arstila, A.U., Jauregui, H.O., Chang, J., and Trump, B.F.: Studies on cellular autophagocytosis. Relationship between heterophagy and autophagy in HeLa cells. Lab. Invest. 24:162–174, 1971.

Arstila, A.U., Shelburne, J.D., and Trump, B.F.: Studies on cellular autophagocytosis. A histochemical study on sequential alterations of mitochondria in the glucagon-induced autophagic vacuoles of rat liver. Lab. Invest. 27:317–323, 1972.

Ashraf, M., White, F., and Bloor, C.M.: Ultrastructural influences of reperfusing dog myocardium with calcium-free blood after coronary artery occlusion. Am. J. Pathol. 90:423–434, 1978.

Baker, P.F.: Transport and metabolism of calcium ions in nerve. Prog. Biophys. Mol. Biol. 24:177–223, 1972.

Barrett, L.A., McDowell, E.M., Harris, C.C., and Trump, B.F.: Studies on the pathogenesis of ischemic cell injury. XV.

Reversal of ischemic cell injury in hamster trachea and human bronchus by explant culture. Beitr. Pathol. *161:*109–121, 1977.

Baue, A.E.: Mitochondrial function in shock. In *The Cell in Shock*, pp. 11–15. The Upjohn Co., Kalamazoo, 1974.

Baue, A.E.: Multiple, progressive, or sequential systems failure. A syndrome of the 1970's. Arch. Surg. *110:*779–781, 1975.

Blaustein, M.P.: The interrelationship between Na and Ca fluxes across cell membranes. Rev. Physiol. Biochem. Pharmacol. *70:*33–82, 1974.

Borle, A.B., and Studer, R.: Effects of calcium ionophores on the transport and distribution of calcium in isolated cells and in liver and kidney slices. J. Membr. Biol. *38:*51–72, 1978.

Brinkley, B.R., Cox, S.M., Pepper, D.A., and Pardue, R.L.: Microtubule assembly sites in cultured mammalian cells: Analysis by tubulin immunofluoresence and electron microscopy. In *37th Annual Proceedings of Electron Microscopy Society of America*, edited by G.W. Bailey, pp. 14–17. San Antonio, 1979.

Brinley, F.J., Jr.: Calcium-buffering in squid axons. Annu. Rev. Biophys. Bioeng. *7:*363–392, 1978.

Bulkley, B., Nunnally, R.L., and Hollis, D.P.: "Calcium paradox" and the effect of varied temperature on its development: A phosphorous nuclear magnetic resonance and morphological study. Lab. Invest. *39:*133–140, 1978.

Cameron, I.L., Smith, N.K.R., Pool, T.B., and Sparks, R.L.: Intracellular concentration of sodium and other elements as related to mitogenesis and oncogenesis in vivo. Cancer Res. *40:*1493–1500, 1980.

Campion, D.S., Lynch, L.J., Rector, F.C., Jr., Carter, N., and Shires, G.T.: Effect of hemorrhagic shock on transmembrane potential. Surgery *66:*1051–1059, 1969.

Carafoli, E.: Mitochondrial uptake of calcium ions and the regulation of cell function. Biochem. Soc. Symp. *39:*89–109, 1974.

Carafoli, E.: The calcium cycle of mitochondria. FEBS Lett. *104:*106, 1979.

Carafoli, E., and Crompton, M.: Calcium ions and mitochondria. Soc. Exp. Biol. Symp. *30:*89–115, 1976.

Champion, H.R., Jones, R.T., Trump, B.F., Decker, R., Wilson, S., Miginski, M., and Gill, W.: A clinicopathologic study of hepatic dysfunction following shock. Surg. Gynecol. Obstet. *142:*657–663, 1976.

Chandler, J.A.: X-ray microanalysis in the electron microscope. In *Practical Methods in Electron Microscopy*, edited by A.M. Glauert, vol. 5, pp. 317–547. North-Holland, Amsterdam.

Chang, S.H., Mergner, W.J., Pendergrass, R.E., Bulger, R.E., Berezesky, I.K., and Trump, B.F.: A rapid method of cryofixation of tissues in situ for ultramicrotomy. J. Histochem. Cytochem. *28:*47–51, 1980.

Cheah, K.S., and Cheah, A.M.: Inclusions in aged mitochondria. J. Bioenerg. Biomembr. *9:*105–115, 1977.

Cheung, Y.W.: Cyclic 3′,5′-nucleotide phosphodiesterases: Demonstration of an activator. Biochem. Biophys. Res. Commun. *33:*533–538, 1970.

Cheung, Y.W.: Calmodulin plays a pivotal role in cellular regulation. Science *207:*19–27, 1980.

Chien, K.R., Abrams, J., Serroni, A., Martin, J.T., and Farber, J.L.: Accelerated phospholipid degradation and associated membrane dysfunction in irreversible, ischemic liver cell injury. J. Biol. Chem. *253:*4809–4817, 1978.

Chien, K.R., Pfau, R.G., and Farber, J.L.: Ischemic myocardial cell injury. Prevention by chlorpromazine of an accelerated phospholipid degradation and associated membrane dysfunction. Am. J. Pathol. *97:*505–529, 1979.

Christensen, A.K.: Frozen thin sections of fresh tissue for electron microscopy with a description of pancreas and liver. J. Cell Biol. *51:*772–804, 1971.

Coleman, S.E., Duggan, J., and Hackett, R.L.: Changes in freeze-fractured nuclei after renal ischemia and reflow in the rat. Exp. Mol. Pathol. *23:*59–69, 1975.

Cone, C.D., Jr.: Unified theory on the basic mechanism of normal mitotic control and oncogenesis. J. Theor. Biol. *30:*151–181, 1971.

Cone, C.D., Jr.: The role of the surface electrical transmembrane potential in normal and malignant mitogenesis. Ann. N.Y. Acad. Sci. *238:*420–435, 1974.

Cowley, R.A., Attar, S., LaBrosse, E., et al.: Some significant biochemical parameters found in 300 shock patients. J. Trauma *9:*926–938, 1969.

Croker, B.P., Jr., Saladino, A.J., and Trump, B.F.: Ion movements in cell injury: Relationship between energy metabolism and the pathogenesis of lethal injury in the toad bladder. Am. J. Pathol. *59:*247–278, 1970.

Crompton, M., Moser, R., Ludi, H., and Carafoli, E.: The interrelations between the transport of sodium and calcium in mitochondria of various mammalian tissue. Eur. J. Biochem. *82:*25–31, 1978.

Cunningham, J.N., Carter, N.W., Rector, R.C., and Seldin, D.W.: Resting transmembrane potential difference of skeletal muscle in normal subjects and severely ill patients. J. Clin. Invest. *50:*49–59, 1971.

Decker, R.S., and Wildenthal, K.: Sequential lysosomal alterations during cardiac ischemia. II. Ultrastructural and cytochemical changes. Lab. Invest. *38:*662–673, 1978.

Decker, R.S., Decker, M.L., and Pool, A.R.: The distribution of lysosomal cathepsin D in cardiac myocytes. J. Histochem. Cytochem. *28:*231–237, 1980.

Dedman, J.R., Brinkley, B.R., and Means, A.R.: Regulation of microfilaments and microtubules by calcium and cyclic AMP. Adv. Cyclic Nucleotide Res. *11:*131–174, 1979.

Donohoe, J.F., Venkatachalam, M.A., Bernard, D.B., and Levinsky, N.G.: Tubular leakage and obstruction after renal ischemia: Structural-functional correlations. Kidney Int. *13:*208–222, 1978.

Elbrink, J., and Bihle, I.: Membrane transport: The relation to cellular metabolic rates. Science *188:*1177–1184, 1975.

Farber, J.L., Martin, J.T., and Chien, K.: Irreversible ischemic cell injury. Am. J. Pathol. *92:*713–732, 1978.

Frank, J.S.: Structure of the freeze-fractured sarcolemma in the normal and anoxic myocardium. Fed. Proc. *39:*276, 1980.

French, S.W., Norum, H.L., Ihrig, T.J., and Todoroff, T.: Effect of phospholipid hydrolysis on the structural and functional integrity of mitochondria. Lab. Invest. *25:*427–434, 1971.

Ginn, F.L., and Trump, B.F.: Ultrastructural changes after ultraviolet irradiation of isolated flounder kidney tubules. Lab. Invest. *22:*496, 1970.

Ginn, F.L., Shelburne, J.D., and Trump, B.F.: Disorders of cell volume regulation. I. Effects of inhibition of plasma membrane adenosine triphosphatase with ouabain. Am. J. Pathol. *53:*1041–1071, 1968.

Glaumann, B., and Trump, B.F.: Studies on the pathogenesis of ischemic cell injury. III. Morphological changes of the proximal pars recta tubules (P_3) of the rat kidney made ischemic in vivo. Virchows Arch. [Cell Pathol.] *19:*303–323, 1975.

Glaumann, B., Glaumann, H., Berezesky, I.K., and Trump, B.F.: Studies on the pathogenesis of ischemic cell injury. II. Morphological changes of the pars convoluta (P_1 and P_2) of the proximal tubule of the rat kidney made ischemic in vivo. Virchows Arch. [Cell Pathol.] *19:*281–302, 1975.

Glaumann, B., Glaumann, H., Berezesky, I.K., and Trump, B.F.: Studies on cellular recovery from injury. II. Ultrastructural studies on the recovery of the pars convoluta of the proximal tubule of the rat kidney from temporary ischemia. Virchows Arch. [Cell Pathol.] *24:*1–18, 1977a.

Glaumann, B., Glaumann, H., and Trump, B.F.: Studies of cellular recovery from injury. III. Ultrastructural studies of the recovery of the pars recta of the proximal tubule (P_3 segment) of the rat kidney from temporary ischemia. Virchows Arch. [Cell Pathol.] *25:*281–308, 1977b.

Goracci, G., Porcellati, G., and Woelk, H.: Subcellular localization and distribution of phospholipases A in liver and brain tissue. Adv. Prostaglandin Thromboxane Res. *3:*55–67, 1978.

Goring, G.G., and Spieckermann, P.G.: Ca^{2+} uptake and release phenomena from cardiac mitochondria under normal and ischemic conditions. Basic Res. Cardiol. *73:*126–132, 1978.

Gritzka, T.L., and Trump, B.F.: Renal tubular lesions caused by mercuric chloride. Electron microscopic observations: Degeneration of the pars recta. Am. J. Pathol. *52:*1225–1277, 1968.

Haljamae, H., Jennische, E., and Medegard, A.: Transmembrane potential measurements as an indicator of heterogeneous distribution of nutritive blood flow in skeletal muscle during shock. Acta Physiol. Scand. *101:*458–464, 1977.

Hanzlikova, V., and Schiaffino, S.: Mitochondrial changes in ischemic skeletal muscle. J. Ultrastruct. Res. *60:*121–133, 1977.

Hawkins, H.K., Ericsson, J.L.E., Biberfeld, P., and Trump, B.F.: Lysosome and phagosome stability in lethal cell injury. Am. J. Pathol. *68:*255–287, 1972.

Hearse, D.J.: Reperfusion of the ischemic myocardium. J. Mol. Cell. Cardiol. *9:*605–616, 1977.

Hearse, D.J., Humphrey, S.M., and Bullock, G.R.: The oxygen paradox and calcium paradox: Two facets of the same problem? J. Mol. Cell Cardiol. *10:*641–668, 1978.

Hochachka, P.W.: *Living Without Oxygen. Closed and Open Systems in Hypoxia Tolerance.* Harvard University Press, Cambridge, MA, 1980.

Jennische, E., Enger, E., Medegard, A., Appelgren, L., and Haljamae, H.: Correlation between tissue pH, cellular transmembrane potentials, and cellular energy metabolism during shock and during ischemia. Circ. Shock *5:*251–260, 1978.

Jones, R.T., Garcia, J.H., Mergner, W.J., Pendergrass, R.E., Valigorsky, J.M., and Trump, B.F.: Effects of shock on the pancreatic acinar cell. Cellular and subcellular effects in humans. Arch. Pathol. *99:*634–644, 1975.

Kahng, M.W., Berezesky, I.K., and Trump, B.F.: Metabolic and ultrastructural response of rat kidney cortex to in vitro ischemia. Exp. Mol. Pathol. *29:*183–198, 1978.

Kakiuchi, S., Yamazaki, R., and Nakajima, H.: Properties of a heat stable phosphodiesterase activating factor isolated from brain extract. Proc. Jpn. Acad. *46:*587–492, 1970.

Karpati, G., Carpenter, S., Melmed, C., and Eisen, A.A.: Experimental ischemic myopathy. J. Neurol. Sci. *23:*129–161, 1974.

Katz, A.M., and Hecht, H.H.: The early "pump" failure of the ischemic heart. Am. J. Med. *47:*479–502, 1969.

Kloner, R.A., Ganote, C.E., Whalen, D.A., and Jennings, R.B.: Effect of transient period of ischemia on myocardial cells. II. Fine structure during the first few minutes of reflow. Am. J. Pathol. *74:*399–422, 1974.

Kretsinger, R.H.: Evolution and functional of calcium-binding proteins. Int. Rev. Cytol. *46:*323–393, 1976.

Laiho, K.U., and Trump, B.F.: Relationship of ionic, water, and cell volume changes in cellular injury of Ehrlich ascites tumor cells. Lab. Invest. *31:*207–215, 1974a.

Laiho, K.U., and Trump, B.F.: The relationship between cell viability and changes in mitochondrial ultrastructure, cellular ATP, ion and water content following injury of Ehrlich ascites tumor cells. Virchows Arch. [Cell Pathol.] *15:*267–277, 1974b.

Laiho, K.U., and Trump, B.F.: Studies on the pathogenesis of cell injury. Effects of inhibitors of metabolism and membrane function on the mitochondria of Ehrlich ascites tumor cells. Lab. Invest. *32:*163–182, 1975a.

Laiho, K.U. and Trump, B.F.: Mitochondria changes, ion and water shifts in the cellular injury of Ehrlich ascites tumor cells. Beitr. Pathol. *155:*237–247, 1975, 1975b.

Laiho, K.U., Shelburne, J.D., and Trump, B.F.: Observations on cell volume, ultrastructure, mitochondrial conformation and vital-dye uptake in Ehrlich ascites tumor cells: Effects of inhibiting energy production and function of the plasma membrane. Am. J. Pathol. *65:*203–30, 1971.

Laiho, K.U., Berezesky, I.K., and Trump, B.F.: Studies on the modification of the cellular response to injury. VII. Effect of the ionophore A23187 on ATP and ion content of Ehrlich ascites tumor cells following anoxia. In preparation, 1981.

Lehninger, A.: Proteins and their biological functions. In *Biochemistry*, edited by A. Lehninger, p. 59. Worth, New York, 1970.

Lipsky, M.M., Hinton, D.E., Goldblatt, P.J., Klaunig, J.E., and Trump, B.F.: Iron negative foci and nodules in safrole-exposed mouse liver made sideroblastic by iron-dextran injection. Pathol. Res. Pract. *164:*178–185, 1979.

Loewenstein, W.R., and Rose, B.: Calcium in (junctional) intercellular communication and a through on its behavior in intracellular communication. Ann. N. Y. Acad. Sci. *307:*285–307, 1978.

Lombardi, B.: Considerations on the pathogenesis of fatty liver. Lab. Invest. *15:*1–20, 1966.

Majno, G., Lagattuta, M., and Thompson, T.: Cellular death and necrosis; chemical, physical and morphological changes in rat liver. Virchows Arch. [Pathol. Anat.] *333:*421–465, 1960.

McDowell, E.M., Becci, P.J., Schurch, W., and Trump, B.F.: The respiratory epithelium. VII. Epidermoid metaplasia of hamster tracheal epithelium during regeneration following mechanical injury. J. Natl. Cancer Inst. *62:*995–1008, 1979.

Means, A.R., and Dedman, J.R.: Calmodulin—An intracellular calcium receptor. Nature *285:*73–77, 1980.

Mergner, W.J., and McDonnell, M.: Phospholipase activity in normal, aged and ischemic mitochondria. Lab. Invest. *38:* 357, 1978.

Mergner, W.J., Smith, M.W., and Trump, B.F.: Structural and functional effects of the negative stains silicotungstic acid, phosphotungstic acid, and ammonium molybdate on rat kidney mitochondria. Lab. Invest. *27:*372–383, 1972.

Mergner, W.J., Smith, M.W., Sahaphong, S., and Trump, B.F.: Studies on the pathogenesis of ischemic cell injury. VI. Accumulation of calcium by isolated mitochondria of ischemic rat kidney cortex. Virchows Arch. [Cell Pathol.] *26:*1–16, 1977a.

Mergner, W.J., Smith, M.W., and Trump, B.F.: Studies on the pathogenesis of ischemic cell injury. XI. P/O ratio and acceptor control. Virchows Arch. [Cell Pathol.] *26:*17–26, 1977b.

Mergner, W.J., Smith, M.W., and Trump, B.F.: Studies on the pathogenesis of ischemic cell injury. IV. Alteration of ionic permeability of mitochondria from ischemic rat kidney. Exp. Mol. Pathol. 26:1–12, 1977c.

Mergner, W.J., Chang, S.H., Marzella, L., Kahng, M.W., and Trump, B.F.: Studies on the pathogenesis of ischemic cell injury. VIII. ATPase of rat kidney mitochondria. Lab. Invest. 40:686–694, 1979.

Meyer, W.L., Fischer, W.H., and Krebs, E.G.: Activation of skeletal muscle phosphorylase b kinase by Ca^{2+}. Biochemistry 3:1033–1039, 1964.

Myers, V.B., and Haydon, D.A.: Ion transfer across lipid membranes in the presence of gramicidin A. II. The ion selectivity. Biochim. Biophys. Acta 274:313–322, 1972.

Nicolson, G.L., Giotta, G., Lotan, R., Neri, A., and Poste, G.: Modifications in transformed and malignant cells. In *International Cell Biology*, edited by B.R. Brinkley and K.R. Porter, pp. 138–148. Rockerfeller University Press, New York, 1977.

Osornio, A.R., Berezesky, I.K., Mergner, W.J., and Trump, B.F.: Mitochondrial membrane fusions in experimental myocardial change in experimental rat myocardial infarction. Fed. Proc. 39:634, 1980.

Osornio-Vargas, A.R., Berezesky, I.K., and Trump, B.F.: Mitochondrial membrane fusions: An early ultastructural change in experimental rat myocardial infarction. In preparation, 1981.

Paul, R.J., Bauer, M., and Prease, W.: Vascular smooth muscle: Aerobic glycolysis linked to sodium and potassium transport processes. Science 206:1414–1416, 1979.

Penttila, A., and Trump, B.F.: Extracellular acidosis protects Ehrlich ascites tumor cells and rat renal cortex against anoxic injury. Science 185:277–278, 1974.

Penttila, A., and Trump, B.F.: Studies on modification of the cellular response to injury. I. Protective effect of acidosis on p-chloromercuribenzene sulfonic acid-induced injury of Ehrlich ascites tumor cells. Lab. Invest. 32:690–695, 1975a.

Penttila, A., and Trump, B.F.: Studies on the modification of the cellular response to injury. II. Electron microscopic studies on the protective effect of acidosis on anoxic injury of Ehrlich ascites tumor cells. Virchows Arch. [Cell Pathol.] 18:1–16, 1975b.

Penttila, A., and Trump, B.F.: Studies on the modification of the cellular response to injury. III. Electron microscopic studies on the protective effect of acidosis on p-chloromercuribenzene sulfonic acid-(PCMBS) induced injury of Ehrlich ascites tumor cells. Virchows Arch. [Cell Pathol.] 18:17–34, 1975c.

Penttila, A., Glaumann, H., and Trump, B.F.: Studies on the modification of the cellular response to injury. IV. Protective effect of extracellular acidosis against anoxia, thermal, and p-chloromercuribenzene sulfonic acid treatment of isolated rat liver cells. Life Sci. 18:1419–1430, 1976.

Polimeni, P.I., and Al-Sadir, J.: Expansion of extracellular space in the nonischemic zone of the infarcted heart and concomitant changes in tissue electrolyte contents in the rat. Circ. Res. 37:725–732, 1975.

Publicover, S.J., Duncan, C.J., and Smith, J.L.: The use of A23187 to demonstrate the role of intracellular calcium in causing ultrastructural damage in mammalian muscle. J. Neuropathol. Exp. Neurol. 37:554–557, 1978.

Rasmussen, H.: Ions as second messenger. Hosp. Pract. 9:99–107, 1974.

Rasmussen, H., and Goodman, D.B.: Relationships between calcium and cyclic nucleotides in cell activation. Physiol. Rev. 57:422–509, 1977.

Reide, U.N., Moore, G.W., and Sandritter, W.A.: Structure and function of peroxisomes and their role in disease processes. In *Pathobiology of Cell Membranes*, edited by B.F. Trump and R.T. Jones, vol. II, pp. 174–222. Academic Press, New York, 1980.

Rubin, R.P.: *Calcium and the Secretory Process*, Plenum, NY, 1974.

Russ, J.C.: Electron probe x-ray microanalysis-principles. In *Electron Probe Microanalysis in Biology*, edited by D.A. Erasmus, pp. 5–36. Chapman and Hall, London, 1978.

Sahaphong, S., and Trump, B.F.: Studies of cellular injury in isolated kidney tubules of the flounder. V. Effects of inhibiting sulfhydryl groups of plasma membrane with the organic mercurials PCMB (parachloromercuribenzoate) and PCMBS (parachloromercuribenzenesulfonate). Am. J. Pathol. 63:277–298, 1971.

Saito, A., Smigel, M., and Fleisher, S.: Membrane junctions in the intermembrane space of mitochondria from mammalian tissues. J. Cell Biol. 60:653–663, 1974.

Saladino, A.J., and Trump, B.F.: Ion movements in cell injury. Effects of inhibition of respiration and glycolysis on the ultrastructure and function of the epithelial cells of the toad bladder. Am. J. Pathol. 52:737–776, 1968.

Saladino, A.J., Bentley, P.J., and Trump, B.F.: Ion movements in cell injury. Effect of amphotericin B on the ultrastructure and function of the epithelial cells of the toad bladder. Am. J. Pathol. 54:421–466, 1969.

Sato, T., Tanaka, J., Kamiyama, Y., Klaunig, J.E., Cowley, R.A., and Trump, B.F.: Serum ornithine carbamoyltransferase (S-OCT) activity and hepatic mitochondria in rats following live E. coli injection. Circ. Shock 7:191, 1980.

Schanne, F.A.X., Kane, A.B., Young, E.E., and Farber, J.L.: Calcium dependence of toxic cell death: A final common pathway. Science 206:700–702, 1979.

Schiaffino, S., Severin, E., and Hanzlikova, V.: Intermembrane inclusions induced by anoxia in heart and skeletal muscle mitochondrial. Virchows Arch. [Cell Pathol.] 31:169–179, 1979.

Shelburne, J.D., Arstila, A.U., and Trump, B.F.: Studies on cellular autophagocytosis, cyclic AMP and dibutyryl cyclic AMP-stimulated autophagy in rat liver. Am. J. Pathol. 72:521–534, 1973.

Shen, A.C., and Jennings, R.B.: Myocardial calcium and magnesium in acute ischemic injury. Am. J. Pathol. 67:417–440, 1972.

Smith, M.W., Collan, Y., Kahng, M.W., and Trump, B.F.: Changes of fatty acids and phospholipids in ischemic rat kidney. Biochim. Biophys. Acta 168:192–201, 1980.

Smuckler, E.A., and Trump, B.F.: Alterations in the structure and function of the rough-surfaced endoplasmic reticulum during necrosis in vitro. Lab. Invest. 18:341–351, 1968.

Somlyo, A.P., Somlyo, A.V., and Shuman, H.: Electron probe analysis of vascular smooth muscle. Composition of mitochondria, nuclei, and cytoplasm. J. Cell Biol. 81:316–335, 1979.

Sun, S.T., Day, E.P., and Ho, J.T.: Temperature dependence of calcium-induced fusion of sonicated phosphatidylserine vesicles. Proc. Natl. Acad. Sci. U.S.A. 75:4325–4328, 1978.

Trump, B.F.: The role of cellular membrane systems in shock. In *The Cell in Shock*, pp. 16–29. The Upjohn Co., Kalamazoo, 1974.

Trump, B.F., and Arstila, A.U.: Cellular reaction to injury. In *Principles of Pathobiology*, edited by R.B. Hill, Jr. and M.F.

La Via, ed. 2, pp. 9–96, Oxford University Press, New York, 1975.

Trump, B.F., and Bulger, R.E.: Studies of cellular injury in isolated flounder tubules. III. Light microscopic and functional changes due to cyanide. Lab. Invest. *18:*721–730, 1968a.

Trump, B.F., and Bulger, R.E.: Studies of cellular injury in isolated flounder tubules. IV. Electron microscopic observations of changes during the phase of altered homeostasis in tubules treated with cyanide. Lab. Invest. *18:*731–739, 1968b.

Trump, B.F., and Ginn, F.L.: The pathogenesis of subcellular reaction to lethal injury. In *Methods and Achievements in Experimental Pathology*, edited by E. Bajusz and G. Jasmin, vol. IV, pp. 1–29. Karger, Basel, 1969.

Trump, B.F., and Harris, C.C.: Human tissues in biomedical research (editorial). Hum. Pathol. *10:*245–248, 1979.

Trump, B.F., and Laiho, K.U.: Studies of cellular recovery from injury. I. Recovery from anoxia in Ehrlich ascites tumor cells. Lab. Invest. *33:*706–711, 1975.

Trump, B.F., and Mergner, W.J.: Cell injury. In *The Inflammatory Process*, edited by B.W. Zweifach, L. Grant, and R.T. McClusky, ed. 2, vol. I, pp. 115–257. Academic Press, New York, 1974.

Trump, B.F., Croker, B.P., Jr., and Mergner, W.J.: The role of energy metabolism, ion, and water shifts in the pathogenesis of cell injury. In *Cell Membranes: Biological and Pathological Aspects*, edited by N. Kaufman and G.W. Richter, pp. 84–128. Williams & Wilkins, Baltimore, 1971.

Trump, B.F., Laiho, K.U., Mergner, W.J., and Arstila, A.U.: Studies on the subcellular pathophysiology of acute lethal cell injury. Beitr. Pathol. *152:*243–271, 1974a.

Trump, B.F., Strum, J.M., and Bulger, R.E.: Studies on the pathogenesis of ischemic cell injury. I. Relation between ion and water shifts and cell ultrastructure in rat kidney slices during swelling at 0–4°C. Virchows Arch. [Cell Pathol.] *16:*1–34, 1974b.

Trump, B.F., Valigorsky, J.M., Jones, R.T., Mergner, W.J., Garcia, J.H., and Cowley, R A.: The application of electron microscopy and cellular biochemistry to the autopsy. Observations on cellular changes in human shock. Hum. Pathol. *6:*499–516, 1975.

Trump, B.F., Berezesky, I.K., Change, S.H., and Bulger, R.E.: Detection of ion shifts in proximal tubule cells of the rat kidney using x-ray microanalysis. Virchows Arch. [Cell Pathol.] *22:*111–120, 1976a.

Trump, B.F., Berezesky, I.K., Collan, Y., Kahng, M. W., and Mergner, W. J.: Recent studies on the pathophysiology of ischemic cell injury. Beitr. Pathol. *158:*363–388, 1976b.

Trump, B.F., Kim, K.M., Jones, R.T., and Valigorsky, J.M.: Pathology of organelles in the human hepatic parenchymal cell. In *Progress in Liver Diseases*, edited by H. Popper and F. Schaffner, pp. 51–68. Grune & Stratton, New York, 1976c.

Trump, B.F., Mergner, W.J., Kahng, M.W., and Saladino, A.J.: Studies on the subcellular pathophysiology of ischemia. Circulation (Suppl. I) *53:*17–26, 1976d.

Trump, B.F., Berezesky, I.K., Pendergrass, R.E., et al: X-ray microanalysis of diffusible elements in scanning electron microscopy of biological thin sections. Studies of pathologically altered cells. Scan. Electron Microsc. *2:*1027–1039, 1978a.

Trump, B.F., Jesudason, M.L., and Jones, R.T.: Ultrastructural features of diseased cells. In *Diagnostic Electron Microscopy*, edited by B.F. Trump and R.T. Jones, vol. I, pp. 1–88. John Wiley & Sons, New York, 1978b.

Trump, B.F., Berezesky, I.K., Mergner, W.J., and Phelps, P.C.: The role of calcium in cell injury. Micron *9:*5–6, 1978c.

Trump, B.F., Berezesky, I.K., Chang, S.H., et al: The role of ion shifts in cell injury. Scan. Electron Microsc. *3:*1–14, 1979a.

Trump, B.F., Laiho, K.U., and Berezesky, I.K.: The role of ion movements in cell injury and shock. Circ. Shock *6:*182, 1979b.

Trump, B.F., Penttila, A., and Berezesky, I.K.: Studies on cell surface conformation following injury. I. Scanning and transmission electron microscopy of cell surface changes following *p*-chloromercuribenzene sulfonic acid (PCMBS)-induced injury of Ehrlich ascites tumor cells. Virchows Arch. [Cell Pathol.] *29:*281–296, 1979c.

Trump, B.F., Penttila, A., and Berezesky, I.K.: Studies on cell surface conformation following injury. II. Scanning and transmission electron microscopy of cell surface changes following anoxic injury in Ehrlich ascites tumor cells. Virchows Arch. [Cell Pathol.] *29:*297–307, 1979d.

Trump, B.F., Phelps, P.C., Shamsuddin, A.M., and Harris, C.C.: Cell surface changes in premalignant and malignant lesions of the colon. Lab. Invest. *40:*289, 1979e.

Trump, B.F., Berezesky, I.K., Laiho, K.U., Osornio, A.R., Mergner, W.J., and Smith, M.W.: The role of calcium in cell injury. A review. Scan. Electron Microsc. *2:*437–462, 1980a.

Trump, B.F., McDowell, E.M., and Arstila, A.U.: Cellular reaction to injury. In *Principles of Pathobiology*, edited by R.B. Hill, Jr. and M.F. LaVia, ed. 3, pp. 20–111. Oxford University Press, New York, 1980b.

Wakabayashi, T., and Green. D.E.: Membrane fusion in mitochondria. I. Ultrastructural basis for fusion. J. Electron Microsc. *26:*305–320, 1977.

Welsh, M.J., Dedman J.R., Brinkley, B.R., and Means, A.R.: Tubulin and calmodulin. Effects of microtuble and microfilaments inhibitors on localization in the mitotic apparatus. J. Cell Biol. *81:*624–634, 1978.

Wildenthal, K.: Lysosomal alterations in ischemic myocardium: Result or cause of myocellular damage? J. Mol. Cell. Cardiol. *10:*595–603, 1978.

Williamson, J.R., Schaffer, S.W., Ford, C., and Safer, B.: Contribution of tissue acidosis to ischemic injury in the perfused rat heart. Circulation (Suppl. 1) *53:*3–14, 1976.

Wolff, D.J., and Siegel, F.: Purification of a calcium-binding phosphoprotein from pig brain. J. Biol. Chem. *247:*4180–4185, 1972.

Wrogemann, K., and Pena, S.D.J.: Mitochondrial calcium overload: A general mechanism for cell necrosis in muscle diseases. Lancet *1:*672–674, 1976.

CHAPTER 2

On the Qualitative Dynamics of Cell Response to Injury

NICHOLAS DeCLARIS

> Virtually all acute responses of cells to injury involve alterations of membrane systems. In order to visualize the effect of lethal or sublethal injury in cellular decay ... we define a reversible phase and an irreversible phase to cell damage, the separation being a "point of no return," or the point of cell death.
>
> Benjamin F. Trump
> The Cell in Shock (1974)

MOTIVATION

Cells, the building blocks of life, as objects of study have been recognized to be complex. In the human body, a cell when alive continuously carries out between 1,000 and 2,000 chemical processes. These processes are not independent; in fact, they are strongly interrelated through feedback mechanisms which ensure by-and-large that the cell will function in its normal manner—homeostasis—most of the time, despite variations in its external environment. While all the details of what takes place all of the time are not there, our knowledge is sufficient to give us a good (in fact, several alternative models) picture of cell homeostatic behavior. However, there are variations in the cell environment known to disrupt the cell processes to the extent that the cell can no longer function as a living unit—the cell dies. In a sense, all cells in the human body (except for neural and other highly specialized cells) cease to exist after a time. Interesting as this process of normal death may be, of greater urgency is the study of the phenomenon of sudden, premature death—abrupt changes in the environment of the cell which bring about premature termination of the life process. In the last few years there have been a number of excellent studies of cell responses to injury. One of the most important (if not *the* most important) results so far is the identification by various experimental biological models of a phase of cell damage (caused by external injury to the cell environment alterations) known as the "point-of-no-return" (Trump, 1974). What has been established so far is that the cell response to deprivation of oxygen and/or substrate with or without removal of metabolism products brings about alterations in the membrane functions that would allow the cell to return to its normal homeostatic state when the insults (deprivations, etc.) are removed. However, the cell in general is not always successful. There are insults that cause the cell to bring about changes to itself which are irreversible (Laiho and Trump, 1974; Morgen et al., 1979; Trump and Arstila, 1975, 1980; Trump, 1974; Trump et al., 1976, 1978). That is, the cell's response to sudden insult is a membrane injury (alterations in membrane function) from which it cannot recover even after the insult has been removed (suddenly or otherwise). To put it in still another way, what has been established is that cell death is not necessarily a driven process—not a gradual forced response—but rather a dynamic event which may take place, once induced, even in the absence of any external forces. That such is the nature of death at the cellular level—involving most certainly unique subcellular biochemical mechanisms, heretofore unsuspected—is an exciting contribution to basic knowledge.

The purpose of this chapter is to illuminate conceptually the mechanism of cell injury and death using a holistic approach which considers gross (large scale) observations rather than microscopic analysis of biochemical experimental data. Such an approach is used in mathematical qualitative analysis (of nonlinear differential equations) and in complex man-made systems when one is interested in illuminating important properties of the mathematical solution or the system responses without actually having to find the exact solutions or responses.

In this chapter a normal mammalian living cell will be viewed as a complex system which functions in a fluid environment by processing energy matter and information. The processing takes place through numerous temporal events, occurring simultaneously, which, depending on the physical mechanisms involved, are classified in traditional scientific language as chemical, electrical, or mechanical. This traditional way of viewing individual cellular events (which are based on the classical law of physics and chemistry) will be departed from and instead an approach which focuses directly on the holistic aspects of the cell response to changes in its environment will be introduced. According to this viewpoint, the cell is a living system—an organized entity whose very existence depends wholly on a structure—of interconnected components (or parts) (Miller, 1978). To be sure, in order to have detailed knowledge of every possible aspect and attribute of the cell's behavior, it is necessary to first acquire complete and detailed knowledge about the components plus complete knowledge about the laws and structure of the interconnection of these components. This is true for a living system (such as the cell of our interest) as it is true for the very complex man-made systems of the last quarter century, such as a fighter, jet plane, or commercial sattelite-based communications network. However, from the man-made systems we have learned that it is possible to understand (or explain) to a satisfactory extent important holistic (or system) features of the behavior of a system without having complete and detailed knowledge of the behavior of the components and their interactions (Kalman and DeClaris, 1971; Miles, 1973). By holistic features we mean those aspects of the behavior which depend in an essential way both on the components of the system *and* on their interconnections. This understanding, in fact, provides the technical basis (in the absence of scientific theory) that enables those charged with the responsibility to manage the system to the extent of successfully modifying its behavior when it becomes necessary to do so in order to maintain its integrity. It is the objective of this presentation to examine cellular reaction to lethal injury as a systemic dynamic phenomenon. In the absence of adequate scientific theory, partial and large scale observations rather than analysis of microscopic biochemical experimental data will provide the basis of the examination. The same applies to testing hypotheses and assessing consequences of possible alternatives for consistency. The approach has its logical foundations in mathematical qualitative analysis frequently employed in the study of nonlinear differential equations (Nemytskii and Stephanov, 1960). Such qualitative analysis provides knowledge for finding the overall features that characterize classes of particular solutions to extremely difficult conceptual problems and very rarely, if ever, furnishes methods for finding the specific solutions themselves. Thus, it is maybe thought of as an approach which provides an intellectual framework for extracting the most essential features of a highly complex mental picture. It does so by employing an economy of thought which focuses on the most essential features needed to identify the picture and ignores or minimizes the role of all other attributes, in much the same way as the cartoonist who, with a few lines, manages to render recognizable a sketch of a particular individual without having to paint the complete and accurate portrait of that person. Admittedly, this is a most difficult job which requires not only talent but specialized training. In mathematical problems this involves abstract concepts and deep insight that takes much time to acquire. Nevertheless, an attempt will be made to bypass these obstacles in the presentation through the use of system concepts and methodology. Thus, we shall first introduce just enough system concepts to enable a discussion of the systemic dynamic aspects of the cell's response to injury on the basis of geometrical arguments of two-dimensional and three-dimensional curves. Clearly this approach has its own limitations, which will be elaborated on later. However, it is important to emphasize from the onset that these limitations do not render invalid the key features found to characterize the cellular death phenomena we started out to comprehend, hypothesis and simplifications notwithstanding. In fact, and it is an excellent indication of the intellectual merit of this approach that, important features of cell reaction to all lethal injury will be identified on the basis of intuitive elementary ideas and simple logical arguments; no biochemical analysis or abstract mathematical terminology will be used.

SYSTEM ASPECTS OF CELLULAR INJURY

One way of viewing a mammalian cell as a system is to consider the energy matter and information transformations that take place in each of its several components and then to attempt to relate them to the overall behavior of the cell. Among the essential components of the cell are the plasma membrane and the organelles, including the nucleus, mitochodria, endoplasmic reticulum, lysosomes, and peroxisomes. In studying the effects of cell injury, the cell components are usually characterized in terms of membrane surfaces and organelle morphogenic parameters (such as volume, density, etc.). In addition, cellular injury involves changes in molecular and ionic concentrations (such as Ca^{2+}, ATP, etc.). All of these quantities and more are related to the injury (as a result of ischemia, for example) directly or indirectly through complex chemoelectromechanical relations (Beers et al., 1972; Braunwald, 1976; Jewett and McCarroll, 1980). The complexity involved and the state of experimental methodology is such that it is very unlikely that one can find, from the incomplete observations alone, a way of simplifying the problem so as to illuminate the basic mechanism that brings about irreversibility. A living cell has a built-in ability to return to its homeostatic normal state when it is disturbed. Thus, much is known: there are injuries after which the cell reassumes its normal function (even after prolonged time periods of exposure to the insult) and there are injuries from which the cell never recovers so as to return to its neostatic state (even if the insult was removed shortly afterward). Is such a phenomenon a consequence of the full complexity of the cell? That is, to understand the mechanism of this irreversible behavior does it require comprehension of the totality of the cell's behavior? We will find the definite answer to these questions by using a basic systems viewpoint, according to which a cell is considered mentally, as an input-output time-dependent map (relation) of appropriate quantities. Given changes in the input quantities (for example, oxygen, substrate, etc.), such a map in theory gives the resulting changes in the output quantities. There is a system notation for writing down this compactly, but it requires defining a set of symbols. Specifically, we let

$E_r^k(t)$ to represent energy matter quantities;
$I_r^k(t)$ represent information variables;
k stand for an index which designates an input quality ($k = i$), or an output quality ($k = 0$);
$r = 1, 2, 3, \ldots, n$ an integer to be assigned to a quantity or variable that has distinct physical identity.

For the simplest cell, one can conceive there will be at least only one kind of energy matter quantity E and only one kind of information quantity I (messenger). Thus, the input and output are considered as (ordered) pairs:

$$\{E^i(t), I^i(t)\}$$

and

$$\{E^0(t), I^0(t)\}.$$

The cell then may be visualized in the most basic way as a system S (an abstraction) which changes the input pair into the output pair. In system notation this is written as

$$\{E^i(t), I^i(t)\} \xrightarrow{S} \{E^0(t), I^0(t)\}. \quad (1)$$

Again in system terminology we have complete knowledge of the behavior of S if we can compile a table (possibly a thick dictionary) of *all* possible corresponding input-output pairs. The classical way of compiling such a lengthy table is to find an algorithm (most likely a mathematical expression) by means of which corresponding pairs can be found when they are needed. Such mathematical expressions (or computer algorithms) are extremely difficult to formulate for living systems, although there have been spectacular successes for special cells under suitably clever hypotheses, e.g., the Hodgkin-Huxley relations for excitable membranes (Cole, 1968). However, there is an alternative.

In the last half of this century, very large scale and complex dynamic systems for processing energy matter and information have been designed and rendered operational by man. The order of complexity of certain of these systems is such that the system can not be conceived in its complete detail by a single mind (even with the help of computers). But because these systems were made deliberately by man (and are not the result of millions of years of evolution as in physiological systems), conceptual tools were developed that allow one to reduce complexity, through systematic simplification techniques, when it is desirable to understand holistic (system) properties of its dynamic behavior. Specifically, it is now recognized that there is a great conceptual advantage in the dynamic characterization of complex man-made systems when a set of specialized variables known as "state variables" is used (Kalman and DeClaris, 1971; Minorsky, 1970). It is the viewpoint of "state space" that is advanced here as the proper methodology, indeed the only one that can illuminate the mechanisms of cell reactions to lethal injuries in the simplest possible conceptual way.

This is done best by introducing state space system concepts and methodology with an example. The example consists of the most elementary cell we believe can possibly be considered. We advance then the hypothesis that the most elementary cell we wish to examine has membrane systems, bioenergetic and bioinformatic processes which in state space techniques are characterized by two sets of relations:

$$dy/dt = g_y(y, x; E^i, I^i; t)$$
$$dx/dt = g_x(y, x; E^i, I^i; t) \quad (2)$$

and

$$E^0 = W(y, x; E^i, I^i; t)$$
$$I^0 = J(y, x; E^i, I^i; t) \quad (3)$$
$$r = f_r(y, x; E^i, I^i; t)$$

In the above equations t stands for time; E^i, I^i, E^0, and I^0 have been defined before; y and x are the state variables and r is any output quantity of interest. This formulation is extremely general. It was necessary to postulate the existence of two state variables, for it will become evident in a subsequent discussion that if only one state variable had been assumed, no matter what assumption was made later on, observed cell reaction to injury cannot be incorporated into this relation.

It is important to note certain features in the form of the postulated set of equations. The first set, equation 2, expresses the fact that the time rate of change (the derivative) of each state variable at a given time depends only on the value of input pair and the value of two state variables (at the given time) in accordance with a relation which holds at the same given time. By contrast, any output quantity r can be computed at a given time directly from the values of these quantities at the given time.

One might question whether actual cells can in fact be described in such a specialized manner. There is no doubt that if a sufficient number of state variables are used, the known dynamics of any living cell can be written in such a form. What information is needed in order to reconcile this formulation with experimental evidence will be discussed in the last section of this chapter. In the remainder of this section, the discussion shall be based solely on the sets of equations 2 and 3. However, in order for the discussion to be effective, it is necessary to introduce greater structure in these equations. Specifically, it is necessary to incorporate (indeed to ascertain that these equations will exhibit) important phenomenological attributes.

As was pointed out earlier, there is a fundamental difference between the two sets of equations. Equation 3 states that the value of any quantity of interest (output quantity) at a specified instant of time t depends solely on the numerical value that the four quantities (input pair and the state variables) have and the relation which exists between them at the time t. This is one of the direct consequences of having chosen y and x as state variables. Equation 3 is known mathematically as an algebraic relation. A digital computer which has been programmed to "simulate the dynamic behavior of a cell" makes use of this property of the state variables when it provides numerical data as a printout or a cathode ray tube (CRT) screen display. Equation 2, on the other hand, relates time-rate changes of the state variables; it is concerned with how y and x change at any given time. Thus, this set of equations incorporates all the important time-dependent characteristics of the cell behavior that are imposed by its own make-up and structure. Herein lies the great significance of the state space techniques. Equation 1 is of the type known in mathematics as first order, nonlinear ordinary differential equation. Such equations have been treated for nearly a century and still furnish some of the most challenging mathematical problems today. However, enough is known about their behavior to enable us to put together consistent bits and pieces of pathophysiological and mathematical observations so as to form a single picture which will tell us a great deal more about the phenomenon of cellular injury than was possible to extract from the pieces alone. In order to keep the discussion simple and to make the ideas available to as wide an audience as possible, we shall not go into the specialized deep knowledge that is required to put together these pieces. Instead, we shall make use of geometrical curves corresponding to the structure imposed on equation 2, and point out the conceptual value of the knowledge thus gained.

For the purposes of discussion then, let us assume that we know the law of the membrane dynamics and bioenergetics of our elementary two-state variable living cell. That means we know the functions $g_y(\ )$ and $g_x(\ )$. Thus, if we specify the input pair E^i, I^i and an (initial) state pair at t, $y^i(t_2)$, $x^i(t_2)$, we can find the resulting response the state variables $x(t)$ and $y(t)$ for all time $t > t_2$. To put it in another way, for each specification consisting of an input pair $\{E^i, I^i\}$ and in initial pair $\{y^i, x^i\}$, the solutions of equation 2 consist of two curves whose general shape is shown in Figure 2.1 and 2.2. These time curves may be written symbolically in the form:

$$y(t; E^i, I^i; y^i, x^i)$$
$$x(t; E^i, I^i; y^i, x^i). \tag{4}$$

The curves corresponding to different choices of the parameters E^i, I^i, y^i, x^i in equation 4 are in fact families of curves. Still another way of viewing equations 4 (for specific choice of parameters) is in a single curve in a three-dimensional space with y, x, and t as coordinates, as shown in Figure 2.3. Such a curve is a solution of equations 2. Figures 2.1 and 2.2 are projections of this solution in the y-t and x-t planes, respectively. We can now see, however, that the solution curve has one more distinct projection on the y-x plane, as shown in Figure

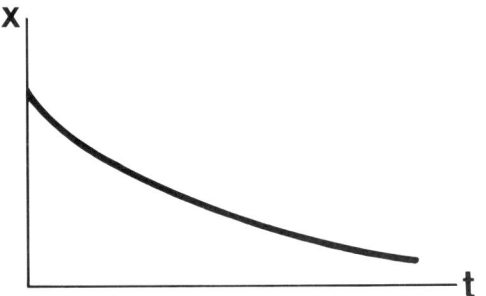

Figure 2.1. Graphic representation of cellular dynamic behavior as a two-dimensional curve.

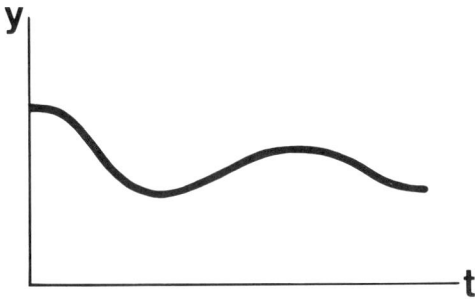

Figure 2.2. Graphic representation of cellular dynamic behavior as a different two-dimensional curve.

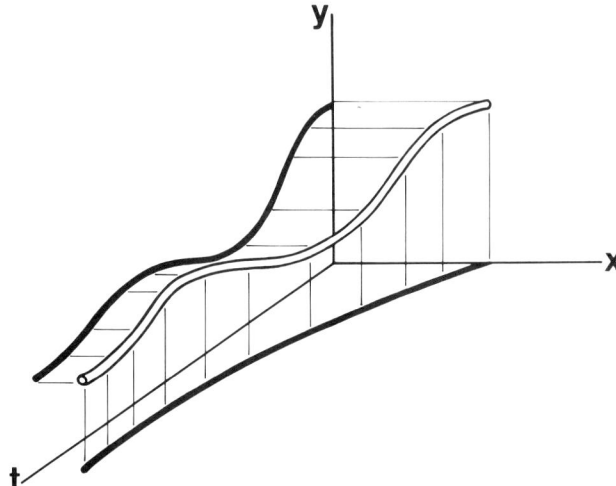

Figure 2.3. Graphic representation of cellular dynamic behavior as a three-dimensional curve.

2.4, which may prove very helpful in our study. Such a curve is known as a "state plane trajectory" and it exhibits all the important features of the dynamic behavior of our elementary cell without having time explicitly appearing in the picture. We may find it helpful to visualize a given state plane trajectory much as a "train-track" with the property that if the cell (with the specified input pair) is considered at a point on this track at time t, then the dynamics of the cell will cause the cell to move to the subsequent points of the track in the direction shown. To put it simply, the cell behaves as if it was

Qualitative Dynamics of Cell Response to Injury

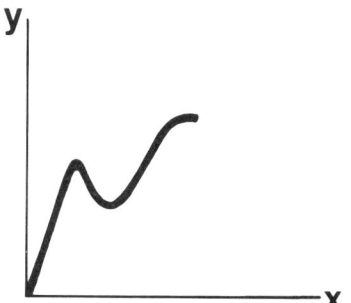

Figure 2.4. State-plane representation of cellular dynamic behavior.

a vehicle constrained (by its structure and make-up) to travel along the specified track in a predetermined direction once it is placed on it. It follows from this observation that if we were given (or were able to somehow determine) all the possible trajectories in appropriate state planes, then from these we can deduce all the qualitative aspects of the dynamic behavior of cellular injury that come about as temporary changes in specified input pairs. To do this, however, we must first ask the crucial question about our elementary cell: "What are the state plane qualitative features that differentiate a normal living cell from a dying cell?" It is extremely doubtful that an actual living cell exists that can be characterized solely in two state variables, but if there was such a cell, we must demand that the dynamics of its two state variables must be such as to enable the cell to carry out what are considered the most basic and important functions. Now the dynamic behavior of all cells fall into one of two categories: cells that undergo a mitotic cycle (liver, lung, etc.) and cells that do not divide (heart, muscle, neuron, etc.) but carry out specialized functions (repetitive contractions, generation of action potentials, etc.). From what we know about important membrane functions and the ADP-ATP bioenergetic cycle, in order to carry out its normal living function it is essential that the cell (however elemental) be able to reach a homeostatic state (which is a state of dynamic equilibrium); only then is it considered a normal living cell. Thus, equilibrium states are the very essence of the life process. As it turns out, state space trajectories which correspond to equilibrium states pretty much determine the structure of all other trajectories (this much is known from the theory of nonlinear differential equations) (Minorsky, 1970). Moreover, under very generous conditions, it can be shown mathematically that states of equilibrium are represented in the state plane either by isolated points or by isolated closed curves. States of equilibrium are frequently referred to as "steady states." Trajectories which correspond to non-equilibrium states are by contrast referred to as "transients." Mathematically, there is a very crucial interdependence of steady-state and transient trajectories in the state plane which has been studied extensively by some of the greatest mathematicians of all times.

This knowledge plus recent cellular pathophysiological findings motivated us to introduce, for the purpose of this discussion, a structure to the elementary cell through a set of postulates. First we postulate that a homeostatic state of our elementary cell (a state of dynamic equilibrium) is represented in the state plane by a simple closed curve. One can easily appreciate the fact that a trajectory which consists only of a single isolated point represents a static equilibrium (the fact that there is no time change in the behavior). For the present discussion, however, it is better to visualize static equilibrium trajectories as initial points on the state plane from which a set of trajectories begin or end points to which a set of trajectories terminates. For reasons which we can not go into now, our elementary living cell must have three static states, S_1, S_2, and S_3, and one homeostatic state Γ (Mitchison, 1971; Strehler, 1962). From the consequence of these requirements (as well as other mathematical (DeClaris and Zadeh, 1966; Heinmets, 1970) and physiological (Chance et al., 1973; Little et al., 1977) arguments) we next postulate state plane trajectories for our elementary cell as shown in Figure 2.5 (for specified constant values of the input pair). The most striking feature of this postulated state plane is the fact that, by construction, very nearly only two states of equilibrium are ultimately reachable by the cell: curve Γ and point S_1. Almost all trajectories lead to Γ and to S_2. What is the meaning of this? Suppose that for the specified input-pair, the dynamics of the cell are such that they are represented by a point on Γ: we then say that the cell is in its homeostatic state. Next, imagine a small temporary disturbance (change in E^i or I^i or both) causing a slight change in the dynamics so that the cell goes into a transient state. If the disturbance is small, as can be seen from Figure 2.5, the transient trajectory will return the cell to Γ; however, if the disturbance is large, the transient behavior of the cell will ultimately lead it to the point of state equilibrium S_1, which corresponds to cell death. Thus, the state plane of Figure 2.5 is divided into two important regions: a region which is characterized by the property that all trajectories lead to a static equilibrium and another region which has the property that all trajectories lead to dynamic equilibrium. The physiological interpretation, of course, is that the first region, representing the dynamic behavior of the cell as it moves (left to its own fate, so to speak) towards certain death, depicts cell death dynamics, while the second region depicts *living dynamics*. But how does the cell find itself in one or the other region?

It was stated earlier that the state plane of Figure 2.5 was postulated for specified constants E^i and I^i. At time t_0, the cell begins its existence as a normal cell with the state variables corresponding to point S_3. As time goes on, and provided there is no change in the input pair, the cell dynamics are depicted by one of the trajectories leading to Γ—the homeostatis state. Notice that, because of the way we have postulated the state plane, as the cell ages, the trajectory that it follows moves closer and closer to Γ and begins to resemble nearly a closed curve almost the same as Γ. At some time $t_1 > t_0$, let us say that there occur sudden changes in the input pair by induced ischemia; now the input pair are $\{E^i - \rho, I^i - \sigma\}$, which

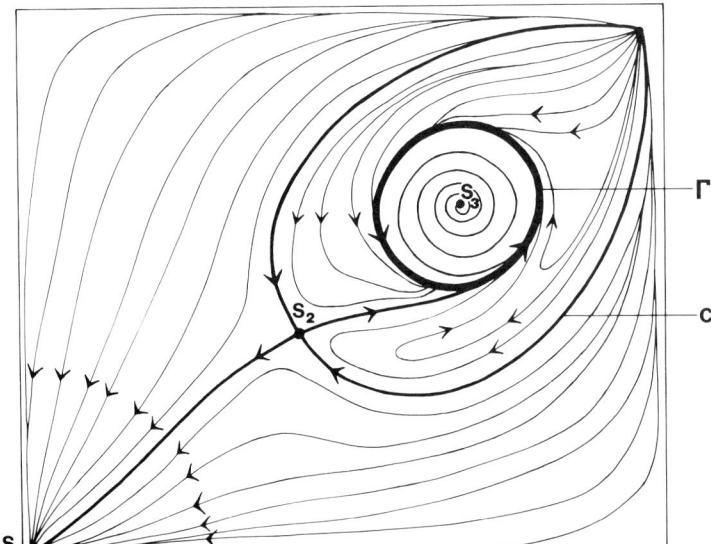

Figure 2.5. State-plane representation of an elementary cell's living dynamics.

we assume to have a constant value until $t_2 > t_1$. Because different values of the input quantities E^I, I^i than those postulated are in effect, in the time interval from t_1 to t_2 the state plane of Figure 2.5 can not be used to study the dynamics of the cell. Nevertheless, there are changes in the state variables and at time t_2 they have now assumed the value $y(t_2)$ and $x(t_2)$. When the original values of the input pair E^i, I^i are returned at t_2 to act on the cell, we return to Figure 2.5 to study the dynamic behavior of the cell, starting with the initial point $y(t_2)$ and $x(t_2)$. If, for example, this point is located in the "living region," then there has been an accelerated or "premature aging" of the cell, but the injured cell ultimately will return to its normal steady state. However, if the states $y(t_2)$ and $x(t_2)$ placed the cell outside of this living region, then the cell has sustained an injury from which it can never recover to assume its normal living function. The curve C which defines the living region is sometimes referred to in mathematics as a *separatrix* (Minorsky, 1970). Is this, therefore, to say that the mechanism of the point-of-no-return in all cell injuries is that of a mathematical separatrix? At this point, it will be a premature conclusion, for cells do not die only as a result of sudden and temporary changes in the input pair. It may well be that the values of the input pair are such that no dynamic equilibrium is possible. That is to say, we must allow a functional dependence in equations 2 such that for certain values of E^e, I^e the only possible dynamics are those which bring about cell necrosis; surely there are values of the input pair with which the cell will never reach homeostatic state (and it is destined for certain death, so to speak). Thus, we present Figure 2.6 as such a state plane representation, intuitively compatible with our previously postulated cell dynamics and assuming that the environment is a constant lethal input pair. Using these two postulated state planes as our elementary cells (Figs. 2.5 and 2.6) we can now see how, theoretically at least, we can predict whether a sudden and temporary insult (a sudden change in the input pair) will prove fatal or not. Let us say that the state plane of Figure 2.6 does correspond to a lethal input pair $\{E^e, I^e\}$. Returning to the previous discussion of the event at time t_2, consisting of small change ρ in the input energy and a small change σ in the input information, we now see how the insult to this cell may bring about death. At the time t_2, there is a sudden change in the input pair so that $E^i - \rho = E^e$ and $I^i - \sigma = I^e$; then we locate the point $\{y(t_2), x(t_2)\}$ $\tau = t_2 - t_1$ seconds later. At time t_2, we return to Figure 2.5 and, using the values $y(t_2)$, $x(t_2)$ we determine which trajectory the cell will follow next. Thus, whether the potentially lethal insult (ρ, σ) will prove fatal to the cell or not depends on several factors, including the time duration τ. In order to study the qualitative dynamics of cell injury, therefore, it is necessary to ask, "How do we describe simply the cell dynamics which bring about the transformation of the state plane of Figure 2.5 so as to become the state plane of Figure 2.6?" The answer to this question, which holds the key to understanding the dynamics of death, will be found in the concept of stability that will be discussed in the next section of this chapter.

STABILITY ASPECTS

While the word stability is very common in every day language, Poincare and Liapounov, two great scientific thinkers, separately and in two distinct parts of the world (France and Russia, respectively), in the turn of this century gave precise meaning to the concept of stability as it pertains to dynamic physical events (LaSale and Lefschetz, 1961; Liapounov, 1974; Poincare, 1874, 1885). It is not possible for us to go deeply here into the beautiful works of Poincare and Liapounov, although they are extremely important. The reader should be aware that almost all modern system treatments concerning stability rest on theories which they founded, and this will certainly prove to be true about the stability aspects of cellular injury dynamics. Our discussion will

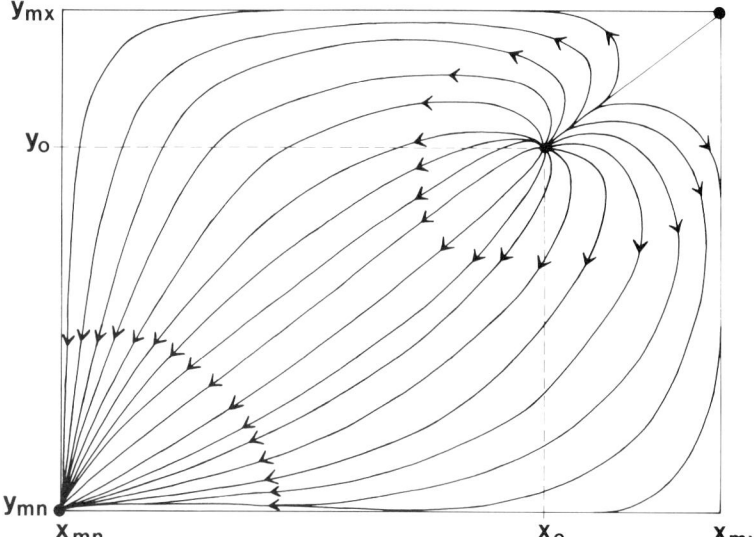

Figure 2.6. State-plane representation of an elementary cell's necrotic dynamics.

draw freely upon their work and upon subsequent results established by their followers (Bogoliubov and Mitropolsky, 1961; Cetaev, 1946; Hayashi, 1974; Minorsky, 1970) without specific references to them. Fortunately, the theories of Poincare and Liapounov are very much in agreement with our common experience and intuition about "stable motion" as a state, with the essential property that "small disturbances, from it, remain small." From this basic requirement of stability, we can see that one can determine whether an equilibrium state (of our elementary cell) is stable or not by examining how the appropriate trajectories behave near that state. For example, the point S_1 in Figure 2.6 (the point trajectory corresponding to death) is a state of stable static equilibrium because all trajectories lead to it. Similarly, the closed curve in Figure 2.5 (corresponding to the living state of homeostasis) is a state of stable dynamic equilibrium, for the cell will return to it after any small disturbance which caused the cell to depart from its dynamic equilibrium state has been removed. However, there is still a qualitative difference between the stability aspects of those two states. Notice that in Figure 2.5, the cell will return to the curve Γ only if the disturbance is sufficiently small, while in Figure 2.6, the cell will return (theoretically, of course) to point S_1, however large the magnitude of the temporary disturbance. Thus, the steady state of cell death (Fig. 2.6) is *globally stable*, whereas the steady state of cell homeostasis (Fig. 2.5) is *locally stable*. In Figure 2.5, the point S_2 represents a point of static equilibrium with the characteristic property that some trajectories lead to it while other trajectories originate from it. However, notice that all trajectories near S_2, no matter how close to S_2 you wish to take them, lead away from S_2. The point S_2 is an unstable state of static equilibrium of the type known as a *saddlepoint*. The state corresponding to the point trajectory S_3 in Figure 2.5, is also clearly unstable; it is of a type known as *unstable focus*. Unstable points of static equilibrium of this type exist in systems which are in an active state—active in

the sense that "free energy" is generated by the dynamics represented by the trajectories near the equilibrium and thereby causing the system to move away from its static state. From stability theory alone, we know that under the postulates made earlier, the existence of the stable isolated closed curve Γ (a *limit cycle* as it is known), preassumes the existence of the unstable point S_3, which again is in agreement with the known facts about cellular physiology. There are many other such qualitative correspondence of mathematical properties of stability and basic holistic dynamic behavior of cells. Perhaps the most important ones involve stability, energy, and morphogenesis.

In "System Aspects of Cellular Injury", the state variables (y, x) were postulated to characterize the dynamics of a simple two-dimensional cell with a known (and constant) input pair E^i, I^i. We can well imagine that since there are chemoelectromechanical events that take place in the cell as the state variables y and x assume different values, we may associate an energy function W with the cell's holistic behavior. W is not necessarily equal to the output E^0 of the cell because what we may consider as output energy may not be the whole story. From what we have said previously about state variables, it follows that it is possible to express W in terms of the state variables and of the input pair E^i, I^i. Symbolically, we have

$$W(y, x; E^i, I^i) \in \text{(real number)} \qquad (5)$$

which says that for a specified input pair for each state variable pair y, x, W assumes a real value. We can visualize this better as a geometrical figure (a surface) in three dimensions (W, y, x). W as a surface may assume very complicated shapes. A good way of getting a mental image of such complicated surfaces is to imagine a plastic sheet which can be stretched and folded on a table top whose coordinate axes are y and x. In such a mental picture W is a point on the plastic sheet and the values of y and x are the coordinates of the point on the table top that form the vertical line (from the table top) W. We wish to emphasize, once again, that the shape of the plastic sheet depends on the function of the cell *and* on the assumed values of the input pair $\{E^i, I^i\}$. Different types of cells may have different shapes of W surfaces for the same values of input pairs $\{E^i, I^i\}$, and on the same cell may have different W surfaces for different values of the input pair $\{E^i, I^i\}$. In our presentation, which is concerned with qualitative aspects of cell dynamics, the exact shape of the W surface is not so important as the overall characteristic features of it. For example, consider W as a surface which is almost flat except for a number of small hill-like lumps in several places. The first most important qualitative feature of our discussion is the fact that W has only an hill-like appearance but no holes or folds. The size of the hills (how wide, how tall, etc.) is of secondary, if any, importance and then only after we know how many hills are there. For you can well see now in this picture, trajectories on the state plane correspond to energy pathways on the surface W (Fig. 2.7). Is this any help to us? Most emphatically, yes. For using our intuitive notions about motion on a surface which may have a moderately complicated shape can help us understand (explain?) the very complicated appearance of the corresponding motion on the flat surface of the state plane. For our elementary cell, the shape of the surface of equation 5 is related, under very mild mathematical assumptions, to the functions $g_y(\ )$ and $g_x(\ )$ of equations 2. Perhaps the most important aspect is that which concerns steady states and transient behavior near them. Mathematically, equilibrium states are characterized by the fact that

$$\dot{y} = 0 = dy/dt$$
$$\dot{x} = 0 = dx/dt. \quad (6)$$

On the state plane, this condition implies the existence of state variables (y_e, x_e) such that the functions g_y and g_x are zero. Symbolically, this is written as

$$g_y(y_e, x_e; E^i, I^i) = 0$$
$$g_e(y_e, x_e; E^i, I^i) = 0. \quad (7)$$

The solutions of equation 7, theoretically at least give us the coordinates of all the equilibrium states $(y_e, x_e)_m$ where $m = 1, 2, 3 \ldots$ If y_e and x_e (for a particular m) are constant numbers, then the equilibrium is static; if there is a fixed relation between y_e and x_e, such that

$$r(y_e, x_e) = 0, \quad (8)$$

this corresponds to a dynamic equilibrium. The same equilibrium states on the energy W surface are characterized by the fact that they correspond to surface locations (points or closed curves) of zero slope. Zero slope locations of a surface are regions of local maxima and/or minima and are referred to mathematically as extrema. Thus, equation 7 is equivalent mathematically to the requirement that the partial derivatives of W with respect to y and x evaluated at the equilibrium states must be equal to zero.

$$\left.\frac{\partial w}{\partial y}\right|_{(y_e, x_e)} = 0 \quad \left.\frac{\partial w}{\partial x}\right|_{(y_e, x_e)} = 0 \quad (9)$$

Symbolically, there is much more to this mathematically, but it involves the so-called Jacobian and Hassian of the W surface and such abstract terminology should be avoided. The point we wish to make, and a very important point it is, is that the W surface gives qualitative information about the steady states of the elementary cell's stability. Points of static equilibrium like S_1 and S_3 of Figure 2.5 correspond to a surface minimum (the bottom of a hole) and a surface maximum (top of a hill).

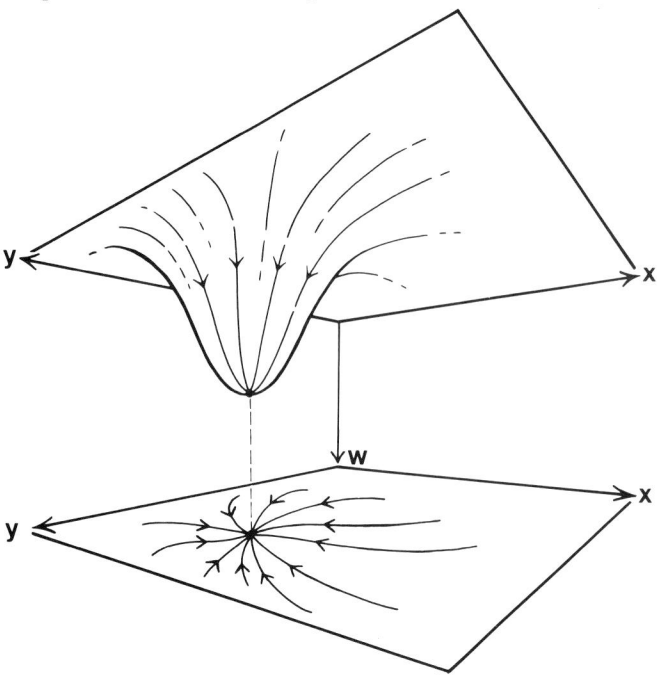

Figure 2.7. Projection of an energy surface on the state-plane.

In fact, this is why S_2 is called a saddle point, because it (and its close neighborhood) is an equilibrium point on a saddle-like surface. To visualize a stable limit cycle, imagine a surface like a Mexican sombrero—somewhere on the rim there exists a single isolated closed curve with zero slope (Fig. 2.8).

With this background information, we can now proceed to take up the most conceptually difficult part of our discussion. We shall again avoid esoteric abstractions and shall appeal to familiar concepts as before, but this time we shall admittedly tax the imagination; herein lies the challenge. It was pointed out in the previous section that Figure 2.5 captured some but not all, of the qualitative aspects of the point-of-no-return phenomenon of cellular injury. For if it did incorporate all aspects, then its mechanism would be totally understood solely in terms of the stability of cell equilibrium (steady states), and this is not the case. It is not the case because in our pictures so far, basic qualitative behavior that pertains to cell control aspects was not considered. True, an input information variable was included in our expressions but it and the input energy variable entered the discussion casually. We postulated two state planes for the elementary cell (Figs. 2.5 and 2.6), and we did carry out a discussion about the lethal (or not) effect of a hypothetical (but very special) cell ischemia-like insult. However, for a wider discussion, a broader range of hypothetical insults are needed, and in order to do that, many more state planes need to be postulated. Why? Let us examine this question. The state-plane of Figure 2.5 corresponds to equation 4 with constants E^i, I^i. It represents the dynamic behavior of the cell as an autonomous system which is bringing about changes to its behavior through controls activated by changes in its own state variables. However, we know that a living cell changes its dynamic behavior through controls brought about by changes in its input. Let us say that we have two identical (in every respect) elementary cells subjected to slightly different input pairs. Using our previously introduced notion for the cell s_1, we have

$$y_1(t; y^i, x^i; E_1^i, I_1^i)$$
$$x_1(t; y^i, x^i; E_1^i, I_1^i)$$

and for the cells s_2, we have

$$y_2(t; y^i, x^i; E_2^i, I_2^i)$$
$$x_2(t; y^i, x^i; E_2^i, I_2^i)$$

Now, although s_1 and s_2 have the identical initial states, y_2, x_2 at time $t = t_2$, and while it may be true that

$$E_1^i - E_2^i = \Delta E^i = 0$$

and

$$I^i - I_2^i = \Delta I^i = 0,$$

the differences

$$y_1 - y_2 = \Delta y$$

and

$$x_1 - x_2 = \Delta x$$

will depend not only on ΔE^i and ΔI^i but also on E^i and I^i, even in a qualitative way. Such dependence is typical of strongly nonlinear behavior, and cellular reaction to injury is indeed highly nonlinear. For this reason, we

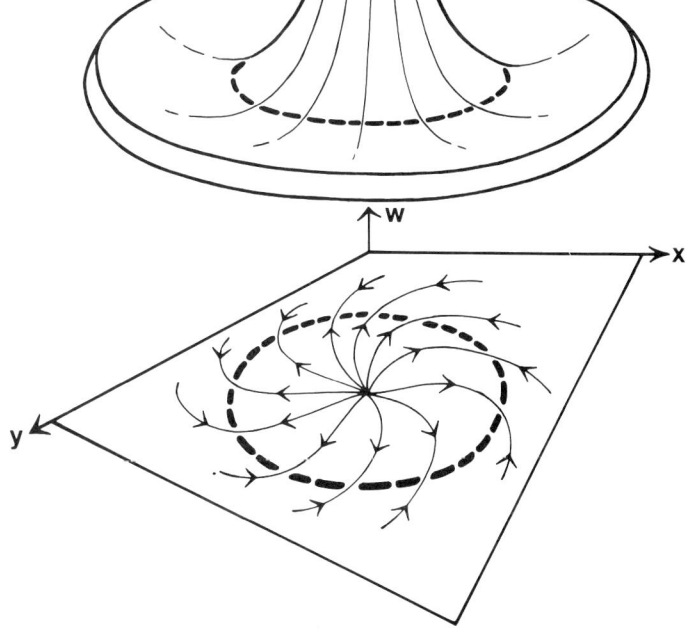

Figure 2.8. Limit cycle as an energy pathway projection.

found it necessary to show explicitly in equation 3 that the rate of change of the state variables is a function of the state variables *and* the input pair. An alternative way, which is more common in physiology (Padilla, 1974; Wright, 1973), is to formulate the law of cell membrane dynamics by means of two sets of equations: 1) a set relating membrane system state variables: $x, y, \ldots$ and membrane morphological parameters (control variables) $a, b, \ldots$; and 2) a set relating control variables $a, b, \ldots$ to the input energy and information. The characterization of our elementary cell in this alternative way is as follows:

Membrane systems:

$$\dot{y} = q_y(y, x; a, b; E^i, I^i)$$
$$\dot{x} = q_x(y, x; a, b; E^i, I^i) \quad (10)$$

Bioenergetics:

$$q_a(a, b; E^i, I^i) = \dot{a}$$
$$q_b(a, b; E^i, I^i) = \dot{b} \quad (11)$$

Two control variables a, b have been postulated for reasons that will be discussed later. Except for the change of symbols, equations 10 and 11 are similar in form. Solving for the control variable a, b in terms of E^i and I^i and then substituting those solutions into equation 10 a new set of equations will emerge which will be in the form of equation 5. But in fact, to study the dynamics of equations 10 and 11 together requires a four-dimensional state space. Visualizing curves in four dimensions is certainly not a familiar experience. However, if we assume, and herein lies the pathophysiological significance of the control variables (Carafoli and Compton, 1978; Kiefer and Sandritter, 1978), that during the duration of the cellular reaction of interest

$$\dot{a} = \dot{b} = 0; \quad (12)$$

then, theoretically at least, from equation 11, we can relate the input pair (E^i, I^i) to the control variables (a, b) and by substitution into equation 10 we can find a new equation

$$f_x(x, y; a, b) = \dot{x}$$
$$f_y(x, y; a, b) = \dot{y} \quad (13)$$

whose dynamics can be studied in a two-dimensional state space since a and b are now constants, according to the assumption of equation 12 (the time rate of change of the control variables during the duration of the cellular reaction is postulated to be zero). Thus, we have succeeded in continuing our discussion of the qualitative aspects of cellular reaction to injury using two-dimensional curves. But now there is a shift in emphasis. Of central importance in the discussion is the question, "How do the state plane trajectories *change* with continuous changes in the control variables?" We have seen earlier that the transient behavior of our elementary cell depends qualitatively in an essential way on steady state behavior—the equilibrium trajectories. Thus, the crucial question now is, "How does the stability of equilibrium states on the state plane depend on the control parameters?" It turns out that the control parameters of some man-made nonlinear systems affected the stability of equilibrium in ways that were totally unexpected. Van der Pol, a great Dutch mathematician and physicist, was the first one to deal, around 1930, with the qualitative aspects of stability of equilibrium through bifurcation theory (Van der Pol; Rabinowitz, 1977). Almost 50 years later, the qualitative aspects of the stability of nonlinear systems are being popularized in a more colorful (but mathematically equivalent) way as catastrophe theory (Thom, 1975; Van der Werff, 1977; Zeeman, 1976). Both of these theories are basic geometrical approaches which require a great deal of mathematical sophistication (Lu, 1976; Callahan, 1974; Dubois and Dufour, 1978) in order to be dealt with in depth. In this part of the discussion, as previously, we shall use simple geometrical pictures (Woodcock and Poston, 1973) and limit it to intuitive arguments.

It was pointed out earlier that the location and the stability of equilibrium trajectories can be qualitatively studied from the characteristics of the energy surface W (equation 5). Under the assumption of slow varying control parameters ($\dot{a} = \dot{b} = 0$) we can replace the input pair in W with expressions involving the control parameters a and b (in exactly the same way as we did to obtain equation 13). In any case, whatever the technique, we can well imagine that the stability aspects of equation 13 can be studied by means of a family of surfaces in a three-dimensional space which shall be designated as

$$\Phi(y, x; a, b) \in \text{(real numbers)}. \quad (14)$$

That is for each value that the control parameter (a, b) can assume the values of Φ lie on a plastic-sheet stretched on a desk top with y and x as coordinate axes. This is still a rather difficult picture to construct in our minds. However, our task can be simplified significantly if instead of examining how *all* trajectories in the state plane behave as the control parameter (a, b) vary, we focus our attention *only* on the steady state trajectories. Recall that steady state trajectories (equilibrium studies) are given by the condition $\dot{y} = \dot{x} = 0$, which is to say, referring to equation 13, that

$$f_x(x, y; a, b) = 0$$
$$f_y(x, y; a, b) = 0. \quad (15)$$

In theory, the solution of the above equation is a family of curves on the $x - y$ plane which gives us the location of the equilibrium states as the control parameters change. One of the most exciting things that can happen with such curves, which is of utmost importance to our discussion, is an unexpected but confirmed (first by Van der Pol) phenomenon corresponding to the abrupt vanishing of certain equilibrium states even though the control variables change smoothly. This is the essence of bifurcation and is a direct consequence of the fact that equation 15 is so highly nonlinear that it includes the possibility of distinct (different) solutions with the same values of control variables. The physical significance of such a nonlinearity is that to a unique set of values of the control variables (a_0, b_0) there may correspond two or more distinct equilibrium states which describes the behavior of the system at any given period of time depending on the past history of the system. Now recall that the notion of the control variables is closely tight up with morphological changes of the Φ surface. One might even say that a good choice of control variables (natural or by man) is one that can bring about major changes in the Φ surface. The most serious effect that the Φ surface can undergo with changes in the control variables is when the number of extrema of the surface changes. This is roughly the mathematical concept of a *catastrophe*. Catastrophes, involving small numbers of control variables and small numbers of state variables have been studied extensively in the last decade. The usual approach is to examine the shape of a surface (in a multidimensional space which includes the control variables as coordinates) consisting of all extrema of the Φ surface. By way of illustration, very artificial in our study, suppose x in equation 15 is a constant (there is only one state variable y). Then the corresponding Φ surface involves four dimensions.

$$\Phi(y; a, b)$$

The changes of extrema of this four-dimensional surface are then studied with the help of an equation of the type

$$\Psi(y; a, b) = 0.$$

Ψ may be visualized as a three-dimensional surface whose coordinates are (y, a, b). In fact, we can visualize this surface as a plastic sheet on a table top whose coordinates are the control variables, as shown in Figure 2.9. The most striking feature of the surface is the existence of a fold. This means that for certain values of the control variables, three steady states are possible. For example, to (a_3, b_3) there corresponds an unstable static equilibrium C_3 which implies a living cell (similar to the point S_3 of Fig. 2.5).

However, because of changes in the energy information input pair (induced by ischemia, let us say) the control variables change to a_2, b_2 and C_3 disappears; in its place there is now a stable static equilibrium C_2 which implies death (similar to that in Fig. 2.6). We further see that if we return the controls to their original values (a_3, b_3), we do not necessarily go back to C_3, but possibly to C_1, depending on the path followed in getting there. In fact, it may well be that once the system is caused (by the controls) to leave the equilibrium state C_2, there exists no physiologically possible sequence of control values that can bring the system to the same equilibrium state. In such a case, as one can well see from Figure 2.9, the values of (a, b) which correspond to the coordinates of the surface fold constitute lines-of-no-return. And this is another aspect of irreversible injury to a cell which is phenomenologically different from the one discussed in "System Aspects of Cellular Injury." The mechanism discussed in this section has to do with the quality of the stability of the states (afforded by means of controls), while the mechanism discussed in the previous section has to do with the quality of the equilibrium of the states.

We conclude with this observation: If the postulates advanced here are correct, then the dynamics of death are multifacet and qualitatively intricately connected to the dynamics of life itself. This is certainly intuitively agreeable.

EXPERIMENTAL ASPECTS AND A FEW CONCLUDING REMARKS

In the previous two sections, we strived to illuminate conceptually how the phase of cellular reaction to injury that Trump (1974) defined as the point-of-no-return comes about when one views the cell as a dynamic system. The presentation was rather specific in the sense that it was carried out with reference to a hypothetical living cell characterized by a postulated two-dimensional state variable and control variable description. It is highly unlikely that such a cell actually exists. Even the simplest of living mammalian cells will involve a state space of much higher dimensions for the description of its behavior (possibly an order or two of magnitude greater). The state space description of dynamic behavior has great intellectual appeal because it has strong geometrical flavor and because the overwhelming number of humans find it satisfying to understand events by means of graphs and pictures. The advantage of pictorial representations, however, in higher dimensions than three is rapidly diminished and soon becomes a burden. This was the principal reason that we limited our discussion to two dimensions and even then, some visualization in three-dimensions was unavoidable. It would have been easier if we could have used one dimension with an occasional reference to two or three. But this was not possible. For it is easily understood that as we lower the dimensionality of the characterization, fewer and fewer

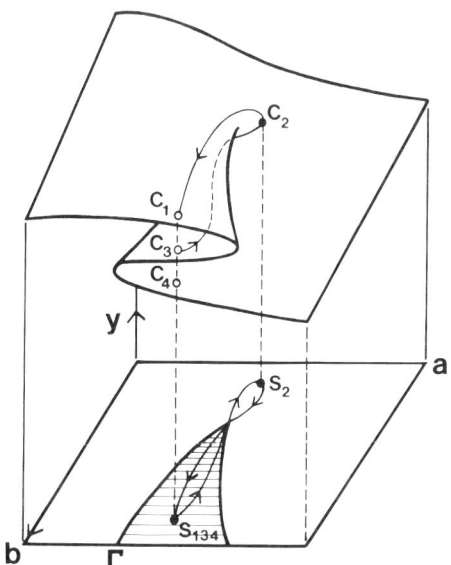

Figure 2.9. Energy surface with a fold.

cellular functions can be induced in the resulting description of the cell. Now there are cell functions that are so basic, so essential to the living processes that they must be included or accounted for in the characterization if the description is to have any validity as a living system. Such is the process of cell homeostasis which we identified as a state of dynamic equilibrium. There is virtually no other more acceptable representation of cell homeostasis in the state plane than that of an isolated closed trajectory, a limit cycle. It is well known that for limit cycles to exist in the behavior of a dynamic system, at least two state variables are required. Thus, a state plane description (two dimensions) was the simplest that we could choose since our discussion is concerned about the dynamics of the impairment of homeostasis. One may then say, "okay, you had to use two dimensions, but are you sure that two are enough and, if indeed they are enough, which ones do you choose?" The answer to this two part question is, and here lies one of the contributions we hope we have made, that to explain the basic aspects of cell necrosis or recovery following ischemia, anoxia and toxic insults, two dimensions are sometimes enough (most likely, it takes four: two state variables and two control variables). We have deliberately avoided attaching any physiological significance to the state variables in our discussion because it simply was not necessary to do so. There was no need for the purposes of this presentation (the illumination of certain observed dynamic behavior) to identify the state variables and the control variables with this or that experimentally measured or calculated quantity. This is not to say that the choice of control variables does not play an important part in the study of the dynamics of cellular injury—it does—and an extremely important role at that. However, in the manner of our presentation, the choice of the variables is a separate problem which fully deserves a separate study of its own. Certain aspects of this problem will be discussed shortly. This is a good place to clarify another intellectual tactic we used in the previous sections. Our discussion was carried out via postulated dynamics of an elementary cell. Only the qualitative holistic features of these dynamics were of importance to our conclusions and much of the postulated trajectory details of Figures 2.5, 2.6, and 2.9 were not necessary. The postulated elementary cell was our way of presenting a theory—a theory which is not limited in its application, as anyone can recognize, to a postulated example but which can be (directly or through suitable generalization) rendered operative to much more complex situations closer to reality.

Scientific reality requires experiments and measurements, not only descriptions and theories. And, this brings us back to the question of the quantification of the cellular behavior we have been discussing. Enormous amounts of data have already been collected (Laiho and Trump, 1974; Morgen et al., 1970) and the amount increases at a fantastic rate, which makes the job of selection and of putting together pieces an extremely difficult undertaking, not to mention the fact that it is also likely that important data, for several reasons, are missing. The value of a qualitative theory (a system approach) like the one we presented here, is that it may be extremely helpful in funding new experiments or in helping analyze the data obtained from the old ones.

In our presentation here, we have suggested a choice of a dual set of variables: one set, the state variables (x_j where $j = 1, 2, \ldots n$), associated with the living cellular membranes, and another set, the control variables (a_j where $j = 1, 2, \ldots m$), associated with the bioenergetics of the internal cellular environment and with the bioinformatics of the cytosol network and cell-to-cell communication. It has been established that the membrane dynamics (not just the static structure) of a living membrane act as regulatory barriers for entry and exit of many kinds of particles and molecules. It has also been established that membrane structural and dynamic properties are linked to events in the internal environment of the cell (such as ATP-ADP-exchange, calcium and ion metabolism, etc.) and events communicated through organelle and cell-to-cell connections and messengers, all of which act as control mechanisms. However, for the systems approach advocated here to serve as a guide to experiment (and ultimately clinical management), there are two additional aspects that need to be studied very extensively. One aspect concerns the relations between state variables, control variables, and those quantities that can be measured directly by experiments. Let us call the experimental determined quantities as "observables" r_j where $j = 1, 2, \ldots$. Some of these observations are molecular concentrations and/or ratios, densities, volume, etc., which consist of numbers obtained during the course of the experiments. In theory, these observables can also be found with a knowledge of the state variables and control variables. The other way around, how to find the state variables and the control variables from a knowledge of the observations is not as easy, even in theory. For one, unless we can be sure from the outset that what is measured is in fact a state variable or a control variable it is unlikely that we will ever find an exact description from measurements alone. For another, much of the observed cellular response to injury is not quantified but is in the form of alterations in electromicroscopic images (Trump et al., 1978). A possible approach is to construct a feedback model estimator algorithm (most likely in the form of a computer program) which will provide estimated values for the state and control variables on the basis of tested and confirmed short-term predictions (Fig. 2.10).

Another aspect that should be mentioned is the matter of the kind of experiments needed to confirm the predicted behavior. Of greatest challenge is the design of experiments for confirming the existence of the high dimensionality folds in the energy surfaces that determine the quality of the stability of the living dynamics. It is highly unlikely, because of the multivalued nature of the surface, that the surface of the folds can be established experimentally without having a good prior insight into the phenomenon. The situation is similar to

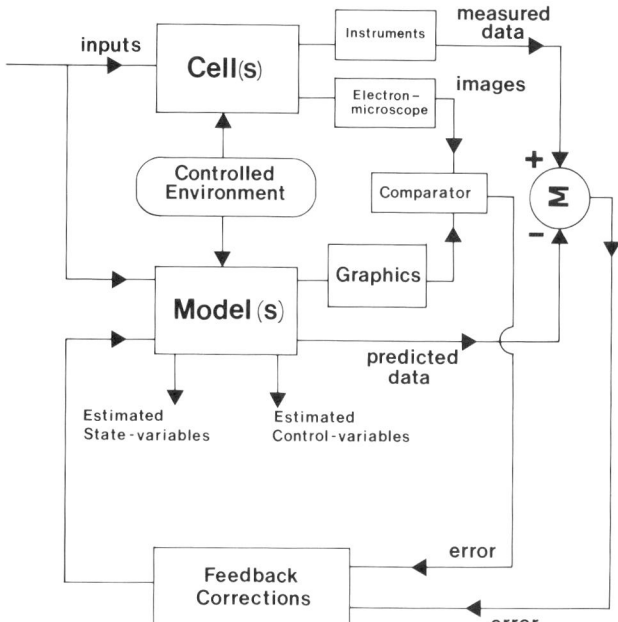

Figure 2.10. A computer based algorithm for state-variable and control-variable estimation.

the voltage clamp experiment which provided the basis for confirming the Hodgkins-Huxley relations for the anoxic excitable membrane (Cole, 1968).

The choice of the variables for making acceptable quantitative predictions of the cellular response to injury and the design of experiments to confirm them are major undertakings. But in time, they will be accomplished. Here we merely presented the elements of a theory, which is distinctly different from the traditional pathophysiological and medical viewpoints. There is a saying which goes like this: "any theory about a natural phenomenon is in a sense a lie, for it is a deliberate attempt to assess importance and to offer justification where none exists." If this is so, we hope we told a good tale, and then no apologies are needed.

References

Beers, R.F., Herriott, R.M., and Tighman, R.C. (Eds.): *Molecular and Cellular Repair Processes*. Johns Hopkins University Press, Baltimore, 1972.

Bogoliubov, N.N., and Mitropolsky, Y.A.: *Asymptotic Methods in the Theory of Nonlinear Oscillations*. Gordon and Breach Science Publications, New York, 1961 (translated from the 1958 Russian edition).

Braunwald, E. (Ed.): Protection of the ischemic myocardium. Circulation (Suppl. 1.), vol. *53*, 1976.

Callahan, J.: Singularities and plane maps. Am. Math. Monthly, vol. *81*, 1974.

Carafoli, E., and Compton, M.: The regulation of intracellular calcium. Curr. Top. Membr. Transp. *10:* 151–216, 1978.

Cetaev, N.G.: *Stability of Motion*. Gostehizdat, Moscow, 1946.

Chance, B., Pye, E.K., Ghosh, A.K., and Hess, B.: *Biological and Biochemical Oscillations*. Academic Press, New York.

Cole, K.S.: *Membranes, Ion and Impulses*. University of California Press, Berkeley, 1968.

DeClaris, N., and Zadeh, L.A. (Eds.): Nonlinear Circuits. IRE Transactions on Circuits, in memory of B. Van der Pol, vol. CT-F, No. 4, pp. 360–553, December, 1960.

Dubois, J.G., and Dufour, J.P.: La théorie des catastrophes transformeés de legendre et theormodynamique. Ann. Inst. Henri Poincare' *29:*161–212, 1978.

Hayashi, C.: *Nonlinear Oscillations in Physical Systems*. McGraw-Hill, New York, 1974.

Heinmets, F.: *Quantitative Biology*. Marcel Dekker, New York, 1970.

Jewett, D.L., and McCarroll, H.R., Jr.: *Nerve Repair and Regeneration*. C. V. Mosby, St. Louis, MO, 1980.

Kalman, R.E., and DeClaris, N. (Eds.): *Aspects of Network and System Theory*, Holt, Reinhart and Winston, New York, 1971.

Kiefer, G., and Sandritter, W.: DNA and the cell cycle. Beitr. Pathol. *158:*332–362, 1978.

Laiho, K.U., and Trump, B.F.: Relationships of ionic, water and cell volume changes in cellular injury of Ehrlich Ascites tumor cells. Lab. Invest. *31:*207–215, 1974.

Little, M., et al. (Eds.): *Mitosis: Facts and Questions*. Springer-Verlag, New York, 1977.

LaSale, J., and Lefschetz, S.: *Stability by Liapounov's Direct Method with Applications*. Academic Press, New York, 1961.

Liapounov, A.M.: Probleme géneral de las stabilite du mouvement. Ann. Math. Studies, vol. *17*, 1974 (reproduction of a 1907 French translation of the 1892 original in Russian).

Lu, Y.C.: *Singularity Theory and an Introduction to Catastrophe Theory*. Springer-Verlag, New York, 1976.

Miles, R.F. (Ed.): *Systems Concepts*. John Wiley & Sons, New York, 1973.

Miller, J.G.: *Living Systems*. McGraw-Hill, New York, 1978.

Minorsky, N.: *Nonlinear Systems*. Van Nostram, New York, 1970.

Mitchison, J.M.: *The Biology of the Cell Cycle*. Cambridge University Press, New Rochelle, NY, 1971.

Morgen, W.J., Garbus, J., Vigonto, R., and Trump, B.F.: Cellular membrane systems in shock and ischemia. In *Acute Respiratory Failure*. Georg Thieme Verlag, Stuttgart, 1979.

Nemytskii, V.V., and Stephanov, V.V.: *Qualitative Theory of Differential Equations*. Princeton University Press, Princeton, NJ, 1960 (edited translation in English from Russian).

Padilla, G.M.: *Cell Cycle Controls*. Academic Press, New York, 1974.

Poincare, H.: Sur les propriétés des fonctions définies par les equations aux differences partielles. Theses de Mathematiques, Paris, Ganthier-Villars, 1879.

Poincare, H.: Sur les courbes definies par les equations differentielles. J. Math. Pures. Appl., vol. *4*, 1885.

Rabinowitz, P.H.: *Applications of Bifurcation Theory*. Academic Press, New York, 1977.

Strehler, B.L.: *Time, Cells and Aging*. Academic Press, New York, 1962.

Thom, R.: *Structural Stability and Morphogenesis*. W. A. Benjamin Inc., New York, 1975 (English translation from the original French 1972 version).

Trump, B.F.: The role of the cellular membrane system in shock. *The Cell in Shock*. The Upjohn Co., Kalamazoo, 1974.

Trump, B.F., and Arstila, A.V. (Eds.): *Pathobiology of Cell Membranes*, vols. I and II. Academic Press, New York, 1975 and 1980.

Trump, B.F., Berezesky, I.K., Collan, Y., Kahng, M.W., and Merger, W.J.: Recent studies on the pathophysiology of ischemic cell injury. Beitr. Pathol. *158:*363–388, 1978.

Van der Pol, B.: *Selected Scientific Papers*, vols. I and II. North-Holland, Amsterdam, 1960.
Van der Werff, T.J.: Catastrophes and bifurcation in biomedical engineering. S. Afr. J. Sci., vol. *73*, 1977.
Woodcock, A.E.R., and Poston, T.: *A Geometrical Study of the Elementary Catastrophes.* Springer-Verlag, New York, 1973.
Wright, B.E.: *Critical Variables in Differentiation.* Prentice-Hall, Englewood Cliffs, NJ, 1973.
Zeeman, E.C.: Catastrophe theory. Scientific American, *234*(No. 4):65–83, 1976.

CHAPTER 3

The Biphasic Hormonal Nature of Stress

SAMUEL P. BESSMAN
V. JAYNE RENNER

This chapter presents an analysis of the metabolic consequences of stress which permits interpretation of the clinical phenomena, allows provision of appropriate therapy, and assists in prognosis. This approach not only identifies the chemical responses to stress, but also relates chemical responses to clinical phenomena such as shock, trauma, postsurgical negative nitrogen balance, starvation, and diabetic ketoacidosis. The theory explains why it is extremely difficult, if not impossible, to reverse acute severe post-traumatic negative nitrogen balance by administration of proteins, fats, carbohydrates, insulin or other hormones, or any combination of these agents. The sensitivity to insulin early, and "resistance" to insulin late in the course of ketoacidosis is also explained. All of these clinical conditions are shown to be the result of the same chemical actions of the stress hormones.

The basis of this theory is that there are two hormonal phases of stress. Phase I, the catecholamine phase, and phase II, the peptide-steroid phase, begin concurrently with the onset of stress, cause similar chemical changes in the blood although through widely different mechanisms, and follow different time courses. It is noteworthy that both these phases are under the regulatory control of the CNS (Porte and Bagdade, 1970; Handbook of Physiology, 1974; Woods and Porte, 1974; Gerich et al., 1976; Reichlin et al., 1976; Schally et al., 1977, 1978; Krieger and Liotta, 1979). The first phase is short and immediate in its biochemical effects, while the second phase takes longer to exert its effects on the organism and is more prolonged, its metabolic consequences able to persist for several hours or days. We thus describe the chemical changes which occur during the release of stress hormones to be BIPHASIC in nature.

The changes produced by the two phases of stress include a rise in blood glucose. This rise in blood glucose evokes a sharp rise in blood insulin in the normal individual. Insulin does not erase or inhibit any reaction stimulated by either phase I or phase II of the stress response. By its anabolic action it causes the return of the small molecules produced by stress reactions, namely, glucose, amino acids, and ketones to glycogen, protein, and fat, respectively (DeSchepper et al., 1965; Bessman, 1966), thereby causing the normalization of the chemical parameters measured clinically. This does not mean that the stress hormone-evoked reactions no longer occur in the individual who can supply appropriate insulin, but merely implies that the common chemical events of stress are no longer visible as changes in the body fluids. In the normal individual, glycogen, fat, and protein do continue to break down, but the end products of these substrates do not accumulate, for the catabolic effects of stress are almost balanced by the anabolic effects of insulin. As will be shown in a later section of this paper, the "almost" in the previous sentence is the basis of postsurgical negative nitrogen balance.

It is worthwhile to consider the evolutionary value of stress reactions and of insulin to the organism. Some primitive animal, lumbering through the jungle or swimming languidly through a warm prehistoric lake was being pursued by another animal. The animal who could secrete epinephrine with its many physiological actions enjoyed a number of obvious advantages. His pupils dilated so he could see better where to go, his heart beat faster and stronger, his blood pressure went up, increasing peripheral circulation, and his gut sphincters closed down, making it unneccessary to occupy himself with problems of elimination. All of these benefits, however, would be minimal if there were no chemical effects produced by epinephrine. These primitive chemical effects will be called phase I, the catecholamine phase of stress. It is necessary to feed the brain to permit effective flight or fight, and the primary food for the brain is glucose (Himwich, 1976a). Earlier reports (Quastel, 1939; Owen et al., 1967; Himwich, 1976b) that the brain can "use" ketones after a period of adaptation have been shown to be irrelevant (Hawkins and Biebuyck, 1979), for the vegetative areas are the major beneficiaries of this primitive capability. Clinically there is no doubt that severe ketoacidosis is accompanied by CNS depression.

The following are the chemical events which occur when epinephrine is released into the blood stream. They are outlined in Table 3.1.

1. *Blood glucose rises.* Epinephrine stimulates production of cyclic AMP (cAMP) by the liver and muscle cells by "turning on" a pre-existing enzyme, adenyl cyclase. cAMP, discovered by Sutherland and his coworkers (Rall and Sutherland, 1958, 1962; Sutherland and Rall, 1958, 1960; Sutherland et al., 1962, 1965; Murad et al., 1962; Klainer et al., 1962; Rabison et al., 1971; Sutherland, 1972) "turns on" a pre-existing, relatively inactive phosphorylase. This enzyme converts glycogen to glucose-1-phosphate, which is rapidly converted to glucose-6-phosphate. In the liver and kidney glucose-6-phosphate is hydrolyzed to free glucose which diffuses out of the cell, entering the plasma and causing the blood glucose to increase. Glucose-6-phosphatase is critical to this liberation of free glucose, for phosphorylated compounds cannot leave the cell (this is the cause of the fasting hypoglycemia of glycogen storage disease, type I).

2. *Blood lactate rises.* Glycogen breaks down in the muscle cells also by the same mechanisms, but the muscle lacks the enzyme, glucose-6-phosphatase. Glucose-6-phosphate continues down the glycolytic path to pyruvate, then to lactate. This is the primary cause of lactatemia of shock and of diabetic ketoacidosis. Lactatemia is generally ascribed to circulatory failure, but it is quite clear that epinephrine produces lactatemia without circulatory failure or peripheral anoxia.

3. *Bicarbonate falls.* The conversion of neutral glycogen to lactic acid in muscle results in the rapid destruction of bicarbonate ion and replacement of bicarbonate by lactate ion, shown by a rise in the anion gap.

4. *pH falls* as a result of the fall in bicarbonate.

5. *Plasma free fatty acids rise.* Epinephrine turns on a lipase in the fat tissues which converts the fats to glycerol and free fatty acids. The free fatty acids diffuse into the plasma and react with bicarbonate, lowering further the bicarbonate and pH.

6. *Plasma ketone acids rise.* Free fatty acids are carried to the liver. The fatty acid oxidizing system of the liver is not "turned on" by epinephrine, so the incomplete oxidation of these fatty acids produces large amounts of ketone acids which destroy more bicarbonate, lowering the pH further and raising the anion gap still more (Engel, 1952; Editorial, 1977).

These six chemical phenomena resulting from epinephrine release include all of the plasma changes seen in diabetic ketoacidosis and starvation. They represent the evolutionary adaptation to release energy substrates, stored fat, and carbohydrate. The animal can fuel his brain and muscles during the extra efforts made to fight or flee.

In the diabetic these changes in the body fluids lead to severe ketosis with CNS depression. This is probably what happened to the primitive animal under severe stress in the stage of evolution prior to insulin. But there is an even greater danger, and that is the wastage of glucose caused by too high an elevation of the blood glucose.

Figure 3.1 is redrawn from Soskin and Levine (1940, 1952; Soskin, 1948). It shows that as the blood glucose rises the muscle uses glucose more and more. The muscle of the animal supplied with insulin uses glucose maximally at a blood level of about 200 mg/100 ml. The animal without insulin increases his muscle utilization of glucose as the blood glucose rises, and when the blood level exceeds about 700 mg/100 ml (40 mmol), the muscle of the diabetic uses glucose as rapidly as the normal animal and *insulin does not increase this usage by either.* Since the diabetic must resemble the primitive animal prior to the appearance of insulin there was a serious danger to the survival of the animal. Epinephrine secretion in stress would be maximal, causing the blood glucose to rise maximally and resulting in the wastage of glucose into the muscle. This follows from the fact that the brain is dependent upon glucose for its metabolism but the muscle is not and the fact that the stores of glycogen in the animal are limited. There is about enough glycogen stored in the whole body of each species to keep its brain supplied with glucose for about 1 day if it were available only to the brain. Since the brain can use glucose maximally when the blood glucose level is about 100 mg% any rise in blood glucose over 100 mg/100 ml increases unnecessarily the consumption of glucose by the muscle. The primitive animal could, therefore, have some advantage to his brain from adrenalin, but within a short time he would succumb because of the wasteful use of his stored glycogen under stress, surviving perhaps for 2–4 hr.

Table 3.1
Epinephrine Effects on Blood Chemistry

1. Glucose ↑
2. Lactate ↑
3. Bicarbonate ↓
4. pH ↓
5. Free fatty acids ↑
6. Ketone acids ↑

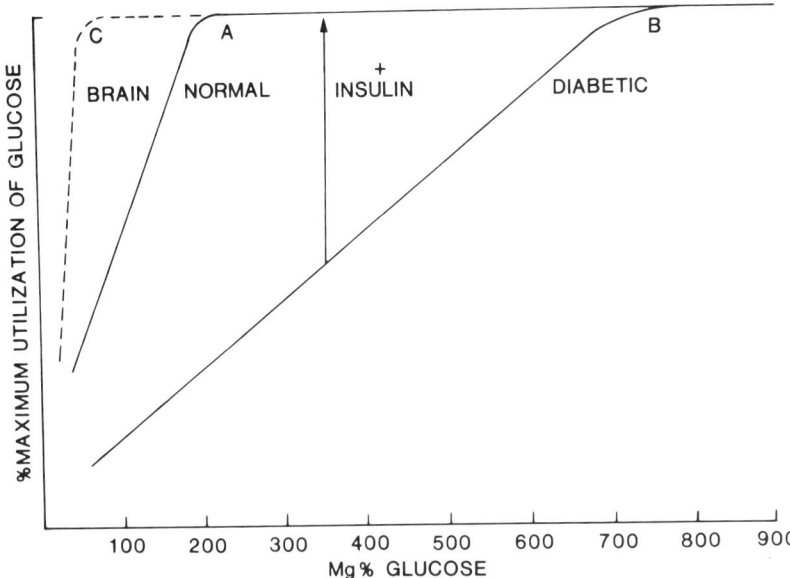

Figure 3.1. Utilization of glucose of normal and diabetic dogs as a function of blood glucose levels.

At this point in evolution, high in the vertebrate scale, insulin appeared (Bentley, 1976). This hormone stimulates the synthesis of all large molecules, particularly glycogen, protein, and fat. Contrary to some belief, insulin does not inhibit any enzyme reaction of glycogenolysis. The evidence is clear that insulin exerts its effect anabolically by stimulating the incorporation of glucose into glycogen, primarily by the liver, by increasing the rate of conversion of acetyl CoA to fatty acids and fatty acids to fats, thereby diminishing the ketosis, and by stimulating the incorporation of amino acids into proteins (DeSchepper et al., 1965; Bessman, 1966) which will be discussed later. These effects are listed in Table 3.2.

The clear evolutionary advantage of these responses to the chemical changes (Table 3.1) produced by adrenalin (note that insulin is secreted primarily when the blood glucose level rises above the level required by the brain) is that the adrenalin-driven excessive breakdown of stored glycogen is counterbalanced by increased resynthesis of glycogen, thereby husbanding the limited glucose for brain metabolism. The early animal with adrenalin and insulin mechanisms operative could, therefore, survive under stress for about a day.

This situation must have lasted for a long while in the development of the vertebrates. Then a fateful evolutionary decision was made—the animal who exhausted his glycogen had no way to supply glucose to his brain except by converting protein to glucose, since there is no mechanism in the higher animal to convert fat to carbohydrate (the step of pyruvate to acetyl CoA is irreversible). There is no stored protein, so this meant that the functional and structural proteins of the body had to be consumed to prolong the survival of the animal by continuing to supply glucose after the glycogen was used up. This trade-off of the animal itself for its survival could not be easily undertaken. The epinephrine effects occur by turning on pre-existing enzymes which are all present but relatively inactive. If the animal turned on

Table 3.2
Insulin Effects

Metabolism	Blood
Glycogen synthesis ↑	Glucose ↓
Protein synthesis ↑	Amino acids ↓
Glucose transport ↑	Glucose ↓
Fatty acid synthesis ↑	Ketones ↓
Fat synthesis ↑	Free fatty acids ↓

enzymes destructive of its structure as frequently and as vigorously as it turned on the adrenalin system it would hardly be an effective mechanism. Every time it ran away its muscles and liver would literally liquify. Such mutations would have little survival value. If, however, the animal had to synthesize extra enzymes to reverse the normal anabolic protein synthesizing process, it would take time to convert the animal to a machine of self-destruction. This was the effective response of evolution, namely, phase II of stress—the peptide-steroid phase. This begins simultaneously with phase I but has little effect on the chemistry of the body fluids till late in stress.

The hormones of phase II are growth hormone, ACTH, and cortisol. These hormones stimulate the synthesis of five enzymes which, when hypertrophied, cause a rapid breakdown of protein and reversal of glycolysis. The term "hypertrophy of enzymes" was first used by Tepperman (1964; Tepperman and Tepperman, 1960). The enzymes are listed in Table 3.3. The synthesis of all of them is stimulated by phase II hormones.

1. *Protease.* This enzyme increases manifold over the course of several hours. It causes increased hydrolysis of protein (Munro, 1979) with an increase in the pool of free amino acids. The nonessential amino acids liberated are converted to pyruvate, aspartate, and glutamate, all of which are glucogenic. Most of the essential amino acids are converted, at least partially, to acetyl CoA, which can only go to ketones or fat or be oxidized. This

Table 3.3
Phase II Hormonal Effects

Metabolism	Blood
Protease ↑	Amino acids, ketones and lactate ↑
G-6-Phosphatase ↑	Glucose ↑
F-1-6-Diphosphatase ↑	Glucose ↑
Pyruvate carboxylase ↑	Glucose ↑
PEP carboxykinase ↑	Glucose ↑

results in the formation of at most 60 g glucose and 15 g ketones from each 100 g protein. It is little recognized that the major ketosis of phase II of stress in diabetic ketoacidosis derives from protein, not from fat. If one looks at the clinical picture of diabetic ketoacidosis, it is not the fat diabetic who gets the worst ketosis, it is the thin one. If fat were the major substrate for ketosis the opposite would be expected. It is clear that ketosis is a necessary part of gluconeogenesis. Gluconeogenesis is an irreversible process because it results in the concomitant destruction of essential amino acids, which can only be replaced exogenously. Although gluconeogenesis is referred to felicitously in most textbooks, in the opinion of these authors it is one of the most destructive processes the organism can undergo. One hundred g of protein are destroyed, equivalent to 410 calories, and recover at best 222 calories as glucose and about 135 calories as fat (ketosis) are recovered, resulting in a net loss of 53 calories, or 13% if the system is perfectly efficient. In the process irreversible destruction of body protein results.

2. *Pyruvate carboxylase (PC) and phosphoenolpyruvate carboxykinase (PEPCK)* increase several fold over a period which varies from 4 to 48 hr, depending on the tissue (Shrago et al., 1963; Lardy et al., 1964; Weber et al., 1965; Foster et al., 1966; Henning et al., 1966; Hanson et al., 1973; Gunn et al., 1975; and Feldman, 1977). Since the pyruvate kinase which converts phosphoenolpyruvate (PEP) to pyruvate is irreversible, there is no direct way for the pyruvate formed from alanine, aspartate, and glutamate to move into the glycolytic cycle. A detour is provided by these two enzymes permitting pyruvate to become oxalacetic acid (OAA); then, using GTP, PEPCK causes synthesis of PEP from the OAA. If the rate of delivery of pyruvate exceeds the capability of these enzymes to use it, the pyruvate goes to lactate. Thus, lactatemia is a component of phase II of stress as well as of phase I.

3. *Fructose 1,6 diphosphatase* is increased (Weber et al., 1961, 1964, 1965; Kuam and Parks, 1960) accelerating the formation of fructose-6-phosphate which is then converted to glucose-6-phosphate.

4. *Glucose-6-phosphatase* increases 2- to 4-fold in 6–12 hr (Weber et al., 1956, 1961, 1964, 1965; Kuam and Parks, 1960; Ashmore and Weber, 1959; Ashmore et al., 1956, 1959).

These enzyme changes result in a marked reversal of the glycolytic pathway, effectively converting carbons from protein to free glucose. Although the literature contains many references to alanine, lactate, and pyruvate as the carbon sources for gluconeogenesis, they are, in fact, all derivatives of protein in this process. Only protein (with an insignificant contribution from glycerol derived from fat) can be the substrate for true gluconeogenesis. The only source of pyruvate and lactate, other than protein, is glycogen or glucose itself. It has been reported that the alanine which is liberated from muscle is greater in amount than the preformed alanine of the muscle (Odessey et al., 1974; Garber et al., 1976). This may be so, but it can only have come (if glycogen is exhausted) from the transamination of protein derived pyruvate.

As the normal organism breaks down under the onslaught of this catabolic system, the anabolic effect of insulin (evoked by the glucose rise in the blood) on protein synthesis causes a return to protein of the amino acids liberated by the proteases, thereby depriving the gluconeogenic pathway of substrate. This is why the diabetic becomes hyperglycemic and ketotic in phase II of stress, but the normal individual does not. Insulin literally "short circuits" the breakdown of protein.

The different time courses of phase I and II are the result of their different mechanisms. Phase I is a "turn-on" or activation of a whole set of pre-existing enzymes. It follows that the metabolic effect can appear rapidly, and also that as soon as the liberation of adrenalin stops, the effects will be reversed by normal metabolism. This is depicted in Figure 3.2A.

The *hatched bar* represents a short-term secretion of epinephrine and the *solid curve* is the metabolic response (changes in the blood levels of glucose, lactate, and ketones). The *open bar* and the *dashed curve* represent the same phenomena during a stress period of several hours. No matter whether the stress is long- or short-term, the development and recrudescence of chemical changes caused by adrenalin have the same rapid time course. The blood level of epinephrine will clearly parallel the chemical signs.

Phase II has a much different time course both for the development of chemical changes and for their disappearance. This is because it takes a long time to synthesize the masses of protein required to change the amounts of the five enzymes described above. Once they are synthesized they have half lives of 6–12 hr quite independent of the presence of the hormones which evoked them.

Figure 3.2B shows the time course of enzyme changes of phase II, as they would be reflected as changes in the formation of ketones, glucose, and lactate.

A short period of phase II hormone secretion causes only a slight increase of the five enzymes and manifests itself as a slight increase in the formation of ketones, lactate, and glucose (seen as blood changes in the diabetic and compensated for by insulin in the normal), but these changes persist for a long time due to the long half-life of the enzymes generated by the stress hormones. The *dotted lines* in Figure 3.2B show the effect of long-term severe stress hormone secretion. The abnormal hypertrophy of the five gluconeogenic enzymes reaches a maximum and their effect is seen as marked changes in the

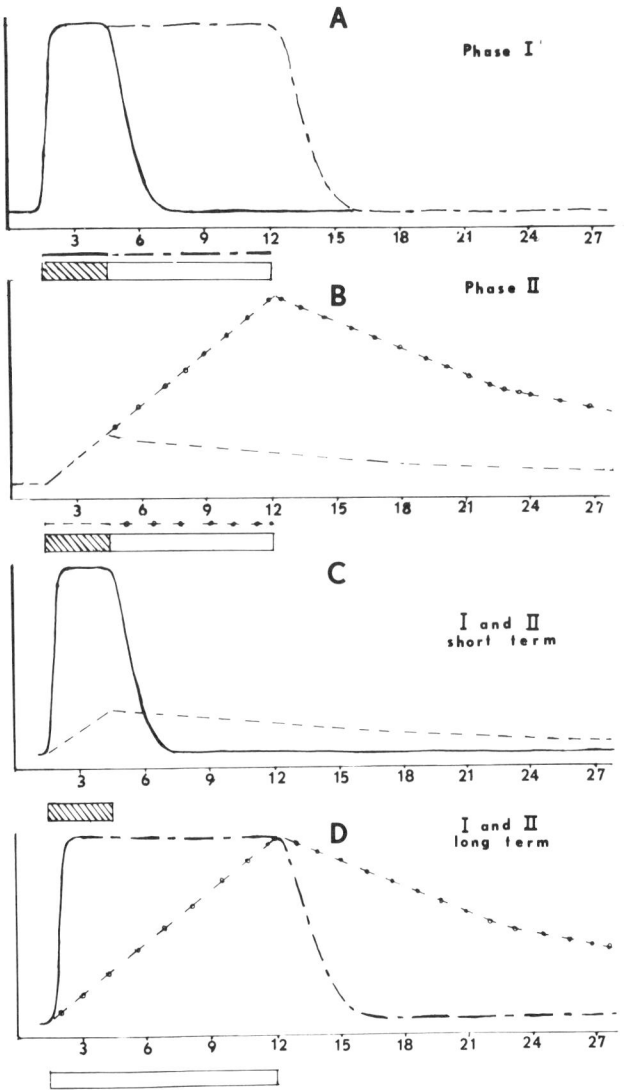

Figure 3.2. Schematic relationship between chemical effects of stress hormones of phase I and II stress and duration of actual stress. The x axis is in hours and the ordinate axis is in the degree of chemical changes in blood. A and B are pure Phases I and II results for stress of short and long duration. C and D show total effect of phases I and II for short- and long-term stress, respectively.

body fluids. When the stress diminishes and the hormone secretion stops, the enzymes do not disappear from the tissues even though the hormones which evoked them are no longer secreted. The enzymes, and the chemical changes which they cause, disappear slowly, over several days. Figure 3.2C and D is a composite of Figure 3.2A and B and shows the combined metabolic effects of both phase I and phase II hormone systems for short-term and long-term stress situations. This lack of correspondence between blood levels of second phase hormones and the changes apparently due to them has led to much confusion among students of stress and diabetes. The best work on the subject has been done by Erika Bruck and her associates (Bruck and MacGillivray, 1975), who showed a good correlation between catecholamine urinary levels and ketones or glucose in diabetics, but a poor correlation between growth hormone, cortisol, and ketones or glucose. The lag in appearance of maximal chemical changes with maximal blood levels of phase II hormones, and the lag in disappearance of the chemical signs (called "resistance to insulin" in the diabetic) are clearly the result of the complex mechanism of action of these hormones.

The relevance of this theoretical discussion of stress lies in the application of these principles to two types of patient: the one with postsurgical negative nitrogen balance, and the trauma patient. Figure 3.2D is a pattern of metabolic changes in a patient who has been under surgical stress for several hours, during which both the first and second phase hormones have been operative. As soon as the stress stops the adrenalin effects will go away, but the protein destruction will continue because the enzymes evoked by the phase II hormones will continue long after the excess hormone secretion stops. Anabolic therapeutic efforts with protein, fats, carbohydrates, insulin, or any combination of nutrients and hormones have relatively little effect because the body is geared up by the phase II hormones to destroy protein.

Perhaps a more rational approach might be to prevent the buildup of the second phase hormones *during* the surgery or during or immediately after trauma.

References

Ashmore, J., and Weber, G.: The role of hepatic glucose-6-phosphatase in the regulation of carbohydrate metabolism. Vitam. and Horm. *17*:91–132, 1959.

Ashmore, J., Hastings, A.B., Nesbett, F.B., and Renold, A.E.: Studies on carbohydrate metabolism in rat liver slice. J. Biol. Chem. *218*:77–88, 1956.

Bentley, P.J.: *Comparative Vertebrate Endocrinology* pp. 93–97. Cambridge University Press, Cambridge, MA, 1976.

Bessman, S.P.: A molecular basis for the mechanism of insulin action. Am. J. Med. *40*:740–749, 1966.

Bruck, E., and MacGillivray, M.H.: Interaction of endogenous growth hormone, cortisol, and catecholamines with blood glucose in children with brittle diabetes mellitus. Pediatr. Res. *9*:535–541, 1975.

DeSchepper, P.J., Toyoda, M., and Bessman, S.P.: A requirement for carbohydrate metabolism for the stimulation of amino acid incorporation into protein by insulin. J. Biol. Chem. *240*:1670–1674, 1965.

Editorial. The anion gap. Lancet *1*:785–786, 1977.

Engel, F.L.: The significance of the metabolic changes during shock. Ann. N.Y. Acad. Sci. *55*:381–393, 1952.

Feldman, D.: Glucocorticoid receptors and regulation of phosphoenolpyruvate carboxykinase activity in rat kidney and adipose tissue. Am. J. Physiol. *233*:E147–E151, 1977.

Foster, D.O., Ray, P.D., and Lardy, H.A.: Studies on the mechanisms underlying adaptive changes in rat liver phosphoenolpyruvate carboxykinase. Biochemistry *5*:555–562, 1966.

Garber, A.J., Karl, I.E., and Kipnis, D.M.: Alanine and glutamine synthesis and release from skeletal muscle. I. Glycolysis and amino acid release. J. Biol. Chem. *251*:826–835, 1976.

Gerich, J.E., Charles, M.A., and Grodsky, G.M.: Regulation of pancreatic insulin and glucagon secretion. Annu. Rev. Physiol. *38:*353–388, 1976.

Greep, R.O., and Astwood, E.B. (Eds.): *Handbook of Physiology, Section 7: Endocrinology, Vol. IV. The Pituitary Gland and its Neuroendocrine Control, Part 2.* American Physiological Society, Washington, DC, 1974.

Gunn, J.M., Hanson, R.W., Meyuhas, O., Reshef, L., and Ballard, F.J.: Glucocorticoids and the regulation of phosphoenolpyruvate carboxykinase (guanosine triphosphate) in the rat. Biochem. J. *150:*195–203, 1975.

Gunn, J.M., Tilghman, S.M., Hanson, R.W., Reshef, L., and Ballard, F.J.: Effects of cyclic adenosine monophosphate, dexamethasone and insulin on phosphoenolpyruvate carboxykinase synthesis in Reuber H-35 hepatoma cells. Biochemistry *14:*2350–2357, 1975b.

Hanson, R.W., Garber, A.J., Reshef, L., and Ballard, F.J.: Phosphoenolpyruvate carboxykinase. II. Hormonal controls. Am. J. Clin. Nutr. *26:*55–63, 1973.

Hawkins, R.A., and Biebuyck, J.F.: Ketone bodies are selectively used by individual brain regions. Science *205:*325–327, 1979.

Henning, H.V., Stumpf, B., Ohly, B., and Seubert, W.: On the mechanism of gluconeogenesis and its regulation. III. The glucogenic capacity and the activities of pyruvate carboxylase and PEP-carboxylase of rat kidney and rat liver after cortisol treatment and starvation. Biochem. Z. *344:*274–288, 1966.

Himwich, H.E.: Foodstuffs of the brain: Glucose. In *Brain Metabolism and Cerebral Disorders*, edited by H.E. Himwich, ed. 2, pp. 11–32. Spectrum Publications, New York, 1976a.

Himwich, H.E.: Foodstuffs of the brain: Ketone bodies. In *Brain Metabolism and Cerebral Disorders*, edited by H.E. Himwich, ed. 2, pp. 33–63. Spectrum Publications, New York, 1976b.

Klainer, L.M., Chi, Y.-M., Freidberg, S.L., Rall, T.W., and Sutherland, E.W.: Adenyl Cyclase. IV. The effects of neurohormones on the formation of adenosine 3',5'-phosphate by preparations from brain and other tissues. J. Biol. Chem. *237:*1239–1243, 1962.

Krieger, D.T., and Liotta, A.S.: Pituitary Hormones in Brain: Where, How, and Why? Science *205:*366–372, 1979.

Kuam, D.C., and Parks, R.E., Jr.: Hydrocortisone-induced changes in hepatic glucose-6-phosphatase and fructose diphosphatase activities. Am. J. Physiol. *198:*21–24, 1960.

Lardy, H.A., Foster, D.O., Shrago, E., and Ray, P.D.: Metabolic and hormonal regulation of phosphopyruvate synthesis. Adv. Enzyme Regul. *2:*39–47, 1964.

Munro, H.M.: Hormones and the metabolic response to injury. N. Engl. J. Med. *300:*41–42, 1979.

Murad, F., Chi, Y.-M., Rall, T.W., and Sutherland, E.W.: Adenyl Cyclase. III. The effect of catecholamines and choline esters on the formation of adenosine 3',5'-phosphate by preparations from cardiac muscle and liver. J. Biol. Chem. *237:*1233–1238, 1962.

Odessey, R., Khairallah, E.A., and Goldberg, A.L.: Origin and possible significance of alanine production by skeletal muscle. J. Biol. Chem. *249:*7623–7629, 1974.

Owen, O.E., Morgan, A.P., Kemp, H.G., Sullivan, J.M., Herrera, M.G., and Cahill, G.F., Jr.: Brain metabolism during fasting. J. Clin. Invest. *46:*1589–1595, 1967.

Porte, D., and Bagdade, J.D.: Human insulin secretion: An integrated approach. Annu. Rev. Med. *21:*219–240, 1970.

Quastel, J.H.: Respiration in the central nervous system. Physiol. Rev. *19:*135–183, 1939.

Rall, T.W., and Sutherland, E.W.: Formation of a cyclic adenine ribonucleotide by tissue particles. J. Biol. Chem. *232:*1065–1076, 1958.

Rall, T.W., and Sutherland, E.W.: Adenyl Cyclase. II. The enzymatically catalyzed formation of adenosine 3',5'-phosphate and inorganic pyrophosphate from adenosine triphosphate. J. Biol. Chem. *237:*1228–1232, 1962.

Reichlin, S., Saperstein, R., Jackson, I.M.D., Boyd, A.E., and Patel, Y.: Hypothalamic Hormones. Annu. Rev. Physiol. *38:*389–424, 1976.

Robison, G.A., Butcher, R.W., and Sutherland, E.W.: *Cyclic AMP.* New York, Academic Press, New York, 1971.

Schally, A.V., Coy, D.H., and Meyers, C.A.: Hypothalamic regulatory hormones. Annu. Rev. Biochem. *47:*89–128, 1978.

Schally, A.V., Kastin, A.J., and Arimura, A.: Hypothalamic Hormones: The link between brain and body. Am. Sci. *65:*712–719, 1977.

Shrago, E., Lardy, H.A., Nordlie, R.C., and Foster, D.O.: Metabolic and hormonal control of phosphoenolpyruvate carboxykinase and malic enzyme in rat liver. J. Biol. Chem. *238:*3188–3192, 1963.

Soskin, S.: *The Endocrines in Diabetes.* Charles C Thomas, Springfield, IL, 1948.

Soskin, S., and Levine, R.: On the mode of action of insulin. Am. J. Physiol. *129:*782–786, 1940.

Soskin, S., and Levine, R.: The mode of action of insulin. In *Carbohydrate Metabolism*, rev. ed., ch. XVI, pp. 196–217. University of Chicago Press, Chicago, 1952.

Sutherland, E.W.: Studies on the mechanism of hormone action. Science *177:*401–408, 1972.

Sutherland, E.W., and Rall, T.W.: Fractionation and characterization of a cyclic adenine ribonucleotide formed by tissue particles. J. Biol. Chem. *232:*1077–1091, 1958.

Sutherland, E.W., and Rall, T.W.: The relation of adenosine 3',5'-phosphate and phosphorylase to the actions of catecholamines and other hormones. Pharmacol. Rev. *12:*265–299, 1960.

Sutherland, E.W., Rall, T.W., and Menon, T.: Adenyl Cyclase. I. Distribution, preparation and properties. J. Biol. Chem. *237:*1220–1227, 1962.

Sutherland, E.W., Øye, I., and Butcher, R.W.: The action of epinephrine and the role of the adenyl cyclase system in hormone action. Recent Prog. Horm. Res. *21:*623–642, 1965.

Tepperman, J.: "Work hypertrophy" and "disuse atrophy" of intracellular enzymes. Physiol. Physicians *2:*1–8, 1964.

Tepperman, J., and Tepperman, H.M.: Some effects of hormones on cells and cell constituents. Pharmacol. Rev. *12:*301–353, 1960.

Weber, G., Allard, C., de Lamirande, G., and Cantero, A.: Liver glucose-6-phosphatase activity and intracellular distribution after cortisone administration. Endocrinology *58:*40–50, 1956.

Weber, G., Banerjee, G., and Bronstein, S.B.: Role of enzymes in homeostasis. III. Selective induction of increases of liver enzymes involved in carbohydrate metabolism. J. Biol. Chem. *236:*3106–3111, 1961.

Weber, G., Singhal, R.L., Stamm, N.B., Fisher, E.A., and Mentendiek, M.A.: Regulation of enzymes involved in gluconeogenesis. Adv. Enzyme Regul. *2:*1–38, 1964.

Weber, G., Singhal, R.L., and Srivastava, S.K.: Action of glucocorticoid as inducer and insulin as suppressor of biosynthesis of hepatic gluconeogenic enzymes. Adv. Enzyme Regul. *3:*43–75, 1965.

Woods, S.C., and Porte, D.: Neural control of the endocrine pancreas. Physiol. Rev. *54:*596–619, 1974.

CHAPTER 4

Intermediary Metabolism

MYONG WON KAHNG

Intermediary metabolism of a cell refers to all enzymatically catalyzed biochemical reactions that take place in the cell; it also encompasses the regulatory processes that maintain normal functions of these reactions. In the intact animal, it includes neurohumoral communication and regulation among the various organs. Intermediary metabolism consists of a series of chemical manipulations that result in the production of biologically available energy; the chemical bond energy thus produced is, in turn, utilized to drive energy-consuming reactions. The exergonic and the endergonic reactions of a cell are always coupled in the cell by the inescapable requirement that the only way an exergonic reaction can drive an endergonic reaction is for the two sets of reactions to share a common intermediate.

In a cell functioning normally, all metabolites are held at appropriate steady state concentrations by homeostatic regulatory processes. Deviations from the normal concentrations of key metabolites are signals for regulatory processes to become operative. The intermediary metabolic processes can function effectively in, and compensate for, many normally occurring perturbations. The large influx of exogenous metabolites during the postabsorptive state, the absence of these during fasting, the sudden, large demand for mechanical work during alarm ("flight or fight")—these are all examples of sudden stresses that are responded to successfully and routinely. Among many lower metazoans (e.g., parasitic nematodes, some bivalve mollusks), prolonged anaerobiosis is a well tolerated metabolic challenge; these animals can be considered facultative anaerobes because they have appropriate physiological responses to anaerobiosis and have alternate metabolic pathways for pyruvate. Many higher vertebrates including mammals are able to endure and function without breathing for long periods; these animals, such as diving turtles and birds and diving mammals, do not possess any new biochemical pathways that enable them to survive but succeed by combinations of anatomical and physiological features such as the increased ability of their tissues to tolerate lactic acidosis or to store oxygen. Terrestrial mammals do not possess any adaptive features that may enable them to withstand sudden anoxia or a sudden deprivation of their aerobic energy production. Nor do they develop any new biochemical pathways when exposed to prolonged sublethal hypoxia; in such a situation the compensatory responses are physiological, such as increased ventilation, increased erythropoeisis, etc. *There are no appropriate and well regulated physiological or biochemical responses on the part of a terrestrial mammal to a sudden and prolonged interruption of its aerobic energy production.*

NORMAL METABOLISM

Energy Metabolism

The quantity of energy produced and utilized may vary over a wide span of time for a given cell. Even a so called "resting cell" utilizes energy continuously for maintaining concentration gradients, compartmentation of metabolites (ions, substrates, cofactors, etc.), repair and maintenance of membrane barriers, etc. Almost all of this energy is produced aerobically by transferring electrons obtained from dehydrogenation reactions to molecular oxygen. The bulk of the energy produced from catabolism is in the form of ATP, synthesized by the phosphorylation of ADP. Since for each mole of oxygen consumed, 6 moles of ATP are generated, it can be calculated that a normally active man will generate nearly his own weight of ATP per day. The human brain, generating ATP at the rate of ~12 Kg (24 moles)/day, has only a total of about 5 mmoles of all species of adenine nucleotides (AMP + ADP + ATP = AXP). It is by the rapid synthesis of and the very prompt utilization of ATP that the tissues can transduce and utilize energy in the quantities needed. No large reservoirs of any energy-rich substances, such as ATP or phosphocreatine (PC) exist in any tissue.

Comparative Metabolism of the Tissues

Normally, the major energy substrate utilized by the body is the free fatty acid(s) (FFA) carried bound to albumin in the blood. The FFA is synthesized for the most part in the adipose tissues from surplus glucose; and the liver is cooperative in converting surplus calories (glucogenic amino acids, etc.) to glucose for this purpose. The FFA are stored as triacylglycerols in the adipose depots, and the FFA are released as needed by hormonal stimulus. The storage of surplus energy as triacylglycerols is compact and efficient. FFA so stored is used solely as fuel, with only a negligible amount being used for synthetic purposes. FFA can be utilized for energy production only aerobically and is a clean fuel, with CO_2 and H_2O as the only end products. It is preferred as a fuel over glucose by most tissues. The brain and the CNS constitute the only, but significant, exception. FFA do not cross the blood-brain barrier and thus are not available.

The brain, which has a mass about 2% of the body weight (1.5 kg/70 kg man) utilizes about 20% of the total oxygen consumption at rest. It derives its energy exclusively by aerobic metabolism of glucose, that is, by glycolysis followed by the tricarboxylic acid (TCA) cycle. The limited catalytic capacity in the brain for utilizing ketone bodies (D-3-hydroxybutyrate and 3-oxybutyrate) is readily adaptively increased during prolonged starvation (Owen et al, 1967). The mitochondrial metabolism of ketone bodies is also obligatorily aerobic. The brain has negligible endogenous reserves of energy (such as glycogen) and does not produce lactate normally. Thus, this very active organ is totally and continuously dependent on uptake of its energy substrates and of oxygen from blood. Normally, the brain is guaranteed its supplies by physiological priorities in blood supply and the sparing of glucose by other tissues.

The liver is at the center of metabolic options available to the organism. The liver receives first the exogenous metabolites, with the exception of chylomicrons, from the intestines via the portal system in the postabsorptive state. Depending on the supply situation, the liver may convert the exogenous surplus glucose to its own glycogen storage or release it as blood glucose. Similarly, during fasting, the liver maintains blood glucose levels at normal values at the expense of its glycogen stores; it receives FFA from adipose depots and converts them to ketone bodies under appropriate conditions. During exercise it receives lactate from skeletal muscle and converts it to glucose. The liver is not only a homeostatic organ for blood glucose but for many other blood constituents. The normal metabolic fuel utilized by the liver is FFA and, hence, it is not an organ expected to function anaerobically. However, in contrast with the brain, the liver does have large glycogen stores and has the potential to derive significant amounts of energy from glycolysis.

The kidney is very similar to the liver in metabolism in that it is also primarily a utilizer of FFA for energy. Some segments of the renal medulla are considered to be dependent on glycolysis for energy, but the kidney on the whole, removes lactic acid from circulation and via gluconeogenesis recovers glucose and, thus, participates in the Cori cycle.

Even though the myocardium has stored glycogen, it utilizes glucose and glycogen sparingly under normal conditions. FFA is the normal fuel, and when glucose (or glycogen) is used, it is utilized with very little production of lactate. The myocardium, like the brain, demands and obtains normally, priorities in blood supply and can use blood lactate as an energy substrate.

The skeletal muscle, particularly the white muscle, is the only major tissue in the body that is adapted for production of energy during temporary inadequacies of oxygen supply. It has a large (~150 g/70 kg man) supply of glycogen that does not participate in the homeostasis of blood glucose and is solely reserved for its energy production. It has a very large reserve supply of glycogen phosphorylase, usually stored in the inactive form, from which it can be activated readily by allosteric modulation or by covalent modification. Thus, for short periods, the skeletal muscle can obtain a significant portion of its energy from glycolysis, subject to the provision that the lactate will be removed by blood for reprocessing via the Cori cycle. Under aerobic conditions, the muscle also utilizes FFA as the preferred fuel.

METABOLISM DURING SHOCK, ISCHEMIA, AND ANOXIA

Anoxia directly affects the delivery of oxygen to the tissues. Ischemia not only interrupts the oxygen supply but also the supply of glucose and other substrates delivered by the blood. In early endotoxin shock, the aerobic metabolism of the tissues is not significantly altered. In later stages of endotoxin shock, and generally in other types of shock (e.g., hemorrhagic shock), the consequences of peripheral vasoconstriction are manifested biochemically as interruptions to the aerobic engery production in those tissues. As may be expected, there are differences in responses among individual tissues and experimental animals and models; however, biochemically shock, ischemia, and anoxia (SIA) are very similar in that the common, primary metabolic abnormality is a rapid and considerable reduction in the aerobic production of energy. Exogenous small molecular weight poisons such as cyanide or fluoroacetate, which produce a shock-like response, also directly interfere with aerobic energy production. *At their normal body temperatures, terrestrial mammals cannot produce enough energy to meet the minimum demands of the tissues in the absence of aerobic pathways.*

Regulation of Metabolism

The *suddenness* of SIA precludes responses that are slowly mobilized. Adaptive biochemical changes such as induction of enzymes have such a long time course, hours to days, to become effective that they do not play a part in the crucial initial stages of SIA; it is only during the prolonged recovery period from trauma and shock that adaptive pathways such as production of ketone bodies by the liver and utilization of these by other tissues, including the brain, may become significant. The rapid regulatory processes that respond to SIA depend directly on changes in concentrations of metabolites and consequent changes in the catalytic properties of preformed enzyme proteins. While neurohumoral interorgan communications do occur, the major part of biochemical regulatory processes that come in to play are local and autonomous. Many of the physiological responses to SIA, such as renal vasoconstriction, would make teleological sense if the proximate causes were transient; in the prolonged and profound hypoxia due to ischemia or hypovolemia, the physiological responses become inappropriate. Similarly, biochemical regulatory responses made during SIA are such that they would and do restore homeostasis following a short ischemic or anoxic episode; when the conditions persist, the regulatory processes themselves lead to irreversible damage.

The primary biochemical alteration in SIA appears to be the disruption of electron transport toward molecular oxygen and consequently production of less energy than needed for minimum maintenance (or performance) in the tissues. The consequences of oxygen deficit are initially felt in the mitochondria, since oxygen utilization by other organelles (peroxisomes, microsomes, etc.) are quantitatively minor pathways.

The reduction in the oxygen availability would leave the intermediates of the electron transport chain in the reduced state in the mitochondrion, including the primary electron acceptors, the flavoproteins and the NAD^+-NADH system. Further dehydrogenation reactions become impossible and, thus, the TCA cycle is stopped. Since electron transport and phosphorylation are tightly coupled in the normal mitochondrion, phosphorylation ceases, even though ATP levels are reduced and ADP (the acceptor for phosphorylation) accumulates. Pyruvate accumulates since pyruvate dehydrogenase (PDH) complex requires NAD^+ as an acceptor; furthermore, unless the TCA cycle resumes functioning, the available CoASH is tied up as acetyl CoA, and CoASH is another cofactor for PDH. Additionally, acetyl CoA is an allosteric negative effector for the PDH complex. Further increases in lactate levels occur in gluconeogenic tissues (liver and kidney) because gluconeogenesis, which is an alternate pathway for pyruvate, is inhibited (see below). The low levels of ATP and citrate (negative effectors for phosphofructokinase) in the cytosol increase the glycolytic rate. The cell shifts to anaerobic metabolism.

The anaerobic metabolism of glucose is the most primitive metabolic pathway and one found in all cells. It is also relatively resistant to exogenous nocuous agents. Fermentation of glucose to pyruvate produces only two moles of ATP and presents the problem of recovering the reducing agent, NAD^+. Usually pyruvate is reduced to the dead-end metabolite, lactate. All alternative metabolic pathways for pyruvate are either aerobic or demand energy in greater amounts than glycolysis can be expected to supply. Under anaerobic conditions, glucose is the only fuel available; it is neither a clean nor an efficient fuel under these conditions.

The abrupt switching from aerobic energy production (about 40% efficient with glucose or FFA as fuels) to glycolysis (about 2% efficient) reduces the energy available to the cell and increases the demand for glucose regardless of the tissue type. The demand for energy is not reduced, and so the ATP/ADP ratio falls precipitously in a few seconds. Concentrations of most intermediates in metabolic pathways in turn are changed and result in the abnormal ratios (reduced/oxidized) of all intracellular redox pairs. Since the metabolic intermediates (e.g., PC, nucleoside triphosphates) are all present only in catalytic amounts, the changes are quick and dramatic. If anoxia or ischemia is transient, as normal conditions of supply are restored, the return of the intracellular concentration of metabolites to normal values is equally rapid, because the altered concentrations and ratios of metabolites trigger compensatory processes of regulation.

Priorities in blood supply spare the brain and the myocardium during hypovolemia; but during myocardial ischemia or brain ischemia, these tissues also switch to anaerobic metabolism. The capacity of a tissue to produce energy anaerobically in adequate amounts, the maintenance of the capacity to resume energy production upon reflow or oxygen uptake, and the ability of the tissue to retain normal vascular responses to reflow— these are the factors that decide the time for irreversible damage to occur. Thus, different tissues have different "points-of-no-return." Tissues that are continuously active and normally obtain guaranteed blood and oxygen supply, namely, the brain and the myocardium, are least tolerant and can endure anoxia for only a few minutes. The point-of-no-return for the kidney during normothermic ischemia is generally considered to be about 1 hr, based on transplantation experience and experimental models. It has been suggested that inability to derive energy from glycolysis is the biochemical feature describing the point of irreversible damage (Kahng et al., 1978). The skeletal muscle can endure much longer periods of ischemia or anoxia.

Degradation of Adenine Nucleotides

The reduction in the concentration of ATP and consequent increases in the concentrations of ADP and AMP following onset of anoxia are so rapid that it is only by in situ freeze-clamping (at liquid N_2 temperature) of tissues that it is possible to obtain normal tissue values for ATP, ADP and AMP. The normal ATP concentrations of tissues are significantly lowered within 3 sec of ischemia or anoxia. The data of Gaja et al. (1973) for liver would be typical for long periods of ischemia (Table 4.1). It should be noted that AMP concentrations decline after an initial rise and that AXP concentrations decline throughout the time periods. Similar changes have been reported for kidney (Fig. 4.1, and Kahng et al., 1978) and other tissues (brain, myocardium, and skeletal muscle) during shock (endotoxemic, hemorrhagic), ischemia, or anoxia.

The reduction of the total adenine nucleotides to very low levels early in ischemia by enzymatic destruction of AMP does not make any teleological sense as an appropriate defensive measure against anoxia; the catabolism of AMP actually makes recovery difficult, if not impossible, upon reflow. The disappearance of AMP is caused by the activities of two pathways (Fig. 4.2). The first one is the major catabolic pathway for AMP by deamination to IMP followed by hydrolysis to hypoxanthine. Hypoxanthine is then oxidized to the catabolic products of the irreversible purine degradation. The second pathway

Intermediary Metabolism

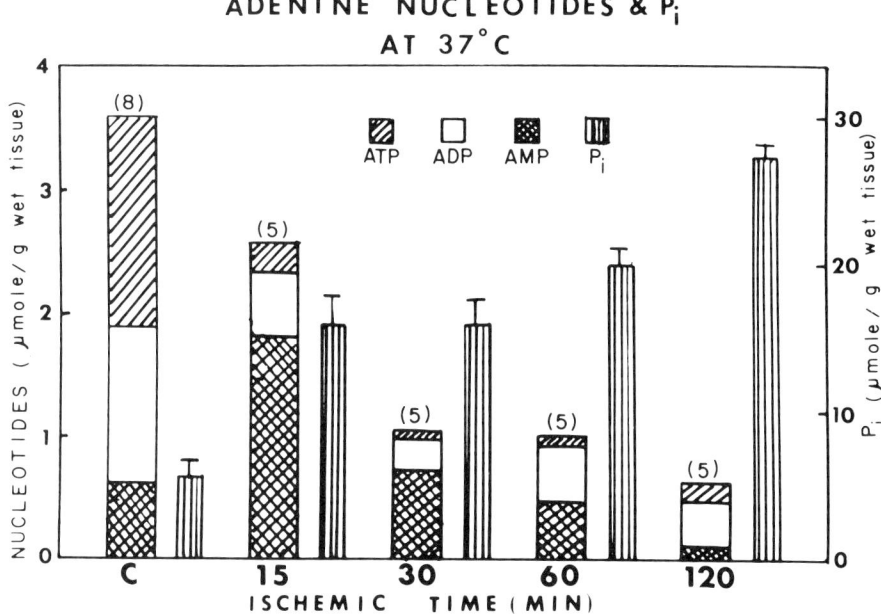

Figure 4.1. Adenine nucleotides in rat kidney during ischemia.

begins with the hydrolysis of AMP to adenosine. The production of adenosine by this pathway is opposed in a substrate cycle (Arch and Newsholme, 1978a) by the enzyme adenosine kinase. Net production of adenosine in this pathway is negligible until the tissue becomes hypoxic.

In normal physiological conditions, the AMP degradation, if it occurs at all, proceeds by the IMP→hypoxanthine pathway. The enzyme AMP deaminase is highly regulated, with very little activity when AMP concentration is low (up to 0.2 mM), and exhibits sigmoidal kinetics with $S_{0.5}$ about 10 mM. ATP (3.0 mM) increases the activity about 200-fold. P_i (in the absence of ATP) and GTP are inhibitors, and a combination of the two inhibits AMP deaminase about 95%. During stress, the increasing AMP levels and the decreasing GTP levels probably compensate for the decreasing ATP levels and increasing P_i levels. Thus, initially there is a substantial reduction in AMP (and hence in AXP) levels. The total obliteration of AXP is prevented when ATP levels fall and the catalytic properties of the enzyme are altered. Chapman and Atkinson (1973) concluded that the enzyme from liver is responsive to adenylate energy charge (see Ch. 5) being most active at the low physiological ranges of energy charge and minimally active at higher ranges or unphysiologically low values. It is suggested that during normal metabolism, when the energy charge is lowered, elimination of AMP restores the en-

Table 4.1
Energy Metabolites in Rat Liver[a,b]

Ischemia	Reflow	ATP	ADP	AMP	AXP	(NAD$^+$)/(NADH)	
						Mito	Cyto
min		μmol/g fresh liver					
Control		2.75	1.08	0.14	3.98	11.2	1084
15		0.58	0.86	1.55	2.77	1.0	14.5
15	15	2.33	0.72	0.07	3.12	20.2	1057
60		0.14	0.53	1.01	1.68	1.5	12.9
60	15	1.31	0.49	0.12	1.93	13.5	783
60	60	2.00	0.93	0.13	3.06	19.4	1188
120		0.15	0.23	0.52	0.89	1.3	15.8
120	15	0.51	0.44	0.15	1.09	—	—
120	120	0.46	0.36	0.11	0.92	5.1	216

[a] From Gaja et al., 1973.
[b] Mito, mitochondria; Cyto, cytosol.

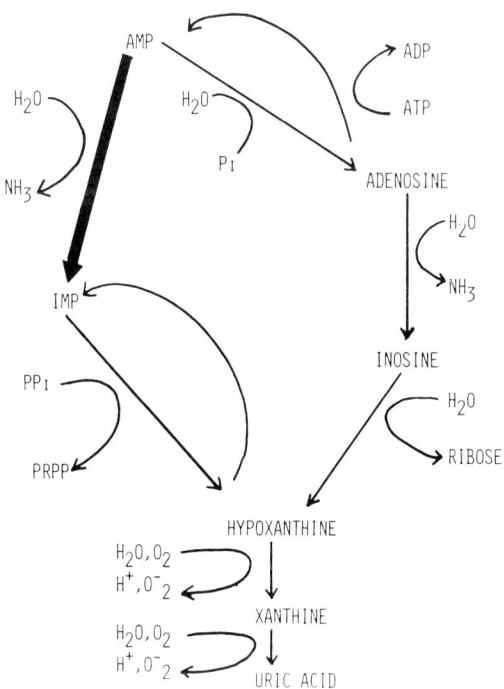

Figure 4.2. Pathways of AMP degradation. IMP, inosine monophosphate; PPi, pyrophosphate; PRPP, phosphoribosyl pyrophosphate.

ergy charge. However, in tissues under stress, the adenylate energy charge falls very rapidly to values far removed from normal physiological values (for example, in rat kidney, energy charge becomes 0.2 in 15 min). Second, in the cardiac muscle, the adenylate deaminase activity does not respond to low energy charge by sparing AMP (Solano and Coffee, 1978). Finally, whatever might be the regulatory role of AMP deaminase in physiological situations, the deamination of AMP in SIA, and consequently, the reduction of the AXP pool is not an appropriate or beneficial response.

The hydrolysis of AMP to adenosine is more understandable because adenosine causes arteriolar vasodilation. Berne and his collaborators (see Arch and Newsholme, 1978b) have studied this role of adenosine and found that during anoxia, the levels (~nM) of adenosine released from anoxic tissues are adequate for such physiological compensation. AMP is cleaved by a phosphatase, 5'-nucleotidase (5'-ribonucleotide phosphohydrolase, E.C. 3.1.3.5); the enzyme is specific for ribonucleoside-5'-phosphates. The most active isoenzyme is plasma membrane-bound and is used as a marker for the plasma membrane fraction. There is another isoenzyme in the lysosomal fraction and a third isoenzyme in the cytosol. The three isoenzymes have not been compared in detail.

Arch and Newsholme (1978a) have studied the properties of 5'-nucleotidase, adenosine kinase, and adenosine deaminase from the livers, muscles, and nerve tissues of a wide variety of vertebrates and invertebrates. The K_m of the nucleotidase in a given tissue was greater than the AMP content of the tissue. In most tissues, the K_m of adenosine kinase for AMP was considerably lower than the K_m of adenosine deaminase in the same tissue. Thus, in the substrate cycle between AMP and adenosine, the kinase is very nearly saturated at low concentrations of adenosine; the 5'-nucleotidase and adenosine deaminase are far from saturation. Thus, small changes in the activity of either enzyme of the cycle can produce large variations in adenosine concentrations in the cell. Since, in many tissues, the maximum catalytic capacity of the nucleotidase was greater than the combined activities of the kinase and deaminase, it was suggested that the nucleotidase was strongly inhibited in vivo to prevent adenosine accumulation. There was a highly significant negative correlation between the glycogen phosphorylase activity of a muscle and its adenosine kinase activity. The maximum catalytic capacity for phosphorylase is a measure of the anaerobic nature of the muscle; these workers concluded that this negative correlation, therefore, supported the theory of Berne and coworkers, that a reduction in the oxygen tension of a muscle leads to the release of adenosine and thus causes vasodilation and reactive hyperemia.

A detailed study of the liver cytosolic nucleotidase is consistent with the above findings (van den Berghe et al., 1977). The cytosolic enzyme, considered to be important in purine catabolism, had hyperbolic kinetics with IMP and most other nucleoside-5'-phosphates, but exhibited low affinity for AMP, with sigmoid kinetics, so that the enzyme was totally inactive towards AMP at physiological concentrations. Low concentrations of IMP (<0.5 mM) had a stimulatory effect on the hydrolysis of AMP, but higher concentrations were inhibitory. The suggestion can be made that low concentrations of IMP indicate the initial consequences of anoxia (increased AMP, substrate for AMP deaminase), and this IMP stimulating production of adenosine is meaningful.

Another source of loss of AXP from the cell is the leak of ATP itself; ATP has been identified as being leaked during work (e.g., by skeletal muscle) under physiological conditions. ATP is also a local vasodilator (Forrester, 1978).

The amounts of adenosine formed and ATP lost are relatively small and, under physiological conditions, cost-effective. (Even in SIA, it is the quantity of AMP lost by the IMP→hypoxathine pathway that accounts for the bulk of AXP loss.) However, the effect of adenosine on the vascular bed of the kidney is a problem. Adenosine has been known to be a vasoconstrictor of the renal vascular bed; it has been established (Osswald et al., 1978) that the effect is mediated through the renin-angiotensin system. This must necessarily exacerbate the problems of the kidney uniquely during SIA. A role for adenosine in renal failure during or after SIA is suggested, and this may be another chemical signal during SIA that is grieviously misdirected or misread.

Glycolysis and Gluconeogenesis

The nature of the insult in SIA is such as to always provoke an epinephrine response. In peripheral tissues, especially muscle, glycogenolysis is induced via cAMP mediated cascade. In the liver, increased glucose output occurs at the expense of stored glycogen. The muscles cannot release glucose from their stored glycogen to the blood because of the absence of glucose-6-phosphate phosphatase (E.C. 3.1.3.9, G6Pase). The hyperglycemia that occurs at the onset of SIA disappears when the hepatic glycogen stores are rapidly exhausted. The tissues become insulin-resistant during this time (Chaudry, 1974; Ryan et al., 1974); it is not conclusive whether the insulin-resistance occurs as a consequence of membrane damage (hence, altered properties of membrane-bound receptor sites) or as a consequence of the confused hormonal-humoral imbalances. Both factors may be operative. Glycolysis dominates during SIA. Glucose is the only substrate for energy production in the absence of oxygen. Peripheral vasoconstriction and epinephrine-induced glycogenolysis in the muscles produce large concentrations of lactate in blood; the persistent production of lactate is not a clinically favorable sign.

The gluconeogenic pathway scavenges hexose from lactate produced by muscle glycolysis or from amino acids obtained from surplus protein calories or protein degradation during fasting. The pathway, by convention, begins with lactate or oxalacetate from TCA cycle and ends with glucose. This cytosolic pathway shares enzymes with glycolysis with only three crucial and regulatory steps being different (Fig. 4.3). Glycolysis produces half as much energy (2 moles ATP/mole glucose) as is needed for converting 2 moles of lactate to glucose by gluconeogenesis. Thus, gluconeogenesis cannot occur when glycolysis is the major source of energy.

The two pathways differ at regulatory points where substrate cycles can occur, between phosphoenolpyruvate (PEP) and pyruvate, between fructose-6-phosphate (F6P) and fructose-1,6-bisphosphate (FDP) and between glucose and G6P. In the liver, glucose is phosphorylated by glucokinase (E.C. 2.7.1.2), which has a Km of ~10 mM. Thus, at normal tissue concentrations (~5 mM) the enzyme converts very little glucose to G6P. The specific enzyme, G6Pase, operates in a substrate cycle and hydrolyzes the little G6P that is formed, thus, feeding very little substrate into glycolysis. The second barrier is at the F6P → FDP point. Phosphofructokinase (E.C. 2.7.1.11, PFK), which synthesizes FDP, is counteracted by D-fructose-1,6-bisphosphate 1-phosphohydrolase (E.C. 3.1.3.11, FDPase). Both enzymes are allosterically regulated. Under physiological concentrations of ATP and citrate, PFK is minimally active, and FDPase, because of low AMP and high ATP concentration, is maximally active. Very little glycolysis takes place in the liver and glucose utilization for fatty acid synthesis is even questionable. The liver, therefore, either deposits exogenous glucose as glycogen or passes it on to the peripheral tissues; it utilizes exogenous lactate for gluconeogenesis and fatty acid synthesis. FFA is, therefore, generally considered to be the metabolic fuel for liver. The kidney cortex, another gluconeogenic tissue, behaves similarily, particularly during prolonged starvation.

During SIA, the conversion of pyruvate to PEP (a component of the third substrate cycle) is not possible. The reactions catalyzed by enzymes, pyruvate carboxylase (E.C. 6.4.1.1), and phosphoenol pyruvate carboxykinase (E.C. 4.1.1.32) are both energy-expending reactions. The low concentrations of ATP and other energy sources, and the high NADH/NAD$^+$ ratio leave no metabolic choice for pyruvate except conversion to lactate. A second block to gluconeogenesis during SIA occurs at the FDP → F6P stage. The low concentrations of ATP and high concentrations of AMP activate PFK and suppress FDPase. The crossover plot of glycolytic intermediates in rat kidney (Fig. 4.4) is typical of the consequences of ischemia. Similar results have been reported for other tissues in various types of SIA (Shoemaker, 1967; Schumer and Erve, 1975).

Lipid Metabolism

Epinephrine-induced lipolytic cascade in adipose tissue is another futile and inappropriate response to SIA. FFA are released from the storage depots, but cannot be utilized by tissues in SIA. The accumulation of FFA contributes to the uncoupling of mitochondrial oxidative phosphorylation. The accumulation of fatty acyl CoA interferes with ADP-ATP translocase in mitochondria (Shrago et al., 1976).

The energy-expending, fatty acid synthesizing pathway cannot remain active during the energy shortage in SIA. Translocation of citrate and the ATP-requiring cleavage of citrate in the cytosol provide the acetyl CoA needed for fatty acid synthesis. The reducing power is

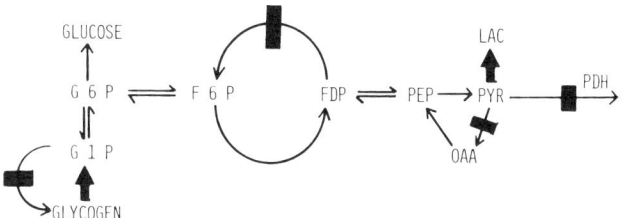

Figure 4.3. Pathways of gluconeogenesis. *LAC*, lactate; *PYR*, pyruvate; *PEP*, phosphoenolpyruvate; *PDH*, pyruvate dehydrogenase; *OAA*, oxalacetic acid; *FDP*, fructose-1,6-bisphosphate; *F6P*, fructose-6-phosphate; *G6P*, glucose-6-phosphate; *G1P*, glucose-1-phosphate.

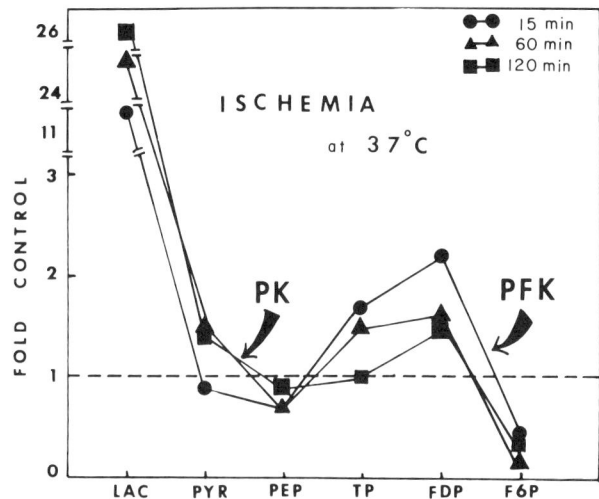

Figure 4.4. Crossover plot of glycolytic intermediates in rat kidney during ischemia. *LAC*, lactate; *PYR*, pyruvate; *PEP*, phosphoenol pyruvate; *TP*, triosephosphate; *FDP*, fructose-1,6-bisphosphate; *F6P*, fructose-6-phosphate; *PK*, pyruvate kinase; *PFK*, phosphofructokinase.

specifically provided by NADPH, which is produced in the cytosol on demand. During SIA, NADPH/NADP$^+$ ratio is very large. This, however, is due to the generally reduced state of all metabolic redox pairs and to nonutilization of NADPH. The generation of NADPH by the phosphogluconate (hexose monophosphate shunt) pathway (and by ancillary reactions such as NADH-NADP$^+$ exchange, malic enzyme-catalyzed reaction, etc.) must cease when all NADPH-NADP$^+$ is trapped as NADPH, that is to say, when the acceptor is no longer available. Even though it has been shown that in vitro many of the enzymes of phosphogluconate pathway remain at normal concentrations, the pathway in vivo must be at a standstill. The lowered concentration of citrate, which is not only the substrate for the production of acetyl CoA but also an indispensable modulator for acetyl CoA carboxylase, would effectively shut off energy-wasting fatty acid synthesis during the energy crisis.

Other Pathways During SIA

The different alterations in other biochemical pathways (based on observed concentrations of metabolites or enzymes, tracer studies, etc.) are consistent with the belief that during SIA, the major metabolic problem is the lack of energy, and that while energy-requiring (endergonic) processes are largely suppressed, many catabolic exergonic processes continue. Normally in the cell there is a turnover of most of the cell components; during SIA, the synthesis of these is stopped, but the degradation continues. The slightly reduced protein content in tissues is thus attributable to a reduced rate of protein synthesis rather than to any increase in degradation. The same is true of the total nucleoside phosphate pools, including AXP. Inability to maintain appropriate compartmentation is due to failure of energy-requiring membrane processes, and this is exacerbated by the concomitant acidosis. The lowered pH and increased lactate appear to offer some protection to the cells in vitro (Penttila et al., 1976). In experimental myocardial ischemia and anoxia, the accumulation of hydrogen ion and lactate contribute to the inhibition of protein degradation (Chua et al, 1979). The leakage of K^+ has been suggested as an early consequence and indicator of damage in SIA (Baue, 1976); ultrastructural studies show that membranes (e.g., mitochondrial, lysosomal) are increasingly damaged as the point-of-no-return for a tissue is approached. The biochemical basis for the damage remains to be elucidated. The catabolic component of turnover is very important in cellular homeostasis (as witness the dire consequences of lysosomal storage diseases for very minor cell components), but the persistence of such catabolism in the absence of balancing synthesis is another inappropriate metabolic response to SIA.

Recovery Phase

There is a unity in the biochemical response to the onset of SIA in that 1) the suddenness of onset and 2) a drastic reduction in aerobic energy production are features common to all types of SIA and all experimental models.

It would be expected that there might be fewer such common denominators during recovery, with respect to experimental models and with organs. The recovery period has not been studied with as much care because of the conception of SIA as an acute condition. The prolonged recovery period from SIA would include 1) a continued need for glucose until the mitochondrial capacity for aerobic energy production is restored, and 2) the accumulation of normal levels of cellular AXP by scavenging, and 3) the utilization of endogenous energy sources until adequate assimilation of exogenous nutrients is restored. During recovery from surgical trauma, there is a phase when exogenous dietary substrates cannot be adequately supplied. In some cases, mobilization of muscle proteins takes place, over and above the loss of protein by turnover problems. In other cases, hepatic ketone body production is stimulated and muscle protein is spared (Munro, 1979). The regulatory processes that lead to these two different options are not understood. During recovery, a major commitment of the metabolic resources is to replenish the glycogen stores that were rapidly depleted during SIA. Following SIA, autophagic vacuoles are seen in many cells (Trump and Arstilla, 1975), indicating that either new substrates (e.g., for gluconeogenesis) are being recycled or deferred repairs are being undertaken. Further studies of this phase of SIA appear warranted.

Ameliorative Agents

The immediate strategy in clinical management is to maintain selective perfusion of brain and myocardium first and kidney next in the face of hypotension, hypovolemia, and a strong tendency for renal vasoconstriction. The experimental data on ameliorative agents other than selective vasoconstrictors come from organ transplant research, principally on renal transplants, although considerable data have been obtained from other models also.

A list of most of these agents reported to protect kidneys during warm ischemia in situ (or during preparation for transplantation) is found in Table 4.2, along with the most probable mode of action of each. Some of these agents like allopurinol and hypoxanthine are in use in renal transplantation. Conflicts in the literature as to the effect of the drugs in various SIA are difficult to resolve because of different models, different experimental protocols, etc. used. In the event, the protective actions of these agents are very imperfectly understood at the molecular level and there is little information on possible synergistic interactions among the agents. Some of these agents may have more than one effect, for example, ATP. Recently Chaudry et al. (1976) reported that one of the modes of action of ATP-$MgCl_2$ is the restoration of insulin sensitivity to tissues. Whether it is a specific

Table 4.2
Protective Agents Against Warm Ischemia

Agent	Probable Mode of Action
1. Allopurinol Hypoxanthine Inosine ATP	Conservation of AXP
2. Corticosteroids Mannitol Trasylol Propranolol ATP	Stabilization of membranes
3. Dihydroxyacetone ATP	Energy source
4. Propranolol	Block of beta-mediated renin release
5. ATP	Vasodilation

AXP = ATP + ADP + AMP

effect on the receptor sites or a general restoration of membrane function remains to be studied. Chaudry et al. (1976) studied rats in hemorrhagic shock. Many other workers have reported on the beneficial effects of ATP, but recently McCaig and Parratt (1979) have found that in the case of endotoxin-shocked cats, ATP-$MgCl_2$ was without any beneficial effect. Further studies of these ameliorative agents and their modes of action and a search for possible synergistic agents appear warranted.

SUMMARY

There are no appropriate physiological or biochemical responses to ischemia and anoxia which deprive the tissues of their capacity for aerobic production of energy. Shock, of whatever origin, ultimately creates a similar constraint, although in some cases it may be delayed or indirectly imposed. Normothermic tissues cannot obtain adequate energy for long by anaerobic pathways and the production of energy by glycolysis leads to the accumulation of lactate. The concentrations of key metabolites and the ratios of the concentrations of paired metabolic effectors (such as ATP/AMP, NAD^+/NADH) become abnormal. These in turn trigger extant, normal regulatory processes that are applied vicariously and inappropriately to perturbations caused by shock, ischemia, or anoxia. The total adenine nucleotides of the tissues are decreased and adenosine is released. Adenosine is an important agent causing reactive hyperemia in most tissues, but it can cause vasoconstriction in the kidney. Most of the energy-requiring reactions, including repair and maintenance are severely restricted, while most of the catabolic reactions continue. The point of irreversible injury is reached when the capacity to generate even the minimal energy by glycolysis is lost due to increasing concentrations of hydrogen ions and decreasing concentrations of electron acceptors.

Further studies on the biochemistry of the tissues during recovery from sublethal injury are warranted. Investigations on the mode of action at the molecular level of ameliorative agents and a systematic search for such agents are also needed.

References

Arch, J.R.S., and Newsholme, E.A.: Activities and some properties of 5'-nucleotidase, adenosine kinase and adenosine deaminase in tissues from vertebrates and invertebrates in relation to the control of the concentration and the physiological role of adenosine. Biochem. J. *174:*965, 1978a.

Arch, J.R.S., and Newsholme, E.A.: The control of the metabolism and the hormonal role of adenosine. In *Essays in Biochemistry*, edited by P.N. Campbell and W.N. Aldridge, vol. 14, pp. 82–122. Academic Press, New York, 1978b.

Baue, A.E.: Metabolic abnormalities of shock. Surg. Clin. North Am. *56:*1059, 1976.

Chapman, A.G., and Atkinson, D.E.: Stabilization of adenylate energy charge by the adenylate deaminase reaction. J. Biol. Chem. *248:*8309, 1973.

Chaudry, I.H.: Insulin resistance in experimental shock. Arch. Surg. *109:*412, 1974.

Chaudry, I.H., Sayeed, M.M., and Baue, A.E.: Insulin resistance and its reversal by in vivo infusion of ATP in hemorrhagic shock. Can. J. Physiol. Pharmacol. *54:*736, 1976.

Chua, B., Kao, R.L., Rannels, E., and Morgan, H.E.: Inhibition of protein degradation by anoxia and ischemia in perfused rat heart. J. Biol. Chem. *254:*6617, 1979.

Forrester, T.: Extracellular nucleotides in exercise: possible effect on brain metabolism. J. Physiol. (Paris) *74:*477, 1978.

Gaja, G., Ferreo, M.E., Piccoletti, R., and Bernelli-Zazzera, A.: Phosphorylation and redox states in ischemic liver. Exp. Mol. Pathol. *19:*248, 1973.

Kahng, M.W., Berezesky, I.K., and Trump, B.F.: Metabolic and ultrastructural response of rat kidney cortex to in vitro ischemia. Exp. Mol. Pathol. *29:*183, 1978.

McCaig, D.J., and Parratt, J.R.: Failure of exogenous ATP and creatine phosphate to modify the course of E. coli endotoxin shock in the cat. Circ. Shock *6:*235, 1979.

Munro, H.N.: Hormones and the metabolic response to injury. N. Engl. J. Med. *300:*41, 1979.

Osswald, H., Schmitz, H. J., and Kemper, R.: Renal action of adenosine: effect on renin secretion in the rat. Arch. Pharmacol. *303:*95, 1978.

Owen, O.E., Morgan, A.P., Kemp, H.G., Sullivan, J.M., Herrera, M.G., and Cahill, G.F., Jr.: Brain metabolism during prolonged starvation. J. Clin. Invest. *46:*1589, 1967.

Penttila, A., Glauman, H., and Trump, B.F.: Studies on the modification of the cellular response to injury. IV. Protective effect of extracellular acidosis against anoxia, thermal, and *p*-chloromercuribenzene sulfonic acid treatment of isolated rat liver cells. Life Sci. *18:*1419, 1976.

Ryan, N.T., George, B.C., Egdahl, D.H., and Egdahl, R.H.: Chronic tissue insulin resistance following hemorrhagic shock. Ann. Surg. *180:*402, 1974.

Schumer, W., and Erve, P.R.: Cellular metabolism in shock. Circ. Shock *2:*109, 1975.

Shoemaker, W.: *Shock: Chemistry, Physiology and Therapy*, 282 pp. Charles C Thomas, Springfield, IL, 1967.

Shrago, E., Shug, A.L., Sul, H., Dittar, N., and Folts, J.D.: Control of energy production in myocardial ischemia. Circ. Res. (Suppl. 1) *38:*I-75, 1976.

Solano, C., and Coffee, C.J.: Differential response of AMP deaminase isozymes to changes in the adenylate energy charge. Biochem. Biophys. Res. Commun. *85:*564, 1978.

Trump, B.F., and Arstila, A.: Cellular reaction to injury. In *Principles of Pathobiology*, edited by M.F. LaVia and R.B. Hill, Jr., ed. 2, pp. 9–96. Oxford University Press, New York, 1975.

van den Berghe, G., van Pottelsberghe, C., and Hers, H.G.: A kinetic study of the soluble 5'-nucleotidase of rat liver. Biochem. J. *162:*611, 1977.

CHAPTER 5

Energy Metabolism

KAZUE OZAWA

The metabolic events in shock have been regarded as secondary to decreased tissue perfusion leading to generalized cellular hypoxia and vital organ damage. The basic characteristic of metabolic regulation in shock is the rapid reorganization of the energy-producing metabolic system. Metabolic disturbances are markedly different in various organs. However, in the various types of shock (hemorrhagic, cardiogenic, vasogenic, or septic), there are basically similar changes in the energy producing pathways of each organ.

Studies on the energy metabolism of the shocked cell as a functional unit are useful for understanding the whole metabolism at the level of the organs. Let us briefly review the changes in the energy pathways in the shock state in a hepatocyte, which has almost all the metabolic pathways and plays a central role in the regulation of the energy-producing homeostasis. The cytoplasm contains the enzymes of the glycolytic cycle. The mitochondria contain the enzymes of the Krebs cycle and of oxidative phosphorylation. In the Krebs cycle, pyruvate is further catabolized to carbon dioxide while generating ATP. In shock, the metabolic pathway for glucose is reorganized by the deficits of oxygen and substrates and controlled by humoral messengers. As oxygen availability inside a cell is decreased by decreased tissue perfusion, the oxidation of NADH to molecular oxygen, through the electron carrier system, decreases, resulting in an inhibition of the Krebs cycle of mitochondria (Drucker et al., 1962; Schumer, 1968). During anaerobic metabolism, glucose is converted to pyruvate and then lactate by the lactate dehydrogenase system. The energy available to the cells is limited to the production of ATP by the glycolytic pathways. The deficits of substrates force gluconeogenesis in the liver. However, the enhanced glycolysis provides a poor yield of ATP, is limited in duration, and puts the life of the cell in danger. With the depletion of ATP, a great number of endergonic biological reactions cease and biological membranes start to malfunction. Thus, the important gradients necessary for the ion pump mechanism of the cellular membrane can no longer be maintained. Sodium moves into the cell with water and potassium moves out. Intracellular acidosis develops. Lactate accumulates in parallel with the severity of shock. Glycolysis ceases with excess accumulation of protons. The cellular metabolism breaks down completely. In the whole body, this noxious lactic acidosis results in myocardial insufficiency, cell swelling, the sludge phenomenon and disseminated intravascular coagulation (DIC), inhibition of the reticuloendothelial system, and the liberation of lysosomal hydrolases. Finally, the energy deficit and acidosis produce irreversible cellular derangements. Ultimately, the summation of such cellular lesions develops into an irreversible failure of the vital organs, leading to death.

RAPID REORGANIZATION OF THE ENERGY PATHWAY IN SHOCKED CELLS

In considering energy metabolism, it is important to clarify the fundamental nature of the derangement of the energy balance initiated by shock. The steady state concentrations of ATP, ADP, and AMP in the cells play an important role as regulatory effectors of many enzymatic reactions and provide the cells with a very sensitive intracellular control mechanism. The concentrations of ATP, ADP, and AMP are especially important elements in allosteric regulation of glycolysis and respiration. It is very convenient to use the concept of the energy charge (ATP + ½ADP)/(ATP + ADP + AMP), which is designated by Atkinson (1966, 1970) as the regulator of the metabolic processes (Fig. 5.1). The energy charge is a major factor in the regulation of pathways that produce and utilize high energy phosphate compounds. The energy charge value reflects the cellular energy balance between the energy generating sequences and the energy-utilizing sequences and is maintained at 0.85–0.90 in normal cells. The regulation of energy generation assures a continuing supply of ATP commensurate with current requirements. In the cells, the glycolytic and Krebs cycles regenerate ATP at a sufficiently rapid rate to maintain a normal energy charge, in spite of many enzymatic reactions that utilize ATP. If the energy charge decreases, the ATP-generating sequences are accelerated and the ATP-requiring sequences are slowed down. If the energy charge increases above the normal level, the reverse changes take place. The energy charge strongly resists any deviations from 0.85. The cellular viability declines with a fall in energy charge (Chapman et al., 1971; Kamiyama et al., 1977; Ozawa et al., 1979).

The concept of the energy charge can be applied to

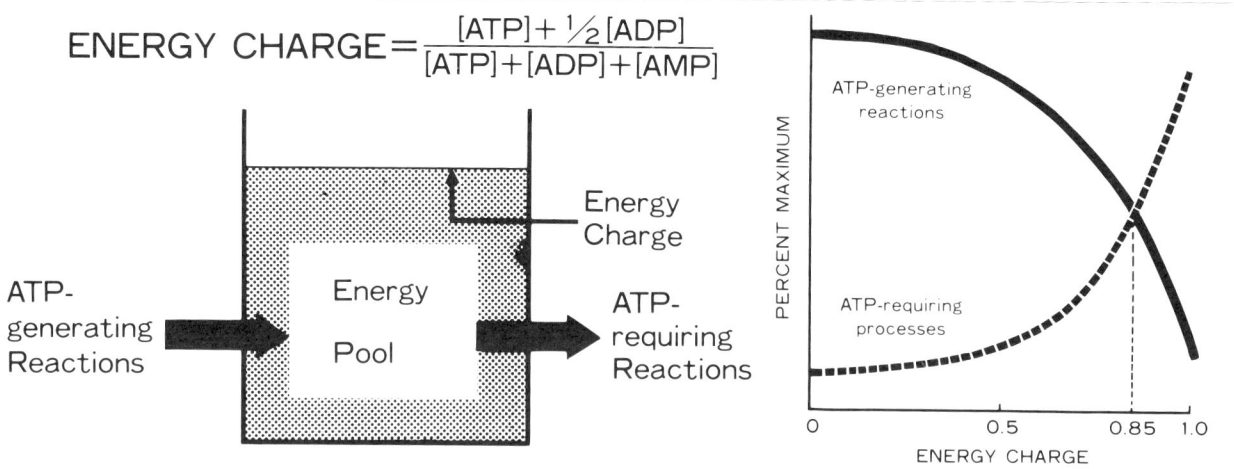

Figure 5.1. The concept of the energy charge (*left*) and the response of ATP-generating and ATP-requiring reactions to the energy charge.

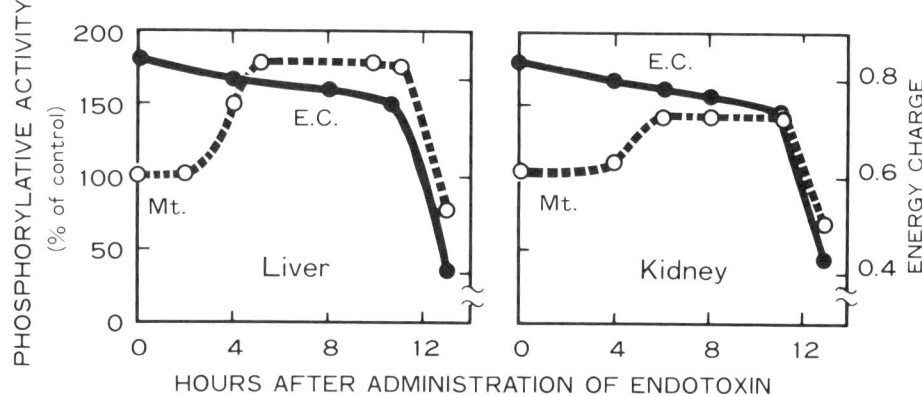

Figure 5.2. Changes in the energy charge and mitochondrial phosphorylative activity in the liver and kidney after the administration of endotoxin.

the shock state. In the liver and kidney, for example, the energy charge is maintained at the normal level by enhanced ATP-generating sequences after the administration of endotoxin of 5 mg/kg in rats, as shown in Figure 5.2. The energy charge was maintained at a higher level than 0.75 until 10 hr, when the blood glucose levels were normal or high. During this period, the mitochondrial phosphorylative activity enhanced markedly. Afterward, the energy charge decreased rapidly with an inhibition of mitochondrial enhancement. The mortality rate elevated remarkably with the severity of the decrease in the energy charge. These results indicate the importance of mitochondrial enhancements for maintaining the energy charge at a normal level in order to maintain life. The fundamental mechanism of mitochondrial enhancement is directly induced by the categoric necessity of responding to the enhanced ATP-utilizing process. This mitochondrial enhancement is encountered in endotoxin shock but is not observed in hemorrhagic shock. Glycolysis enhances in hemorrhagic shock as described below. Both the enhancement of mitochondrial phosphorylative activity and the enhancement of glycolysis act to restore the decreased energy charge in shock. Complete aerobic oxidation forms 36 mol of ATP/mol of glucose. In the absence of oxygen, a net of only 2 mol of ATP/mol of glucose is obtained by anaerobic glycolysis. So, in order to generate ATP by glycolysis at the same rate as aerobically, glycolysis must be enhanced by a multiple of 18. Thus, mitochondrial enhancement effectively prevents a decrease in the energy charge, while hyperglycolysis is not effective. In hemorrhagic shock, the hepatic energy charge decreases rapidly, because enhanced glycolysis is not effective in restoring the decreased energy charge (Fig. 5.6). These findings are consistent with the observations of Blackwood et al. (1973) that in hemorrhagic shock the liver ATP drops markedly, while there is little change in the corresponding ATP levels in endotoxin shock. Lactic acid is higher in all tissues in hemorrhagic shock than in endotoxin shock. Anaerobic metabolism appears to be a more important component of hemorrhagic shock than it is of endotoxin shock.

How does the hepatic energy charge change in hypoxia and ischemia? In hypoxia, the hepatic energy charge starts to decrease when the arterial PO_2 (PaO_2) is reduced below about 50 mm Hg and then decreases rapidly with further decreasing PaO_2 (Fig. 5.3) (Ukikusa et al., 1979). One of the first consequences to be expected of a decrease

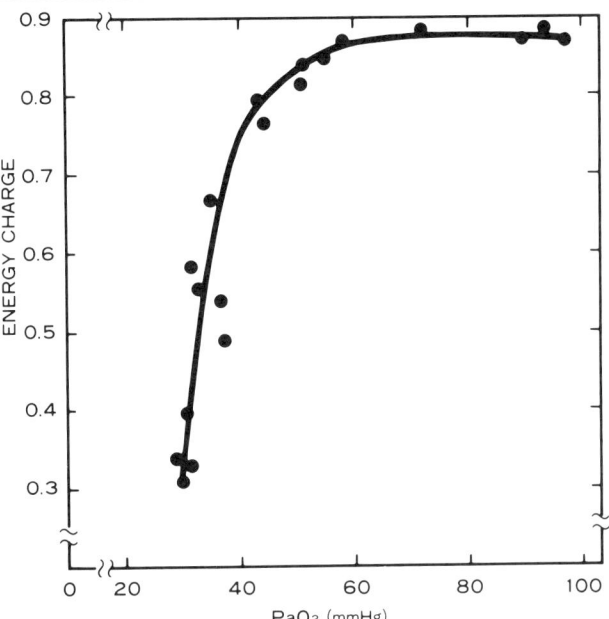

Figure 5.3. Changes in the hepatic energy charge related to the arterial PO_2 in hypoxia with the oxygen content varied in steps from 7–20%.

in PaO_2 would be a corresponding decrease in electron transfer along the respiratory chain at the mitochondrial level of the cell. This in turn would lead to a fall in oxidative phosphorylation of ADP to ATP and a decrease in energy charge levels. By contrast, in hemorrhagic hypotension at 40 mm Hg arterial blood pressure, the hepatic energy charge falls rapidly within 1 hr, although the PaO_2 remains essentially normal or higher (Fig. 5.4). However, there is a striking decrease in liver oxygen tension as measured by a microelectrode technique (Mela et al., 1973). This is due to peripheral circulation disturbances, with inadequate transport of oxygen at the microcirculatory and cellular levels. The disturbed PO_2 gradient between capillary blood and tissue appears to be insufficient to induce oxidative phosphorylation, since isolated mitochondria can go down maximally to or even below a PaO_2 level of 1–3 mm Hg. The changes in the energy charge in hemorrhagic shock are similar to those in pure hypoxia in the presence of adequate tissue perfusion. The cellular biochemical disorders in hemorrhagic shock are obviously produced by attendant hypoxia.

Is there a close correlation between the hepatic energy charge and the mortality rate in hemorrhagic shock? The relationship was studied in rats subjected to acute blood loss according to Swan's model (Swan et al., 1959). The volume of the shed blood relative to mortality was calculated by the following formula. With a high mortality rate at which 69 of 70 rats died, **v = 2.80-1/750 (B.W. −230)**; with a moderate mortality rate at which 35 of 70 rats died, **v = 2.65-1/575 (B.W. −240)**; and with a low mortality rate at which 2 of 85 rats died, **v = 2.50-1/850 (B.W. −245)** (where v = blood volume withdrawn; B.W. = body weight) (Kamiyama et al., 1979). At 15 min after acute blood loss, the hepatic energy charge had decreased significantly to 0.592 in the rats with a low mortality rate ($p < 0.001$), to 0.399 in those with a moderate mortality rate ($p < 0.001$), and to 0.304 in those with a high mortality rate ($p < 0.001$). The hepatic energy charge level negatively correlated with the volume of shed blood ($r = -0.728, p < 0.01$) (Fig. 5.5). These results suggest that changes in the hepatic energy charge play an important role in determining the survival of hemorrhagic-shocked animals.

Let us review the changes in the energy metabolism of the liver following the induction of hemorrhagic hypotension in more detail. The changes in the energy charge and the mitochondrial and cytoplasmic redox states of the liver after hemorrhagic shock were studied in normal rats as models of reversible shock and in jaundiced rats

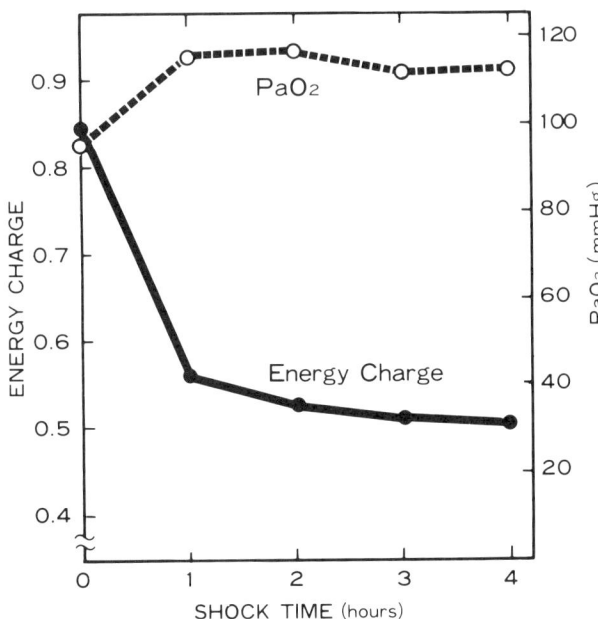

Figure 5.4. Changes in the hepatic energy charge related to the arterial PO_2 in hemorrhagic shock.

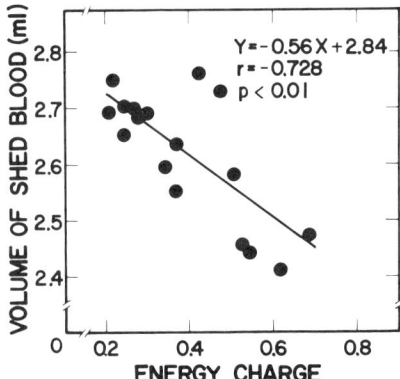

Figure 5.5. Relationship of the hepatic energy charge to the withdrawn blood volume after acute blood loss.

Energy Metabolism

as models of irreversible shock (Fig. 5.6). The systemic arterial blood pressure was maintained at 40 mm Hg by bleeding according to Wiggers's model (Werle et al., 1942; Wiggers, 1950). More than 50% of the jaundiced rats died within 2 hr following the induction of shock despite the return of all their shed blood. However, all of the jaundiced rats survived when the shed blood was returned within 30 min after the induction of shock. In normal rats, the energy charge decreased from 0.84 to 0.56 within 1 hr after the induction of shock and remained at the same level during the next hour. Following the reinfusion of the shed blood, the energy charge returned to the control level within 2 min (Ozawa et al., 1976). The mitochondrial and cytoplasmic redox states decreased gradually to half of the control within 2 hr after shock. After the reinfusion of the shed blood they increased rapidly to higher levels than the control. By contrast, in jaundiced rats the hepatic energy charge dropped to 0.49 within 1 hr after the induction of shock and remained unchanged in the surviving jaundiced rats during the next hr (Yamamoto et al., 1978). After the reinfusion of 5 ml/200 g of the reserved blood the energy charge did not recover to the preshock level. The mitochondrial and cytoplasmic redox states decreased markedly within 1 hr after the induction of shock and did not recover to half of the preshock level after the reinfusion of the reserved blood.

The sequence and kinetics of the electron transport chain are closely related to the arrangement of the redox system on the mitochondrial cristae. The lowering of oxygen availability in the electron transport chain induces a marked decrease in the mitochondrial $NAD^+/NADH$ ratio. In shocked normal and jaundiced rats, the mitochondrial and cytoplasmic redox states become reduced as shock progresses. Presumably this change is the result of a lower rate of oxidative phosphorylation and thus of a restricted mitochondrial reoxidation of NADH through inhibition of the electron carrier system. The accumulations of NADH depress the citrate synthase which decides the turnover rate of the Krebs cycle (Fig. 5.7) (Newsholme and Start, 1973). Also, the decrease in the mitochondrial redox state induces a decrease in the ratio of oxaloacetate to malate, which results in an inhibition of the Krebs cycle. A highly reduced mitochondrial redox state causes a decrease in the $NAD^+/NADH$ ratio in the cytosol. NAD is required for an important action of the pyruvate dehydrogenase complex which catalyzes the oxidative decarboxylation of pyruvate to acetyl CoA (White et al., 1978). Conversely, NADH is required by lactic dehydrogenase for the reduction of pyruvate to lactate. Thus, a decrease of $NAD^+/NADH$ in the cytosol results in a decrease in the rate of pyruvate conversion to acetyl CoA and an increase in the rate of lactate production, which leads to an increase in pyruvate and lactate.

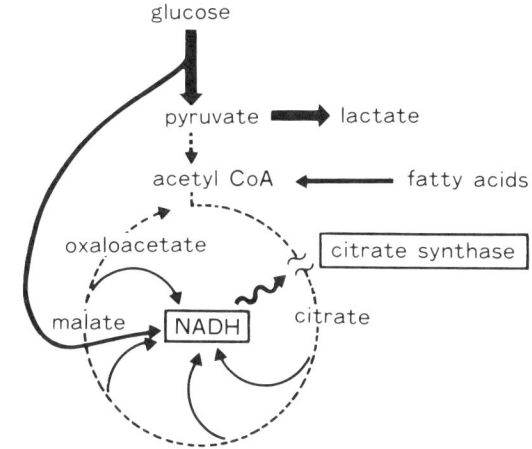

Figure 5.7. Blocking of the Krebs cycle by accumulated NADH in shock.

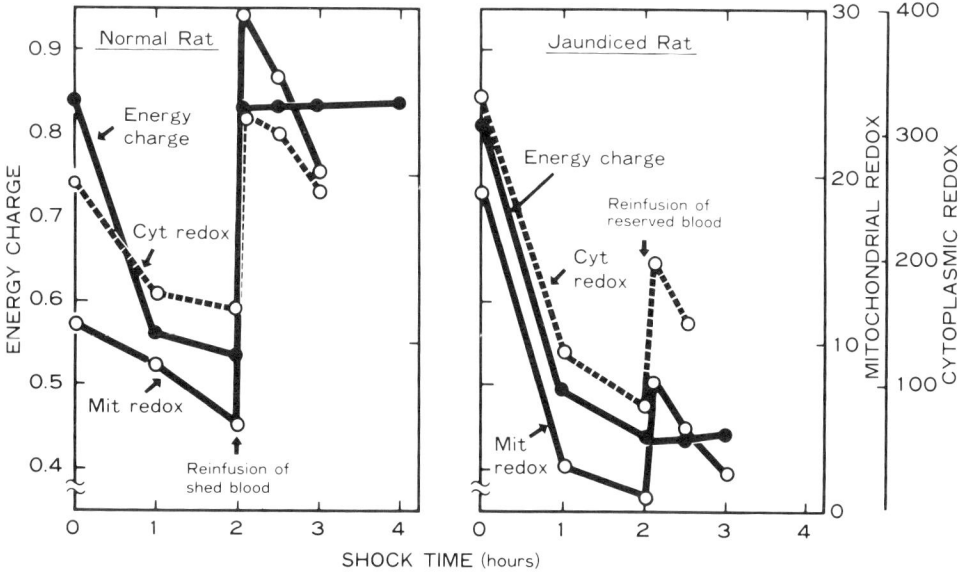

Figure 5.6. Changes in the energy charge and redox states in the liver after the induction of hemorrhagic shock in normal (*left*) and jaundiced (*right*) rats.

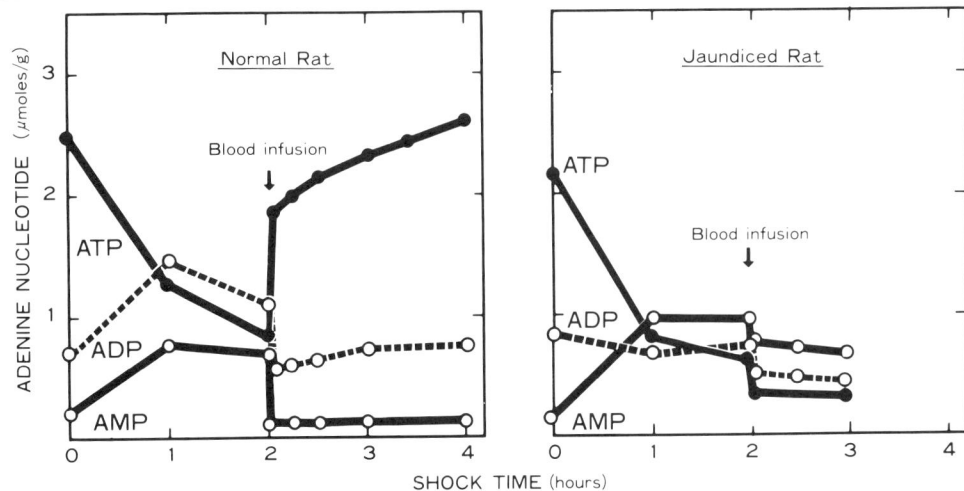

Figure 5.8. Changes of ATP, ADP, and AMP levels in the livers of normal (*left*) and jaundiced (*right*) rats in hemorrhagic shock.

On the other hand, the decline in the energy charge levels is dependent on the decrease in ATP contents accompanying the increases in ADP and AMP. As shown in Figure 5.8, the ADP increased significantly after the induction of shock but decreased immediately after the reinfusion of the shed blood. The increased ADP pool in shock indicates the decrease of the ADP-phosphorylating reactions catalized by the mitochondria with a lowering of the available oxygen. On the other hand, the increase in the energy charge levels after the reinfusion of the shed blood was accompanied by the rapid increase of ATP and the rapid decrease of ADP and AMP, indicating the phosphorylation of ADP by the mitochondria.

By contrast, in jaundiced rats the ADP did not increase after shock and remained unchanged after the reinfusion of the reserved blood. These results suggest that in jaundiced rats, the mitochondrial phosphorylative activity is already damaged irreversibly during shock. Actually, as shown in Figure 5.9, the phosphorylative activity of the isolated liver mitochondria in normal rats remained unchanged after shock. Tissue hypoxia alone is not an etiologic factor in mitochondrial dysfunction. While, in jaundiced rats, though the mitochondrial phosphorylative activity was not significantly different from that in normal rats before the induction of shock, it decreased markedly within 1 hr after the induction of shock. Then, within the next hour the uncoupling of oxidative phosphorylation was seen in more than 80% of the surviving rats. After reinfusion of the reserved blood the mitochondrial phosphorylative activity was restored only slightly. There is controversy as to whether irreversible mitochondrial injury is actually the inception of irreversible cellular damage or a later manifestation of cell death (Baue and Sayeed, 1970; Depalma et al., 1970; Mela et al., 1971; Rhodes et al., 1977). However, even if the energy charge slows down, in so far as the mitochondria are not impaired, restoration from shock is very easy. By contrast, when the mitochondria are damaged, shock is irreversible.

When the mitochondrial function is inhibited, glycolysis is increased. Let us discuss this mechanism. In shock, a marked decrease in the energy charge is accompanied by a massive increase of AMP and inorganic phosphate. As a rule the ratio of AMP to ATP in normal cells is from 1:10 to 1:100. A slight reduction in ATP brings about a massive increase in AMP concentrations. The accumulated AMP stimulates phosphofructokinase, which is an allosteric enzyme, stimulates phosphorylase, and blocks phosphoenolpyruvate carboxykinase, which is a key enzyme in gluconeogenesis, and fructosediphosphatase (Fig. 5.10). AMP is also the foremost factor in increasing the permeability of the membrane for glucose. On the other hand, the decrease in the energy charge

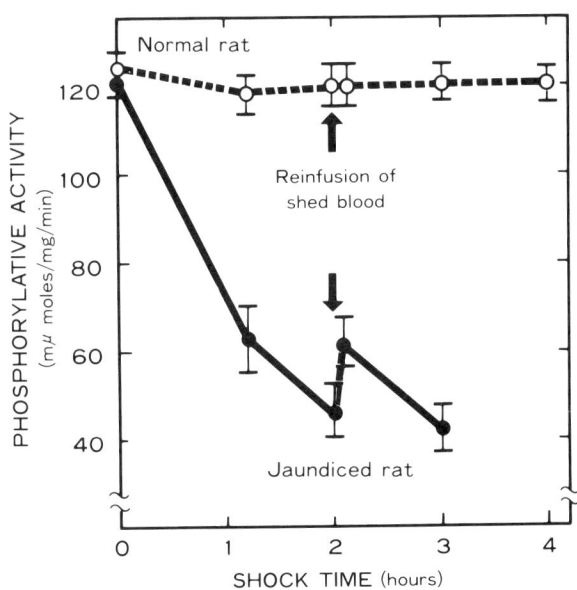

Figure 5.9. Changes in mitochondrial phosphorylative activity in normal and jaundiced rats after hemorrhagic shock.

brings about an excess of inorganic phosphate. Increased inorganic phosphate stimulates phosphofructokinase and phosphorylase. These accelerated enzymes increase glycolysis, consequently augmenting pyruvate and lactate contents.

Figure 5.11 shows the changes in pyruvate and lactate in the liver of normal and jaundiced rats after hemorrhagic shock. The marked increase in lactate and pyruvate in both kinds of rats indicates an enhancement of glycolysis in shock. In normal rats, pyruvate increased in parallel with lactate for a prolonged period after shock, while in jaundiced rats pyruvate decreased markedly after 1 hr. The changes in pyruvate in the liver are consistent with those in the blood glucose levels. In normal rats, the blood glucose level is normal or higher for a prolonged period after shock (Fig. 5.12). In jaundiced rats, hypoglycemia develops after 1 hr of shock, with decreasing contents of hepatic pyruvate. A positive correlation exists between blood glucose levels and survival time. In irreversible shock, the substrates utilized by enhanced glycolysis appear to deplete rapidly. The blood glucose level is an important indicator of survival in shocked animals.

The blood glucose and stored glycogen are preferentially first used for enhanced glycolysis. The rate of intracellular utilization of blood glucose in shock is very high owing to the hyperactivity of hexokinase, which is closely correlated with enhanced phosphofructokinase activity. When stored glycogen depletes, gluconeogenesis is promoted from lactate, amino acids, and glycerol. Since it does require ATP, gluconeogenesis occurs when the hepatic energy charge is not so low. But, as shock progresses, gluconeogenesis declines with the lowering of ATP supplies and the accumulation of AMP and inorganic phosphate. At this stage, all the cytoplasmic and intramitochondrial metabolites are directed toward the formation of pyruvate and then lactate. Extramitochondrial oxaloacetate, for instance, is acted upon by phosphoenolpyruvate carboxykinase to yield phosphoenolpyruvate and increase the amount of pyruvate, which then turns into lactate.

However, in the late stages of shock hypoglycemia develops, following both depletion of glycogen in the liver and muscle, and the arrest of gluconeogenesis.

Aside from hypoglycemia, in the terminal stage of shock, the enhanced glycolysis in cells brings about the accumulation of huge and irreducible amounts of lactate and NADH with the continuing reduction of NAD^+ by glyceraldehyde 3-phosphate deriving from glucose, though the reconversion of NADH to NAD^+ is enhanced by lactic dehydrogenase. Normally the restoration of NAD^+ is assured by the glycerol and malate-asparate shuttles, effecting the net transfer of reducing, equivalent from NADH in the cytoplasm to NAD^+ in the mito-

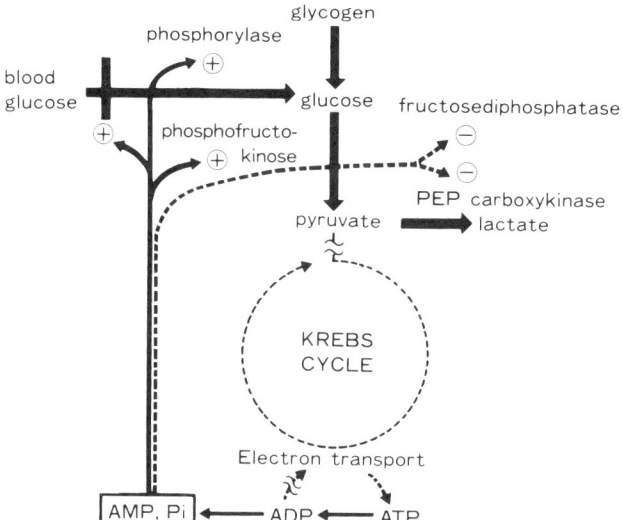

Figure 5.10. Acceleration of glycolysis by accumulated AMP and P_i in shock.

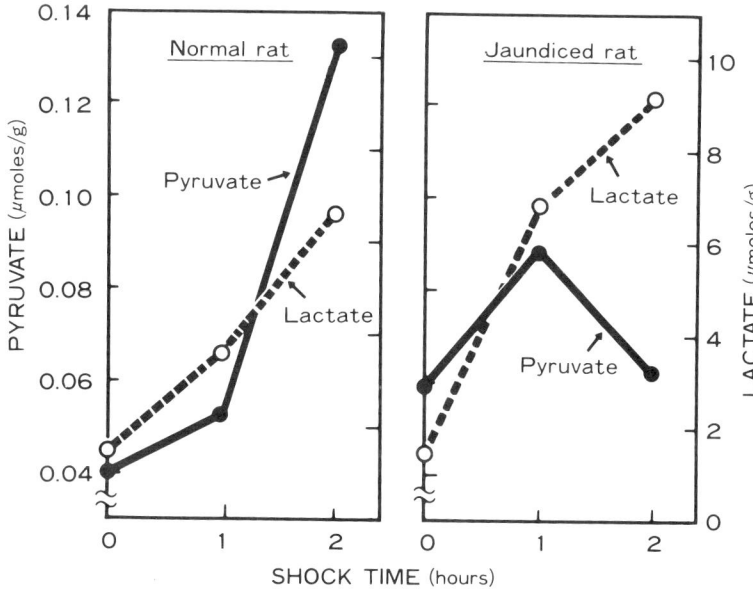

Figure 5.11. Changes in the contents of pyruvate and lactate in the liver of normal (*left*) and jaundiced (*right*) rats after the induction of hemorrhagic shock.

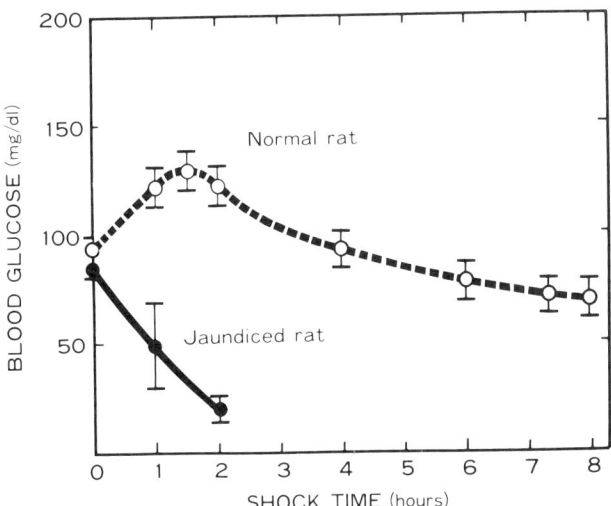

Figure 5.12. Changes of blood glucose of normal and jaundiced rats after the induction of hemorrhagic shock.

chondria, which depends on molecular oxygen. These shuttles are not operative in shock. Thus, recuperation of NAD^+ becomes impossible. Finally, the accumulated NADH inhibits glycolysis through the inhibition of phosphofructokinase. Citrate, also, accumulates extramitochondrially, resulting in an inhibition of phosphofructokinase. The inhibition of phosphofructokinase inhibits hexokinase, resulting in the prevention of the entrance of blood glucose into cells. These events stop the production of lactate and the last energy generation of cells.

INTERPLAY OF ENERGY METABOLISM BETWEEN ORGANS IN SHOCK

In shock, energy disturbances precede alterations of the biological homeostasis and clinical symptoms. The changes in blood metabolites such as lactate, inorganic phosphate, and plasma α-amino acid precede those of pH, PaO_2, and $PaCO_2$, which come before the clinical hemodynamic signs expressed by the pulse rate, blood pressure, and central venous pressure (Kinney, 1967; Schumer, 1966). Temperature also reflects reliably the functional energy-yielding capacity of the body, being closely correlated with intensity and severity of shock. A fall in temperature is indicative of a reduced energy metabolism.

Each specialized organ is functionally connected with all the others by a metabolic regulating system. The efficient exchange of energy and substrates between the organs is important for the most favorable steady state to maintain life. In the first stage of hemorrhagic shock, the decrease in the energy charge, indicating exhaustion of the energy store, is one of the essential critical events in shock. Alterations in the energy charge do not, however, occur to the same degree in the different organs. The organs most affected are the liver and kidney; the lung and muscle are much less affected (Fig. 5.13). In gastric mucosa, the energy charge falls rapidly to a level low enough to cause cellular necrosis in hemorrhagic shock (Menguy and Masters, 1974a and b). The heart and brain remain relatively unchanged until a critical stage, though both extract more oxygen from blood than do other organs. The ability of the brain and heart to protect their energy reserve depends upon circulatory adjustments by catecholamine to maintain blood flow. In hypovolemic shock the central circulation of the heart and brain is maintained as much as possible by reflex vasoconstriction of muscle, adipose tissue, kidney, liver, and splanchnic bed. Moreover, in hypoxic myocardium there are several bypaths by means of which ATP can still be produced under shock conditions, for instance, a preponderance of free fatty acid (FFA) oxidation rather than glucose oxidation as energy substrates and a high activity of the hexokinase system resulting in a prevalent use of exogenous glucose. When the heart receives fatty acids as substrates it is able to respond to increased work activity with smaller changes in the phosphate potential than with glucose as substrate (Neely et al., 1976). In addition, the decrease in the energy charge is accompanied by a fall in adenine nucleotide levels. This breakdown of nucleotides releases free adenosine, which has a direct coronary-dilating effect and augments coronary flow. Cerebral blood flow also tends to remain constant over a wide range of blood pressure. During hemorrhage, cerebrovascular resistance falls commensurately with the decline in blood pressure. Unless arterial pressure falls below the lower limits of cerebrovascular autoregulation in severe hemorrhage, cerebral blood flow is maintained (Kovach and Sandor, 1976). A critical change of the energy metabolism of the brain occurs when shock affects cardiovascular function by a fall in blood pressure.

The liver is becoming recognized increasingly as a critical organ in the pathogenesis of a variety of types of circulatory shock (Cowley et al., 1969; Nolan, 1975; White et al., 1973). One of the reasons for the increased interest in the liver during shock is the clearance of the

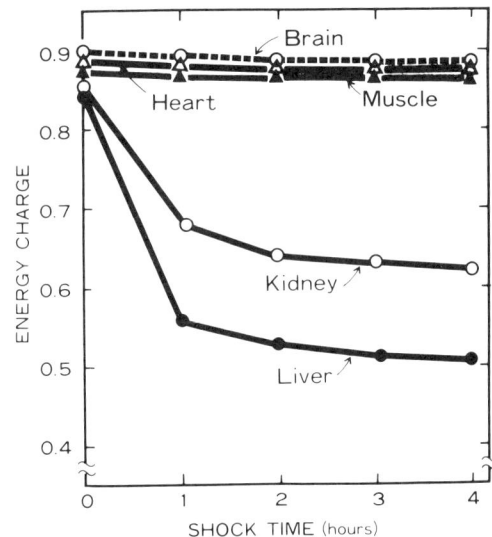

Figure 5.13. Changes in the energy charge in various organs after hemorrhagic shock.

portal venous and hepatic arterial blood by the Kupffer cells. This phagocytosis is dependent upon an intact and normally functioning liver, because 85% of the reticuloendotherial system (RES) of the whole body resides in the liver, approximately 10% is in the spleen, and the rest is distributed in the lymph nodes, endocrine glands, blood vessel walls, and a number of other locations (Biozzi and Stiffel, 1965). In hemorrhagic shock, splanchnic hypotension increases intestinal mucosal permeability and reduces the phagocytic capacity of the Kupffer cell to remove particulate matter from the blood (Blattberg and Levy, 1962; Hershey and Altura, 1969; Rhodes et al., 1973; Zweifach and Benacerraf, 1958). Phagocytosis is sustained by the energy produced by glycolysis and the pentose pathway. In the first stage of shock, glycolysis is stimulated, resulting in the stimulation of the RES. Lactate, as well as concomitantly accumulated NADH, blocks glycolysis. Phagocytic activity of the RES rapidly collapses with a worsening of the state of shock (Altura and Hershey, 1970; Rutenburg et al., 1960). The collapse of the RES functions also affects the coagulolytic system, for which the RES is the clearance organ. Hepatic clearance failure is a major predisposing factor to the development of pulmonary insufficiency, renal failure, septicemia, and DIC. In the terminal stage, cardiovascular failure reaches a circulatory point of no return after which death results, regardless of volume restoration. In this period, the energy charge levels of the heart and brain decrease irreversibly.

A characteristic pattern of the cellular metabolism exists in shock. To clarify the apparent abnormalities of fuel substrate utilization in the metabolism of energy production during shock, it is of great importance to evaluate the complex hormonal interaction among catecholamine, corticoids, and glucagon in the regulation of glycogenolysis, gluconeogenesis, and lipolysis in shock. There are metabolic and hemodynamic divergences between hypovolemic and septic shock (Garcia-Barreno and Balibrea, 1978). Hypovolemic shock refers to a hypodynamic circulatory condition with a decreased cardiac output and an increase in the total peripheral vascular resistance. Catecholamine is released, resulting in an increase of glycogenolytic and lipolytic response and a decrease in the release of insulin. In addition to glycogenolysis by catecholamine, the release of glucocorticoids provokes an increase in gluconeogenesis (Wiener and Spitzer, 1974) resulting in a hyperglycemic state. The secretion of glucagon is inhibited because the glucagon secretion by catecholamine and alanine is inhibited by hyperglycemia. Energy production during hypovolemic shock in the whole organism shifts primarily to an enhancement of anaerobic glycolysis by means of stored glycogen and blood glucose, resulting in hyperlactacidemic acidosis. This enhanced glycolysis rapidly depletes the stores of glucose as energy substrate. The gluconeogenesis of the liver is enhanced to maintain the blood glucose at normal levels. A great amount of lactate readily leaves the muscle and red blood cells, major sources of lactate production in shock, and reaches the liver, where it is reconverted into glucose (Cori cycle).

This newly formed glucose is released into the blood and is offered indirectly to the neurons. At this stage blood glucose is not taken up by the muscle, but the muscle is using FFA mobilized from the adipose tissue (Randle cycle) (Randle et al., 1963). In advanced shock, the lactate accumulates remarkably and can not be metabolized adequately by the liver, due to an inhibition of gluconeogenesis by lactate, leading to marked intracellular acidosis and extracellular acidemia. After the exhaustion of the substrates, the cell is forced to struggle on with only the breakdown of its own fatty and amino acids for the production of energy.

The initial response to septic shock represents a hyperdynamic state characterized by an elevated cardiac output and reduced peripheral resistance. The relationships of energy deficits to glucose and insulin have been explored (Clowes, 1974; Cryer et al., 1971; Griffiths et al., 1973; Hinshaw et al., 1974, 1975, 1977; Holper, 1973; Weisul, 1975). Blood glucose is normal or high with hyperinsulinemia at an initial stage. In order to satisfy the energy fuel deficit, proteolysis is enhanced in the muscle because of the low availability of fat and ketone from adipose tissue due to hyperinsulinemia. Only branched chain ketogenic amino acids can be oxidized in the cell. The other amino acids are transported to the liver for gluconeogenesis. This series of responses is a defence mechanism for the vital brain and cardiovascular system to transport glucose into the cells. Also, there is no significant elevation in lactate levels. Recent results from our laboratory show that an elevated level of insulin available to the cell enhances the oxidative and phosphorylative activities of the mitochondria (Ida et al., 1976; Ozawa et al., 1974a and b, 1979). This leads us to the supposition that energy production in the hyperdynamic state depends mainly upon mitochondrial function. However, the resulting circulatory insufficiency after continued high cardiac output in septic shock results in hypoglycemia and hypoinsulinemia. This hypoglycemia is based on a lessened ability of hepatic gluconeogenesis and increased glucose utilization peripherally (Hinshaw, 1976). Hypoinsulinemia is based on the alpha-adrenergic effect of catecholamine with a subsequent suppression of pancreatic insulin secretion and deficient blood perfusion of the pancreas. Hypoinsulinemia is associated with cardiovascular insufficiency, which characterizes the hypodynamic circulatory state. At this stage, amino acids are released by the catabolic effect of the corticosteroids on the proteins. The alanine level in the blood is raised because of a failure in gluconeogenesis, stimulating increasingly the secretion of glucagon. Siegel (1971) reported that the gravity of septic shock is always correlated with the biochemical parameters and seldom with hemodynamic ones.

In hypovolemic shock, the mortality of patients under anaerobic conditions correlates with lactate or excess lactate levels in the blood. The progress of acidosis is a reliable marker of the severity of shock. Lactate values of over 7–8 mEq are always critical (Peretz et al., 1964; Peretz et al., 1965). On the other hand, energy metabolism in the liver changes first after hemorrhagic shock, and the mitochondrial phosphorylative activity of the liver plays an important role in recovering from shock. A clinical indicator for hypovolemic shock should, therefore, represent the energy status of the liver more exactly. The ratio of acetoacetate to β-hydroxybutyrate in the liver is in equilibrium with the free $NAD^+/NADH$ ratio in the mitochondria. Since acetoacetate and β-hydroxybutyrate freely penetrate cell membranes, the ratio of acetoacetate to β-hydroxybutyrate in the blood reflects the mitochondrial free $NAD^+/NADH$ ratio. In hemorrhagic shock in rabbits, the changes in the acetoacetate/β-hydroxybutyrate ratio in the arterial blood reflect the mitochondrial redox state and are correlated with hepatic energy charge levels rather than with the lactate/pyruvate ratio (Fig. 5.14) (Yamamoto et al., 1980). This is due to the fact that glycolysis occurs not only in the liver but also in other organs, while the liver is the only organ that makes a net contribution of ketone bodies to the blood stream. The blood ketone body ratio can signify the severity of the impairment of the hepatic energy status.

Most of the studies of the last 10 years deal with the cellular metabolic response to shock. Because of space limitations, it is impossible to describe many other worthy achievements in this field. However, the major progress is to be expected from the basic studies aimed at a better understanding of cellular energy status in shock. Derangements of energy metabolism occur a long while before they become clinically apparent. Therefore, the clinician must be always aware of the cellular energy status in shock by monitoring the biochemical parameters most reliable for assessing the severity of impaired energy metabolism in shock. The basis for more effective therapeutic regimens than those currently used will be offered by developing such an accurate parameter.

References

Altura, B.M., and Hershey, S.G.: Effects of glyceryl trioleate on the reticuloendothelial system and survival after experimental shock. J. Pharmacol. Exp. Ther. *175:*555, 1970.

Atkinson, D.E.: The energy charge of the adenylate pool as a regulatory parameter interaction with feedback modifiers. Biochemistry *7:*4030, 1966.

Atkinson, D.E.: Enzymes as control elements in metabolic regulation. In *The Enzymes*, edited by P.D. Boyer, ed. 3, vol. 1, p. 461. Academic Press, New York, 1970.

Baue, A.E., and Sayeed, M.M.: Alteration in the functional capacity of mitochondria in hemorrhagic shock. Surgery *68:* 40, 1970.

Biozzi, G., and Stiffel, C.: The physiopathology of the reticuloendothelial cells of the liver and spleen. In *Progress in Liver Diseases*, edited by H. Popper and F. Schaffner, vol. 2, p. 166. William Heinemann Medical Books, London, 1965.

Blackwood, J.M., Fewel, J., Rush, B.F., et al.: Tissue metabolites in endotoxin and hemorrhagic shock. Arch. Surg. *107:* 181, 1973.

Blattberg, B., and Levy, M.N.: Mechanism of depression of reticuloendothelial system in shock. Am. J. Physiol. *203:*111, 1962.

Chapman, A.G., Fall, L., and Atkinson, D.E.: Adenylate energy charge in Escherichia coli during growth and starvation. J. Bacteriol. *108:*1072, 1971.

Clowes, G.H.A., O'Donnell, T.F., Ryan, N.T., et al.: Energy metabolism in sepsis: treatment based on different patterns in shock and high output stage. Ann. Surg. *179:*684, 1974.

Cowley, R.A., Attar, S., La Brosse, E., et al.: Some significant biochemical parameters found in 300 shock patients. J. Trauma *9:*926, 1969.

Cryer, P.E., Herman, C.M., and Sode, J.: Carbohydrate metabolism in the baboon subjected to gram-negative E. Coli septicemia-I. hyperglycemia with depressed plasma insulin concentrations. Ann. Surg. *174:*91, 1971.

Depalma, R.G., Levey, S., and Holden, W.D.: Ultrastructure and oxidative phosphorylation of liver mitochondria in experimental hemorrhagic shock. J. Trauma *10:*122, 1970.

Drucker, W.R., Craig, J., Kingsburg, B., et al.: Citrate metabolism during surgery. Arch. Surg. *85:*557, 1962.

Garcia-Barreno, P., and Balibrea, J.L.: Metabolic response in shock. Surg. Gynecol. Obstet. *146:*182, 1978.

Griffiths, J., Groves, A.C., and Leung, F.Y.: Hypertriglyceridemia and hypoglycemia in gram-negative sepsis in the dog. Surg. Gynecol. Obstet. *136:*897, 1973.

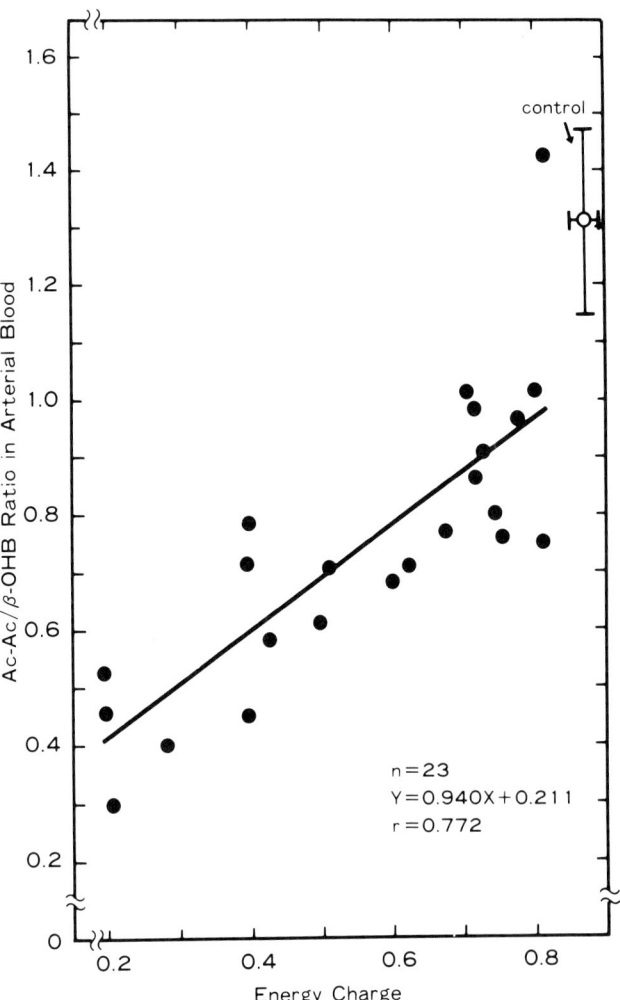

Figure 5.14. Relation between the hepatic energy charge and the acetoacetate/β-hydroxybutyrate ratio in arterial blood during 2 hr of hemorrhagic shock in rabbits.

Hershey, S.G., and Altura, B.M.: Function of the reticuloendothelial system in experimental shock and combined injury. Anesthesiology 30:138, 1969.

Hinshaw, L.B.: Concise review: The role of glucose in endotoxin shock. Circ. Shock 3:1, 1976.

Hinshaw, L.B., Peyton, M.D., Archer, L.T., et al.: Prevention of death in endotoxin shock by glucose administration. Surg. Gynecol. Obstet. 139:851, 1974.

Hinshaw, L.B., Benjamin, B., Coalson, J.J., et al.: Hypoglycemia in lethal septic shock in subhuman primates. Circ. Shock 2:197, 1975.

Hinshaw, L.B., Benjamin, B., Holmes, D.D., et al.: Responses of the baboon to live Escherichia coli organisms and endotoxin. Surg. Gynecol. Obstet. 145:1, 1977.

Holper, K., Trejo, R.A., Brettschneider, L., et al.: Enhancement of endotoxin shock in the lead-sensitized subhuman primate. Surg. Gynecol. Obstet. 136:593, 1973.

Ida, T., Sato, M., Yamaoka, Y., et al.: Effect of insulin on mitochondrial oxidative phosphorylation and energy charge of the perfused guinea pig liver. J. Lab. Clin. Med. 87:925, 1976.

Kamiyama, Y., Takeda, H., Ohshita, H., et al.: Hepatic metabolic changes following energy deprivation by ammonium in jaundiced patients and rabbits. Surg. Gynecol. Obstet. 145:33, 1977.

Kamiyama, Y., Ukikusa, M., Jones, R.T., et al.: Pathophysiology of shock. II. Anoxic metabolism of the liver after acute blood loss. Circ. Shock 6:196, 1979.

Kinney, J.M.: The effect of injury on metabolism. Br. J. Surg. 57:435, 1967.

Kovach, A.G.B., and Sandor, P.: Cerebral blood flow and brain function hypotension and shock. Physiol. Rev. 38:571, 1976.

Mela, L., Bacalzo, L.V., and Miller, L.D.: Defective oxidative metabolism of rat liver mitochondria in hemorrhagic and endotoxin shock. Am. J. Physiol. 220:571, 1971.

Mela, L., Miller, L., Bacalzo, L.V., et al.: Role of intracellular variations of lysosomal enzyme activity and oxygen tension in mitochondrial impairment in endoxemia and hemorrhage in the rat. Ann. Surg. 178:727, 1973.

Menguy, R., and Masters, Y.F.: Gastric mucosal energy metabolism and "stress ulceration." Ann. Surg. 180:538, 1974a.

Menguy, R., and Masters, Y.F.: Mechanism of stress ulcer. III. Effects of hemorrhagic shock on energy metabolism in the mucosa of the antrum, corpus, and fundus of the rabbit stomach. Gastroenterology 66:1168, 1974b.

Neely, J.R., Whitmer, K.M., and Mochizuki, S.: Effects of mechanical activity and hormones on myocardial glucose and fatty acid utilization. Circ. Res. (Suppl. 1) 38:22, 1976.

Newsholme, E.A., and Start, C.: Regulation in Metabolism. John Wiley & Sons, New York, 1973.

Nolan, J.P.: The role of endotoxin in liver injury. Gastroenterology 69:1346, 1975.

Ozawa, K., Yamada, T., and Honjo, I.: Role of insulin as a portal factor in maintaining the viability of liver. Ann. Surg. 180:716, 1974a.

Ozawa, K., Yamaoka, Y., Nanbu, H., et al.: Insulin as the primary factor governing changes in mitochondrial metabolism leading to liver regeneration and atrophy. Am. J. Surg. 127:669, 1974b.

Ozawa, K., Ida, T., Kamano, T., et al.: Different response of hepatic energy charge and adenine nucleotide concentrations to hemorrhagic shock. Res. Exp. Med. 169:145, 1976.

Ozawa, K., Kamiyama, Y., Kimura, K., et al.: Comparison of subcutaneous and intraportal insulin administrations on adenylate energy charge of the liver in diabetic rats. J. Lab. Clin. Med. 89:937, 1977.

Ozawa, K., Tanaka, J., Ukikusa, M., et al.: Early metabolic disturbances in the liver following hepatic or common bile duct ligation in rabbits. Eur. Surg. Res. 11:61, 1979.

Peretz, D.I., McGregor, M., and Dossetor, J.B.: Lactic acidosis: a clinically significant aspect of shock. Can. Med. Assoc. J. 90:673, 1964.

Peretz, D.I., Scott, H.M., Duff, J., et al.: The significance of lacticacidemia in the shock syndrome. Ann. N.Y. Acad. Sci. 119:1133, 1965.

Randle, P.J., Garland, P.B., Newsholme, E.A., et al.: The glucose fatty acid cycle. Its role, insulin sensitivity and metabolic disturbances of diabetes mellitus. Lancet 1:785, 1963.

Rhodes, R.S., Depalma, R.G., and Robinson, A.V.: Intestinal barrier function in hemorrhagic shock. J. Surg. Res. 14:305, 1973.

Rhodes, R.S., Depalma, R.G., and Druet, R.L.: Reversibility of ischemically induced mitochondrial dysfunction with respiration. Surg. Gynecol. Obstet. 145:719, 1977.

Rutenburg, S.H., Schweinburg, F.B., and Fine, J.: In vitro detoxification of bacterial endotoxin by macrophages. J. Exp. Med. 112:801, 1960.

Schumer, W.: Lactic acid as a factor in the production of irreversibility in oligohaemic shock. Nature 212:1210, 1966.

Schumer, W.: Localization of the energy pathway block in shock. Surgery 64:55, 1968.

Siegel, J.H., Goldwyn, R.M., and Friedman, H.P.: Pattern and process in the evolution of human septic shock. Surgery 70:232, 1971.

Swan, H., Blavier, J., Marchioro, T., et al.: Experimental hemorrhage. Prediction of mortality following acute measured hemorrhage in dogs. Arch. Surg. 79:176, 1959.

Ukikusa, M., Ida, T., Ozawa, K., et al.: The influence of hypoxemia and ischemia upon adenylate energy charge and bile flow in rats. Surg. Gynecol. Obstet. 149:346, 1979.

Weisul, J.P., O'Donnell, T.F., Jr., Stone, M.A., et al.: Myocardial performance in clinical septic shock; effects of isoproterenol and glucose potassium insulin. J. Surg. Res. 18:357, 1975.

Werle, J.M., Cosby, R.S., and Wiggers, C.J.: Observations on hemorrhagic hypotension and hemorrhagic shock. Am. J. Physiol. 136:401, 1942.

White, R.R., Mela, L., Bacalzo, L.V., Jr., et al.: Hepatic ultrastructure in endotoxemia, hemorrhage, and hypoxia: Emphasis on mitochondrial changes. Surgery 73:525, 1973.

White, A., Handler, P., Smith, E.L., et al.: *Principles of Biochemistry*, 340 pp. McGraw-Hill Kogakusha, Tokyo, 1978.

Wiener, R., and Spitzer, J.J.: Lactate metabolism following severe hemorrhage in the conscious dog. Am. J. Physiol. 227:58, 1974.

Wiggers, C.J.: *The Physiology of Shock*. Commonwealth Press, New York, 1950.

Yamamoto, M., Sato, M., Ida, T., et al.: Obstructive jaundice and hemorrhagic shock. Circ. Shock 5:235, 1978.

Yamamoto, M., Tanaka, J., Ozawa, K., et al.: Significance of acetoacetate/β-hydroxybutyrate ratio in arterial blood as an indicator of the severity of hemorrhagic shock. J. Surg. Res. 28:124, 1980.

Zweifach, B.W., and Benacerraf, B.: Effect of hemorrhagic shock on the phagocytic function of Kupffer cells. Circ. Res. 6:83, 1958.

CHAPTER 6

Mitochondrial Function in Shock, Ischemia, and Hypoxia

LEENA MELA

In mammalian tissues cellular energy is supplied by energy-rich products of carbohydrate, fatty acid, and ketone body metabolism. A major fraction of cellular energy is supplied by glucose metabolism through its various steps, glycolysis in the cytoplasm and Krebs cycle and electron transfer activities coupled to oxidative phosphorylation in the mitochondria. The steps involving mitochondrial electron transfer and oxidative phosphorylation are by far the most efficient cellular reactions producing energy-rich compounds such as ATP. For each molecule of glucose utilized, 36 mol of ATP are synthesized in the mitochondria, while only 2 mol of ATP/mol glucose can be produced through anaerobic glycolysis in the cytoplasm.

These considerations concerning energy production indicate the importance of intact, continuously operating mitochondrial metabolic reactions for the well-being of mammalian cells. The energy requirements of different cell types vary depending on their level of functional activity. Continuous demands of cellular energy are dictated by cellular and subcellular membrane ion pumps, by protein synthesis, especially in cells with high rate of turnover of cellular proteins, and by mechanical work such as muscle contraction in cardiac, smooth, and skeletal muscle. The energy reserves of cells are low. They last only seconds to minutes at a level necessary to support normal cellular functions. Cell functions can continue only when supported by uninterrupted mitochondrial energy production. Mitochondrial reactions depend on continuous supplies of oxygen and reducing equivalents, the latter derived mostly from glucose metabolism via the glycolytic pathway. Stores of glucose and oxygen in mammalian tissues are low or nonexistent, thus requiring effective tissue perfusion to provide the metabolic pathways with the essential nutrients. Thus, any conditions compromising tissue perfusion either at macro or microcirculatory levels would tend to alter secondarily the capabilities of mitochondria to produce energy due to the lack of substrates for their enzyme reactions.

In this chapter current literature is reviewed on mitochondrial functional consequences of tissue hypoxia, ischemia, and conditions imposed on tissues by alterations of perfusion by systemic circulatory shock, either hemorrhagic or septic in origin. Special emphasis is paid to primary and secondary mitochondrial alterations and the possible causes of these alterations, direct or indirect. Where precise cause-and-effect relationships are not known, sequences of interrelated events are emphasized. The mitochondrial alterations are characterized in terms of specific reactions responsible for the overall functional changes.

ISCHEMIC INJURY

Complete Tissue Ischemia

Complete tissue ischemia implies total shutdown of the flow of necessary nutrients into the cells. As a result, cellular oxygen and glucose stores are completely depleted within a short time. Oxygen supply lasts only a few seconds. In the brain, tissue PO_2 falls to 0 in less than 30 sec (Silver, 1977). After this interval, oxidative metabolism ceases. The electron transfer chain components become reduced and electron flow and oxidative metabolism stop (Harbig et al., 1976). Cellular pyridine nucleotides (NAD) are completely reduced in the distribution of the middle cerebral artery within seconds after ligation of the artery in the cat, as shown by in vivo measurements (Fig. 6.1) (Ginsberg et al., 1976). As a result of the mitochondrial shutdown, tissue ATP level drops. Five minutes of complete ischemia is sufficient to lower brain ATP practically to 0 (Lowry et al., 1964; Ljunggren et al., 1974; Welsh et al., 1977, 1978a and b). In seconds, brain lactate levels increase moderately (Ljunggren et al., 1974; Siesjo and Nordstrom, 1977) and maximal lactate levels are reached within 3 min. In the heart, however, tissue ATP is still half-normal after 30 min of complete ischemia, although creatine phosphate declines by 90% during that time period (Isselhard et al., 1976).

Lack of oxygen induces reduction of the respiratory chain components and cessation of electron flow. As

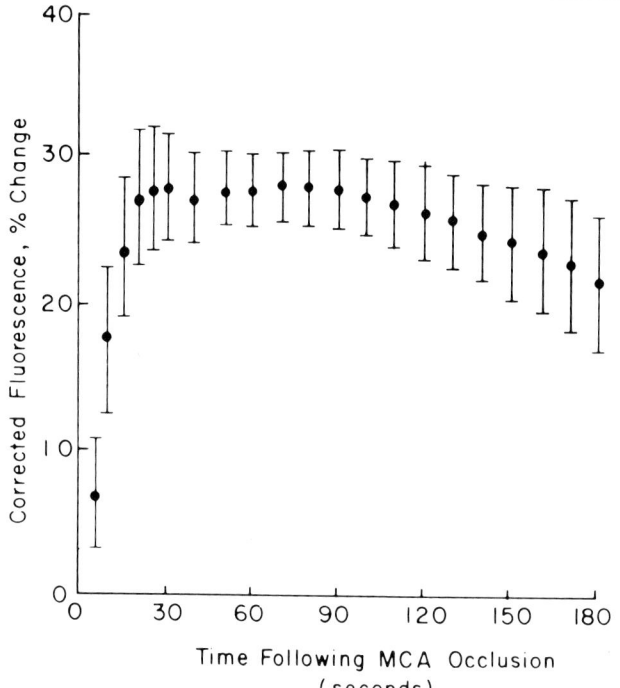

Figure 6.1. Rate of reduction of cerebral cortical NAD after occlusion of middle cerebral artery in cat. (Data from Ginsberg et al., 1976.)

long as mitochondrial membranes have not become permanently damaged, replenishment of the oxygen supply reactivates electron transfer and utilization of oxygen and substrates to resynthesize ATP. Mitochondrial membranes and other cellular membranes are sensitive to long-term ischemia, however, and eventually permanent membrane damage occurs if ischemia continues beyond a critical time period.

Isolated mitochondria have been studied to characterize functional membrane damage after tissue ischemia. Mitochondria isolated after several minutes of complete ischemia are not capable of utilizing substrates and oxygen at maximal rates in the presence of ADP (Mela et al., 1979a). The extent of inhibition of O_2 consumption and ATP synthesis rates depends on the length of prior ischemia and varies from organ to organ. Similarly, mitochondrial calcium transport activity becomes severely reduced. Brain mitochondria appear particularly sensitive. Only a few minutes of ischemia are required to damage their ATP synthetic and calcium transport capacities. Kidney mitochondria show more resistance to ischemic injury. Much longer time is required to achieve a 50% inhibition—30 min as compared to 5–15 min in the brain (Mela et al., 1979a). In the heart, 20–30 min of complete ischemia are required to lower O_2 utilization rates during oxidative phosphorylation to 50% of normal (Lindenmayer et al., 1977).

Incomplete Tissue Ischemia

Since the glucose requirements of tissues for oxidative phosphorylation can be satisfied at a lower level of flow than their oxygen requirements, severe incomplete ischemia induces shutdown of mitochondrial function while allowing a low level of anaerobic glycolytic activity to continue. This activity provides some ATP synthesis at the expense of severely increased levels of cellular lactate and, thus, a larger decrease in cell pH than is observed during complete ischemia (Nordström et al., 1976, 1978).

Inhibition of mitochondrial ATP synthetic and calcium transport functions occurs to the same extent as in complete ischemia (Ginsberg et al., 1977). Kinetically, however, the appearance of these changes in incomplete ischemia depends on the level of remaining tissue perfusion and the organ in question. In severe incomplete ischemia with only 5–10% of blood flow remaining, brain mitochondrial ATP synthesis is inhibited about 40% after 30 min (Rehncrona et al., 1979b). A 60–70% inhibition of mitochondrial ATP synthesis occurs after 90 min of hypovolemia in the cat at mean arterial blood pressure of 55 mm Hg, a condition that induces a significant reduction of mean blood flow to the brain and a 30% increase of reduced mitochondrial pyridine nucleotides (NADH) (Mela et al., 1975a, 1978a). In other organs, a longer period of incomplete ischemia is required to reach the same level of inhibition of mitochondrial ATP synthetic capacity. In the liver a 50% inhibition is reached after 2–3 hr at 30 mm Hg mean arterial blood pressure in the rat (Mela et al., 1971).

The described in vitro studies of mitochondria isolated after certain periods of tissue ischemia, complete or partial, can be used only to indicate remaining mitochondrial capacity to synthesize ATP or perform other energy-linked functions. These studies do not indicate directly what level of activity the mitochondria exhibit in situ during the ischemic period. Reliable methods for direct monitoring of mitochondrial ATP synthetic or ion transport activities in situ are not available. Various types of experiments providing indirect estimates of in situ mitochondrial function, however, have been performed. The increased fluorescence of mitochondrial reduced pyridinenucleotides indicates that cessation of blood flow to the brain induces complete reduction of NAD in seconds (Ginsberg et al., 1976). Increased reduction of NAD in incomplete ischemia occurs in parallel with the decline in blood flow (Welsh et al., 1977b; Welsh and O'Connor, 1978). NADH redox level is sensitive to two independent but often simultaneous cellular alterations, a change in tissue oxygenation, *and* a change in mitochondrial electron transfer or energy transduction activity. Thus the interpretation of the in situ redox changes of NADH in terms of mitochondrial activity is difficult.

Extracellular K^+ ion activities and pH have been recorded simultaneously and separately in the ischemic brain. These recordings provide information on the consequences of rapid mitochondrial shutdown in ischemia, resulting in severely reduced (below K_m for cell membrane sodium-potassium ATPase) or 0 levels of tissue ATP. Adequate amounts of tissue ATP to support the cell membrane sodium-potassium pump activity as shown by the kinetics of increased extracellular K^+

activities in complete cerebral ischemia are preserved for only seconds after induction of ischemia (Fig. 6.2) (Silver, 1977; Crowe et al., 1979; Mayevsky et al., 1980). Within less than 1 min of complete ischemia, extracellular K^+ reaches its maximum concentration of 30 mM. Similar events occur in brain anoxia (Silver, 1977), indicating that anaerobic metabolism cannot provide adequate amounts of ATP to support cell membrane ion-pumping activity at a level necessary for the maintenance of normal cellular ion balance. In complete ischemia of the brain, induced by hypovolemic shock, brain extracellular K^+ concentration increases gradually as soon as the mean arterial blood pressure has been lowered to 40 mm Hg in the rat (Mela et al., 1975a, 1978a). A slowly progressing linear increase continues for hours without a sudden increase in extracellular K^+. Eventually the animal reaches a level of vascular insufficiency at which the mean arterial blood pressure starts to decline further, if no fluid replacement is provided. At this point, as the mean arterial blood pressure approaches 25 mm Hg, a sudden large increase of brain cortical extracellular K^+ occurs (up to 60 mM), indicating equilibration of K^+ across the cell membrane, collapse of the membrane potential and, thus, total cessation of the ion pumping activity. Parallel with the increasing extracellular K^+, intracellular Na^+ and Cl^- activities have been shown to increase in the brain and the liver (Dora and Zeuthen, 1976; Sayeed and Baue, 1973; Sayeed et al., 1974, 1975a and b).

In severe incomplete ischemia, large regional heterogeneity appears in the level of mitochondrial respiratory chain reduction, as measured by three-dimensional scanning of NADH fluorescence in frozen brain. Welsh et al. (1977b, 1978a) identified several regions of the cerebrum exhibiting greater sensitivity to lowered blood flow than the rest of the brain. The ischemic insult was induced by occlusion of both common carotid arteries and the midbasilar artery in combination with mild hypotension in the cat. This procedure leads to variable regional changes in brain blood flow, with a reduction of cerebral cortical flow ranging from 14–60% (Ginsberg et al., 1978). Marked heterogeneity in brain metabolic response occurs. Tissue NADH fluorescence and ATP and lactate levels all exhibit varying regional responses.

Reversibility of Mitochondrial Metabolic Responses to Ischemia

Using their model of oligemia of the brain, Welsh et al. (1977b, 1978a and b) and Ginsberg et al. (1978) showed that recirculation of the brain after 30 min of ischemia results in great regional variability of flow recovery. Areas remaining severely ischemic as well as hyperemic areas are found. Total mean cortical blood flow remains somewhat below normal. Metabolite studies show generally lower than normal levels of ATP in most studies of the brain after recirculation. Particularly low values are found in the medial gyrus and the sulci (Welsh et al., 1978a and b). NADH levels remain above normal in most areas except in the white matter and the sulci. In the sulci total NAD and NADH after recirculation are below normal. These findings suggest severe ischemic damage of mitochondria and cellular membranes in some areas of the brain, resulting in cellular leakage and washout of mitochondrial components such as NAD.

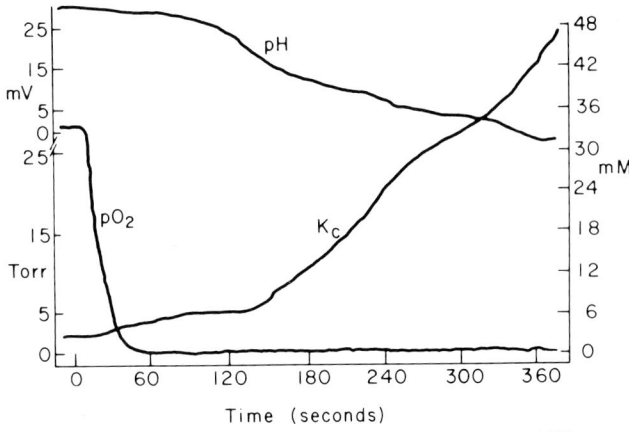

Figure 6.2. Brain cortical PO_2, pH, and extracellular K^+ activity as recorded by microelectrodes after induction of complete ischemia of the rat brain cortex. (Data from Silver, 1977.)

These data on oligemia are consistent with the findings of Nordström et al. (1976, 1978), indicating that during recirculation, cellular energy metabolites and the energy charge do not recover after incomplete ischemia of the brain, although complete recovery occurs after 30 min of complete ischemia. The irreversibility of mitochondrial damage after incomplete ischemia has been verified by direct mitochondrial studies (Fig. 6.3) (Rehncrona et al., 1979b). Complete recovery of mitochondrial capacity to synthesize ATP occurs after 30 min of complete ischemia followed by 30 min of recirculation. After 30 min of severe incomplete ischemia, however, a 30-min period of recirculation induces further mitochondrial inhibition rather than improved function. The precise factors contributing to these differences of mitochondrial responses to complete and incomplete ischemia are not known. The possibility of secondary damage during the recirculation period, however, should be considered. This suggestion might be explained by the findings of Demopoulos and associates (1977), indicating reduced levels of free radical scavengers such as ascorbic acid after brain ischemia. The possibility of damaging effects by excessive amounts of oxygen free radicals forming during the recirculation period exists. This is verified by the findings of Majewska et al. (1978), who showed increased breakdown of mitochondrial membrane phospholipid components occurring in parallel with increased free radical oxidation processes of unsaturated fatty acids. These changes are inhibited by barbiturate anesthesia, which also prevent irreversible metabolic damage of the brain in incomplete ischemia (Nordström et al., 1978; Majewska et al., 1978).

In the ischemic heart, propanolol, which reduces infarct size, specifically decreases mitochondrial swelling and structural damage (Kloner et al., 1978). In endotoxemia, glucocorticoid treatment, which reduces mortality and protects against reduction in organ blood flow, also preserves mitochondrial functional integrity (Emerson and Bryan, 1977; Mela, 1979-see details below). Similarly, glucocorticoids protect the mitochondria against ischemic damage in the kidney (Mela et al., 1979a). These findings indicate the important role of mitochondrial functional damage in the pathophysiology of ischemic cell injury.

Septic Shock

As described above, studies on experimental animals have demonstrated that loss of blood flow to organs induces a rapid depletion of tissue energy metabolites.

In rats, cats, and dogs, simultaneously with falling ATP levels, tissue lactate concentrations and lactate/pyruvate ratios increase and pH falls (Lowry et al., 1964; Silver, 1977; Effros et al., 1975). Similar metabolic alterations have been demonstrated in experimental animals as a result of septic or endotoxic shock. Significantly lowered tissue ATP and increased lactate values are found after several hours of endotoxemia in the brain, liver, and kidney but not in the cardiac or skeletal muscle of the animals studied (Schmahl, 1973; Pappova et al., 1971; Blackwood et al., 1973; Holtzmann and Balderman, 1977; and Staples et al., 1969). These alterations in tissue metabolite levels indicate metabolic failure in the vital organs of animals in septic and endotoxin shock. Investigations of tissue samples obtained at autopsy from shock patients confirm the vulnerability of brain, liver, and kidney mitochondria—the sites of oxidative energy metabolism (Trump et al., 1975).

The demonstrated lack of recovery of brain energy stores in animals after the occurrence of oligemia indicates an irreversible inhibition of mitochondrial energy-synthesizing mechanisms in shock. In studies of mitochondria isolated at the time of death of animals due to endotoxin or septic shock, these findings have been confirmed and the alterations carefully characterized.

In the vital organs, liver, kidney and brain, mitochondria have been shown consistently to become functionally damaged in endotoxemia and hemorrhagic shock (Baue and Sayeed, 1970; Baue et al., 1972; Mela et al., 1970, 1971, 1972, 1973; Moss et al., 1969; Sayeed and Baue, 1971; Schumer et al., 1970, 1971a; White et al., 1973). Brain mitochondria are particularly sensitive to live *Escherichia coli* septicemia in the dog (Fig. 6.4) (Mela, 1979a; Mela et al., 1979b). At the time of the animal's death due to septic shock, 60% of brain mitochondrial ATP synthetic capacity are inhibited, whereas the inhibitory effects on kidney mitochondria isolated

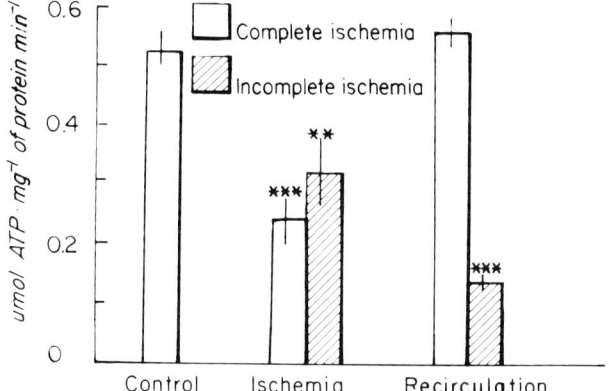

Figure 6.3. Brain mitochondrial ATP synthetic capacity as measured in mitochondria isolated after 30 min of complete or incomplete cerebral ischemia and after 30 min of recirculation. (Data from Rehncrona et al., 1979b.)

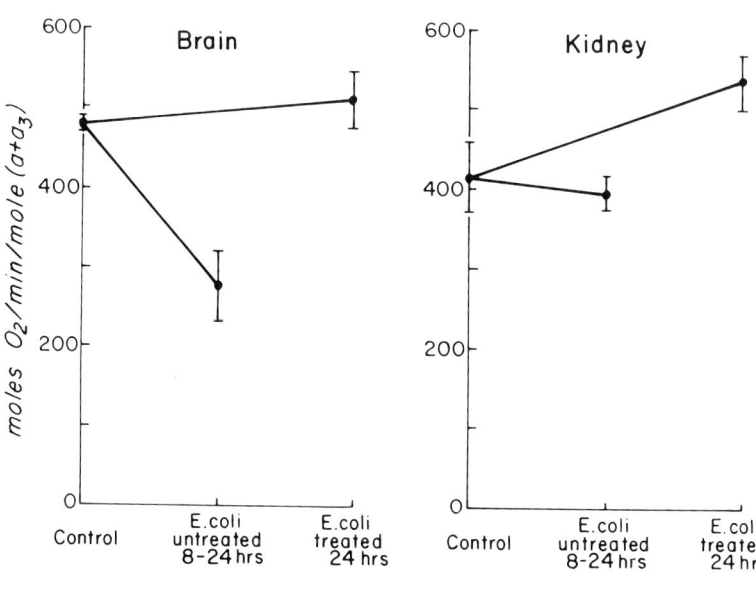

Figure 6.4 Dog brain and kidney mitochondrial maximal respiratory capacity after live *E. coli* septicemia in untreated and in methylprednisolone and gentamicin-treated animals. (Data from Mela, 1979a.)

from the same animals are much milder (values 30% below normal). The inhibition of kidney mitochondrial function seems to lag several hours behind the inhibition of brain mitochondrial function in septicemia.

Studies of mitochondria isolated from skeletal and cardiac muscle of animals have yielded conflicting results. At the time of cardiac failure, some investigations have shown dog heart mitochondrial function to be normal, although opposite findings in other investigations have been reported (Mela, 1975; Mela et al., 1975c; Reed et al., 1970; Schumer et al., 1971b; Schumer and Erve, 1971). Similarly, deleterious alterations in the mitochondrial capacity to synthesize ATP were not found in skeletal muscle of dogs at the time when liver and kidney mitochondrial function was severely damaged (Mela, 1975).

The appearance of mitochondrial inhibition in different organs of animals in septic or endotoxic shock seems to follow a definite time course. The earliest changes occur in the brain and are followed soon by changes in the liver and kidney, and only very late, if at all, by changes in the cardiac and skeletal muscles. These data indicate the importance of diminished organ flow in the precipitation of cellular shock and injury at the mitochondrial level. Brain, liver, and kidney blood flows in dogs and subhuman primates are diminished significantly in shock (Cavanagh and Rao, 1969; Emerson and Bryan, 1977; Imamura and Clowes, 1975; Lillehei et al., 1964; Linder et al., 1974; Parker and Emerson, 1977; Reichgott et al., 1973; Selmyer et al., 1973); however, only slight alterations, if any, in the coronary flow in these animals occur (Hinshaw et al., 1971, 1974; Reichgott et al., 1973).

The lack of mitochondrial inhibition in skeletal muscle of experimental animals in shock is surprising since it is unlike the responses of other tissues to ischemia. Measurements of tissue PO_2 indicate that blood flow to the skeletal muscle is reduced to a very low level (Mela et al., 1973). In spite of tissue PO_2 of practically 0, skeletal muscle mitochondria remain functionally intact in shock. This is compatible with the high capacity of anaerobic glycolysis in that tissue to provide adequate amounts of ATP.

Specific Mitochondrial Alterations Induced by Ischemia and Septic Shock

Several specific sites of the complex mitochondrial enzyme system are affected by tissue ischemia and septic shock. In the mitochondria isolated from the liver and kidney of animals in endotoxin shock, the respiratory enzymes, namely cytochromes, remain intact (Fig. 6.5; Table 6.1) (Mela et al., 1973; Mela, 1975). The electron-transfer reaction from pyruvate, malate, α-ketoglutarate, or succinate to oxygen functions normally. However, the components of oxidative phosphorylation and other energy-linked functions, such as Ca^{2+} transport, are inhibited severely. At late stages of endotoxemia, a 60–70% inhibition of mitochondrial adenosine triphosphatase (ATPase) occurs. In addition to the inhibition of ATPase, adenine nucleotide translocase is incapable of transport-

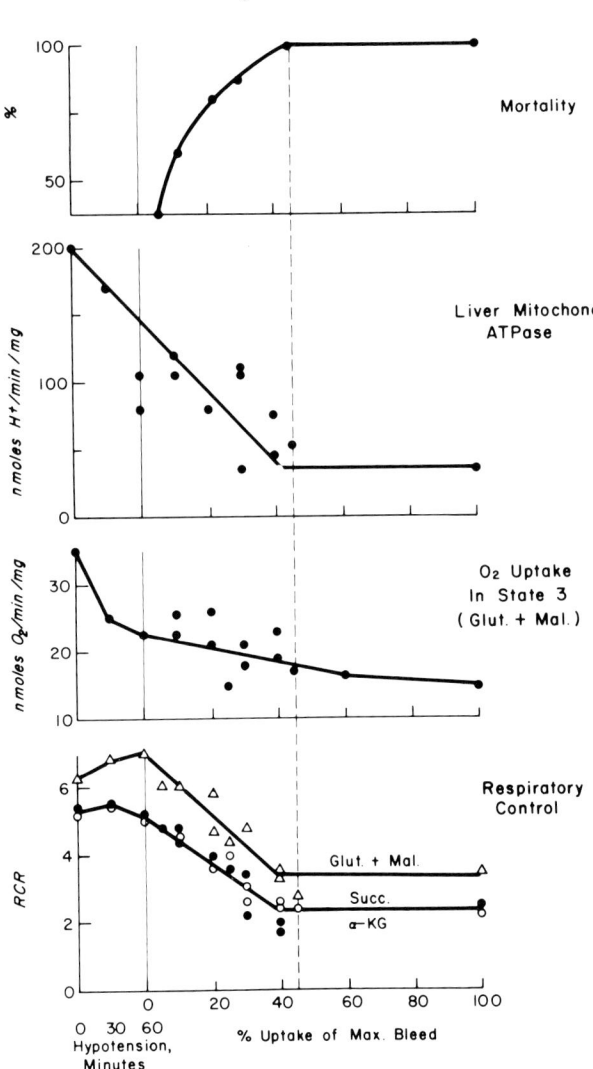

Figure 6.5. Liver mitochondrial decreasing ATPase and respiratory activity and respiratory control as related to increasing mortality of the animals due to hemorrhagic shock. (Data from Mela et al., 1974b.)

ing adenosine diphosphate (ADP) or ATP across the mitochondrial membrane, thus inducing inhibition of ATP synthesis (Mela et al., 1972, 1973; Mela, 1975). Inhibition of adenine nucleotide translocase also occurs in heart mitochondria after myocardial ischemia (Bittar et al., 1976), and inhibition of ATPase is found in kidney mitochondria after ischemia (Mergner et al., 1979).

Accumulation of Ca^{2+} is the energy-linked function of mitochondrial membranes most sensitively affected by endotoxemia and ischemia (Mela et al., 1974b, 1979a; Nicholas et al., 1974; Mergner et al., 1977). The consequences of this inhibition could be very damaging to the cell by way of increased levels of intracellular free Ca^{2+} (Mela, 1977). The severe inhibition of mitochondrial adenine nucleotide translocase and calcium transport indicates that the two specific membrane-bound carrier

Table 6.1
Effects of Terminal Endotoxemia on Rat Liver Mitochondria [a]

Mitochondrial Reaction	Measured Parameter	Unit	Control	Endotoxic	Change
					%
Electron transfer	State 4, succinate	nmoles O_2/min/mg	7.5	10.0	+33
	State 4, glutamate + malate	nmoles O_2/min/mg	5.0	10.0	+50
	Cytochrome b redox, succinate	% of total	53	40	−24
Oxidative phosphorylation	RCR glutamate + malate		7.0	1.5	−79
	State 3, glutamate + malate	nmoles O_2/min/mg	35	15	−57
	ATPase, rate	nmoles H^+/min/mg	175	60	−61
	ATP hydrolyzed	nmoles/mg in 2 min	125	60	−52
	ADP utilization, rate	nmoles/min/mg	160	0	−100
	Cytochrome b oxidation, ADP	% of succinate reduced	40	0	−100
Energy-linked transport	Ca^{2+} uptake (−Pi)	nmoles/min/mg	400	150 → 0	−63 → 100
	K^+ uptake, spontaneous (−Pi)	nmoles/mg	85	165	+94
	Mg^{2+} concentration	nmoles/mg	30	18	−40

[a] Data from Mela, 1975.

systems responsible for these transport functions are particularly vulnerable in low perfusion states.

The currently available experimental evidence does not indicate whether the described mitochondrial alterations are primary or secondary cellular targets of ischemic or shock injury. When necessary supplies of oxygen and substrates are unavailable to the cell, a shutdown of mitochondrial function occurs. Diminished cell ATP levels result, and a multitude of other cellular alterations are initiated because of insufficient energy stores. The concentration of intracellular K^+ decreases, and the intracellular concentrations of Na^+ and Cl^- increase. Intracellular free Ca^{2+} increases, and Mg^{2+} decreases. Because of the presence of metabolic acidosis, cell pH drops. Alterations in lysosomal enzyme activities occur simultaneously with the mitochondrial alterations (Mela et al., 1973). Similarly, free radical oxidation of mitochondrial phospholipids occurs during brain ischemia (Majewska et al., 1978). It is not clear whether these extramitochondrial alterations, which are induced by lowered mitochondrial activity and cellular ATP, can secondarily damage mitochondrial membranes, thereby inducing irreversible inhibition of their function. In vitro studies have indicated this possibility (Mela et al., 1972, 1973). No conclusive studies exist to prove directly a cause-and-effect relationship between extramitochondrial alterations and damage to mitochondrial membranes. It is clear, however, that cells whose energy-producing machinery has been irreversibly damaged cannot recover.

Protection Against Mitochondrial Damage in Septic Shock

Recent studies on endotoxic and septicemic animals and in humans in septic shock have shown clearly that glucocorticoids improve survival significantly (Balis et al., 1978; Emerson and Raymond, 1979; Ch. 16 and Hinshaw et al., 1979; Mela, 1979a; Mela et al., 1979b; Schumer, 1976). Rao and colleagues (1974) studied the effects of glucocorticoids in the subhuman primate during endotoxic shock. Renal blood flow in treated endotoxic animals was significantly higher than in untreated animals. Emerson and collaborators (1977, 1979) reported protection against the drop in cerebral blood flow in different regions of the brain in dogs by the early administration of glucocorticoids in conjunction with endotoxin. The cerebral blood flow was improved in spite of lowered mean arterial blood pressure in the treated animals. Hinshaw and his collaborators (Ch. 16 and Hinshaw et al., 1979), however, showed significant protection against shock-induced drop of mean arterial blood pressure by early antibiotic and glucocorticoid combination treatment in dogs and monkeys made septic by live E. coli organisms. Balis and coworkers (1978) indicated that improved liver microcirculation may be an important protective component of glucocorticoid therapy. Schumer and Nyhus (1970) have shown that corticosteroid therapy in human oligemic and septic shock diminishes metabolic acidosis. Thus, the development of tissue ischemia of vital organs so characteristic of endotoxic shock can be prevented by proper treatment.

Studies have been performed in my laboratory (Mela, 1979a; Mela et al., 1974a, 1979a and b) to ascertain whether the use of glucocorticoids may protect against mitochondrial functional deterioration in experimental animals under two conditions—E. coli entoxemia and live E. coli septic shock. A LD_{60} dose of E. coli endotoxin in the rat induces severe inhibition of liver and kidney mitochondrial ATP synthesis and Ca^{2+} transport in 18–24 hr. Parallel with the mitochondrial changes, liver and kidney lysosomal enzyme activity increases by 50%. An intraperitoneal injection of 100 mg of methylprednisolone sodium succinate per kilogram body weight, together with endotoxin, completely protects against the mitochondrial and lysosomal alterations and diminishes mortality from 60% to 0. Combined treatment with gentamicin and methylprednisolone sodium succinate gives protection against the inhibition of brain and kidney mitochondrial ATP synthetic and Ca^{2+} transport functions in live *E. coli* septicemia in the dog (Fig. 6.6). After an LD_{100} dose of live *E. coli* organisms given intravenously, early treatment is fully protective. Brain mitochondria of untreated animals exhibit 50–60% inhibition of their rates of ATP synthesis, and 40–50% inhibition of their Ca^{2+} transport activity at 12–24 hr. In treated animals sacrificed at 24 hr, brain mitochondria possess normal or supranormal activities of energy-linked functions. Kidney mitochondria are only slightly affected in the untreated septic animals at the time of death, but they also exhibit normal and supranormal activities in treated animals. The hemodynamic and metabolic effects achieved by treatment are higher arterial glucose (particularly early hyperglycemia), higher mean arterial blood pressure (≥ 100 mm Hg), higher arterial pH (~ 7.4), lower hematocrit, and higher leukocyte counts.

It is not clear whether the sole improvement of the hemodynamic and microcirculatory status of the animals can protect against damage to mitochondrial functions. The stabilizing effect of glucocorticoids on the cellular membranes has been suggested as a possible additional mechanism for cellular protection. No evidence exists to indicate whether these stabilizing effects could be directed specifically to mitochondrial membranes or whether the protection is indirect via protection against damage of other cellular membrane components. Direct evidence to support a specific mechanism of protection would help uncover the mechanism of shock-induced cellular damage and cell death.

ADAPTATION TO SUBLETHAL TISSUE HYPOXIA

The K_m for oxygen measured in isolated mitochondria is extremely low, less than 0.1 μM (Chance, 1965). Applied directly to the in vivo situation, this means that the cellular oxygen concentration would have to be lowered below 0.1 μM before any appreciable decline in cellular respiration could occur.

Sublethal hypoxia of the brain, induced by lowering the arterial PO_2 from 100 to 24 mm Hg, results in a compensatory increase in cerebral blood flow (Johannsson and Siesjö, 1974, 1975). It has been proposed that this change is initiated by increased parenchymal lactate levels (Kogure et al., 1970). The increased lactate results from the increased glycolytic rate during the first 2 min of hypoxia, which occurs without any change in cerebral oxygen utilization (Borgström et al., 1976; Norberg et al., 1975; Johannsson and Siesjö, 1974, 1975). Thus, compensatory protective increases in cerebral blood flow and the rate of glycolysis are activated rapidly in acute hypoxia. After 15 min of hypoxia, the glycolytic rate returns to normal level (Borgström et al., 1976). During acute hypoxia only minor changes occur in brain phosphocreatine, ATP, ADP, and AMP (Norberg et al., 1975), although lactate/pyruvate ratios increase significantly. These data and the normal cerebral oxygen utilization during acute hypoxia indicate that this condition, at the tissue level, is very different from ischemia. No inhibition of oxidative metabolism seems to develop. However, hypoxic conditions inducing tissue oxygena-

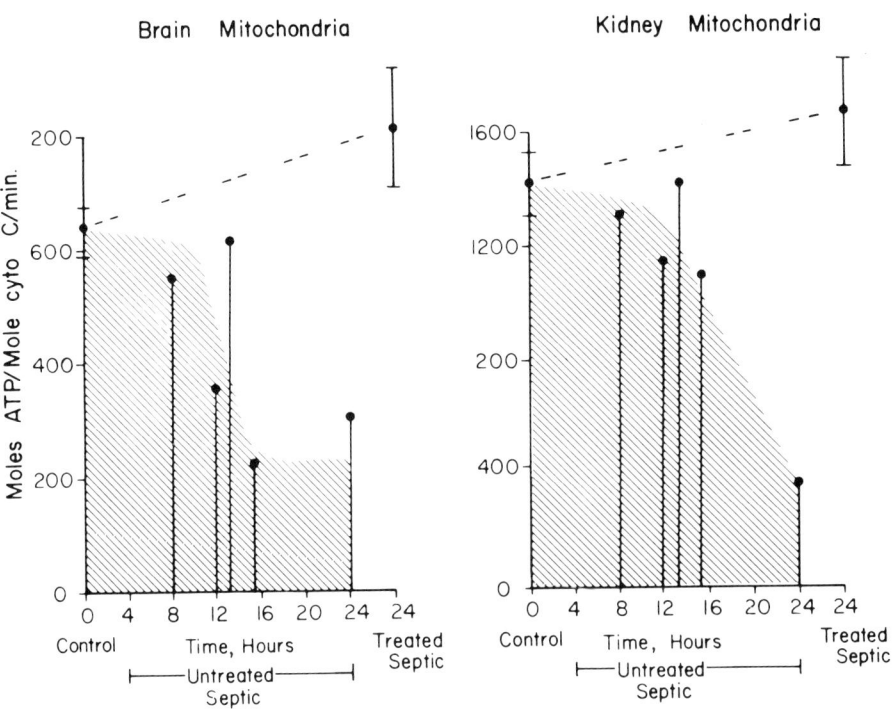

Figure 6.6. Glucocorticoid-antibiotic protection against brain and kidney mitochondrial deterioration in live *E. coli* septicemia in dog. (Data from Mela, 1979a.)

tion below the critical level required for effective ATP synthesis by mitochondria lead to cell injury similar to that found in ischemia (Nakazawa and Nunokawa, 1977).

Adaptation of Mitochondrial Function to Acute Hypoxia

Direct studies of mitochondria isolated after tissue hypoxia have shown that adaptive changes occur in the mitochondrial enzyme system. The first change, within minutes after initiation of systemic hypoxia at the level of approximately 30 mm Hg arterial PO_2 in the rat, is an increased capacity of mitochondria to respire and synthesize ATP (Mela et al., 1973, 1975b, 1976, 1977). Within 30–60 min, state 3 respiratory activities in liver, kidney, heart, and brain mitochondria reach a new steady state of respiration at twice normal activities. State 4 respiratory activities are very low, resulting in high respiratory control ratios. Thus, the increased state 3 rates cannot be explained on the basis of uncoupling.

Parallel with the increased respiratory capacity in state 3, there is an increase in the maximal rates of uncoupler activated respiration (Mela et al., 1976, 1977). Maximal Ca^{2+} transport activity, supported by substrate oxidation, increases similarly and reaches twice normal activities (Mela et al., 1976, 1977). These findings indicate that under all conditions of increased energy drain in the respiratory chain, the electron transfer capacity is enhanced above normal level after acute in vivo hypoxia.

Chronic Hypoxia

Continued in vivo hypoxia for several days induces additional mitochondrial changes. Changes in mitochondrial respiratory enzyme concentrations during the development of chronic hypoxia have been followed only in the heart. With 3–5 days of chronic hypoxia at 40 mm Hg arterial PO_2, dog heart mitochondrial cytochrome b, c, and $a + a_3$ concentrations all decrease (Mela et al., 1975b, 1976, 1977). Cytochrome oxidase concentration per milligram of total mitochondrial protein falls by almost 50%, cytochrome c by 38%, and cytochrome b by 30%. These values compare well with concentrations of cytochromes in heart mitochondria isolated from chronically acyanotic and cyanotic children. The heart mitochondria from acyanotic children contain about twice as many molecules of cytochrome oxidase per milligram of mitochondrial protein as mitochondria from cyanotic children, whose arterial oxygen tensions are about 40 mm Hg (Park et al., 1973). The maximally stimulated (state 3 or uncoupled) respiratory activities, however, remain above control levels per milligram of mitochondrial protein (Fig. 6.7). Thus, in chronic hypoxia, mitochondrial respiratory capacities are very high, in spite of the low concentrations of cytochromes. Calculations of the enzymatic turnover of cytochrome oxidase during state 3 respiration indicate that the maximal turnover of the respiratory chain in mitochondria from chronically hypoxic tissues is as much as three to five times higher than normal mitochondrial respiratory chain turnover.

An example of mitochondrial adaptation to severe chronic oxygen deficiency can be found in the neonate at birth. Prior to the change of fetal arterial PO_2 (10–25 mm Hg) at birth to adult values, the respiratory capacities of brain and heart mitochondria in the newborn dog, sheep, and guinea pig are about 300% of adult levels (Mela et al., 1976, 1977, 1978b; and Mela, 1979b). Immediately after birth mitochondrial respiratory capacity "adapts" and reaches normal adult levels within 10–14 days. This occurs in parallel with the increasing oxygenation of the arterial blood (PaO_2 increases during the first few days to adult level) and the tissues (see Fig. 6.7).

The adult respiratory chain has adapted to operate during normoxia at a level much below its maximal

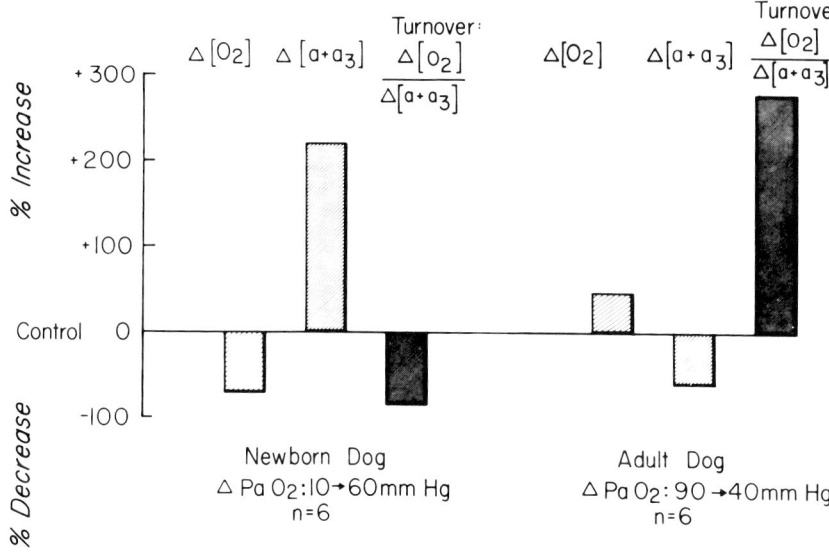

Figure 6.7 Changes in dog heart mitochondrial oxygen utilization rates and cytochrome oxidase concentration during chronic changes in tissue oxygenation in the newborn and adult. (Data from Mela et al., 1976, 1977.)

capacity. Maximal capacity can be achieved quickly via acute adaptation under conditions of stress such as tissue hypoxia. The adult respiratory chain thus possesses a considerable amount of reserve. This reserve is lacking in the newborn, whose respiratory chain operates at a high activity with limited cytochrome concentrations (Mela, 1979b). An adaptation of the newborn respiratory enzyme system to an increased level of tissue oxygenation occurs during the first 2 weeks of life (Mela et al., 1976, 1977; Mela, 1979b). This adaptation presumably is required in the development of the newborn tissues to achieve the flexibility of energy metabolism seen in the adult. The respiratory capacities of mitochondria in the newborn, at very low systemic arterial PO_2 of 10–25 mm Hg, and in the normoxic adult, at 90 mm Hg PO_2, set the extreme limits within which varying levels of in vivo oxygen availability can regulate the activity of mitochondrial electron transfer in an adaptive manner.

Mechanism of Mitochondrial Adaptive Response

The level of tissue oxygenation appears to control both the respiratory chain enzyme concentrations and activities. The fact that higher than normal respiratory chain activities can be achieved in hypoxia at lower than normal cytochrome concentrations eliminates the cytochrome concentrations and their activities as possible rate-limiting and regulating sites of this adaptation. Since uncoupled respiration and Ca^{2+} transport as well as state 3 respiration are increased in hypoxia, specific carrier systems involved in these reactions, such as the adenine nucleotide translocase, the phosphate carrier, and the Ca^{2+} carrier, also can be excluded as possible regulators. Indirect evidence suggests that the various mitochondrial dehydrogenases are responsible for oxygen-induced control of respiratory activity. Succinic dehydrogenase activities several-fold above normal have been demonstrated in mitochondria isolated after both acute and chronic hypoxia (Goodwin et al., 1978; Mela et al., 1976; Purshottam and Ghosh, 1975; Skertzer and Cascarano, 1972; Sivaramakrishnan and Ramasarma, 1975). Thus, it appears that via some unknown mechanism the altered state of cellular oxygenation can trigger changes in the level of activation of latent mitochondrial dehydrogenases to the extent needed for the adaptive increases or decreases in respiratory chain electron transfer capacity. It is not known at present whether some intracellular but extramitochondrial, regulatory changes are required to trigger the mitochondrial adaptive responses.

SUMMARY

Mitochondria show different responses to in vivo tissue ischemia, including low flow states induced by circulatory shock, and to tissue hypoxia. Cessation or reduction of organ blood flow induces damage of the mitochondrial membrane-associated enzyme systems responsible for energy-linked reactions, such as ATP synthesis and ion transport. These mitochondrial functions thus become inhibited, resulting in lowering of the efficiency of energy production and of cellular energy stores. Tissue hypoxia at a sublethal level, however, does not induce inhibition of mitochondrial energy-linked reactions. Under hypoxic conditions mitochondria can adapt their electron transfer functions to an increased level of efficiency.

These two opposite changes are mechanistically different. The inhibitory changes induced by ischemia result from the deterioration of mitochondrial adenine nucleotide and calcium carrier functions as well as of the inhibition of mitochondrial ATPase and coupling factors. The adaptive responses inducing increased efficiency of energy-linked reactions, in contrast, seem to be regulated by adaptive fluctuations of the dehydrogenase enzyme activities in an oxygen sensitive manner.

References

Balis, J.U., Paterson, J.F., Shelley, S.A., Fareed, J., and Gerber, L.I.: Glucocorticoid and antibiotic effects on hepatic microcirculation and associated host responses in lethal gram-negative bacteremia. Circ. Shock 5:225–226, 1978.

Baue, A.E., and Sayeed, M.M.: Alterations in the functional capacity of mitochondria in hemorrhagic shock. Surgery 68: 40–47, 1970.

Baue, A.E., Wurth, M.A., and Sayeed, M.M.: The dynamics of altered ATP-dependent and ATP-yielding cell processes in shock. Surgery 72:94–101, 1972.

Bittar, N., Shug, A.L., Koke, J.R., et al.: Inhibited adenine nucleotide translocation in mitochondria isolated from ischemic myocardium. Recent Adv. Stud. Cardiac Struct. Metab. 7:137–143, 1976

Blackwood, J.M., Hsieh, J., Fewel, J., and Rush, B.F.: Tissue metabolites in endotoxin and hemorrhagic shock. Arch. Surg. 107:181–185, 1973.

Borgström, L., Norberg, K., and Siesjö, B.K.: Glucose consumption in rat cerebral cortex in normoxia, hypoxia and hypercapnia. Acta Physiol. Scand. 96:569–574, 1976.

Cavanagh, D., and Rao, P.S.: Endotoxin shock in the subhuman primate. Arch. Surg. 99:107–112, 1969.

Chance, B.: Reaction of oxygen with the respiratory chain in cells and tissues. J. Gen. Physiol. 49:163–188, 1965.

Crowe, W., Mayevsky, A., and Mela, L.: The dynamics of K^+ leakage and recovery in cerebral ischemia. Adv. Shock Res. 1:221–232, 1979.

Demopoulos, H., Flamm, E., Seligman, M., Power, R., Pietronigro, D., and Ransohoff, J.: Molecular pathology of lipids in CNS membranes. In *Oxygen and Physiological Function*, edited by F.F. Jöbsis, pp. 491–508. Professional Information Library, Dallas, 1977.

Dora, E., and Zeuthen, T.: Brain metabolism and ion movements in the brain cortex of the rat during anoxia. In *Ion and Enzyme Electrodes in Biology and Medicine*, edited by M. Kessler, L.C. Clark, D.W. Lubbers, I.A. Silver, and W. Simon, pp. 294–298. Urban & Schwarzenberg, Munchen, 1976.

Effros, R.M., Haider, B., Ettinger, P.O., Ahmed, S.S., Oldewurtel, H.A., Marold, K., and Regan, T.: In vivo myocardial cell pH in the dog. Response to ischemia and infusion of alkali. J. Clin. Invest. 55:1100–1110, 1975.

Emerson, T.E., and Bryan, W.J.: Regional cerebral blood flows in endotoxin shock with methylprednisolone treatment. Proc. Soc. Exp. Biol. Med. 156:378–381, 1977.

Emerson, T.E., and Raymond, R.M.: Prevention of cerebral hemodynamic and metabolic disorders during endotoxic shock in the dog by methylprednisolone. Surg. Gynecol. Obstet. *148:*361–366, 1979.

Ginsberg, M.D., Reivich, M., Frinak, S., and Harbig, K.: Pyridine nucleotide redox state and blood flow of the cerebral cortex following middle cerebral artery occlusion in the cat. Stroke *7:*125–131, 1976.

Ginsberg, M., Mela, L., Wrobel-Kuhl, K., and Reivich, M.: Mitochondrial metabolism of normal and ischemic brains from urethane anesthetized gerbils. Ann. Neurol. *1:*519–527, 1977.

Ginsberg, M.D., Budd, W.W., Welsh, F.A.: Diffuse cerebral ischemia in the cat. I. Local blood flow during severe ischemia and recirculation. Ann. Neurol. *3:*482–492, 1978.

Goodwin, C.W., Mela, L., and Miller, L.D.: Adaptive activation of succinic dehydrogenase in chronic systemic hypoxia. Fed. Proc. *37:*414, 1978.

Harbig, K., Chance, B., and Kovach, A.G.B.: In vivo measurements of pyridine nucleotide fluorescence during reduced cortical perfusion pressure from the cat brain surface. J. Appl. Physiol. *41:*480–488, 1976.

Hinshaw, L.B., Archer, L.T., Greenfield, L.J., and Guenter, C.A.: Effects of endotoxin on myocardial hemodynamics, performance and metabolism. Am. J. Physiol. *221:*504–510, 1971.

Hinshaw, L.B., Archer, L.T., Black, M.R., Elkins, R.C., Brown, P.P., and Greenfield, L.J.: Myocardial function in shock. Am. J. Physiol. *226:*357–366, 1974.

Hinshaw, L.B., Beller, B.K., Archer, L.T., Flournoy, D.J., White, G.L., and Phillips, R.W.: Recovery from lethal *Escherichia coli* shock in dogs. Surg. Gynecol. Obstet. *149:*545–553, 1979.

Holtzmann, S., and Balderman, S.C.: Comparison of lactate and pyruvate during endotoxin shock. Surg. Gynecol. Obstet. *145:*677–681, 1977.

Imamura, M., and Clowes, G.H.A.: Hepatic blood flow and oxygen consumption in starvation, sepsis and septic shock. Surg. Gynecol. Obstet. *141:*27–34, 1975.

Isselhard, W., Geppert, E., Menge, M., Lauterjung, K.L., Vogel, W., Witte, J., and Heugel, E.: Effect on myocardial metabolic pattern of local complete and incomplete ischemia. Recent Adv. Stud. Cardiac Struct. Metab. *7:*231–236, 1976.

Johannsson, H., and Siesjö, B.K.: Blood flow and oxygen consumption of the rat brain in profound hypoxia. Acta Physiol. Scand. *90:*281–282, 1974.

Johannsson, H., and Siesjö, B.K.: Cerebral blood flow and oxygen consumption in the rat in hypoxic hypoxia. Acta Physiol. Scand. *90:*269–276, 1975.

Kloner, R.A., Fishbein, M.C., Braunwald, E., et al.: Effect of propanolol on mitochondrial morphology during acute myocardial ischemia. Am. J. Cardiol. *41:*880–886, 1978.

Kogure, K., Scheinberg, P., Reinmuth, O.M., Fujishima, M., and Busto, R.: Mechanisms of cerebral vasodilatation in hypoxia. J. Appl. Physiol. *29:*223–229, 1970.

Lillehei, R.C., Longerbeam, J.K., Bloch, J.H., and Manax, W.G.: The nature of irreversible shock: Experimental and clinical observations. Ann. Surgery *160:*682–710, 1964.

Linder, M.M., Hartel, W., Alken, P., and Muschaweck, R.: Renal tissue oxygen tension during the early phase of canine endotoxin shock. Surg. Gynecol. Obstet. *138:*169–173, 1974.

Lindenmayer, G.E., Steer, R.G., and Newman, W.H.: Myocardial ion transport in hypoxia and ischemia. In *Oxygen and Physiological Function*, edited by F.F. Jöbsis, pp. 434–443. Professional Information Library, Dallas, 1977.

Ljunggren, B., Schutz, H., and Siesjö, B.K.: Changes in energy state and acid-base parameters of the rat brain during complete compression ischemia. Brain Res. *73:*277–289, 1974.

Lowry, O.H., Passonneau, J.V., Hasselberger, F.X., and Schulz, D.W.: Effect of ischemia on known substrates and cofactors of the glycolytic pathway in brain. J. Biol. Chem. *239:*18–30, 1964.

Majewska, M.D., Strosznajder, J., and Lazarewicz, J.: Effect of ischemic anoxia and barbiturate anesthesia on free radical oxidation of mitochondrial phospholipids. Brain Res. *158:*423–434, 1978.

Mayevsky, A., Crowe, W., and Mela, L.: Interrelation between brain oxidative metabolism and extracellular potassium in the unanesthetized gerbil. Neurol. Res. *1:*213–225, 1980.

Mela, L.: Mitochondrial metabolic alterations in experimental circulatory shock. In *Gram-Negative Bacterial Infections and Mode of Endotoxin Actions*, edited by B. Urbaschek, R. Urbaschek, and E. Neter, pp. 288–295. Springer-Verlag, New York, 1975.

Mela, L.: Mechanism and physiological significance of calcium transport across mammalian mitochondrial membranes. In *Current Topics in Membranes and Transport*, edited by F. Bronner and A. Kleinzeller, vol. 9, pp. 321–366. Academic Press, New York, 1977.

Mela, L.: Reversibility of mitochondrial metabolic response to circulatory shock and tissue ischemia. Circ. Shock (Suppl.) *1:*61–67, 1979a.

Mela, L.: Development of the newborn to meet its own energy requirements. Proc. Am. Philosophical Soc. *123:*293–297, 1979b.

Mela, L., Bacalzo, L.D., Jr., White, R.R., IV, and Miller, L.D.: Shock-induced alterations of mitochondrial energy-linked functions. Surg. Forum *21:*6–8, 1970.

Mela, L., Bacalzo, L.V., and Miller, L.D.: Defective oxidative metabolism of rat liver mitochondria in hemorrhagic and endotoxin shock. Am. J. Physiol. *220:*571–577, 1971.

Mela, L., Miller, L.D., and Nicholas, G.G.: Influence of cellular acidosis and altered cation concentrations on shock-induced mitochondrial damage. Surgery *72:*102–110, 1972.

Mela, L., Miller, L.D., Bacalzo, L.V., Olofsson, K., and White, R.R.: Role of intracellular variations of lysosomal enzyme activity and oxygen tensions in mitochondrial impairment in endotoxemia and hemorrhage. Ann. Surg. *178:*727–735, 1973.

Mela, L., Nicholas, G.G., Laskowski, R., and Miller, L.D.: Glucocorticoid protection against endotoxin induced cellular shock. Surg. Forum *25:*74–75, 1974a.

Mela, L., Nicholas, G.G., and Miller, L.D.: Inhibition of mitochondrial energy metabolism in hypovolemic and endotoxic shock. In *Steroids and Shock*, edited by T.M. Glenn, pp. 301–313. University Park Press, Baltimore, 1974b.

Mela, L., Crowe, W., Harbig, K., Wrobel-Kuhl, K., and Kovach, A.G.B.: Inhibition of brain mitochondrial function and changes of tissue H^+ and K^+ concentration in hemorrhagic shock. Surg. Forum *26:*51–53, 1975a.

Mela, L., Goodwin, C.W., and Miller, L.D.: Correlation of mitochondrial cytochrome concentration and activity to oxygen availability in the newborn. Biochem. Biophys. Res. Commun. *64:*384–390, 1975b.

Mela, L., Hinshaw, L.B., and Coalson, J.J.: Correlation of cardiac performance, ultrastructural morphology and mitochondrial function in endotoxemia in the dog. Circ. Shock *1:*265–272, 1975c.

Mela, L., Goodwin, C.W., and Miller, L.D.: In vivo control of mitochondrial enzyme concentrations and activity by oxygen. Am. J. Physiol. *231:*1811–1816, 1976.

Mela, L., Goodwin, C.W., and Miller, L.D.: In vivo adaptation of O_2 utilization to O_2 availability. Comparison of adult and newborn mitochondria. In *Oxygen and Physiological Function*, edited by F.F. Jöbsis, pp. 285–291. Professional Information Library, Dallas, 1977.

Mela, L., Crowe, W., Wrobel-Kuhl, L., and Miller, L.D.: Brain mitochondrial activity after tissue hypoxia and circulatory shock. In *Pathophysiological, Biochemical and Morphological Aspects of Cerebral Ischemia and Arterial Hypertension*, edited by M.J. Mossakowski, I.B. Zelman, and H. Kroh, pp. 96–98. Polish Medical Publishers, Warsaw, 1978a.

Mela, L., Delivoria-Papadopoulos, M., and Miller, L.D.: Fetal and neonatal mitochondrial electron transfer chain. In *Fetal and Newborn Cardiovascular Physiology*, edited by L.D. Longo and D.D. Reneau, vol. 2, pp. 81–88. Garland, New York, 1978b.

Mela, L., Burrows, A., Knee, A., and Wrobel-Kuhl, K.: Ischemic injury of brain and kidney mitochondria in endotoxin shock. Circ. Shock 6:183, 1979a.

Mela, L., Hinshaw, L.B., Archer, L.T., Beller, B.K., and Wrobel-Kuhl, K.: Protection against metabolic failure of the brain in *E. coli* septicemia by antibiotic-glucocorticoid treatment. Fed. Proc. 38:1262, 1979b.

Mela, L., Laskowski, R., and Miller, L.D.: Glucocorticoid protection against mitochondrial and lysosomal alterations in endotoxemia. Circ. Shock, in press, 1980.

Mergner, W.J., Smith, M.W., Sahaphong, S., and Trump, B.F.: Studies on the pathogenesis of ischemic cell injury. VI. Accumulation of calcium by isolated mitochondria of ischemic rat kidney cortex. Virchows Arch. [Cell Pathol.] 26:1–16, 1977.

Mergner, W.J., Chang, S-H., Marzella, L., et al.: Studies on the pathogenesis of ischemic cell injury. VIII. ATPase of rat kidney mitochondria. Lab. Invest. 40:686–694, 1979.

Moss, G.S., Erve, P.P., and Schumer, W.: Effect of endotoxin on mitochondrial respiration. Surg. Forum 20:24–25, 1969.

Nakazawa, T., and Nunokawa, T.: Energy transduction and adenine nucleotides in mitochondria from rat liver after hypoxic perfusion. J. Biochem. 82:1575–1583, 1977.

Nicholas, G.G., Mela, L., and Miller, L.D.: Early alterations in mitochondrial membrane transport during endotoxemia. J. Surg. Res. 16:373–383, 1974.

Norberg, K., Quistorff, B., and Siesjö, B.K.: Effects of hypoxia of 10–45 seconds duration on energy metabolism in the cerebral cortex of unanesthetized and anesthetized rats. Acta Physiol. Scand. 95:301–310, 1975.

Norström, C-H., Rehncrona, S., Siesjö, B.K.: Restitution of cerebral energy state after complete and incomplete ischemia of 30 min duration. Acta Physiol. Scand. 97:270–272, 1976.

Nordström, C-H., Rehncrona, S., Siesjö, B.K.: Effects of phenobarbital in cerebral ischemia. Part two: Restitution of cerebral energy state, as well as of glycolytic metabolites, citric acid cycle intermediates and associated amino acids after pronounced incomplete ischemia. Stroke 9:335–343, 1978.

Pappova, E., Urbaschek, B., Heitmann, L., Oroz, M., Streit, E., Lemeunier, A., and Lundsgaard-Hansen, P.: Energy-rich phosphates and glucose metabolism in early endotoxin shock. J. Surg. Res. 11:506–512, 1971.

Park, C.D., Mela, L., Wharton, R., Reilly, J., Fishbein, P., and Aberdeen, E.: Cardiac mitochondrial activity in acute and chronic cyanosis. J. Surg. Res. 14:139–146, 1973.

Parker, J.L., and Emerson, T.E.: Cerebral hemodynamics, vascular reactivity, and metabolism during canine endotoxin shock. Circ. Shock 4:41–53, 1977.

Purshottam, T., and Ghosh, N.C.: Effect of acute hypoxia on the enzymes involved in the metabolic and nervous functioning of rat brain. Env. Physiol. Biochem. 5:73–77, 1975.

Rao, P.S., Cavanagh, D., Gaston, L.W., Tung, K., and Bhagat, B.D.: Endotoxin shock in the subhuman primate: Some effects of methylprednisolone and low molecular weight Dextran administration. In *Steroids and Shock*, edited by T.M. Glenn, pp. 177–201. University Park Press, Baltimore, 1974.

Reed, P.C., Erve, P.R., Das Gupta, T.K., and Schumer, W.: Endotoxemic effect of *Escherichia coli* on cardiac and skeletal muscle mitochondria. Surg. Forum 21:13–14, 1970.

Rehncrona, S., Mela, L., and Chance, B.: Cerebral energy state, mitochondrial function and redox state measurements in transient ischemia. Fed. Proc. 38:2489–2492, 1979a.

Rehncrona, S., Mela, L., and Siesjö, B.: Recovery of brain mitochondrial function in the rat after complete and incomplete cerebral ischemia. Stroke 10:437–446, 1979b.

Reichgott, M.J., Melmon, K.L., Forsyth, R.P., and Greineder, D.: Cardiovascular and metabolic effects of whole or fractionated gram-negative bacterial endotoxin in the unanesthetized Rhesus monkey. Circ. Res. 33:346–352, 1973.

Sayeed, M.M., and Baue, A.E.: Mitochondrial metabolism of succinate, β-hydroxybutyrate and α-ketoglutarate in hemorrhagic shock. Am. J. Physiol. 220:1275–1281, 1971.

Sayeed, M.M., and Baue, A.E.: Na-K transport in rat liver slices in hemorrhagic shock. Am. J. Physiol. 224:1265–1270, 1973.

Sayeed, M.M., Wurth, M.A., Chaudry, I.H., and Baue, A.E.: Cation transport in the liver in hemorrhagic shock. Circ. Shock 1:195–207, 1974.

Sayeed, M.M., Chaudry, I.H., and Baue, A.E.: Na^+-K^+ transport and adenosine nucleotides in the lung in hemorrhagic shock. Surgery 77:395–402, 1975a.

Sayeed, M.M., Senior, R.M., Caudry, I.H., and Baue, A.E.: Characteristics of sodium and potassium transport in the lung. Am. J. Physiol. 229:1073–1079, 1975b.

Schmahl, F.W.: Effects of endotoxic shock on the oxygen supply and the levels of energy-rich phosphates of the cerebral cortex. In *Oxygen Supply*, edited by M. Kessler, D.F. Bruley, L.C. Clark, D.W. Lubbers, I.A. Silver, and J. Strauss, pp. 256–264. University Park Press, Baltimore, 1973.

Schumer, W.: Steroids in the treatment of clinical septic shock. Ann. Surg. 184:333–341, 1976.

Schumer, W., and Erve, P.R.: Bovine serum albumin effect on endotoxin-challenged mitochondria. Surgery 69:699–701, 1971.

Schumer, W., Nyhus, L.M.: Corticosteroid effect on biochemical parameters of human oligemic shock. Arch. Surg. 100:405–408, 1970.

Schumer, W., Das Gupta, T.K., Moss, G.S., and Nyhus, L.M.: Effect of endotoxemia on liver cell mitochondria in man. Ann. Surg. 171:875–882, 1970.

Schumer, W., Das Gupta, T.K., Moss, G.S., Nyhus, L.M., and Erve, P.R.: Effect of endotoxemia on liver cell mitochondria in man. Z. Exp. Chir. 4:379–387, 1971a.

Schumer, W., Erve, P.R., and Obernolte, R.P.: Endotoxemic effect on cardiac and skeletal muscle mitochondria. Surg. Gynecol. Obstet. 133:433–436, 1971b.

Selmyer, J.P., Reynolds, D.G., and Swan, K.G.: Renal blood flow during endotoxin shock in the subhuman primate. Surg. Gynecol. Obstet. 137:3–6, 1973.

Skertzer, H.G., and Cascarano, J.: Mitochondrial alterations in heart, liver and kidney of altitude-acclimated rats. Am. J. Physiol. 223:632–636, 1972.

Siesjö, B.K., Nordstrom, C.H.: Brain metabolism in relation to oxygen supply. In *Oxygen and Physiological Function*, edited by F. F. Jöbsis, pp. 459–479. Professional Information Library, Dallas, 1977.

Silver, I.A.: Changes in pO_2 and ion fluxes in cerebral hypoxia-ischemia. In *Tissue Hypoxia and Ischemia*, edited by M. Reivich, R. Coburn, S. Lahiri, and B. Chance, pp. 299–312. Plenum Press, New York, 1977.

Sivaramakrishnan, S., and Ramasarma, T.: Oxidation of succinate in heart, brain and kidney mitochondria in hypobaria and hypoxia. Environ. Physiol. Biochem. *5:*189–200, 1975.

Staples, D., Topuzlu, C., and Blair, E.: A comparison of adenosinetriphosphate levels in hemorrhagic and endotoxic shock in the rat. Surgery *66:*883–885, 1969.

Trump, B.F., Valigorsky, J.M., Jones, R.T., Mergner, W.J., Garcia, J.H., and Cowley, R.A.: The application of electron microscopy and cellular biochemistry to the autopsy. Observations on cellular changes in human shock. Human Pathol. *6:*499–516, 1975.

Welsh, F.A., and O'Connor, M.J.: Patterns of microcirculatory failure during incomplete cerebral ischemia. Adv. Neurol. *20:*133–139, 1978.

Welsh, F.A., Durity, F., and Langfitt, T.W.: The appearance of regional variations in metabolism at a critical level of diffuse cerebral oligemia. J. Neurochem. *28:*71–79, 1977a.

Welsh, F.A., O'Connor, M.J., and Langfitt, T.W.: Regions of cerebral ischemia located by pyridine nucleotide fluorescence. Science *198:*951–953, 1977b.

Welsh, F.A., Ginsberg, M.D., Rieder, W., and Budd, W.W.: Diffuse cerebral ischemia in the cat. II. Regional metabolites during severe ischemia and recirculation. Ann. Neurol. *3:* 493–501, 1978a.

Welsh, F.A., O'Connor, M.J., and Marcy, V.R.: Effect of oligemia on regional metabolite levels in cat brain. J. Neurochem. *31:*311–319, 1978b.

White, R.R., Mela, L., Olofsson, K., Bacalzo, L.R., and Miller, L.D.: Hepatic ultrastructure in endotoxemia, hemorrhage and hypoxia: Emphasis on mitochondrial changes. Surgery *73:*525–534, 1973.

CHAPTER 7

Membrane Transport and the Regulation of the Cell Calcium Levels

ERNESTO CARAFOLI

The observation by Ringer (1883) that isolated hearts did not beat in absence of Ca^{2+} offers the first important indication that the role of Ca^{2+} in biology is not just structural. In retrospect, it is easy to understand why Ca^{2+} was essentially regarded as an inert element, since in the human body over 99% of it is present in the bones. The observation by Ringer, however, was followed by a series of observations on different tissues which were not logically connected with each other but which pointed unmistakably to a role of Cs^{2+} as a biological messenger. Nowadays, the messenger function of Ca^{2+} is an established concept. It represents an interdisciplinary area of research which spans from chemistry to medicine and in which experimental approaches coming from different directions merge. Basically, it is now clear that Ca^{2+} has the unique role of transmitting the "signals" from the area of their generation, which is the plasma membrane, to a large number of target functions inside the cell. In addition, it is now established that Ca^{2+} may even interfere directly with the process of signal generation at the level of the plasma membrane.

The number of intracellular functions which are sensitive to Ca^{2+} is continuously expanding, and the list presented in Table 7.1 will certainly need updating in a short time. As can be seen, it covers a large spectrum of biological activities, and it is necessary to stress at this point that all of the activities listed in Table 7.1 are sensitive to Ca^{2+} in the μM activity range. This is an important concept. Several intracellular enzymes are sensitive to Ca^{2+} at much higher activity ranges, and for this reason they cannot be considered as targets for the messenger function of Ca^{2+}. Ca^{2+}-modulated (enzyme) functions are those which are switched on and off by variations of the Ca^{2+} activity in a narrow range, around

Table 7.1
Ca²⁺-Dependent Reactions in Cells

- Activation of enzyme systems
    - Glycogenolysis (phosphorylase-*b* kinase)
    - Lipases and phospholipases
    - α-Glycerophosphate dehydrogenase
    - Pyruvate dehydrogenase
    - Isocitric dehydrogenase
    - Synthesis of some phospholipids
    - NADH dehydrogenase (plant mitochondria)
    - Light emission
    - Decision to divide
- Activation of contractile and motile systems
    - Muscle myofibrils
    - Cilia and flagella
    - Microtubules and microfilaments
    - Cytoplasmic streaming
    - Pseudopod formation
- Hormonal regulation
    - Formation and/or function of cAMP (GH, LH, TSH, MSH, PTH)
    - Release of insulin, steroids, vasopressin, oxytocin, catecholamines, thyroxine, and progesterone
- Membrane-linked functions
    - Excitation secretion coupling at nerve endings
    - Excitation contraction coupling in muscles
    - Exocrine secretion (pancreas, salivary glands, and HCl in the stomach)
    - Aggregation of platelets
    - Action potential (nerve and muscle cells)
    - Na^+, K^+,-ATPase of several membranes
    - Tight junctions and gap junctions
    - Cell contact and cell-cell communication

μM. They must, therefore, have a very high affinity for Ca^{2+}.

The messenger function requires that Ca^{2+} be kept inside cells, where the target activities are present, at a very low activity level, and that it be allowed to fluctuate widely and rapidly around this low activity level to switch the targets on and off. This is achieved essentially in two ways: 1) by complexing the Ca^{2+} that has entered the cell down its concentration (and its electrical) gradient from the extracellular space, and 2) by transporting the Ca^{2+} reversibly across various membrane systems, to enrich, or impoverish, various cell compartments in it. An interesting consideration at this point is that Ca^{2+} is the only ion for which a very large number of specific ligands and a multiplicity of membrane transporting systems have been developed. This underscores the importance of the messenger function of Ca^{2+} and the resulting necessity of regulating its activity inside cells with utmost efficiency and precision. Perhaps it would be good at this point to discuss the reasons, or at least to speculate on what the reasons may have been, for the evolutionary selection of Ca^{2+} as a biological messenger. This, evidently, is an area which cannot offer final proof for any of the speculations that may be made. It seems reasonable, however, as has been discussed extensively elsewhere (Williams, 1975, 1976; Carafoli and Crompton, 1978), to suggest that the choice of evolution has been oriented by the particular versatility of Ca^{2+} as a ligand, a fact that offered obvious advantages in developing, e.g., specific molecular systems for complexing it, and transporting it across membrane boundaries. In looking at the coordination chemistry of Ca^{2+} and in comparing it, for example, to that of Mg^{2+} or other cations present in abundant amounts in the original environment, one important consideration emerges. The polarizing power of Ca^{2+}, resulting from its charge and ionic radius, enables it to space the six to eight coordinating oxygen atoms around it at variable bond lengths and angles, thus permitting Ca^{2+} to accept cavities of very irregular geometries, as are those normally offered by complex biological ligands. By contrast, Mg^{2+}, which has a considerably smaller size and therefore a higher polarizing power, requires that the coordinating oxygen atoms be spaced around it at regular bond lengths and angles. The resulting regular octahedral cavity is naturally a very unlikely event in complex biological molecules, a fact that is reflected in the very infrequent occurrence of specific Mg^{2+} ligands.

Some last general considerations are in order on the messenger function of Ca^{2+}. In most cases, the type of interaction between Ca^{2+} and the target molecule is not known. It has become clear in the last few years, however, that one important factor in mediating the transmission of the Ca^{2+} signal and its interaction with the target functions is a small molecular weight acidic protein, which has been termed "calmodulin." This molecule is now recognized as ubiquitous, and its importance in the messenger function of Ca^{2+} is growing continuously. It will, therefore, be covered in a later section somewhat more extensively.

Finally, in these introductory remarks on the role of Ca^{2+} as a messenger, its interplay with the other recognized biological messenger, cyclic AMP (cAMP), must be briefly discussed. The nature of this interplay has been debated extensively (see Rasmussen, 1970; Rasmussen et al., 1972; Kretsinger and Nelson, 1976 for reviews), but at the present moment very little can be said in addition to the fact that such an interplay does indeed exist. The basic problem is that in most instances it is not known whether Ca^{2+} and cAMP work in series or in parallel. Interest and complications are added to the issue by the discovery that Ca^{2+}, via calmodulin (see above), activates two key enzymes having opposite functions in the metabolism of cAMP: adenylate cyclase (Teo and Wang, 1973; Brostrom et al., 1976), and phosphodiesterase (Wang et al., 1975).

THE INTERACTION OF Ca²⁺ WITH BIOLOGICAL MEMBRANES

One interesting point can be made concerning the interaction of Ca^{2+} and biological membranes preliminarly to a discussion of the various transporting systems. The molecular architecture, the stability, and the functional properties of biological membranes are influenced by Ca^{2+} in a very peculiar way. For example, several lines of evidence indicate that Ca^{2+}, very likely by virtue of its ability to interact with (and to dehydrate) various membrane components, has a profound influence on the stability of membranes (see Manery, 1966; Carafoli, 1975, for reviews). Träuble and Eibl (1974) have shown that the transition from the fluid to the ordered state of the paraffinic chains of the phospholipids of (model) membranes occurs at a different temperature in the presence of Ca^{2+}, implying that the latter can influence the fluid → ordered transition at a constant temperature. The interactions of hydrophilic proteins with relatively apolar regions of the membrane domain may also be regulated and promoted by Ca^{2+}, either by the formation of "bridges" between negative charges on the proteins and the polar heads of the phospholipids or by an ion pair mechanism. Experiments by Gitler and Montal (1972) and Azzi et al. (1975) suggest this possibility for cytochrome c, whereas experiments by Prestipino et al (1974) and Carafoli (1975) indicate that this might be the case for the mitochondrial Ca^{2+}-binding glycoprotein. The Ca^{2+}-promoted, reversible interaction of proteins with the lipid bilayer is indeed an attractive possibility, which is in line with the modern dynamic conceptions of the architecture of biological membranes. Finally, it is worth mentioning in this context that the unequal distribution of Ca^{2+} in the media bathing the two faces of biological membranes may be an important factor in maintaining the asymmetric distribution of phospholipids in the two monolayers of the membranes (Williams, 1975). Of the phospholipids normally encountered in biological membranes, one, diphosphatidyl-glycerol (cardiolipin), has a high affinity for Ca^{2+}. It is, perhaps, not a coincidence that the membrane that contains the highest proportion of phospholipids is the inner mitochondrial membrane, whose inner monolayer faces an ambient (the mitochondrial matrix) of high Ca^{2+} concentration. Recent work (Krebs et al., 1979) has shown that cardiolipin is predominantly distributed in the inner monolayer of the inner mitochondrial membrane.

Some consideration must be given at this point to the matter of the intracellular Ca^{2+} concentration as compared to intracellular Ca^{2+} activity. It has been mentioned repeatedly that the concentration of ionized Ca^{2+} inside cells is at least 1000 times lower than that in the extracellular environment. In fact, *direct* measurements of ionized intracellular Ca^{2+} are difficult and available only for a comparatively small number of cells. They range between 0.13 and 1.3 μM, although indirect methods may yield higher values (Table 7.2) (Baker et al., 1971; Di Polo et al., 1976; Meech and Standen, 1975; Rose and Loewenstein, 1976; Ridgway and Durham, 1976). By contrast, the *total* concentration of Ca^{2+} in cells may reach values as high as 8 or 9 mM (Wacker and Williams, 1968), i.e., in the same range as in the extracellular fluids. The question at this point arises regarding the respective contribution of membrane-enclosed intracellular compartments and "soluble" cytoplasmic ligands to the very large difference between the ionized and total Ca^{2+} inside cells. This is an important point, since methods for the estimates of ionized intracellular Ca^{2+} are based on the introduction of indicators, or of specific electrodes, in the cytoplasmic space. Clearly, any Ca^{2+} that may be enclosed in membrane-bound compartments will not be "visible" in these measurements and will thus artifactually increase the nonionized cellular Ca^{2+} pool. In fact, the proportion of cell Ca^{2+} that may be present in intracellular, membrane-bound organelles may be very high, but it is necessary to realize that not all of the organelle-enclosed Ca^{2+} is necessarily nonionized. It can be concluded, therefore, that in all likelihood the proportion of intracellular (i.e., cytoplasmic *plus* organellar) Ca^{2+} that is ionized is underestimated by current measurements. The cytoplasm, however, contains a variety of Ca^{2+} ligands which undoubtedly contribute to reducing the ionized Ca^{2+} concentration. Small molecular weight molecules like phosphate, citrate, pyridine nucleotides and adenine nucleotides are obvious candidates, and it is even possible to speculate that their effectiveness may be modulated by metabolic activity, which is an interesting possibility, since it may afford a way to influence the Ca^{2+}-requiring enzymes in synchrony with the demands of metabolism. As an example, one may quote here the K_d for Ca^{2+} of ADP and ATP, since their respective levels are obviously influenced by the metabolic state of the cell: 4.5×10^{-4} M for the former and 3.1×10^{-5} M (O'Sullivan and Perrin, 1964) for the latter. Higher molecular weight Ca^{2+} ligands, e.g., proteins, are currently the focus of very active research and have afforded significant advances in the understanding of the molecular aspects of the binding of Ca^{2+} by complex molecules. Of particular interest are the studies on parvalbumin (Kretsinger, 1977) and troponin C, the Ca^{2+} receptor in the troponin molecule (Ebashi and Endo, 1968). The most actively investigated molecule at the moment, however, is calmodulin, which will be covered in a separate section in view of its general significance for the regulation of intracellular Ca^{2+} and for its messenger function.

GENERAL CONSIDERATIONS ON THE TRANSPORT OF Ca^{2+} ACROSS BIOLOGICAL MEMBRANES

Three membrane systems have been shown to be able to transport Ca^{2+}: the plasma membrane, the endoplasmic and sarcoplasmic reticulum and the mitochondrion. Before discussing in detail their respective roles in the regulation of intracellular Ca^{2+}, one general consideration which was made before must be repeated and re-emphasized. Ca^{2+} is the only ion for which a variety of different transport modes have been developed in the course of evolution, a fact that reflects the paramount importance of its messenger function, which evidently requires control by a multiplicity of independent transport systems. At the moment, the following systems have been described: electrophoretic Ca^{2+} uniport systems; channels (possibly gated by potentials); Ca^{2+} specific, and possibly different, ATPases; Na^+-Ca^{2+} antiport systems, which may also be in different membranes; and Ca^{2+}-H^+ antiport systems. In the section to follow, some of these transport systems will be discussed as they are encountered in the various cellular membranes. At this point, however, it is of interest to consider another aspect of the transport of Ca^{2+} across cellular membranes, namely, the respective contribution of the three membrane systems mentioned above to the overall regulation of the cellular Ca^{2+} balance. Here, one point must be made clear at the outset, and that is the fact that the long-term maintenance of the gradient of Ca^{2+} between intracellular milieu and external medium requires the continuous ejection of Ca^{2+} across the plasma membrane. This is obvious if one considers that Ca^{2+} diffuses continuously from the medium into the cell down a chemical (and electrical) gradient. However, the *rapid* regulation of intracellular Ca^{2+}, as demanded by metabolism, is almost certainly best achieved by reversible transport across the membranes of intracellular organelles. This is so because the proportion of total surface of cellular membranes capable of transporting Ca^{2+}, at least in the cells so far analyzed morphometrically, greatly favors the intracellular organelles (Table 7.3). The plasma membrane represents only between 1 and 10% of the total Ca^{2+} transporting area, suggesting very strongly indeed that the intracellular Ca^{2+} transporting membranous network predominates over the plasma membrane in the *rapid* regulation of cellular Ca^{2+}. The kinetic parameters of the Ca^{2+} transporting systems in the various membranes are of importance in this respect. Indeed, the consideration made above is only valid if the transport in the plasma membrane and in the intracellular organelles operates with approximately equivalent efficiency. This seems indeed to be the case if one compares Ca^{2+} transporting velocities, at least under optimal conditions (Schatzmann, 1975; Carafoli and Crompton, 1976; Reeves and Sutko, 1979; Pitts, 1979).

THE TRANSPORT OF Ca^{2+} ACROSS THE PLASMA MEMBRANE

The Influx of Ca^{2+}

Probably, the mode of Ca^{2+} penetration is different in excitable and nonexcitable tissues. In the former, specific channels gated by electrical potentials (see Reuter, 1974; Baker, 1975) allow the penetration of Ca^{2+}. This generates an inward current which is slow with respect to that generated by Na^+ ("slow Ca^{2+} channel"). The Na^+ and Ca^{2+} channels can be discriminated by the use of appropriate inhibitors. The former is blocked by tetrodotoxin, the latter by verapamil, D-600, and Cd^{2+} (Fleckenstein et al., 1969; Kohlhardt et al., 1972; Kostyuk and Krishtal, 1978). The old observation by Ringer mentioned at the opening of this article and more recent observations by others (Bailey and Dresel, 1968; Rich and Langer, 1975; Shine et al., 1971) indicate that the Ca^{2+} that enters heart cells on the slow channel is essential for contractility, since the beating of heart cells stops in its absence. However, the penetrating extracellular Ca^{2+} does not acitvate troponin C directly. Possibly, the essential role of Ca^{2+} influx from the extracellular spaces is linked to the phonomenon of Ca^{2+}-induced Ca^{2+} release from sarcoplasmic reticulum (see below). The molecular as-

Table 7.2
Some Representative Values for the Ionized Ca^{2+} in the Cytoplasm[a]

Squid axoplasms	20–500 nM	Baker et al. (1971); DiPolo et al. (1976)
Erythrocyte	0.73–4 μM	Schatzmann (1973); Quist and Roufogalis (1975); Pfleger and Wolf (1975); Scharff (1976); Ferreira and Lew (1976).
Muscle	0.1–1.0 μM	Felo et al. (1965); Ebashi and Endo (1968); Weber (1966); Solaro et al. (1974); Portzehl et al. (1964); Hagiwara and Nakajima (1966).
Helix aspersa neurons	30–80 μM	Meech and Standen (1975)
Chironomus salivary gland	20 μM	Rose and Loewenstein (1976)
Physarum polycephalum	0.1 μM	Ridgway and Durham (1976)

[a] From Carafoli and Crompton, 1978.

Table 7.3
Total Area of Ca^{2+}-Transporting Membranes in Some Representative Cells[a,b]

Cell	Area		
	Plasma Membrane	Mitochondria	Endo- or Sarcoplasmic Reticulum
	m^2/g tissue		
Erythrocyte	1.66 (100%)	0	0
Liver	0.55 (11.4%)	2.65 (54.8%)	1.63 (33.7%)
Heart	0.10 (0.8%)	10.60 (87%)	1.48 (12.1%)

[a] The data on erythrocytes are based on an area of 145 μm²/erythrocyte (Davson, 1970), on a hematocrit of 44.5% (Ganong, 1973), and on an erythrocyte content of 5.1 × 10⁶/mm³ (Ganong, 1973). The data on liver are derived from morphometric measurements carried out by E. R. Weibel (personal communication). Only the inner mitochondrial membrane and the smooth endoplasmic reticulum are considered, since the outer membrane and rough endoplasmic reticulum are not involved in the transport of Ca^{2+} (see text). The total area of liver cell membranes is 8.2 m²/g tissue. The data on heart plasma membrane are derived from Winegrad and Shanes (1962). For those on heart mitochondria and sarcoplasmic reticulum, the following two assumptions have been made: 1) the inner membrane represents 50% of the total mitochondrial protein in heart; and 2) the ratio of protein content to area is the same in rat liver mitochondrial inner membrane, heart mitochondrial inner membrane, and heart sarcoplasmic reticulum. The total mitochondrial content is 50 mg protein/g wet wt in rat liver (Reith et al., 1976) and 100 mg protein/g wet wt in rat heart (Scarpa and Graziotti, 1973); the total content of the sarcoplasmic reticulum in heart is 7 mg protein/g wet wt (Solaro and Briggs, 1974).

[b] From Carafoli and Crompton, 1978.

pects of the operation of the slow Ca^{2+} channel are completely obscure. One interesting observation is the stimulation of the influx of Ca^{2+} into excited cardiac cells by catecholamines (Grossmann and Furchgott, 1964; Reuter, 1965), which may be related to the observation by Wollenberger et al. (1975) of a cAMP-dependent phosphorylation of sarcolemmal protein. The phosphorylation increases the affinity for Ca^{2+} of specific binding sites in the sarcolemma.

No potential gated slow Ca^{2+} channels have been described in nonexcitable tissues. In these, Ca^{2+} apparently diffuses passively from the extracellular spaces. The possibility of a hormonal control of the process has been suggested (Borle, 1970, 1975), with parathyroid hormone accelerating and calcitonin inhibiting the influx of Ca^{2+}. A role in the penetration of Ca^{2+} in at least some nonexcitable tissues is, in all likelihood, played by a water-soluble protein of MW 28,000, which is synthesized under the influence of vitamin D. This protein was first described in intestinal mucosa by Wasserman and Taylor (1966) but is now known to be present in various other tissues. It binds Ca^{2+} at two types of sites, four of which per mole have a rather high affinity (K_d, 4 μM). The evidence linking this protein to the penetration of Ca^{2+} into intestinal mucosa (and other cells) is indirect, but rather convincing. Its mode of action in aiding the penetration of Ca^{2+}, however, is completely obscure.

The Efflux of Ca^{2+}

Two systems mediate the transfer of Ca^{2+} across the plasma membrane from the intracellular milieu to the environment. One is a Ca^{2+} specific ATPase, the other a specific Na^+-Ca^{2+} exchange system. Until recently, the generalization was made that the former system represented the mode of Ca^{2+} ejection from nonexcitable cells and the latter from excitable cells. This concept, however, now appears to be an oversimplification, since the two systems seemingly coexist in several excitable and nonexcitable cell systems.

The Ca^{2+} ATPase was discovered by Schatzmann and Vincenzi (1969) in the plasma membrane of erythrocytes (see Schatzmann, 1975, for a review) and later found in other cell types as well: liver (van Rossum, 1970), kidney (Gmaj, et al., 1979), L-cells (Lamb and Lindsay, 1971). Of particular interest is the finding of a Ca^{2+} specific ATPase in the plasma membrane of the excitable tissue heart (Caroni and Carafoli, 1980) and the observation that in the basal lateral membrane of kidney tubular cells, *both* a Ca^{2+} specific ATPase, and a Na^+-Ca^{2+} exchange system are present (Gmaj et al., 1979).

The Ca^{2+} specific ATPase has been studied essentially in erythrocytes, where most of its kinetic parameters have been established. It is a transmembrane protein, which splits ATP at the inner side of the inner membrane, becoming phosphorylated in the process. The affinity for Ca^{2+} is rather high (K_d, about 1 μM) but the ATP-Ca^{2+} stoichiometry is still being debated. Schatzmann and Vincenzi (1969) and Schatzmann (1975) have reported values of 1; others (Quist and Roufogalis, 1975; Ferreira and Lew, 1976; Sarkadi et al., 1977), values of 2. The maximal rate of Ca^{2+} transport lies between 85 and 200 μmoles of Ca^{2+} per liter of cells per min at 37°C (Ferreira and Lew, 1976; Sarkadi et al., 1977), and can be stimulated two to four times by calmodulin (Bond and Clough, 1973; Luthra et al., 1976; Gopinath and Vincenzi, 1977; Jarrett and Penniston, 1978). The stimulation by calmodulin and its Ca^{2+}-dependent interaction with the ATPase (Niggli, et al., 1979b) have been successfully exploited to purify the latter from erythrocyte ghosts, using an affinity chromatography approach (Niggli et al., 1979a). The ATPase enzyme has a MW of 138,000, is phosphorylated by ATP, and can be reconstituted into artificial phospholipid bilayer membranes (Peterson et al., 1978; Gietzen et al., 1979; Niggli et al., 1981).

The other system responsible for the ejection of Ca^{2+} from cells is the Na^+-Ca^{2+} exchange, which, as mentioned, has so far been studied mainly in excitable tissues. In squid axons, the system is probably responsible for the largest portion of the total Ca^{2+} ejection (Baker, 1976; Mullins, 1976; Blaustein, 1976). It displays a sigmoidal dependence on the external Na^+ concentration, with half-maximal velocity at 120 mM Na^+. On the basis of these kinetic data, the suggestion has been made that at least 3 Na^+ ions are exchanged per 1 Ca^{2+} ion (Baker and McNaughton, 1976; Blaustein et al., 1974; Mullins and Brinley, 1975), leading to the net movement of positive charges into the cell. Accordingly, the Na^+-Ca^{2+} exchange is inhibited by depolarization. It has also been found that low amounts of ATP activate the exchange from within the axon, transforming the kinetics of the Na^+ dependence from sigmoidal to hyperbolic and lowering the concentration of ionized Ca^{2+} required for half-maximal activation from about 10 μM to about 0.2 μM (Baker and Glitsch 1973; Baker and McNaughton, 1976).

The other membrane system in which the Na^+-Ca^{2+} exchange has been studied in detail is heart sarcolemma. The original observations by Jundt et al. (1975) on intact heart tissue led to the proposal of an electroneutral exchange, responsible for the re-extrusion of Ca^{2+} that had entered heart sarcoplasma during excitation on the "slow Ca^{2+} channel." More recent experiments on vesicular preparations derived from heart sarcolemma (Reeves and Sutko, 1979; Pitts, 1979; Caroni and Carafoli, 1980), however, have indicated that the exchange in the heart is also probably electrogenic, extruding 1 Ca^{2+} per 3 Na^+ that enter the heart cell (Pitts, 1979). The work on sarcolemmal vesicles has shown that the system exchanges about 600 μmoles of Ca^{2+} per mg of protein per hr at 37°C, with a K_m for Ca^{2+} of about 20 μM and for Na^+ of about 18 mM (Reeves and Sutko, 1979; Pitts, 1979; Caroni and Carafoli 1980).

A Na^+-Ca^{2+} exchange has been described also in nonexcitable tissues. In kidney tubular cells, the basal lateral membrane contains a Na^+-Ca^{2+} exchange which seems to function electrogenically, like its axon or heart counterparts (Gmaj, et al., 1979) and which is absent from the brush-border membrane. A Na^+-Ca^{2+} exchange has also been described in the plasma membrane of toad bladder epithelia (Taylor et al., 1978). In addition, indirect evidence for its presence has been obtained by Terepka et al. (1976) for the case of the luminal and basal portion of the chick chorioallantoic membrane and the plasma membrane of small intestine. As mentioned above, a specific Ca^{2+} ATPase and a Na^+-Ca^{2+} exchange seem to coexist in the plasma membranes of some excitable cells (Caroni and Carafoli, 1980; Di Polo, 1978; Di Polo et al., 1979). The problem then arises of their respective roles in the ejection of Ca^{2+} from these cells. Since the ATPase seems to have a lower K_m (about 0.2 μM) for Ca^{2+} and a slower V_{max} of transport (8.5 μmoles per mg of protein per hr) than the Na^+-Ca^{2+} exchange (Caroni and Carafoli, 1980), it is possible that the former system is responsible for the maintenance of the low Ca^{2+} activity inside resting cells, whereas the latter system would be responsible for the rapid ejection of the extra Ca^{2+} that has entered the cell during excitation.

THE TRANSPORT OF Ca^{2+} BY ENDOPLASMIC AND SARCOPLASMIC RETICULUM

Sarcoplasmic Reticulum

The ability of sarcoplasmic reticulum (SR) to accumulate Ca^{2+} varies from muscle to muscle. It is a reflection not only of the variable content of different muscles in this organelle but also of the intrinsic different abilities of SR to accumulate Ca^{2+} in different muscles. In heart, for example, the organelle is less active than in skeletal muscle (Suko and Hasselbach, 1976; Carafoli, 1975). The uptake of Ca^{2+} by SR is catalyzed by an ATPase which is activated by Ca^{2+} and which transports it with a stoichiometry of 2 Ca^{2+} to 1 ATP. The enzyme has been extracted from the membrane environment, where it represents between 60 and 90% of the total protein content (Meissner, 1975) and has been purified to homogeneity (Martonosi, 1968; McLennan, 1970; Ikemoto et al., 1971; Warren et al., 1974; Meissner et al., 1973). Its MW is about 105,000, it binds 2 moles of Ca^{2+} per mole of enzyme with high affinity, and becomes phosphorylated by ATP during the transport of Ca^{2+} with the formation of an aspartyl-phosphate residue at the active site (Degani and Boyer, 1973). Makinose (1973) has shown that the discharge of Ca^{2+} to the interior of the vesicle membrane occurs prior to the dephosphorylation of the enzyme. The kinetic parameters of the ATPase are different in fast as opposed to slow and cardiac muscle. In the former, the enzyme transports Ca^{2+} with a V_{max} of between 0.4 and 3.6 μmoles per mg of vesicle protein per min (Table 7.4); in the latter, of between 0.1 and 0.15. Partial or total charge compensation during the influx of Ca^{2+} occurs by mechanisms that are still debated. Kanazawa and Boyer (1973) have proposed 1 Ca^{2+} per 1 Mg^{2+} or 2 K^+ exchange, but it must be stressed that the SR membrane is permeable to anions (Martonosi and Feretos, 1964; Duggan and Martonosi, 1970). The penetration of oxalate, indeed, is frequently exploited to increase the total amount of Ca^{2+} accumulated, since oxalate precipitates Ca^{2+} in the intravesicular space.

The Ca^{2+} ATPase has been reconstituted in phospholipid bilayer vesicles (Racker, 1972). Reconstitution in planar bilayers has required its previous transformation into a water-soluble form through alkylation (see Shamoo and Goldstein, 1977, for a review) or its proteolytic fragmentation. The latter work has permitted discrimination of the Ca^{2+} ionophoric portion of the molecule from the portion responsible for the formation of the phosphoenzyme.

Sarcoplasmic reticulum contains two more proteins able to bind Ca^{2+}: one with low affinity (calsequestrin—McLennan and Wong, 1971) and one with both high and low affinity (Meissner et al., 1973; Ikemoto et al., 1972; Ostwald et al., 1974). The former protein is thought to be responsible for the storing of Ca^{2+} inside the vesicles, particularly in the terminal cisternae (Meissner, 1975; Shamoo and Goldstein, 1977).

The ATP-dependent accumulation of Ca^{2+} by SR can be reversed (Barlogie et al., 1971) in the presence of ADP, P_i, and Mg^{2+}. However, the process has a rather slow time course and occurs only when the extravesicular

Table 7.4
Properties of Active Ca^{2+} Transport in Isolated Sarcoplasmic Reticulum[a]

Sarcoplasmic Reticulum Preparation	Oxalate	Maximal Uptake	V_{max}	K_m for Ca^{2+} (μM)	Reference
White skeletal muscle microsomes	Present	—	0.4–0.9	0.1–1.0	Weber (1966)
	Absent	0.17	—	—	Weber (1966)
	Present	6.0	1.8	—	Sreter (1969)
	Absent	0.25	1.8	—	Sreter (1969)
	Absent	0.14	3.6	—	Inesi and Scarpa (1972)
	Present	—	2.8	10	Worsfold and Peter (1970)
	Absent	—	—	3	Martonosi (1975)
	Absent	0.14	—	0.03	Fiehn and Migala (1971)
Reconstituted pump from white skeletal muscle microsomes	Absent	—	—	25	Knowles and Racker (1975)
Red skeletal muscle microsomes	Present	1.2	0.15	—	Sreter (1969)
	Absent	0.04	0.15	—	Sreter (1969)
Cardiac microsomes	Absent	0.07	0.12	—	Besch and Schwartz (1971)
	Present	0.30	0.10	—	Fanburg et al. (1964)
	Present	0.42	—	—	Baskin and Deamer (1969)

[a] From Carafoli and Crompton, 1978.

concentrations of ADP and Ca^{2+} are extremely low. As a result, the likelihood of the occurrence of a reversal of the ATP-dependent Ca^{2+} pumping system under physiological conditions seems rather remote. This then introduces the problem of the release of Ca^{2+} from SR, an essential phenomenon if the organelle, as is universally accepted, is to regulate *both* the relaxation and the contraction of the myofibrils. At the present time, two mechanisms have been proposed. One is triggered by inducing a membrane potential, positive outside, across the vesicle membrane (Constantin and Podolsky, 1967; Endo and Thorens, 1975; Nakajima and Endo, 1973). However, the results of these experiments have been criticized since osmotic damage is induced to the vesicles by the conditions employed (Meissner and McKinley, 1976). The other mechanism that has been proposed is the so-called "Ca^{2+}-induced Ca^{2+} release" (Ford and Podolsky, 1970, 1972a and b; Endo et al., 1970), in which an increase in extravesicular Ca^{2+} would induce a massive Ca^{2+} release. In skeletal muscle, however, this has been shown to occur at concentrations of external Ca^{2+} that are orders of magnitude higher than the physiological range. In skinned heart fibers and in isolated heart SR, on the other hand, Ca^{2+} may be released from SR upon variations in the external concentration that are in the physiological range (Fabiato and Fabiato, 1975; Katz et al., 1977).

At the moment, therefore, the mechanism of Ca^{2+} release is the major area of uncertainty in considering skeletal muscle sarcoplasmic reticulum from the standpoint of the overall regulation of Ca^{2+}. On the other hand, in heart, and probably slow muscles, a major problem may be the total extent of Ca^{2+} accumulation. In heart and slow muscles, the rate of Ca^{2+} removal and the total amount of sarcoplasmic reticulum present in the tissue are considerably lower than in fast muscles (Fanburg et al., 1964; Besch and Schwartz, 1971; Chiesi, 1978; Solaro and Briggs, 1974; Carafoli and Crompton, 1978) and may fall short of the total requirements for myofibril contraction (Solaro et al., 1974).

It is interesting, however, that the rate of Ca^{2+} uptake by SR of heart and slow skeletal muscles can be stimulated by the cAMP-dependent phosphorylation of a serine residue of a 21,000 MW membrane protein (Tada et al., 1974; Tada et al., 1975a and b; Kirchberger et al., 1974; Kirchberger and Tada, 1976; Schwartz et al., 1974, 1976). Of interest is also the finding that calmodulin stimulates the rate of Ca^{2+} transport in heart [Katz and Remtulla, 1978; LePeuch et al., 1979; Malmström and Carafoli (unpublished data)], and other SR muscles [Malmström and Carafoli (unpublished data)].

Endoplasmic Reticulum

That endoplasmic reticulum (ER) fragments from several tissues can take up Ca^{2+} has now been known for some years (Table 7.5) (Otsuka et al., 1965; Robinson and Lust, 1968; Selinger et al., 1970; DeMeis et al., 1970; Alonso et al., 1971; Robblee et al., 1973; Moore et al., 1974; Moore et al., 1975; Blaustein et al., 1978). In general, the uptake process resembles that of SR, except that the efficiency of the uptake reaction seems to be considerably lower. The system has a rather high affinity for Ca^{2+} and seems to be concentrated in smooth ER. Its role in the cellular homeostasis of Ca^{2+} is now being considered with increasing attention. Blaustein et al. (1978) have offered indications for a participation of ER in the regulation of Ca^{2+} at the low concentrations physiologically present inside nerve endings.

THE TRANSPORT OF Ca^{2+} BY MITOCHONDRIA

General Concepts

That mitochondria can accumulate Ca^{2+} against a concentration gradient utilizing energy made available by the operation of the respiratory chain was first shown by Vasington and Murphy in 1962. The process has now been studied in great detail in a number of laboratories and shown to be present in mitochondria from a large variety of tissues (see Lehninger et al., 1967; Carafoli, 1974; Carafoli and Crompton, 1976, 1978; Bygrave, 1977, for reviews). Although the basic characteristics of the process seem to be the same in most cases, in at least two tissues (Carafoli et al., 1970, 1971) the process exhibits peculiar properties.

Table 7.5
Properties of Active Ca^{2+} Transport in Isolated Endoplasmic Reticulum[a]

Source	Oxalate	Maximal Capacity	K_m for Ca^{2+}	Inhibitors	Reference
		nmoles/mg protein	μM		
Brain	No stimulation	~50	—	SH reagents, oligomycin, amytal	Robinson and Lust (1968)
	No stimulation	~50	—	—	Otsuka et al. (1965)
	No stimulation	~65	50–100	—	DeMeis et al. (1970)
Salivary gland	Stimulates	2750	—	Salyrgan	Selinger et al. (1970)
	Stimulates	150	100	—	Alonso et al. (1971)
Kidney	Stimulates	~50	20	—	Moore et al. (1974)
Liver	Stimulates	~400	4.6	SH reagents, oligomycin	Moore et al. (1975)
Platelets	Stimulates	350	100	—	Robblee et al. (1973)
Nerve endings	Stimulates	—	0.35	Tetracaine	Blaustein et al. (1978)

[a] Energy source, ATP; Mg^{2+} required.

During the last few years, it has become evident that the overall process by which mitochondria transport Ca^{2+} consists of two separate reactions: one responsible for the uptake, the other for the releases of the cation (Carafoli, 1979). The uptake pathway transports Ca^{2+} inside the organelle at the expense of the transmembrane electrical potential maintained by respiration (or by ATP hydrolysis). The release pathway returns Ca^{2+} to the environment (the cytosol) in a reaction which is presumbly electrically neutral. As a result, Ca^{2+} becomes available again to the uptake pathway, establishing what has been termed a "Ca^{2+} cycle" (Carafoli, 1979).

The Uptake of Ca^{2+} by Mitochondria

During the period following its discovery, the process of Ca^{2+} uptake by mitochondria was essentially studied under conditions that emphasized the accumulation of massive amounts of the cation, rather than the mechanism and regulation of the process. The so-called "matrix loading" (Lehninger et al., 1967) was made possible by the inclusion in the medium, and by the accumulation, of inorganic phosphate, and resulted in the precipitation of large amounts of calcium phosphate salts inside mitochondria, which could be documented by electron microscopy. Clearly, the matrix-loading process has limited significance in the physiology of most tissues, since mitochondrial calcification in vivo would require the sustained presence of concentrations of Ca^{2+} far exceeding those normally present in most cytosols. However, in tissues specialized in the transport of Ca^{2+}, and thus presumably exposed to large fluctuations of its cytosolic level, mitochondria can undergo massive loading in vivo. Large precipitates of Ca^{2+} and phosphate have been described within the mitochondrial profiles in a number of specialized tissues (Table 7.6), and it is of interest that the amounts of Ca^{2+} endogenously present in mitochondria may be very large even in some tissues not directly involved in the transport of unusually large amounts of Ca^{2+} (Malmström and Carafoli, 1977; Gómez-Puyou et al., 1979). These findings underscore the importance of mitochondria as cellular Ca^{2+} buffers and their role in preventing large deviations of Ca^{2+} cytosolic activity from the level that is optimal for its messenger function. Related to this point is the matter of the role of mitochondria as Ca^{2+}-buffering structures in cells experimentally or spontaneously injured. Since the pioneering observation and suggestions of Judah and associates (1964), it is widely accepted that an early manifestation of cell injury is the increased permeability of the cell membrane to the ambient Ca^{2+}. Very recently, the interesting observation was made (Schanne et al., 1979) that various toxic agents able to produce cell injury require the penetration of Ca^{2+} inside the cell for their expression. It is, therefore, of great importance that mitochondria in a large number of injured cells (Table 7.7) have been shown to contain large amounts of Ca^{2+} and phosphate. Since it has now become clear (discussed above) that mitochondria can function in a relatively normal way even after the accumulation of large amounts of Ca^{2+}

Table 7.6
Massive Uptake of Ca^{2+} by Mitochondria in Situ[a]

Condition	Location	Reference
Osteoclasts in healing bone fractures	Bone	Gonzales and Karnovsky (1961)
Chondrocytes in calcifying epiphysial cartilage	Cartilage	Martin and Matthews (1969)
Calciferous gland of the earthworm	Epithelium	Crang et al. (1968)
Egg shell gland	Epithelium	Homan and Schraer (1966)
Toad urinary bladder exposed to high Ca^{2+} concentration	Epithelium and smooth muscle	Peachey (1964)
Dog heart perfused with high Ca^{2+} concentrations	Heart	Legato et al. (1968)

[a] From Carafoli, 1974.

Table 7.7
Massive Loading of Mitochondria with Ca^{2+} and Phosphate in Spontaneous and Experimental Pathology[a]

	Tissue	Reference
Spontaneous pathology		
Coronary occlusion	Heart	Herdson et al. (1965)
Tumor calcinosis	Tumor	Lafferty et al. (1965)
Renal failure	Heart	Woodhouse and Burston (1969)
Tetanus	Muscle	Zacks and Sheff (1964)
Cardiac surgery	Heart	D'Agostino and Chiga (1970)
Intoxications		
Thioacetamide	Liver	Gallagher et al. (1956)
Carbon tetrachloride	Liver	Thiers et al. (1960); Carafoli and Tiozzo (1968)
Plasmocid	Heart, muscle	D'Agostino (1963)
2-Fluorocortisol and sodium phosphate	Heart	D'Agostino (1964)
Papain	Heart	Ruffolo (1964)
Isoproterenol	Heart	Bloom and Cancilla (1969)
Iodoform	Liver	Sell and Reynolds (1969)
Uranium	Kidney	Carafoli et al. (1971b)
Dietary errors		
Mg^{2+} deficiency	Heart	Heggtveit et al. (1964)
Hormonal and vitamin inbalances		
Vitamin E deficiency	Muscle	Van Vleet et al. (1968)
Excess of vitamin D	Kidney	Scarpelli (1965)
Excess of parathyroid hormone	Kidney	Caulfield and Schrag (1964)

[a] From Carafoli, 1974.

and phosphate (Malmström and Carafoli, 1977; Vallieres, et al., 1975; Gómez-Puyou et al., 1979) and since at least some of the pathological conditions listed in Table 7.7 are reversible if the injuring condition is removed, it is evident that the Ca^{2+}-buffering function of mitochondria is an essential component in the prevention of toxic cell death (see Carafoli, 1974, for discussion). Essentially, the question of cell death or survival may depend on whether the injuring condition is removed before or after the maximal capacity of mitochondria for Ca^{2+} accumulation is exceeded.

Important as it may be as a cell defense mechanism, the process of matrix loading with Ca^{2+} and phosphate has been less useful for studying the mechanism and other essential characteristics of the uptake reaction than the so-called "membrane-loading" process. During membrane loading, mitochondria accumulate limited amounts of Ca^{2+} in the absence of permeating complexing anions and do not store it semi-irreversibly in the matrix as insoluble salts. In a large series of studies on membrane loading carried out in several laboratories, the properties of the process of Ca^{2+} uptake have been documented (Table 7.8). Of particular interest among the properties listed in Table 7.8 is the affinity of the process for Ca^{2+}. The K_m of between 5 and 10 μM places mitochondria on the border of the activity range where the regulation by Ca^{2+} of some important cell processes (e.g., the contraction and relaxation of muscle) takes place and indicates that their role may be that of overall intracellular Ca^{2+} buffers rather than of fine regulators of cytosolic Ca^{2+} at very low Ca^{2+} activities. Another point worth emphasizing is the electrophoretic mechanism of the uptake reaction, which a series of studies (Rottenberg and Scarpa, 1974; Heaton and Nicholls, 1976; Crompton and Heid, 1978) has shown to occur without charge compensation. Taken together with the accepted existence of a transmembrane electrical potential, negative inside, of about 180 mV, these observations indicate that the process of Ca^{2+} uptake is essentially irreversible and operates as a one-way pump. Release of the accumulated Ca^{2+} must therefore occur, in respiring mitochondria, by a way independent of the uptake route (Carafoli and Crompton, 1976). Conclusive support for the existence of a separate route for releasing Ca^{2+} has come from the use of the inhibitor ruthenium red, which is mentioned in Table 7.8. This polycation inhibits the uptake of Ca^{2+} at very low concentrations by interacting specifically with a component that is essential for the uptake reaction (Niggli et al., 1978). Very likely, this component is a water-soluble glycoprotein which has been purified to homogeneity and shown to be involved in the uptake of Ca^{2+} some years ago (Sottocasa et al., 1972; Carafoli and Sottocasa, 1974; Prestipino et al., 1974; Panfili et al., 1976).

The Release of Ca^{2+} from Mitochondria

That ruthenium red has no inhibitory effect on the release of Ca^{2+} from respiring mitochondria was first shown by Rossi et al. (1973). This observation provided an important indication for the existence of separate Ca^{2+} uptake and release routes and has provided an essential experimental approach to the identification of the latter. Indeed, in the presence of concentrations of ruthenium red which block the uptake pathway completely, release of Ca^{2+} must of necessity occur by a separate route. So far, an independent pathway for the release of Ca^{2+} has been characterized in mitochondria from heart and a large number of other tissues (Crompton et al., 1976; Crompton et al., 1978) and shown to be mediated by a specific Na^+-Ca^{2+} exchange carrier, the characteristics of which are summarized in Table 7.9. In some tissues, however, mitochondria are Na^+-insensitive and release Ca^{2+} by a different, and still obscure, mechanism. Several compounds have been recently proposed as participants in the process of Ca^{2+} release from mitochondria that are Na^+-insensitive (e.g., liver, kidney). Phosphate (Wehrle and Pedersen, 1979; Lötscher et al., 1979) has been shown to induce uptake of Ca^{2+} because liver submitochondrial particles have an inverted membrane polarity. This system should correspond to the release of Ca^{2+} in intact mitochondria, and it has been proposed (Lötscher et al., 1979a) that phosphate could be transported out of mitochondria electrophoretically, thus triggering the release of Ca^{2+} for reasons of charge compensation.

In kidney mitochondria (Roman et al., 1979), it has been shown that a rapid Ca^{2+} release can be induced by polyunsaturated fatty acids. It has been known for a long time that fatty acids may act as uncouplers of oxidative phosphorylation, but in the observations by Roman et al. (1979), they act as concentrations which are below the minimal ones required to uncouple. Also interesting, in view of the previously mentioned effect of Na^+ in re-

Table 7.8
The Energy-Linked Uptake of Ca^{2+} by Mitochondria[a]

Requirements	An energy source (respiration of ATP)
Inhibited by (indirectly)	Inhibitors of energy conservation
Inhibited by (directly)	Lanthanides, ruthenium, red, Mg^{2+}
Total capacity	100–150 nmoles Ca^{2+}/mg protein (without phosphate), up to 3 μmoles Ca^{2+}/mg protein (with phosphate)
Rate	3–10 nmoles Ca^{2+}/mg protein/sec
K_m	About 10 μM
Mechanism	Electrophoretic, charge uncompensated

[a] From Carafoli and Crompton, 1978.

Table 7.9
General Properties of the Na^+-Induced Release of Ca^{2+}

Monovalent cation specificity	In addition to Na^+, Li^+ has some releasing effects; K^+, Rb^+, Cs^+, no effect
K_m (Na^+)	About 8 mM
K_m (Ca^{2+}, from outside)	About 13 μM
Kinetics	Strongly sigmoidal
V_{max}	About 0.2 nmoles/Ca^{2+}/mg protein/sec
Inhibited by	La^{3+} (at high concentrations)
Present in mitochondria from	Heart, brain, skeletal muscle, exocrine and endocrine tissues
Absent in mitochondria from	Liver, kidney, lung

[a] From Carafoli and Crompton, 1978.

leasing Ca^{2+} from some mitochondrial types, is the fact that the Ca^{2+}-releasing effect of polyunsaturated fatty acids is inhibited by Na^+. As to the mechanism by which fatty acids induce Ca^{2+} release, two possibilities can be considered: either a direct ionophoric effect, or an increase in the permeability of the inner membrane mediated by an increased fluidity of its phospholipid phase. Lehninger and associates (1978) have recently observed that the redox ratio of mitochondrial pyridine nucleotides has a profound influence on the maintenance of Ca^{2+}, conditions that lead to an increase in oxidation resulting in its release. The mechanism by which the redox ratio of mitochondrial pyridine nucleotides may control the Ca^{2+} maintenance is obscure. Lötscher et al. (1980) have found that the leakage of Ca^{2+} induced by conditions that lead to the oxidation of pyridine nucleotides is accompanied by the loss of nicotinamide from mitochondria.

CONTROL AND REGULATION OF Ca^{2+} TRANSPORT ACROSS THE PLASMA AND THE INTRACELLULAR MEMBRANES

That the traffic of Ca^{2+} across the various cellular membranes must be precisely regulated is an obvious conclusion from the data discussed in the preceding sections. The information available on this subject, however, is fragmentary and incomplete, so it is impossible at the present stage to extract a logical pattern from it or to present a reasonable generalized model.

The effect of vitamin D in mediating the influx of Ca^{2+} into the cells of intestinal mucosa, and in other epithelial cells, has been mentioned already, but it must be emphasized again here that no clues are available at the moment as to the possible mechanism by which vitamin D exerts its function. As mentioned, calcitonin and parathormone (Borle, 1970, 1975) have also been suggested as playing a role in the transfer of Ca^{2+} across the plasma membrane; the former has been claimed to stimulate the efflux of Ca^{2+} (Parkinson and Radde, 1971). Also in these cases, however, no clues as to the possible mechanism of action are available. That catecholamines and cAMP increase the permeability of cells to Ca^{2+} is a widely held notion which has been experimentally demonstrated in some cases (Reuter, 1965; Wollenberger et al., 1975). One recent and potentially very important observation is the stimulation by calmodulin of the outwardly directed Ca^{2+}-pumping ATPase of the plasma membrane (Gopinath and Vincenzi, 1977; Jarrett and Penniston, 1978). This type of work has now been extended to include some molecular aspects of the interaction between the ATPase and calmodulin, and it is likely to lead to the development of important concepts in terms of regulation of the Ca^{2+} fluxes in and out of cells.

At the level of intracellular organelles, the problem of the regulation of the fluxes of Ca^{2+} is even more obscure. Since mitochondria represent the most abundant membrane system in most cells (see Table 7.3), it is logical to suggest that they will be important targets for natural control mechanisms. However, the type of fine and rapid regulation normally provided by hormones or similar substances, so far, has not been demonstrated in mitochondria. Situations have been described where the ability of mitochondria to transport Ca^{2+} can be altered by hormonal influences, but the effects are of the long-term type and are probably indirect. Among the hormones that have been shown to influence the Ca^{2+} transporting system of mitochondria are steroids (Kimberg and Goldstein, 1966, 1967; Kimura and Rasmussen, 1977), insulin, and glucagon (Dorman et al., 1975; Yamazaki, 1975; Hughes and Barritt, 1977). Reports of a direct and rapid stimulatory effect of cAMP on the release of Ca^{2+} from mitochondria (Borle, 1975; Matlib and O'Brien 1974) have lately been discounted (Scarpa et al., 1976). Worth mentioning is the finding that calmodulin may have no effect on either the uptake or release of Ca^{2+} from mitochondria (Malmström and Carafoli, unpublished data). This however needs further study. Probably, the short-term regulation of the Ca^{2+} balance in mitochondria is achieved kinetically and rests on the level of cytosolic Ca^{2+}, which is affected by the activity of the plasma membrane-transporting systems, and on the levels of intramitochondrial Ca^{2+}. The uptake and release legs of the previously mentioned Ca^{2+} cycle will be differently privileged depending on the activity of Ca^{2+} at the two faces of the inner membrane. Cytosolic Mg^{2+}, however, may also play a role, since it inhibits quite substantially the electrophoretic influx of Ca^{2+} (Jacobus et al., 1975; Sordahl, 1974; Åkerman, 1977).

One possibility that may be considered, at least in cells that possess Na^+-sensitive mitochondria, is the integration of the Na^+ fluxes across the plasma membrane (e.g., during action potentials) with the release of Ca^{2+} from mitochondria. One could envisage a situation where the increased penetration of Na^+ from the environment would trigger the Na^+-dependent Ca^{2+}-releasing mechanism in mitochondria. This could in turn trigger, or take part in the triggering of, Ca^{2+}-dependent reactions like muscle contraction or secretion. It is of interest in this context that the release of the neurotransmitter (Rahamimoff et al., 1978) and the secretion of insulin (Lowe et al., 1976) can be induced by the penetration of Na^+ into nerve endings and β-Langherans cells.

The regulation of the transport of Ca^{2+} in SR by a cAMP-dependent phosphorylation process has already been mentioned. Considering the great interest presently focused on calmodulin research, the previously mentioned observations of a stimulation of the transport of Ca^{2+} in SR of heart and other muscles by calmodulin deserve to be emphasized again.

CALMODULIN IN THE INTRACELLULAR TRANSMISSION AND TRANSLATION OF THE Ca^{2+} MESSAGE

Calmodulin has been mentioned repeatedly in the preceding sections of this article, and it has been emphasized that calmodulin research is in a phase of explosive growth. In view of this and of the obvious implications of calmodulin in many aspects of the field of Ca^{2+}-directed metabolic regulation, its chemical and biochemical properties will be reviewed here in some detail (see Cheung, 1980, for a recent review).

The protein was discovered by Cheung (1967) during studies of the activation of phosphodiesterase and is now known to be present in all eukaryotes examined (Cheung, 1980). It has a MW of 16,700 and is thermostable and acidic, since about 30% of its amino acids consist of asparatate and glutamate. It contains no cysteine or tryptophan but does contain the unusual amino acid trimethyllysine at position 115. Its complete amino acid sequence has been determined (Watterson et al., 1980) and is shown in Figure 7.1.

Calmodulin contains four Ca^{2+}-binding sites, with dissociation constants ranging from 4 to 18 μM (Lin et al., 1974). Of interest is the observation that the binding of Ca^{2+} induces conformational changes in the molecule (Richman and Klee, 1979; Krebs and Carafoli, unpublished data). Calmodulin can be subdivided into four domains having a homologous sequence. This is particularly evident if one compares domains 1 (residues 8–40) and 3 (residues 81–113), and domains 2 (residues 44–76) and 4 (residues 117–148) (Fig. 7.2). The homologies of calmodulin with two other Ca^{2+}-binding proteins,

parvalbumin and troponin C, are impressive. The crystal structure of parvalbumin is known, and on its basis, Kretsinger and Barry (1975) have identified in its domains the putative Ca^{2+}-binding sites. On the basis of the extensive amino acid homologies, they have also predicted the three-dimensional structure of troponin C and identified its putative Ca^{2+}-binding sites. By analogy, it is now possible to assign tentatively the residues that bind Ca^{2+} in the calmodulin sequence (Cheung, 1980). They are indicated with an *asterisk* in Figure 7.2.

As mentioned, the first enzyme shown to be activated by calmodulin was phosphodiesterase. In the course of the years, phosphodiesterase was followed by adenylate cyclase and then by many other enzymes and cellular processes (see Cheung, 1980). To date, the activities known to be influenced by calmodulin are more than a dozen, as can be seen in Figure 7.3. It is of interest that calmodulin seems to interact differently with different target activities, as evidenced by the fact that in some cases it can be easily dissociated from the enzyme by chelating agents (Niggli et al., 1979b), whereas in other cases it appears to be more tightly bound. Of particular interest is the case of phosphorylase b kinase (Cohen et al., 1978), which in its active form is a hexadecamer consisting of 5α, 4β, 4γ, and 4δ subunits. Calmodulin appears to be the δ subunit, and remains bound to the holoenzyme throughout the purification procedure. In

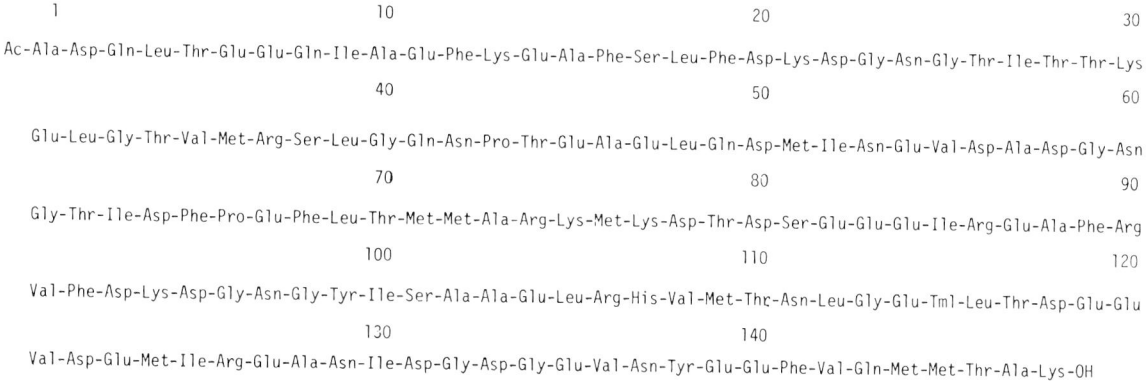

```
                   1                                 10                                    20                                    30
Ac-Ala-Asp-Gln-Leu-Thr-Glu-Glu-Gln-Ile-Ala-Glu-Phe-Lys-Glu-Ala-Phe-Ser-Leu-Phe-Asp-Lys-Asp-Gly-Asn-Gly-Thr-Ile-Thr-Thr-Lys
                                                    40                                    50                                    60
Glu-Leu-Gly-Thr-Val-Met-Arg-Ser-Leu-Gly-Gln-Asn-Pro-Thr-Glu-Ala-Glu-Leu-Gln-Asp-Met-Ile-Asn-Glu-Val-Asp-Ala-Asp-Gly-Asn
                                                    70                                    80                                    90
Gly-Thr-Ile-Asp-Phe-Pro-Glu-Phe-Leu-Thr-Met-Met-Ala-Arg-Lys-Met-Lys-Asp-Thr-Asp-Ser-Glu-Glu-Glu-Ile-Arg-Glu-Ala-Phe-Arg
                                                   100                                   110                                   120
Val-Phe-Asp-Lys-Asp-Gly-Asn-Gly-Tyr-Ile-Ser-Ala-Ala-Glu-Leu-Arg-His-Val-Met-Thr-Asn-Leu-Gly-Glu-Tml-Leu-Thr-Asp-Glu-Glu
                                                   130                                   140
Val-Asp-Glu-Met-Ile-Arg-Glu-Ala-Asn-Ile-Asp-Gly-Asp-Gly-Glu-Val-Asn-Tyr-Glu-Glu-Phe-Val-Gln-Met-Met-Thr-Ala-Lys-OH
```

Figure 7.1. Amino acid sequence of bovine brain calmodulin. (Reprinted with permission from W. Y. Cheung: Science 207:19–27, 1980.)

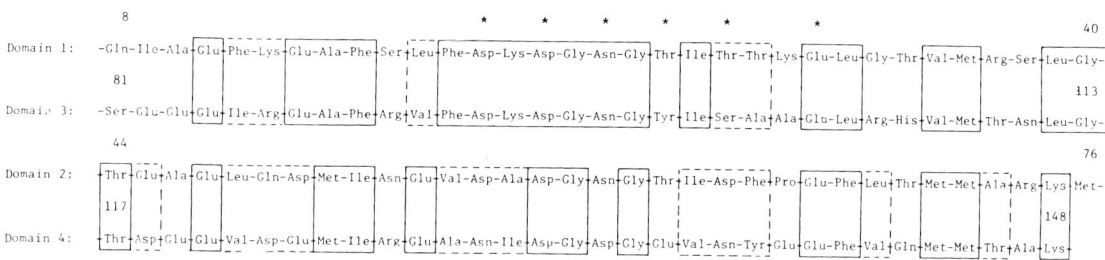

Figure 7.2. Internal sequence homology in calmodulin. (Reprinted with permission from W. Y. Cheung: Science 207:19–27, 1980.)

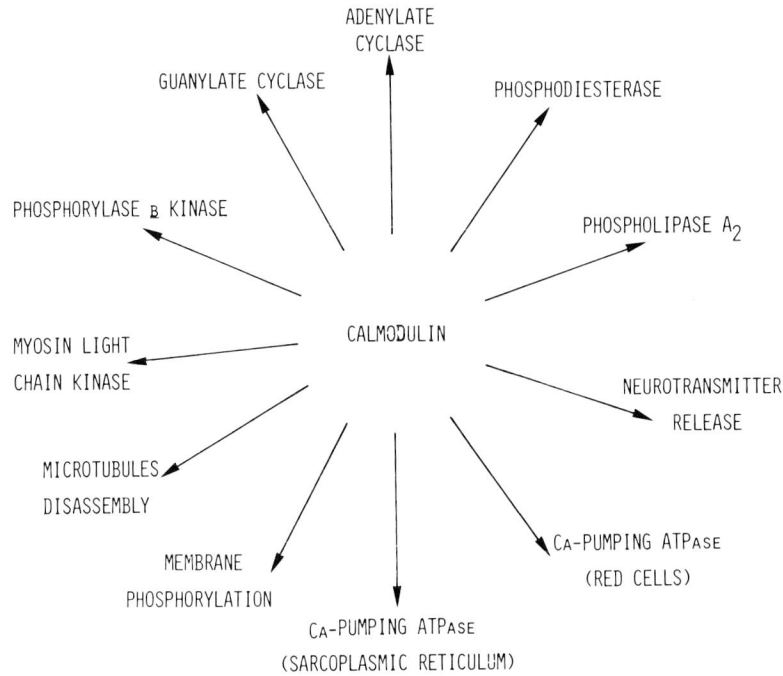

Figure 7.3. Calmodulin-regulated enzymes or cellular processes. (From Cheung, 1980, slightly modified.)

general, it is assumed that calmodulin per se is inactive, its active form being the calmodulin-Ca^{2+} complex, which binds reversibly to the target enzyme.

CONCLUSIONS

One important feature of the metabolic regulation by Ca^{2+} is that it occurs in a very low (around μM), and frequently very narrow, activity range. This underscores once again the necessity of controlling the cytosolic Ca^{2+} concentration efficiently and precisely and rationalizes the existence of the above described multiplicity of Ca^{2+} transporting and complexing systems. The role of non-membranous ligands in controlling the Ca^{2+} activity in the cytosol has not been considered in detail in this paper, since it is not easy to imagine their response to Ca^{2+}-related regulation signals. However, the work on calmodulin and its presence often in large amounts in all eukaryotic cytoplasms has indicated that soluble ligands may play an important role as transient reservoirs for cellular Ca^{2+}. How they may bind or release Ca^{2+} in synchrony with regulation demands will predictably be the subject of intensive research in the future.

It is perhaps surprising that the unique role of Ca^{2+} as a biological regulator, already indicated very clearly by the observations of Ringer of almost a century ago, has been fully appreciated only in relatively recent times. The reasons for this may be manifold, but the result has been the maintenance of this exceptionally important field in a state of hibernation well into the modern area of research in metabolic regulation. That the period of hybernation is over should have become clear from the data and the discussions presented in this paper. It is a safe prediction that the field is now on its way to becoming one of the most exciting in modern biology.

References

Åkerman, K.E.O.: Effect of Mg^{2+} and spermine on the kinetics of Ca^{2+}-transport in rat-liver mitochondria. J. Bioenerg. Biomembr. 9:65–72, 1977.

Alonso, G.L., Bazerque, P.M., Arrigo, D.M., and Tumiliasci, O.R.: Adenosine triphosphate-dependent calcium uptake by rat submaxillary gland microsomes. J. Gen. Physiol. 58:340–350, 1971.

Azzi, A., Sorgato, C.M., and Montecucco, C.: Effect of calcium ions on the interaction between cytochrome c and the mitochondrial membrane. In *Calcium Transport in Contraction and Secretion*, edited by E. Carafoli, F. Clementi, W. Drabikowski, and A. Margreth, pp. 35–44. North-Holland, Amsterdam, 1975.

Bailey, L.E., and Dresel, P. E.: Correlation of contractile force with a calcium pool in the isolated cat heart. J. Gen. Physiol. 52:969–982, 1968.

Baker, P.F.: Transport and metabolism of calcium in nerve. In *Calcium Movements in Excitable Cells*, edited by P.F. Baker and H. Reuter, pp. 7–53. Pergamon, Oxford, 1975.

Baker, P.F.: The regulation of intercellular calcium. Symp. Soc. Exp. Biol. 30:67–69, 1976.

Baker, P.F., and Glitsch, H.G.: Does metabolic energy participate directly in the sodium-dependent extrusion of calcium from squid giant axons. J. Physiol. (Lond.) 233:44, 1973.

Baker, P.F., and McNaughton, P.A.: Kinetics and energetics of calcium efflux from intact squid axons. J. Physiol. (Lond.) 259:103–144, 1976.

Baker, P.F., Hodgkin, A.L., and Ridgway, E.B.: Depolarization and calcium entry in squid axons. J. Physiol. (Lond.) 218:709–755, 1971.

Barlogie, B., Hasselbach, W., and Makinose, M.: Activation of calcium efflux by ADP and inorganic phosphate. FEBS Lett. 12:267–268, 1971.

Baskin, R.J., and Deamer, D.W.: Comparative ultrastructure and calcium transport in heart and skeletal muscle microsomes. J. Cell Biol. 43:610–617, 1969.

Besch, H.R., and Schwartz, A.: Initial calcium binding rates of canine cardiac relaxing systems (sarcoplasmic reticulum fragments) determined by stopped flow spectrophotometry. Biochem. Biophys. Res. Commun. 45:286–292, 1971.

Blaustein, M.P.: The ins and outs of calcium transport in squid axons: Internal and external ion activation of calcium efflux. Fed. Proc. 35:2574–2578, 1976.

Blaustein, M.P., Russell, J.M., and De Weer, P.: Calcium efflux from internally dialyzed squid axons: The influx of external and internal cations. J. Supramol. Struct. 2:558–581, 1974.

Blaustein, M.P., Ratzlaff, W., and Kendrick, N.K.: The regulation of intracellular calcium in presynaptic nerve terminals. Ann. N.Y. Acad. Sci. U.S.A. 307:195–211, 1978.

Bloom, S., and Cancilla, P.A.: Myocytolysis and mitochondrial calcification in rat myocardium after low doses of isoproterenol. Am. J. Pathol. 54:373–391, 1969.

Bond, G.H., and Clough, D.L.: A soluble protein activation of $(Mg^{2+} + Ca^{2+})$-dependent ATPase in human red cell membranes. Biochim. Biophys. Acta 323:592–599, 1973.

Borle, A.: Kinetic analysis of Ca^{2+} movements in cell cultures: III. Effects of Ca^{2+} and of parathyroid hormone in kidney cells. J. Gen. Physiol. 55:163–186, 1970.

Borle, A.: Regulation of cellular Ca^{2+} metabolism and Ca^{2+} transport by calcitonin. J. Membr. Biol. 21:125–146, 1975.

Brostrom, M.A., Brostrom, C.O., Breckenridge, B.M., and Wolff, D.J.: Regulation of adenylate cyclase from glial tumor cells by calcium and a calcium-binding protein. J. Biol. Chem. 251:4744–4750, 1976.

Bygrave, F.L.: Mitochondrial calcium transport. Curr. Top. Bioenerg., 6:259–318, 1977.

Carafoli, E.: Mitochondrial uptake of calcium ions and the regulation of cell function. Biochem. Soc. Symp. 39:89–109, 1974.

Carafoli, E.: Mitochondria, Ca^{2+}-transport and the regulation of heart contraction and metabolism. J. Mol. Cell. Cardiol. 7:83–89, 1975.

Carafoli, E.: The calcium cycle of mitochondria. FEBS Lett. 104:1–5, 1979.

Carafoli, E., and Crompton, M.: Calcium ions and mitochondria. Symp. Soc. Exp. Biol. 30:89–115, 1976.

Carafoli, E., and Crompton, M.: The regulation of intracellular calcium. Curr. Top. Membr. Transp. 10:151–216, 1978.

Carafoli, E., and Sottocasa, G.L.: The Ca^{2+} transport system of the mitochondrial membrane and the problem of the Ca^{2+}-carrier. In *Dynamic of Energy-Transducing Membranes*, edited by L. Ernster, R.W. Estabrook, and E.C. Slater, pp. 453–469. Elsevier, New York, 1974.

Carafoli, E., and Tiozzo, R.: A study of energy-linked calcium transport in liver mitochondria during CCl_4 intoxication. Exp. Mol. Pathol. 9:131–140, 1968.

Carafoli, E., Balcavage, W.X., Lehninger, A.L., and Mattoon, J.R.: Ca^{2+} metabolism in yeast cells and mitochondria. Biochim. Biophys. Acta 205:18–26, 1970.

Carafoli, E., Hansford, R.G., Sacktor, B., and Lehninger, A.L.: Interaction of Ca^{2+} with blowfly flight muscle mitochondria. J. Biol. Chem. 246:964–972, 1971a.

Carafoli, E., Tiozzo, R., Pasquali-Ronchetti, I., and Laschi, R.: A study of Ca^{2+} metabolism in kidney mitochondria during acute uranium intoxication. Lab. Invest. 25:516–527, 1971b.

Caroni, P., and Carafoli, E.: An ATP-dependent Ca^{2+}-pumping system in dog heart sarcolemma. Nature 283:765–767, 1980.

Caulfield, J.B., and Schrag, B.A.: Electronmicroscopic study of renal calcification. Am. J. Pathol. 44:365–380, 1964.

Cheung, W.Y.: Phosphodiesterase: Pronounced stimulation by snake venom. Biochem. Biophys. Res. Commun. 29:478–482, 1967.

Cheung, W.Y.: Calmodulin plays a pivotal role in cellular regulation. Science 207:19–27, 1980.

Chiesi, M.: Characteristics of cardiac sarcoplasmic reticulum and of its Ca^{2+}-pumping enzyme; a comparative study with fast skeletal muscle. Ph.D. Thesis. Swiss Federal Institute of Technology (ETH), Zurich, Switzerland, 1978.

Cohen, P., Burchell, A., Foulkes, J.G., Cohen, P.T.W., Vanaman, T.C., and Nairn, C.: Identification of the Ca^{2+}-dependent modulator protein as the fourth subunit of rabbit skeletal muscle phosphorylase kinase. FEBS Lett. 92:287–293, 1978.

Constantin, L.L., and Podolsky, R.J.: Depolarization of the internal membrane system in the activation of frog skeletal muscle. J. Gen. Physiol. 50:1101–1124, 1967.

Crang, R.E., Holsen, R.C., and Hitt, J.B.: Calcite production in mitochondria of earthworm calciferous glands. Am. Inst. Biol. Sci. Bull. 18:299–301, 1969.

Crompton, M., and Heid, I.: The cycling of calcium, sodium and protons across the inner membrane of cardiac mitochondria. Eur. J. Biochem. 91:599–608, 1978.

Crompton, M., Capano, M., and Carafoli, E.: The sodium induced efflux of calcium from heart mitochondria. A possible mechanism for the regulation of mitochondrial calcium. Eur. J. Biochem. 69:453–462, 1976.

Crompton, M., Moser, R., Lüdi, H., and Carafoli, E.: The interrelations between the transport of sodium and calcium in mitochondria of various mammalian tissues. Eur. J. Biochem. 82:25–31, 1978.

D'Agostino, A.N.: An electron microscopic study of skeletal and cardiac muscle of the rat poisoned by plasmocid. Lab. Invest. 12:1060–1071, 1963.

D'Agostino, A.N.: An electron microscopic study of cardiac necrosis produced by fluorocortisol and sodium phosphate. Am. J. Pathol. 45:633–645, 1964.

D'Agostino, A.N., and Chiga, M.: Mitochondrial mineralization in human myocardium. Am. J. Clin. Pathol. 53:820–824, 1970.

Davson, M.: A textbook of general physiology. Churchill, London, 1970.

Degani, C., and Boyer, P.D.: A borohydride reduction method for characterization of the acyl phosphate linkage in proteins and its application to sarcoplasmic reticulum adenosine triphosphatase. J. Biol. Chem. 248:8222–8226, 1973.

DeMeis, L., Rubin-Altschul, B.M., and Machado, R.D.: Comparative data of Ca^{2+} transport in brain and skeletal muscle microsomes. J. Biol. Chem. 245:1883–1889, 1970.

DiPolo, R.: Ca pump driven by ATP in squid axons. Nature 274:390, 1978.

DiPolo, R., Requena, J., Brinley, F.J., Mullins, L.J., Jr., Scarpa, A., and Tiffert, T.: Ionized calcium concentrations in squid axons. J. Gen. Physiol. 67:433–467, 1976.

DiPolo, R., Rojas, H.R., and Beaugé, L.A.: Vanadate inhibits uncoupled Ca efflux but not Na-Ca exchange in squid axons. Nature 281:228, 1979.

Dorman, D.M., Barritt, G.J., and Bygrave, F.L.: Stimulation of hepatic mitochondrial calcium transport by elevated plasma insulin concentrations. Biochem. J. 50:389–395, 1975.

Duggan, P.F., and Martonosi, A.: Sarcoplasmic reticulum. IX.

The permeability of sarcoplasmic reticulum membranes. J. Gen. Physiol. *56:*147–167, 1970.

Ebashi, S., and Endo, M.: Calcium ion in muscle contraction Prog. Biophys. Mol. Biol. *18:*123–183, 1968.

Endo, M., and Thorens, S.: Mechanism of release of calcium from sarcoplasmic reticulum. In *Calcium Transport in Contraction and Secretion*, edited by E. Carafoli, F. Clementi, W. Drabikowski, and A. Margreth, pp. 359–366. North-Holland, Co., Amsterdam, 1975.

Endo, M., Tanaka, M., and Ogawa, Y.: Calcium-induced release of calcium from the sarcoplasmic reticulum of skeletal muscle fibres. Nature (Lond.) *288:*34–36, 1970.

Fabiato, A., and Fabiato, F.: Contractions induced by a calcium-triggered release of calcium from the sarcoplasmic reticulum of single skinned cardiac cells. J. Physiol. (Lond.) *249:*469–495, 1975.

Fanburg, B.L., Finkel, R.M., and Martonosi, A.: The role of calcium in the mechanism of relaxation of cardiac muscle. J. Biol. Chem. *239:*2298–2306, 1964.

Felo, R.S., Bohr, D.F., and Ruegg, J.C.: Glycerinated skeletal and smooth muscle:Calcium and magnesium dependence. Science *147:*1581–1583, 1965.

Ferreira, H.G., and Lew, V.L.: Use of ionophore A23187 to measure cytoplasmic Ca^{2+} buffering and activation of the Ca^{2+} pump by internal Ca^{2+}. Nature (Lond.) *259:*47–49, 1976.

Fiehn, W., and Migala, A.: Calcium binding to sarcoplasmic membranes. Eur. J. Biochem. *20:*245–248, 1971.

Fleckenstein, A., Tritthart, H., Fleckenstein, B., Herbst, A., Grün, G.: Eine neue Gruppe kompetitiver Ca^{2+} antagonisten (roveratril, D. 600, Prenylamin) mit starken Hemmeffekten auf die elektromechanische Kopplung Warmblütermyokard. Pflüegers Arch. *397:*25–38, 1969.

Ford, L.E., and Podolsky, R.J.: Regenerative calcium release within muscle cells. Science *167:*58–59, 1970.

Ford, L.E., and Podolsky, R.J.: Calcium uptake and force development by skinned muscle fibres in EGTA buffered solution. J. Physiol. (Lond.) *223:*1–19, 1972a.

Ford, L. E., and Podolsky, R.J.: Intracellular calcium movements in skinned muscle fibers. J. Physiol. (Lond.) *223:*21–33, 1972b.

Gallagher, C.M., Gupta, D.N., Judah, J.D., and Rees, K.R.: Biochemical changes in liver in acute thioacetamide intoxication. J. Pathol. Bacteriol. *72:*193–201, 1956.

Ganong, W.F. *Review of Medical Physiology*. Lange, Los Altos, 1973.

Gietzen, K., Seiler, S., Fleischer, S., and Wolf, H.U.: Ca^{2+}-transport by reconstituted high-affinity Ca^{2+}-ATPase of human erythrocytes. In *Function and Molecular Aspects of Biomembrane Transport*, edited by E. Quagliariello, F. Palmieri, S. Papa, and M. Klingenberg, pp. 519–522. North-Holland, Co., Amsterdam, 1979.

Gitler, C., and Montal, M.: Formation of decane-soluble proteolipids: Influence of monovalent and divalent cations. FEBS Lett. *28:*329–332, 1972.

Gmaj, P., Murer, H., and Kinne, R.: Calcium ion transport across plasma membranes isolated from rat kidney cortex. Biochem. J. *178:*549–557, 1979.

Gómez-Puyou, A., Tuena de Gómez-Puyou, M., Klipp, M., and Carafoli, E.: The effect of calcium on the translocation of adenine nucleotides in rat liver mitochondria. Arch. Biochem. Biophys. *194:*399–404, 1979.

Gonzales, F., and Karnovsky, M.J.: Electron microscopy of osteoclasts in healing fractures of rat bone. J. Cell. Biol. *9:*299–361, 1961.

Gopinath, R.M., and Vincenzi, F.F.: Phosphodiesterase protein activator mimics red blood cell cytoplasmic activator of (Ca^{2+} + Mg^{2+}) ATPase. Biochem. Biophys. Res. Commun. *77:*1203–1209, 1977.

Grossmann, A., and Furchgott, R.F.: The effects of various drugs on calcium exchange in the isolated guinea-pig left muscle. J. Pharmacol. Exp. Ther. *145:*162–172, 1964.

Hagiwara, S., and Nakajima, S.: Effects of intracellular calcium ion concentration on the excitability of the muscle fibre of a barnacle. J. Gen. Physiol. *49:*807–818, 1966.

Heaton, G.M., and Nicholls, D.G.: The calcium conductance of the inner membrane of rat liver mitochondria and the determination of the calcium electrochemical gradient. Biochem. J. *156:*635–646, 1976.

Heggtveit, A.M., Herman, L., and Mishra, R.R.: Cardiac necrosis and calcification in experimental magnesium deficiency. Am. J. Pathol. *45:*757–782, 1964.

Herdson, P.B., Sommers, M.M., and Jennings, R.B.: A comparative study of the fine structure of normal and ischemic dog myocardium with special reference to early changes following temporary occlusion of a coronary artery. Am. J. Pathol. *46:*367–386, 1965.

Homan, W., and Schraer, H.: The intracellular distribution of calcium in the mucosa of the avian shell gland. J. Cell. Biol. *30:*317–331, 1966.

Hughes, B.P., and Barritt, G.J.: The effects of glucagon adrenalin, and dibutyryl adenosine 3'5, monophosphate on calcium transport in rat liver mitochondria. Proc. Aust. Biochem. Soc. *10:*36–45, 1977.

Ikemoto, N., Bhatnagar, G.M., and Gergely, J.: Fractionation of solubilized sarcoplasmic reticulum. Biochem. Biophys. Res. Commun. *44:*1510–1515, 1971.

Ikemoto, N., Bhatnagar, G.M., Nagy, B., and Gergely, J.: Interaction of divalent cations with the 55'000 dalton protein component of the sarcoplasmic reticulum. Studies of fluorescence and circular dichroism. J. Biol. Chem. *247:*7835–7837, 1972.

Inesi, G., and Scarpa, A.: Fast kinetics of adenosine triphosphate dependent Ca^{2+} uptake by fragmented sarcoplasmic reticulum. Biochemistry *11:*356–359, 1972.

Jacobus, W.E., Tiozzo, R., Lugli, G., Lehninger, A.L., and Carafoli, E.: Aspects of energy linked Ca^{2+} accumulation by rat-heart mitochondria. J. Biol. Chem. *250:*7863–7870, 1975.

Jarrett, H.W., and Penniston, J.T.: Purification of the Ca^{2+} stimulated ATPase activator from human erythrocytes. J. Biol. Chem. *253:*4676–4682, 1978.

Judah, J.D., Ahmed, K., and McLean, A.E.M.: Possible role of ion shifts in liver injury. In *Ciba Foundation Symposium on Cellular Injury*, edited by A.V.S.de Rueck and J. Knight, pp. 187–205. Churchill, London, 1964.

Jundt, H., Porzig, H., Reuter, H., and Stucki, J.W.: The effect of substances releasing intracellular calcium ions on sodium-dependent calcium efflux from guinea-pig auricles. J. Physiol. (Lond.) *246:*229–253, 1975.

Kanazawa, T., and Boyer, P.D.: Occurrence and characteristics of a rapid exchange of phosphate oxygens catalyzed by sarcoplasmic reticulum. J. Biol. Chem. *248:*3163–3172, 1973.

Katz, S., and Remtulla, M.A.: Phosphodiesterase protein activator stimulates calcium transport in cardiac microsomal preparations enriched in sarcoplasmic reticulum. Biochem. Biophys. Res. Commun. *83:*1373–1379, 1978.

Katz, A.M., Repke, E.I., Dunnett, J., and Hasselbach, W.: Dependence of calcium permeability of sarcoplasmic vesicles on external and internal ion concentrations. J. Biol. Chem. *252:*1950–1956, 1977.

Kimberg, D.V., and Goldstein, S.A.: Binding of calcium by liver mitochondria of rats treated with steroid hormones. J. Biol. Chem. *241*:95–103, 1966.

Kimberg, D.V., and Goldstein, S.A.: Binding of calcium by liver mitochondria: An effect of steroid hormones in vitamin D-depleted and parathyroidectomized rats. Endocrinology *80*:89–98, 1967.

Kimura, S., and Rasmussen, H.: Adrenal glucocorticoids, adenine nucleotide translocation and mitochondrial calcium accumulation. J. Biol. Chem. *252*:1217–1225, 1977.

Kirchberger, M.A., and Tada, M.: Effects of adenosine 3':5'-monophosphate-dependent protein kinase on sarcoplasmic reticulum isolated from cardiac and slow and fast contracting muscle. J. Biol. Chem. *251*:725–719, 1976.

Kirchberger, M.A., Tada, M., and Katz, A.M.: Adenosine 3':5'-monophosphate-dependent protein kinase catalyzed phosphorylation reaction and its relationship to calcium transport in cardiac sarcoplasmic reticulum. J. Biol. Chem. *249*:6166–6173, 1974.

Knowles, A.F., and Racker, E.: Properties of a reconstituted calcium pump. J. Biol. Chem. *250*:3538–3544, 1975.

Kohlhardt, M., Bauer, B., Krause, H., and Fleckenstein, A.: Differentiation of the transmembrane Na and Ca channels in mammalian cardiac fibres by the use of specific inhibitors. Pflüegers Arch. *355*:309–322, 1972.

Kostyuk, P.G., and Krishtal, O.A.: Ionic and gating currents in the membrane of nerve cells. In *Membrane Transport Process*, edited by D.C. Tosteson, Yu.A. Ovchinnikov, and R. Latorre, vol. 2, pp. 101–123. Raven Press, New York. 1978.

Krebs, J.J.R., Hauser, H., and Carafoli, E.: Asymmetric distribution of phospholipids in the inner membrane of beef heart mitochondria. J. Biol. Chem. *254*:5308–5316, 1979.

Kretsinger, R.H.: Evolution of the formational role of calcium in eukaryotes. In *Calcium Binding Proteins and Calcium Functions*, edited by R.H. Wasserman, R.A., Corradino, E. Carafoli, R.H. Kretsinger, D.H. MacLennan, and F.L. Sigel, pp. 63–72. North-Holland, Amsterdam, 1977.

Kretsinger, R.H., and Barry, C.D.: The predicted structure of the calcium-binding component of troponin. Biochem. Biophys. Acta *405*:40–52, 1975.

Kretsinger, R.H., and Nelson, D.J.: Calcium in biological systems. Coordination Chemistry Reviews *18*:29–124, 1976.

Lafferty, F.W., and Reynolds, E.S., and Pearson, O.H.: Tumoral calcinosis. A metabolic disease of obscure etiology. Am. J. Med. *38*:105–117, 1965.

Lamb, J.F., and Lindsay, R.: Effect on Na, metabolic inhibitors and ATP on Ca movements in L cells. J. Physiol. (Lond.) *218*:691–708, 1971.

Legato, M.J., Spiro, D., and Langer, G.A.: Ultastructural alterations produced in mammalian myocardium by variation in perfusate ionic composition. J. Cell. Biol. *37*:1–12, 1968.

Lehninger, A.L., Rossi, C.S., and Carafoli, E.: Energy linked ion-movements in mitochondrial systems. Adv. Enzymol. *29*:259–320, 1967.

Lehninger, A.L., Vercesi, A., and Bababunmi, E.A.: Regulation of Ca^{2+} release from mitochondria by the oxidation-reduction state of pyridine nucleotides. Proc. Natl. Acad. Sci. U.S.A. *79*:1690–1694, 1978.

Le Peuch, C.J., Maiech, J., and Demaille, J.G.: Concerted regulation of cardiac sarcoplasmic reticulum calcium transport by cardiac adenosine monophosphate dependent and calcium calmodulin-dependent phosphorylation. Biochemistry *18*:5150–5157, 1979.

Lin, Y.M., Liu, Y.P., and Cheung, W.Y.: Cyclic 3':5'-Nucleotide phosphodiesterase:Purification, characterization and active form of the protein activator from bovine brain. J. Biol. Chem. *249*:4943–4954, 1974.

Lötscher, H.R., Schwerzmann, K., and Carafoli, E.: The transport of Ca^{2+} in a purified population of inside-out vesicles from rat liver mitochondria. FEBS Lett. *99*:194–198, 1979a.

Lötscher, H.R., Winterhalter, K.H., Carafoli, E., and Richter, C.: Hydroperoxides can modulate the redox state of pyridine nucleotides and the calcium balance in rat liver mitochondria. Proc. Natl. Acad. Sci. U.S.A. *76*:4340–4344, 1979b.

Lötscher, H.R., Winterhalter, K.H., Carafoli, E., and Richter, C.: Hydroperoxide-induced loss of pyridine nucleotides and release of calcium from rat liver mitochondria. J. Biol. Chem. *255*:9325–9330, 1980.

Lowe, D.A., Richardson, B.P., Taylor, P., and Donatsch, P.: Increasing intracellular sodium triggers calcium release from bound pools. Nature *260*:337–338, 1976.

Luthra, M.G., Hildenbrandt, G.R., and Hanahan, D.J.: Studies on an activator of the ($Ca^{2+} + Mg^{2+}$)-ATPase of human erythrocyte membrane. Biochim. Biophys. Acta *419*:164–179, 1976.

Makinose, M.: Possible functional states of the enzyme of the sarcoplasmic calcium pump. FEBS Lett. *37*:140–143, 1973.

Malmström, K., and Carafoli, E.: The interaction of Ca^{2+} with mitochondria from human myomerium. Arch. Biochem. Biophys. *182*:657–666, 1977.

Manery, J.F.: Effects of Ca ions on membranes. Fed. Proc. *25*:1804–1810, 1966.

Martin, J.H., and Matthews, J.L.: Mitochondrial granules in chondrocytes. Calcif. Tissue Res. *3*:184–193, 1969.

Martonosi, A.: Sarcoplasmic reticulum. IV. Solubilization of microsomal adenosine triphosphatase. J. Biol. Chem. *243*:71–81, 1968.

Martonosi, A.: The mechanism of calcium transport in sarcoplasmic reticulum. In *Calcium Tranport in Contraction and Secretion*, edited by E. Carafoli E. Clementi, W. Drabikowski, and A. Margreth, pp. 313–327. North-Holland, Amsterdam, 1975.

Martonosi, A., and Feretos, R.: Sarcoplasmic reticulum. I. The uptake of Ca^{2+} by sarcoplasmic reticulum fragments. J. Biol. Chem. *239*:648–658, 1964.

Matlib, A., and O'Brien, J.P.: Adenosine 3':5'-cyclic monophosphate stimulation of calcium efflux. Biochem. Soc. Trans. *2*:997, 1974.

McLennan, D.H.: Purification and properties of an adenosine triphosphatase from sarcoplasmic reticulum. J. Biol. Chem. *245*:4508–4518, 1970.

McLennan, D.H., and Wong, P.T.S.: Isolation of a calcium-sequestering protein from the sarcoplasmic reticulum. Proc. Natl. Acad. Sci. U.S.A. *68*:1231–1235, 1971.

Meech, R.W., and Standen, N.B.: Potassium activation in Helix aspersa neurones under voltage-clamp. J. Physiol. (Lond.) *249*:211–239, 1975.

Meissner, G.: Isolation and characterization of two types of sarcoplasmic reticulum vesicles. Biochim. Biophys. Acta *389*:51–68, 1975.

Meissner, G., and McKinley, D.: Permeability of sarcoplasmic reticulum membrane. The effect of changed ionic environments of Ca^{2+} release. J. Membr. Biol. *30*:79–80, 1976.

Meissner, G., Conner, G.E., and Fleischer, S.: Isolation of sarcoplasmic reticulum by zonal centrifugation and purification of Ca^{2+} pump and Ca^{2+}-binding proteins. Biochim. Biophys. Acta *298*:246–269, 1973.

Moore, L., Fitzpatrick, D.F., Chen, T.S., and London, E.J.: Calcium pump activity of the renal plasma membrane and renal microsomes. Biochim. Biophys. Acta 345:405–418, 1974.

Moore, L., Chen, T.S., Knapp, H.P., and Landon, E.J.: Energy-dependent calcium sequestration activity in rat liver microsomes. J. Biol. Chem. 250:4562–4568, 1975.

Mullins, L. J.: Steady state calcium fluxes: Membrane versus mitochondrial control of ionized calcium in axoplasm. Fed. Proc. 35:2583–2588, 1976.

Mullins, L. J., and Brinley, F.J.: Sensitivity of calcium efflux from squid axons to change in membrane potential. J. Gen. Physiol. 65:135–152, 1975.

Nakajima, Y., and Endo, M.: Release of calcium by depolarization of the sarcoplasmic reticulum membrane. Nature 246:216–218, 1973.

Niggli, V., Gazzotti, P., and Carafoli, E.: Experiments on the mechanism of the inhibition of mitochondrial Ca^{2+} transport by La^{3+} and ruthenium red. Experientia 34:1136–1137, 1978.

Niggli, V., Penniston, J. T., and Carafoli, E.: Purification of the Ca^{2+}, Mg^{2+} ATPase from human erythrocyte membranes using a calmodulin affinity column. J. Biol. Chem. 254:9955–9958, 1979a.

Niggli, V., Ronner, P., Carafoli, E., and Penniston, J.T.: Effects of calmodulin on the ($Ca^{2+} + Mg^{2+}$)-ATPase partially purified from erythrocyte membranes. Arch. Biochem. Biophys. 198:124–130, 1979b.

Niggli, V., Adunyah, E. S., Penniston, J.T., and Carafoli, E.: Purified (Ca^{2+}-Mg^{2+})-ATPase of the erythrocyte membrane. Reconstitution and effect of calmodulin and phospholipids. J. Biol. Chem. 256:395–401, 1981.

Ostwald, T.J., McLennan, D. H., and Dorrington, K.H.: Effects of cation-binding on the conformation and the high affinity calcium-binding proteins of sarcoplasmic reticulum. J. Biol. Chem. 249:5867–5871, 1974.

O'Sullivan, W.J., and Perrin, D.D.: The stability constants of metal-adenine nucleotide complexes. Biochemistry 3:18–26, 1964.

Otsuka, M., Ohtsuki, I., and Ebashi, S.: ATP-dependent Ca-binding of brain microsomes. J. Biochem. (Tokyo) 58:183–190, 1965.

Panfili, E., Sandri, G., Sottocasa, G.L., Lunazzi, G., Liut, G., and Graziosi, G.: Specific inhibition of mitochondrial Ca^{2+}-binding glycoprotein. Nature 264:185–186, 1976.

Parkinson, D.K., and Radde, I.C.: Properties of a Ca^{2+}- and Mg^{2+}-activated ATP-hydrolyzing enzyme in rat kidney cortex. In Cellular Mechanism for Calcium Homeostasis, edited by G. Nicholls, Jr. and R.H. Wasserman, pp. 506–511. Academic Press, New York, 1971.

Peachey, L.D.: Electron microscopic observations on the accumulation of divalent cations in intramitochondrial granules. J. Cell Biol. 20:95–111, 1964.

Peterson, S.W., Ronner, P., and Carafoli, E.: Partial purification and reconstitution of the ($Ca^{2+} + Mg^{2+}$)-ATPase of erythrocyte membranes. Arch. Biochem. Biophys. 186:202–210, 1978.

Pfleger, H., and Wolf, H.U.: Activation of membrane-bound high affinity calcium ion-sensitive adenosine triphosphatase of human erythrocytes by divalent metal ions. Biochem. J. 147:359–361, 1975.

Pitts, B.J.R.: Stoichiometry of sodium-calcium exchange in cardiac sarcolemmal vesicle. J. Biol. Chem. 254:6232–6235, 1979.

Portzehl, M., Caldwell, P.C., and Rüegg, J.C.: The dependence of contraction and relaxation of muscle fibers of the crab Maia squinado on the internal concentrations of free calcium ions. Biochim. Biophys. Acta 74:581–591, 1964.

Prestipino, G., Ceccarelli, D., Conti, F., and Carafoli, E.: Interactions of a mitochondrial Ca^{2+}-binding glycoprotein with lipid bilayer membranes. FEBS Lett. 45:99–103, 1974.

Quist, E.E., and Roufogalis, B.P.: Determination of the stoichiometry of the calcium pump in human erythrocytes lanthanum as a selective inhibitor. FEBS Lett. 50:135–139, 1975.

Racker, E.: Reconstitution of a calcium pump with phospholipids and a purified Ca^{2+} adenosine triphosphatase from sarcoplasmic reticulum. J. Biol. Chem. 247:8198–8200, 1972.

Rahamimoff, R., Meiri, H., Erulkar, S.D., and Barenholz, Y.: Changes in transmitter release induced by ion-containing liposomes. Proc. Natl. Acad. Sci. U.S.A. 75:5214–5216, 1978.

Rasmussen, H.: Cell communication, calcium ion, and cyclic adenosine monophosphate. Science 170:404–411, 1970.

Rasmussen, H., Goodman, D.B.P., and Tenenhouse, A.: The role of cAMP and calcium in cell activation. C.R.C. Crit. Rev. Biochem. 1:95–148, 1972.

Reeves, J.P., and Sutko, J.L.: Sodium-calcium exchange in cardiac membrane vesicles. Proc. Natl. Acad. Sci. U.S.A. 76:590–594, 1979.

Reith, A., Barnard, T., and Rohr, H.P.: Sterology of cellular reaction patterns. C.R.C. Crit. Rev. Toxicol. 4:219–169, 1976.

Reuter, H.: Ueber die Wirkung von Adrenalin auf den Cellulären Ca-Umsatz des Meerschweinchenvorhofs. Naunyn-Schmiedebergs Arch. Exp. Pathol. Pharmacol. 251:401–412, 1965.

Reuter, H.: Exchange of calcium ions in the mammalian myocardium. Mechanism and physiological significance. Circ. Res. 34:399–605, 1974.

Rich, T.L., and Langer, G.A.: A comparison of excitation contraction coupling in heart and skeletal muscle: An examination of "calcium induced calcium release." J. Mol. Cell Cardiol. 7:747–765, 1975.

Richman, P.G., and Klee, C.B.: Specific perturbation by Ca^{2+} of tyrosyl residue 138 of calmodulin. J. Biol. Chem. 254:5372–5376, 1979.

Ridgway, E.B., and Durham, A.C.H.: Oscillation of calcium concentration in physarum polycepharum. J. Cell. Biol. 69:223–226, 1976.

Ringer, S.: Regarding the action of hydrate of soda, hydrate of ammonia, and hydrate of potassium on the ventricle of the frog's heart. J. Physiol. 3:195–202, 1883.

Robblee, L.S., Shepro, D., and Belamarich, F.A.: Calcium uptake and associated ATPase activity of isolated platelets membranes. J. Gen. Physiol. 61:462–481, 1973.

Robinson, J.D., and Lust, W.D.: Adenosine triphosphate dependent calcium accumulation by brain microsomes. Arch. Biochem. Biophys. 125:286–294, 1968.

Roman, I., Gmaj, P., Nowicka, C., and Angielski, S.: Regulation of Ca^{2+} efflux from kidney and liver mitochondria by unsaturated fatty acids and Na^+ ions. Eur. J. Biochem. 102:615–623, 1979.

Rose, B., and Loewenstein, W.R.: Permeability of a cell junction and the local cytoplasmic fee ionized calcium concentration. A study with aequorin. J. Membr. Biol. 28:87–119, 1976.

Rossi, C.S., Vasington, F.D., and Carafoli, E.: The effects of ruthenium red on the uptake and release of Ca^{2+} by mitochondria. Biochem. Biophys. Res. Commun. 50:846–852, 1973.

Rottenberg, H., and Scarpa, A.: Calcium uptake and membrane potential in mitochondria. Biochemistry 13:4811–4819, 1974.

Ruffolo, P.R.: The pathogenesis of necrosis. I. Correlated light and electron microscopic observations of the myocardial necrosis induced by the intravenous injection of papain. Am. J. Pathol. *45:*741–749, 1964.

Sarkadi, B., Szász, I., Gerlóczy, A., and Gárdos, G.: Transport parameters and stoichiometry of active calcium ions extrusion in intact human red cells. Biochem. Biophys. Acta *464:* 92–107, 1977.

Scarpa, A., and Graziotti, P.: Mechanism for intracellular calcium regulation in heart. J. Gen. Physiol. *62:*756–772, 1973.

Scarpa, A., Malmström, K., Chiesi, M., and Carafoli, E.: On the problem of the release of mitochondrial calcium by cyclic AMP. J. Membr. Biol. *29:*205–208, 1976.

Scarpelli, D.G.: Experimental nephrocalcinosis. A biochemical and morphological study. Lab. Invest. *14:*123–141, 1965.

Schanne, F.A.X., Kane, A.B., Young, E.E., and Farber, J.L.: Calcium dependence of toxic cell death: a final common pathway. Science *209:*700–702, 1979.

Scharff, O.: Ca^{2+} activation of membrane-bound (Ca^{2+} + Mg^{2+})-dependent ATPase from human erythrocytes prepared in the presence or absence of Ca^{2+}. Biochim. Biophys. Acta *443:*206–218, 1976.

Schatzmann, H.J.: Dependence on Ca^{2+} concentration and stoichiometry of the Ca^{2+} pump in human red cells. J. Physiol. (Lond.) *235:*551–569, 1973.

Schatzmann, H.J.: Active calcium transport and Ca^{2+}-activated ATPase in human red cells. Curr. Top. Membr. Transp. *6:* 126–168, 1975.

Schatzmann, H.J., and Vincenzi, F.F.: Ca^{2+} movements across the membrane of human red cells. J. Physiol. (Lond.) *201:* 369–395, 1969.

Schwartz, A., Entman, M.L., Kaniike, K., and Bornet, E.: Phosphorylase *b* kinase and c-AMP-dependent protein kinase effects on sarcoplasmic reticulum: Cardiac, fast and slow skeletal muscle (abstract). Fed. Proc. *33:*1583, 1974.

Schwartz, A., Entman, M.L., Kaniike, K., Lane, L.K., van Winkle, W.B., and Bornet, E.P.: The rate of calcium uptake into sarcoplasmic reticulum of cardiac muscle and skeletal muscle. Effects of cyclic AMP-dependent protein kinase and phosphorylase *b* kinase. Biochim. Biophys. Acta *426:*57–72, 1976.

Selinger, Z., Nains, E., and Lasser, M.: ATP-dependent calcium uptake by microsomal preparations from rat parotid and submaximillary glands. Biochim. Biophys. Acta *203:*326–334, 1970.

Sell, D.A., and Reynolds, E.S.: Liver parenchymal cell injury VIII. Lesions of membranous cellular components following iodoform. J. Cell. Biol. *41:*736–752, 1969.

Shamoo, A., and Goldstein, D.A.: Isolation of ionophores from ion transport systems and their role in energy transduction. Biochim. Biophys. Acta *472:*13–53, 1977.

Shine, K.I., Serena, S.P., and Langer, G.A.: Kinetic localization of contractile calcium in rabbit myocardium. Am. J. Physiol. *221:*1408–1417, 1971.

Solaro, R.J., and Briggs, F.N.: Estimating the functional capabilities of sarcoplasmic reticulum in cardiac muscle. Circ. Res. *34:*531–540, 1974.

Solaro, R.J., Wise, R.M., Shiner, J.S., and Briggs, E.N.: Calcium requirements for cardiac myofibrillar activation. Circ. Res. *34:*525–530, 1974.

Sordahl, L.A.: Effects of magnesium, ruthenium red and the antibiotic ionophore A23187 on initial rates of calcium uptake and release by heart mitochondria. Arch. Biochem. Biophys. *167:*104–115, 1974.

Sottocasa, C.L., Sandri, G., Panfili, E., de Bernard, B., Gazzotti, P., Vasington, F., and Carafoli, E.: Isolation of a soluble Ca^{2+} binding glycoprotein from ox liver mitochondria. Biochem. Biophys. Res. Commun. *47:*808–813, 1972.

Sreter, F.A.: Temperature, pH and seasonal dependence of Ca^{2+}-uptake and ATPase activity of white and red muscle microsomes. Arch. Biochem. Biophys. *134:*25–33, 1969.

Suko, J., and Hasselbach, W.: Characterization of cardiac sarcoplasmic reticulum ATP-ADP phosphate exchange and phosphorylation of the calcium transport adenosine triphosphatase. Eur. J. Biochem. *64:*123–130, 1976.

Tada, M., Kirchberger, M.A., Repke, D.I., Katz, A.M.: The stimulation of calcium transport in cardiac sarcoplasmic reticulum by adenosine 3',5'-monophosphate-dependent protein kinase. J. Biol. Chem. *249:*6174–6180, 1974.

Tada, M., Kirchberger, M.A., and Katz, A.M.: Phosphorylation of a 22,000 dalton component of the cardiac sarcoplasmic reticulum by adenosine 3':5'-monophosphate-dependent protein kinase. J. Biol. Chem. *250:*2640–2647, 1975a.

Tada, M., Kirchberber, M.A., Li, H.C., and Katz, A.M.: Interrelationship between calcium and cyclic AMP in the mammalian heart. In *Calcium Transport in Contraction and Secretion,* edited by E. Carafoli, F. Clementi, W. Drabikowski, and A. Margreth, pp. 373–382. North-Holland, Amsterdam, 1975b.

Taylor, A., Eich, E., and Pearl, M.: Cytosolic calcium and action of vasopressin in toad bladder. In *Proceedings of the International Union of Physiological Sciences,* edited by Pitié-Salpetriére, vol. XIII, abstract 2217. Paris, 1978.

Teo, T.S., and Wang, J.H.: Mechanism of activation of a cyclic adenosine 3':5'-monophosphate phosphodiesterase from bovine heart by calcium ions. Identification of the protein activator as Ca^{2+} binding protein. J. Biol. Chem. *248:*5950–5955, 1973.

Terepka, A.R., Coleman, J.R., Armbrecht, H.J., and Gunter, T.E.: Transcellular transport of calcium. Symp. Soc. Exp. Biol. *30:*117–140, 1976.

Thiers, R.E., Reynolds, E.S., and Vallee, B.L.: The effect of carbon tetrachloride poisoning on subcellular metal distribution in rat liver. J. Biol. Chem. *235:*2130–2133, 1960.

Träuble, H., and Eibl, H.: Electrostatic effects on lipid phase transition: Membrane structure and ionic environment. Proc. Natl. Acad. Sci. U.S.A. *71:*214–219, 1974.

Valliéres, J., Scarpa, A., and Somlyo, A.P.: Subcellular fractions of smooth muscle. Isolation, substrate utilization and calcium transport by main pulmonary artery and mesenteric vein mitochondria. Arch. Biochem. Biophys. *170:*659–669, 1975.

van Rossum, G.D.V.: Net movements of Ca^{2+} and Mg^{2+} in slices of rat liver. J.Gen. Physiol. *55:*18–32, 1970.

van Vleet, J.F., Hall, B.V., and Simon, J.: Vitamin E deficiency: A sequential light and electron microscopic study of skeletal muscle degeneration in weanling rabbits. Am. J. Pathol. *52:* 1067–1079, 1968.

Vasington, F.D., and Murphy, J.V.: Ca^{2+} uptake by rat kidney mitochondria and its dependence on respiration and phosphorylation. J. Biol. Chem. *237:*2670–2672, 1962.

Wacker, W.E.C., and Williams, R.J.P.: Magnesium/calcium balances and steady state of biological systems. J. Theor. Biol. *20:*65–78, 1968.

Wang, J.H., Teo, T.S., Ho, H.C., and Stevens, F.C.: Bovine heart protein activator of cyclic nucleotide phosphodiesterase. Adv. Cyclic Nucleotide Res. *5:*179–194, 1975.

Warren, G.B., Toon, P.A., Birdsall, N.J.M., Lee, A.G., and Metcalfe, J.C.: Reconstruction of a calcium pump using defined membrane components. Proc. Natl. Acad. Sci. U.S.A. 71:622–626, 1974.

Wasserman, R.H., and Taylor, A.N.: Vitamin D_3-induced calcium binding protein in chick intestinal mucosa. Science 152:791–793, 1966.

Watterson, D.M., Sharief, F.W., and Vanaman, T.C.: The complete amino acid sequence of the Ca^{2+}-dependent modulation protein (calmodulin) of bovine brain. J. Biol. Chem. 255:962–975, 1980.

Weber, A.: Energized calcium transport and relaxing factors. Curr. Top. Bioenerg. 1:203–254, 1966.

Wehrle, J.P., and Pederson, P.L.: Phosphate transport in rat liver mitochondria. Properties of a Ca^{2+}-activated uptake process in inverted inner membrane vesicles. J. Biol. Chem. 254:7269, 1979.

Williams, R.J.P.: The binding of metal ions to membranes and its consequences. In *Biological Membranes: Twelve Assays of Their Organization, Properties, and Functions*, edited by D.S. Parson, pp. 106–121. Oxford University Press (Charendon), London, 1975.

Williams, R.J.P.: Calcium chemistry and its relation to biological function. Symp. Soc. Exp. Biol. 30:1–17, 1976.

Winegrad, S., and Shanes, A.M.: Calcium flux and contractility in guinea-pig atria. J. Gen. Physiol. 45:371–394, 1962.

Wollenberger, A., Will, H., and Krause, E.G.: Adenosine 3'-5'-monophosphate, the myocardial cell membrane, and calcium. Recent Adv. Stud. Cardiac Struct. Metab. 51:81–93, 1975.

Woodhouse, M.A., and Burston, J.: Metastatic calcification of the myocardium. J. Pathol. 97:733–736, 1969.

Worsfold, M., and Peter, J.B.: Kinetics of calcium transport by fragmented sarcoplasmic reticulum. J. Biol. Chem. 245:5545–5552, 1970.

Yamazaki, R.K.: Glucagon stimulation of mitochondrial respiration. J. Biol. Chem. 250:7924–7930, 1975.

Zacks, S.I., and Sheff, M.F.: Studies on tetanous toxin 1. Formation of intramitochondrial dense granules in mice acutely poisoned with tetanus toxin. J. Neuropathol. Exp. Neurol. 23:323, 1964.

CHAPTER 8

Membrane Na^+-K^+ Transport and Ancillary Phenomena in Circulatory Shock

MOHAMMED M. SAYEED

The continued existence of the cell is dependent on its ability to transform and transduce energy to support endergonic cellular processes such as the active transport of ions and molecules and macromolecular synthesis. The plasma membrane of animal cells actively transports a variety of ions and molecules (Na^+, K^+, H^+, Ca^{2+}, Cl^-, sugars, and amino acids). Virtually all of these active transport processes are involved in the control of vital cellular functions.

Active sodium transport out of cells (sodium pump), which appears to be ubiquitous throughout the animal kingdom, is concerned with: 1) maintenance of low sodium and high potassium concentration in the cytosol, 2) maintenance of a transmembrane electric gradient, and 3) regulation of water flux across the plasma membrane (Lowe, 1971; Baker, 1972). Each of these sodium pump-related functions in turn support vital cellular processes. Appropriate intracellular concentrations of Na^+ and K^+ are required for protein biosynthesis (Pestka, 1971), optimal activation of enzymes (Lowe, 1971), and the uphill transmembrane transport of other ions and molecules (Ca^{2+}, glucose, and some amino acids) (Baker, 1972). Sodium pump-dependent transmembrane potentials support membrane excitability found in nerves and muscles. By regulating transmembrane flux of water, the sodium pump prevents an otherwise inevitable swelling and lysis of animal cells due to intracellular colloid osmotic pressure.

The aforementioned considerations indicate that important cellular functions would not be possible without the sodium pump and that cell viability would be threatened by a failure of the sodium pump mechanism.

Although we do not know what eventually causes cell death in any pathological condition, critical changes in the plasma membrane functions could undoubtedly play an important role. The plasma membrane-bound sodium pump mechanism with its implications in the maintenance of cell volume and metabolism may well constitute the Achilles heel of the plasma membrane.

The failure of the sodium pump in the cell injury of anoxia, ischemia, and shock is a tenable hypothesis. To date, many investigators have studied the effect of shock on the electrolyte and water distribution in a variety of tissues. They have evaluated electrolyte and fluid disturbances in tissues by measuring tissue ion and fluid content, net ion movements, Na^+, K^+ fluxes, cell volume regulation, or membrane potentials. Whereas many of these studies indicate gross alterations in the sodium-potassium transport mechanism, there are also indications that electrolyte disturbances may be related to altered permeabilities of membranes to ions.

In this chapter, studies dealing with transmembrane sodium potassium transport and ancillary "reactions" such as resting potentials and the transport enzyme, (Na^+ + K^+)-ATPase, in circulatory shock are described and discussed. Studies in the liver are emphasized, as membrane transport studies in other organ systems (cardiac and skeletal muscle and kidney) with shock, anoxia, and/or ischemia are discussed elsewhere in this book. Before proceeding with the discussion of studies on the effect of shock, the basic knowledge of the characteristics and mechanisms of the membrane sodium-potassium transport in general and in particular in the hepatic tissue are summarized. Basic topics have been selected which either have been emphasized in shock research or have prospects of being implicated in the physiopathology of shock, anoxia, and/or ischemia.

ION GRADIENTS AND RESTING POTENTIALS

Liver cells maintain a low ratio of $[Na^+]/[K^+]$ inside the cells in the face of a high $[Na^+]/[K^+]$ ratio in the extracellular fluid. The hepatic intracellular sodium concentration ranges from 15 to 28 mmoles/liter cell water in tissue samples excised immediately after sacrificing the animals. The values for hepatic ion content and the hepatic intracellular ion concentrations obtained by several investigators are summarized in Table 8.1. The extracellular $[Na^+]$, as estimated from concentrations in plasma water is approximately 6–10 times higher than the intracellular sodium concentrations. The potassium concentration inside the hepatic cell is 130–160 mmoles/liters cell water, which is 25–35 times the concentration in the extracellular fluid. Like sodium, the chloride concentration in the extracellular fluid is 5 times higher than the intracellular concentrations. Since the transmembrane concentration gradient of K^+, $\Delta[K^+]$, is directed outward and that of Na^+ and Cl^- inward, one would expect a flux of K^+ out of cells and fluxes of Na^+ and Cl^- into the cells as a result of passive movement of ions. Such passive fluxes would dissipate the transmembrane gradients of ions, $\Delta[Na^+]$, $\Delta[K^+]$, and $\Delta[Cl^-]$. The question must then be asked, are passive movements due to concentration gradients in equilibrium with opposing passive movements due to any electric charge ($\Delta\psi$) so that there is no net passive movement of an ion? The gradient of electric charge which will support the existing transmembrane gradient of $[K^+]$ is the potassium equilibrium potential ($\Delta\psi_K$) and can be calculated from the Nernst equation, as follows:

$$\Delta\psi_K = -\frac{RT}{FZ_K} \ln\left(\frac{[K^+]_i}{[K^+]_e}\right)$$

where $\Delta\psi$ is the electrical potential in millivolts,

R = gas content = 8.314 J/(°A × mole),
T = temperature in °A,
Z_K = valence of K^+,
F = Faraday's constant = 96,504 coul/mole, and
$[K]_i$ and $[K]_e$ represent intracellular and extracellular K^+ concentrations, respectively.

Sodium and chloride equilibrium potentials ($\Delta\psi_{Na^+}$ and $\Delta\psi_{Cl^-}$, respectively) can be calculated similarly as $\Delta\psi_{K^+}$ from the Nernst equation with slight modifications of the equation which take into account the direction of the gradient and the sign of the charge on the ion.

Table 8.2 gives values of ion equilibrium potentials calculated from the hepatic $\Delta[Na^+]$, $\Delta[K^+]$, and $\Delta[Cl^-]$. Table 8.2 also shows values of actually measured gradients of electric charge across the hepatic cell membrane as reported by several investigators. The transmembrane gradients of electric charge, or the so-called resting membrane potentials ($\Delta\psi_m$), were measured by means of an intracellular glass microelectrode. The calculated $\Delta\psi_{Cl}$ is

Table 8.1
Total Ion Content and Intracellular Ion Concentrations in the Rat Liver

Total Ion Content			Intracellular Ion Conc.			Authors
Na	K	Cl	Na^+	K^+	Cl^-	
mmoles/kg wet wt			mmoles/liter intracellular water			
12 ± 3	80 ± 3	50 ± 4	16.4	113.0	25.5	Claret and Mazet (1972)
34 ± 1	100 ± 1	24 ± 1	29 ± 2	166 ± 1	19 ± 1	Williams et al. (1971)
30 ± 2	86 ± 3	22 ± 2	29 ± 5	175 ± 6	23 ± 2	Sayeed et al. (1980)

Table 8.2
Ion Equilibrium Potentials ($\Delta\psi_{ion}$) and the Resting Membrane Potentials ($\Delta\psi_m$) in the Liver

	$\Delta\psi_{ion}$			$\Delta\psi_m$	Authors
	K^+	Na^+	Cl^-		
	mV				
Rat liver, isolated-perfused	−80	—	−35	−34	Claret and Mazet (1972)
Rat liver, in vivo	−94	+43	−47	−44	Williams et al. (1971)
Rat liver, in vivo	−94	−42	−30	−40	Sayeed et al. (1980)

comparable to the measured $\Delta\psi_m$ value. Thus, it becomes obvious that as far as transmembrane distribution of chloride is concerned, it is a result of a balance between $\Delta[Cl^-]$ and $\Delta\psi_{Cl}$, i.e., the combined electrochemical gradient of Cl^- ($\Delta\bar{\mu}_{Cl^-}$). The comparison of $\Delta\psi_m$ with $\Delta\psi_{Na^+}$ or $\Delta\psi_{K^+}$ values shows that both Na^+ and K^+ are distributed away from their electrochemical gradients. In the case of K^+, hepatic $\Delta\psi_m$ (resting membrane potential) is clearly less negative than the $\Delta\psi_{K^+}$ (-40 versus -90 mV). Therefore, at the steady state of $\Delta\psi_m$, passive $\Delta\psi_m$ would promote greater passive efflux of K^+ than the passive influx. Conversely, $\Delta\psi_m$ is more negative than $\Delta\psi_{Na^+}$; this would promote a greater influx of Na^+ than its efflux. Thus, passive movements of Na^+ and K^+, but not Cl^-, due to electrochemical gradients ($\Delta\bar{\mu}_{ions}$) which exist across the liver cell membrane, would cause a net efflux of K^+ and a net influx of Na^+. These net fluxes must then be balanced by movements of Na^+ and K^+ against electrochemical gradients of these ions ($\Delta\bar{\mu}_{Na^+}$ and $\Delta\bar{\mu}_{K^+}$). Such a balancing of fluxes is necessary for the steady states of $\Delta[Na^+]$ and $\Delta[K^+]$ which exist across the hepatic cell membrane not only under in vivo conditions but under proper in vitro conditions for a period of several hours.

ACTIVE Na^+ AND K^+ FLUXES

Whereas the passive movements of ions are spontaneous processes and occur with a decrease in free energy, movements against electrochemical gradients must necessarily depend upon input of free energy such as cellular metabolic energy. Extrusion of sodium out of cells against an electrochemical gradient was first proposed and termed as active transport by Dean (1941). Such an active transport system was subsequently investigated in giant squid axon by Hodgkin and Keynes (1955). These investigators found that the "uphill" movement of sodium out of cells depended on the presence of energy-yielding substrates, but the "downhill" movement of sodium was not affected by the inhibition of cell metabolism. Active sodium extrusion has been investigated in detail in other nerve and skeletal muscle cells (Caldwell, 1968), in smooth muscle cells (Casteels, 1970), in cardiac muscle cells (Page and Storm, 1965), and in red blood cells (Dunham and Glynn, 1961). Active transport is apparently present in the plasma membrane of all animal cells which maintain a low intracellular Na^+/K^+ ratio in the presence of high Na^+/K^+ ratio in the extracellular fluid.

One of the first demonstrations of active Na^+ and K^+ movements in the liver tissue was made by Flink et al. (1950). They incubated liver tissue slices in an oxygenated medium at 38°C and showed that, although Na^+ increased and K^+ decreased in the slices during the initial 15 min of incubation, the ion changes were subsequently reversed. Further evidence of the ability of liver slices to actively transport Na^+ and K^+ was obtained by Elshove and van Rossum (1963) and McLean (1963). In these experiments, the investigators cooled liver slices at 0°C for 35–90 min in 150 mM saline or Ringer's solution and then rewarmed the slices in oxygenated Ringer's solution at 37°C. The chilling-induced increase in tissue sodium and decrease in tissue potassium were reversed by rewarming of slices. Since cooling suppresses metabolism, it would suppress energy-dependent ion movements while allowing passive movements to occur. Such passive movements at 0.5°C would dissipate ion gradients. Measurement of tissue sodium and potassium after 90 min of chilling did indicate substantial loss of cellular potassium (up to 75% of prechilling values); tissue sodium increased to levels to the point that Na^+ concentration in cell water was roughly equal to the extracellular Na^+ concentration. Then with rewarming, the reversal of cation changes was due to movement of ions against concentration gradients. Since resting membrane potentials ($\Delta\psi_m$) were not measured, it cannot be unequivocally concluded that ion reversals with rewarming were movements of ions against electrochemical gradients. Elshove and van Rossum (1963) did demonstrate that ion reversals with rewarming were inhibited by inhibitors of oxidative metabolism (dinitrophenol or cyanide) or an ATP inhibitor (oligomycin).

The cardiotonic steroid ouabain, which is known to inhibit the Na^+-K^+ pump (Schatzmann, 1953), also effectively prevented reversal of ions with rewarming of slices. Figure 8.1 shows data on liver slice ion contents with chilling and rewarming of the tissue as well as the effect of ouabain. These data obtained from the author's laboratory are in agreement with the earlier studies of Elshove and van Rossum (1963) and van Rossum (1966). Van Rossum (1966) also reported values of total ^{24}Na efflux measured in liver slices which were previously labeled with the isotope. Efflux of ^{24}Na was measured during incubation of slices in media containing ^{23}Na. This procedure simultaneously evaluated bidirectional fluxes of Na^+: 1) ^{23}Na influx which is a passive process only, and 2) ^{24}Na efflux which includes both passive and active movements. These studies demonstrated that about two-thirds of the cellular sodium efflux was due to passive sodium movement and one-third was due to active, ouabain, or dinitrophenol inhibitable efflux. Claret and Mazet (1972) measured K^+ and Na^+ fluxes in isolated perfused livers. They designed their experiments to primarily quantitate passive ion fluxes and to estimate membrane permeabilities to ions from measured values of fluxes. ^{24}Na efflux and ^{42}K effluxes were estimated during washout of ^{24}Na and ^{42}K from perfused livers which were previously loaded with the isotopes. We can estimate from the data of Claret and Mazet values of both passive and active Na^+ fluxes. Active K^+ flux could not be ascertained because total K^+ influx (7 pmoles × cm^{-2} × sec^{-1}) was measured, without identifying the active component of this K influx. The total efflux of ^{24}Na was about 13 pmoles × cm^{-2} × sec^{-1}. Of this value about 6 pmoles of the efflux were due to ouabain-inhibitable Na^+ extrusion and about 3 pmoles due to exchange diffusion of Na^+ (Na^+-Na^+ exchange). This suggests that about 30% of total efflux was due to the Na^+ pump. This estimation is comparable to that of van Rossum (1966), who studied ^{24}Na efflux in liver slices.

Recently, there have been reports of K^+ flux measure-

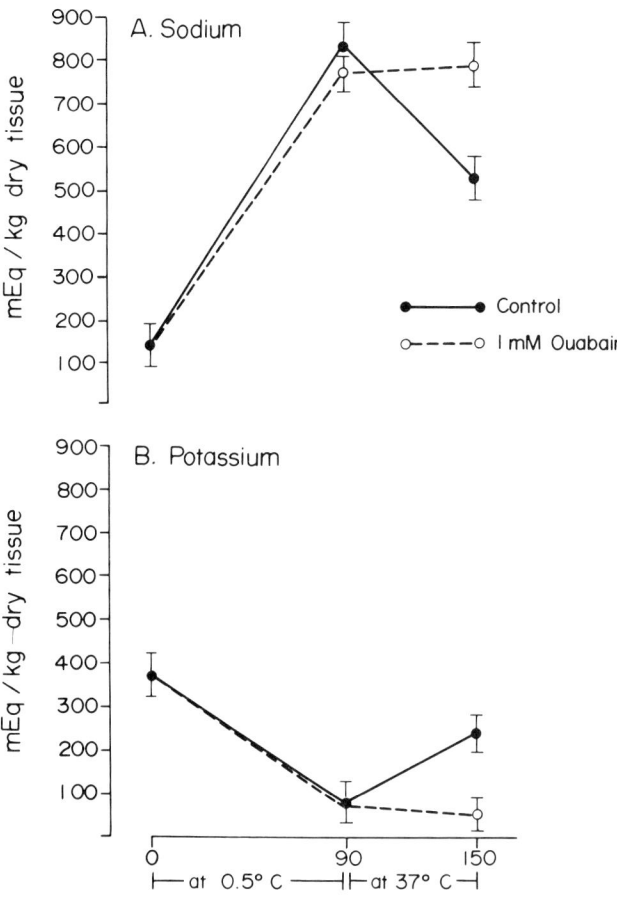

Figure 8.1. Net cation movements in liver slices in vitro in the presence or absence of ouabain. The slices were chilled for 90 min at 0.5°C and then transferred to a 37°C medium. Graphs A and B show changes in liver slice Na and K contents, respectively.

ments in isolated liver cell preparations. Barnabei et al. (1974) and Tomasi et al. (1975), from the same laboratory, have studied active K^+ uptake by rat liver cells isolated by the method of Berry and Friend (1969). As pointed out by Barnabei et al. (1974), the isolated cell preparation, although it retains normal glycolytic activity and a normal ability to respond to hormones, contains only 40% of tissue K^+ found in intact liver. The liver slice preparation has been repeatedly shown to retain normal tissue potassium under in vitro conditions (McLean, 1963; Van Rossum, 1963a, 1964, Seidman and Cascarano, 1966; Sayeed and Baue, 1973; Sayeed et al., 1974). Nevertheless, isolated liver cells lose and gain K^+ by chilling and rewarming and thus exhibit active transport of K^+. Barnabei et al. (1974) reported a 25% inhibition of K^+ uptake in the presence of ouabain. On the other hand, Tomasi et al. (1975) reported that more than 50% of active uptake was inhibited by ouabain. Berg and Iversen (1976) have estimated K^+ fluxes by measuring ^{42}K exchanges in isolated liver cells. They estimated ^{42}K influx to be 8 pmoles $\times$ cm^{-2} $\times$ sec^{-1}. We do not know from the data of Berg and Iversen the proportion of the K^+ influx which represents the active component.

Claret et al. (1973) have estimated ouabain-sensitive Na^+ efflux and K^+ influx in isolated perfused rat livers. They corrected total Na^+ efflux and K^+ influx for passive fluxes due to ouabain-insensitive diffusional flux and for the self-exchange of ions. The K^+ efflux was diminished by about 70% in the presence of ouabain and the active flux amounted to about 4.5 pmoles $\times$ cm^{-2} $\times$ sec^{-1}. The mean value of ouabain-sensitive Na^+ efflux was 7.3 pmoles $\times$ cm^{-2} $\times$ sec^{-1}. The latter value has a SE of $\pm$ 1.9, which is in good agreement with values previously reported from that laboratory (Claret and Mazet, 1972).

The data on passive and active fluxes measured in the liver cells are depicted in Figure 8.2.

IONIC REGULATION OF Na^+ AND K^+ TRANSPORT

If the Na^+ pump is to maintain low intracellular $[Na^+]$, it seems reasonable that pump activity would be affected by changes in intracellular $[Na^+]$. This is the case in several of the cell systems that have been studied. For example, Na efflux increased following an increase in $[Na^+]_i$ in the squid axons (Baker et al., 1962), skeletal muscle (Keynes and Steinhardt, 1968; Sjodin and Beauge, 1968), and cardiac muscle (Page and Storm, 1965). The kinetic course of Na^+ efflux as a function of $[Na^+]_i$ is like a first order reaction. With the intracell $[Na^+]$ in the physiological range, which will vary from one cell type to another, a steady state exists with the Na^+ extrusion balancing the Na^+ influx so that intracell Na^+ remains relatively constant. If the Na^+_i content decreases, for example, due to a decrease in $[Na^+]$ in the extracellular fluid, then Na^+ efflux decreases more pre-

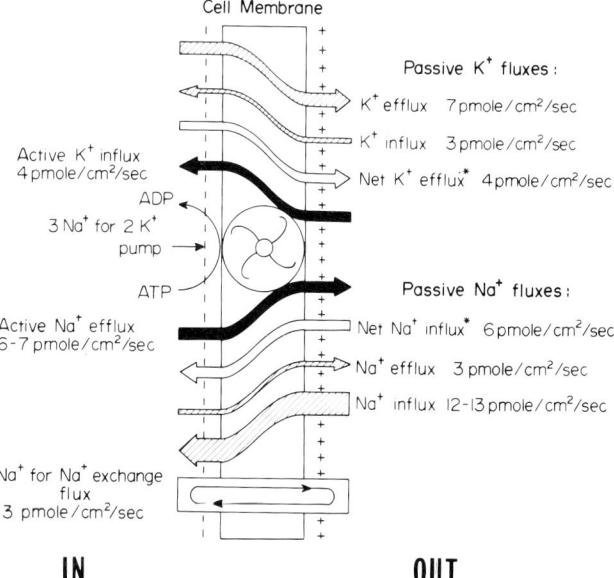

Figure 8.2. Membrane fluxes of Na^+ and K^+ in the liver.

cipitously than the decrease in efflux in the "physiological" range of $[Na^+]_i$. With an increase in intracellular Na^+ beyond the physiological range, the increase in Na^+ efflux is linearly related to the cube of $[Na^+]_i$ (Keynes, 1965).

The intracellular $[Na^+]$ may increase with increased leakiness of membranes to Na^+. This is the probable course of events in the hereditary disease spherocytosis—the red cells become spherical and fragile (Jacobs, 1966). The increased $[Na^+]_i$ is associated with an increased Na^+-K^+ transport enzyme and a release of metabolic control over red cell glycolysis; this could cause an increased phospholipid breakdown and a decrease in cell surface with consequent spherocytosis and red cell fragility. In spherocytosis, there is a pertinent example of a clinical observation which contributes to a better understanding of the molecular basis of cation transport and vice versa, i.e., better understanding of a clinical observation on the basis of understanding the mechanism of basic membrane transport function.

Alternatively, intracellular $[Na^+]$ can increase when extracellular $[K^+]$ is diminished, as is known to occur in skeletal muscle fibers (Fozzard and Kipnis, 1967). An increase in $[K^+]$ in the extracellular fluid can enhance Na^+ efflux when $[Na^+]_i$ is high (Conway et al., 1961). Page and Storm (1965) have shown that cat papillary muscle, which was previously chilled, contained high $[Na^+]_i$ and extruded Na^+ at faster rates at higher extracellular $[K^+]$ than at the normal extracellular $[K^+]$.

In rat liver slices, Elshove and van Rossum (1963) found that sodium extrusion was sensitive to changes in the $[Na^+]$ and $[K^+]$ in the medium. Changes in medium $[Na^+]$ and $[K^+]$ affected both Na^+ extrusion and K^+ uptake. The intracellular $[Na^+]$ was varied by incubating tissue slices at $1°C$ in media containing 10–147 mM Na^+ by substituting Li^+ for Na^+. At the end of 90 min of chilling, Na^+ content varied from 44 to 170 mmol/kg tissue water. With the rewarming of liver slices, Na^+ extrusion increased from 70 mmoles/kg fat free dry wt at a medium $[Na^+]$ of 20 mM to 180 mmoles/kg fat free dry wt at the medium $[Na^+]$ of 80 mM. There seemed to be no further increase in Na^+ extrusion when $[Na^+]$ in the medium was increased from 80 to 120 mmol. This is likely due to the saturation of the Na^+ transport mechanism in the "physiological" range of $[Na^+]_i$. Concomitant increases in K^+ uptake with increasing tissue Na^+ contents, however, were linear throughout the entire range of medium $[Na^+]$. The effect of increasing $[K^+]$ in the medium from 0 to 20 mM was clearly stimulatory with saturation of both Na^+ extrusion and K^+ uptake occurring at about 10 mM K^+. Claret and associates (1973) have shown that Na^+ efflux was reversibly diminished when K^+ was removed from the medium. These observations support activation of the Na^+ pump in the liver by external K^+. Experiments of Elshove and van Rossum (1963) also provided evidence that liver cells could not extrude Li^+. Thus, Na^+ was specifically required by the pumping mechanism. A particularly interesting effect of Li^+ is that it enters cells but is not pumped out by the Na^+ pump mechanism. Entrance of Li^+ into the cell would continue until it is distributed across the membrane in accordance with the membrane potential ($\Delta\psi_m$). The more negative the intracellular environment, the more Li^+ would enter the cells. The increase in intracellular Li^+ would cause loss of intracellular K^+ and concomitant depolarization of cells. Such a Li^+-induced depolarization in nerve cells interferes with functioning of the nervous system. This may account for the therapeutic usefulness of Li^+ in mental disorders.

COUPLING OF Na^+ AND K^+ TRANSPORT

In this chapter so far, active Na^+ efflux and K^+ influx have been considered as processes which occur independently of each other. The dependence of Na^+ efflux on the extracell $[K^+]$, however, indicates that there is a linkage between Na^+ and K^+ movements. Earlier studies in the frog muscle (Keynes, 1954) and in the giant squid axon (Hodgkin and Keynes, 1955) had supported the concept of 1:1 coupling between Na^+ transported out to K^+ transported in the cell. Later, Post and Jolly (1957) showed that in red blood cells 3 Na^+ were extruded in exchange for 2 K^+ which were transported into the cells.

In liver slices, Elshove and van Rossum (1963) indicated that for the most part the ratio of net Na^+ extrusion to K^+ uptake was near unity. However, they did observe some net extrusion of Na^+ in the absence of K^+ uptake. The overall interpretation was that the coupling between Na^+ and K^+ movement was close to unity but not absolute. The ratio of ouabain-sensitive Na^+ and K^+ fluxes, as measured by Claret et al. (1973), was 3:2.

At the outset, the question of whether Na^+-K^+ transport occurs with a stoichiometric ratio of 1:1 or 3:2 appears to be of an academic nature. However, this concept becomes less evident as we look into potentially different roles the transport mechanism could play in the two stoichiometric modes. With the Na^+/K^+ ratio of 1:1, the pump would operate as an electroneutral mechanism. This implies that movement of ions across the plasma membrane via Na^+-K^+ pump would proceed without affecting the membrane gradient of electric charge ($\Delta\psi_m$), i.e., the resting membrane potential. This would indirectly support the view that resting membrane potential is primarily dependent upon passive ionic diffusional forces. The concept of resting membrane potential resulting from ion diffusional forces will be returned to later. For the time being we are confronted with the issue of whether or not Na^+-K^+ directly affects the resting membrane potential. The ratio of active movement of Na^+/K^+ of 1:1 seemingly cannot contribute to the membrane potential. On the other hand, if the Na^+-K^+ pump were to transport an excess of Na^+ over K^+, as it would with the Na^+/K^+ transport ratio of 3:2, the pump would directly contribute to the resting potential. The excess sodium flux causes an outward sodium current. This presumes that excess sodium flux is not accompanied by an equivalent quantity of anions such as chloride. The extent of contribution of the excess Na^+ flux to the resting potential would depend on the ratio of Na^+ transport to K^+. The higher the ratio the greater the active transport-dependent component of the resting membrane potential. When contributing to the resting membrane potential, an ion pump is referred to as electrogenic.

The physiological implications of an electroneutral versus electrogenic Na^+-K^+ pump in nonexcitable cells such as liver cells must remain restricted to hypothetical considerations. However, since an electrogenic coupling of the Na^+ to K^+ transport directly affects the resting membrane potential, modulations and/or alterations of an electrogenic Na^+-K^+ pump would cause a more rapid change in the resting membrane potential than would occur if the Na^+-K^+ pump was electroneutral. This would mean that an electrogenic pump could cause a more rapid activation or inhibition of a membrane potential-dependent cellular process. As a result the pump can be involved in "fast" physiological responses. To illustrate the electrogenic action of the Na^+-K^+ pump in the liver, we could consider a relationship between the liver gluconeogenic process and the pump. There is some evidence that the Na^+-K^+ pump-dependent hyperpolarization of liver cell membrane accompanies the action of gluconeogenic hormones on these cells (Dambach and Friedmann, 1974). This is an example of a situation where an electrogenic Na^+-K^+ pump may provide for the regulation of hepatic gluconeogenesis on a short-term basis under physiological conditions. With a breakdown of an electrogenic pump, liver cells may not respond to the gluconeogenic hormones.

Another aspect of the Na^+-K^+ pump coupling ratio which may be important in assessing altered pump activity is the release of Na^+ efflux from its dependency on K^+. A number of studies have supported the concept that under conditions which augment cellular ADP supply, there is Na^+ efflux in the absence of K^+ in the extracellular medium (Caldwell et al., 1960; DeWeer, 1974). Na^+ efflux in the absence of extracellular K^+ acquires a new dependency on extracellular Na^+. This Na^+ efflux, which retains its sensitivity to ouabain, has been shown to be an electroneutral Na/Na exchange mechanism. These studies suggest the possibility that when cellular metabolism is affected under pathological conditions so that there is an increase in the ADP/ATP ratio, the Na^+-K^+ pump may switch to a Na^+ for Na^+ exchange process.

RELATIONSHIP BETWEEN THE Na^+-K^+ PUMP AND THE RESTING MEMBRANE POTENTIAL

As indicated in the above section, a "tight" 1:1 coupling between Na^+ and K^+ transport would not directly contribute to the resting membrane potential. Under this circumstance, the resting membrane potential would be determined by passive ionic diffusional forces which depend on the ionic gradients ($\Delta[Na^+]$, $\Delta[K^+]$, $\Delta[Cl^-]$) and permeability of the membrane to these ions. Ob-

viously if the membrane was impermeable to an ion, there would be no diffusional contribution by that ion to the membrane potential. The relationship between the resting membrane potential ($\Delta\psi_m$) and the diffusional forces of ions is described by the Goldman-Hodgkin-Katz equation (GHK equation) as follows:

$$\Delta\psi_m = \frac{RT}{F} \ln \frac{P_{K^+}[K^+]_e + P_{Na^+}[Na^+]_e + P_{Cl^-}[Cl^-]_i}{P_{K^+}[K^+]_i + P_{Na^+}[Na^+]_i + P_{Cl^-}[Cl^-]_e}$$

where P_{K^+}, P_{Na^+}, P_{Cl^-} are permeability constants (cm/sec) for ions K^+, Na^+, and Cl^-, respectively; other symbols are same as used on page 113.

The GHK equation can be reduced to the following form if the chloride ion is distributed passively across the cell membrane.

$$\Delta\psi_m = \frac{RT}{F} \ln \frac{P_{K^+}[K^+]_e + P_{Na^+}[Na^+]_e}{P_{K^+}[K^+]_i + P_{Na^+}[Na^+]_i}$$

or

$$\Delta\psi_m = \frac{RT}{F} \ln \frac{[K^+]_e + (P_{Na^+}/P_{K^+})[Na^+]_e}{[K^+]_i + (P_{Na^+}/P_{K^+})[Na^+]_i}.$$

The modified form of the GHK equation is applicable to the liver, as in this tissue chloride is distributed in accordance to the membrane potential. The modified forms of the GHK equation indicate that the resting membrane potential ($\Delta\psi_m$) primarily depends on the permeability of the membrane to Na^+ and K^+. Thus, with electroneutral coupling (1:1) of Na^+ to K^+ transport, the hepatic resting membrane potential is determined primarily by membrane permeabilities to Na^+ and K^+ and only secondarily by the pump. This means if the Na^+-K^+ pump stops, transmembrane ion gradients dissipate first and then there is a change in the resting membrane potential, i.e., depolarization. When the resting membrane potential is altered in this manner, there may not be any change in permeability of the membrane to Na^+ and K^+. On the other hand membrane permeability might change first and affect membrane potential without any effect on the membrane Na^+-K^+ pump. A finding of altered resting membrane potential alone does not indicate whether the change was due to the pump or the permeabilities. A direct analysis of both the pump and the membrane permeability characteristics are fundamental to assessment of the integrity of the membrane in its handling of Na^+ and K^+ transport. The resting membrane potential alterations indicate either a pump-related or a permeability-related membrane dysfunction.

In the case of an electrogenic Na^+-K^+ pump, not only passive diffusional forces but a Na^+ current would also contribute to the resting membrane potential. The diffusional forces operate because of partial coupling between the Na^+ and K^+ movements. Mullins and Noda (1963) have developed an equation which relates the resting membrane potential to diffusional forces as well as the contribution of electrogenic Na^+ extrusion (unaccompanied by K^+) to the potential. This equation is very similar to the modified form of GHK except that it takes into account the ratio of coupling between Na^+ and K^+

transport. The Mullins and Noda equation (MN equation) is:

$$\Delta\psi_m = \frac{RT}{F} \ln \frac{\gamma[K^+]_o + (P_{Na^+}/P_{K^+})[Na^+]_o}{\gamma[K^+]_i + (P_{Na^+}/P_{K^+})[Na^+]_i}$$

where

$$\gamma = \frac{\text{active } Na^+ \text{ efflux}}{\text{active } K^+ \text{ influx}}$$

other symbols are the same as in the previous equation.

Thus, if we determine the Na^+-K^+ pump coupling ratio experimentally and have the knowledge of permeabilities to Na^+ and K^+ (derived from passive fluxes) and the ionic gradients, we can calculate the resting membrane potential. An agreement between the calculated resting membrane potential and the measured membrane potential confirms the electrogenic nature of the Na^+-K^+ pump.

Unlike the electroneutral pump, the electrogenic pump when altered directly affects the membrane potential as well as the ion gradients. Thus, the electrogenic pump affects both membrane potential-dependent and ion gradient-dependent cellular functions without any alteration in the permeability of membranes to ions.

Membrane Na^+ and K^+ Permeabilities in the Liver

As pointed out in the section, Ion Gradients and Resting Potentials, the resting membrane potential in the liver is less than the equilibrium potential for K^+ ($\Delta\psi_{K^+}$). Williams et al. (1971) pointed out that the measured hepatic resting potential ($\Delta\psi_m$) would correspond to the Na^+-K^+ diffusional potential (as calculated by the GHK equation) if we assume the value of the ratio of membrane permeability to Na^+ and K^+ (P_{Na^+}/P_{K^+}) to be about 0.2. This value is about 20 times higher than that found in excitable cells such as the nerve and muscle cells. According to Williams (1970), the discrepancy between the resting membrane potential and the K^+ equilibrium potential is due primarily to higher permeability to Na^+ relative to K^+ in the liver than in nerve and muscle. When we calculate the value of the ratio P_{Na^+}/P_{K^+} from permeability constants (P_{Na^+}, P_{K^+}) derived from passive Na^+ and K^+ flux, as reported by Claret and Mazet (1972), it turns out to be greater than 0.2. Thus, the membrane Na^+ permeability relative to permeability to K^+ is innately higher in the liver than in the excitable cells.

Electrogenic Na^+-K^+ Pumping in the Liver

There is some evidence that the Na^+-K^+ pump is electrogenic in the liver. Williams et al. (1971) showed that an increase in $[K^+]_e$ caused a hyperpolarization of the hepatic resting membrane potential by about 5–6 mV. This is contrary to what would be predicted by the GHK equation and by the presence of a tightly coupled Na^+-K^+ pump. Williams et al. interpreted that K^+-induced hyperpolarization was due to the presence of electrogenic Na^+ pumping. The measurement of ouabain-sensitive Na^+ efflux and K^+ influx in the liver in the ratio of 3:2 by Claret et al. (1973) provided direct proof for the electrogenic nature of the pump. Further evidence for the hepatic electrogenic Na^+-K^+ transport can be derived from measurements of hepatic membrane conductance and pump current. The total membrane conductance across the liver is 52 μmhos × cm^{-2} (Claret and Mazet, 1971). The value of Na^+ pump current, obtained by multiplying the ouabain-sensitive Na^+ efflux value (3 pmoles × cm^{-2} × sec^{-1}, Claret and coworkers, 1973) by the Faraday, is 0.3 μA × cm^{-2}. The potential generated by the pump would be equal to current divided by membrane conductance and 5.8 mV. This value is equal to the K^+-induced hyperpolarization of the hepatic cell membrane (Williams et al., 1971).

DIFFUSIBILITY OF INTRACELLULAR Na^+ AND K^+

In considering passive and active fluxes of Na^+ and K^+ and the relationship between these fluxes and the resting membrane potential, it is presumed that ions are present intracellularly to a large extent in a free diffusible form. According to some investigators (Ling, 1962; Troshin, 1966), ion distribution and the membrane potential in the cells are due to selective adsorption of ions to fixed negative charges within the cells. Ling's theory involves a near complete association of living protoplasm with ions and a near complete absence of free intracellular ions in solution. However, the most widely accepted view with regards to the intracellular distribution of ions is that it results from selective permeability of the membrane for the ions and from the transmembrane active transport. Nevertheless, there is evidence that the cytoplasmic activity coefficient of an ion differs from the activity coefficient of that ion in the extracellular medium (Lev and Armstrong, 1975).

Although definitive data on hepatic intracellular activity coefficients for Na^+, K^+ or Cl^- are not available at present, measurements in other tissues (nerve, skeletal, and cardiac muscle, and intestinal mucosal) showed that the apparent activity coefficient for potassium is about 0.77 and 0.33–0.49 for sodium (Lev and Armstrong, 1975). Since the cytoplasmic mean K^+ activity coefficient was about equal to the apparent cellular potassium activity coefficient, intracellular potassium would appear to be mainly in the free diffusible form. We can reach a similar conclusion with regard to intracellular chloride. However, free cellular sodium appears to be about 50% of total in frog oocytes and frog intestinal epithelium.

ENERGETICS OF Na^+-K^+ TRANSPORT

In general, there have been more extensive studies of the energetics and membrane-linked molecular mechanisms of active Na^+ and K^+ transport than of any other transport process across the plasma membrane. Whereas some ion transport processes may depend on free energy derived from redox reactions, there is little doubt at the present time that Na^+-K^+ transport utilizes ATP synthesized during oxidative reaction and glycolysis.

At 37°C, the energy cost of transporting a monovalent ion against a concentration gradient with a concentration ratio of 10 is about 5.9 kJ/mole. Since the $[Na^+]_e/$

[Na$^+$]$_i$ ratio is 8–10 and the [K$^+$]$_i$/[K$^+$]$_o$ ratio is about 25, and since each Na$^+$-K$^+$ pump cycle transports 3 Na$^+$ out and 2 K$^+$ in the liver cells, the energy costs would be equal to 17.7 kJ/mole for Na$^+$ transport and 15.5 kJ/mole for K$^+$ transport. The total energy required to transport Na$^+$ and K$^+$ would be 32.2 kJ/cycle. The free energy change for the hydrolysis of ATP under the usual physiological conditions is in the neighborhood of -30 to -33 kJ/mole. It is sufficient to drive the Na$^+$-K$^+$ pump. The molar ratio of Na$^+$ and K$^+$ transport to ATP consumed has been computed to be 3 Na$^+$:2 K$^+$:1 ATP in human red cells (Sen and Post, 1964).

One of the direct evidences which link Na$^+$-K$^+$ transport to the hydrolysis of ATP is provided by the experiments of Garrahan and Glynn (1967). They demonstrated synthesis of ATP from inorganic phosphate when they reversed the Na$^+$-K$^+$ pump activity in the red cells. They made Δ[Na$^+$] and Δ[K$^+$] steeper than normal and promoted larger than normal "downhill" fluxes of Na$^+$ and K$^+$ in the red cells. This resulted in an increased incorporation of ^{32}P-labeled inorganic phosphate into ATP. That ATP is undoubtedly better than any other energy-rich phosphate compound in supporting Na$^+$ transport has also been shown in squid axons (Brinley and Mullins, 1968).

In cells that contain mitochondria, Na$^+$ transport depends on oxidative phosphorylation. In cells which were highly engaged in anaerobic glycolysis, such as the seminal vesicular mucosal cells, there was no reduction of Na$^+$ transport, although ATP production was reduced to 25% of the aerobic level (Breuer and Whittam, 1957). This observation suggests that in cells with potential for glycolysis, aerobic ATP is far in excess of that required for cellular Na$^+$ extrusion. A similar observation was made by van Rossum (1963a and b) in liver cells from the 21-day rat fetus. In the adult rat liver, Na$^+$-K$^+$ transport depended on respiration and decreased with decreased respiratory activity. However, the oxidative ATP had to decrease to very low levels before active Na$^+$ movements would cease (Judah et al, 1966; van Rossum, 1972a). Judah et al. (1966) showed that in male rats poisoned with ethionine in vivo, liver ATP decreased to 75–80%, and yet there was virtually no change in the ionic composition of the liver. van Rossum (1972a) reduced the rate of respiration and thus ATP formation to varying levels in rat liver in vitro by the addition of varying concentrations of amytal. The rate of respiration had to be reduced from 12 (μliters/mg protein/hr) to about 5 and ATP was reduced from 9 (μmoles/g protein) to 2.0 before a significant decrease in active Na$^+$ extrusion could be demonstrated. van Rossum (1972a) indicated that since O$_2$ consumption by liver slices could not be reduced by amytal below 3 (μliters/mg protein/hr), the residual O$_2$ consumption was probably due to the liver's mixed functional oxidase system. This would indicate that the level of ATP present in the tissue with only a residual O$_2$ consumption probably was due to glycolysis and that active Na$^+$ extrusion was inhibited only when aerobic oxidation was switched to the anaerobic levels. The data of van Rossum (1972b), shown in Figure 8.3, clearly suggest that the Na$^+$-K$^+$ transport mechanism of the liver is protected against reduction of metabolic energy from mitochondria and that Na$^+$-K$^+$ transport competes successfully with the other energy requiring processes of the liver in the face of limited ATP supply. The latter suggestion implies that the K$_m$ of Na$^+$ transport has a high affinity for ATP. The data on the dependency of Na$^+$ transport on ATP in the liver support the concept that decreased ATP alone can not be taken to indicate significant suppression of Na$^+$-K$^+$ transport unless ATP is decreased to critical anaerobic levels.

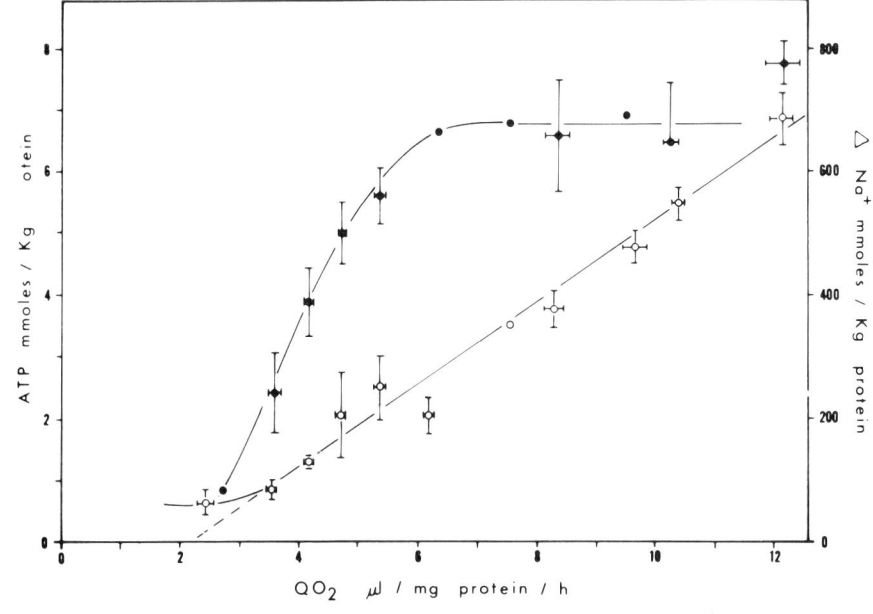

Figure 8.3. Relation of Na$^+$ transport and ATP content to the varying rates of respiration induced by different concentrations of Amytal in rat liver slices. At the end of the incubation period, the slices were put into 10% perchloric acid/40% ethanol at $-20°$C, homogenized, and centrifuged. Protein was determined on the precipitate by a biuret method, while Na$^+$ and ATP were analyzed in the supernatant (the latter by an enzymic method). (Reprinted with permission from G.D.V. van Rossum: In *Hibernation and Hypothermia, Perspectives and Challenges*. Elsevier, New York, 1972b.)

($Na^+ + K^+$)-ADENOSINE TRIPHOSPHATASE

Skou (1957) originally presented evidence that a "microsomal" fraction of crab nerve homogenate contained an ATP-hydrolyzing enzyme which was specifically activated by Na^+ and K^+. Since that time, Mg^{2+}-dependent, ($Na^+ + K^+$)-activated adenosine triphosphatase [($Na^+ + K^+$)-ATPase] has been considered to be an integral part of the molecular mechanism of the Na^+-K^+ transport in the cell membrane. This enzyme concomitantly accomplishes hydrolyzing of ATP and an asymmetric translocation of Na^+ and K^+ across the cell membrane. Na^+-K^+ ATPase has been isolated from plasma membranes of several tissues (Bonting, 1970). The Na^+-K^+ ATPase activity is closely parallel to the Na^+ and K^+ pumping activity of a variety of tissues. The enzyme reacts with Mg^{2+}, Na^+, and Ca^{2+} and ATP at the cytoplasmic surface of the membrane and with K^+ at the outer surface. Studies with ^{32}P-labeled ATP show that ATP hydrolysis and the transport of ions by the enzyme involve a cycle of phosphorylation and dephosphorylation of an aspartyl residue on a polypeptide chain of the enzyme protein (Dahl and Hokin, 1974). Internal (intracellular) Na^+ stimulates phosphorylation and external (extracellular) K^+ stimulates dephosphorylation. Outward movement of Na^+ presumably occurs concomitantly with phosphorylation and K^+ inward movement with dephosphorylation. Transport of ions is presumably due to the cyclic changes in the conformations of the enzyme proteins. The change in conformation of the pump enzyme protein is demonstrated with exposure to Na^+ or K^+. A schema of the action of the enzyme and its structural characteristics are shown in Figure 8.4. The enzyme molecule always possesses two types of polypeptide chains. The larger polypeptide ("catalytic unit" or α chain) has a MW of 100,000 and is phosphorylated and dephosphorylated at the aspartyl residue. The smaller chain (β chain) is a glycopeptide with a MW of 50,000.

An important link in the functional identity of the Na^+-K^+ ATPase and the Na^+-K^+ pumping is established by studies of the effect of the cardiotonic steroids. These steroids inhibit Na^+-K^+ transport in a variety of tissues (Glynn, 1964). Soon after the discovery of Na^+-K^+ ATPase, the enzyme was also found to be inhibited by the cardiotonic steroid (Post et al., 1960).

Na^+-K^+ ATPase interacts with the cardiotonic steroid, ouabain, at the outer side of the plasma membrane (Hokin and Dahl, 1972). Since the larger polypeptide of the Na^+-K^+ ATPase molecule possesses both the internally oriented phosphorylation site and the externally exposed ouabain-sensitive, K^+-dependent dephosphorylation site, it appears that the larger polypeptide component spans the thickness of the plasma membrane.

The effectiveness of ouabain in inhibiting the Na^+-K^+ ATPase is progressively decreased as K^+ concentration is increased (Baker, 1972). This observation is of clinical interest, as cardiotonic steroids, which are used normally to augment the cardiac contractile force, occasionally cause an exaggerated response due to an overdose of the steroid. If K^+ can decrease the binding of ouabain to the Na^+-K^+ ATPase site via a competitive antagonism between K^+ and the ligand, then K^+ may serve as an antidote to overdose of cardiotonic steroids. Studies with HeLa cells have shown that K^+ shifted to the right the dose-response curve of Na^+-K^+ ATPase inhibition by ouabain and that there was a competitive type of interaction between K^+ and ouabain (Baker, 1972). However, the concept of competitive inhibition is not supported by the studies of Schwartz and coworkers (1974), who have presented rather convincing data that ouabain and K^+ interact at different binding sites on the Na^+-K^+ ATPase preparations from the cardiac tissue. Schwartz and his colleagues have shown that ouabain inhibition was due neither to a direct nor an indirect displacement of potassium at the potassium site but rather that the inhibition was due to binding of ouabain at a site different from the potassium-binding site. They suggested that ouabain interferes with the phosphorylated form of Na^+-K^+ ATPase and presumably has no effect on the dephosphorylation step. Since the phosphoenzyme is augmented by Na^+ and by ATP-dependent phosphorylation and reduced by K^+-dependent dephosphorylation, it seems logical that an increase in intracellular Na^+ will potentiate inhibition by ouabain by providing more phosphoenzyme substrate for ouabain binding and that K^+ will decrease the ouabain interference with the phosphoenzyme by the dephosphorylation process.

Another aspect of the enzymic mechanism of Na^+-K^+ transport which may be of some interest in physiopathologic condition is concerned with a K^+-dependent phosphatase activity associated with the Na^+-K^+ ATPase (Ahmed and Judah, 1964; Rega et al., 1968). The K^+ phosphatase action hydrolyzes phosphate esters such as paranitrophenyl phosphate, carbamyl phosphate, or acetyl phosphate. The K^+-dependent hydrolysis of phosphate esters occurs in the absence of Na^+ and is sensitive

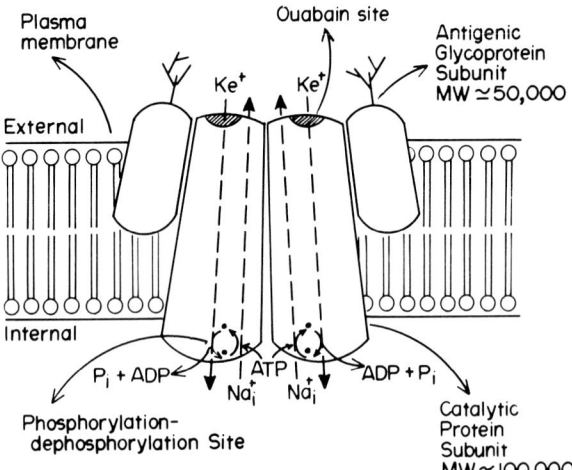

Figure 8.4. Schematic representation of structural and functional components of the cell membrane-bound transport enzyme, ($Na^+ + K^+$)-adenosine triphosphatase. K^+_e, extracellular K^+; Na^+_i, intracellular Na^+; P_i inorganic phosphate. ATP and ADP have their usual meaning.

to ouabain. The close relationship between the Na$^+$-K$^+$ ATPase and K$^+$-dependent phosphatase suggested that the latter enzymic activity may be involved in the final step (dephosphorylation) of the transport enzyme. However, recent studies with an antibody to brain Na$^+$-K$^+$ ATPase have indicated that Na$^+$-K$^+$ ATPase activity and Na$^+$-dependent phosphorylation, but not the K$^+$-dependent phosphatase, of brain can be inhibited by the antibody (Askari, 1974).

The liver possesses a substantial quantity of the enzyme Na$^+$-K$^+$ ATPase (Emmelot et al., 1964). Judah and Ahmed (1964) reported that the liver ATPase is 100 times less sensitive to ouabain than to the brain enzyme but that the liver enzyme was strongly inhibited by chlorpromazine.

FUNCTIONAL ASPECTS OF Na$^+$-K$^+$ TRANSPORT

Active Na$^+$-K$^+$ transport fulfills many functional needs of mammalian cells. A detailed account of Na$^+$ pump-related cellular functions is provided in a review by Baker (1972). This section briefly accounts some of the better known cellular phenomena of active Na$^+$-K$^+$ transport. Clearly, the fact must be appreciated that active transport of electrolytes from either the extracellular to the intracellular compartment or from the intracellular to the extracellular side would be of little functional value to cells if passive movements in opposite directions were not under control or "normal." Thus, the efficacy of Na$^+$-K$^+$ transport in cell function is dependent upon cell membrane permeability to ions Na$^+$ and K$^+$.

Regulation of Cell Volume

A tenable hypothesis in regard to the most primitive organism living in a watery environment is that it needed to maintain constant concentrations of proteins and nucleic acids within its membrane-bound domain. Such a constancy of internal environment was likely threatened because of permeability of the membrane. To counteract the protein osmotic pressure and to resist changes in the volume of protoplasm appear to have been the most logical functions attributable to active transport in that primitive organism.

The characteristic of living cells that they contain a concentration of membrane impermeable negatively charged macromolecules is just as important today as it was to the most primitive life. The osmotic force due to the intracellular macromolecules is in excess of that present in most extracellular environments. Animal cell volume is not fixed. Therefore, according to the osmotic gradient, animal cells would swell as water entered the cells. Obviously, some mechanism must exist under in vivo and under favorable in vitro conditions which protects cells against swelling. Under abnormal in vitro conditions, such as incubation of tissues with metabolic inhibitors or at low temperatures, cells slowly swell. Along with swelling, cell K$^+$ decreases and cell Na$^+$ increases. The swelling process can be hastened by increasing membrane permeability to Na$^+$ and K$^+$. For example, treatment of red cells with surface active agents such as digitonin causes a significant increase in the rate of swelling (Davson and Danielli, 1952). Leaf (1956) postulated that although sodium could permeate the cell membrane, it was effectively restricted to the extracellular compartment because passive influx of Na$^+$ was balanced by the active extrusion via the Na$^+$-K$^+$ pump. Thus, extracellular sodium could balance the intracellular protein osmotic pressure and account for a stable cell volume in metabolically active tissue. With cessation of metabolism, the Na$^+$ pump would cease to operate. Consequently, the check against the intracellular protein osmotic pressure would disappear, and this would lead to cellular swelling. The consequence of a failure of an Na$^+$ pump, whether it is electroneutral or electrogenic, would be an eventual decrease in the resting membrane potential ($\Delta\psi_m$). In the case of failure of an electrogenic Na$^+$ pump, the decrease in $\Delta\psi_m$ would follow immediately and prior to changes in ion gradients. A failure of the electroneutral Na$^+$-K$^+$ pump would first affect ion gradients and then secondarily affect depolarization. Whether the $\Delta\psi_m$ decreases directly or indirectly, the eventual depolarization causes a shift of chloride, from the extracellular to the intracellular side to be followed by the entrance of additional Na$^+$ into cells. The increased intracellular NaCl would lead to increased cell water and cell swelling.

There is little doubt that decreased sodium pumping would lead to cell swelling. Whether or not ouabain-sensitive Na$^+$-K$^+$ transport is involved in the maintenance of cell volume is less clear (MacKnight and Leaf, 1977). It has been argued that inhibition of a tightly coupled, ouabain-sensitive Na$^+$-K$^+$ pump only produces equivalent changes in intra- and extracellular Na$^+$ and K$^+$ concentrations. A decrease in membrane potential may not effect an increase in intracellular chloride in cells which accumulate chloride intracellularly against its electrochemical gradient. Such chloride uptake may decrease with depolarization. There is evidence for the distribution of intracellular chloride against its electrochemical gradient in the kidney (MacKnight and Leaf, 1977). But in the liver, where there is evidence (discussed earlier) that Cl is distributed passively, the failure of an electroneutral Na$^+$-K$^+$ pump would lead to cell swelling.

There is increasing evidence that Ca^{2+} plays an important role in the regulation of membrane permeability to Na$^+$ and K$^+$ as well as in Na$^+$-K$^+$ pumping. The extracellular Ca^{2+} is essential for stabilizing cell membrane permeability (Shanes, 1958). Without extracellular Ca^{2+}, cells lose K$^+$ and gain Na$^+$ (Kleinzeller et al., 1968; Whitembury et al., 1960). In liver slices, active K$^+$ uptake is delayed until intracellular calcium is decreased (van Rossum, 1970). Clearly, Ca^{2+}-related alterations in membrane permeability or pumps could alter cell volume regulation.

Regulation of Cell Metabolism

The metabolic role of the Na$^+$-K$^+$ pump in the liver is evident from the observation that gluconeogenic substrates, pyruvate, lactate, alanine, and fructose can hyperpolarize the hepatic cell membrane via potentiation of active Na^+-K^+ transport (Dambach and Friedmann, 1974). An increase in hepatic membrane potential also occurs in the presence of cyclic AMP, glucagon (Friedmann et al, 1971), or alpha adrenergic agonists (Jenkinson and Koller, 1977). The hormone responses may be related to redistribution of ions subsequent to changes in membrane permeability.

In addition, Na^+-K^+ transport is apparently involved in the tonic regulation of the formation of cellular ATP via generation of ADP through the ATPase action of the pump (Whittam, 1970). A number of studies in the liver support the concept of control of respiration via Na^+-K^+ transport. First of all, it has been shown that ouabain inhibition of the pump decreases respiration by about 30% (Sayeed and Baue, 1971). Secondly, it has been shown that K^+ effects increased transport of Na^+ and a concomitant increase in the activation of the citric acid cycle in the salt gland of the herring gull (van Rossum, 1970). Addition of K^+ stimulated NADPH oxidation and reduction of cytochrome c and a. Furthermore, the changes in electron carriers (toward state 3) were reversed by ouabain. Studies by van Rossum (1966) have also shown that state 3 to state 4 transitions could be seen by activation and inhibition of Na^+-K^+ transport in liver slices. The experiments on the activation of electron carriers and their reversal by ouabain support the view that Na^+-K^+ transport at the plasma membrane controls respiratory ATP formation.

One overt consequence of the Na^+-K^+ pump action is high intracellular $[K^+]$ relative to $[Na^+]$. K^+ has been implicated in the activation of glycolytic as well as gluconeogenic enzymes (Soling and Kleineke, 1976). These observations further demonstrate the metabolic significance of the Na^+-K^+ transport process. The importance of pump-related maintenance of high intracellular K^+ is also evident from the role of K^+ in protein biosynthesis (Pestka, 1971). The overall process of peptide bond formation appears to be dependent on K^+. It is a reasonable supposition that Na^+-K^+ transport not only regulates ATP formation directly but also may exert an indirect regulatory influence on ATP formation via control of the cell's energy-regulating protein synthetic process.

In addition to regulating cell volume and metabolic activity, Na^+-K^+ transport plays important roles in regulating membrane transport of other substances and excitability in nerve and muscle cells. However, in liver there is no evidence at the present time to link Na^+-K^+ transport to membrane transport of other substances.

ALTERATION IN CELLULAR FUNCTIONS IN SHOCK

The term circulatory shock refers to the condition of impending tissue hypoperfusion which often prevails after severe trauma, sepsis, or hemorrhage. The hypoperfusion-induced dysfunction in the vital organs can be reversed to normal function if tissue perfusion is restored in the initial stages. An inability to reverse the vital organ dysfunction with restored perfusion must necessarily mean damage to cells in these organs. The depression of myocardium (Guyton, 1963; Lefer, 1970), the loss of vascular tone (Bond et al., 1973), the altered nervous system function (Kovach and Fonyo, 1960), the respiratory insufficiency (Demling, 1980), and the altered metabolic and REF functions of the liver (Fine et al., 1959; Filkins and Cornell, 1974) are the various vital functional deficits that have been demonstrated in prolonged circulatory shock. These must represent altered cellular function in the respective organs. Initially, the cellular functions are affected by the diminished oxygen and nutrient supply. As hypoperfusion persists, altered concentrations of normal metabolic substances in blood (glucose, amino acids, H^+, K^+, P_i) and appearance of "abnormal" metabolites (lactate, adenine nucleotide breakdown products) and neuroendocrine substances (catecholamines, histamine, kinins and prostaglandins, etc.) in the extracellular fluid compartment could also adversely affect cellular functions. In short, there can be a complete breakdown of the regulation of the milieu intérieur in shock. The cellular effects of the altered milieu intérieur may include alterations in a wide spectrum of subcellular activities such as the cytosolic intermediary metabolism of lipids, proteins, and carbohydrates; the mitochondrial energy synthesis; the endoplasmic reticular-microsomal macromolecular biosynthesis; the membranogenic process in the Golgi apparatus; the nuclear process of transcription of the genetic code; and membrane transport of ions and molecules. Additionally, the cells' latent functions such as the lysosomal release of proteolytic and lipolytic enzymes may also be activated. Alterations in these various cellular functional capabilities may be closely related to structural changes of the various organelles. To date, studies have examined the role of intermediary metabolism (see Ch. 4), mitochondrial energy synthesis (see Ch. 6), and membrane transport in the cell injury of shock. There is relatively little or no information on the effect of shock on the DNA-mediated transcriptive process or the biosynthetic and the membranogenic processes.

Membrane Ion Transport Alterations

Rosenthal and Tabor (1945) and Fox and Baer (1947) demonstrated sodium as the cause for critical fluid loss from the systemic circulation in shock produced by trauma and burn. The injured area of the body was shown to be the site of absorption of electrolytes and subsequently of fluid to the point that fluid was abstracted from the vascular and extracellular spaces in noninjured areas. This resulted in the condition of circulatory collapse. In normal animals, circulatory collapse could be produced after sodium depletion but not after fluid depletion alone (Darrow and Yannet, 1935). Furthermore, associated with sodium depletion in shocked animals was an eight-fold increase in shock sensitivity to potassium (Tabor and Rosenthal, 1947). Studies of Fuhrman and Crismon (1951) provided further insight into electrolyte changes in shock. They showed that injured muscle in shocked animals not only gained sodium and fluid but also lost potassium. Later on, Fuhrman (1960) raised the question of whether or not the sodium potassium shifts in the muscle tissue in animals subjected to tourniquet shock was due to failure of the metabolically dependent sodium pump. This appears to be the first time an active transport failure was implicated as the mechanism for the deranged distribution of sodium and potassium in the muscle in shock.

The observation that injured tissues in shock take up extracellular sodium and fluid and lose potassium is comparable to tissue sodium and potassium shifts that were demonstrated in skeletal muscle subjected to anoxia (Calkin et al., 1954; Paul, 1961). Similar electrolyte shifts occur in the anoxic liver (Flink et al., 1951). Petterson et al. (1974) have studied the effects of ischemia on the potassium and sodium contents and on the $(Na^+ + K^+)$-ATPase activity in dog kidney slices. In these experiments, there was evidence of loss of active Na^+-K^+ transport, as both active net movements of ions and ouabain-sensitive $(Na^+ + K^+)$-ATPase were measured in the kidney slices. Studies of Trump and his colleagues (Saladino et al., 1968; Croker et al., 1970; Sahaphong and Trump, 1971) in epithelial tissues (toad bladder and kidney tubules) have shown altered Na^+, K^+ movements after inhibition of glycolysis and respiration or after treating tissues with sulfhydryl inhibitors. These studies provide insights into the effect of a primary change in membrane permeability opposed to a primary effect of cellular energy deficit on alterations in the ion movements. Ionic shifts occurred faster after altered membrane permeability than after blocking of glycolytic and respiratory ATP formation. These studies as well as the studies on the effects of anoxia in various tissues support the concept that ion movements across plasma membranes are affected secondarily to altered ATP formations.

Studies by Haljamäe (1967, 1970a and b) and Hagberg et al. (1968) demonstrated ionic alterations in skeletal muscle and tissue fluids in hemorrhagic shock. These authors employed single muscle cell preparations for the determination of in situ changes in cell sodium and potassium as well as for the in vitro assessment of K^+ transport. The extracellular electrolyte changes with shock were presumably measured in the extravascular-intercellular spaces by means of a micropipet. The intracellular potassium in skeletal muscle decreased by 26% in dogs subjected to hemorrhagic shock (45 mm Hg hypotension for 135 min). The tissue fluid potassium concentration increased from 4.5 to 10 mEg/liter after shock. The muscle cell sodium increased and tissue fluid sodium decreased simultaneously with potassium changes. The in vitro potassium transport was quantitated by measuring the ion in isolated muscle cells during incubation. During in vitro incubation muscle potassium initially decreased and then reaccumulated. The reaccumulation of potassium was considered an active transport process. However, since skeletal muscle transmembrane distribution of $[K^+]$ is such that the potassium equilibrium potential ($\Delta\psi_{K^+}$) is very close to the measured resting transmembrane potential ($\Delta\psi_m$) and since Haljamae (1970a and b) did not measure skeletal muscle resting membrane potential, we do not know if K^+ uptake measurements under in vitro conditions represented movement of K^+ against an electrochemical gradient.

Campion et al. (1969) and Trunkey et al. (1973) reported measurements of resting transmembrane potential in the skeletal muscle in animals subjected to hemorrhage. In the former study, the resting membrane potential in the skeletal muscle cells decreased progressively from about -90 to -60 mV during 50 min bleeding in the rat. A similar change in the membrane potential occurred with hemorrhage in the dog. The decrease in membrane potential was parallel to decrease in blood pressure. After assuming a passive transmembrane distribution of chloride, the authors could estimate the intracellular chloride in shock muscles from a solution of the Nernst equation after substituting values of the measured membrane potential and the extracellular $[Cl^-]$. With depolarization, intracellular chloride increases and would be followed by an increase in intracell sodium and fluid contents. Whether or not active Na^+ pumping was affected could not be ascertained, as a membrane potential change could occur due to a primary change in membrane permeability. Trunkey et al. (1973) measured membrane potential in the skeletal muscle of the monkey during 3 hr of hemorrhagic shock and the effect of resuscitation of animals for several hours to several days after shock. The membrane potential decreased from about -90 to -60 mV and with resuscitation recovered to control level, along with recovery of blood pressure. The intracellular chloride concentration and extracellular space values were calculated from solution of the Nernst equation. The extracellular space values were used to estimate intracellular $[Na^+]$ and $[K^+]$. These estimations revealed an increase in intracellular Na^+ and a decrease in intracellular $[K^+]$. Again, since ion data were derived from membrane potential measurements, studies of Trunkey et al. (1973) indicate an interference with either the Na^+-K^+ pump or membrane Na^+ and K^+ permeability in shock.

HEPATIC Na^+-K^+ TRANSPORT IN SHOCK

In our laboratory, we have measured the capability of the liver to support active ion transport in experimental hemorrhagic shock (Sayeed et al., 1974, 1981). We evaluated the overall ability of the liver to transport Na^+ and K^+ by measuring 1) in vivo hepatic intracellular concentrations of Na^+ and K^+; 2) net active and passive movements of Na^+ and K^+ in vitro; 3) unidirectional isotopic fluxes in vitro; and 4) hepatic resting membrane potential in vivo. Additionally, we evaluated the relative membrane permeability for Na^+ to that for K^+, (P_{Na^+}/P_{K^+}). A previous study also determined the hepatic $(Na^+ + K^+)$-ATPase in hemorrhagic shock (Wurth et al., 1972). These studies suggested an early progressive failure of the active Na^+-K^+ transport function in shock.

The experimental shock model, which was used in the

study of hepatic Na^+-K^+ transport mechanisms, consisted of bleeding rats to a mean arterial pressure of 40 mm Hg. The animals were referred to as early shock animals when a decrease in blood pressure to 40 mm Hg was first observed. Intermediate shock was designated when the blood pressure was maintained at 40 mm Hg by a gradual reinfusion of 25–30% of shed blood which required about 1 hr. Late shock referred to the stage of shock when 60–70% of the shed blood was returned to maintained pressure at 40 mm Hg; it usually took about 2 hr from the initiation of bleeding. Animals in early or intermediate shock were killed before or after rapid infusion of the shed blood (or the remaining shed blood) plus 3–4 ml of Ringer's lactate solution. For the assessment of intracellular concentrations of ions in vivo, liver was excised immediately after sacrificing the animals and analyzed for sodium, potassium, and chloride. We estimated the extracellular space of the liver by measuring the inulin accessible space within the liver in situ. The concentrations of Na^+, K^+, and Cl^- in the plasma water were used to make corrections for the extracellular ions in the liver tissue and to estimate the intracellular ion concentrations. Changes in hepatic intracellular and plasma ion concentration in shocked animals are shown in Figures 8.5–8.7. There were no demonstrable differences in plasma K^+, Na^+ of Cl^- concentrations of control and shocked animals except that plasma $[K^+]$ was higher

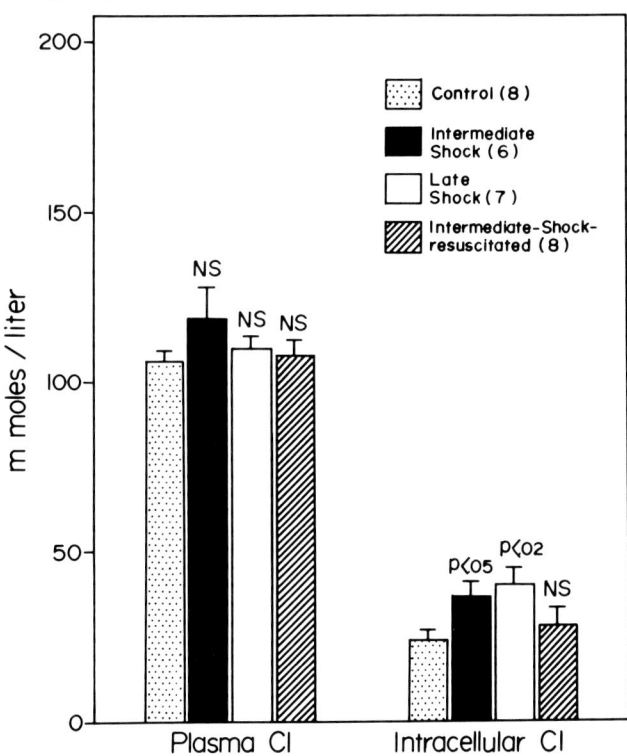

Figure 8.6. Hepatic intracellular and plasma Cl^- concentrations in shock animals. (Reprinted with permission from M.M. Sayeed, R.J. Adler, I.H. Chandry et al.: American Journal of Physiology 240:R211, 1981.)

in the late shock animals as compared with control or intermediate shock groups. The hepatic intracellular $[Na^+]$ of shocked animals was higher than controls. The accompanying decrease in K^+ and Cl^- could be due to a disturbance in coupled Na^+-K^+ movement plus an impairment of uphill movement of NaCl. Russo et al. (1977) have demonstrated a net outward transport of Na^+ to depend on a ouabain-sensitive coupled Na^+-K^+ movement as well as on an ouabain-insensitive coextrusion of Na^+ and Cl^-. While the Na^+-K^+ exchange pump operates across the plasma membrane, the Na^+ and Cl^- coextrusion was indicated to occur via exocytic process (Russo et al., 1977). Resuscitation of rats after intermediate shock resulted in a complete recovery of cell $[K^+]$ and $[Cl^-]$ but not $[Na^+]$. This may indicate recovery of the putative equally coupled Na^+-K^+ pump and the NaCl extrusion process with continued inhibition of an electrogenic sodium pump in the liver. Changes in intracellular $[K^+]$ and $[Na^+]$ with shock may alternatively be due to altered membrane permeability.

Transmembrane movements of Na^+ and K^+ were determined in vitro during incubations of thin liver slices (0.3–0.5 mm) in an oxygenated Krebs-Ringer media. Net passive movements were measured by incubating liver slices either at 0.5°C or at 37°C in the presence of 1.0 mM ouabain. Under both of these incubation conditions there is cessation of active Na^+ and K^+ movements without any interruption of passive ion movements.

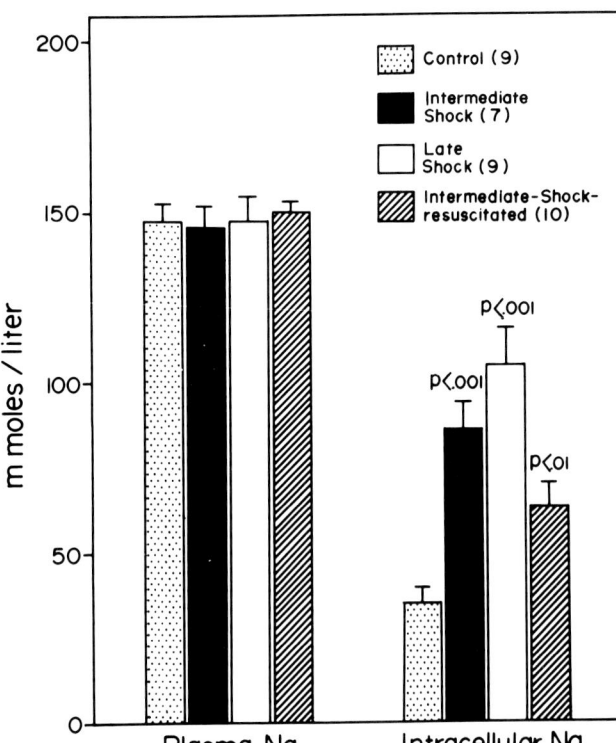

Figure 8.5. Hepatic intracellular and plasma Na^+ concentrations in shock animals. (Reprinted with permission from M.M. Sayeed, R.J. Adler, I.H. Chandry et al.: Amerian Journal of Physiology 240:R211, 1981.)

Table 8.3 shows measurements of passive loss of K⁺ by liver tissue slices. As can be seen, measurements of loss of K⁺ at 0.5°C were comparable to measurements of net ion movements at 37°C in the presence of the inhibitor of active transport (ouabain). These data validate the measurements of passive K⁺ efflux at 0.5°C. Figures 8.8 and 8.9 show a lack of effect of intermediate shock on the passive Na⁺ and K⁺ transport in the liver.

To measure net active movements of ions, we initially incubated liver slices at 0.5°C to cause dissipation of transmembrane gradients of ions. Subsequently, chilled (0.5°C) liver slices were transferred to 37°C and net active ion movements were quantitated. Figure 8.10 shows the effect of late shock on net active movements of Na⁺ and K⁺. In both control and shocked rat liver slices, Na⁺ increased and K⁺ decreased with chilling. With rewarming, whereas there was a reversal of the chilling-induced changes in Na⁺ and K⁺ in the controls, Na⁺ continued to increase and K⁺ was unaltered in the shocked rats. It is possible that the increase in liver sodium represented an increase that becomes bound or immobile intracellularly. Figures 8.11 and 8.12 show net active Na⁺ and K⁺ movements in livers of early shock and intermediate shock animals. These figures also show the effect of treatment or resuscitation of the animals. As can be seen, although Na⁺ and K⁺ active transport was inhibited in early shock, these processes could be restored to control levels with resuscitation. However, the recovery with resuscitation became limited in the intermediate shock animals. Thus, the intermediate shock stage would appear to be a "point of no return" for the Na⁺-K⁺ transport impairment in shock. In summary, in vitro measurements of net ion movements indicated that net active but not passive movements were affected with shock.

The unidirectional Na⁺ efflux was measured in liver slices which were initially incubated in a Krebs-Ringer medium containing a trace quantity of ^{24}Na. Isotopically labeled slices were subsequently washed in media containing nonradioactive Krebs-Ringer solutions. The washout of ^{24}Na into the medium measured the efflux activity. Figures 8.13 and 8.14 show ^{24}Na efflux in liver

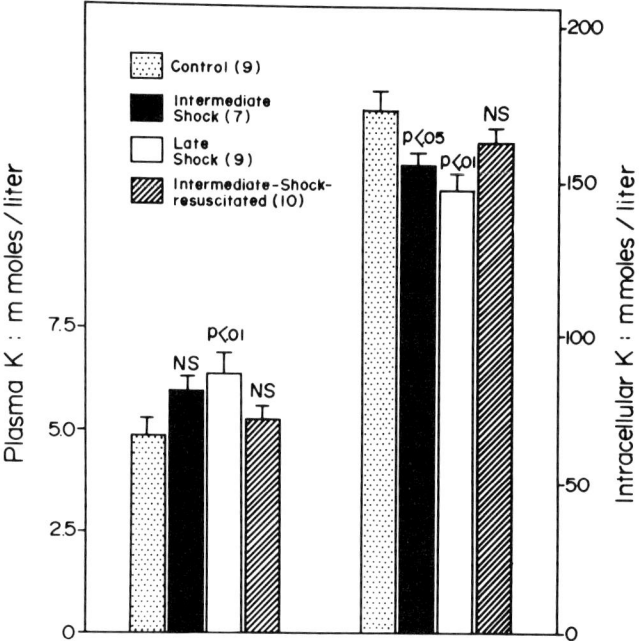

Figure 8.7. Hepatic intracellular and plasma K⁺ concentrations in shock animals. (Reprinted with permission from M.M. Sayeed, R.J. Adler, I.H. Chandry et al.: American Journal of Physiology 240:R211, 1981.)

Table 8.3
Loss of Liver Slice Potassium during Incubation of Slices at 0.5°C or Incubation With Ouabain (1 mM) at 37°C

Time	Incubated at 0.5°C	Incubated with Ouabain at 37°C
min	mmoles/kg dry tissue	
0	330 ± 6[a]	342 ± 8[a]
5	164 ± 5	167 ± 6
15	142 ± 6	136 ± 9
25	125 ± 3	124 ± 3
40	118 ± 3	100 ± 3
60	109 ± 2	99 ± 5

[a] Mean ± SE.

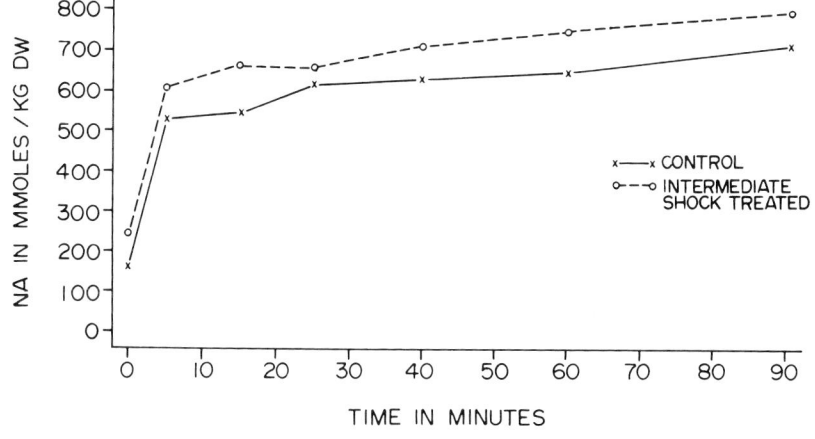

Figure 8.8. Passive influx of Na⁺ in rat liver slices during 0.5°C incubation.

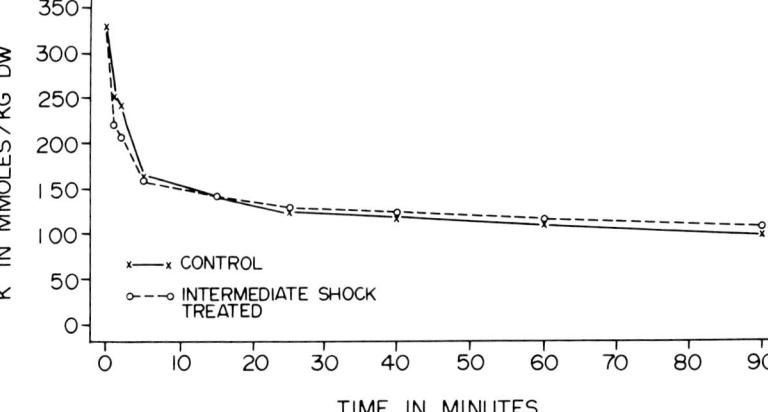

Figure 8.9. Passive efflux of K⁺ in rat liver slices during 0.5°C incubation.

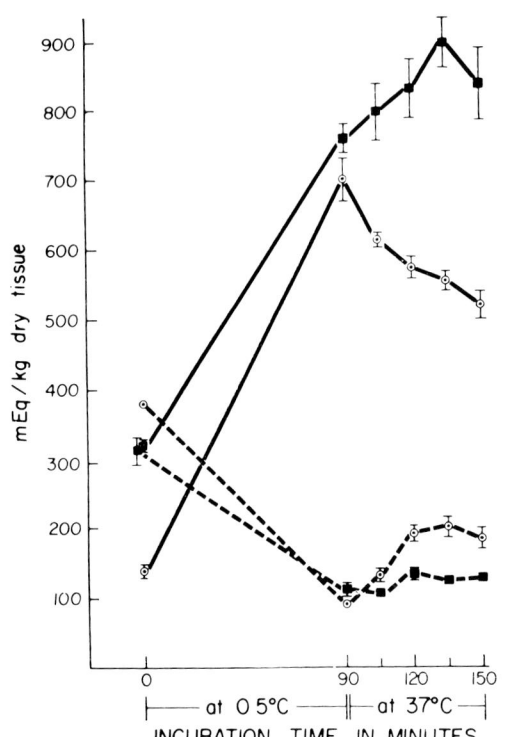

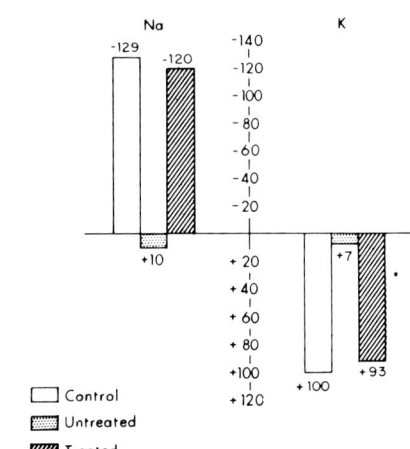

Figure 8.11. The transport capability of liver slices from control, untreated, and treated animals in early shock is expressed as the mEq·kg dry wt of Na extruded (−) and K reincorporated (+) after incubation at 37°C for 60 min preceded by chilling to 0.5°C for 90 min. In untreated shock, Na was + and K was only +7, indicating lack of active transport. (Reprinted with permission from A.E. Baue, M.A. Wurth, and M.M. Sayeed: Annals of Surgery 178:412, 1973.)

Figure 8.10. Na (———) and K (- - -) contents of rat liver slices from control (⊙) and shocked (■) animals at end of chilling at 0.5°C and during rewarming at 37°C. Cation contents given for *time 0* were determined in freshly prepared slices. Means ± SE of *n* samples (2 samples per animal) are shown. Control, *n* = 6; shock, *n* = 10. SEM values less than 5 are not shown on this figure. (Reprinted with permission from M.M. Sayeed and A.E. Baue: American Journal of Physiology 224:1265, 1973.)

slices of control rats and of rats in intermediate shock. The initial rapid loss of ^{24}Na represented a loss of isotope from the extracellular space. This was followed by the slower loss of ^{24}Na representing efflux from the intracellular space. The rate of efflux, expressed in terms of log cpm/0.5 hr in liver slices from shocked rats, was about one-half of that found in controls. Furthermore, it was shown that whereas ouabain inhibited the cellular efflux of ^{24}Na to about 50% in controls, there was no significant inhibition of ^{24}Na efflux by ouabain in liver slices from rats in intermediate shock. These data clearly show an inhibition of ouabain-sensitive Na⁺ transport in shock.

Another aspect of altered Na⁺ transport in livers of shocked rats was discovered during unidirectional flux measurements. We discovered that whereas ouabain-sensitive Na⁺ transport was not sensitive to changes in extracellular [Na⁺] in liver slices of control animals, shock animal liver slices exhibited a dependency of Na⁺ efflux on extracellular [Na⁺]. This would suggest an emergence of a Na⁺-for-Na⁺ exchange process in the shocked animal livers. As discussed in one of the preceding sections, the shift of the Na⁺ pump from the Na⁺-K⁺

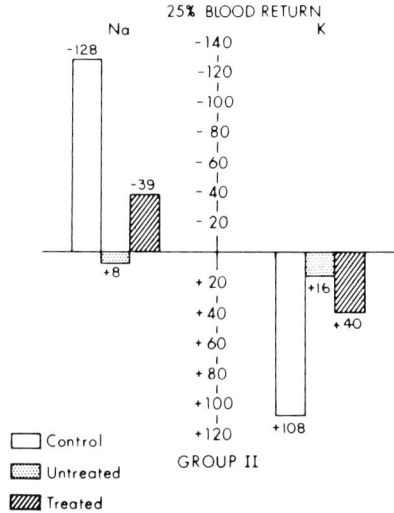

Figure 8.12. Plot of the differences in Na and K content of slices at 0.5°C for 90 min followed by 60 min at 37°C. Normal transport is present in controls, none with untreated shock animals and minimal transport 1 hr after treatment. (Reprinted with permission from A.E. Baue, M.A. Wurth, and M.M. Sayeed: Annals of Surgery 178:412, 1973.)

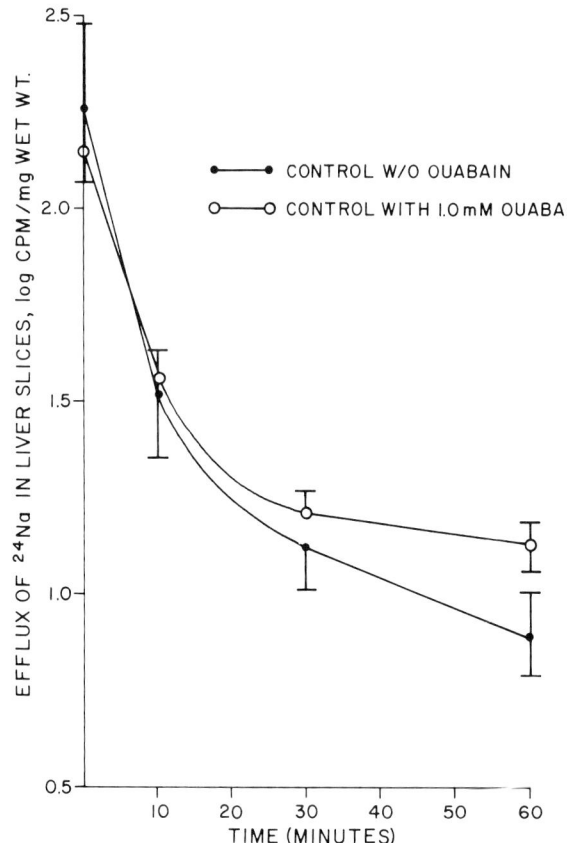

Figure 8.13. Active Na^+ efflux in control animal liver slices.

exchange to a Na^+-Na^+ exchange mode might be indicative of possible loss of the electrogenicity of Na^+ pump.

We determined the extent of membrane depolarization in hepatic cells which accompanied shock. Hepatic resting membrane potentials ($\Delta\psi_m$) were measured in situ in the livers of control and shocked rats by means of intracellular glass microelectrodes. Table 8.4 shows the

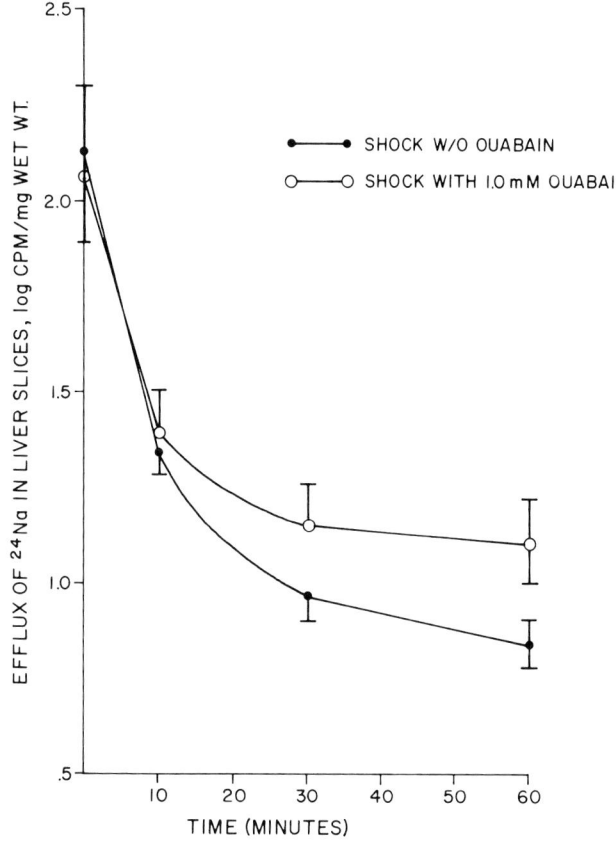

Figure 8.14. Active Na^+ efflux in shock animal liver slices.

Table 8.4
Transmembrane Potential (E_m) and Cl Equilibrium Potential (E_{Cl}) in the Rat Liver[a]

	E_m[b]	E_{Cl}
	mV	mV
Control	-40.4 ± 0.4 (90)[b]	-39.5 ± 2.1
	$n = 21$	$n = 8$
Intermediate shock	-30.9 ± 2.0 (36)[c]	-32.1 pm 1.2
	$n = 8$	$n = 6$
Late shock	-18.8 ± 0.4 (64)[c]	-26.6 ± 1.5[d]
	$n = 11$	$n = 7$
Intermediate shock-resuscitated	-36.3 ± 1.0 (38)[c]	-33.6 ± 1.8
	$n = 8$	$n = 8$

[a] From Sayeed et al., 1980.
[b] All values are means ± SE; N, number of animals; values given in parentheses are number of cell penetrations, 4–5 penetrations/animal. Mean and SE were calculated with values from all penetrations.
[c] Significantly different ($p < .05$), control versus shock.
[d] Significantly different ($p < .05$) from E_m in late shock.

values of hepatic $\Delta\psi_m$ in control and shocked animals. The loss of Na^+ transport activity in the livers of intermediate shock animals was associated with a depolarization of the membrane by about 10 mV. A further depolarization was noted in late shock. With resuscitation of rats in intermediate shock, there was a partial recovery of the $\Delta\psi_m$. The change in $\Delta\psi_m$ with shock definitely indicates an in vivo disturbance in membrane Na^+-K^+ transport. However, like changes in intracellular ion concentrations, $\Delta\psi_m$ changes could be due either to altered an Na^+-K^+ pump or an altered membrane permeability to Na^+ and K^+. Since we measured both the intracellular and the intracellular (plasma) concentrations of Na^+, K^+ and Cl^- and the membrane potentials in situ in the livers of various control and shock animals, we could estimate the ratio of membrane permeability to Na^+ relative to K^+ by using the GHK or the MN equations, which were discussed in earlier sections. The chloride ion must be distributed passively across the liver cell membrane as it remained at the electrochemical equilibrium across the membrane (see Table 8.4). We could use the MN equation (p. 118) to calculate P_{Na^+}/P_{K^+} in control livers, as the coupling ratio of Na^+ to K^+ transport in these livers was 3:2. The P_{Na^+}/P_{K^+} in livers of intermediate shock animals before and after resuscitation could be calculated only by using the GHK equation (p. 117), as in the livers of shocked animals the coupling ratio was 1:1. The calculated values of P_{Na^+}/P_{K^+} in shocked animals was 0.3, which is similar to that found in controls. This estimation indicates that gross changes in cell permeability to Na^+ ralative to K^+ did not occur, at least in the intermediate stage of shock.

This would mean that gross alterations in hepatic intracellular Na^+ and K^+ were probably due to failure of active Na^+-K^+ transport. Furthermore, it appears that the decrease in membrane potential with intermediate shock was due to failure of an electrogenic Na^+ pump. These data support the concept that hemorrhagic shock primarily alters an electrogenic component of the Na^+-K^+ pump and this preceeds the membrane depolarization and shifts in intracellular ion concentrations. The extent of depolarization due only to cessation of electrogenic pump, however, remains unresolved. A failure of electrogenic Na^+ pumping in the liver would cause a more rapid alteration of transmembrane gradients of potentials and ion concentrations and of cellular processes which are dependent on these gradients than that caused by an impairment of an electroneutral Na^+ pump.

The in vivo failure of the hepatic Na^+-K^+ pump in shock is supported by in vitro measurements of net Na^+ and K^+ movements and unidirectional ouabain-sensitive Na^+ effluxes in liver slices from animals in shock.

HEPATIC $(Na^+ + K^+)$-ATPASE IN SHOCK

Another aspect of the Na^+-K^+ transport that has been studied in shock is the activity of the transport enzyme, $(Na^+ + K^+)$-ATPase (Wurth et al., 1972). A decreased pumping of Na^+ and K^+ would be associated with a decreased activity of the $(Na^+ + K^+)$-ATPase. In our studies, the $(Na^+ + K^+)$-ATPase activity increased in the liver in shock when Na^+-K^+ transport was shown to be decreased (Fig. 8.15). We can only speculate as to how the transport of Na^+ and K^+ and the ATP hydrolyzing activity of the Na^+ pump mechanism were affected in a paradoxical manner. One possible explanation would be that Na^+ efflux was increased, as was the ATPase activity, in response to an increased inward leak of Na^+, but the increased efflux could not compensate for the inward leaking of Na^+. This would suggest an uncompensated increase in ion conductance to be a primary membrane alteration in shock. However, this is not tenable since we have actually measured the ouabain-sensitive Na^+ efflux activity and found it to be depressed in shock. It is plausible that the Na^+-for-Na^+ exchange process, which we found in shock but not in control livers, may be related to increased $(Na^+ + K^+)$-ATPase. A second possible explanation for the increased $(Na^+ + K^+)$-ATPase in the face of decreased Na^+ pumping would be an "uncoupling" of the ATP hydrolyzing activity of the enzyme from the work of translocation of ions. This would presumably be due to an increase in the Na^+-sensitive phosphorylation of the $(Na^+ + K^+)$-ATPase, at the expense of ATP, on the internal surface of the plasma membrane without the subsequent dephosphorylation of the enzyme or the uphill translocation of Na^+ and K^+. Further research would be required to resolve this possibility.

HEPATIC CELL VOLUME REGULATION IN SHOCK

The method of chilling and rewarming of liver slices was also employed to study the regulation of cell volume

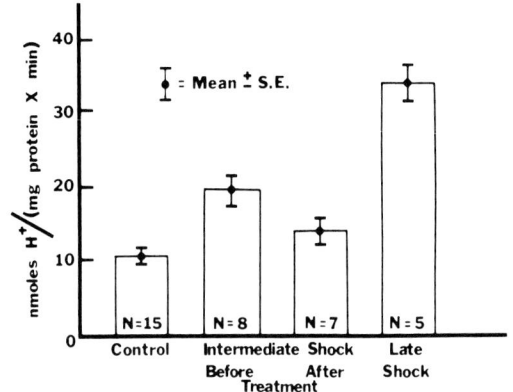

Figure 8.15. (Na + K)-ATPase activity in livers of rats in intermediate and late shock. N, number of animals. The values in intermediate shock and late shock were significantly higher ($p < 0.001$) than control values. The activity after treatment in intermediate shock was significantly lower ($p < 0.05$) than the activity before treatment. (Reprinted with permission from M.M. Sayeed, M. Wurth, I.N. Chandry, and A.E. Baue: Circulatory Shock 1:195, 1974.)

regulation in vivo. It was previously shown by Elshove and van Rossum (1963) that during chilling of control liver slices, total tissue water increased and then partially decreased in rewarming. This indicated the ability of control liver slices to regulate cell volume. The increase in tissue water after chilling and the decrease after rewarming were actually caused by an increase and decrease in intracellular water (Sayeed and Baue, 1973). The results of measurements of total water content in liver slices from control animals are presented in Table 8.5. Liver slices from control animals were swollen with suppression of metabolism at 0.5°C but cell volume recovered after restoration of metabolism at 37°C. Liver slices from shocked animals failed to do so. Furthermore, we have determined that hepatic cell volume regulation is not restored after resuscitation of the animals in intermediate shock. Shock-related alterations in hepatic cell volume regulation were parallel to changes in electrogenic Na^+ pumping, as both processes were affected in early shock and became irreversible after the intermediate stage of shock. Alterations in cell volume regulation may be secondary to changes in electrogenic Na^+ pumping.

HEPATIC CELLULAR ATP AND Na^+-K^+ TRANSPORT IN SHOCK

An important question that should be raised regarding the shock-induced alteration in active Na^+-K^+ transport is whether or not this is due primarily to decreased cellular ATP synthesis. The loss of active transport function after ischemia or anoxia in kidney and skeletal muscle cells has been shown to be due to ATP depletion in these cells. However, two factors suggest that this may not be true in the case of hemorrhagic shock-induced derangement of Na^+-K^+ pump. First of all, hemorrhagic shock does not cause an ischemic type of insult in the liver, as blood flow to liver is reduced only partially—to about 50% of the preshock level (Blahitka and Rakusan, 1977). Second, as pointed out elsewhere in this chapter ("Energetics of the Na^+-K^+ Transport"), the energy requirements of hepatic Na^+-K^+ transport are very low. About one-half of maximal Na^+-K^+ transport activity persisted when ATP synthesis was reduced from aerobic levels to just above the anaerobic level. There is also indication that Na^+-K^+ transport has a higher affinity for cellular ATP than other energy-dependent cellular processes. Experimental data concerning hepatic mitochondrial energy metabolism in hemorrhagic shock also support the concept that hepatic cellular ATP depletion may not primarily contribute to active Na^+-K^+ transport. We found that liver mitochondrial metabolism, although it was depressed in the intermediate shock stages, was restored to control levels after resuscitating animals at this stage. Both respiratory control and ADP-stimulated respiration by isolated mitochondria were restored to near control levels (Sayeed and Baue, 1971). A similar protocol of resuscitation as was used in the study of mitochondrial metabolism failed to restore the Na^+-K^+ pump activity (Sayeed et al., 1980). Thus, active Na^+-K^+ transport could not be restored even after the recovery of mitochondrial mechanisms which are responsible for the ATP synthesis. Measurements of tissue adenine nucleotide content of liver showed a decrease in hepatic ATP from 1.80 ± 0.03 (mean $\pm$ SE, μmole/g) in controls to 0.35 ± 0.04 in intermediate shock (Sayeed et al., 1974). The decreased level of ATP in the liver in intermediate shock was above the K_m value of hepatic Na^+-K^+ transport for ATP which was reported to be 0.20 μmole/g (van Rossum, 1972b). Although we do not have direct evidence for Na^+-K^+ transport failure to occur before ATP changes in shock, the foregoing consideration suggests that membrane active Na^+-K^+ transport is affected in the absence of significant alterations in hepatic ATP. There is also a possibility that ATP alterations occur secondarily to an impairment of active Na^+-K^+ transport. A transport-related change in the cytoplasmic cationic milieu can adversely affect mitochondrial respiration; increased intracellular Na^+ has a detrimental effect on the respiratory control of rat liver mitochondrial (Gómez-Puyou et al., 1969). At present, the most tenable hypothesis which can account for the altered hepatic Na^+-K^+ transport in shock is that of an irreversible alteration in the membrane-bound molecular transport apparatus, i.e., the $(Na^+ + K^+)$-ATPase.

Table 8.5
In Vitro Cell Volume Regulation in Liver Slices[a]

	Control	Early shock	Intermediate shock	Late shock
Fresh tissue	2.09 ± 0.05[b]	2.42 ± 0.12	2.74 ± 0.13	2.48 ± 0.15
	(16)	(6)	(5)	(9)
Tissue chilled for 90 min	3.89 ± 0.08	4.16 ± 0.16	4.21 ± 0.17	4.04 ± 0.17
	(18)	(6)	(5)	(11)
	$p < 0.001$[c]	N.S.[d]	$p < 0.01$	$p < 0.01$
Tissue chilled for 90 min and rewarmed for 60 min	3.25 ± 0.08	4.42 ± 0.11	5.14 ± 0.07	4.64 ± 0.10
	(18)	(6)	(5)	(11)

[a] From Sayeed et al., 1974.
[b] Mean $\pm$ SE values in units of liters of water/kg dry tissue. Parentheses indicate number of animals; change in fresh tissue water contents: control versus early shock, $p < 0.02$, control versus intermediate shock, $p < 0.001$; control vs. late shock, $p < 0.02$.
[c] Significance of change in H_2O contents during tissue rewarming.
[d] Not significant ($p > 0.05$).

Acknowledgment. I thank Dr. Diane Klein for reading the manuscript and making suggestions to improve its style. Thanks are also due to Ms. Vivian Rogala for her expert typing of the manuscript. At the time of the writing of this chapter, author's research was supported by National Institutes of Health Grants, HL 20878 and HL 08682.

References

Ahmed, K., and Judah, J.D.: Preparation of lipoproteins containing cation-dependent ATPase. Biochim. Biophys. Acta *93:*603, 1964.

Askari, A.: The effects of antibodies to Na^+, K^+-ATPase on the reactions catalyzed by the enzyme. Ann. N.Y. and Acad. Sci. *242:*372–388, 1974.

Baker, P.F.: The sodium pump in animal tissues and its role in the control of cellular metabolism and function. In *Metabolic Pathways* edited by L. E. Hokin, ed. 3, vol. 6, ch. 7. Academic Press, New York, 1972.

Baker, P.F., Hodgkin, A.L., and Shaw, T.I.: The effects of changes in internal concentrations on the electrical properties of perfused giant axons. J. Physiol. (Lond.) *164:*355, 1962.

Barnabei, O., Leghissa, G., and Tomasi, V.: Hormonal control of the potassium level in isolated rat liver cells. Biochim. Biophys. Acta *362:*316, 1974.

Berg, T., and Iversen, J.G.: K^+ transport in isolated rat liver cells stimulated by glucagon and insulin in vitro. Acta Physiol. Scand. *97:*202, 1976.

Berry, M.N., and Friend, D.S.: High-yield preparation of isolated rat liver parenchymal cells. A biochemical and fine structural study. J. Cell Biol. *43:*506, 1969.

Blahitka, J., and Rakusan, K.: Blood flow in rats during hemorrhagic shock: Differences between surviving and dying animals. Circ. Shock *4:*79, 1977.

Bond, R.F., Manning, E.S., Gonzales, N.M., et al.: Myocardial and skeletal muscle responses to hemorrhage and shock during α-adrenergic blockage. Am. J. Physiol. *225:*247, 1973.

Bonting, S.L.: Sodium-potassium activated adenosine triphosphatase and cation transport. In *Membranes and Ion Transport*, edited by E.E. Bittar, pp. 257–363. John Wiley & Sons, New York, 1970.

Breuer, H., and Whattam, R.: Ion movements of seminal vesicle mucosa. J. Physiol. (Lond.), *135:*213, 1957.

Brinley, F.J., and Mullins, L.J.: Sodium fluxes in internally dialyzed squid axons. J. Gen. Physiol. *52:*181, 1968.

Caldwell, P.C.: Factors governing movements and distribution of inorganic ions in nerve and muscle. Physiol. Rev. *48:*1, 1968.

Caldwell, P.C., Hodgkin, A.L., Keynes, R.D., et al.: Partial inhibition of the active transport of cations in the giant axons of loligo. J. Physiol. *752:*591, 1960.

Calkins, E., Taylor, I.M., and Hastings, B.A.: Potassium exchange in the isolated rat diaphragm; effect of anoxia and cold. Am. J. Physiol. *177:*211, 1954.

Campion, D.S., Lynch, L.J., Rector, F.C., Jr., et al.: Effect of hemorrhagic shock on transmembrane potential. Surgery *66:*1051, 1969.

Casteels, R.: The relation between the potential and the ion distribution in smooth muscle cells. In *Smooth Muscle*, edited by E. Bülbring, A. Brading, A. Jones, and T. Tomita, ed. 1, ch. 2. Williams & Wilkins, Baltimore, 1970.

Claret, M., and Mazet, J.L.: Ionic fluxes and permeabilities of cell membranes in rat liver. J. Physiol. (Lond.) *223:*279, 1972.

Claret, B., Claret, M., and Mazet, J.L.: Ionic transport and membrane potential of rat liver cells in normal and low-chloride solutions. J. Physiol. *230:*87, 1973.

Conway, E.J., Kernan, R.P., and Zadunaisky, J.A.: The sodium pump in skeletal muscle in relation to energy barriers. J. Physiol. (Lond.) *155:*263, 1961.

Croker, B.P., Saladino, A.J., and Trump, B.F.: Ion movements in cell injury: Relationship between energy metabolism and the pathogenesis of lethal injury in the toad bladder. Am. J. Pathol. *59:*247, 1970.

Dahl, J.L., and Hokin, L.E.: The sodium-potassium adenosinetriphosphatase. Annu. Rev. Biochem. *43:*327, 1974.

Dambach, G., and Friedmann, N.: Substrate-induced membrane potential changes in the perfused rat liver. Biochim. Biophys. Acta *367:*366, 1974.

Darrow, D.C., and Yannet, H.: The changes in the distribution of body water accompanying increase and decrease in extracellular electrolytes. J. Clin. Invest. *14:*266, 1935.

Davson, H., and Danielli, J.F.: *The Permeability of Natural Membranes*, 365 pp. MacMillan, New York, 1952.

Dean, R.B.: Theories of electrolyte equilibrium in muscle. Symp. Soc. Exp. Biol. *3:*331, 1941.

Demling, R.H.: Lung fluid and protein dynamics during hemorrhagic shock, resuscitation, and recovery. Circ. Shock *7:*149, 1980.

DeWeer, P.: Na^+, K^+ exchange and Na^+, Na^+ exchange in the giant axon of the squid. Ann. N.Y. Acad. Sci. *242:*435–444, 1974.

Dunham, E.T., and Glynn, I.M.: Adenosinetriphosphatase activity and the active movements of alkali metal ions. J. Physiol. (Lond.) *156:*274, 1961.

Elshove, A., and van Rossum, G.D.V.: Net movements of sodium, potassium and their relationships to respiration in slices of rat liver incubated in vitro. J. Physiol. (Lond.) *168:*531, 1963.

Emmelot, P., Bos, C.J., Benedetti, E.L., et al.: Studies on plasma membranes. I. Chemical composition and enzyme content of plasma membranes isolated from rat liver. Biochim. Biophys. Acta *90:*126, 1964.

Filkins, J.P., and Cornell, R.P.: Depression of hepatic gluconeogenesis and the hypoglycemia of endotoxin. Am. J. Physiol. *227:*778, 1974.

Fine, J., Rutenburg, S., and Schweinburg, F.B.: The role of the reticuloendothelial system in hemorrhagic shock. J. Exp. Med. *110:*547, 1959.

Flink, E.B., Hastings, A.B., and Lowry, J.K.: Changes in potassium and sodium concentrations in liver slices accompanying incubation in vitro. Am. J. Physiol. *163:*598, 1950.

Fox, C.L., and Baer, H.: Redistribution of potassium, sodium and trauma, and its relation to the phenomena of shock. Am. J. Physiol. *151:*155, 1947.

Fozzard, H.A., and Kipnis, D.M.: Regulation of intercellular sodium concentrations in rat diaphragm muscle. Science *156:*1257, 1967.

Friedmann, N., Somlyo, A.V., and Somlyo, A.P.: Cyclic adenosine and guanosine monophosphate and glucagon: Effect on liver membrane potentials. Science *171:*400, 1971.

Fuhrman, F.A.: Electrolytes and glycogen in injured tissues. In *The Biochemical Response to Injury*, edited by H.B. Stoner and C.J. Threlfall, pp. 5–21. Charles C Thomas, Springfield, IL, 1960.

Fuhrman, F.A., and Crismon, J.M.: Early changes in the distribution of sodium, potassium, and water in rabbit muscles following release of tourniquets. Am. J. Physiol. *166:*424, 1951.

Garrahan, P.J., and Glynn, I.M.: The incorporation of inorganic phosphate into adenosine triphosphate by reversal of the sodium pump. J. Physiol. *192:*237, 1967.

Glynn, I.M.: The action of cardiac glycosides on ion movements. Pharmacol. Rev. *16:*381, 1964.

Gómez-Puyou, A., Sandoval, T., Pena, A., et al.: Effect of sodium and potassium on mitochondrial respiratory control, oxygen uptake, and adenosine triphosphatase activity. J. Biol. Chem. *244:*5339, 1969.

Guyton, A.C.: *Circulatory Physiology: Cardiac Output and Its Regulation,* 347 pp. W.B. Saunders, Philadelphia, 1963.

Hagberg, S., Haljamäe, H., and Rockett, H.: Shock reactions in skeletal muscle. III. The electrolyte content of tissue fluid and blood plasma before and after induced hemorrhagic shock. Ann. Surg. *168:*243, 1968.

Haljamäe, H.: Shock reactions in skeletal muscle. A method for determining the potassium content of single skeletal muscle cells. Acta Cir. Scand. *133:*259, 1967.

Haljamäe, H.: Sampling of nanoliter volumes of mammalian subcutaneous tissue fluid and ultra-micro flame photometric analyses of the K^+ and Na^+ concentrations. Acta Physiol. Scand. *78:*1, 1970a.

Haljamäe, H.: Effects of hemorrhagic shock and treatment with hypothermia on the potassium content and transport of single mammalian skeletal muscle cells. Acta Physiol. Scand. *78:*189, 1970b.

Hodgkin, A.L., and Keynes, R.D.: Active transport of cations in giant axons from sepia and loliga. J. Physiol. (Lond.) *128:*28, 1955.

Jacobs, H.S.: Abnormalities in the physiology of erythrocyte membrane in hereditary spherocytosis. Am. J. Med. *41:*734, 1966.

Jenkinson, D.H., and Koller, K.: Interactions between the effects of α- and β-adrenoceptor agonists and adenine nucleotides on the membrane potential of cells in guinea-pig liver slices. Br. J. Pharmacol. *59:*163, 1977.

Judah, J.D., and Ahmed, K.: The biochemistry of sodium transport. Biol. Rev. *39:*160, 1964.

Judah, J.D., Ahmed, K., McLean, A.E.M., et al.: Ion transport in ethionine intoxication. Lab. Invest. *15:*167, 1966.

Keynes, R.D.: The ionic fluxes in frog muscle. Proc. R. Soc. Lond. (Biol.) *142:*359, 1954.

Keynes, R.D.: Some further observations on the sodium efflux in frog muscle. J. Physiol. *178:*305, 1965.

Keynes, R.D., and Steinhardt, R.A.: The components of the sodium efflux in frog muscle. J. Physiol. (Lond.) *198:*581, 1968.

Kleinzeller, A., Knotkova, A., and Nedvidkova, J.: The effects of calcium ions on the steady state ionic distribution in kidney cortex cells. J. Gen. Physiol. (Suppl.) *51:*326, 1968.

Kovach, A.G.B., and Fonyo, A.: Metabolic responses to injury in cerebral tissues. In *The Biochemical Response to Injury,* edited by H.B. Stoner and C.J. Threfall, pp. 129–160. Charles C Thomas, Springfield, IL, 1960.

Leaf, A. On the mechanism of fluid exchange of tissues in vitro. Biochem. J. *62:*241, 1956.

Lefer, A.M.: Role of myocardial depressant factor in the pathogenesis of circulatory shock. Fed. Proc. *29:*1836, 1970.

Lev, A.A., and Armstrong, W.M.: Ionic activities in cells. In Curr. Top. Membr. Transp. *6:*59–123, 1975.

Ling, G.N.: *A Physical Theory of the Living State: The Association-Induction Hypothesis.* Blaisdell, New York, 1962.

Lowe, A.G.: Functional aspects of active cation transport. In *Membranes and Ion Transport,* edited by E.E. Bittar, ed. 1, ch. 8. Wiley-Interscience, New York, 1971.

MacKnight, A.D.C., and Leaf, A.: Regulation of cellular volume. Physiol. Rev. *57:*510, 1977.

McLean, A.E.M.: Ion transport in rat liver slices. Biochem. J. *87:*161, 1963.

Mullins, L.J., and Noda, K.: The influence of Na-free solutions on membrane potential of frog muscle fibres. J. Gen. Physiol. *47:*117, 1963.

Page, E., and Storm, S.R.: Cat heart muscles in vitro. VII. Active transport of sodium in papillary muscles. J. Gen. Physiol. *48:*957, 1965.

Paul, D.H.: The effects of anoxia on the isolated rat phrenic-nerve- diaphragm preparation. J. Physiol. (Lond.) *155:*358, 1961.

Pestka, S.: Protein biosynthesis: Mechanism, requirements, and potassium dependency. In *Membranes and Ion Transport,* edited by E.E. Bittar, ch. 9. Wiley-Interscience, London, 1971.

Petterson, S., Gelin, L.E., Jonsson, O., et al.: Effects of warm ischemia on the potassium and sodium contents and on the sodium-potassium-ATPase activity in dog kidney slices. Eur. Surg. Res. *6:*330, 1974.

Post, R.L., and Jolly, P.C.: The linkage of sodium, potassium and ammonium active transport across the human erythrocyte membrane. Biochim. Biophys. Acta *25:*118, 1957.

Post, R.L., Merrit, C.R., Kinsolving, C.R., et al.: Membrane adenosinetriphosphate as a participant in the active transport of sodium and potassium in the human erythrocyte. J. Biol. Chem. *235:*1796, 1960.

Rega, A.F., Garrahan, P.J., and Pouchan, M.I.: Effect of ATP and Na^+ on K^+ activated phosphatase from red blood cell membranes. Biochim. Biophys. Acta *150:*742, 1968.

Rosenthal, S.M., and Tabor, H.: Electrolyte changes and chemotherapy in experimental burn and traumatic shock and hemmorhage. Arch. Surg. *51:*244, 1945.

Russo, M.A., van Rossum, G.D.V., and Galeotti, T.: Observations on the regulation of cell volume and metabolic control in vitro; changes in the composition and ultrastructure of liver slices under conditions of varying metabolic and transporting activity. J. Membr. Biol. *31:*267, 1977.

Sahaphong, S., and Trump, B.F.: Studies of cellular injury in isolated kidney tubules of the flounder. V. Effects of inhibiting sulfhydryl groups of plasma membrane with the organic mercurials PCMB (parachloromercuribenzoate) and PCMBS (parachloromercuribenzenesulfonate). Am. J. Pathol. *63:*277, 1971.

Saladino, A.J., Hawkins, H.K., and Trump, B.F.: Ion transport and cell injury. Alterations in ultrastructure and ion flux in toad bladder epithelium after treatment with surfactants. Lab. Invest. *18:*333, 1968.

Sayeed, M.M., and Baue, A.E.: Mitochondrial metabolism of succinate, β-hydroxybutyrate, and α-ketoglutarate in hemorrhagic shock. Am. J. Physiol. *220:*1275, 1971.

Sayeed, M.M., and Baue, A.E.: Na-K transport in rat liver slices in hemorrhagic shock. Am. J. Physiol. *224:*1265, 1973.

Sayeed, M.M., Wurth, M., Chaudry, I.H., and Baue, A.E.: Cation transport in the liver in hemorrhagic shock. Circ. Shock *1:*195, 1974.

Sayeed, M.M., Alder, R.J., Chaudry, I.H., et al.: Effect of hemorrhagic shock on hepatic transmembrane potentials and intracellular electrolytes, in vivo. Am. J. Physiol. *240:*R211, 1981.

Schatzmann, J.H.: Herzglykoside als Hemmstoffe für den aktiven Kalzium und Natriumtransport durch die erythrocytenmembrane. Helv. Physiol. Pharmacol. Acta *1:*346, 1953.

Schwartz, A., Lindenmayer, G.E., Allen, J.C., et al.: The nature of the cardiac glycoside enzyme complex: Mechanism and kinetics of binding and dissociation using a high-activity heart Na$^+$, K$^+$-ATPase. Ann. N.Y. Acad. Sci. *242:*577, 1974.

Seidman, I., and Cascarano, J.: Anaerobic cation transport in rat liver slices: Effect of metabolites and inhibitors. Am. J. Physiol. *211:*1165, 1966.

Sen, A.K., and Post, R.L.: Stoichiometry and localization of adenosine triphosphate dependent sodium and potassium transport in the erythrocyte. J. Biol. Chem. *239:*345, 1964.

Shanes, A.M.: Electrochemical aspects of physiological action in excitable cells. I. The resting cell and its alteration by extrinsic factors. Pharmacol. Rev. *10:*59, 1958.

Sjodin, R.A., and Beaugé, L.A.: Coupling and selectivity of sodium and potassium transport in squid giant axons. J. Gen. Physiol. (Suppl.) *51:*152, 1968.

Skou, J.C.: The influence of some cations on the adenosine triphosphatase from peripheral nerves. Biochim. Biophys. Acta *23:*394, 1957.

Soling, H.D., and Kleineke, J.: *Species Dependent Regulation of Hepatic Gluconeogenesis in Higher Animals*, 369 pp. John Wiley & Sons, New York, 1976.

Tabor, H., and Rosenthal, S.M.: Body temperature and oxygen consumption in traumatic shock and hemorrhage in mice. Am. J. Physiol. *149:*449, 1947.

Tomasi, V., Poli, A., Ferretti, E., et al.: Hormone and prostaglandin E, control of potassium and cyclic AMP levels in isolated rat liver cells. Adv. Enzyme Regul. *13:*189, 1975.

Troshin, A.S.: *Problems of Cell Permeability*. Pergamon Press, Oxford, 1966.

Trunkey, D.D., Illner, H., Wagner, I.V., et al.: The effect of hemorrhagic shock on intracellular muscle action potentials in the primate. Surgery *74:*241, 1973.

van Rossum, G.D.V.: Net sodium and potassium movements in liver slices prepared from rats of different foetal and postnatal ages. Biochim. Biophys. Acta *74:*1, 1963a.

van Rossum, G.D.V.: Respiration and glycolysis in liver slices prepared from rats of different foetal and post-natal ages. Biochim. Biophys. Acta *74:*15, 1963b.

van Rossum, G.D.V.: Simultaneous measurement of ^{24}Na$^+$ efflux and pyridine nucleotides in slices of rat liver. Biochim. Biophys. Acta *122:*312, 1966.

van Rossum, G.D.V.: Relation of intracellular Ca$^+$ to retention of K$^+$ by liver slices. Nature *225:*638, 1970.

van Rossum, G.D.V.: The relation of sodium and potassium ion transport to the respiration and adenine nucleotide content of liver slices treated with inhibitors of respiration. Biochem. J. *129:*427, 1972a.

van Rossum, G.D.V.: The metabolic coupling of ion transport. In *Hibernation and Hypothermia, Perspectives and Challenges*, edited by F.E. South, J.P. Hannon, J.R.Willis, E.T. Pengelley, and N.R. Alpert, ed. 1, pp. 191–218. Elsevier, New York, 1972b.

Whittam, R.: *Enzymatic Aspects of the Sodium Pump*, 235 pp. Wiley-Interscience, New York 1970.

Whittembury, G., Sugino, N., and Solomon, A.K.: Effect of antidiuretic hormone and calcium on the equivalent pore radius of kidney slices from necturus. Nature *187:*699, 1960.

Williams, J.A.: Origin of transmembrane potentials in nonexcitable cells. J. Theor. Biol. *28:*287, 1970.

Williams, J.A., Withrow, C.W., and Woodbury, D.M.: Effects of ouabain and diphenylhydantoin on transmembrane potentials, intracellular electrolytes, and cell pH of rat muscle and liver in vivo. J. Physiol. *212:*101, 1971.

Wurth, M.A., Sayeed, M.M., and Baue, A.E.: (Na$^+$ + K$^+$)-ATPase activity in the liver with hemorrhagic shock. Proc. Soc. Exp. Biol. Med. *139:*1238, 1972.

CHAPTER 9

Ion and Water Shifts, Cellular

KEITH A. REIMER
ROBERT B. JENNINGS

Cell swelling and altered ion transport long have been known to accompany a variety of pathologic states. However, the potential role of altered ion transport and/or volume regulation in the pathogenesis of cell injury and death in ischemic or anoxic states has received widespread attention only during the last 15 years. There are now two major aspects to this general subject. The first is the potential role of cell swelling or abnormal ion transport on the process of cell injury, per se. For example, cell swelling could potentially become a lethal event if it resulted in rupture of the cell membrane or in the distortion of internal structural relationships essential for subcellar function. Alternatively, calcium overload has been implicated to the development of cell death in several types of injury.

The second major aspect to this general subject is the possibility that cell swelling may cause capillary compression and thereby limit microvascular perfusion. Thus transient episodes of hypoxia or ischemia, insufficient in severity to cause parenchymal cell death, could nevertheless be lethal through the secondary development of persistent ischemia.

Before considering these aspects of defective ion transport and cell volume regulation, we shall review briefly the mechanisms of normal cell volume regulation and ion transport. Both of these topics are very broad and a thorough review is beyond the scope of this chapter. Thus, we will try to summarize the current concepts of these processes and refer the reader to several extensive reviews for more in-depth analysis (Macknight and Leaf, 1977; Baker, 1972; Glitsch, 1979; Glynn and Karlish, 1975; Hokin, 1976; Skou, 1965).

CHARACTERISTICS OF CELL VOLUME REGULATION AND ION TRANSPORT

It is now generally accepted that the cell membrane is permeable to water and the small molecular weight solutes of the extracellular fluid including sodium, chloride, and potassium ions. It is also well known that the extracellular fluid has a relatively low colloid content, whereas the intracellular fluid contains proteins and organic phosphates which exert a considerable oncotic pressure. In the absence of opposing forces, this oncotic pressure would draw fluid and electrolytes into the cell causing progressive cell swelling. Plant cells resist this oncotic pressure with a thick cell wall but animal cells lack this protective mechanism. In the first half of this century, it was hypothesized that cell volume was maintained by energy-dependent extrusion of water from the cell to maintain intracellular osmolality greater than that of the extracellular fluid. However, the energy necessary to continuously pump water from the cell would be inordinate, and it has subsequently been established that osmolality is equivalent inside and outside the cell. This equivalence of osmotic forces is achieved by the active extrusion of sodium to balance the internal content of impermeant solutes. This extrusion of sodium also results in a membrane potential so that the interior of the cell is electronegative compared to the exterior.

In the steady state, the ionic constituency of the cell is maintained by the counterbalancing effects of this sodium extrusion and the diffusion of ions and molecules down their electrochemical gradients. Diffusion is modulated by the permeability of the membrane to various solutes, to the presence of specific ion exchange pathways, and, in excitable tissues, to the presence of ion specific channels which can be opened or closed to modulate ion conductance.

In effect, a double Donnan system is established in which the positively charged sodium ion balances the osmotic force of the negatively charged impermeant anions (Fig. 9.1) (Leaf, 1970). Chloride is largely excluded from the cell by the membrane potential and the high intracellular potassium content also is a consequence primarily, but not entirely, of its electrochemical equilibrium.

The extrusion of sodium from the cell is achieved by at least one and perhaps two or more membrane pumps which are fueled by ATP. The most widely studied sodium pump is the $(Na^+ + K^+)$-activated ATPase, which has been identified in many types of cells and has been characterized in considerable detail (Hokin, 1976; Skou, 1965; Schwartz et al., 1975). This enzyme complex spans the cell membrane and is composed of two catalytic subunits and a glycoprotein which have a combined mw of 250,000 (Hokin, 1976).

Present evidence indicates that the pump is electrogenic, i.e., Na^+ extrusion exceeds K^+ intake and contributes directly to the maintenance of the membrane potential (Glitsch, 1979). Na^+-K^+ exchange is stimulated by high internal Na^+ concentration or high external K^+ and is inhibited by high internal Ca^{2+}, ouabain, and the absence of external K^+.

The pump cannot operate in the absence of sarcoplasmic ATP to provide the energy for Na^+-K^+ ex-

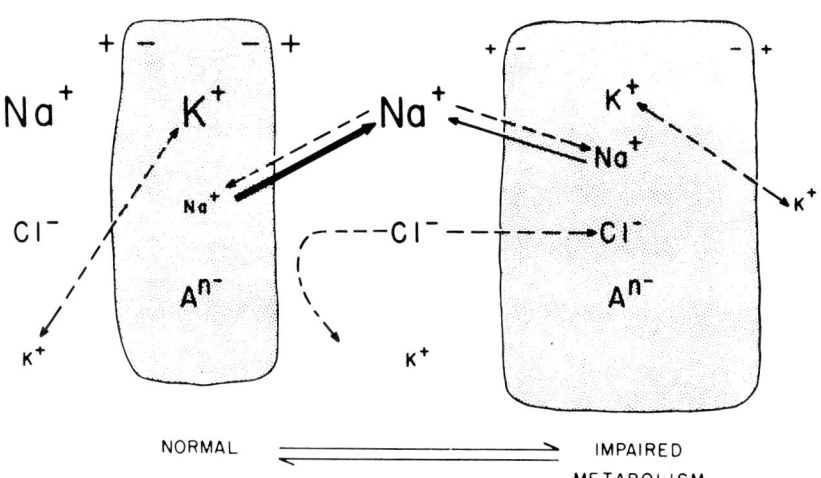

Figure 9.1 This schematic diagram illustrates ion fluxes associated with normal cell volume regulation (*left*) and the effects of metabolic inhibition on ion flux and cell volume regulation (*right*) (see text). (Reprinted with permission from A. Leaf: Regulation of intracellular fluid volume and disease. American Journal of Medicine 49:291–295, 1970.)

change. ATP is bound and split on the internal side of the enzyme complex and phosphorylation of the enzyme complex occurs as an intermediate step. It has been estimated that as much as one-third of basal energy utilization of the cell is devoted to maintenance of this Na^+-K^+ exchange (Hokin, 1976).

Some evidence for a second sodium pump which is not inhibited by ouabain and does not involve exchange with K^+ has been obtained in kidney, myocardium, and uteri (Whittembury and Proverbio, 1970; Pine et al., 1979a; Daniel and Robinson, 1971). Slices of these tissues, when swollen in the cold and then rewarmed in oxygenated medium, have been shown to extrude some NaCl and water even when the Na^+-K^+ ATPase pump is inhibited by ouabain. However, the existence of a second pump has not been proven, and little is known about the characteristics of this type of sodium extrusion.

Although calcium does not have a major direct role in cell volume regulation, in most types of cells, its internal concentration may have a crucial indirect role in the regulation of sodium and potassium flux (MacKnight and Leaf, 1977; Glitsch, 1979; Skou, 1965). In addition, calcium can either potentiate or interfere with the energy metabolism of the cell. Calcium overload has been considered to be a lethal event or a contributing factor in several diverse forms of cell injury including myocardial and liver cell ischemia (Chien et al., 1978; Fleckenstein et al., 1974; Shen and Jennings, 1972a and b; Shine et al., 1978).

The intracellular concentration of calcium is normally maintained at very low levels compared to its extracellular concentration. The mechanism for this calcium gradient is now believed to be dependent, in many cells including cardiac myocytes, on a sodium-calcium exchange pathway in which the uphill extrusion of calcium is coupled to, and driven by the downhill influx of sodium (Glitsch, 1979; Mullins, 1979; DiPolo, 1977). This process requires ATP as an allosteric cofactor for

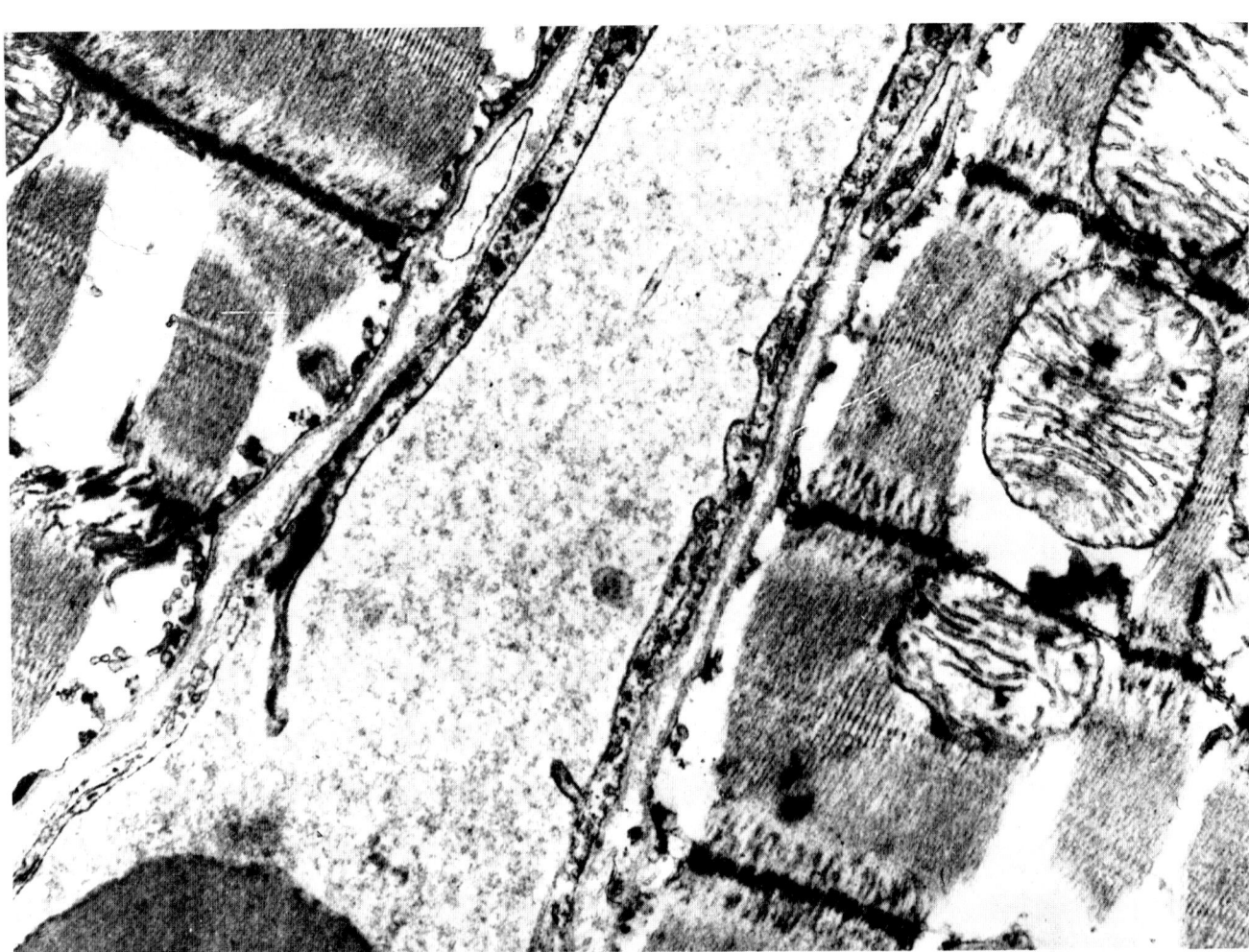

Figure 9.2. The effects of 60 min of severe ischemia in vivo on myocardial ultrastructure is illustrated. Parts of two myocytes and an intervening capillary are shown. Mitochondria and the sarcoplasm of both myocytes are moderately swollen and the mitochondria contain amorphous matrix densities. Glycogen is absent. The capillary is structurally intact. ×20,600. (Reprinted with permission from C.E. Ganote, R.B. Jennings, M.L. Hill, and E. C. Growchowski: Journal of Molecular and Cellular Cardiology 8:189–204, 1976).

activation but ATP is not split in this transport process. Nevertheless, ATP indirectly provides the energy for this exchange by maintaining the high sodium gradient.

EFFECTS OF METABOLIC INHIBITION, HYPOXIA, OR ISCHEMIA ON ION FLUX AND CELL VOLUME REGULATION

Inhibition of all metabolism by incubation of tissues in a cold medium results in marked cell swelling (Fig. 9.1) (Grochowski et al., 1976; Mudge, 1951; Sayeed and Baue, 1973; Robinson, 1961). The failure to actively extrude sodium results in net influx of sodium. The membrane potential is thereby reduced, and chloride enters and potassium leaves the cell. In addition, because the sodium gradient no longer counterbalances the osmotic force of intracellular anions, sodium and chloride are drawn into the cell in excess of the potassium loss in accord with the classic Donnan equation. Water is simultaneously drawn into the cell to maintain osmotic equilibrium.

The immediate effects of specifically inhibiting energy metabolism, by hypoxia, ischemia, or metabolic inhibitors, on ion transport and cell volume regulation are less clear cut. The onset of ischemia or hypoxia in vivo has been associated with an almost immediate efflux of potassium in many tissues but the heart and brain are particularly sensitive organs (Silver, 1977; Case, 1971–1972; Hill and Gettes, 1980). In myocardium, for example, potassium efflux has been detected in coronary sinus blood concomitantly with the onset of decreased contractile function, ST segment elevation, and anaerobic

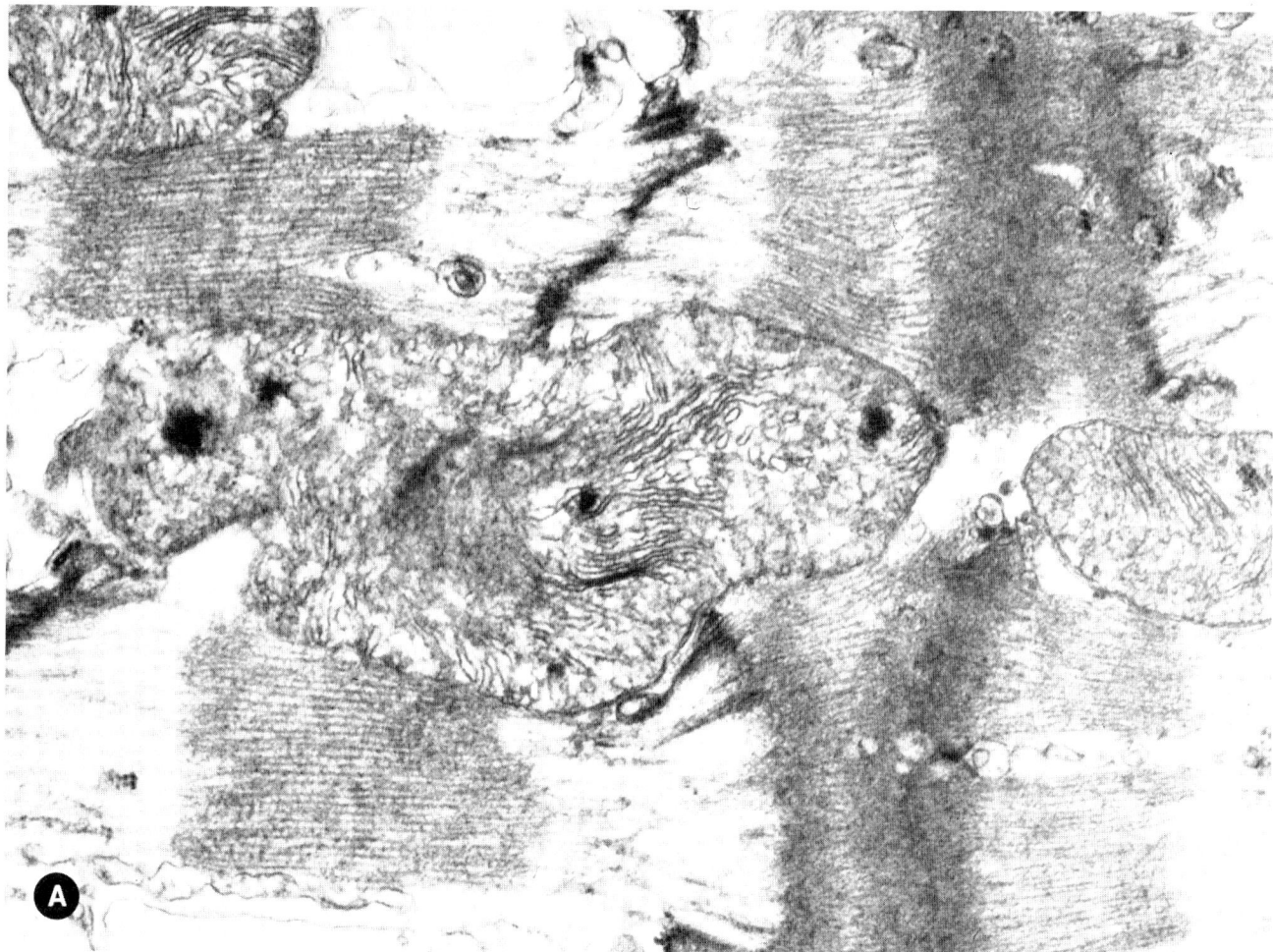

Figure 9.3. The effects of 60 min of severe ischemia in vivo followed by preparation of slices and aerobic incubation in vitro is illustrated. The changes are similar to those associated with reperfusion in vivo and include the changes illustrated in Figure 9.2 plus: A, subsarcolemmal blebs over which the plasma membrane of the sarcolemma has been completely disrupted. Small circular profiles of plasmalemma are still attached to the glycocalyx. ×36,000. B, myofibrillary disruption characterized by the formation of contraction bands which are composed of aggregates of two or more sarcomeres. ×28,800. (Reprinted with permission from R.B. Jennings, H.K. Hawkins, J.E. Lowe, M.L. Hill, S. Klotman, and K.A. Reimer: American Journal of Pathology 92:187–214, 1978.)

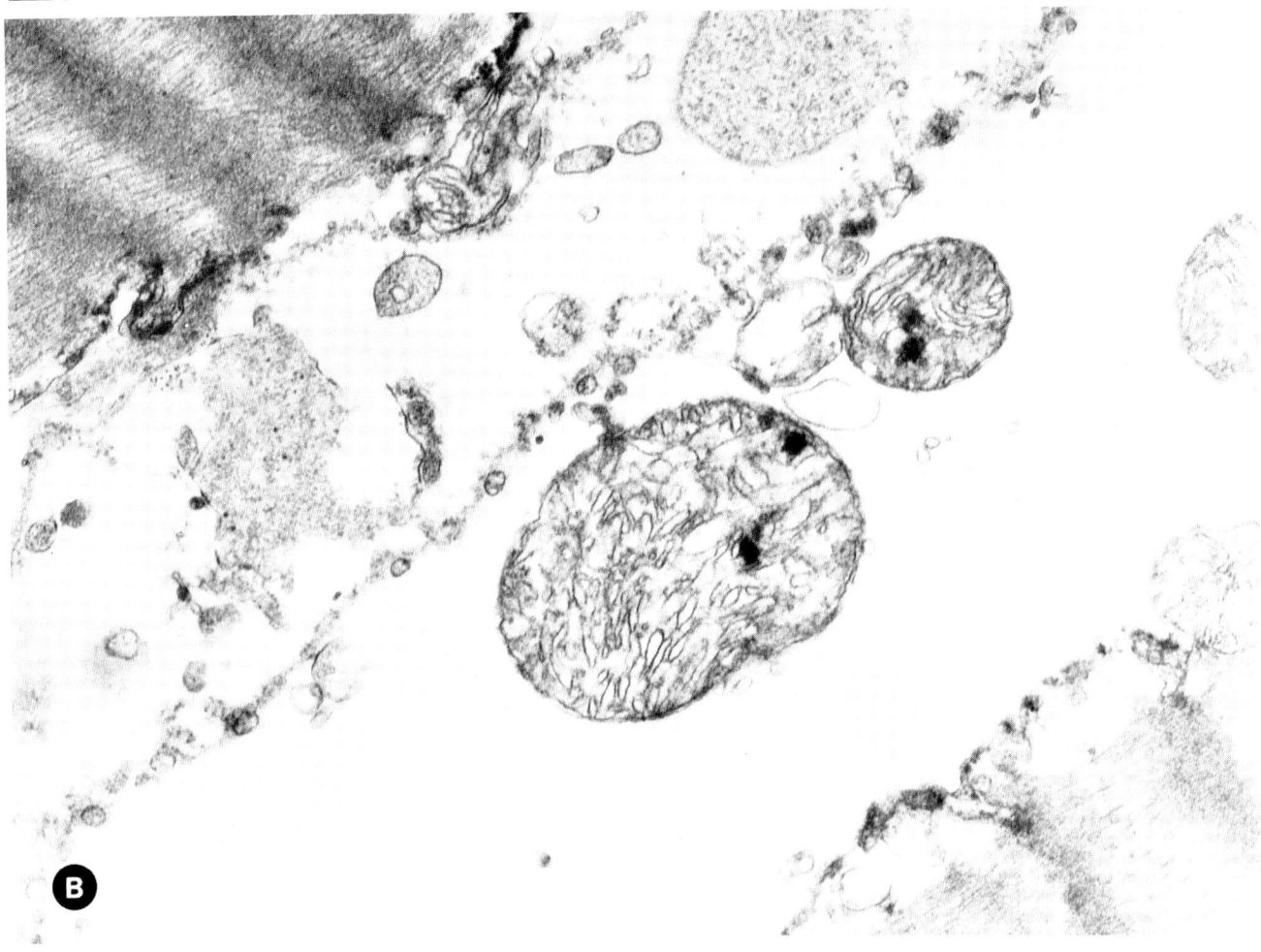

Figure 9.3B

metabolism as indicated by lactate efflux (Case, 1971–1972). The exact mechanism of this early potassium loss during ischemia or hypoxia has not been completely established. If it is related to low levels of HEP needed to run the Na^+-K^+ ATPase of the sarcolemma, it would have to be due to low levels of ATP in the sarcoplasm adjacent to the pumps. CP is low at this time, but overall tissue ATP content is normal. Nevertheless, an increase in tissue AMP is detectable and indicates that alterations in the local concentration of ATP cannot be eliminated as a cause of the K^+ loss. Studies of unidirectional potassium flux in isolated cat papillary muscles has shown that potassium influx is not inhibited by anoxia until the tissue ATP levels are markedly depleted (Goerke and Page, 1965). Similar studies in an isolated, blood perfused rabbit septum preparation have shown that the onset of ischemia is associated with an increased rate of efflux rather than a decreased rate of influx (Rau et al., 1977). Similar results have been observed much earlier in isolated rat diaphragm subjected to anoxia (Calkins et al., 1954). The mechanism of increased K^+ efflux has not been established. It may reflect an increase in the membrane permeability to potassium, perhaps effected by decreased pH, increased calcium, or anoxia per se, or may simply be the result of a reduced membrane potential and consequent increased electrochemical K^+ gradient across the cell membrane.

Sodium-potassium exchange and cell volume regulation are variably affected by metabolic blockade depending on the tissue type and specific experimental conditions. Several studies in the 1950s established that cell swelling occurred in slices of renal cortex subjected to anoxia and/or metabolic blockade (Deyrup, 1953; Mudge, 1951; Robinson, 1950; Whittam and Davies, 1953). Cell swelling was also found to be a prominent ultrastructural feature of renal ischemia in vivo (Reimer et al., 1972). Such studies suggested that cell volume regulation by the kidney is highly dependent on aerobic metabolism and ATP production. Other studies, however, have shown that cold-induced swelling of slices of renal cortex could be reversed when rewarming was done in an anaerobic medium (MacKnight, 1968). In contrast, brain slices have been shown to swell markedly during anoxic incubation (Franck et al., 1968). Furthermore, a transient period of cerebral ischemia in vivo for as little as 5–7 min, caused microvascular defects (Kowada et al., 1968) which were associated in part with swelling of glial and capillary endothelial cells (Chiang et al., 1968).

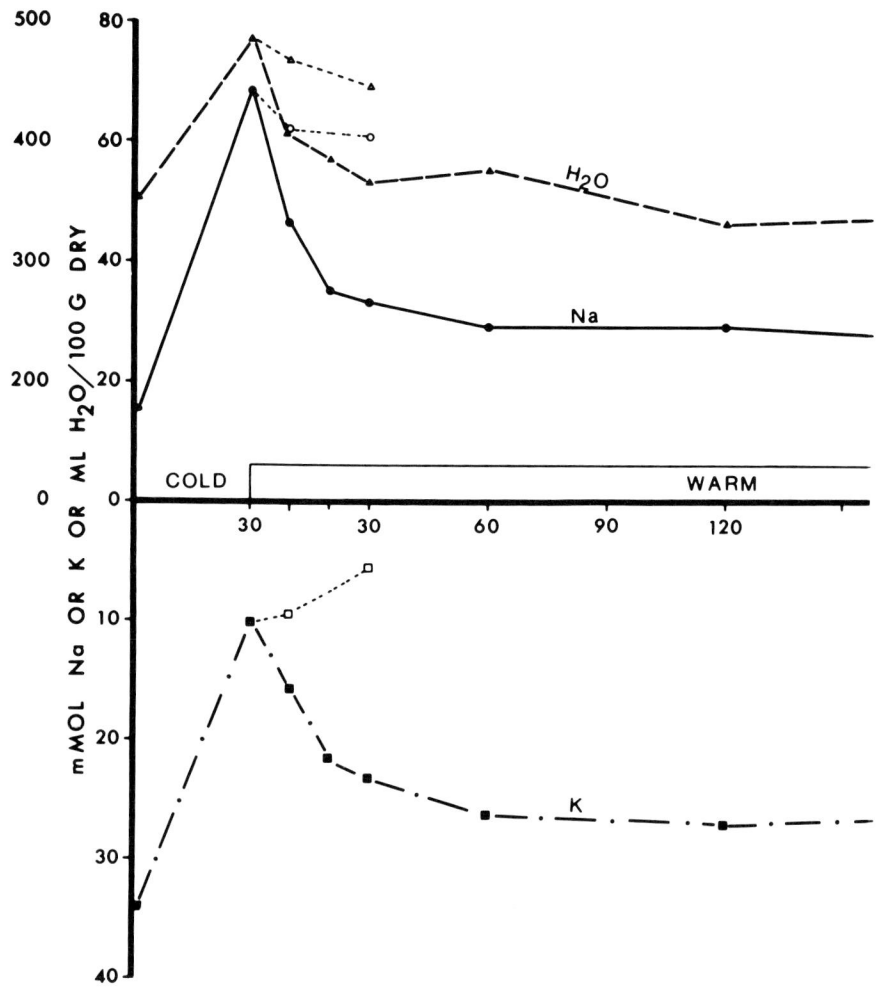

Figure 9.4. The effects of cold-induced swelling and subsequent warm incubation on slices of normal myocardium is illustrated. Cold incubation resulted in massive efflux of K^+ and influx of Na^+ and water. These changes were largely reversible by subsequent rewarming in an oxygenated medium (*closed points*). Rewarming in the presence of ouabain (*open points*) caused additional K^+ efflux and prevented most of the extrusion of Na^+ and water.

In other organs such as the liver, retina, and myocardium, cell volume regulation has been found to be relatively insensitive to changes in energy metabolism. For example, liver slices incubated in the presence of various concentrations of inhibitors of respiration such as cyanide, amytal, or oligomycin have shown no reduction of Na^+-K^+ exchange until respiration was reduced to less than 50% of control rates and ATP levels were markedly depressed. Thus, ion transport in liver is apparently less sensitive to metabolic inhibition compared to other functions such as protein synthesis or compared to ion transport in brain or kidney (van Rossum, 1972). Ethionine intoxication results in marked reduction of hepatic ATP levels because of the formation of S-adenosyl ethionine but does not increase the tissue water content, supporting the conclusion that cell volume regulation by liver cells is relatively insensitive to overall tissue ATP content (Judah et al., 1966). However, energy production by respiration is not impaired in the latter system. Rabbit retina subjected to hypoxia and glucose deprivation have shown no loss of cell volume regulation until 30 or more min of injury (Parks et al., 1976).

Cell volume regulation by myocardium also appears to be relatively insensitive at least initially, to inhibition of energy production. Myocardial ischemia in vivo has been associated with only moderate degrees of cell swelling during the first 40–60 min despite the rapid depletion of high energy phosphates (Jennings and Ganote, 1974; Jennings et al., 1975; Jennings et al., 1978). On the other hand, changes in volume in severely ischemic myocardium may not be detectable early because the low arterial flow of ischemia provides insufficient new extracellular fluid to allow the detection of either swelling or loss of ion gradients. The data of Hill and Gettes (1980) indicate that ion gradients are reduced early and lend credence to the idea that volume and ion gradients are sensitive to inhibition of energy production even though changes are difficult to detect in zones of low flow ischemia.

Some of the variation noted among different tissues relative to the effects of inhibition of energy production on cell volume regulation and ion gradients may be due to differences in experimental conditions or in metabolic peculiarities among the various tissues. For example, in nonworking myocardial slices, anaerobic glycolysis provides enough energy at 37°C to maintain volume and significant ion gradients for 1 hr, but not for 2–3 hr. However, inhibition of anaerobic glycolysis by iodoacetate greatly accelerates the loss of gradients. These results suggest that ATP production via anaerobic glycolysis is adequate to maintain cell volume regulation in the nonworking slice (K.A. Reimer, R.B. Jennings, and M.L. Hill, unpublished data). In contrast, Pine et al. (1978 and 1979b) have shown in working isolated rat papillary muscle or dog right ventricular trebeculae that the combination of hypoxia plus glycolytic blockade with iodoacetate for 1 hr caused contractile failure but no change in tissue water. Thus, while energy is required to maintain volume, the relationship between inhibition of energy production and the onset of depressed cell volume regulation has not yet been established.

The variable capacity of cells to temporarily resist swelling during ischemia or anoxia has two probable explanations. The first is that the sodium-potassium pump has a relatively high affinity for ATP and can continue to operate after more specialized cellular functions have been inhibited. The second is that, although cell volume regulation ultimately depends on metabolic energy, cell swelling will not occur as long as potassium efflux equals or exceeds sodium influx (Hughes and Macknight 1977). Thus, as long as ion gradients persist, the severity of cell swelling may be related more to relative membrane permeability to sodium and potassium than to metabolic conditions within the cell.

ROLE OF CELL SWELLING AND/OR DEFECTIVE CELL VOLUME REGULATION IN THE PATHOGENESIS OF IRREVERSIBLE CELL INJURY

The early cell swelling associated with ischemic or hypoxic injury, especially in brain and kidney, led to the hypothesis that cell swelling per se could contribute to the onset of irreversible cell injury and death either directly or by further limiting microvascular perfusion (Leaf, 1970). The latter possibility will be considered below. A direct link between cell swelling and lethal injury has been sought by a number of investigators in models of myocardial ischemia or hypoxia. Christodou-

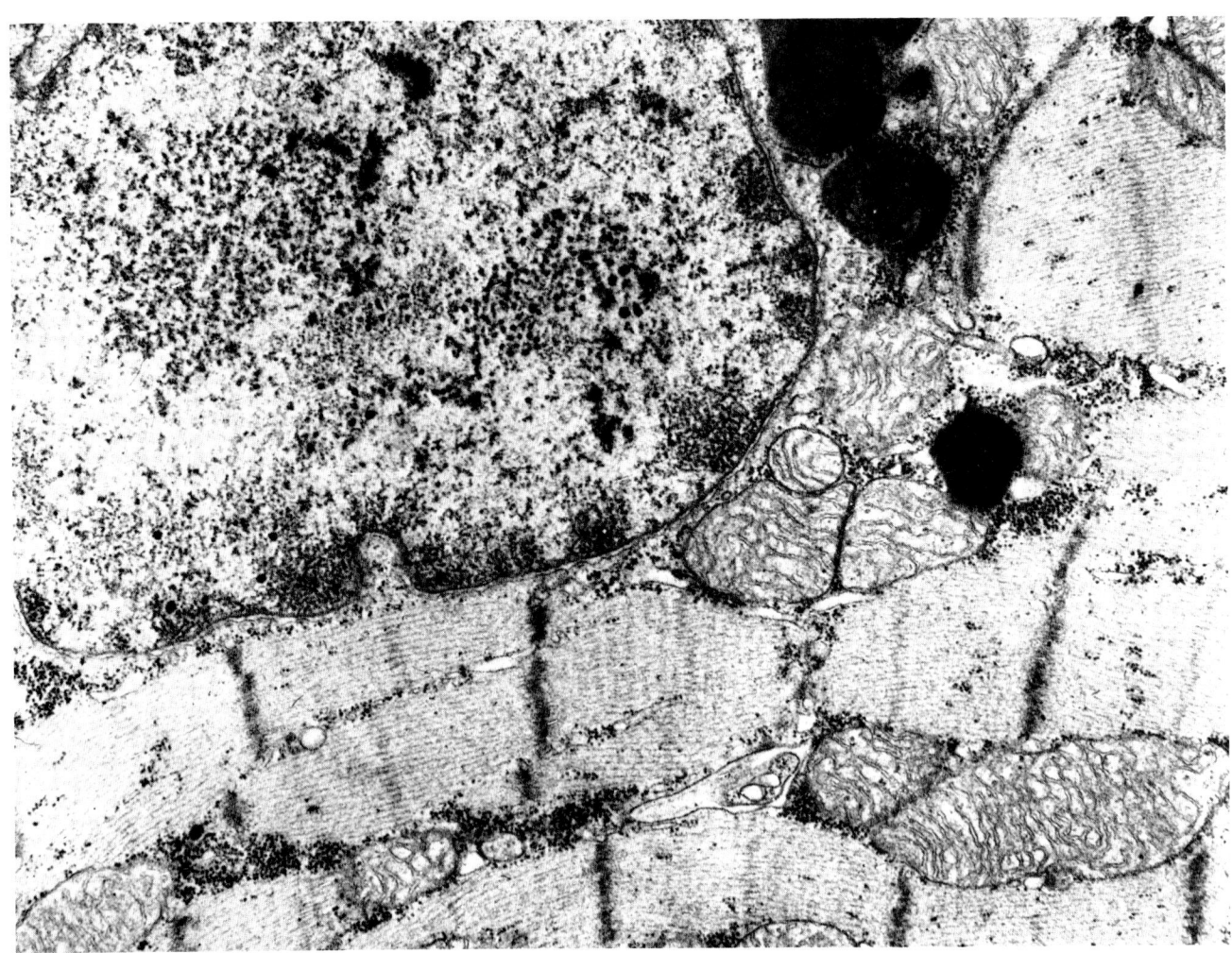

Figure 9.5. Part of a myocyte from a slice of normal myocardium incubated in an oxygenated medium for 1 hr is illustrated. Nuclear, myofibrillar, and mitochondrial structure is intact. Glycogen is still abundant. ×24,800. (Reprinted with permission from E.C. Grochowski, C.E. Ganote, M.L. Hill, and R.B. Jennings: Journal of Molecular and Cellular Cardiology 8:173–187, 1976.)

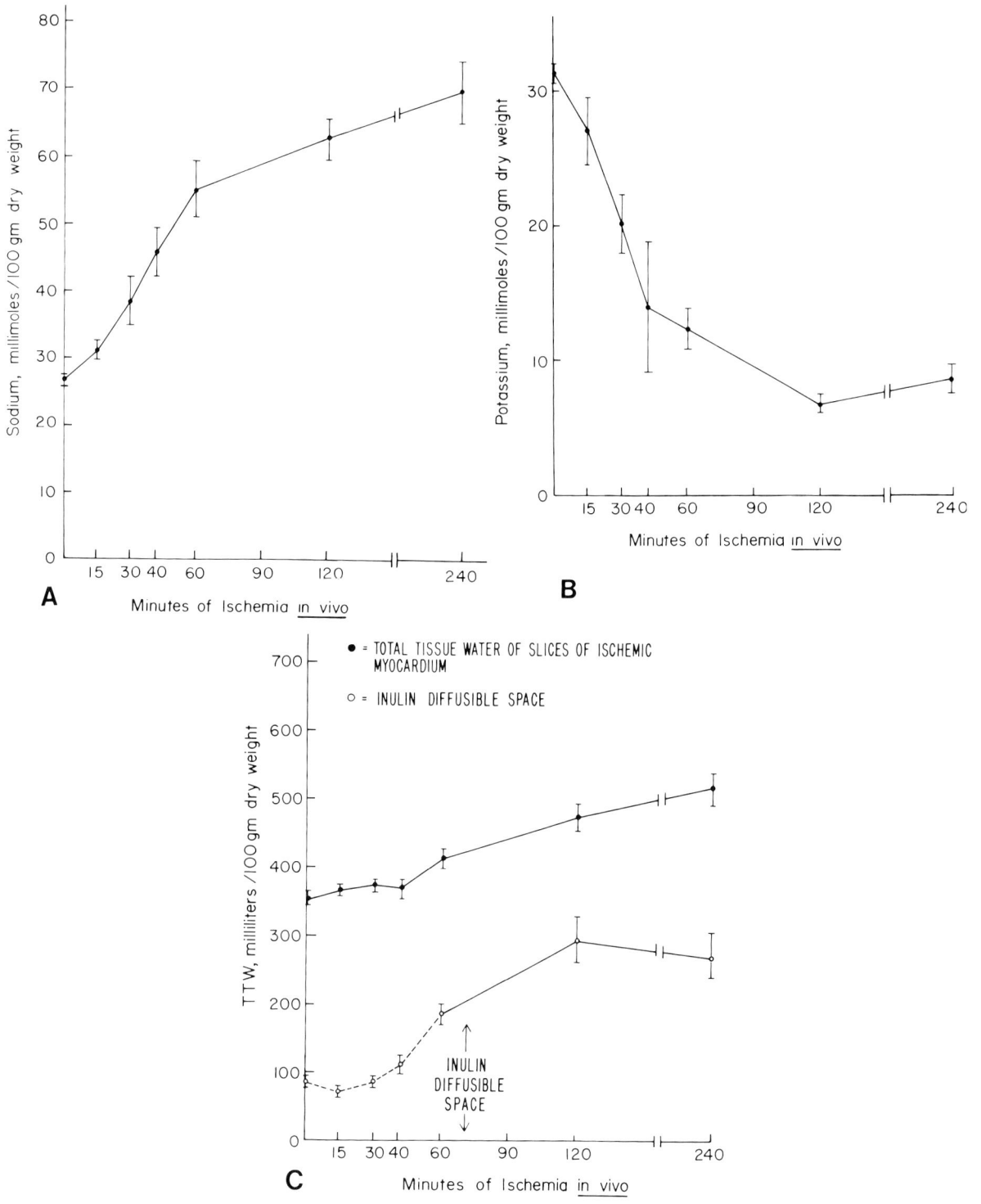

Figure 9.6. The effects of various periods of ischemia (37°C) in vivo on the ability of incubated slices to maintain sodium (Na) (A), potassium (K) (B), and total tissue water (TTW) and inulin diffusible space (C) are illustrated. After 30 min or more of ischemia, injured slices contained more Na and less K than control slices, and after 40 min or more, the inulin diffusible space also increased, indicating abnormal plasmalemmal permeability. (Reprinted with permission from R.B. Jennings, H.K. Hawkins, J.E. Lowe, M.L. Hill, and K.A. Reimer: High energy phosphate and cell volume control in lethal ischemic injury. Government Printing Office, in press.)

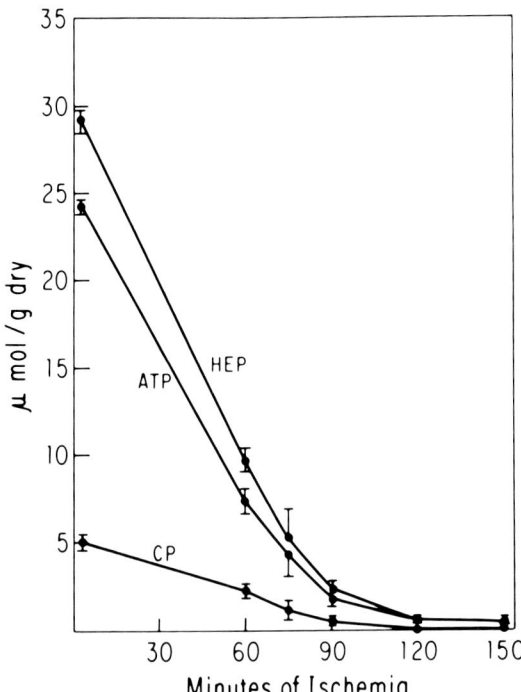

Figure 9.7. The effect of total ischemia at 37°C in vitro (autolysis) on high energy phosphates (HEP = ATP + CP) is illustrated. Marked loss of creatine phosphate occurred even prior to the first sampling at about 3 min after extirpation of the heart. ATP content remained normal during the first 3 min but then decreased at a relatively constant rate until 90 min. At this time, only 7.5% of the control high energy phosphates remained.

Iou, et al (1975) and Powell et al. (1976) have shown that hypoxic perfusion of isolated rat hearts followed by reoxygenation caused ultrastructural evidence of mitochondrial and myofibrillar damage associated with extensive cell swelling. Inclusion of hypertonic mannitol in the perfusate significantly reduced both the cell swelling and other ultrastructural evidence of cell injury. We also have shown that mannitol can delay the development of irreversible ischemic injury and thereby reduce the amount of necrosis produced by a 40-min period of temporary coronary occlusion followed by reperfusion (Kloner et al., 1976). However, whether the apparent protective effect of mannitol in these studies was causally related to reduced cell swelling has not been established.

The fact that cell swelling can be induced by incubation of a variety of tissues in cold medium and can be reversed by rewarming, indicates that cell swelling, per se, does not immediately cause irreversible damage to the cell membrane or ion transport systems (Grochowski, 1976; Sayeed and Baue, 1973; Robinson, 1961). Nevertheless, it has been shown (Ginn et al., 1968; Trump and Ginn, 1968) that inhibition of Na^+-K^+ transport with ouabain or replacement of extracellular sodium with potassium resulted in marked swelling of isolated flounder kidney tubules and subcellular organelles, which was eventually followed by a sequence of events terminating in disruption of the cell membrane and intracellular organelles.

We became interested in the role of cell swelling and ion transport in myocardial ischemia because of the observation that, although severely ischemic myocardial cells did not become markedly swollen during 40 min of ischemia induced by coronary occlusion in vivo (Fig. 9.2), reperfusion of the ischemic region with arterial blood was associated with "explosive cell swelling" (Fig. 9.3) (Whalen et al., 1974; Kloner et al., 1974). This explosive cell swelling developed almost immediately and was characterized by marked cellular and subcellular swelling and development of subsarcolemmal blebs. This generalized cell swelling was associated with the massive influx of calcium, the development of myofibrillar contraction bands and mitochondrial accumulation, and the deposition of calcium phosphate. The glycocalyx of the cell membrane was intact by ultrastructural appearance but the plasmalemma of the sarcolemma was disrupted and often converted to small vesicular profiles attached to the glycocalyx. This phenomenon suggested that defective cell volume regulation was an early feature of myocardial ischemic injury. However, whether the explosive cell swelling was caused by loss of ATP to drive ionic pumps, by damage to the ionic pumps per se, or by increased membrane permeability to ions was not known.

To assess ion exchange and cell volume regulation by ischemic myocardium in more detail, an in vitro system was designed in which thin slices of control or injured myocardium were incubated in oxygenated Krebs-Ringer's phosphate medium (Growchowski et al., 1976). Thin slices were cut by hand using a razor blade from the papillary muscles of dog hearts. The slices were cut parallel to the long axis of the papillary muscle so that muscle fibers ran longitudinally within the slice. This orientation is important to minimize the number of cut cells in a slice. Slice thickness by this technique varied from about 15 to 40 cells. The uncut fibers within these slices demonstrated ion transport and volume control. Cold incubation of such slices resulted in influx of Na^+ and water and efflux of K^+ (Fig. 9.4). Rewarming resulted in the extrusion of Na^+ and water and reaccumulation of potassium. Addition of ouabain to the medium caused continued loss of potassium and largely, although not completely, inhibited the extrusion of sodium and water. The ultrastructural appearance of cells within control slices was well maintained during incubation (Fig. 9.5).

In contrast, slices cut from the posterior papillary muscle following various periods of ischemia in vivo and incubated in oxygenated medium for 1 hr, in vitro showed a progressive loss of ion and cell volume regulation (Fig. 9.6) (Jennings et al., 1978; Ganote et al., 1976). With increasing duration of injury, slices lost the capacity to maintain potassium or extrude sodium. Sodium influx was associated with increased tissue water. In order to distinguish between cell swelling and extra-

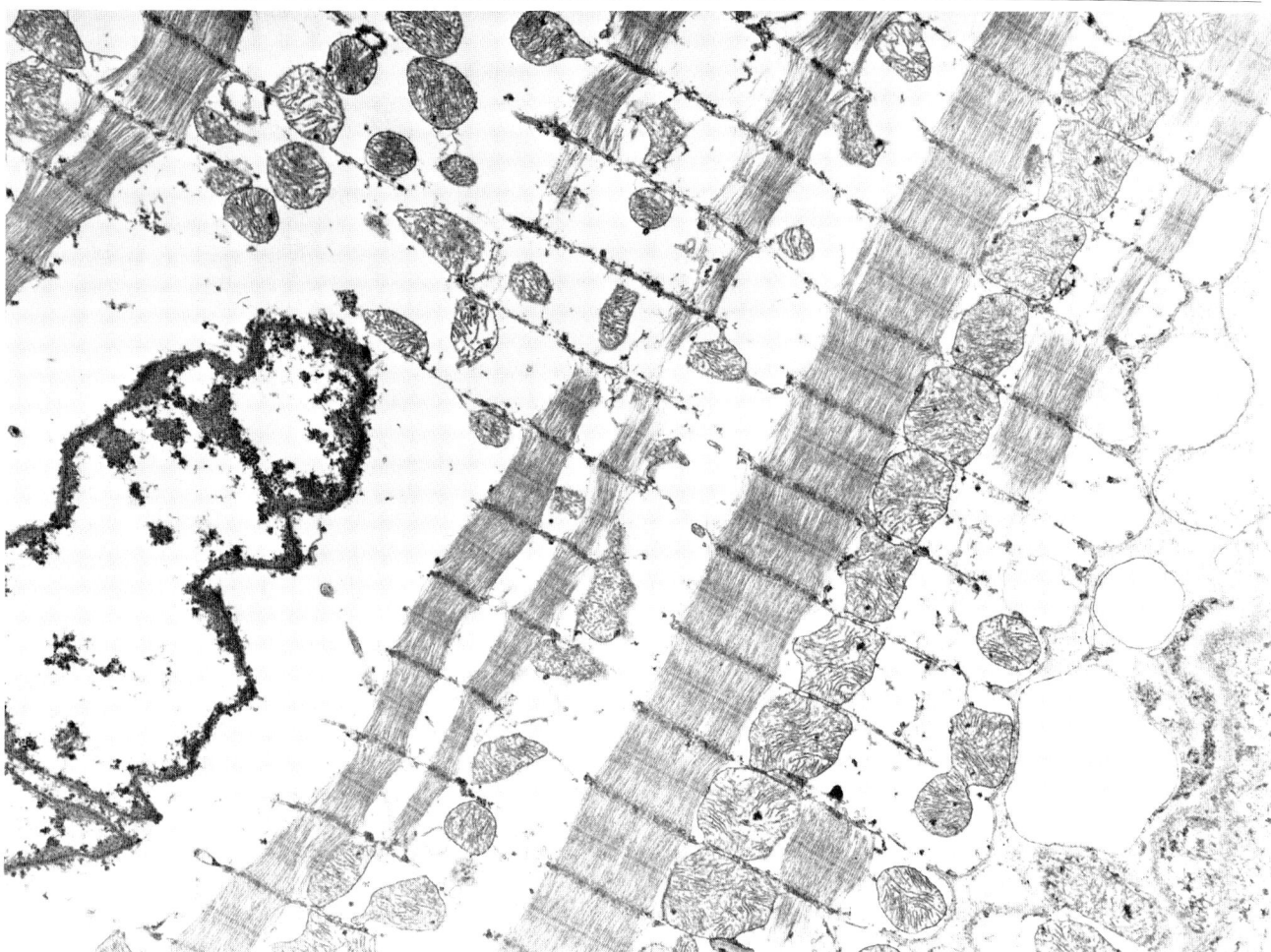

Figure 9.8. Part of a myocyte injured by total ischemia in vitro is illustrated. The sarcoplasm is markedly swollen, presumably indicating a redistribution of fluid from the extra to intracellular space. Mitochondria are moderately swollen and contain amorphous matrix densities. Clumping of nuclear chromatin and loss of glycogen are also evident. ×11,500. (Photographed by Dr. Hal K. Hawkins.)

cellular edema, inulin, a 5000-MW molecule which does not penetrate the normal cell membrane was added to the media to estimate the extracellular space. An increased inulin diffusible space (IDS) was observed in all slices after 40 or more min of ischemia in vivo (Fig. 9.6). Taken at face value, the increased IDS suggested extracellular edema with shrinkage of the intracellular compartment. However, this was clearly not the case because electron microscopy of these slices showed marked cell swelling with no apparent interstitial edema. In fact, many of the features of explosive cell swelling observed after reperfusion in vivo had been reproduced by reoxygenation of slices in vitro. Massive cell swelling was associated with breaks in the cell membrane and other features of irreversible cell injury including myofibrillar contraction bands and mitochondrial swelling with amorphous matrix densities. As observed in vivo, cell membrane damage was characterized by an intact glycocalyx but with areas devoid of the trilaminar unit membrane which had broken and reformed small vesicles. Based on these ultrastructural findings, the only logical explanation for the increased IDS of slices was that inulin had gained access to the interior of cells from which it is normally excluded. Thus, these studies provided functional as well as structural evidence for cell membrane damage as one of the earliest features of irreversible myocardial ischemic cell injury.

Nevertheless, the pathogenesis of membrane damage and defective cell volume regulation is unknown. It is possible that cell volume regulation fails either because of insufficient ATP to fuel the ionic pumps or damage to the pumps and that membrane damage is a secondary phenomenon. Conversely, structural damage to the cell membrane could increase membrane permeability and permit more rapid loss of ion gradients.

We have shown that high energy phosphate depletion occurs rapidly during severe ischemia in vivo (Jennings et al., 1978). By 40 min, when many cells have been irreversibly injured, ATP levels were already decreased to 10% or less of control levels.

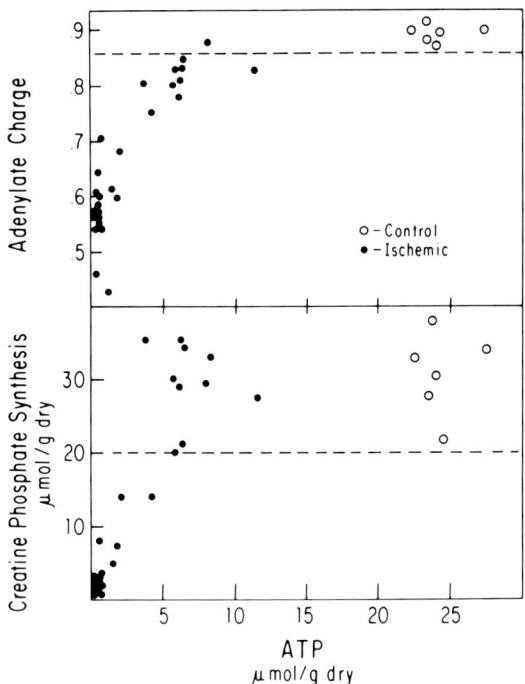

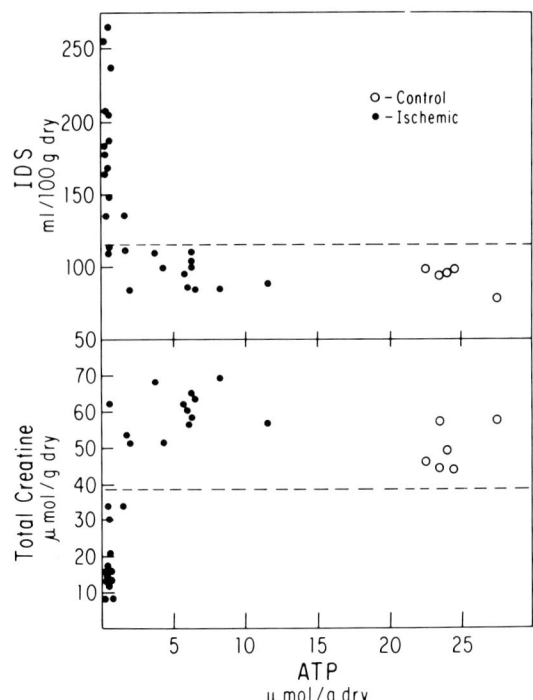

Figure 9.9. The ability of incubated slices to restore the adenylate charge or resynthesize creatine phosphate after various periods of total ischemia is illustrated. Slices of injured myocardium are plotted with respect to the ATP content of the ischemic tissue at the time the slices were prepared and without regard for the duration of ischemia (which ranged from 60 to 150 min). The *dotted lines* indicate 2 SD from the control means. The ability to restore high energy phosphates was invariably lost once the tissue ATP content decreased to 4.0 μmoles/g or less. (Reprinted with permission from K.A. Reimer, R.B. Jennings, and M.L. Hill: Circulation Research, in press, 1981.)

Figure 9.10. The ability of incubated slices to exclude inulin and retain creatine after various periods of total ischemia is illustrated. Slices of injured myocardium are plotted with respect to the ATP content of the ischemic tissue at the time the slices were prepared, without regard for the duration of ischemia (which ranged from 60 to 150 min). The *dotted lines* indicate 2 SD from the control means. The integrity of the plasmalemma, as measured by inulin entry to, and creatine loss from the cells, was maintained until the tissue ATP level decreased to 2.0 μmoles/g dry weight or less. There was a lag time of about 30 min between the loss of high energy phosphate resynthesis and loss of membrane integrity as measured by these two indices. (Reprinted with permission from K.A. Reimer, R. B. Jennings, and M.L. Hill: Circulation Research, in press, 1981.)

On the other hand, the Na^+-K^+ ATPase has been isolated and studied following myocardial ischemia by several groups who have shown either no change or mild loss of enzymatic activity (Beller et al., 1976; Schwartz et al., 1973; Willerson et al., 1977). Thus, the Na^+-K^+ pump itself, seems to be relatively resistant to ischemic injury.

In order to assess more precisely the associations between tissue ATP content, loss of cell volume regulation, and altered membrane permeability, an in vitro model of total ischemia was employed to produce large samples of uniformly injured myocardium (Reimer et al., 1981). This was accomplished by incubating blocks of myocardium containing the papillary muscles in sealed jars maintained at 37°C. Variables present in vivo, such as collateral blood flow and the continued contraction of surrounding myocardium were thus eliminated.

At times from 0 to 150 min after the onset of total ischemia, slices were cut for measurement of high energy phosphates. Additional slices were incubated in oxygenated medium to assess the capacity of the injured cells to 1) resynthesize high energy phosphate compounds, 2) resume cell volume regulation, and 3) exclude inulin.

The rate of high energy phosphate depletion during total in vitro ischemia varied among experiments. However, ATP levels averaged less than 10% of control by 90 min of total ischemia (Fig. 9.7). At this time, despite the complete absence of perfusion, myofibers showed ultrastructural evidence of cell swelling presumably mediated by redistribution of fluid from the extracellular to the intracellular space (Fig. 9.8).

Irrespective of the duration of total ischemia, depletion of ATP to less than 5.0 μmoles/g dry weight was always associated with the failure of slices to restore the adenylate charge ratio [(ATP + ½ADP)/(ATP + ADP + AMP)] or to resynthesize creatine phosphate (Fig. 9.9). These results indicate that mitochondrial failure had

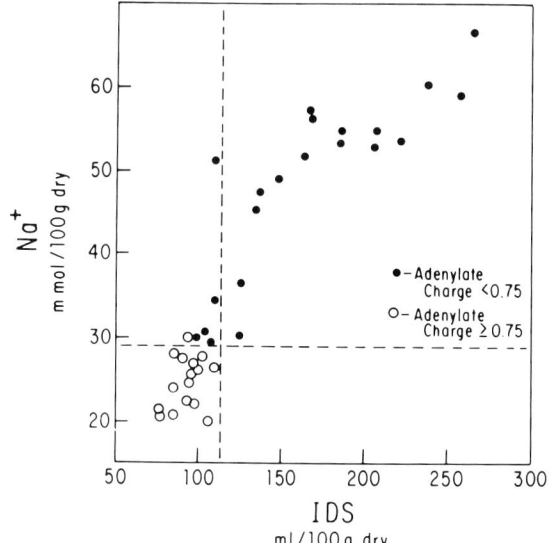

Figure 9.11. The ability of incubated slices of ischemically injured myocardium to extrude sodium is plotted with respect to the inulin diffusible space, without regard to the duration of total ischemia prior to incubation. The *dotted lines* indicate 2 SD from the control means. As expected, every slice with an increased inulin space also had an increased Na^+ content. However, some slices with cells which were still able to exclude inulin also had an increased Na^+ content, which indicated the loss of cell volume regulation prior to the development of overt membrane damage. The loss of cell volume regulation coincided with the loss of high energy phosphate resynthesis as defined by an adenylate charge of less than 0.75. (Reprinted with permission from K.A. Reimer, R.B. Jennings, and M.L. Hill: Circulation Research, in press, 1981.)

occurred either because of insufficient substrate or cofactors or because of mitochondrial damage per se. Experiments to establish whether substrate or cofactor repletion could restore high energy phosphates have not yet been completed.

Evidence of overt membrane damage developed somewhat later. The IDS of the slices was never increased until the initial ATP content of the tissue had decreased to 2.0 or less per gram dry tissue and occasionally even lower ATP levels were not associated with an increased IDS (Fig. 9.10). Creatine loss from the slices provided an independent measure of altered membrane integrity and paralleled the increased IDS (Fig. 9.10). Cell volume and ionic regulation were impaired simultaneous with the evidence of depressed mitochondrial function and preceded the increased IDS (Fig. 9.11).

Sayeed and associates (Sayeed and Baue, 1973; Sayeed et al., 1974) have shown a similar correlation between ATP depletion, reduction in the adenylate charge ratio, and the failure of cell volume regulation in liver slices following hemorrhagic shock in rats. In their studies, in slices with depressed cell volume regulation, slice oxygen consumption was similar in the presence and absence of ouabain, indicating the absence of any respiration associated with ion transport.

The close linkage between the loss of energy metabolism and defective cell volume regulation, in tissue slices incubated aerobically after different durations of total ischemia, has at least two possible explanations: 1) the inability of the cell to resume ATP production could impair cell volume and ionic regulation, and 2) conversely, loss of ionic gradients, and specifically excess calcium within the cell, could uncouple oxidative phosphorylation and cause mitochondrial dysfunction. To date, it has not been possible to differentiate between these two possibilities. Since the data available indicate that membrane damage, detectable with inulin, was not present in the slices at the time that altered cell volume regulation first was detected, membrane damage does not appear to play a role in the early failure of volume regulation. On the other hand, whenever significant membrane damage was detected, massive cell swelling and loss of ion gradients invariably were present. Thus, membrane damage contributes to the loss of volume control and ion gradients and the detection of membrane damage is an objective sign of the presence of lethal injury.

The mechanism of membrane disruption is still unknown. The membrane damage may occur because of activation of membrane bound or lysosomal phospholipases followed by depletion of membrane phospholipids (Chien et al., 1978). This possibility is of particular interest because membrane phospholipids are responsible for the normal impermeability of the cell membrane to calcium. Thus, phospholipid degradation could permit the massive influx of calcium which is associated with ischemic cell death. Activation of phospholipases could be induced either by calcium, following gradual calcium influx (Chien et al., 1978), or as a direct consequence of ATP depletion through failure to phosphorylate inhibitory proteins. Progressive depletion of membrane phospholipids has been observed in ischemic liver cells along a time course which paralleled the development of irreversible cell injury (Chien et al., 1978). In that study, chlorpromazine delayed both the phospholipid depletion and the onset of irreversible cell injury.

However, mechanisms of membrane damage other than phospholipase activation, e.g., cell swelling due to loss of cell volume regulation, or lipid peroxidation also may occur. Regardless of the mechanism of overt membrane disruption, detectable by an increased IDS in total myocardial ischemia, this phenomenon appears to be preceded by defective cell volume regulation and depressed energy metabolism (Reimer et al., 1981).

CELL SWELLING AND THE "NO-REFLOW PHENOMENON"

The very early development of a "no-reflow phenomenon" was first documented in the brain by the extensive studies of Ames and coworkers (Kowada et al., 1968; Ames et al., 1968; Chiang et al., 1968). They showed that

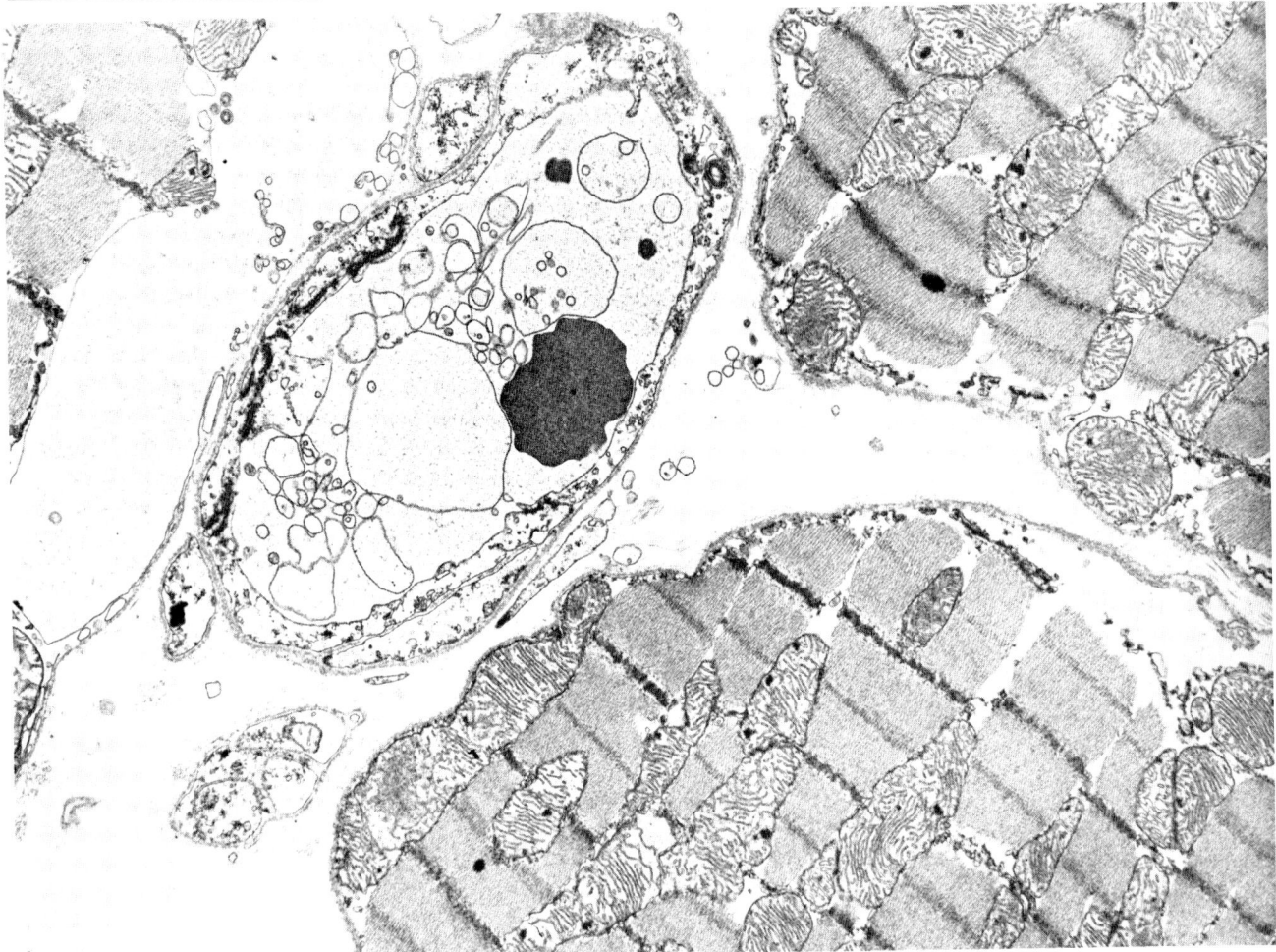

Figure 9.12. The effects of 3 hr of ischemic injury on myocyte and capillary ultrastructure is illustrated. Myocytes are moderately swollen and mitochondria contain amorphous matrix densities. The capillary endothelium is swollen and the capillary lumen is obstructed in large part by swollen blebs of endothelial cytoplasm. ×12,000. (Reprinted with permission from R.B. Jennings and H.K. Hawkins: *Ultrastructural Changes of Acute Myocardial Ischemia*. Elsevier, New York, in press, 1981.)

after as little as 5 min of cerebral ischemia, reperfusion was patchy. Widespread perfusion defects could be readily demonstrated by perfusing the vasculature with carbon black. This no-reflow phenomenon initially was related to capillary obstruction due to glial swelling and capillary endothelial blebs. Subsequent studies have shown that increased blood viscosity, red cell aggregates, and platelet thrombi also play a role in this phenomenon (Fischer and Ames, 1972; Waltz and Sundt, 1967). Prevention of the microvascular perfusion defects has prolonged the duration of cerebral anoxia required to cause irreversible loss of neuronal function (Neely and Youmans, 1963). Thus, it seems likely that the exquisite sensitivity of the cerebral cortex to ischemic or anoxic injury may be due more to the microvascular obstruction than to sensitivity of the neurons.

Subsequently, the no-reflow phenomenon has been documented in other organs including kidney (Flores et al., 1972; Summers and Jamison, 1971) and heart (Kloner et al., 1974a; Krug et al., 1966) and again has been related, at least in part, to parenchymal or capillary cell swelling. However, a role of this no-reflow phenomenon in the further progression of parenchymal ischemic injury has not been demonstrated in these organs. On the contrary, mannitol was shown to prevent the no-reflow phenomenon following renal ischemia but did not prevent or reduce the proximal tubular necrosis produced by 60 min of renal artery occlusion followed by reperfusion in the rat (Franklin et al., 1974).

The no-reflow phenomenon occurs in dog myocardium following 90 min of severe ischemia in vivo, where it is associated with capillary blebs and red cell plugs (Fig. 9.12) (Kloner et al., 1974b). However, this phenomenon has not been demonstrated after 40 min of ischemia (Kloner et al., 1974b; Willerson et al., 1977) when much of the subendocardial ischemic region has already been irreversibly injured by biologic, ultrastructural, and metabolic criteria (Jennings et al., 1975; Jennings and Reimer, 1979). At this earlier time, perfusion of the ischemic region with dyes such as thioflavin S or carbon black have not revealed perfusion defects (Kloner et al., 1974b). In addition, regional blood flow in the presence of maximal vasodilation by adenosine has not been reduced by 40 min of ischemia (Willerson et al., 1977). Furthermore, capillary structure has been well preserved in areas showing severe myocyte injury. Thus, although the no-reflow phenomenon has been demonstrated in several organs, only in the brain has it been convincingly shown to have a primary contributory role in the pathogenesis of ischemic or anoxic cell death. The no-reflow phenomenon appears to be a later, secondary event in myocardial ischemia in the dog.

SUMMARY AND CONCLUSIONS

Cell volume regulation in all animal cells is dependent on the continued extrusion of sodium from the cell by membrane bound pumps, including the ouabain-sensitive sodium-potassium ATPase. This process is directly dependent on ATP and consumes as much as one-third of the basal oxidative metabolism of the cell. In conditions of ischemia or anoxia, whether induced by asphyxia, shock, or arterial occlusion, potassium loss occurs quickly. Sodium influx and cell swelling also occur quickly in some anoxic tissues such as brain and kidney, whereas cardiac myocytes develop cell swelling more slowly. Nevertheless defective cell volume regulation becomes an early feature of ischemic injury in heart as well as in other tissues.

Defective cell volume regulation may contribute to the development of lethal cell injury in two general ways: Cell swelling or ionic imbalance could be important factors leading directly to the onset of irreversibility. On the other hand, cell swelling could cause microvascular compression and perfusion defects which could further exacerbate anoxia or prevent reperfusion of ischemic areas and thereby potentiate parenchymal cell injury. This no-reflow phenomenon occurs early in brain and may be an important determinant of the extent of cerebral anoxic or ischemic injury but appears to be a later phenomenon in other organs such as the heart.

On the other hand, defective cell volume regulation is an early component of myocyte injury following myocardial ischemia. Defective cell volume regulation invariably occurs despite reoxygenation of totally ischemic dog myocardium after the myocardial ATP content has been depleted below 5.0 μmoles/g dry tissue weight. This defective cell volume regulation is associated with the loss of high energy phosphate production. Whether depressed energy metabolism is the cause or the consequence of the loss of ion transport is unknown. Each defect could contribute to the exacerbation of the other. Nevertheless, the development of these defects is quickly followed by overt disruption of the cell membrane and cell death.

References

Ames, A., Wright, L., Kowada, M., Thurston, J.M., and Majno, G.: Cerebral ischemia. II. The no-reflow phenomenon. Am. J. Pathol. 52:437–454, 1968.

Baker, P.F.: The sodium pump in animal tissues and its role in the control of cellular metabolism and function. In *Metabolic Pathways*, ed. 3, vol. 6 (Metabolic Transport), pp. 243–268. Academic Press, New York, 1972.

Beller, G.A., Conroy, J., and Smith, T.W.: Ischemia-induced alterations in myocardial ($Na^+ + K^+$)-ATPase and cardiac glycoside binding. J. Clin. Invest. 57:341–350, 1976.

Calkins, E., Taylor, I.M., and Hastings, A.B.: Potassium exchange in the isolated rat diaphragm; effect of anoxia and cold. Am. J. Physiol. 177:211–218, 1954.

Case, R.B.: Ion alterations during myocardial ischemia. Am. J. Cardiol. 56:245–262, 1971–1972.

Chiang, J., Kowada, M., Ames, A., Wright, R.L., and Majno, G.: Cerebral ischemia. III. Vascular changes. Am. J. Pathol. 52:455–476, 1968.

Chien, K.R., Abrams, J., Serroni, A., Martin, J.T., and Farber, J.L.: Accelerated phospholipid degradation and associated membrane dysfunction in irreversible, ischemic liver cell injury. J. Biol. Chem. 253:4809–4817, 1978.

Christodoulou, J., Erlandson, R., Smithen, C., Killip, T., and Brachfeld, N.: Effects of mannitol on cardiac ultrastructure and microcirculation following anoxia. Am. J. Physiol. 229:853–860, 1975.

Daniel, E.E. and Robinson, K.: Effects of inhibitors of active transport on ^{22}Na and ^{42}K movements and on nucleotide levels in rat uteri at 25°C. Can. J. Physiol. Pharmacol. 202:178–204, 1971.

Deyrup, I.: A study of the fluid uptake of rat kidney slices in vitro. J. Gen. Physiol. 36:739, 1953.

DiPolo, R.: Characterization of the ATP-dependent calcium efflux in dialyzed squid giant axons. J. Gen. Physiol. 69:795–813, 1977.

Fischer, E.G., and Ames, A.: Studies on mechanisms of impairment of cerebral circulation following ischemia: Effect of hemodilution and perfusion pressure. Stroke 3:538–542, 1972.

Fleckenstein, A., Janke, J., Doring, H.J., and Leder, O.: Myocardial fiber necrosis due to intracellular Ca overload—A new principle in cardiac pathophysiology. Recent Adv. Stud. Cardiac Struct. Metab. 4:563–580, 1974.

Flores, J., Dibona, D.R., Beck, C.H., and Leaf, A.: The role of cell swelling in ischemic renal damage and the protective effect of hypertonic solute. J. Clin. Invest. 51:118–126, 1972.

Franck, G., Cornette, M., and Schoffeniels, E.: The cationic composition of incubated cerebral cortex slices. J. Neurochem. 15:843–857, 1968.

Franklin, W., Ganote, C.E., and Jennings, R.B.: Blood reflow after renal ischemia. Effects of hypertonic mannitol on reflow and tubular necrosis after transient ischemia in the rat. Arch. Pathol. 98:106–111, 1974.

Ganote, C.E., Jennings, R.B., Hill, M.L., and Grochowski, E.C.: Experimental myocardial ischemic injury. II. Effect of in vivo ischemia on dog heart slice function in vitro. J. Mol. Cell. Cardiol. 8:189–204, 1976.

Ginn, F.L., Shelburne, J.D., and Trump, B.F.: Disorders of cell volume regulation. I. Effects of inhibition of plasma membrane adenosine triphosphatase with ouabain. Am. J. Pathol. 53:1041–1059, 1968.

Glitsch, H.G.: Characteristics of active Na transport in intact cardiac cells. Am. J. Physiol. 236:H189–199, 1979.

Glynn, I.M., and Karlish, S.J.D.: The sodium pump. Annu. Rev. Physiol. *37:*13–55, 1975.

Goerke, J. and Page, E.: Cat heart muscle in vitro. VI. Potassium exchange in papillary muscles. J. Gen. Physiol. *48:*933–948, 1965.

Grochowski, E.C., Ganote, C.E., Hill, M.L., and Jennings, R.B.: Experimental myocardial ischemic injury. I. A comparison of Stadie-Riggs and free-hand slicing techniques on tissue ultrastructure, water and electrolytes during in vitro incubation. J. Mol. Cell. Cardiol. *8:*173–187, 1976.

Hill, J.L. and Gettes, L.S.: Effect of acute coronary artery occlusion on local myocardial extracellular K^+ activity in swine. Circulation *61:*768–778, 1980.

Hokin, L.E.: The molecular machine for driving the coupled transports of Na^+ and K^+ is an $(Na^+ + K^+)$-activated ATPase. Trends Biochem. Sci. *1:*233–237, 1976.

Hughes, P.M., and Macknight, A.D.C.: Effects of replacing medium sodium by choline, caesium, or rubidium, on water and ion contents of renal cortical slices. J. Physiol. 267:113–136, 1977.

Jennings, R.B., and Ganote, C.E.: Structural changes in myocardium during acute ischemia. Circ. Res. (Suppl.) *34, 35:* III-156-III-172, 1974.

Jennings, R.B., and Reimer, K.A.: Biology of experimental, acute myocardial ischaemia and infarction. In *Enzymes in Cardiology. Diagnosis and Research,* edited by D.J. Hearse and J. DeLeiris, ch. 2, pp. 21–57. John Wiley & Sons, New York, 1979.

Jennings, R.B., Ganote, C.E., and Reimer, K.A.: Ischemic tissue injury. Am. J. Pathol. *81:*179–198, 1975.

Jennings, R.B., Hawkins, H.K., Lowe, J.E., Hill, M.L., Klotman, S., and Reimer, K.A.: Relation between high energy phosphate and lethal injury in myocardial ischemia in the dog. Am. J. Pathol. *92:*187–214, 1978.

Judah, J.D., Ahmed, K., McLean, A.E.M., and Christie, G.S.: Ion transport in ethionine intoxication. Lab. Invest. *15:*167–175, 1966.

Kloner, R.A., Ganote, C.E., and Jennings, R.B.: The "no-reflow" phenomenon after temporary coronary occlusion in the dog. J. Clin. Invest. *54:*1496–1508, 1974a.

Kloner, R.A., Ganote, C.E., Whalen, D., and Jennings, R.B.: Effect of a transient period of ischemia on myocardial cells. II. Fine structure during the first few minutes of reflow. Am. J. Pathol. *74:*399–422, 1974b.

Kloner, R.A., Reimer, K.A., Willerson, J.T., and Jennings, R.B.: Reduction of experimental myocardial infarct size with hyperosmolar mannitol. Proc. Soc. Exp. Biol. Med. *151:*677–683, 1976.

Kowada, M., Ames, A., Majno, G., and Wright, L.: Cerebral ischemia. I. An improved experimental method for study; cardiovascular effects and demonstration of an early vascular lesion in the rabbit. J. Neurosurg. *28:*150, 1968.

Krug, A., Rochemont, W., and Korb, G.: Blood supply of the myocardium after temporary coronary occlusion. Circ. Res. *19:*57–62, 1966.

Leaf, A.: Regulation of intracellular fluid volume and disease. Am. J. Med. *49:*291–295, 1970.

Macknight, A.D.C.: Regulation of cellular volume during anaerobic incubation of rat renal cortical slices. Biochim. Biophys. Acta *163:*557, 1968.

Macknight, A.D.C., and Leaf, A.: Regulation of cellular volume. Physiol. Rev. *57:*510–573, 1977.

Mudge, G.H.: Electrolyte and water metabolism of rabbit kidney slices: Effect of metabolic inhibitors. Am. J. Phys. *167:*206, 1951.

Mullins, L.: The generation of electric currents in cardiac fibers by Na/Ca exchange. Am. J. Physiol. *236:*C103-C110, 1979.

Neely, W.A., and Youmans, J.R.: Anoxia of canine brain without damage. J.A.M.A. 183:1085, 1963.

Parks, J.M., Shay, J., and Ames, A.: Cell volume and permeability of oxygen-and glucose-deprived retina in vitro. Arch. Neurol. *33:*709–714, 1976.

Pine, M.B., Bing, O.H.L., Brooks, W.W., and Abelmann, W.H.: Changes in in vitro myocardial hydration and performance in response to transient metabolic blockade in hypertonic, isotonic, and hypotonic media. Cardiovasc. Res. *12:*569–577, 1978.

Pine, M.B., Bing, O.H.L., Weintraub, R., and Abelmann, W.H.: Dissociation of cell volume regulation and sodium-potassium exchange pump activity in dog myocardium in vitro. J. Mol. Cell. Cardiol. *11:*585–590, 1979a.

Pine, M.B., Caulfield, J., Bing, O., Brooks, W., and Abelmann, W.: Resistance of contracting myocardium to swelling with hypoxia and glycolytic blockade. Cardiovasc. Res. *13:*215–224, 1979b.

Powell, W.J., Jr., DiBona, D.R., Flores, J., Frega, N., and Leaf, A.: Effects of hyperosmotic mannitol in reducing ischemic cell swelling and minimizing myocardial necrosis. Circulation *53:*I-45-I-49, 1976.

Rau, E.E., Shine, K.I., and Langer, G.A.: Potassium exchange and mechanical performance in anoxic mammalian myocardium. Am. J. Physiol. *232(1):*H85-H94, 1977.

Reimer, K.A., Ganote, C.E., and Jennings, R.B.: Alterations in renal cortex following ischemic injury. III. Ultrastructure of proximal tubules after ischemia or autolysis. Lab. Invest. *26:* 347–363, 1972.

Reimer, K.A., Jennings, R.B., and Hill, M.L.: Total myocardial ischemia, in vitro. 2. High energy phosphate depletion and associated defects in energy metabolism, cell volume regulation, and sarcolemmal integrity. Circ. Res., in press, 1981.

Robinson, J.R.: Osmoregulation in surviving slices from the kidneys of adult rats. Proc. Roy. Soc. London *137:*378, 1950.

Robinson, J.R.: Exchanges of water and ions by kidney slices determined by a balance method. J. Physiol. *158:*449, 1961.

Sayeed, M.M., and Baue, A.E.: Na-K transport in rat liver slices in hemorrhagic shock. Am. J. Physiol. *224:*1265–1270, 1973.

Sayeed, M.M., Wurth, M.A., Chaudry, I.H., and Baue, A.E.: Cation transport in the liver in hemorrhagic shock. Circ. Shock *1:*195–207, 1974.

Schwartz, A., Wood, J.M., Allen, J.C., Barnet, E.P., Entman, M.L., Goldstein, M.A., Sordahl, L.A., and Suzuki, M.: Biochemical and morphologic correlates of cardiac ischemia. I. Membrane systems. Am. J. Cardiol. *32:*46–61, 1973.

Schwartz, A., Lindenmayer, G.E., and Allen, J.C.: The sodium-potassium adenosine triphosphatase: Pharmacological, physiological and biochemical aspects. Pharmacol. Rev. *27:*3–134, 1975.

Shen, A.C., and Jennings, R.B.: Myocardial calcium and magnesium in acute ischemic injury. Am. J. Path. *67:*417–440, 1972a.

Shen, A.C., and Jennings, R.B.: Kinetics of calcium accumulation in acute myocardial ischemic injury. Am. J. Pathol. *67:*441–452, 1972b.

Shine, K.I., Douglas, A.M., and Ricchiuti, N. V.: Calcium, strontium, and barium movements during ischemia and reperfusion in rabbit ventricle. Implications for myocardial preservation. Circ. Res. *43:*712–720, 1978.

Silver, A.: Ion fluxes in hypoxic tissues. Microvasc. Res. *13:* 409–420, 1977.

Skou, J.C.: Enzymatic basis for active transport of Na⁺ and K⁺ across cell membrane. Physiol. Rev. *45:*596–617, 1965.

Summers, W.K., and Jamison, R.L.: The no-reflow phenomenon in renal ischemia. Lab. Invest. *25:*635–643, 1971.

Trump, B.F., and Ginn, F.L.: Studies of cellular injury in isolated flounder tubules. II. Cellular swelling in high potassium media. Lab. Invest. *18:*341–351, 1968.

van Rossum, G.D.V.: The relation of sodium and potassium ion transport to the respiration and adenine nucleotide content of liver slices treated with inhibitors of respiration. Biochem. J. *129:*427–438, 1972.

Waltz, A.G., and Sundt, T.M.: The microvasculature and microcirculation of the cerebral cortex after arterial occlusion. Brain *70:*681–696, 1967.

Whalen, D.A., Hamilton, D.G., Ganote, C.E., and Jennings, R.B.: Effect of a transient period of ischemia on myocardial cells. I. Effects on cell volume regulation. Am. J. Pathol. *74:*381–397, 1974.

Whittam, R., and Davies, R.E.: Active transport of water, sodium, potassium and α-oxogluterate by kidney-cortex slices. Biochem. J. *55:*880, 1953.

Whittembury, G., and Proverbio, F.: Two modes of Na extrusion in cells from guinea pig kidney cortex slices. Pflügers Arch. *316:*1-25, 1970.

Willerson, J., Scales, F., Mukherjee, A., Platt, M., Templeton, G., Fink, G., and Buja, M.: Abnormal myocardial fluid retention as an early manifestation of ischemic injury. Am. J. Pathol. *87:*159–188, 1977.

CHAPTER 10

Regulation and Roles of Cyclic Nucleotides

FERID MURAD

Subsequent to the discovery of adenosine 3',5'-monophosphate (cyclic AMP) by Sutherland and Rall (Rall et al., 1957; Sutherland and Rall, 1958), it has become apparent that this cyclic nucleotide mediates a variety of hormone and drug-induced responses in numerous tissues (Robison et al., 1971). These investigators and their associates were examining the mechanism of epinephrine and glucagon-induced hyperglycemia. Utilizing liver slices and extracts they found that the rate-limiting step in the conversion of glycogen to glucose was catalyzed by phosphorylase and that the hyperglycemic agents increased the activity of this enzyme. Glucagon and epinephrine increased the formation of a heat stable factor that was identified as cyclic AMP (Rall et al., 1957; Sutherland and Rall, 1958). The increased formation of cyclic AMP with hormones in intact cells or cell free systems of liver resulted in the activation of phosphorylase kinase and phosphorylase with glycogen hydrolysis.

In the past 20 years, work by these and many other investigators has demonstrated that most but not all hormones produce a host of physiological and biochemical effects in a diverse list of tissues through the altered formation of cyclic AMP. The concept has evolved that cyclic AMP represents a "second messenger" or "intracellular messenger" to transmit information to intracellular enzymes and pathways which are regulated by extracellular hormones and drugs (Fig. 10.1). Hormones such as catecholamines, polypeptides, etc., interact with specific membrane recognition sites (receptors). Through what appear to be very complicated and unknown events this hormone-receptor interaction leads to the activation of adenylate cyclase and the formation of cyclic AMP from ATP. There is at least one membrane macromolecule and perhaps several that are required to couple the receptor to adenylate cyclase (Ross et al., 1978). Once cyclic AMP accumulates, a cascade of secondary events ensue, as discussed below. The primary specificity of this information transfer process probably resides in the specificity of the hormone-receptor interaction and the differentiated functions of the tissue that can be influenced by cyclic AMP. In one tissue the major effect observed when cyclic AMP levels are increased might be glycogenolysis, while in another tissue altered muscle motility or secretion could occur.

Most of the effects of cyclic AMP are mediated through the activation of cyclic AMP-dependent protein kinase (Greengard, 1971). This enzyme catalyzes the transfer of the terminal (gamma) phosphate of ATP to various protein substrates. As a result of the phosphorylation or dephosphorylation of these proteins their functional activities (enzymatic or perhaps structural) are altered (discussed below).

The intracellular pool of cyclic AMP is a function of its rate of hydrolysis and inactivation as well as its rate of synthesis. Tissues contain several enzymes referred to as cyclic nucleotide phosphodiesterases which hydrolyze cyclic AMP to 5'-AMP (Butcher and Sutherland, 1962). The activity of these enzymes can be influenced by a number of drugs, most notably methylxanthines such as caffeine and theophylline and these effects may explain the mechanism of action of these drugs and their ability to mimic various hormone-induced responses.

Another cyclic nucleotide has also been described in urine and most tissues (see Murad et al., 1979, and references therein). The formation and hydrolysis of guanosine 3',5'-monophosphate (cyclic GMP) resembles that of cyclic AMP in many respects (Fig. 10.2). While it is clear that the formation and hydrolysis of cyclic GMP are unrelated to cyclic AMP, interactions of these systems cannot be excluded. Although separate cyclases, phosphodiesterases, and protein kinases exist for cyclic AMP and cyclic GMP metabolism, these enzymes are not totally specific, as described below. A major difficulty at present is the assignment of some physiological functions to cyclic GMP. It has been proposed that cyclic GMP may be involved in a number of processes. However, only several of these have withstood the test of time and additional experiments. The more promising effects of cyclic GMP on smooth muscle relaxation and intestinal secretion are discussed later. With few exceptions, most tissues contain all of the enzymes and components of each of the cyclic nucleotides systems.

SYNTHESIS OF CYCLIC NUCLEOTIDES

Adenylate Cyclase

In the case of cyclic AMP the appropriate hormone-receptor interaction results in the activation of adenylate cyclase in the plasma membrane. The enzyme which is located predominantly in the plasma membrane of mammalian tissues catalyzes the formation of cyclic AMP and phyrophosphate from ATP (Robison et al., 1971). While the enzyme complex prefers Mg^{2+} as its cation cofactor, the catalytic unit of the complex can use Mn^{2+} as cofactor. The mechanism of coupling hormone recep-

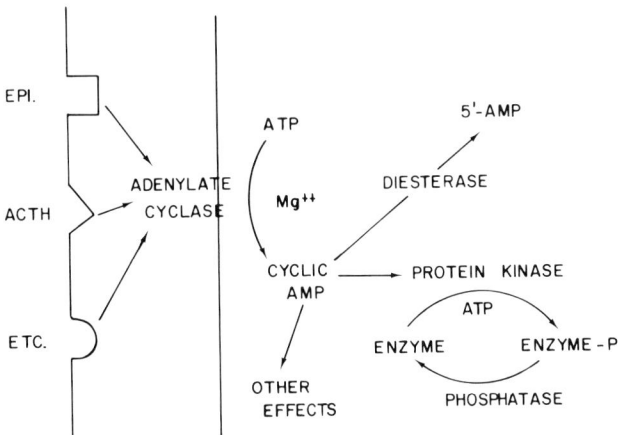

Figure 10.1. Second messenger concept of cyclic AMP. Various hormones interact with specific cell membrane receptors that result in adenylate cyclase activation and cyclic AMP synthesis.

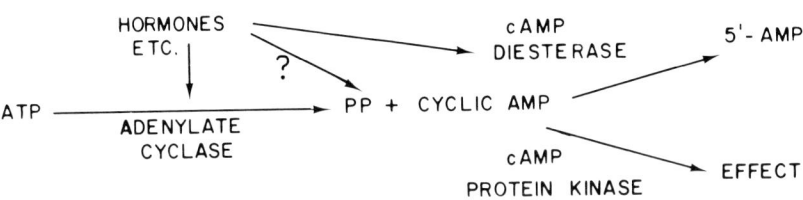

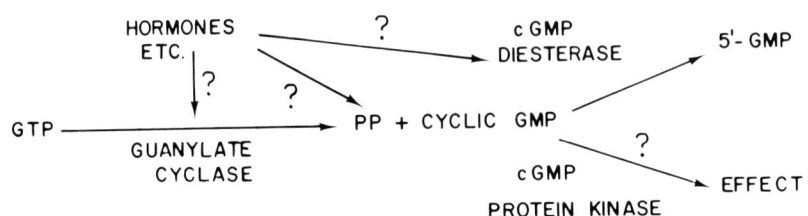

Figure 10.2. Similarities of the cyclic AMP and cyclic GMP systems.

tors to adenylate cyclase is not completely understood. Recent studies with partially purified fractions and their reconstitution as well as genetic variants of cell cultures indicate that another macromolecule is required to couple and transmit information from hormone-receptor binding to adenylate cyclase activation (see Ross et al., 1978, and references therein). This protein macromolecule is referred to as the G/F factor, which interacts with guanyl nucleotides and fluoride. The interaction of this protein with the catalytic subunit of adenylate cyclase leads to its activation and permits the enzyme to utilize Mg^{2+} as cofactor.

The addition of the appropriate hormone to a tissue results in a rapid accumulation of cyclic AMP. Cyclic AMP levels generally reach a peak within several minutes and then decline, in spite of the continued presence of the hormone (Manganiello et al., 1971). The increase in cyclic AMP is frequently much greater than the amount required to give a maximal physiological response. The reasons for this "overshoot effect" are unknown. While it may represent an insignificant artifact of in vitro experiments with excessively high concentrations of hormone, it has been suggested that this is a "fail safe" mechanism to ensure the transfer of information. The decline in cyclic AMP with the continued presence of hormone is an interesting phenomenon that is called refractoriness or desensitization (Manganiello et al., 1971). It is observed in many tissues with a variety of hormones (Perkins et al., 1978). Explanations for this phenomenon have included decreased hormone receptors, decreased coupling of receptors to adenylate cyclase, decreased adenylate cyclase activity, and increased cyclic AMP hydrolysis by phosphodiesterase. In many systems the desensitization or refractoriness is cyclic AMP-dependent, in that addition of exogenous cyclic AMP or its analogues leads to a similar phenomenon, and inhibition of cyclic AMP accumulation can overcome the refractoriness. Thus, the accumulation of cyclic AMP in tissues can probably influence its own rate of synthesis and hydrolysis.

Although adenylate cyclase has been purified to homogeneity from bacteria (Takai et al., 1974), the enzyme and other components of the receptor-adenylate cyclase system have not been purified from mammalian sources (Neer, 1978; Ross et al. 1978).

Guanylate Cyclase

In contrast to adenylate cyclase, guanylate cyclase is found in both soluble and particulate fractions of tissue homogenates (Kimura and Murad, 1975a). The kinetic and physical properties of the soluble and particulate forms of the enzyme are quite different and the forms are readily separable (Kimura and Murad, 1975b). It is not possible at present to determine if the two forms of the enzyme represent dissimilar proteins (isoenzymes) or if their different properties are due to other conditions or constituents in assays. The particulate enzyme is found in plasma membranes, endoplasmic reticulum, and Golgi with liver and other preparations (see Kimura and Murad, 1975a, and references therein). There is some evidence that the particulate forms of the enzyme also have somewhat different properties. Thus, there may be a variety of forms of guanylate cyclase in tissues that can exist in their inactive and active states.

The reaction catalyzed by guanylate cyclase is the formation of cyclic GMP and pyrophosphate from GTP. The native enzyme prefers Mn^{2+} as cation cofactor with Mg^{2+} about 5-20% as effective. The apparent preference for Mn^{2+} has always been perplexing in view of the low concentrations of Mn^{2+} normally present in tissues. However, when the enzyme is activated (see below), it can utilize either cation as effectively as the other and the physiological cofactor may be Mg^{2+} (Kimura et al., 1976). Interestingly, the activated enzyme can also catalyze the formation of cyclic AMP from ATP (Mittal and Murad, 1977; Mittal et al., 1979). The significance of this alternate pathway for the synthesis of cyclic AMP is unknown. The rate of formation of cyclic AMP by activated guanylate cyclase is about 1-15% of the rate of cyclic GMP formation. Perhaps the effects of some hormones and drugs on cyclic AMP levels in tissues could result from the activation of guanylate cyclase and/or adenylate cyclase.

The soluble enzyme from rat liver and lung has recently been purified to homogeneity (Braughler et al., 1979; Garbers, 1979). The soluble enzyme has a MW of 150,000 daltons and contains two identical subunits. Estimates of the size of the particulate form of the enzyme after detergent solubilization have been about twice this size using gel filtration techniques (Murad et al., 1979). While the particulate enzyme has been purified from sea urchin sperm (Garbers, 1976), the particulate mammalian enzyme has not been purified to homogeneity to permit comparisons of the soluble and particulate forms.

Although a number of hormones including choline esters, α-adrenergic agents, prostaglandins, histamine, etc., increase cyclic GMP levels in tissues, hormones have not activated guanylate cyclase in cell free preparations (Murad et al., 1979). The few effects of hormones on guanylate cyclase that have been reported may be due to interesting artifacts or nonenzymatic formation of cyclic GMP. As noted below nitroso compounds, fatty acids, and other compounds activate the enzyme in broken cell preparations and increase cyclic GMP levels in intact cells (Murad et al., 1979, and references therein).

HYDROLYSIS BY PHOSPHODIESTERASES

When tissue extracts are chromatographed on DEAE columns, usually three peaks of cyclic nucleotide phosphodiesterase activity can be obtained (Gain and Appleman, 1978). One form has a high affinity for cyclic GMP; one form has a high affinity for cyclic AMP; and another form hydrolyzes both cyclic AMP and cyclic GMP. The cyclic GMP phosphodiesterase is activated by calcium in the presence of a protein factor calmodulin (Cheung et al., 1978). The activity of the cyclic AMP phosphodiesterase in adipose tissue and liver is increased with insulin (Kono et al., 1977; Loten and Sneyd, 1970; Thompson et al., 1973). All forms of the phosphodiesterase are inhibited by methylxanthines such as caffeine or theophylline and in some tissues some agents exhibit some partial selectivity for inhibiting one form of the phosphodiesterase. It has also been reported that phenothiazine inhibition of phosphodiesterase is due to the interaction of this class of drugs with calmodulin (Weiss and Levin, 1978).

The ratios of the different forms of phosphodiesterase and the subcellular distribution in soluble and particulate fractions vary in different tissues. While interconversion of these multiple enzyme forms might provide additional mechanisms to regulate intracellular cyclic nucleotide levels, there are no data to support or refute this hypothesis.

The effects of insulin on phosphodiesterase activity indicate that the enzyme is regulatable in cells. Furthermore, the synthesis and activity of phosphodiesterase can be influenced by other hormones such as steroids and prostaglandins (Manganiello and Vaughan, 1972; Strada and Thompson, 1978). The inhibition of phosphodiesterases by methylxanthines and the effects of these drugs on cyclic nucleotide levels and potentiation of various hormone effects have been interpreted as their mechanism of action. However, methylxanthines also block adenosine receptors in tissues and perhaps some of their pharmacological effects are mediated through this latter mechanism (see Rall, 1980, and discussion therein).

PROTEIN KINASES

Many and perhaps all of the effects of cyclic AMP in eukaryotes appear to be mediated through the activation of cyclic AMP-dependent protein kinase. This enzyme is a tetramer of 190,000 daltons composed of two cyclic AMP binding subunits of 55,000 daltons each and two catalytic subunits of 40,000 daltons each, as depicted in Figure 10.3 (see Corbin and Lincoln, 1978, and references therein). The holoenzyme is inactive and upon the binding of cyclic AMP to the regulatory subunits the enzyme dissociates, resulting in activation of the catalytic subunit. The catalytic subunit can transfer the terminal phosphate of ATP to serine residues of various protein substrates. The protein substrates for cyclic AMP-dependent protein kinase are quite diverse and include several enzymes such as phosphorylase kinase, glycogen synthase, hormone sensitive lipase, as well as membrane, structural and contractile proteins, etc. Tissues also contain phosphoprotein phosphatases that remove the serine phosphate from these proteins (Curnow and Larner, 1979). Through the cyclic phosphorylation and dephosphorylation of these proteins, their catalytic and/or functional activities are increased or decreased. Both types of examples exist where either the phosphorylated enzyme or the dephosphorylated enzyme is more active.

Some effects of cyclic AMP in bacteria do not require activation of protein kinase and another binding protein for cyclic AMP that influences messenger RNA and protein synthesis has been described (Anderson et al., 1972). Thus, not all of the effects of cyclic AMP are mediated through activation of a protein kinase and protein phosphorylation.

$$R_2C_2 + 2\,cAMP \rightleftharpoons R_2cAMP_2 + 2C$$
$$\text{(INACTIVE)} \qquad\qquad \text{(ACTIVE)}$$

$$C_2 + 2\,cGMP \rightleftharpoons C_2cGMP_2$$

Figure 10.3. Activation of cyclic AMP (cAMP) and cyclic GMP (cGMP) dependent protein kinases.

Cyclic GMP-dependent protein kinase has also been described in numerous tissues (Corbin and Lincoln, 1978). This enzyme is 160,000 daltons with two similar subunits, (Fig. 10.3). The binding of 2 moles of cyclic GMP per mole of enzyme leads to activation without dissociation of the protein. To date the protein substrates for both cyclic AMP-dependent and cyclic GMP-dependent protein kinases have unfortunately been quite similar. Whether or not the physiological effects of cyclic GMP involve the phosphorylation of the same or different proteins is unknown. It has been presumed that the identification of specific protein substrates for cyclic GMP-dependent protein kinase should lead to an understanding of some functions of cyclic GMP. However, to date this approach and plan has not materialized and led to a definition of some roles for this nucleotide.

HORMONAL AND DRUG REGULATION OF CYCLIC NUCLEOTIDE LEVELS

In the early studies catecholamines and glucagon increased cyclic AMP synthesis and accumulation in preparations from liver and heart (Sutherland and Rall, 1958; Murad et al., 1962; Robison et al., 1965). These and subsequent studies led to the proposal that beta-adrenergic effects in tissues were the result of adenylate cyclase activation and cyclic AMP formation. This hypothesis has been examined with relative potencies of catecholamines, effects of adrenergic blocking agents, etc., in a number of systems and this proposal continues to hold up.

Sutherland and his associates (1968) have developed several criteria to be met in order to implicate cyclic AMP in the mechanism of action of a hormone or drug. These include: 1) the demonstration in broken cell preparations of a tissue an adenylate cyclase system whose activity can be enhanced by the hormone in question and prevented with appropriate pharmacological blocking agents or antagonists; 2) the hormone response should be enhanced or potentiated with inhibitors of phosphodiesterases such as methylxanthines; 3) increased cyclic AMP levels in the tissue with hormone treatment should occur prior to or coincident with the biochemical or physiological response regulated by the hormone; 4) cyclic AMP or an active analogue of the nucleotide should mimic the response of the hormone. Although these criteria have been useful, the effects of some hormones and agents have been erroneously included or excluded from the list of agents that work through cyclic AMP when the criteria are used in the strictest sense. Applying these criteria, reports from many laboratories have described hormone-tissue interactions which are thought to be mediated by cyclic AMP.

Most hormones, with few exceptions, increase cyclic AMP formation in the appropriate target tissues. The list of effective hormones is quite diverse, as is the list of tissues affected (see Robison et al., 1971; and references therein). Thus, a number of very dissimilar types of agents appear to utilize this information transfer system of adenylate cyclase—cyclic AMP.

Alpha-adrenergic agents can decrease cyclic AMP formation in platelets and other tissues (Salzman and Levine, 1971), and perhaps some agents mediate some of their effects by decreasing cyclic AMP synthesis. While choline esters increase cyclic GMP levels in many tissues (see below), muscarinic agents decrease adenylate cyclase activity and cyclic AMP levels in heart and other tissues (Murad et al., 1962). Insulin and prostaglandins decrease cyclic AMP in liver and adipose tissue (Butcher and Sutherland, 1967).

Clearly some hormones do not alter cyclic AMP formation acutely and their physiological effects are probably not mediated through this system. These agents include steroids, thyroid hormone, growth hormone, and others.

Several hormones also increase cyclic GMP levels in tissues (Goldberg et al., 1973; Murad et al., 1979). These agents include choline esters, histamine, some prostaglandins, insulin, and α-adrenergic agents. However, it is not known if the effects of these hormones or autocoids are mediated through cyclic GMP or not. The effects of choline esters in smooth muscle on muscle motility occur before increases in cyclic GMP can be detected (Katsuki and Murad, 1977). Thus, it appears unlikely that these effects of choline esters can be mediated through changes in cyclic GMP levels.

Bacterial toxins also utilize the cyclic nucleotide systems to produce their effects in tissues. The first toxin with a described effect on cyclic nucleotides was cholera toxin, which has since been found to increase cyclic AMP in most tissues (see Perkins et al., 1978; and references therein). Some strains of *Escherichia coli* secrete a heat-stable enterotoxin that produces diarrhea in animals and man, activates intestinal mucosa guanylate cyclase, and increases cyclic GMP levels in intestine (Hughes et al., 1978). The effects of the toxin on fluid secretion are also mimicked with 8-bromo cyclic GMP. One of the functions of cyclic GMP may be to regulate fluid and electrolyte transport and secretion in the intestine and this area is receiving more attention. It is of interest that cyclic AMP has apparently similar effects on intestinal secretion. The effects of both cyclic nucleotides to increase intestinal secretion and to relax some smooth muscle preparations are excellent examples where both nucleotides lead to similar physiological effects. Clearly cyclic AMP and cyclic GMP do not necessarily have antagonistic effects and functions as proposed several years ago (Goldberg et al., 1973).

While hormones have generally failed to activate guanylate cyclase in cell free systems, a variety of nitroso compounds and nitric oxide precursors can activate the enzyme and increase cyclic GMP in intact tissues (see Murad et al., 1979, and references therein). These agents have included azide, hydroxylamine, nitrite, nitroglycerin, nitroprusside and other materials that can form the reactive free radical nitric oxide (Fig. 10.4). These and other studies have indicated that guanylate cyclase and

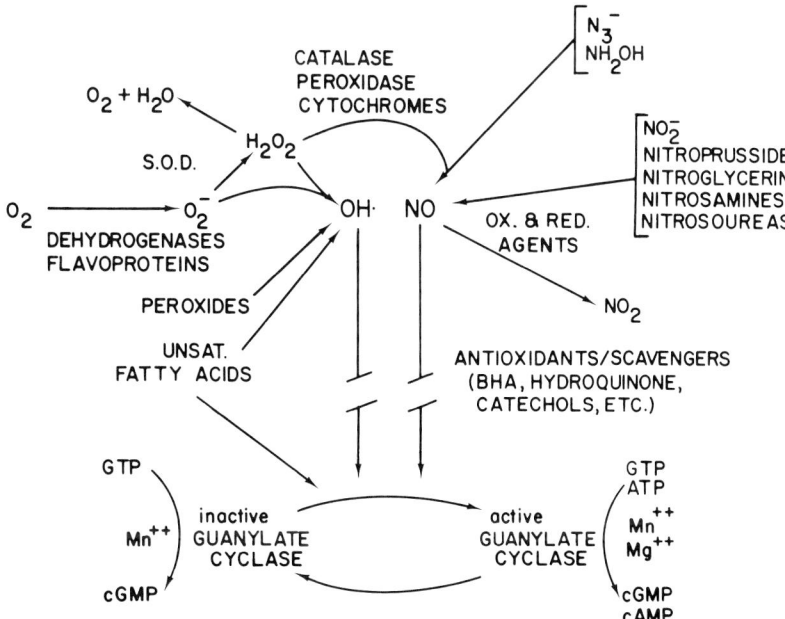

Figure 10.4. Mechanisms of nitric oxide and hydroxyl free radical formation and guanylate cyclase activation.

cyclic GMP are regulated by oxidation and reduction events in tissues (Mittal and Murad, 1977). These effects on cyclic GMP may be the mechanism of action of the nitro compound smooth muscle relaxants and vasodilators (see Murad et al., 1979).

SOME CLINICAL STUDIES WITH CYCLIC NUCLEOTIDES

The fundamental role of cyclic nucleotides in the mechanism of action of many hormones and drugs indicates that defects or perturbations of these systems could explain the pathophysiology of some disorders and may be used to diagnose some diseases. This has indeed been the case with some endocrine and metabolic disorders (Murad, 1973; Broadus, 1977). The most promising areas for diagnostic applications have been with parathyroid and calcium disorders. Parathyroid hormone increases cyclic AMP levels in the kidney and also in urine. Approximately one-half of the cyclic AMP in urine is derived from plasma filtration and about one-half comes from the kidney under the influence of parathyroid hormone. In hyperparathyroidism urinary cyclic AMP and cyclic GMP are increased about twofold and their analysis has proven useful in the diagnosis of this disorder (Murad and Pak, 1972). When urinary cyclic AMP is normalized for urinary creatinine or for the renal contribution of urinary cyclic AMP (nephrogeneous portion), this simple diagnostic test is highly specific and is used widely to evaluate calcium disorders (Murad, 1973; and Broadus, 1977). With the removal of adenomatous or hyperplastic parathyroid glands, urinary cyclic AMP and cyclic GMP return to normal and can be used to assess surgical therapy and/or recurrence (Table 10.1).

Urinary cyclic nucleotides may be altered in a variety of other endocrine and metabolic disorders. The alterations observed are in part due to the methods used to normalize urinary levels and are observed in cystic fibrosis, thyroid disorders, pheochromocytoma, syndrome of inappropriate antidiuretic hormone secretion, carcinoid, glucagon-secreting tumors, manic depressive disorders, etc.

Plasma cyclic nucleotides or the metabolism of cyclic nucleotides in tissue specimens have also been used in some clinical studies successfully. Readers are referred to articles by Murad (1973), Murad et al. (1977), and Broadus (1977) for a more detailed discussion of clinical studies with cyclic nucleotides.

SUMMARY

The formation and hydrolysis of cyclic nucleotides and more notably cyclic AMP are involved in a very fundamental way in the transmission of information between cells. Many examples exist where chemical messengers or membrane signals and perturbations lead to some biochemical or physiological response as a result of the alteration of cyclic nucleotide metabolism. Obviously not all hormones utilize this system of information transfer. Furthermore, in many instances cyclic nucleotides should be considered in a regulatory capacity and not as essential intermediates in the control of metabolic and physiological processes. Many processes that are influenced by cyclic nucleotides can also be influenced by calcium, other ions, and nucleotides, etc. Thus, cyclic nucleotides serve to modulate or "fine tune" some events that are also controlled in other ways.

Cyclic nucleotide metabolism can also be influenced indirectly through the availability of ion cofactors, substrate levels, etc., and in some instances the altered levels of cyclic nucleotides that occur in tissues are secondary and unrelated to the primary effects of hormones and drugs. This can be a difficult issue to resolve. It may be extremely difficult in complicated in vivo models and clinical studies to determine whether cyclic nucleotides are causally and primarily related to an event or occur as a later unrelated event. Precise dose-response and temporal relationships are usually required to test correlations of cyclic nucleotides to the regulation of some process. Since it is often quite difficult to meet these criteria in clinical and in vivo animal studies, the role of cyclic nucleotides in some models of disease and pathophysiology are difficult to assess. However, the examination of cyclic nucleotide metabolism, when possible with existing or new methods, could provide investigators and clinicians important information with regard to normal or abnormal tissue function.

Table 10.1
Cyclic Nucleotide Excretion With Various Calcium Disorders[a]

Diagnosis	Cyclic AMP	Cyclic GMP
	μmoles/g creatinine	
Normals	2.75 ± 0.13 (27)[b]	0.45 ± 0.08 (23)[b]
Primary hyperparathyroidism	5.86 ± 0.31 (54)[c]	0.90 ± 0.15 (12)[c]
Suspected hyperparathyroidism	6.73 ± 0.74 (16)[c]	1.17 ± 0.21 (3)[b]
"Ectopic PTH-tumor"	8.99 ± 2.36 (4)[c]	—
After surgery for hyperparathyroidism	2.79 ± 0.36 (14)	0.62 ± 0.08 (8)
Hypoparathyroidism	1.81 ± 0.19 (20)[c]	0.53 ± 0.06 (13)
Osteoporosis	3.48 ± 0.28 (10)[c]	0.71 ± 0.10 (9)[c]
Nephrolithiasis	2.98 ± 0.24 (25)	0.64 ± 0.12 (18)

[a] From Murad et al., 1977.
[b] Values are the mean ± SE daily excretion of cyclic nucleotide normalized for urinary creatinine. Number of patients are designated in parentheses.
[c] Significantly different from normal values ($p < 0.05$).

References

Anderson, W.B., Perlman, R.L., and Pastan, I.: Effect of adenosine 3',5'-monophosphate analogues on the activity of cyclic adenosine 3',5'-monophosphate receptor in *Escherichia coli*. J. Biol. Chem. 247:2717, 1972.

Braughler, J.M., Mittal, C.K., and Murad, F.: Purification of soluble guanylate cyclase from rat liver. Proc. Natl. Acad. Sci. USA 76:219, 1979.

Broadus, A.E.: Clinical cyclic nucleotide research. Adv. Cyclic Nucleotide Res. 8:509, 1977.

Butcher, R.W., and Sutherland, E.W.: Purification and properties of cyclic 3′,5′-nucleotide phosphodiesterase and use of this enzyme to characterize adenosine 3′,5′-monophosphate in human urine. J. Biol. Chem. *237*:1244, 1962.

Butcher, R.W., and Sutherland, E.W.: The effects of catecholamines, adrenergic blocking agents, prostaglandin E_1, and insulin on cyclic AMP levels in rat epididymal fat pad in vitro. Ann. N.Y. Acad. Sci. *139*:849, 1967.

Cheung, W.Y., Lynch, T.J., and Wallace, R.W.: An endogenous Ca^{2+}-dependent activation protein of brain adenylate cyclase and cyclic nucleotide phosphodiesterase. Adv. Cyclic Nucleotide Res. *9*:233, 1978.

Corbin, J.D., and Lincoln, M.: Comparison of cAMP- and cGMP-dependent protein kinases. Adv. Cyclic Nucleotide Res. *9*:159, 1978.

Curnow, R.T., and Larner, J.: Hormonal and metabolic control of phosphoprotein phosphatase. Biochem. Act. Horm. *6*:77, 1979.

Gain, K.R., and Appleman, M.M.: Distribution and regulation of the phosphodiesterases of muscle tissues. Adv. Cyclic Nucleotide Res. *9*:221, 1978.

Garbers, D.L.: Sea urchin sperm guanylate cyclase: purification and loss of cooperativity. J. Biol. Chem. *251*:4071, 1976.

Garbers, D.L.: Purification of soluble guanylate cyclase from rat lung. J. Biol. Chem. *254*:240, 1979.

Goldberg, N.D., O'Dea, R.F., and Haddox, M.K.: Cyclic GMP. Adv. Cyclic Nucleotide Res. *3*:155, 1973.

Greengard, P.: On the reactivity and mechanism of action of cyclic nucleotides. Ann. N.Y. Acad. Sci. *185*:18, 1971.

Hughes, J., Murad, F., Chang, B., and Guerrant, R.: The role of cyclic GMP in the mechanism of action of the heat-stable enterotoxin of *E. coli*. Nature *271*:755, 1978.

Katsuki, S., and Murad, F.: Regulation of cyclic 3′,5′-adenosine monophosphate and cyclic 3′,5′-guanosine monophosphate levels and contractility in bovine tracheal smooth muscle. Molec. Pharmacol. *13*:330, 1977.

Kimura, H., and Murad, F.: Subcellular localization of guanylate cyclase. Life Sci. *17*:837, 1975a.

Kimura, H., and Murad, F.: Two forms of guanylate cyclase in mammalian tissues and possible mechanisms for their regulation. Metabolism *24*:439, 1975b.

Kimura, H., Mittal, C.K., and Murad, F: Appearance of magnesium guanylate cyclase activity in rat liver with sodium azide activation. J. Biol. Chem. *251*:7769, 1976.

Kono, T., Robinson, F.W., Sarver, J.A., Vega, F.V., and Pointer, R.H.: Actions of insulin rat—Effects of low temperature, uncouplers of oxidative phosphorylation, and respiratory inhibitors. J. Biol. Chem. *252*:2226, 1977.

Loten, E.G., and Sneyd, J.G.T.: An effect of insulin on adipose tissue adenosine 3′,5′-monophosphate phosphodiesterase. Biochem J. *120*:187, 1970.

Manganiello, V., and Vaughan, M.: An effect of dexamethasone on adenosine 3′,5′-monophosphate content and adenosine 3′,5′-monophosphate phosphodiesterase activity of cultured hepatoma cells. J. Clin. Invest. *51*:2763, 1972.

Manganiello, V., Murad, F., and Vaughan, V.: Effects of lipolytic and antilipolytic agents on cyclic 3′,5′-adenosine monophosphate in fat cells. J. Biol. Chem. *246*:2195, 1971.

Mittal, C.K., Braughler, J.M., Ichihara, K., and Murad, F.: Synthesis of adenosine 3′,5′-monophosphate by guanylate cyclase, a new pathway for its formation. Biochim. Biophys. Acta *585*:333, 1979.

Mittal, C.K., and Murad, F.: Properties and oxidative regulation of guanylate cyclase. J. Cyclic Nucleotide Res. *3*:381, 1977.

Murad, F.: Clinical studies and applications of cyclic nucleotides. Adv. Cyclic Nucleotide Res. *3*:335, 1973.

Murad, F., and Pak, C.: Urinary excretion of adenosine 3′,5′-monophosphate and guanosine 3′,5′-monophosphate. N. Engl. J. Med. *286*:1382, 1972.

Murad, F., Chi, Y.M., Rall, T.W., and Sutherland, E.W.: The effect of catecholamines and choline esters on the formation of adenosine 3′,5′-monophosphate by preparations from cardiac muscle and liver. J. Bio. Chem. *237*:1233, 1962.

Murad, F., Weitzman, R., and Taylor, A.: Use of cyclic nucleotides to evaluate calcium disorders. In *Clinical Aspects of Cyclic Nucleotides*, edited by L. Volicer, pp. 1–18. Spectrum, New York, 1977.

Murad, F., Arnold, W.P., Mittal, C.K., and Braughler, J.M.: Properties and regulation of guanylate cyclase and some proposed functions for cyclic GMP. Adv. Cyclic Nucleotide Res. *11*:175, 1979.

Neer, E.J.: Physical and functional properties of adenylate cyclase from mature rat testes. J. Biol. Chem. *253*:5808, 1978.

Perkins, J.P., Johnson, G.L., and Harden, T.K.: Drug-induced modification of the responsiveness of adenylate cyclase to hormones. Adv. Cyclic Nucleotide Res. *9*:19, 1978.

Rall, T.W.: *Methylxanthines in the Pharmacological Basis of Therapeutics*, edited by L. Goodman, A. Gilman, and A.G. Gilman, ed. 6. Macmillian, New York, 1980.

Rall, T.W., Sutherland, E.W., and Berthet, J.: Relationship of epinephrine and glucagon to liver phosphorylase. IV. Effect of epinephrine and glucagon on the reactivation of phosphorylase in liver homogenate. J. Biol. Chem. *224*:463, 1957.

Robison, G.A., Butcher, R.W., Oye, I., Morgan, H.E., and Sutherland, E.W.: The effect of epinephrine on adenosine 3′,5′-monophosphate levels in the isolated perfused rat heart. Mol. Pharmacol. *1*:168, 1965.

Robison, G.A., Butcher, R.W., and Sutherland, E.W.: *Cyclic AMP*. Academic Press, New York, 1971.

Ross, E.M., Haga, T., Howlett, A.C., Schwarzmeier, J., Schleifer L.S., and Gilman, A.G.: Hormone-sensitive adenylate cyclase: Resolution and reconstitution of some components necessary for regulation of the enzyme. Adv. Cyclic Nucleotide Res. *9*:53, 1978.

Salzman, E.W., and Levine, I.: Cyclic 3′,5′-adenosine monophosphate in human blood platelets II. Effect of N^6-2^1-0-dibutyryl cyclic 3′,5′-adenosine monophosphate on platelet function. J. Clin. Invest. *50*:131, 1971.

Strada, S.J., and Thompson, W.J.: Multiple forms of cyclic nucleotide phosphodiesterases: Anomalies or biologic regulators. Adv. Cyclic Nucleotide Res. *9*:265, 1978.

Sutherland, E.W., and Rall, T.W.: Fractionation and characterization of a cyclic adenine ribonucleotide formed by tissue particles. J. Biol. Chem. *232*:1077, 1958.

Sutherland, E.W., Robison, G.A., and Butcher, R.W.: Some aspects of the biological role of adenosine 3′,5′-monophosphate. Circulation *37*:279, 1968.

Takai, K., Kurashina, Y., Suzuki-Hori, C., Okamoto, H., and Hayaishi, O.: Adenylate cyclase from Brevibacterium liquefaciens: I. Purification, crystallization and some properties. J. Biol. Chem. *249*:1965, 1974.

Thompson, W.J., Little, S.A., and Williams, R.H.: Effect of insulin and growth hormone on rat liver cyclic nucleotide phosphodiesterase. Biochemistry *12*:1889, 1973.

Weiss, B., and Levin, R.M.: Mechanism of selectively inhibiting the activation of cyclic nucleotide phosphodiesterase and adenylate cyclase by antipsychotic agents. Adv. Cyclic Nucleotide Res. *9*:285, 1978.

PART 2

ALTERATIONS IN THE MICROCIRCULATION

EDITORS' SUMMARY

The microcirculation is the major circulation in the body system and the least studied because of the difficulties involved in the development of excellent techniques. In contrast, the greater and lesser circulation can readily be examined by more familiar techniques.

Examination of the microcirculation involves two major methods:

1. Microscopic Techniques. These involve personal observation and, therefore, these techniques tend to be semiquantitative, e.g., how red is red, are the cells hypoxic or not, and are the tissues pink or white? Problems also exist in determining presence and degree of constricted capillaries and arterioles and presence and degree of shunts. All of these are relative to the observer, his training, and his attempts to communicate the results. This has limited our ability to critically study the microcirculation by direct observation. It would be helped by newer techniques of cinematography and newer electronic techniques using television and image processing, where several people could watch the same screen and come to a concerted group evaluation; moreover, better quantitation could be performed.

2. Biochemical Techniques. The other techniques for measuring the microcirculation involve biochemical and metabolic methods. One example is the study of lactate, which is increased with poor circulation at the tissue level. One limitation of standard microcirculatory techniques is that observations are usually limited to the surface vessels.

In the chapter by McCuskey, the problems with the terminology of the microcirculation are discussed; it is evident that the terminology still needs improvement. Another recent review of the subject appears in a chapter by Mason and Balis (1980). The role of the cytoskeleton, especially contractile filaments and microtubules, as well as both myo-myo and myoendothelial cell junctions seems to be especially important in the precapillary arterioles. Presently, much more is being learned about the role of contractile filaments in the regulation of cell movement and cell shape in all types of cells. In the microvascular system this is especially important. Loss of control of ionized calcium within the cell following anoxia and/or ischemia could, as discussed elsewhere in this volume, exert many important effects, including the "no reflow" phenomenon through defective ion regulation, which may well be an important control point in this type of injury. Although much more needs to be learned about the controls effected on the microvasculature, both myogenic and metabolic control mechanisms are discussed and these can easily be interrelated through the effects of failure to control ionized calcium. In addition, many chemical modulators are affected in shock and anoxia, including corticosteroids, serotonin, and histamine. It should also be noted that inflammatory cells resulting from tissue injury can result in a variety of additional effects.

The effects of anoxia on the endothelium also contribute to changes in vascular permeability, presumably through the changes in cell shape and modification of cell junction permeability. This can be of particular significance in the shock lung. The effects of injury on the endothelium are somewhat similar to those in cells elsewhere (see Ch. 1) but in this case result not only in changes in the endothelium but also in changes of vascular permeability. In the case of septic and endotoxin shock, the presence of microorganisms can result in a great enhancement of tissue damage to the endothelium with marked accentuation of all factors mentioned above.

In his chapter, Lefer reviews some major vascular mediators, including the renin-angiotensin system, the prostacycline-thromboxane system and lysosomal hydrolases. These newly discovered vascular mediators may play a very important role in the initiation as well as in the perpetuation of ischemia and shock. These mediators are of potential importance because some of them are susceptible to therapeutic modification and thus could result in amelioration of cell injury. Lefer considers that among the mechanisms which can be involved in this mediation are severe vasoconstriction or vasospasm, induction of platelet aggregation and thrombus formation, increased capillary permeability, and redistribution of blood flow away from vital tissues. This chapter thus logically extends that of McCuskey. The major vasoactive agents discussed include angiotensins II and III, thromboxane A_2, and the myocardial depressant factor. These are all potent naturally occurring constrictors that clearly can contribute to or directly produce a state of shock or serious cardiovascular decompensation. These mediators are all either peptides or lipids and thus have many other actions in addition to their severe vasoconstrictive effects, including enhanced capillary leakage, thromboxane-induced platelet aggregation, MDF-induced decreased myocardial contractility and altered reticuloendothelial function. Several inhibitors of the formation of all three vascular mediators are discussed. Experiments and clinical trials are now underway in several centers to determine if such modification can improve the therapeutic response.

In their chapter, Webb and Brunswick stress the principle that, in addition to appropriate fluid replacement, attention must be given to the microvasculature in terms of reducing vascular resistance, of course in the presence of appropriate monitoring of cardiovascular parameters. Increased vascular volume must be compatible with the pressure and tone of the vessels in order to maintain these in equilibrium as the diminished volume of cardiac output and increased vascular tone return to normal. This has received particular attention in the lung but these changes in the microvasculature have effects in many other organs as well, though the venous system particularly, stressed in this chapter, is often overlooked. The capillaries, venules, and veins act as a capacitance system which contains some 60% of the total blood volume and if maximally dilated could contain greater than the normal circulating volume. Thus, the status of this capacitance system is extremely important in determining cardiac output. In general, the veins remain responsive in ischemia and anoxia after the arterioles have lost tone and dilated. Another little understood factor is the observation that atelectasis in the lung markedly increases resistance by collapsing capillaries and venules, causing local hypoxia. In our program at the University of Maryland, School of Medicine, careful attention to respiratory therapy has greatly modified the incidence and severity of shock lung, suggesting that primary vascular injury may not be responsible.

In his chapter, Hardaway discusses the concept of disseminated intravascular coagulation (DIC) which he innovated. DIC is said to be relatively common but is often not diagnosed. In our own experience, it is severe in only a few cases, usually associated with sepsis, and only minor degrees occur, at least as seen in our patients and at autopsy. It may well be that more than one exposure to endotoxin is needed because of the generalized Schwartz-Mann phenomenon. Therefore, we still need more information concerning this potentially serious complication. More experiments are needed with treatment using fibrinolysin or other agents which could modify the progress of DIC without increasing the risk of serious hemorrhage. It is evident, however, that a large number of clinical syndromes in a variety of serious diseases is associated with shock and can result in DIC.

Reference

Mason, R.G., and Balis, J.U.: In *Pathobiology of Cell Membranes*, edited by B.F. Trump, and A.U. Arstila, vol. II, pp. 425–460. Academic Press, New York, 1980.

CHAPTER 11

Microcirculation—Basic Considerations

ROBERT S. McCUSKEY

Sustaining an optimal microcirculation is a requirement for the maintenance and survival of virtually all vertebrate cells, tissues, and organs. Failure to maintain an optimal microcirculation results in tissue hypoxia or anoxia, lack of nutrition, accumulation of metabolic products, and cellular death. Since the lack of oxygen delivery to the vital cells and tissues of organs is one of the major and fundamental causes of death, the purpose of this chapter is to review briefly some of the basic principles of the microvascular system, especially as they are related to an inadequate microcirculation during hypoxia, ischemia, and shock.

DEFINITIONS AND BASIC CONCEPTS

The term "microvascular system" has been introduced into the literature as a generic term that includes all blood vessels, their contents, and associated structures which are visible only by microscopic examination, i.e., blood vessels smaller than 300 μm (Bloch, 1966; Baez, 1977). The use of the term "microcirculation" should be restricted only to the blood flowing within these vessels. Unfortunately, microcirculation frequently is used incorrectly in the literature to refer to the vessels as well as to the flow within them (Bloch, 1966; Baez, 1977).

The majority of the microvascular system consists of arterioles, capillaries, and venules. In addition, sinusoids and arteriovenous shunts exist in some tissues and organs. While there are many structural and functional similarities between the microvascular beds of various organs and tissues, enough dissimilarities exist that extrapolation of data from one site to another frequently is impossible. As a result, to date, no totally adequate unified nomenclature has been developed to further classify most of these vessels, although certain morphological and functional subclassifications have been suggested. Nevertheless, a few generalizations about the microvascular system can be made.

Arterioles are afferent vessels that supply the capillary bed. Such vessels are tapered and have a lumen with a decreasing bore as the capillaries are approached (Jeffords and Knisely, 1956; Bloch, 1962). The tunica media of precapillary arterioles is composed of smooth muscle cells wrapped circularly around the endothelial tube lining these vessels (Rhodin, 1967). In contrast, the smooth muscle cells in larger arterioles and in small arteries are helically arranged with a pitch sometimes exceeding 45° (Rhodin, 1967). The number of layers of smooth muscle cells decreases as the capillary bed is approached, becoming a single layer of continuous to discontinuous cells at the arteriolar-capillary junction. At this junction, the bore is often less than that of the capillary as well as less than the diameter of individual erythrocytes (Bloch, 1956, 1966a). Thus, such vessels frequently produce a "bottleneck effect" which, coupled with their tapering bore, is responsible for the bulk of the "peripheral resistance" as evidenced by the large drop in systemic blood pressure that occurs along the course of these vessels (Jeffords and Knisely, 1956; Rappaport et al., 1959; Bloch, 1962; Richardson and Zweifach, 1970; Zweifach, 1974a, and b; Fronek and Zweifach, 1975; Gore and Bohlen, 1975; Bohlen and Gore, 1977). Because precapillary arterioles supply numerous capillaries, variations in the internal arteriolar diameter can regulate simultaneously the flow of blood through a large segment of the capillary bed.

Myo-myo and myo-endothelial contacts (direct contacts between the membranes of adjacent smooth muscle cells and between the membranes of smooth muscle cells and adjacent endothelial cells) are more numerous in precapillary arterioles than in larger vessels (Rhodin, 1967). Such contacts suggest a morphologic mechanism for impulse transmission and the rapid diffusion of pharmacodynamic substances since normally a basement membrane tends to isolate individual muscle cells from each other and from the endothelium (Rhodin, 1962, 1967). This may help explain the high sensitivity of these vessels to vasoactive substances (Altura, 1971).

In some tissues and organs (e.g., skeletal and cardiac muscle, mesentery, kidney, exocrine pancreas) vascular smooth muscle cells frequently surround the orifices of capillaries that originate from precapillary arterioles. Such groups of cells have been termed "precapillary sphincters" (Fulton and Lutz, 1940; Weideman, 1963; Rhodin, 1967; McCuskey, 1971). In contrast to the precapillary arterioles, the sphincteric action of these cells can serve to regulate flow to smaller portions of the capillary bed, i.e., blood flow into individual or small numbers of capillaries. The morphology of the smooth muscle cells of the sphincter is very similar to that of the media of precapillary arterioles, and such cells have been considered to be extensions from the arteriolar tunica media (Rhodin, 1967). Physiologically, however, the precapillary sphincters can respond independently of the musculature of adjacent arterioles (Lutz and Fulton, 1958) and may be more sensitive to vasoactive substances (Altura, 1971). This may be a reflection of the morphology of the site since myoendothelial membrane contacts are very numerous at the sites of precapillary sphincters (Rhodin, 1967).

The majority of arterioles have adrenergic innervation and in some sites also possess cholinergic innervation (Siggins, 1970; Siggins and Weitsen, 1971; Burnstock, 1975; Rosell, 1978). The distribution of sensory nerves to the vascular wall, especially in the microvasculature system, is ill defined. In general, adrenergic innervation provides a degree of vascular tone in the arterioles, while cholinergic innervation, when it exists, generally is dilatory. The amount of "resting" tone in these vessels varies from site to site in the body. This contributes to the variability in the responsiveness of vessels in different sites, as do differences in the distribution and types of pharmacologic receptor sites (Vanhoutte, 1978; Bevan, 1979) and heterogeneity in vascular smooth muscle metabolism (Granger et al., 1976; Cook et al., 1977).

The capillaries are cylindrical tubes, lined by endothelium, not surrounded by smooth muscle, and with only a minimal connective tissue investment. Due to the thinness of their walls and their lumens being approximately the diameter of a single erythrocyte, capillaries are the principal site of exchange between the blood and extravascular tissue. The ultrastructure of the endothelial walls of capillaries varies along sequential segments of the microvasculature from tissue to tissue and between various organs (Wolff, 1977; Simionescu and Simionescu, 1977; Simionescu et al., 1978a and b; Thorgeirsson and Robertson, 1978). Differences are found in the numbers of pinocytotic vesicles, intercellular junctions, and fenestrae or pores in the endothelium. In addition, depending on the site, the thickness and continuity of the basal lamina may vary. All of these differences are thought to be related to the functional requirements of the tissue or organ being served by a particular capillary (Wolff, 1977; Renkin, 1979).

Sinusoids are a special type of capillary whose internal diameter generally is larger than that of an individual erythrocyte and whose walls have been modified for the passage of large molecules and/or blood cells as well as for phagocytosis (Simionescu and Simionescu, 1977).

Such vessels are found in the spleen (Weiss, 1977a), bone marrow (Weiss, 1977b), and liver (Wisse, 1977). The internal diameters of these vessels under normal conditions may vary so that a cylindrical appearance as seen in capillaries may not be exhibited (McCuskey et al., 1971; McCuskey and McCuskey, 1977; McCuskey et al., 1979).

Endothelial cells have been found in some internal organs to act as sphincters that regulate the flow of blood through individual capillaries or sinusoids (McCuskey, 1971). Endothelial sphincters have been studied most extensively in the liver, where they form the inlet and outlet sphincters of the sinusoids as well as the sphincters in intersinusoidal sinusoids (McCuskey, 1966). Like muscular precapillary sphincters, endothelial sphincters open and close the lumen of the sinusoids, apparently in response to local metabolic requirements and are responsive to various vasoconstrictor and vasodilator substances (McCuskey, 1966, 1967a and b, 1968; McCuskey et al., 1979). Similar cells have been seen in the sinusoids of the spleen and bone marrow, in the alveolar capillaries of the lung, and in the acinar and islet tissue of the pancreas (Bloch, 1965; McCuskey and Chapman, 1969; McCuskey et al., 1971; McCuskey, 1971; McCuskey and McCuskey, 1977). They also may exist in other internal organs that have not yet been examined in detail by high resolution in vivo microscopic methods (Bloch, 1966a; McCuskey, 1970; McCuskey and McCuskey, 1977).

Several lines of evidence suggest that endothelial cells are capable of active contraction and are not simply responding to changes in intracellular osmolarity by passively swelling. In addition to observation of the rapid response to vasoactive substances (McCuskey, 1966, 1967a and b, 1968; McCuskey and Chapman, 1969; Reilly and McCuskey, 1977; McCuskey et al., 1979), microfilaments and microtubules have been demonstrated by electron microscopy in the cytoplasm of these cells; the presence of these organelles suggests contractile activity (Bensch et al., 1964; Majno et al., 1967; Rhodin, 1967, Röhlich and Oláh, 1967; Phelps and Luft, 1969; Burkel, 1970). The fibrils generally are oriented parallel to the axis of the vessel; thus, if contractile, they could cause the endothelial cell to bulge into the lumen, which has been reported in vivo. More convincingly, however, is the demonstration of contractile protein in endothelium using immunofluorescent and histochemical methods (Puchtler et al., 1968; Becker and Murphy, 1969; Becker and Nachman, 1973).

Venules are efferent vessels which collect blood from the capillary bed. As the diameter of venules increases, their walls acquire a discontinuous investment of vascular smooth muscle which becomes progressively more continuous in larger vessels (Wolff, 1977; Simionescu and Simionescu, 1977). With the acquisition of smooth muscle, innervation also is acquired, which is sparse when compared to arterioles (Burnstock, 1975). It should be noted that a significant amount of transvasculature exchange occurs in the nonmuscular (pericytic) postcapillary venules; and, because of the less structured nature of their walls, venules are more fragile and subject to injury than are their accompanying arterioles (Berman et al., 1955; Majno et al., 1967; Zweifach, 1973; Simionescu et al., 1978a and b).

Arteriovenous anastomoses (AVA) provide direct communication between the arterial and venous system and have been found in most tissues and organs (Clark, 1938; Clara, 1956). Thus, AVA provide a mechanism for shunting blood around the capillary network. Histologically, the tunica media of AVA in some sites contains significant numbers of smooth muscle cells which serve to regulate the flow through the lumen. The transition from the arterial to the venous portion of these AVA usually is marked by an abrupt loss of muscle cells and the appearance of a thin walled vessel containing few if any smooth muscle cells. Blood flow through these shunts is intermittent and depends upon the functional requirements of the surrounding tissue. In contrast, some shunts are of capillary dimensions with scattered smooth muscle cells embracing the endothelium. In the mesentery they have been termed "thoroughfare" or "preferential" channels since blood is continuously flowing through these vessels while flow through the capillaries is intermittent (Chambers and Zweifach, 1944; Zweifach and Metz, 1955). However, these channels generally have not been found in other locations (Weideman, 1963), and in most sites, such as in the liver, blood flow through arterioportal anastomoses is intermittent and appears to depend upon the functional activity of the hepatic parenchyma (McCuskey, 1966).

Finally, the overall morphology and patterns of blood flow of the microvascular bed varies from organ to organ and appears related not only to the organization of the parenchyma but also to the functional requirements of each organ or tissue. For example, striking differences are seen in the pancreas where capillaries abut several sides of each endocrine cell in the islets, whereas in the exocrine tissue the number of capillaries is dramatically reduced and only the base of each acinar cell is in contact with a capillary. The longitudinal arrangement of capillaries in parallel with skeletal muscle fibers contrasts strikingly with the tortuous loops found in the renal glomerulus. The microvasculature of the liver, spleen, lung, etc., all differ from each other and that of other organs. Such differences probably are significant and must be considered in the final analysis of blood flow in each organ or tissue (Sobin and Tremer, 1977). Only now are serious attempts (Schmid-Schoenbein et al., 1977) being made to evaluate the functional significance of these differences in health and disease, especially as they are related to adequate oxygenation of the tissues and cells involved.

CHARACTERISTICS OF OPTIMAL BLOOD FLOW

Based on extensive studies in both man and experimental animals, blood flow through the microvasculature is characterized as optimal (Figs. 11.1–11.4) when the following criteria are met (Bloch, 1956, 1966b): 1) erythrocytes, leukocytes and platelets are distributed relatively

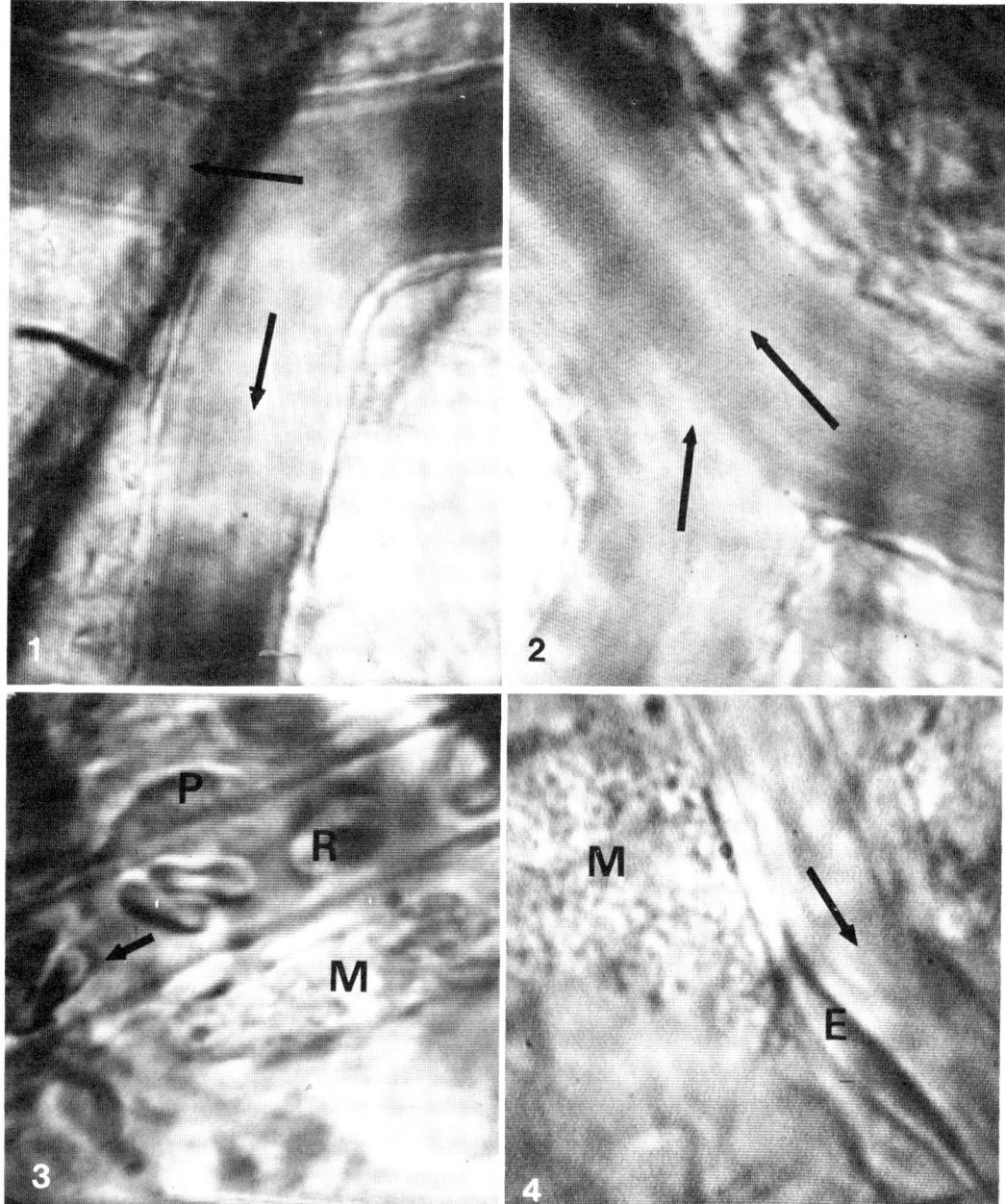

Figure 11.1. Arteriole containing optimal blood flow. Flow appears streamlined and no cells are adherent to the endothelium. *Arrows* indicate direction of flow.

Figure 11.2. Venule containing optimal blood flow. Flow appears streamlined and no cells are adherent to the endothelium. *Arrows* indicate direction of flow.

Figure 11.3. Capillary containing optimal blood flow which is slow enough to detect individual cells. *Arrow* indicates direction of flow. *P*, pericyte; *R*, red blood cell; *M*, mast cell.

Figure 11.4. Capillary containing optimal blood flow which, in contrast to Fig. 11.3, is too rapid to detect individual cells. *Arrow* indicates direction of flow. *M*, mast cell; *E*, endothelium.

homogeneously in the circulating blood; 2) the formed elements adhere neither to each other nor to the endothelium upon making random contact (Figs. 11.1–11.4); 3) the velocity of flow in arterioles and venules is such that individual cells are not resolved optically and the flow appears streamlined (Figs. 11.1 and 11.2); 4) when individual erythrocytes are seen, e.g., in capillaries, they exhibit a sharp outline and have no visible coating on their surface (Fig. 11.3); and 5) the viscosity and composition of the blood is normal with respect to cellular composition and plasma constituents. As a result, the vascular walls are adequately nourished and their permeability is such that neither tissue edema nor hemoconcentration occurs. Failure of any of the above criteria to be met can lead to a suboptimal or pathologic microcirculation and resultant ischemia or hypoxia of cells, tissues, or organs.

The physiological mechanisms for regulating blood flow through the microvasculature in order to maintain an optimal microcirculation are poorly understood, especially in organs. There appear to be four basic mechanisms (Rodbard, 1971; Altura, 1978; Johnson, 1978): 1) neural, 2) humoral, 3) myogenic, and 4) local metabolic. All may be operative in various degrees at any given moment; and one may predominate over the others, depending upon the circumstances as well as the tissue or organ involved.

As indicated previously, most arterioles and, to a lesser extent, venules have adrenergic innervation. The distribution of cholinergic, sensory, and nerves having aminergic substances other than norepinephrine as their neurotransmitter is less clear. In general, adrenergic stimulation leads to vasoconstriction mediated through alpha receptors on the vascular wall. Norepinephrine produces similar effects. In most organs, a certain degree of arteriolar basal tone is maintained which can be abolished by alpha blockade or acute denervation; in some organs alpha blockade unmasks a vasodilatory effect of adrenergic stimulation or norepinephrine which is mediated through beta receptors on the vascular wall. In contrast, cholinergic stimulation usually results in vasodilation, which in some organs is thought to be the indirect effect of altered metabolism or the formation of kinins. In other sites a direct effect on the vascular wall is postulated. While neural mechanisms probably are responsible for major readjustments in blood flow through organs, the moment-to-moment regulation of flow through the microvasculature probably is largely controlled by local mechanisms.

Two basic local mechanisms of microvascular control have been identified—myogenic and metabolic. Both appear to be operative in most sites to greater or lesser degrees in order to maintain an optimal, nutritive microcirculation. In response to elevations or decreases in intraluminal pressure, arterioles in many microvascular beds dilate or constrict. As a result, volumetric flow and pressure within the capillary bed is maintained relatively constant due to the myogenic response of the smooth muscle in walls of the afferent and efferent vessels of the bed. Microvascular tone also is affected by the presence of vasoactive substance(s) released from surrounding parenchymal cells as a result of normal metabolism or when blood flow falls below nutritive levels. Adenosine, carbon dioxide, lactic acid, and potassium are examples of such substances. As nutritive blood flow and tissue oxygenation falls or metabolism and/or the need for oxygen increases, one or more metabolites may be released which cause vasodilation and the re-establishment of optimal nutritive flow and tissue oxygenation.

The neural and local regulatory mechanisms can be modulated or modified by other substances which are synthesized in the tissue or circulating in the blood (Altura, 1978; Altura and Altura, 1978). Circulating steroids, for example, modify the responsiveness of microvasculature to vasoactive substances. Other locally produced substances are vasoactive, such as serotonin, which is present in circulating platelets and, like histamine, also in perivascular mast cells. Prostaglandins, thromboxane, and kinins are tissue-derived substances which are themselves vasoactive or which can modify vascular responses to other stimuli. Circulating neurohypophyseal hormones, catecholamines, angiotensin, etc., also have effects in the microvasculature.

In summary, it is clear that the moment-to-moment regulation of blood flow through the microvascular system is dependent upon a number of interacting factors—morphologic as well as physiologic. The precise functional relationships of all of these mechanisms is not completely known and requires more investigation. What is clear, however, is that the utilization of the mechanisms varies and is not the same for any two tissues or organs. Thus, extrapolation of data derived from one vascular bed is not applicable to another where the structure, function, and metabolic requirements of the surrounding parenchyma differ. The questions that must be asked for each site are what mechanisms are operative, when are they operative, and under what circumstances are they operative?

FACTORS JEOPARDIZING OPTIMAL BLOOD FLOW

A large number of factors can jeopardize an optimal microcirculation. Among these are physical, hemodynamic, hematologic, immune, chemical and pathologic factors which acting alone or in combination can compromise oxygen delivery leading to ischemia or hypoxia of vital tissues and organs. The penultimate event is anoxia, microvascular collapse, shock, and death. Of these factors, compression or obstruction of microvasculature due to diseased tissue or severe trauma and low flow due to hemorrhage are the most obvious. Less apparent are the common responses of microvasculature to mild trauma, blood-borne foreign particulate or toxic substances, and vasoactive substances released from hypoxic or infected tissue or from mast cells as the result of immune, humoral, or toxic reactions. Depending upon the type of stimulus, the microvascular responses to all of these factors may be focal or widely disseminated; and they may vary in their intensity and duration. However, there are no basic differences in the responses (Bloch, 1956, 1966b).

Even the slightest degree of injury to the endothelium results in the adhesion of platelets and their aggregation along with fibrin to form thrombi (Berman and Fulton, 1961; Zweifach, 1973; Thorgeirsson and Robertson, 1978). Concomitant with injury, an inflammatory response generally occurs, evidenced by leukocytes sticking to and paving the endothelial wall, particularly in venules (Figs. 11.5–11.8) (Bloch, 1956, 1966b; Zweifach, 1973; Thorgeirsson and Robertson, 1978; Goodman et

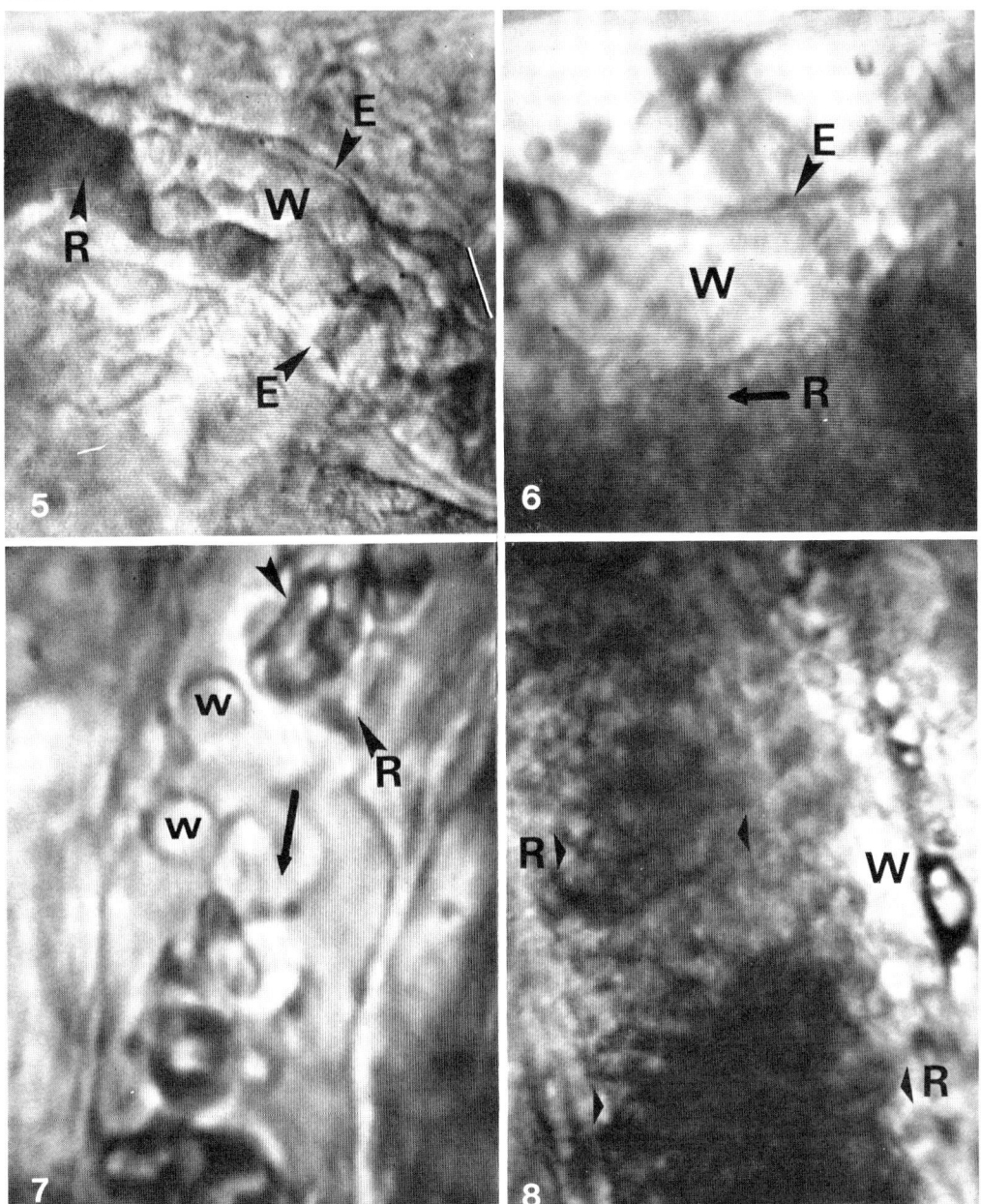

Figure 11.5. Postcapillary venule during anaphylactic shock. Note white blood cells adhering to the endothelium (E), plugging the lumen, and blocking the passage of red blood cells (R).

Figure 11.6. Venule during anaphylactic shock. Note formation of a thrombus (W) composed of platelets and some white blood cells. Arrow indicates the direction of flow of red blood cells (R), which is reduced in velocity.

Figure 11.7. Postcapillary venule during initial stage of anaphylactic shock. Two white blood cells (W) have adhered to the endothelium. Occasionally, aggregates of loosely bound red blood cells (R) are seen. Arrow indicates direction of flow.

Figure 11.8. Venule during later stage of anaphylactic shock containing larger aggregates of red blood cells (R). Note adherence of white blood cells and platelets to endothelium. Flow is very slow and pulsatile; and individual red blood cells can be distinguished.

al., 1979; Urbaschek and Urbaschek, 1979). Most of the inflammatory events are chemically mediated; histamine, serotonin, prostaglandins, kinins, complement components, etc., have been implicated (Wilhelm, 1973; Urbaschek and Urbaschek, 1979). Initially such reactions do not produce microvascular obstruction, due in part, to a transient increased flow rate through the microvascular bed, resulting from arteriolar dilation. However, as the numbers of adhering cells increase so does venular resistance with a concomitant reduction in flow. Depending upon the severity or duration of the inflammatory response, tissue hypoxia may result which may further aggravate the initial insult by effecting further adhesion of leukocytes and platelets to the endothelial wall. Continued adhesion, aggregation, and thromboembolism within a microvascular bed may render the tissue ischemic. Not only is the tissue in jeopardy but so is the integrity of the vascular wall; and in response to the increased venular pressure, the presence of chemical mediators and hypoxia, the capillaries and postcapillary venules become more permeable, the tissue edematous, and the blood hemoconcentrated. If prolonged, this culminates in total loss of integrity of the vascular wall and hemorrhage. At the ultrastructural level these changes are evidenced by disruptions of tight junctions between adjacent endothelial cells, focal ballooning and rarefication of endothelial cells, and, ultimately, lysis of these cells, exposing the basal lamina and interstitial tissue to the vascular space (Wilson, 1972; Harrison et al., 1977; Asano et al., 1979). Associated with these changes leukocytes, erythrocytes, and platelets are observed with disrupted limiting membranes, extracellular granules and lysosomes, and edematous interstitial tissue with disoriented collagen fibers.

In addition to and concomitant with the above changes, the normal responsiveness of the microvasculature to hormonal and neural stimuli is altered or lost (Hutchins et al., 1973; Zweifach, 1973). In short, there is a failure of normal compensatory mechanisms to provide adequate perfusion of the affected tissues or organs. This failure exacerbates the loss of integrity of normal structural-functional relationships at the site(s) of injury.

In many disease states, including low flow states, the cellular elements in the circulating blood, particularly erythrocytes, may aggregate and produce masses of cells of varying degrees of rigidity (Figs. 11.7 and 11.8) (Knisely et al., 1945; Bloch, 1956, 1959, 1966b). The mechanisms involved in this process are unclear but a hyaline coating on the erythrocyte membrane has been demonstrated (Bloch et al., 1956). The nature of this coating that alters the normally repulsive nature of erythrocytes to each other is not yet known. Such masses may intermittently or permanently embolize arterioles with concomitant reactions of the vessel walls such as constriction, dilation, or sacculation. Whether transient or permanent, such plugging of afferent vessels reduces flow through the capillary bed and leads to tissue hypoxia. Extensive erythrocytic aggregation results in sedimentation or "sludging" (Knisely et al., 1945) of the cellular masses in larger vessels, particularly venules and veins, reduces the number of circulating erythrocytes, and impairs the ability of the system to provide adequate tissue oxygenation.

Hematologic changes (Murphy, 1973) such as altered erythrocytic deformability, altered concentrations of cellular elements in the blood or plasma constituents, altered erythrocytic and blood chemistries all have marked effects on the ability of the microvasculature to perform its functions. Alterations in the clotting mechanisms can lead to disseminated intravascular coagulation and can result in plugging of the microvasculature and ischemia, as can increased rigidity of erythrocytes. The latter may result from disease such as sickle cell anemia or spherocytosis or from altered blood chemistry, e.g., a fall in blood pH varies the deformability of erythrocytes. Changes in blood pH and ion concentrations also may affect normal vascular tone and permeability, lead to failure of normal regulatory mechanisms (Altura and Altura, 1978), and impair blood flow through the microvasculature. Alterations in viscosity due to abnormal concentrations of cells (anemia, polycythemia, leukemia) or plasma components (hyperglobulinemia) can adversely affect microvascular perfusion and oxygen delivery to vital tissues. Abnormalities in the circulating platelets probably are of high significance since platelets are thought to be important in maintaining the integrity of the endothelial lining (D'Amore, 1978; Thorgeirsson and Robertson, 1978; Gingrich and Hoak, 1979). In addition, abnormal erythrocyte chemistry, e.g., shifts in 2, 3-DPG, may effect oxygen exchange with the tissue and render it hypoxic.

Various vascular pathologies clearly affect microvascular function either through a physical reduction of flow to the capillary bed due to structural changes (atherosclerosis), altered vascular reactivity due to autonomic neuropathy or abnormal smooth muscle metabolism (diabetes mellitus), or altered permeability characteristics of the exchange vessels (e.g., diabetes mellitus). Any or all of these changes ultimately can affect the distribution of oxygen to tissues and organs.

CONCLUSIONS

What have been described above are the general sequelae of responses observed in the microvascular system that contribute to ischemia, hypoxia and/or anoxia, and microvascular collapse. It is beyond the scope of this chapter to discuss in detail all of the factors that initiate or contribute to these responses; many of these are discussed in detail in other chapters of this book. It should be remembered, however, that in addition to the injurious substances that are blood-borne or released locally in tissues as the result of low flow states, injury, or disease, hematologic factors and vascular pathology also can cause impairment of an optimal microcirculation and exacerbate the microvascular responses to low flow, disease, or injury. If compensatory responses fail or are inadequate to maintain adequate perfusion and tissue oxygenation, the resultant hypoxia may initiate the sequelae of cellular adhesion, aggregation, thromboemboli, edema and hemoconcentration, stasis, ischemia, hypoxia and/or anoxia, and cellular death.

References

Altura, B.M.: Chemical and humoral regulation of blood flow through the precapillary sphincter. Microvasc. Res. 3:361–384, 1971.

Altura, B.M.: Humoral, hormonal, and myogenic mechanisms in microcirculatory regulation. In *Microcirculation*, edited by G. Kaley and B.M. Altura, vol. 11, pp. 431–502. University Park Press, Baltimore, 1978.

Altura, B.T., and Altura, B.M.: Factors effecting vascular responsiveness. In *Microcirculation*, edited by G. Kaley and B.M. Altura, vol. 11, pp. 547–616. University Park Press, Baltimore, 1978.

Asano, G., Ohkubu, K., Hoshino, M., Yamada, N., and Aihara, K.: Early changes in the arterial endothelium under various pathological correlations: An electron histochemical study with visualization of altered permeability using electron microscopic tracers. Acta Pathol. Jpn 29:21–34, 1979.

Baez, S.: Microvascular terminology. In *Microcirculation*, edited by G. Kaley and B.M. Altura, vol. 1, pp. 23–34. University Park Press, Baltimore, 1977.

Becker, C.G., and Murphy, G.E.: Demonstration of contractile protein in endothelium and cells of the heart valves, endocardium, intima, arteriosclerotic plaques, and Aschoff bodies of rheumatic heart disease. Am. J. Pathol. 55:1–37, 1969.

Becker, C.G., and Nachman, R.L.: Contractile proteins of endothelial cells, platelets and smooth muscle. Am. J. Pathol. 71:1–22, 1973.

Bensch, K.G., Gordon, G.B., and Miller, L.: Fibrillar structures resembling myofibrils in endothelial cells of mammalian pulmonary blood vessels. Z. Zellforsch. Mikrosk. Anat. 63:759–766, 1964.

Berman, H.J., and Fulton, G.P.: Platelets in the peripheral circulation. In *Henry Ford Hospital International Symposium, Blood Platelets*, edited by S.A. Johnson, Little, Brown, Boston, 1961.

Berman, H.J., Fulton, G.P., Lutz, B.R., and Pierce, D.L.: Susceptibility to thrombosis in normal young, aging, cortisone-treated, heparinized, and x-irradiated hamsters as tested by topical application of thrombin. Blood 10:831–840, 1955.

Bevan, J.A.: Some bases of differences in vascular response to sympathetic activity. Circ. Res. 45:161–171, 1979.

Bloch, E.H.: Microscopic observations of the circulating blood in the bulbar conjunctiva in man in health and disease. Ergeb. Anat. Entwicklungogeschicte 35:1–98, 1956.

Bloch, E.H.: Visual changes in the living microvascular system in man and experimental animals as they are related to thrombosis and embolism. Angiology 10:421–425, 1959.

Bloch, E.H.: A quantitative study of the hemodynamics in the living microvascular system. Am. J. Anat. 110:125–153, 1962.

Bloch, E.H.: The dynamic histology of organs in situ. II. The lung, liver and kidney. Anat. Rec. 151:498, 1965.

Bloch, E.H.: Television microphotometry of organs in situ. Methods Med. Res. 11:228–232, 1966a.

Bloch, E.H.: Principles of the microvascular system. Invest. Ophthalmol. 5:250–255, 1966b.

Bloch, E.H., Powell, A., Merryman, H.T., Warner, R., and Kafig, E.: A comparison of the surfaces of human erythrocytes from health and disease by in vivo light microscopy and in vitro electron microscopy. Angiology 7:479–494, 1956.

Bohlen, H.G., and Gore, R.W.: Comparisons of pressures and diameters in the innervated and denervated microcirculation of rat intestine. Microvasc. Res. 14:251–264, 1977.

Burkel, W.W.: The fine structure of the terminal branches of the hepatic arterial system of the rat. Anat. Rec. 167:329–350, 1970.

Burnstock, G.: Innervation of vascular smooth muscle: Histochemistry and electron microscopy. Clin Exp. Pharmacol. Physiol. (Suppl. 2) 2:7–20, 1975.

Chambers, R., and Zweifach, B.W.: Topography and function of the mesenteric circulation. Am. J. Anat. 75:173–202, 1944.

Clara, M.: *Die Arterio-venosen Anastomosem*, 315 pp. Springer-Verlag, Wien, 1956.

Clark, E.R.: Arterio-venous anastomoses. Physiol. Rev. 18:229–247, 1938.

Cook, B.H., Granger, H.J., and Taylor, A.E.: Metabolism of coronary arteries and arterioles. A histochemical study. Microvasc. Res. 14:145–159, 1977.

D'Amore, P.: Platelet-endothelial interaction and the maintenance of the microvasculature. Microvasc. Res. 15:137–145, 1978.

Fronek, K., and Zweifach, B.W.: Microvascular pressure distribution in skeletal muscle and the effect of vasodilation. Am. J. Physiol. 228:791–796, 1975.

Fulton, G.P., and Lutz, B.R.: The neuromotor mechanism of small blood vessels of the frog. Science 92:223–224, 1940.

Gingrich, R.D., and Hoak, J.C.: Platelet-endothelial cell interactions. Semin. Hematol. 16:208–220, 1979.

Goodman, M.L., Way, B.A., and Irwin, J.W.: The inflammatory response to endotoxin. J. Pathol., 128:7–14, 1979.

Gore, R.W., and Bohlen, H.G.: Pressure regulation in the microcirculation. Fed. Proc. 34:2031–2037, 1975.

Granger, D.N., Cook, B.H., and Taylor, A.E.: Histochemistry of microvascular smooth muscle in the gastrointestinal tract. Microvasc. Res. 12:157–168, 1976.

Harrison, M.W., Connell, R.S., Campbell, J.R., and Webb, M.C.: Microcirculatory changes in the lung of the hypoxic and hypovolemic puppy. An electron microscope study. Ann. Surg. 185:311–317, 1977.

Hutchins, P.M., Goldstone, J., and Wells, R.: Effects of hemorrhagic shock on the microvasculature of skeletal muscle. Microvasc. Res. 5:131–140, 1973.

Jeffords, J.G., and Knisely, M.H. Concerning the geometric shapes of arteries and arterioles. A contribution to the biophysics of health, disease and death. Angiology 7:105–136, 1956.

Johnson, P.C.: Principles of peripheral circulatory control. In *Peripheral Circulation*, edited by P.C. Johnson, pp. 111–139. John Wiley & Sons, New York, 1978.

Knisely, M.H., Eliot, T.S., and Bloch, E.H.: Sludged blood in traumatic shock. I. Microscopic observations of the precipitation and agglutination of blood flowing through vessels in crushed tissues. Arch. Surg. 51:220–236, 1945.

Lutz, B.R., and Fulton, G.P.: Smooth muscle and blood flow in small blood vessels. In *Factors Regulating Blood Flow*, edited by G.P. Fulton and B.W. Zweifach, pp. 13–24. American Physiology Society, Washington, DC, 1958.

McCuskey, R.S.: A dynamic and static study of hepatic arterioles and hepatic sphincters. Am. J. Anat. 119:455–478, 1966.

McCuskey, R.S.: Dynamic microscopic anatomy of the fetal liver. II. Effect of pharmacodynamic substances on the microcirculation. Bibl. Anat. 9:71–75, 1967a.

McCuskey, R.S.: Erythropoietin: Effect on the living fetal hepatic microvascular system in situ. Life Sci. 6:2129–2133, 1967b.

McCuskey, R.S.: Dynamic microscopic anatomy of the fetal liver. III. Erythropoeisis. Anat. Rec. 161:267–279, 1968.

McCuskey, R.S.: Microscopic methods for evaluating drug action at the cellular level in living organs in situ. Symposium on the effects of drugs on sequential segments of the peripheral vasculature. *Proceedings of the 4th International Congress on Pharmacology, Basel, Switzerland (July 14–18, 1969)*, vol. v, pp. 333–337. Schwake and Co., Basel, 1970.

McCuskey, R.S.: Sphincters in the microvascular system. Microvasc. Res. 2:428–433, 1971.

McCuskey, R.S., and Chapman, T.M.: Microscopy of the living

pancreas in situ. Am. J. Anat. *126:*395–408, 1969.
McCuskey, R.S., and McCuskey, P.A.: In vivo microscopy of the spleen. Bibl. Anat. *16:*121–125, 1977.
McCuskey, R.S., McClugage, S.G., and Younker, W.J.: Microscopy of living bone marrow in situ. Blood *38:*87–95, 1971.
McCuskey, R.S., Reilly, F.D., McCuskey, P.A., and Dimlich, R.V.W.: In vivo microscopy of the hepatic microvascular system. Bibl. Anat. *18:*73–76, 1979.
Majno, G., Gilmore, V., and Leventhal, M.: On the mechanism of vascular leakage caused by histamine-type mediators. Circ. Res. *21:*833–847, 1967.
Murphy, J.R.: Hematology disorders: Hematology and the microcirculation. In *The Microcirculation in Clinical Medicine*, edited by R. Wells, pp. 227–252. Academic Press, New York, 1973.
Phelps, P.C., and Luft, J.H.: Electron microscopical study of relaxation and constriction in frog arterioles. Am. J. Anat. *125:*399–428, 1969.
Puchtler, H., Sweat, F., Terry, M.S., and Conner, H.M.: Investigation of staining, polarization and fluorescence-microscopic properties of myoendothelial cells. J. Microsc. *89:*95–104, 1968.
Rappaport, M.G., Bloch, E.H., and Irwin, J.W.: A manometer for measuring dynamic pressures in the microvascular system. J. Appl. Physiol. *14:*651–655, 1959.
Reilly, F.D., and McCuskey, R.S.: Studies of the hemopoietic microenvironment. VI. Regulatory mechanisms in the splenic microvascular system of mice. Microvasc. Res. *13:*79–90, 1977.
Renkin, E.M.: Relation of capillary morphology to transport of fluid and large molecules: a review. Acta Physiol. Scand. (Suppl.) *463:*81–91, 1979.
Rhodin, J.A.G.: Fine structure of vascular walls in mammals. Physiol. Rev. *42:*48–81, 1962.
Rhodin, J.A.G.: The ultrastructure of mammalian arterioles and precapillary sphincters. J. Ultrastruct. Res. *18:*181–233, 1967.
Richardson, D.R., and Zweifach, B.W.: Pressure relationships in macro- and microcirculation of the mesentery. Microvasc. Res. *2:*474–488, 1970.
Rodbard, S.: Local regulation of blood flow. Monograph Nr. 33, 158 pp. American Heart Association, New York, 1971.
Röhlich, P., and Oláh, I.: Cross-striated fibrils in the endothelium of the rat myometrical arterioles. J. Ultrastruct. Res. *18:*667–676, 1967.
Rosell, S.: Nervous control of the microcirculation. In *Microcirculation*, edited by G. Kaley and B.M. Altura, vol. 11, pp. 371–400. University Park Press, Baltimore, 1978.
Schmid-Schoenbein, G.W., Zweifach, B.W., and Kovalcheck, S.: The application of stereological principles to morphometry of the microcirculation in different tissues. Microvasc. Res. *14:*303–317, 1977.
Siggins, G.R.: Some aspects of humoral and neuromotor control of the microvascular system. In *Microcirculation, Perfusion and Transplantation of Organs*, edited by T.I. Malinin, B.S. Linn, A.B. Callahan, and W.D. Warren, pp. 59–74. Academic Press, New York, 1970.
Siggins, G.R., and Weitsen, H.A.: Cytochemical and physiological evidence for cholinergic, neurogenic vasodilation of amphibian arterioles and precapillary sphincters. I. Light microscopy. Microvasc. Res. *3:*308–322, 1971.
Simionescu, N., and Simionescu, M.: The cardiovascular system. In *Histology*, edited by L. Weiss and R.O. Greep, ed. 4, pp. 373–432. McGraw-Hill, New York, 1977.

Simionescu, N., Simionescu, M., and Palade, G. E.: Structural basis of permeability in sequential segments of the microvasculature. I. Bipolar microvascular fields in the diaphragm. Microvasc. Res. *15:*1–16, 1978a.
Simionescu, N., Simionescu, M., and Palade, G.E.: Structural basis of permeability in sequential segments of the microvasculature. II. Pathways followed by microperoxidase across endothelium. Microvasc. Res. *15:*17–36, 1978b.
Sobin, S.S., and Tremer, H.M.: Three dimensional organization of microvascular beds as related to function. In *Microcirculation*, edited by G. Kaley and B.M. Altura, vol. 1, pp. 43–67. University Park Press, Baltimore, 1977.
Thorgeirsson, G., and Robertson, A.L.: The vascular endothelium-pathobiologic significance. Am. J. Pathol. *93:*803–848, 1978.
Urbaschek, B., and Urbaschek, R.: The inflammatory response to endotoxins. Bibl. Anat. *17:*74–104, 1979.
Vanhoutte, P.M.: Heterogeneity in vascular smooth muscle. In *Microcirculation*, edited by G. Kaley and B.M. Altura, vol. 11, pp. 181–310. University Park Press, Baltimore, 1978.
Weideman, M.P.: Patterns of the arteriovenous pathways. In *Handbook of Physiology, Section 2: Circulation, Vol. 11*, edited by W.F. Hamilton and P. Dow, pp. 891–933. American Physiological Society Washington, DC, 1963.
Weiss, L.: Bone marrow. In *Histology*, edited by L. Weiss and R.O. Greep, ed. 4, pp. 487–502. McGraw-Hill, New York, 1977a.
Weiss, L.: The spleen. In *Histology*, edited by L. Weiss and R.O. Greep, ed. 4, pp. 545–573. McGraw-Hill, New York, 1977b.
Wilhelm, D.L.: Chemical mediators. In *The Inflammatory Process*, edited by B.W. Zweifach, L. Grant, and R.T. McCluskey, vol. 11, pp. 251–301. Academic Press, New York, 1973.
Wilson, J.W.: Leukocyte segmentation and morphologic augmentation in the pulmonary network following hemorrhagic shock and related forms of stress. Adv. Microcirc. *4:*197–232, 1972.
Wisse, E.: Ultrastructure and function of Kupffer cells and other sinusoidal cells in the liver. In *Kupffer Cells and Other Sinusoidal Cells*, edited by E. Wisse and D.L. Knook, pp. 33–60. Elsevier, New York, 1977.
Wolff, J.R.: Ultrastructure of the terminal vascular bed as related to function. In *Microcirculation*, edited by G. Kaley and B.M. Altura, vol. 1, pp. 95–130. University Park Press, Baltimore, 1977.
Zweifach, B.W.: Microvascular aspects of tissue injury. In *The Inflammatory Process*, edited by B.W. Zweifach, L. Grant and R.T. McCluskey, ed. 2, vol. 11, pp. 3–46, Academic Press, New York, 1973.
Zweifach, B.W.: Quantitative studies of microcirculatory structure and function. I. Analysis of pressure distribution in the terminal vascular bed in cat mesentery. Circ. Res. *34:*843–857, 1974a.
Zweifach, B.W.: Quantitative studies of microcirculatory structure and function. II. Direct measurement of capillary pressure in splanchnic mesenteric vessels. Circ. Res. *34:*858–866, 1974b.
Zweifach, B.W., and Metz, D.G.: Selective distribution of blood through the terminal vascular bed of mesenteric structures and skeletal muscle. In *Vascular Patterns as Related to Function*, edited by G.P. Fulton, pp. 282–289. Williams & Wilkins, Baltimore, 1955.

CHAPTER 12

Vascular Mediators in Ischemia and Shock

ALLAN M. LEFER

CONCEPT OF VASCULAR MEDIATORS

Vascular mediators are becoming increasingly more intimately involved in the pathogenesis of ischemia and shock as more information on the actions of some important humoral systems is obtained. Thus, some newly discovered vascular mediators appear to play a key role in the initiation of ischemia as well as in the development of circulatory shock (Lefer, 1978, 1979; Lefer and Trachte, 1980). A variety of vascular mediators can be involved in the pathophysiology of ischemia. These vasoactive agents can contribute to the genesis of shock by virtue of three or four major mechanisms:
1. severe vasoconstriction or vasospasm;
2. induction of platelet aggregation and thrombus formation;
3. increased capillary permeability; and
4. redistribution of blood flow away from vital tissues.

Vasoconstriction

Vasoconstriction can promote ischemia when it occurs regionally in selected vascular beds. Thus, norepinephrine or angiotensin II can severely constrict regional beds (e.g., mesenteric, renal). These agents can constrict virtually all vasculatures to some extent, although catecholamines in general do not constrict the cerebral and coronary beds. In the case of the heart, catecholamines stimulate cardiac contractile force and hence increase myocardial metabolism which secondarily dilates the coronary vessels (Wexler, 1979). Many vascular mediators are either metabolized by the brain or do not cross the blood-brain barrier and thus do not influence the cerebral circulation under normal conditions. In some cases (i.e., thromboxane A_2), the vasoconstriction is so severe that it induces vasospasm in certain vessels. This is known to occur in the coronary circulation during angina, where it may contribute to the onset of myocardial ischemia (Lewy et al., 1979).

Platelet Aggregation

Another mechanism of vascular mediation of ischemia and shock is the stimulation of platelet aggregation (e.g., by epinephrine). Aggregating platelets can then release other vasoconstrictors (i.e., serotonin, TxA_2). In addition to the release of vasoconstrictors by aggregating platelets, the aggregates themselves tend to stick to the endothelium of the blood vessels and thus restrict flow of blood within the lumen of small vessels (Blaisdell, 1972). In fact, if the extent of aggregation is great enough, thrombosis can occur and large arteries as well as veins can be totally obstructed, leading to localized infarcts. This can be particularly dangerous in the heart and lungs.

Increased Capillary Permeability

A third mechanism of vascular mediation of ischemia and shock is increased capillary permeability. Although they may have other vascular effects, certain agents including bacterial endotoxins, myocardial depressant factor (MDF), histamine, bradykinin, and PGE_1 promote the loss of fluid from the intravascular space. Among these substances, endotoxin is thought not to have direct vasoactivity, MDF is a constrictor, and histamine, bradykinin, and PGE_1 are generally vasodilators. The major consequence of the enhanced capillary permeability is the promotion of loss of vascular fluid and protein; leading to hypovolemia, which is serious in itself since it leads to shock and impairs the effectiveness of the circulatory system (Greenbaum, 1969). However, it also leads to reflex activation of the sympathetic nervous system, which tends to aggravate the situation by further promoting vasoconstriction and tachycardia.

Redistribution of Blood Flow

Finally, vascular mediators can produce redistribution of blood flow within a given vascular bed. Thus, angiotensin causes a shift in renal blood flow from cortical to medullary regions, and other vasoactive agents like kinins and prostaglandins shift blood from the endocardium of the heart to the subepicardial layers (Smith et al., 1978). Sometimes, severe shifts of this type can exert untoward effects. In this regard, potent vasodilator agents (i.e., isoproterenol, glucagon) can result in a "cardiac steal," whereby a severe shift of blood flow to the subepicardium produces a subendocardial ischemia (Hoffman and Buckberg, 1978).

Table 12.1 summarizes the basic information on the major naturally ocurring vasoconstrictor agents that may be involved in the pathogenesis of ischemia and shock. Three of the most interesting of these systems have been selected for further discussion: 1) the renin-angiotensin system, 2) the thromboxane-prostacyclin system, and 3)

Table 12.1
Naturally Occurring Vasoconstrictor Agents Playing a Role in Shock

Vasoconstrictor	Major Sources	Site of Action	Means of Controlling
Norepinephrine	Sympathetic NS and adrenal medullae	Systemic	α-Adrenergic, β-blockers, ganglionic blockers
Epinephrine	Adrenal medullae	Systemic	α-Adrenergic, β-blockers, ganglionic blockers
Angiotensin II	Kidneys, blood, brain	Systemic, mesenteric	Converting enzyme inhibitors, receptor antagonists
Antidiuretic hormone (ADH)	Posterior pituitary	Systemic	[1-Deaminopenacillamine 4 valine, 8-D-arginine], vasopressin
Thromboxane A_2	Platelets	Cardiac, pulmonary, others	Tx synthetase inhibitors, Tx antagonists
Myocardial depressant factor (MDF)	Pancreas	Systemic	Membrane stabilizers, protease inhibitors
Serotonin (5-HT)	Platelets	Systemic	Anti-serotonergic agents
Prostaglandin $F_{2\alpha}$ ($PGF_{2\alpha}$)	Platelets and smooth muscle	Local and systemic	Cyclo-oxygenase inhibitors

the lysosomal hydrolase-myocardial depressant factor system. These three systems have been selected since considerable information is known about them. They all represent diverse and interesting mechanisms, all of which have been brought to light in the past 5–10 years, and, thus, newer mechanisms which have not been extensively reviewed for their role in shock. Finally, all three systems appear to play a key role in the pathogenesis of circulatory shock.

THE RENIN-ANGIOTENSIN SYSTEM

The renin-angiotensin system is a complex humoral system with important components in the plasma, the kidney, and perhaps in the brain. The system generates a variety of potent peptides (i.e., angiotensin I, angiotensin II, and angiotensin III). These peptides exert major cardiovascular effects including: vasoconstriction systemically, positive inotropic effect, and increased capillary permeability.

In general, angiotensin II is the most potent of these peptides, although angiotensin III is comparable or slightly less potent than angiotensin II, and angiotensin I is much less potent than the other two angiotensins.

Formation of Angiotensins

Angiotensins I, II, and III are deca-, octa-, and heptapeptides, respectively, formed by the hydrolytic action of various enzymes cleaving the small peptides from large protein substrates. Figure 12.1 summarizes the major biochemical mechanisms for the formation of the biologically active angiotensins. Angiotensin I (the decapeptide) is formed by the hydrolytic action of activated renin upon the large protein substrate angiotensinogen. This peptide is not very active, but is rapidly transformed into either a very active octapeptide (i.e., angiotensin II) by the action of converting enzyme, or to a slightly active nonpeptide (i.e., des-Asp^1-angiotensin I) by the action of an aminopeptidase (Needleman and Marshall, 1976).

Both angiotensin II and des-Asp^1-angiotensin I can be further hydrolyzed to the heptapeptide angiotensin III by the reciprocal action of converting enzyme (i.e., on des-Asp^1-angiotensin I) or aminopeptidase (i.e., on angiotensin II). Angiotensin III is a potent peptide which, in addition to exerting vasoconstrictor and positive inotropic effects, is capable of stimulating the release of aldosterone from the zona glomerulosa of the adrenal cortices (Devynck et al., 1977). Angiotensin II also has a potent steroidogenic effect. Both angiotensin II and III also stimulate the adrenal medullae to release catecholamines (e.g., epinephrine and norepinephrine) (Peach and Ackerly, 1978).

Angiotensin III is further hydrolyzed by nonspecific peptidases to inactive peptide fragments that have essentially no cardiovascular activity and at present are not considered to be involved as vascular mediators of ischemia and shock.

Cardiovascular Actions

The following is a synopsis of the cardiovascular effects of the three angiotensin peptides.

ANGIOTENSIN I

Angiotensin I, which has some biological activity in certain vascular beds, exerts a positive inotropic effect in isolated rabbit atria of about 60% at 10^{-6} M (Bonnardeaux and Regoli, 1973). Right atrial myocardial tissue exhibited a greater sensitivity to the decapeptide than did left atrial tissue. The positive inotropic effect was reduced after application of converting enzyme inhibition, indicating a dependency on conversion to angiotensin II for biological activity (Ackerly and Peach, 1975). Inotropic actions of angiotensin I, however, were not reduced by converting enzyme blockade in isolated right ventricular cat papillary muscles (Trachte and Lefer, 1979d). Angiotensin I produced moderate increases in active tension development (i.e., maximal stimulation 50%), being the least potent angiotensin inotropically in ventricular myocardial tissue.

Angiotensin I has been reported to constrict the coronary vasculature. However, both Gerlings and Gilmore (1974) and Britton and DiSalvo (1973) observed reduced coronary vascular responses to angiotensin I after converting enzyme blockade in dogs, indicating angiotensin II is the primary coronary constrictor of the two sub-

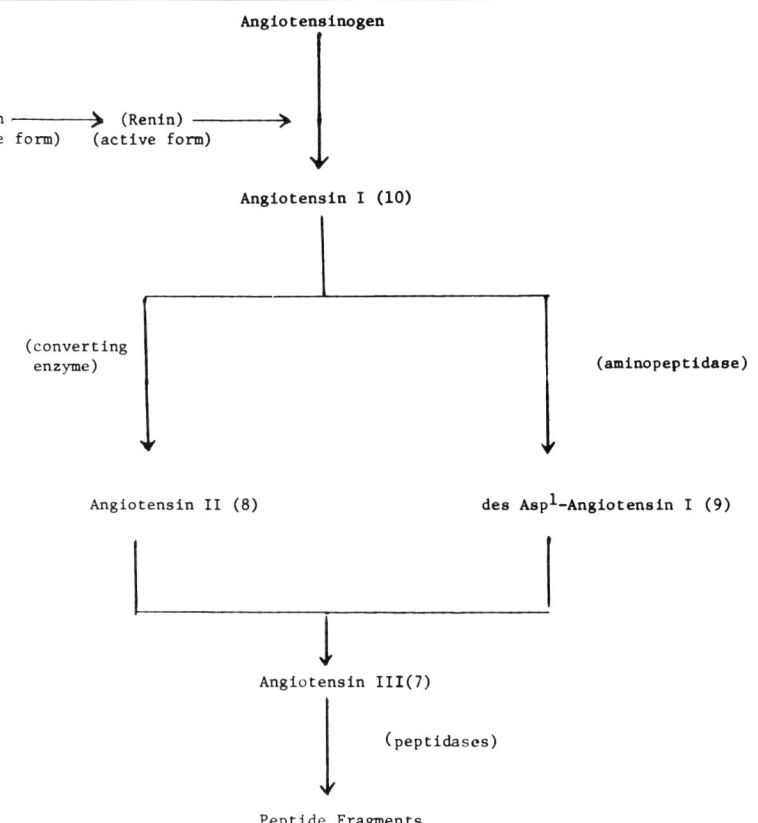

Figure 12.1. Formation of angiotensins. Two pathways exist for angiotensin III formation. Numbers in parentheses are the numbers of amino acids in the peptide.

stances. Recent data in isolated cat coronary arteries also show a reduced vasoconstriction in response to angiotensin I after converting enzyme inhibition (Trachte and Lefer, 1979d). The results suggest a slight direct action of angiotensin I on the coronary vasculature with the majority of the decapeptide action being due to angiotensin II formation.

ANGIOTENSIN II

Angiotensin II is the most potent of the angiotensins regarding cardiac actions. Angiotensin II increases contractility of cardiac tissue in a variety of preparations including isolated cat hearts (Hill and Andrus, 1941), cat papillary muscles (Koch-Weser, 1964; Lefer, 1967), isolated cat and rabbit atria (Bonnardeaux and Regoli; 1973; Koch-Weser, 1964), and dog heart-lung preparations (Mayer et al., 1970). The maximal stimulation occurred at 10^{-6} M and produced a 100% increase in active tension development. Koch-Weser (1965) found the maximal increase in contractility to angiotensin II to be less than that of norepinephrine (i.e., 100 versus 190%). Thus, while angiotensin II is a stronger inotropic stimulus than other angiotensins or pancreatic hormones, it is not as potent as the catecholamines.

The threshold for inotropic responses to angiotensin is about 1 nM. Circulating physiological levels of angiotensin II, however, usually do not exceed 100 nM (Trachte and Lefer, 1978), probably indicating no major role of angiotensin II in physiological regulation of cardiac contractility. However, during hemorrhage, circulating angiotensin II plasma concentrations exceed 1 nM (Trachte and Lefer, 1978; Lorber, 1942), a concentration greater than that required for myocardial activity. Therefore, angiotensin II may influence cardiac contractility during certain situations, particularly if the formation of angiotensin continues over a prolonged period of time and is not just a transient phenomenon.

Angiotensin II constricts all vascular beds including the coronary vasculature. Lorber (1942) and Hill and Andrus (1941) noted a constrictor action of angiotensin II in isolated cat hearts, as did Gerlings and Gilmore (1974) in isolated dog hearts. Trachte and Lefer (1980) found that angiotensin II constricts isolated perfused coronary arteries in concentrations above 1 ng/ml. The degree of constriction was similar to that of angiotensin III but was much more potent than angiotensin I.

The coronary constrictor activity of angiotensin II may be of significance in control of coronary blood flow in vivo. Gavras et al. (1978a) found an increased coronary blood flow after administration of an angiotensin-converting enzyme inhibitor (e.g., SQ-20881, teprotide) in sodium-depleted dogs. However, it had no effect in animals having normal sodium balance. Sodium depletion stimulates renin release, which increases angiotensin II production. The increased coronary flow after converting enzyme inhibition probably indicates a coronary constriction induced by angiotensin II in sodium-depleted animals (Gavras et al., 1978b). Interpretation of these results, however, is complicated by bradykinin-potentiating activities of teprotide, bradykinin being a vasodilator (Murthy et al., 1977).

In this regard, Trachte and Lefer (1979c) showed that at hypotensive pressures similar to that existing during hemorrhagic shock, converting enzyme inhibitors (e.g., SQ-14,225, captopril) do not potentiate the vascular effects of bradykinin, although they still effectively block conversion of angiotensin II. Thus, it is primarily the blockade of angiotensin II and angiotensin III formation that protects in shock, rather than the potentiation of bradykinin actions.

Cardiac actions of angiotensin II may be classified as positive inotropic and coronary constrictor with variable chronotropic effects. The direct inotropic response is relatively large and independent of catecholamines. Angiotensin II also influences cardiac tissue by potentiating the sympathetic nervous stimulation of myocardial contractility. Constrictor activity of angiotensin II is produced by direct stimulation of the angiotensin II receptor in coronary vascular smooth muscle.

These actions of angiotensin II make it highly unsuitable for use in ischemic heart disease or circulatory shock. This agent decreases myocardial blood supply by constricting the coronary vasculature and increases myocardial oxygen demand by increasing contractility, two actions which would further compromise myocardial function in ischemia states. Angiotensin II also increases total peripheral resistance, which increases the amount of cardiac work required to pump blood. Gavras et al. (1971) have found a prolonged infusion of angiotensin II to produce myocardial infarctions in rabbits, further emphasizing the deleterious actions of high levels of angiotensin II on cardiac function.

Recently, Trachte and Lefer (1979a) reported that prolonged infusion of angiotensin II produces lesions in the heart which are characterized by petechial hemorrhages. These foci are much smaller than those seen after coronary ligation and were found to result from enhanced permeability and increased incidence of pinocytotic vesicles in coronary microvessels (Trachte and Lefer, 1979a).

Patients suffering from chronic heart failure have responded positively to inhibition of angiotensin-converting enzyme (Gavras et al., 1978b). Many of these patients exhibited improved cardiac output and lowered left ventricular end-diastolic pressures after enzyme inhibition, indicating improved cardiac function. Saralasin, an angiotensin II receptor antagonist, also produced similar changes in 45% of the patients with chronic heart failure tested (Turini et al., 1978). The improvement in cardiac function was attributed to reduced afterload, indicating that angiotensin II influences cardiac function by systemic as well as direct myocardial effects.

ANGIOTENSIN III

Angiotensin III generally produces cardiac effects similar to those of angiotensin II. Bonnardeaux et al. (1973) observed angiotensin III to be equipotent to angiotensin II in increasing tension development in isolated rabbit atria. However, Trachte and Lefer (1979d) found angiotensin III to be less potent than angiotensin II in isolated cat papillary muscles. In ventricular tissue, angiotensin III is intermediate in inotropic activity between angiotensin I and II.

Trachte and Lefer (1979d) also found angiotensin III to constrict isolated cat coronary arteries. The constriction induced by angiotensin III was only slightly less than that observed in response to angiotensin II. Angiotensin III, therefore, constricts the coronary vasculature with a potency comparable to angiotensin II.

Angiotensin III induces inotropic and coronary constrictor actions closely related to those of angiotensin II. Angiotensin III produces undesirable effects in ischemic or failing hearts for the same reasons as angiotensin II. Converting enzyme inhibitors have been demonstrated to decrease angiotensin III production in addition to blocking angiotensin II formation (Freeman et al., 1978). The beneficial actions of converting enzyme inhibitors in chronic heart failure, therefore, may involve elimination of angiotensin III in addition to angiotensin II.

Renin-Angiotensin System in Shock

The concept that endogenous angiotensin II is involved in the pathogenesis of circulatory shock has gained support since the original study of Errington and Rocha e Silva (1974), who employed a converting enzyme inhibitor to improve the hemodynamic state of hemorrhagic shock. Subsequently, other investigators also found that converting enzyme inhibition substantially improved the status of animals in shock (Trachte and Lefer, 1978; Morton et al., 1977). In these studies, however, one could not differentiate between a reduction in angiotensin II concentrations and other effects of the converting enzyme inhibitor, including accumulation of angiotensin I and potentiation of kinins (Cushman et al., 1978). Moreover, this converting enzyme inhibitor (i.e., captopril) possesses intrinsic lysosomal-stabilizing and antiprotease activities, actions which are of potential value in circulatory shock (Trachte and Lefer, 1978). Therefore, converting enzyme inhibitors cannot exclusively implicate the prevention of angiotensin II formation as its major beneficial effect in shock.

Angiotensin receptor antagonists (e.g., saralasin) have also been used to specifically eliminate direct effects of angiotensin II by blocking effects on its receptors, thus clarifying the role of angiotensin II in hemorrhage (Trachte and Lefer, 1979b). Elimination of angiotensin actions succeeded in improving conditions that follow a severe hemorrhage. Systemic blood pressure and superior mesenteric artery flow of shocked cats receiving saralasin were significantly normalized compared to cats receiving only vehicle (Trachte and Lefer, 1979b). It therefore seems probable that angiotensin II contributes to the decline of circulatory function in hemorrhagic shock by virtue of its cardiovascular effects.

Angiotensin II blockade did not diminish cathepsin D release during oligemia or in the postreinfusion period (Trachte and Lefer, 1979b). Therefore, angiotensin does not appear to be directly involved in lysosomal labilization in shock. However, plasma amino-nitrogen values, an indicator of proteolysis, were significantly reduced by saralasin, although in vivo studies revealed no direct antiproteolytic action of saralasin (Trachte and Lefer, 1979b). Therefore, the lowered degree of proteolysis in shock animals probably can be attributed to improved splanchnic blood flow or to some other action [e.g., preventing formation of a myocardial depressant factor (MDF)]. Plasma MDF activities were also reduced by saralasin. These differences cannot be attributed to differing severities of hemorrhage because maximum reservoir volumes of all groups were almost identical, indicating that they were bled to an equivalent degree.

Shock Inducing Actions of Angiotensin

Cardiovascular actions of angiotensin II appear to be responsible for the enhanced circulatory dysfunction observed when angiotensin II is present in shocked animals. Two potential sites of angiotensin action are the splanchnic vasculature and the heart. The splanchnic vasculature constricts in response to angiotensin II, but under ordinary circumstances, the constriction is not permanent, due to autoregulatory escape. In hemorrhagic shock, angiotensin II is not essential to the sustained constriction of the splanchnic vasculature because a similar reduction in mesenteric flow occurred in the presence and absence of saralasin (Trachte and Lefer, 1979b). However, angiotensin may play a role in impairing the postoligemic recovery of mesenteric blood flow. Thus, angiotensin II may contribute along with other factors (e.g., catecholamines, vasopressin, thromboxane release, or stimulation of sympathetic vasoconstrictor fibers) to the secondary decline in mesenteric blood flow observed after reinfusion of the shed blood.

An additional potential site of angiotensin action in shock is in the heart. Gavras et al. (1978a) and Giacomelli et al. (1976) have reported damaged myocardial tissue and myocardial vessels after angiotensin II infusion. Because angiotensin II levels are elevated during hemorrhage (Trachte and Lefer, 1978; Morton et al., 1977), the myocardium appears to be another important circulatory site of the deleterious action of angiotensin II in hemorrhagic shock. Since saralasin eliminates the cardiac damage resulting from an angiotensin II accumulation in blood during hemorrhage, it adds further support to the concept of angiotensin II contributing to the circulatory collapse observed in hemorrhagic shock.

The cardiac microcirculatory effects of angiotensin are now well known (Trachte and Lefer, 1979a; Giacomelli et al., 1976; Miller et al., 1964; Robertson and Khairallah, 1971). An increase in capillary permeability has been confirmed by a variety of techniques including horseradish peroxidase leakage from the vasculature (Giacomelli et al., 1976), increase in cardiac lymph flow (Miller et al., 1964), and increase in the number of pinocytotic vesicles in endothelial cells of myocardial capillaries (Robertson and Khairallah, 1971). Trachte and Lefer (1979a) have provided recent histological and ultrastructural findings to indicate an alteration in endothelial cell appearance characterized by leakage of formed elements from the vasculature. The effect only occurred in hemorrhaged cats or those given angiotensin II. The basis of this process was the increased pinocytotic vacuoles in capillaries located in both the epicardium and endocardium, observed by electron microscopy. This alteration in the physical properties of the microvasculature is another deleterious action attributable to angiotensin II and may be responsible in large part for the overall cardiac pathology observed, since it may be indicative of microcirculatory stasis in the myocardium. In addition, angiotensin II is a well known coronary vasoconstrictor agent (Bohr and Uchida, 1967; Drimal et al., 1969; Cohen and Kirk, 1973) that produces a significant reduction in coronary blood flow which can override the primary positive inotropic effect of angiotensin (Lefer, 1967; Koch-Weser, 1965), resulting in a decrease in myocardial contractility (Drimal et al., 1969). These effects would be deleterious in hemorrhagic, endotoxic, and cardiogenic shock, where MDF accumulates to toxic levels (Lefer, 1974) and severely depresses myocardial performance. Table 12.2 summarizes the major cardiovascular effects of the angiotensins as they relate to ischemia and shock.

In summary, angiotensin II and III qualify as vascular mediators in shock since they exert a series of detrimental effects during shock. Their major effect appears to be induction of intense systemic vasoconstriction, resulting in mesenteric, renal, and coronary ischemia, and summating with the intense sympathetically mediated vasoconstriction. In addition, angiotensin inappropriately stimulates the already weakened myocardium, further depleting its exhausted reserve capacity. Finally, high concentrations of angiotensin enhance fluid leakage by increasing capillary permeability in the heart and other sites and, if prolonged, can result in petechial hemorrhages and ultimately in cardiac lesions.

THE PROSTACYCLIN-THROMBOXANE SYSTEM

Recent developments in the field of prostanoid research have elucidated some of the important factors responsible for the control of blood vessel function which would be of importance in ischemia and shock. Until 1975, attention was focused on the classical prostaglandins (PG), particularly PGE_1, PGE_2, and $PGF_{2\alpha}$. Previously, it was generally thought that E-type prostaglandins were usually vasodilator and F-type prostaglandins were vasoconstrictor in action. There were exceptions to this rule with regard to species and vessels, but the main concept was valid. Moreover, it was generally accepted that the monoenoic and bisenoic prostaglandins were the primary prostanoids concerned with regulation of vascular homeostasis, and were important in autoregulation of blood flow. These concepts have rapidly changed over the last 5 years. There now are three major recognized pathways of prostaglandin generation, not just the classical monoenoic and bisenoic pathways originating from dihomo-γ-linolenic and arachidonic acids, respectively. Needleman and coworkers (1979) have recently elucidated the trienoic pathway, originating from eicosapentaenoic acid.

Formation of Prostacyclin and Thromboxanes

Figure 12.2 outlines the three major prostaglandin synthetic pathways starting with the membrane-bound fatty acid released by appropriate phospholipases (e.g., phospholipase A_2). The fatty acid is then converted into an endoperoxide having the designation PGG or PGH. These endoperoxides act as controlling substances directing and shunting substrates into one of three major sub-pathways (Needleman et al., 1976b). One of the alternate sub-pathways to the classical prostaglandins was discovered by Hamberg and colleagues (1975) and termed thromboxanes. In the bisenoic pathway, thromboxane A_2 (TxA_2) is the primary thromboxane. Thromboxane A_2 (TxA_2) is a very potent vasoconstrictor and inducer of platelet aggregation and thus is a powerful thrombogenic substance (Needleman et al., 1976a). Thromboxane A_2 is formed primarily by platelets (Hamberg et al., 1975; Gryglewski et al., 1977), although it may be formed elsewhere to a lesser degree (i.e., lungs, spleen). The other major sub-pathway of the bisenoic PG series leads to the formation of prostacyclin (PGI_2), discovered and synthesized in 1976 by Vane and coworkers (Bunting et al., 1976; Moncada et al., 1976; Moncada and Vane, 1979; Johnson et al., 1976). PGI_2 is a very potent vasodilator and inhibitor of platelet aggregation (Bunting et al., 1976; Moncada and Vane, 1979; Dusting et al., 1977) and thus is an important antithrombotic substance. It is formed primarily by the vascular endothelium of blood vessels (Armstrong et al., 1978; Herman et al., 1977), although it is also produced in gastric mucosa and perhaps elsewhere. Prostacyclin is now viewed as a vascular humor protecting the integrity and function of blood vessels, by preventing thrombus formation and even dissolving formed thrombi (Moncada and Vane, 1979; Armstrong et al., 1978).

Less is known about the other primary pathways of prostaglandin generation. The monoenoic pathway appears to be less well understood and perhaps less well developed. It, too, originates with a membrane bound fatty acid (i.e., dihomo-γ-linolenic acid) and is converted to endoperoxides (i.e., PGG_1 and PGE_1) (Marcus, 1978). The major prostaglandin to be formed from this system appears to be PGE_1. Although PGE_1 is a potent vasodilator and inhibitor of platelet aggregation, it is only $\frac{1}{5}$–$\frac{1}{10}$ as potent as PGI_2 (Hutton et al., 1973). Apparently, human platelets do not produce TxA_1 (Dyerberg et al., 1978) to any appreciable extent, nor is PGI_1 a major factor in vascular dynamics, if it is indeed produced.

The trienoic pathway, however, is different. It originates with the membrane-bound fatty acid, eicosapentaenoic acid, which is converted to the endoperoxides PGG_3 and PGH_3. These endoperoxides are in turn converted to a prostacyclin-like compound, PGI_3, and a thromboxane, TxA_3. PGI_3 is much like PGI_2 in that it is

Table 12.2
Cardiovascular Effects of the Renin-Angiotensin System

Hormone	Inotropic Effect	Effect on Vascular Permeability	Vasoactive Effects	Action on Ischemic Myocardium
Renin	None	None	None	No direct effect
Angiotensin I	Moderate positive effect	Probably no major effect	Slight constriction	Deleterious
Angiotensin II	Large positive effect	Large increase in permeability	Large constriction	Aggravates myocardial ischemia
Angiotensin III	Significant positive effect	Unknown	Large constriction	Aggravates myocardial ischemia

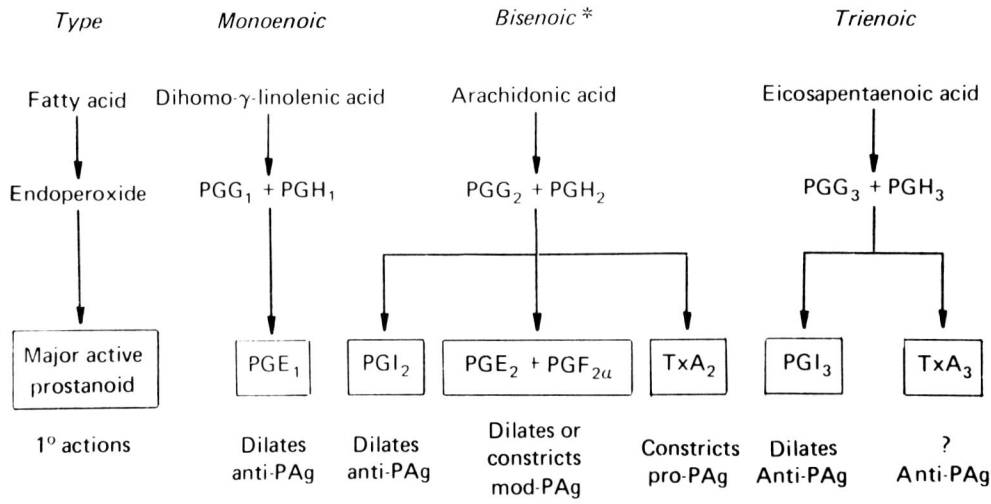

Figure 12.2. Three separate pathways of prostaglandin generations: monoenoic, bisenoic, and trienoic. The major active prostanoids are boxed in at the bottom. *PA*g, platelet aggregation; *PG*, prostaglandin; *Tx*, thromboxane.

a potent vasodilator and inhibitor of platelet aggregation (Needleman et al., 1976a, 1979). However, TxA_3 is not totally analogous to TxA_2, since it increases cyclic AMP levels in platelets and thus antagonizes platelet aggregation (Needleman et al., 1976a). Although TxA_3 appears to be a prominent vasoconstrictor, it is usually accompanied by formation of PGD_3, which is a vasodilator that largely offsets the constrictor action of TxA_3. The net result is an antithrombotic action of this primary pathway, in contrast to that of the bisenoic pathway which is strongly prothrombotic. This may have physiologic significance since certain Eskimos develop a shift to the trienoic pathway due to their dietary intake, which may have a significant bearing on their lack of ischemic circulatory disease (Dyerberg et al., 1978; Gubdjarmason, 1978).

Figure 12.3 illustrates in more detail the complexities of the bisenoic prostaglandin pathway (i.e., the "arachidonic acid cascade"). It can be seen that in addition to the cyclo-oxygenase shunting of arachidonic acid to endoperoxides, there is a lipoxygenase pathway that is not inhibited by nonsteroidal anti-inflammatory agents (i.e., indomethacin, meclofenamate, aspirin), which are classical inhibitors of cyclo-oxygenase (Flower and Vane, 1974). This pathway leads to the formation of hydroperoxides (e.g., HPETE), which are potent vasoconstrictors, and can further be reduced to HETE, a substance that increases the adhesiveness of platelets to their own and other surfaces, and thus contributes to the development of thrombosis (Marcus, 1978). The availability of substances increase after aspirin administration (Marcus), which may be a hazard of regular chronic aspirin usage.

Figure 12.3 also indicates the enzymes and metabolites involved in the bisenoic pathway. It is now clear that PGG_2 is converted to PGH_2 by a peroxidase, and that PGH_2 is the pivotal endoperoxide that shunts substances to one of three sub-pathways: 1) prostacyclin, 2) bisenoic prostaglandins, and 3) thromboxane A_2. It appears that the bisenoic prostaglandins (e.g., PGA_2, PGD_2, PGE_2, and $PGF_{2\alpha}$) are basically metabolites which are not primary determinants of vessel-platelet homeostasis. In addition, the two primary agents, PGI_2 and TxA_2, are very unstable substances that are rapidly converted to other substances. Thus, prostacyclin has a half-life of about 3 min (Cho and Allen, 1978), whereas TxA_2 has a half-life of only 30 sec (Hamberg et al., 1975). Thromboxane A_2 is converted to the largely but not totally inactive substance TxB_2, also called PHD. Prostacyclin spontaneously decomposes to 6 keto-$PGF_{1\alpha}$ (Cho and Allen) and is metabolically degraded by a prostaglandin dehydrogenase to 15-keto-PGI_2. However, these metabolites can be converted to 6-keto-PGE_1, a mimic of PGI_2, but with a lower potency (Hong, 1981). Most of these metabolites are stable and specific for the parent com-

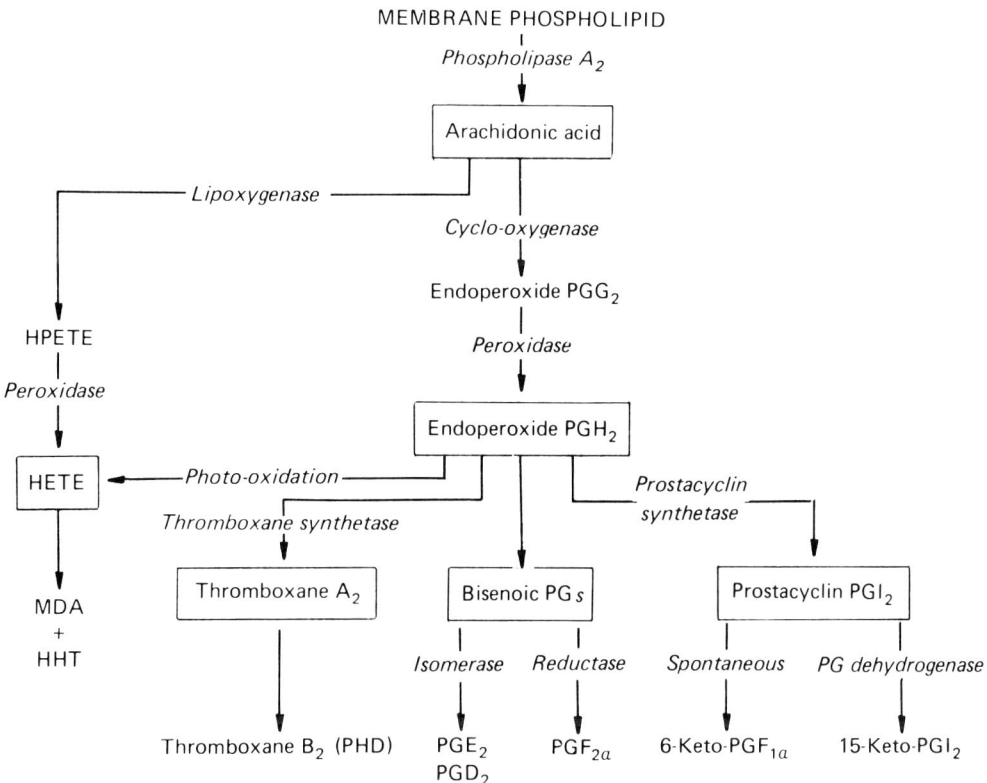

Figure 12.3. Arachidonic acid cascade of prostanoids from membrane-bound phospholipid to arachidonic acid via the two major subpathways, the cyclo-oxygenase and the lipoxygenase routes. Active substances are boxed in, substances below the boxed-in products are major metabolites.

pound and thus form the basis for measurement of PGI_2 and TxA_2, either by direct chemical or radioimmunoassay techniques.

Cardiovascular Actions

The crucial relationships of the prostanoid system relevant to myocardial ischemia and circulatory shock are illustrated in Figure 12.4. This diagram is a schematic representation of a blood vessel with an inner endothelium and outer muscular layer and platelets circulating within a plasma matrix in the lumen of the vessel. Platelet A is in midstream, and if stimulated by hypoxia, ischemia, ADP, collagen, thrombin, or any other stimulus that tends to produce extrusion of thromboxane A_2-containing granules, it releases thromboxane A_2. However, if this phenomenon is localized, the TxA_2 released will diffuse downstream and soon be inactivated. In platelet B, which is located close to the endothelium of the vessel, the released TxA_2 can come in contact with the vessel wall to stimulate severe vasoconstriction. If it is a healthy vessel, the prostaglandin formed will counteract the vasoconstriction, by the potent direct vasodilation of PGI_2 (Lefer et al., 1978). PGI_2 also tends to curtail TxA_2 formation (Lefer et al., 1978) and thus secondarily prevent vasoconstriction and platelet aggregation (Moncada and Vane, 1979; Armstrong et al., 1978; Lefer et al., 1978).

In the case of platelet C, which is adjacent to a damaged area of endothelium, the released thromboxane A_2 can promote the aggregation and further release of additional TxA_2 since it is unopposed by PGI_2, which either is not capable of being synthesized or is trapped within the vessel wall and cannot exert its important protective effects at the endothelium-blood interface. Thus, prostacyclin is thought to be a "defensive humor" of the vasculature (Moncada and Vine, 1978) since it protects the vessel from thrombosis and vasoconstriction induced by the thromboxanes (Bourgain, 1978; Higgs et al., 1978). TxA_2 is therefore considered to be a dangerous thrombogenic substance which has recently been shown not only induce vasospasm (Shimamoto, 1977; Terashita et al., 1978; Ellis et al., 1976) in coronary and other arteries, but which can also directly lead to myocardial ischemia and myocardial infarction (Morooka et al., 1979; Ogletree et al., 1978). Recently, a thromboxane A_2 analog, carbocyclic thromboxane A_2, more potent than any purified thromboxane analog, has been found to produce sudden cardiac death when injected intravenously into rabbits (Lefer et al., 1980). The major manifestation of the sudden death appears to be a severe coronary constriction to the point of inducing acute myocardial ischemia. These findings show the shock-inducing capacity of thromboxanes.

Production in Shock and Ischemia

Recently, TxA_2 generation was confirmed in the early stages of myocardial ischemia (Smith et al., 1979; Schrör et al., 1980) as well as in traumatic shock (Lefer et al., 1980a). The degree of TxA_2 formation, as assessed by specific radioimmunoassay for TxB_2, correlated well with the severity of the shock state.

The major peak of thromboxane release occurred about 2 hr after coronary artery ligation in myocardial ischemia (Smith et al., 1979) and 4–5 hr after induction of trauma in traumatic shock (Lefer et al., 1980a). However, in endotoxin shock, circulating thromboxane values peaked 5–15 min after injection of endotoxin and was largely cleared from the blood by 2 hr. Thus, each type of ischemia or shock has a different pattern of thromboxane formation and accumulation. Moreover, inhibitors of thromboxane synthetase, including imidazole (Moncada et al., 1979) and pinane thromboxane A_2, PTA_2 (Nicolaou et al., 1979), dramatically prevented TxB_2 appearance and sharply curtailed the extension of the ischemic damage experienced after abrupt coronary artery occlusion (Smith et al., 1979; Schrör et al., 1980).

Therapy in Shock

PTA_2 is a thromboxane A_2 receptor antagonist as well as a thromboxane synthetase inhibitor (Nicolaou et al., 1979) and by virtue of these effects is dramatically effective in improving survival and protecting against the consequences of myocardial ischemia (Schrör et al., 1980) and trauma in Noble-Collip drum trauma shock (Lefer et al., 1979c).

Not only does thromboxane inhibition protect in ischemia and shock, but intravenous infusion of prostacyclin is also protective in both situations (Ogletree et al., 1979; Lefer et al., 1979). PGI_2 at low dose rates (i.e., 0.5 nmoles $\cdot kg^{-1} \cdot min^{-1}$) preserved myocardial cell integrity as well as prevented the extension of ischemic damage in acute myocardial ischemia (Ogletree et al., 1979; Jugdult et al., 1979). Moreover, PGI_2 was more effective in myocardial ischemia than other prostaglandins including $PGF_{2\alpha}$, PGE_2 and PGE_1 (Ogletree and Lefer, 1978). PGI_2 was also effective in improving survival and lessening the severity of traumatic (Lefer et al., 1979) and endotoxin (Fletcher and Ramwell, 1980; Smith et

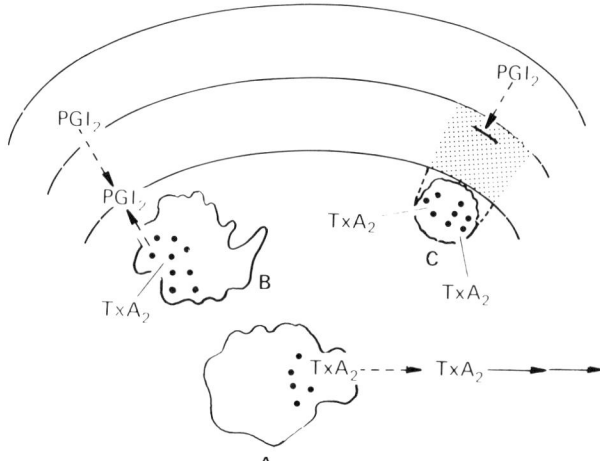

Figure 12.4. Platelet endothelial interrelationships. Platelet A in midstream; platelet B near normal endothelium; platelet C near diseased endothelium. PGI_2, prostacyclin; TxA_2, thromboxane A_2.

1980) shock. Therefore, PGI$_2$ appears to have considerable promise in the treatment of ischemic disorders (Szczeklik et al., 1979; Lefer and Smith, 1979) including shock and atherosclerosis (Gryglewski et al., 1978).

Knowledge of the prostaglandin-thromboxane system is becoming increasingly important for investigators in the field of circulatory shock since the prostanoids appear to be involved in the pathogenesis of ischemia and shock. This system promises to be a very fruitful one in helping to understand fundamental processes in the pathophysiology of shock as well as in applying these principles toward the study of therapeutic agents in shock and ischemia.

THE LYSOSOMAL HYDROLASE—MYOCARDIAL DEPRESSANT FACTOR (MDF) SYSTEM

Humoral toxic agents have been found in a variety of types of circulatory shock (Lefer, 1973b). Several of these substances fulfill the criteria necessary to qualify as a toxic factor in shock (Lefer, 1973b). One of the best known shock factors is MDF, which occurs in the plasma of animals and humans in several types of circulatory shock. MDF was initially discovered in 1966 in the plasma of cats in hemorrhagic shock (Lefer, 1979). Since the initial discovery of MDF in the blood during circulatory shock, the observation has been confirmed in many other laboratories around the world (Baxter et al., 1966; Fisher et al., 1973; Haglund and Lundgren, 1973; Okuda et al., 1973; Williams et al., 1969; Rogel and Hilewitz, 1978).

Thus far, MDF has been found in hemorrhagic, endotoxic, cardiogenic, splanchnic ischemic, pancreatitis, burn, and traumatic shock. Moreover, MDF has been found in the plasma of cats, dogs, rabbits, rats, baboons, and man during shock (Lefer, 1973b, 1974). This suggests that MDF may represent a common denominator in many types of circulatory shock and in many mammalian species.

Considerable data have been obtained recently on the chemical and physical properties of MDF. MDF has been purified from the plasma of dogs and cats in hemorrhagic and splanchnic ischemia shock and has been differentiated from either salt or pentobarbital contamination (Lefer and Inge, 1973; Lefer and Glenn, 1974). The molecular weight of MDF is about 500 (Lefer and Martin, 1970); it is water-soluble, relatively insoluble in methylene chloride; the plasma concentration during shock is on the order of 0.1–1 ng/ml (Greene et al., 1977). MDF is inactivated by ashing (Lefer and Spath, 1974), trypsinization (Litvin et al., 1973), and addition of the nonspecific protease pronase (Lefer, 1970) and possesses free amino groups (Lefer, 1970). On the basis of these and other findings, MDF has been identified as a peptide containing three to four amino acid residues (Greene et al., 1977); no sulfur-containing amino acids are present in the peptide. Although the amino acid composition of MDF is known (Greene et al., 1977), the exact amino acid sequence of the peptide is unclear. This is due to the fact that one of the four residues in MDF is not an amino acid but rather a complex organic substance having a free amino group. Furthermore, the MDF that has been analyzed is one of two MDF substances that are closely related to each other (Greene et al., 1977). Thus, there are at least two MDF entities which further complicate the chemical identification.

Formation of MDF

MDF accumulates in the plasma during shock and reaches toxic levels approximately 2–7 hr after the onset of shock. The common factor in these shock states is not the mean arterial blood pressure but rather the magnitude of the hypoperfusion to the splanchnic region. The critical step in MDF production appears to be splanchnic hypoperfusion. Figure 12.5 outlines the pathophysiologic mechanisms responsible for the formation of MDF. The

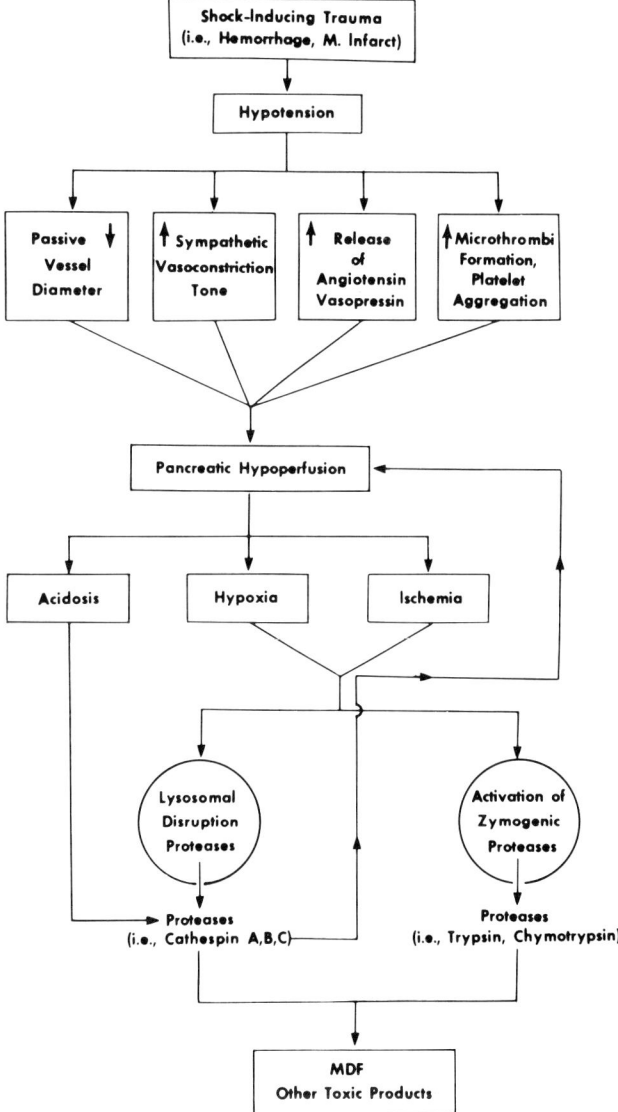

Figure 12.5. Mechanism of the formation of myocardial depressant factor (MDF), from the initial hypotension to the proteolysis. These events occur primarily within pancreatic acinar cells.

shock-inducing event (e.g., hemorrhage, myocardial infarction, septicemia, etc.) usually results in hypotension, which then induces hypoperfusion of the splanchnic region, especially the pancreas.

Pancreatic blood flow decreases abruptly in hemorrhagic shock. Thus, 30 min after a hemorrhage to 45 mm Hg in the dog, pancreatic flow decreases 70% (Lefer and Spath, 1974; Forsyth et al., 1970). Two hours later, there is a 80–85% decrease in pancreatic blood flow (Spath et al., 1974). This pancreatic hypoperfusion occurs in anesthetized and conscious animals as well as in man during shock. The pancreatic vasculature appears to be sensitive to alterations in cardiovascular performance, and uniformly responds to shock and trauma states with marked decreases in blood flow. Pancreatic hypoperfusion often occurs without severe degrees of hypotension as in splanchnic ischemia or hemorrhagic pancreatitis.

The major mechanisms for the shock-induced pancreatic hypoperfusion appear to be: 1) passive decrease in vessel lumen diameter in response to a reduced perfusion pressure; 2) active increase in sympathetic tone to the splanchnic resistance vessels leading to a vasoconstriction; 3) release of humoral vasoconstrictor agents such as angiotensin II, thromboxane A_2 and vasopressin; and 4) physical obstruction of the microcirculatory vessels by the formation of microthrombi and platelet aggregation. The primary consequence of these events is reduced perfusion to the pancreas and, to a lesser extent, other splanchnic viscera. This hypoperfusion results in acidosis, hypoxia, and ischemia to the pancreas. Hypoxia and ischemia are potent stimuli for lysosomal disruption and for activation of zymogenic enzymes (i.e., conversion of trypsinogen to trypsin and chymotrypsin to chymotrypsin). The result is the release of large amounts of proteolytic enzymes into the cytoplasm of pancreatic acinar cells. Acidosis does not appear to be directly involved in activation of these enzymes but rather enhances the activity of the lysosomal proteases once they are released from the lysosomes (Glenn and Lefer, 1971a). The zymogenic and lysososmal proteases released during the shock process appear to accelerate proteolysis and thereby stimulate MDF production (Lituin et al., 1973; Lefer and Barenholz, 1972). Presumably, other peptides are also formed as a direct consequence of increased proteolysis occurring in the ischemic pancreas during shock.

One of the more striking events in circulatory shock is the release of lysosomal enzymes into the circulation. The major source of these acid hydrolases is the ischemic splanchnic region, particularly the liver and pancreas (Glenn and Lefer, 1971a). Evidence obtained in the isolated perfused cat pancreas indicates that lysosomal enzyme release is closely associated with MDF production (Ferguson et al., 1972). The pancreas was the only possible source of MDF in this preparation since the perfusion fluid contained only inorganic ions and glucose with no plasma proteins or blood cells. Moreover, this preparation allowed the independent control of blood flow, pH, and oxygenation. After 150 min of perfusion with normal flow, tissue β-glucuronidase was only slightly reduced from normal values of 100 U/mg protein. However, ischemia or hypoxia reduced the tissue activity of this hydrolase to 40–50% of control values. Perfusate samples were studied to determine if the enzyme activity was lost from the tissue by inactivation or decreased protein synthesis. High perfusate activity was found with low tissue activity and vice versa (i.e., perfusate activity mirrors tissue activity). These data confirm the loss of tissue lysosomal enzyme activity and the simultaneous increase in MDF activity in the perfusate in the ischemia and hypoxic preparations. These data closely show that the pancreas is a major source of MDF during circulatory shock and that lysosomal disruption is intimately linked to MDF production.

The mechanism of MDF transport from the pancreatic acinar cell to the circulation is not completely known. It

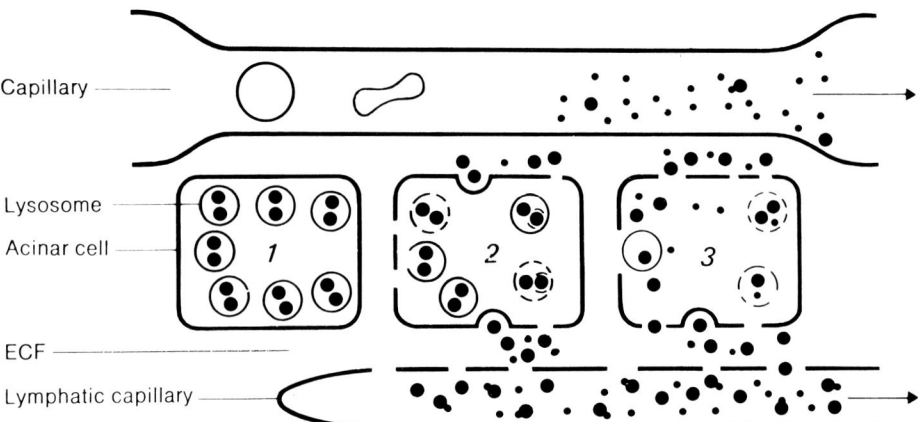

Figure 12.6. Lymphatic transport of myocardial depressant factor (*MDF*) from extracellular fluid (*ECF*) surrounding pancreatic acinar cells to the systemic circulation. Lysosomes are large circles containing large dots (proteolytic enzymes), small dots are the peptide, *MDF*. *MDF* that is bound to protein is transported via the lymphatic capillary to the central circulation. Free *MDF* is transported primarily via the systemic capillary but also to some extent by the lymphatic capillary to the central circulation.

appears that MDF is released from acinar cells through damaged cell membranes (Fig. 12.6). The peptide may bind to large carrier proteins in the extracellular fluid or it may remain as a free peptide (Lefer, 1973a; Glenn and Lefer, 1970). Much of the bound MDF as well as the lysosomal enzymes are taken up by lymphatic capillaries and transported via lymphatic vessels to the systemic circulation (Glenn and Lefer, 1970). Some of the free MDF as well as other small molecules can be transported directly by capillaries, since unbound MDF presumably diffuses across the capillary membrane. The kinetics of the binding of MDF to carrier material is not clear at present. This process may play a key role in the distribution of MDF in the circulation. At present, most of the MDF can be obtained in the free form in peripheral blood, but the degree of protein binding is not known.

Thus, MDF is generated in the ischemic and hypoxic pancreas during circulatory shock. It is formed as a product of proteolysis in or around the acinar cell by the combined autolytic action of lysosomal and zymogenic proteases (Lefer and Barenholz, 1972). Once formed, the peptide is either transported by the capillaries or bound in a carrier protein and transported by the lymphatics to the circulation where it is able to exert its deleterious effects.

Cardiovascular Actions of MDF

MDF has been shown to exert a variety of pathophysiological effects in the intact animal as well as in isolated organs or tissues. Table 12.3 summarizes these biological actions. The best known action of MDF is its negative inotropic effect (i.e., the depression of myocardial contractility). MDF was discovered by virtue of its ability to impair developed tension in isolated cat papillary muscles. This dramatic effect occurs within 5–10 min in the isolated papillary muscle preparation (Lefer, 1970) and within 1–2 min in perfused hearts.

Even more dramatic is the negative inotropic effect of MDF in the intact animal. MDF has been shown to depress the heart during hemorrhagic shock in the dog (Wangensteen et al., 1970). Moreover, exogenously injected MDF has been shown to impair myocardial contractility in the normal animal (Glenn and Lefer, 1971a). Control ventricular function curves were obtained 2 hr apart in control cats. Cardiac performance, expressed as maximal left ventricular power, declined by only 5% over this time period. In contrast, intravenous injection MDF, to yield circulating titers present in shock animals, exerted a progressive impairment of cardiac performance so that maximal left ventricular power was depressed 54% within 60 min; circulatory shock occurred at this time (Glenn and Lefer, 1971a). Thus, MDF appears to be responsible for a significant portion of the myocardial depression observed in shock states.

In addition to its negative inotropic effect, MDF participates in other positive feedback actions which tend to undermine circulatory homeostasis and which are of negative survival value. One of these actions is constriction of the resistance vessels within the splanchnic area.

Table 12.3
Biological Actions of MDF

Negative inotropic effect
  Isolated papillary muscles
  Isolated perfused heart
  Intact animal
Splanchnic vasoconstrictor effect
  Isolated vessel strips
  Isolated perfused pancreas
Depression of phagocytosis by reticuloendothelial system
  Occurs in fixed macrophages
  Does not occur in leukocytes

MDF constricts isolated superior mesenteric artery strips but apparently not other strips (e.g., carotid, aortic, or femoral) (Glucksman and Lefer, 1971). The constrictor effect occurs in the absence of any vasoactive agent as well as in the presence of potent constrictor concentrations of norepinephrine or angiotensin II (Glucksman and Lefer, 1971). The net effect of this constrictor effect is to further compromise blood flow to the vital splanchnic organs and thus promote conditions which favor the continued production of MDF. However, MDF does not induce platelet aggregation (Bridenbaugh and Lefer, 1976) so that its vasoconstrictor effect is primarily by stimulation of vascular smooth muscle, even though it may promote increased capillary permeability (Ferguson et al., 1972). The severe vasoconstrictor action of MDF may help explain the failure of autoregulatory mechanisms to restore splanchnic blood flow to normal during prolonged circulatory shock.

Another positive feedback loop in which MDF may participate during shock is depression of the reticuloendothelial system (RES). Apparently MDF impairs phagocytosis (Lefer and Blattberg, 1968) in fixed macrophages (i.e., Kupffer cells of the liver) but not in leukocytes (Williams et al., 1970). The result of this depression of phagocytosis is to impair further the already depressed RES, perhaps by a combination of reduced liver blood flow, depletion of plasma opsonins, and the presence of a reticuloendothelial depressing substance (RDS) (Blattberg and Levy, 1962). Biological and chemical evidence indicates that MDF may be identical with RDS (Lefer and Levy, 1962). Biological and chemical evidence indicates that MDF may be identical with RDS (Lefer and Blattberg, 1968), a finding which could clarify our understanding of this pathophysiologic aspect of shock. The net result of the reticuloendothelial depression is to inactivate one of the primary avenues of clearance of foreign or native toxic materials from the blood, such as MDF and lysosomal enzymes. Since renal function is also usually impaired during shock, the organism has few viable options with which to clear toxic factors such as MDF from the circulatory system.

Pharmacologic Prevention of Antagonism of MDF

Intensive investigation has been directed toward preventing the formation of MDF or preventing the actions of MDF once it is formed. Table 12.4 lists several pharmacologic interventions and summarizes their

Table 12.4
Pharmacologic Modulation of the Lysosomal Hydrolase-MDF System

Agent	Potential Beneficial Action	Difficulty or Deleterious Side Effects
Glucocorticoids (e.g., dexamethasone, methylprednisolone)	Stabilizes lysosomal membranes, prevents MDF formation	None (acutely)
Protease inhibitors (e.g., aprotinin)	Antagonizes zymogenic proteases; prevents MDF formation	None (acutely)
Prostacyclin (PGI$_2$)	Stabilizes membranes, vasodilates, prevents platelet aggregation; prevents MDF formation	Must be infused slowly, effects transient
Thromboxane inhibitors (PTA$_2$, imidazole)	Prevents thromboxane synthesis and/or action, stabilizes membranes, Prevents MDF formation	Must be constantly infused
Local anesthetics (e.g., lidocaine)	Partially prevents splanchnic ischemia, prevents MDF formation	Must be given locally, effects transient
Dopamine	Dilates splanchnic bed, partially prevents and counteracts MDF	Increases cardiac oxygen demand, constricts at high doses
Glucagon	Positive inotropic effect, partially counteracts effects of MDF	Disrupts lysosomal membranes
Isoproterenol	Positive inotropic effect, partially counteracts effect of MDF	Exerts strong systemic vasodilators, blood pressure difficult to maintain
Digitalis glycosides	Positive inotropic effect, partially counteracts effect of MDF	Severe splanchnic constriction, induces arrhythmias
Calcium ion	Strong positive inotropic effect, counteracts effect of MDF	Constricts blood vessels, overwhelms neuromuscular control

mechanism of action on the MDF system as well as lists several potential hazards in their usefulness as therapeutic agents in shock. By far, the most successful therapeutic agent in preventing the formation of MDF is the synthetic glucocorticoid. The most widely used glucocorticoids are methylprednisolone and dexamethasone, which are available as water-soluble derivatives. If given early in the course of shock in pharmacologic doses, glucocorticoids are very effective in enhancing survival as well as in preventing MDF formation in animals as well as man (Lefer and Glenn, 1974; Glenn and Lefer, 1971b). Moreover, glucocorticoids have a high margin of safety and at high doses have no serious side effects or toxic action when given acutely. Their remarkable safety is of considerable virtue in the treatment of shock. Their major protective mechanism appears to be the stabilization of cellular and subcellular membranes, especially of the lysosomes (Lefer and Glenn, 1974; Glenn and Lefer, 1971b).

In this regard, glucocorticoids have been shown to prevent the leakage of acid hydrolases (e.g., cathepsin D and β-glucuronidase) into the circulation from the ischemic pancreas and liver (Glenn and Lefer, 1971a; Ferguson et al., 1972). High doses of glucocorticoids also prevent the increase in percentage free activity of these enzymes in tissue homogenates (Lefer and Barenholz, 1972). In addition, glucocorticoids prevent the swelling and vacuolization of lysosomes in liver and pancreas cells (Lefer and Barenholz). This has recently been found to be the case in the ischemic region of the myocardium in acute myocardial ischemia. Figure 12.7 illustrates the protective effect of methylprednisolone on cardiac lysosomes in the ischemic cat heart. This glucocorticoid dramatically prevented the swelling and vacuolization of cardiac lysosomes during the first 5 hr after myocardial ischemia. This is direct positive evidence of the lysosomal stabilizing effect of glucocorticoids in ischemia and shock.

Another agent that appears to be effective in preventing MDF formation as well as in improving survival in shock is the protease inhibitor, aprotinin (Trasylol) (Lefer and Martin, 1970; Lefer and Barenholz, 1972; Glenn et al., 1973). The major action of this agent in preventing the formation of MDF appears to be inhibition of phospholipase A and kallikrein from pancreatic zymogen granules and cathepsin B for lysosomes (Lefer and Barenholz, 1972). MDF activity as well as cathepsin B activity are both reduced approximately 40–50% in pancreatic large granule fractions by aprotinin. The decrease in the cathepsin B activity may be related to the reduced kallikrein activity in these fractions. Aprotonin is also effective in vivo and improves survival in other types of shock, such as that produced by acute pancreatitis (Trapnell et al., 1974). Also, aprotinin, if given slowly in appropriate doses, does not exert appreciable undesirable hemodynamic or metabolic effects.

Recently, prostacyclin (PGI$_2$), a prostanoid produced by the endothelium of the vasculature, has been found to possess a variety of actions which are useful in shock. Prostacyclin is a very potent inhibitor of platelet aggregation, a vasodilator, and is a good membrane stabilizer (Armstrong et al., 1978; Lefer et al., 1978). It has been found to prevent MDF formation in traumatic (Lefer et al., 1979) and endotoxin (Smith et al., 1980) shock. Similarly, thromboxane synthetase inhibitors, (e.g., imidazole) has been found to prevent the formation of thromboxane A$_2$ by platelets and thus diminish the vasoconstrictor and proaggregating actions of thromboxane A$_2$ (Lefer et al., 1978).

Imidazole and a new thromboxane inhibitor [i.e.,

pinane thromboxane A_2 (PTA$_2$)], which is also an antagonist of the aggregating and vasoconstrictor actions of thromboxane A_2, has been found to effectively prevent MDF formation in traumatic (Lefer et al., 1980a) and endotoxin shock (Smith et al., 1979).

Local anesthetics have been found to be of limited value in the prevention of MDF. Thus, agents such as lidocaine, infiltrated locally into the celiac ganglia, prevented much of the decrease in splanchnic blood flow and consequently diminished MDF formation in endotoxic shock (Wangensteen et al., 1971). However, the agent is only effective if given locally and is only active for a few hours. This type of pharmacologic intervention is obviously not the method of choice in clinical shock.

A series of inotropic agents, such as dopamine, digitalis glycosides, glucagon, isoproterenol, and calcium, have been used extensively in clinical shock to counteract myocardial depression, although not with any notable degree of success in improving survival (Lefer et al., 1971). Moreover, these agents do not prevent MDF production due to deleterious side effects of these inotropic agents. These findings suggest that treatment of shock should focus on basic cellular defects as well as hemodynamic alterations. Thus, there are a variety of pharmacologic agents that can either prevent MDF formation or antagonize its cardiotoxic effects.

SUMMARY AND CONCLUSIONS

Evidence has been presented that certain vasoactive agents (e.g., angiotensins II and III, thromboxane A_2, and MDF) are potent naturally occurring vasoconstrictors that clearly contribute to the pathogenesis of circulatory shock. In fact, all these agents have been shown to produce a state of shock or serious cardiovascular decompensation when injected directly into normal animals (Trachte and Lefer, 1979a; Shimamoto et al., 1977; Morooka et al., 1979; Glenn and Lefer, 1971a).

These vascular mediators of ischemia and shock are either peptides or lipids. They have a diversity of actions in addition to their severe vasoconstrictor effects. Thus, angiotensin II or III stimulates the myocardium and enhances capillary leakage. Thromboxane A_2 induces platelet aggregation without any significant inotropic activity. MDF severely decreases myocardial contractility and reticuloendothelial function without affecting platelet aggregation.

These vascular mediators are very potent, all exerting effects in the nanomolar range. Moreover, they are all small molecules (i.e., 300–1000) so that they are transported readily to different loci. They are all different in their biological stability. Thromboxane A_2 has a half-time of about 30 sec, angiotensin several minutes, and MDF apparently several hours during shock.

There are inhibitors of the formation of all three vascular mediators. Converting enzyme inhibitors (e.g., captopril, teprotide) prevent angiotensin II formation, thromboxane synthetase inhibitors (e.g., imidazole, PTA$_2$) prevent thromboxane A_2 formation, and glucocorticoids (e.g., dexamethasone, methylprednisolone) and protease inhibitors (e.g., aprotinin) prevent MDF formation. There are receptor antagonists available for angiotensin II (e.g., saralasin) and thromboxane A_2 (e.g., PTA$_2$), but none exist for MDF.

These vascular mediators are thought to play a vital

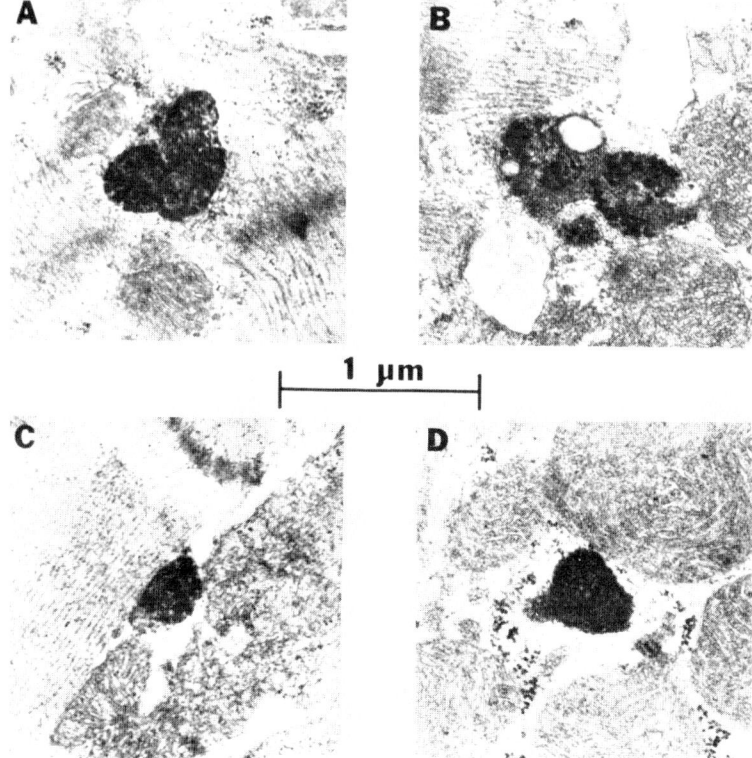

Figure 12.7. Electron micrographs of lysosomes (darkly stained with cathepsin D as a marker) from A, control myocardium; B, ischemic myocardium; C, normal myocardium plus methylprednisolone (30 mg/kg); and D, ischemic myocardium plus methylprednisolone (30 mg/kg). × 42,000. In myocardial ischemia, the lysosome is enlarged and has a large clear vacuole. These changes are prevented by methylprednisolone.

role in propagation of ischemia and in development of circulatory shock. As knowledge accumulates in this key area, we will achieve a greater understanding of the pathophysiology and therapeutics of ischemia and shock.

Acknowledgment. A contribution of the Ischemia-Shock Research Center of Thomas Jefferson University.

References

Ackerly, J.A., and Peach, M.J.: Metabolism of angiotensins in the rabbit myocardium. Pharmacologist *17:*327, 1975.

Armstrong, J.M., Dusting, G.J., Moncada, S., and Vane, J.R.: Cardiovascular actions of prostacyclin (PGI_2), a metabolite of arachidonic acid which is synthesized by blood vessels. Circ. Res. *43:*112–119, 1978.

Baxter, C.R., Cook, W.A., and Shires, G.T.: Serum myocardial depressant factor of burn shock. Surg. Forum *17:*1–2, 1966.

Blaisdell, F.W.: The role of thromboembolism in shock. In *Shock in Low and High Flow States,* edited by B.K. Forschev, pp. 172–180. Excerpta Medica, Amsterdam, 1972.

Blattberg, G., and Levy, M.N.: A humoral reticuloendothelial-depressing substance in shock. Am. J. Physiol. *203:*409–411, 1962.

Bohr, D. F., and Uchida, E.: Individualities of vascular smooth muscles in response to angiotensin. Circ. Res. (Suppl. II) *21:*135–143, 1967.

Bonnardeaux, J.L., and Regoli, D.: Action of angiotensin and analogues on the heart. Can. J. Physiol. Pharmacol. *52:*50–60, 1973.

Bourgain, R.H.: Inhibition of PGI_2 (Prostacyclin) synthesis in the arterial wall enhances the formation of white platelet thrombi in vivo. Haemostasis *7:*252–255, 1978.

Brand, E.D., and Lefer, A.M.: Myocardial depressant factor in the plasma of cats in irreversible postoligemic shock. Proc. Soc. Exp. Biol. Med. *122:*200–203, 1966.

Bridenbaugh, G.A., and Lefer, A.M.: Influence of humoral shock factors *in vitro* aggregation of dog platelets. Thrombosis Res. *8:*599–606, 1976.

Britton, S., and DiSalvo, J.: Effects of angiotensin I and angiotensin II on hindlimb and coronary vascular resistance. Am. J. Physiol. *225:*1226–1231, 1973.

Bunting, S., Gryglewski, R., Moncada, S., and Vane, J.R.: Arterial walls generate from prostaglandin endoperoxides a substance (prostaglandin X) which relaxes strips of mesenteric and coeliac arteries and inhibits platelet aggregation. Prostaglandins *12:*897–913, 1976.

Cho, M.J., and Allen, M.A.: Chemical stability of prostacyclin (PGI_2) in aqueous solutions. Prostaglandins *15:*943–954, 1978.

Cohen, M.V., and Kirk, E.S.: Differential response of large and small coronary arteries to nitroglycerin and angiotensin. Circ. Res. *33:*445–453, 1973.

Cushman, D.W., Cheung, H.S., Sabo, E.F., and Ondetti, M.A.: Design of new anti-hypertensive drugs: potent and specific inhibitors of angiotensin-converting enzyme. Prog. Cardiovasc. Dis. *3:*176–182, 1978.

Devynck, M.A., Pernollet, M.G., Matthews, P.G., Khosla, M.C., Bumpus, F.M., and Meyer, P.: Specific receptors for des-Asp^1-angiotensin II ("angiotensin III") in rat adrenals. Proc. Natl. Acad. Sci. U.S.A. *74:*4029–4032, 1977.

Drimal, J., Pavek, K., and Selecky, F.V.: Primary and secondary effects of angiotensin on the coronary circulation. Cardiologia *54:*1–15, 1969.

Dusting, G.J., Moncada, S., and Vane, J.R.: Prostacyclin (PGX) endogenous metabolite responsible for relaxation of coronary arteries induced by arachidonic acid. Prostaglandins *13:*3–15, 1977.

Dyerberg, J., Bang, H.O., Stoffersen, E., Moncada, S., and Vane, J.R.: Eicosapentaenoic acid: prevention of thrombosis and atherosclerosis? Lancet *ii:*117–119, 1978.

Ellis, E. F., Oelz, O., Roberts, L. G., Payne, M.A., Sweetman, B.J., Nies, A.S., and Oates, J.A.: Coronary arterial smooth muscle contraction by a substance released from platelets; evidence that it is thromboxane A_2. Science *193:*1135–1137, 1976.

Errington, M.L., and Rocha e Silva, M.: On the role of vasopressin and angiotensin in the development of irreversible haemorrhagic shock. J. Physiol. (Lond.) *242:*119–141, 1974.

Ferguson, W.W., Glenn, T.M., and Lefer, A.M.: Mechanisms of production of circulatory shock factors in the isolated perfused pancreas. Am. J. Physiol. *222:*450–457, 1972.

Fisher, W.D., Heimbach, D.W., McArdle, C.S., Maddern, M., Hutcheson, M.M., and Ledingham, I.McA.: A circulating depressant effect following canine hemorrhagic shock. Br. J. Surg. *60:*392–393, 1973.

Fletcher, J.R., and Ramwell, P.W.: Indomethacin treatment following baboon endotoxin shock improves survival. In *Advances In Shock Research,* edited by W. Schumer, J.J. Spitzer, and B. Marshall, vol. 4, pp. 103–111. Alan R. Liss, Inc., New York, 1980.

Flower, R.J., and Vane, J.R.: Inhibition of prostaglandin biosynthesis. Biochem. Pharmacol. *23:*1439–1450, 1974.

Forsyth, R.P., Hoffbrand, B.I., and Melmon, K.L.: Redistribution of cardiac output during hemorrhage in the unanesthetized monkey. Circ. Res. *27:*311, 1970.

Freeman, R.H., Davis, J.O., and Khosla, M.C.: Renal and adrenal responses to [des-Asp^1] angiotensin I in the dog. Am. J. Physiol. *234:*F130–F134, 1978.

Gavras, H., Brown, J. J., Lever, A.F., Macadam, R.F., and Robertson, J.J.S.: Acute renal failure, tubular necrosis and myocardial infarction induced in the rabbit by intravenous angiotensin II. Lancet *2:*19–22, 1971.

Gavras, H., Faxon, D.P., Berkoben, J., Brunner, H.R., and Ryan, T.J.: Angiotensin converting enzyme inhibition in patients with congestive heart failure. Circ. Res. *58:*770–776, 1978a.

Gavras, H., Liang, C.S., and Brunner, H.R.: Redistribution of regional blood flow after inhibition of the angiotensin-converting enzyme. Circ. Res. *43:*I59–I62, 1978b.

Gerlings, E.D., and Gilmore, J.P.: Evidence for myocardial conversion of angiotensin I. Basic. Res. Cardiol. *69:*222–227, 1974.

Giacomelli, F., Anversa, P., and Wiener, P.: Effect of angiotensin-induced hypertension on rat coronary arteries and myocardium. Am. J. Pathol. *84:*111–128, 1976.

Glenn, T.M., and Lefer, A.M.: Protective effect of thoracic lymph diversion in hemorrhagic shock. Am. J. Physiol. *219:*1305–1310, 1970.

Glenn, T.M., and Lefer, A.M.: Significance of splanchnic proteases in the production of a toxic factor in hemorrhagic shock. Circ. Res. *29:*338–349, 1971a.

Glenn, T.M., and Lefer, A.M.: Anti-toxic action of methylprednisolone in hemorrhagic shock. Eur. J. Pharmacol. *13:*230–238, 1971b.

Glenn, T.M., Herlihy, B.L., and Lefer, A.M.: Protective action of a protease inhibitor in hemorrhagic shock. Arch. Int. Pharmacodyn. Ther. *203:*292–304, 1973.

Glucksman, E.E., and Lefer, A.M.: Effects of a myocardial

depressant factor on isolated vascular smooth muscle. Am. J. Physiol. *220:*1581–1585, 1971.

Greenbaum, R.: The blood and transfusion fluids in shock. In *Physiological and Practical Aspects of Shock*, edited by J. Freeman, vol. 7, pp. 775–797. Little, Brown, Boston, 1969.

Green, L.J., Shapanka, R., Glenn, R.M., and Lefer, A.M.: Isolation of myocardial depressant factor (MDF) from plasma of dogs in hemorrhagic shock. Biochim. Biophys. Acta *491:*275–285, 1977.

Gryglewski, R.J., Zmuda, A., Korbut, R., Krecioch, E., and Bieron, K.: Selective inhibition of thromboxane A_2 biosynthesis in blood platelets. Nature *267:*627–628, 1977.

Gryglewski, R.J., Dembinska-Kiec, A., Zmuda, A., and Gryglewska, T.: Prostacyclin and thromboxane A_2 biosynthesis capacities of heart, arteries and platelets at various stages of experimental artherosclerosis in rabbits. Atherosclerosis *31:* 385–394, 1978.

Gubdjarnason, S., Oskarsdottir, G., Doell, B., and Hallgrimsson, J.: Myocardial membrane lipids in relation to cardiovascular disease. Adv. Cardiol. *25:*130–144, 1978.

Haglund, U., and Lundgren, O.: Cardiovascular effects of blood borne material released from the cat small intestine during simulated shock conditions. Acta Physiol. Scand. *89:* 558–565, 1973.

Hamberg, M., Svensson, J., and Samuelsson, B.: Thromboxanes: A new group of biologically active compounds derived from prostaglandin endoperoxides. Proc. Nat. Acad. Sci. U.S.A. *72:*2994–2998, 1975.

Herman, A.G., Moncada, S., and Vane, J.R.: Formation of prostacyclin (PGI_2) by different layers of the arterial wall. Arch. Int. Pharmacodyn. Therap. *227:*162–163, 1977.

Higgs, E.A., Higgs, G.A., Moncada, S., and Vane, J.R.: Prostacyclin (PGI_2) inhibits the formation of platelet thrombi in arterioles and venules of the hamster cheek pouch. Br. J. Pharmacol. *63:*535–539, 1978.

Hill, H.P., and Andrus, E.L.: The cardiac factor in the "pressor" effects of renin and angiotonin. J. Exp. Med. *72:*91, 1941.

Hoffman, J.I., and Buckberg, G.D.: The myocardial supply: Demand ratio—A critical review. Am. J. Cardiol. *41:*327–332, 1978.

Hong, P.: Metabolism of prostacyclin. In *Prostaglandin and Microcirculatory Function*, edited by G. Kaley. In press, 1981.

Hutton, I., Parratt, J.R., and Lawrie, T.D.: Cardiovascular effects of prostaglandin E_1 in experimental myocardial infarction. Cardiovas. Res. *7:*149–155, 1973.

Johnson, R.A., Morton, D.R., Kinner, J.H., Gorman, R.R., McGuire, J.R., Sun, F.F., Whittaker, N., Bunting, S., Salmon, J.A., Moncada, S., and Vane, J.R.: The chemical structure of prostaglandin X (prostacyclin). Prostaglandins *12:*915–928, 1976.

Jugdutt, B.I., Hutchins, G.M., Bulkley, B.H., and Becker, L.C.: Infarct size reduction by prostacyclin after coronary occlusion in conscious dogs. Clin. Res. *27:*177A, 1979.

Koch-Weser, J.: Myocardial actions of angiotensin. Circ. Res. *14:*337–344, 1964.

Koch-Weser, J.: Nature of the inotropic action of angiotensin on ventricular myocardium. Circ. Res. *16:*230–237, 1965.

Lefer, A.M.: Influence of mineralocorticoids and cations on the inotropic effect of angiotensin and norepinephrine in isolated cardiac muscle. Am. Heart J. *73:*674–680, 1967.

Lefer, A.M.: Role of a myocardial depressant factor in the pathogenesis of circulatory shock. Fed. Proc. *29:*1836–1847, 1970.

Lefer, A.M.: Role of a myocardial depressant factor in shock states. Mod. Concepts Cardiovasc. Dis. *42:*59–64, 1973a.

Lefer, A.M.: Blood borne humoral factors in the pathophysiology of circulatory shock. Circ. Res. *32:*129–139, 1973b.

Lefer, A.M.: Myocardial depressant factor and circulatory shock. Klin. Wochenschrift *52:*358–370, 1974.

Lefer, A.M.: Properties of cardio-inhibitory factors produced in shock. Fed. Proc. *37:*2734–2740, 1978.

Lefer, A.M.: Role of prostaglandin-thromboxane system in vascular homeostasis during shock. Circ. Shock *6:*297–303, 1979.

Lefer, A.M., and Barenholz, Y.: Pancreatic hydrolases and the formation of a myocardial depressant factor in shock. Am. J. Physiol. *223:*1103–1109, 1972.

Lefer, A.M., and Blattberg, B.: Comparison of the effects of two factors present in plasma of shocked animals. J. Reticuloendothel. Soc. *5:*54–60, 1968.

Lefer, A.M., and Glenn, T.M.: Corticosteroids and the lysosomal protease-MDF system; In *Glenn Corticosteroids in the Therapy of Shock*, edited by T.M. Glenn, pp. 233–251. University Park Press, Baltimore, 1974.

Lefer, A.M., and Inge, T.M.: Differentiation of a myocardial depressant factor present in shock plasma from known plasma peptides and salts. Proc. Soc. Exp. Biol. Med. *142:* 429–433, 1973.

Lefer, A.M., and Martin, J.: Relationship of plasma peptides to the myocardial depressant factor in hemorrhagic shock in cats. Circ. Res. *26:*59–69, 1970.

Lefer, A.M., and Smith, E.F., III: Protective action of prostacyclin in myocardial ischemia and trauma. In *Prostacyclin*, edited by J.R. Vane and S. Bergström, pp. 339–347. Raven Press, New York, 1979.

Lefer, A.M., and Spath, J.A., Jr.: Pancreatic hypoperfusion and the production of a myocardial depressant factor in hemorrhagic shock. Ann. Surg. *179:*868–876, 1974.

Lefer, A.M., and Trachte, G.J.: Effects of hormones on heart. In *Hearts and Heart-like Organs*, edited by G.H. Bourne, vol. 2, pp. 1–40. Academic Press, New York, 1980.

Lefer, A.M., Glenn, T.M., Lopez-Rasi, A.M., Kiechel, S.F., Ferguson, W.W., and Wangensteen, S.L.: Mechanism of the lack of a beneficial response to inotropic agents in hemorrhagic shock. Clin. Pharmacol. Ther. *12:*506–516, 1971.

Lefer, A.M., Ogletree, M.L., Smith, J.B., Silver, M.J., Nicolaou, K.C., Barnette, W.E., and Gasic, G.P.: Prostacyclin: profile of a potentially valuable agent for preserving jeopardized myocardial tissue in acute myocardial ischemia. Science *200:* 52–54, 1978.

Lefer, A.M., Sollott, S.J., and Galvin, M.J.: Beneficial actions of prostacyclin in traumatic shock. Prostaglandins *17:*761–767, 1979.

Lefer, A.M., Araki, H., Smith, J.B., Nicolaou, K.C., and Magolda, R.: Protective effects of a novel thromboxane analog in lethal traumatic shock. Prostaglandins Med. *3:*139–146, 1979.

Lefer, A.M., Smith, E.F. III, Araki, H., Smith, J.B., Aharony, D., Claremon, D.A., Magolda, R.L., and Nicolaou, K.C.: Dissociation of vasoconstrictor and platelet aggregatory activities of thromboxane by carbocyclic thromboxane A_2, a stable analog of thromboxane A_2. Proc. Natl. Acad. Sci. *77:* 1706–1710, 1980.

Lewy, I., Smith, J.B., Silver, M.J., Saia, J., Walinsky, P., and Wiener, L.: Detection of thromboxane B_2 in peripheral blood of patients with Prinzmetal's angina. Prostaglandins Med. *5:* 243–248, 1979.

Litvin, Y., Leffler, J.H., Barenholz, Y., and Lefer, A.M.: Factors influencing the *in vitro* production of a myocardial depressant factor. Biochem. Med. *8:*199–212, 1973.

Lorber, V.: The action of angiotonin on the completely isolated mammalian heart. Am. Heart J. *23:*37–42, 1942.

Marcus, A.J.: The role of lipids in platelet function: with particular reference to the arachidonic acid pathway. J. Lipid Res. *19:*793–826, 1978.

Mayer, S.E., Namm, D.H., and Rice, L.: Effect of glucagon on cyclic 3'5'-AMP, phosphorylase activity and contractility of heart muscle of the rat. Circ. Res. *26:*225–234, 1970.

Miller, A.J., Ellis, A.B., and Hirsch, L.J.: Effects of increased left ventricular resistance loads on flow and composition of cardiac lymph in the dog. Proc. Soc. Exp. Biol. Med. *116:* 392–394, 1964.

Moncada, S., and Vane, J.R.: Prostacyclin, platelet aggregation, and thrombosis. In *Platelets: A Multidisciplinary Approach*, edited by G. deGaetano and S. Garattini, pp. 239–258. Raven Press, New York, 1978.

Moncada, S., and Vane, J.R.: The role of prostacyclin in vascular tissue. Fed. Proc. *38:*66–71, 1979.

Moncada, S., Gryglewski, R.J., Bunting, S., and Vane, J.R.: An enzyme isolated from arteries transforms prostaglandin endoperoxides to an unstable substance that inhibits platelet aggregation. Nature *263:*663–665, 1976.

Moncada, S., Bunting, S., Mullane, K., Thorogood, P., and Vane, J.R.: Imidazole: A selective inhibitor of thromboxane synthetase. Prostaglandins *13:*611–618, 1979.

Morooka, S., Kobayashi, M., Takahashi, T., Takashima, Y., Sakamoto, M., and Shimamoto, T.: Experimental ischemic heart disease—Effects of synthetic thromboxane A_2. Exp. Mol. Pathol. *30:*449–457, 1979.

Morton, J.J., Semple, P.F., Ledingham, I.M., Stuart, B., Tehrani, M., Garcia, A., and McGarrity, G.: Effect of angiotensin-converting enzyme inhibitor (SQ 20881) on plasma concentration of angiotensin I, angiotensin II, and arginine vasopressin in the dog during hemorrhagic shock. Circ. Res. *41:*301–308, 1977.

Murthy, V.S., Waldron, T.L., Goldberg, M.E., and Vollmer, R.R.: Inhibition of angiotensin converting enzyme by SQ 14,225 in conscious rabbits. Eur. J. Pharmacol. *46:*207–212, 1977.

Needleman, P., and Marshall, G.R.: Angiotensin antagonists: Overview and projection. Fed. Proc. *35:*2486–2487, 1976.

Needleman, P., Minkes, M., and Raz, A.: Thromboxanes: Selective biosynthesis and distinct biological properties. Science *193:*163–165, 1976a.

Needleman, P., Moncada, S., Bunting, S., and Vane, J.R.: Identification of an enzyme in platelet microsomes which generate thromboxane A_2 from prostaglandin endoperoxides. Nature *261:*558–560, 1976b.

Needleman, P., Raz, A., Minkes, M.S., Ferrendelli, J.A., and Sprecher, H.: Triene prostaglandins: Prostacyclin and thromboxane biosynthesis and unique biological properties. Proc. Natl. Acad. Sci. U.S.A. *76:*944–948, 1979.

Nicolaou, K.C., Magolda, R.L., Smith, J.B., Aharony, D., Smith, E.F., III, and Lefer, A.M.: Synthesis and biological properties of pinane-thromboxane A_2 (PTA_2). A selective inhibitor of coronary artery constriction, platelet aggregation and thromboxane formation. Proc. Nat. Acad. Sci. U.S.A. *70:*2566–2570, 1979.

Ogletree, M.L., and Lefer, A.M.: Prostaglandin induced preservation of the ischemic myocardium. Circ. Res. *42:*218–224, 1978.

Ogletree, M.J., Smith, J.B., and Lefer, A.M.: Actions of prostaglandins on isolated perfused cat coronary arteries. Am. J. Physiol. *235:*H400–H406, 1978.

Ogletree, M.L., Lefer, A.M., Smith, J.B., and Nicolaou, K.C.: Studies on the protective effect of prostacyclin in acute myocardial ischemia. Eur. J. Pharmacol. *56:*95–103, 1979.

Okuda, M., Yamada, T., and Hosono, K.: Characterization of a myocardial depressant factor isolated from cardiogenic shock. Jpn. Circ. J. *37:*1009–1017, 1973.

Peach, M.J., and Ackerly, J.A.: Angiotensin antagonists and the adrenal cortex and medulla. Fed. Proc. *35:*2502–2507, 1978.

Robertson, A., and Khairallah, P.A.: Angiotensin II: Rapid localization in nuclei of smooth and cardiac muscle. Science *172:*1138–1139, 1971.

Rogel, S., and Hilewitz, H.: Cardiac impairment and shock factors. Fed. Proc. *37:*2718–2723, 1978.

Schrör, K., Smith, E.F.III, Bickerton, M., Smith, J.B., Nicolaou, K.C., Magolda, R., and Lefer, A.M.: Preservation of the ischemic myocardium by pinane thromboxane. Am. J. Physiol. *238:*H87–H92, 1980.

Shimamoto, T., Kobayashi, M., Takahashi, T., Motomiya, T., Numano, F., and Morooka, S.: Heart attack induced experimentally with thromboxane A_2. Proc. Jpn. Acad. *53:*38–42, 1977.

Smith, E.F.,III, Ogletree, M.L., Sherwin, J.R., and Lefer, A.M.: Effects of prostaglandins on distribution of blood flow in the cat. Prostaglandins Med. *1:*411–418, 1978.

Smith, E.F.,III, Smith, J.B., and Lefer, A.M.: Role of arachidonic acid products in early myocardial ischemia. Fed. Proc. *38:*1037, 1979.

Smith, E.F.,III, Tabas, J.H., and Lefer, A.M.: Beneficial actions of imidazole in endotoxin shock. Prostaglandins Med. *4:* 215–225, 1980.

Spath, J.A., Jr., Gorczynski, R.J., and Lefer, A.M.: Pancreatic perfusion in the pathophysiology of hemorrhagic shock. Am. J. Physiol. *226:*443–451, 1974.

Szczeklik, A., Gryglewski, R.J., Nizankowski, R., Skawinski, S., Szcseklik, J., and Gluszki, P.: Treatment of peripheral artery disease with prostacyclin. *Proceedings of the 4th International Prostaglandin Conference*, p. 114. 1979.

Terashita, Z., Fukui, H., Nishikawa, K., Hirata, M., and Kikuchi, S.: Coronary vasospastic action of thromboxane A_2 in isolated, working guinea pig hearts. Eur. J. Pharmacol. *53:* 49–56, 1978.

Trachte, G.J., and Lefer, A.M.: Beneficial action of a new angiotensin converting enzyme inhibitor (SQ 14,225) in hemorrhagic shock. Circ. Res. *43:*577–582, 1978.

Trachte, G.J., and Lefer, A.M.: Cardiac and splanchnic vascular consequences of angiotensin II infusion in cats. Fed. Proc. *38:*114, 1979a.

Trachte, G.J., and Lefer, A.M.: Effect of angiotensin II receptor blockade by (Sar^1, Ala^8) angiotensin II (Saralasin) in hemorrhagic shock. Am. J. Physiol. *236:*280–285, 1979b.

Trachte, G.J., and Lefer, A.M.: Mechanism of the protective effect of angiotensin-converting enzyme inhibition in hemorrhagic shock. Proc. Soc. Exp. Biol. Med. *162:*54, 1979c.

Trachte, G.J., and Lefer, A.M.: Inotropic and vasoactive effects of the naturally occurring angiotensins in isolated cat cardiac muscle and coronary arteries. Res. Commun. Chem. Pathol. Pharmacol. *25:*419, 1979d.

Trachte, G.J., and Lefer, A.M.: Prostaglandin-mediated angiotensin induced vasoconstriction in isolated cat arteries. Blood Vessels *17:*196–201, 1980.

Trapnell, J.E., Rigby, C.C., Talbot, C.H., and Duncan, E.H.L.: A controlled trial of Trasylol in the treatment of acute pancreatitis. Br. J. Surg. *61:*177–182, 1974.

Turini, G.A., Brunner, H.R., Ferguson, R.K., Rivier, J.L., and Gavras, H.: Angiotensin II blockade in congestive heart failure. Arch. Int. Pharmacodyn. Ther. *233:*166–176, 1978.

Wangensteen, S.L., deHoll, J.D., Kiechel, S.F., Martin, J., and Lefer, A.M.: Influence of hemodialysis on a myocardial depressant factor in hemorrhagic shock. Surgery 67:935–943, 1970.

Wangensteen, S.L., Geissinger, W.T., Lovett, A.L., Glenn, T.M., and Lefer, A.M.: Relationship between splanchnic blood flow and a myocardial depressant factor in endotoxin shock. Surgery 69:410–418, 1971.

Wexler, B.C.: Opposing effects of deoxycorticosterone and spironolactone on isoprenaline-induced myocardial infarction. Cardiovasc. Res. 13:119–126, 1979.

Williams, L.F., Goldberg, A.H., Polansky, B.J., and Byrne, J.J.: Myocardial effects of acute intestinal ischemia. Surgery 66: 138–144, 1969.

Williams, A.D., Mandell, G.L., and Lefer, A.M.: Phagocytosis and bactericidal activity of leucocytes in hemorrhagic shock. Infec. Immunity 2:345–346, 1970.

CHAPTER 13

Microcirculation in Shock—Clinical Review

WATTS R. WEBB
RICHARD A. BRUNSWICK

The microcirculation is rarely primary in the development of shock but in its reactive role plays a most important part in the development and perpetuation of shock states. Regulation of perfusion to the tissues is controlled in vessels less than 300 μ, and often becomes the dominant theme regardless of the initiating factor. The "major" systemic vascular and "minor" pulmonary vascular systems often respond quite differently to the same agents. Similarly, there are more forces operating on the pulmonary vascular tree than on the systemic vessels.

Resistance in the microcirculation can be approximated by evaluation of the tone of the arterioles, capillaries, and veins. Resistance is, of course, altered by blood flow, viscosity, particulate obstruction (produced by such things as the platelet or red or white cell aggregates), and the architectural arrangements of the microvessels. The major control of resistance is achieved through regulation of local tone. The constrictor-dilator mechanisms are controlled primarily by the nervous system but, likewise, are influenced by local tissue metabolites and the circulating vasoactive substances.

In addition, there are local factors regulating the different regions and organs of the body. As a general statement, however, it can be said that in shock, blood flow is preserved primarily in the heart and brain at the expense of virtually all other organs. Similarly, blood flow is better preserved in the low pressure portal system than in the kidney or other abdominal organs. For a more complete understanding of various organ differences in microcirculation there are excellent reviews, such as the symposium, *Microcirculation as Related to Shock* (Sapro and Fulton, 1968).

ARTERIOLES

Vascular tone of microcirculation is controlled primarily by the smooth muscle cells associated with the peripheral blood vessels—the arterioles, precapillary sphincters, and venules. The arterioles constitute about 80% of total peripheral resistance in the normal state, though in low flow states or other abnormalities the venous resistance may constitute more than half of the peripheral resistance. Regulation of blood flow to the exchange vessels is determined both by the tone of the arterioles and the precapillary sphincters. These latter are only one or two smooth muscle cells wrapped around the arterioles at the origin of the capillaries. Their action controls the effective capillary surface and endocapillary distance and, thus, the network surface available for metabolic change. In response to hypovolemia, the arteriolar resistance vessels respond to sympathetic vasoconstrictor nerve activity. The most sensitive element appears to be the precapillary sphincters which, within a few minutes of anoxia, lose their response to nerve stimulation. The decreased response appears to be due to diminished local blood flow with its relative ischemia and anoxia (Stevens, 1979). Other factors known to change the tone of the arterioles are listed in Table 13.1. The catecholamines released by the sympathetic nerves locally are the most important factor but even these are modified by interreaction with various local humoral, rheologic, and extrinsic toxic factors.

Histamine, bradykinin, and serotonin are known to be released from damaged tissue, mast cells, and platelets. The effect of serotonin can be prevented, or at least decreased, by thrombocytopenia (Bredenberg et al., 1977) and massive doses of heparin, lysergic acid diethyl amide, or methysergide. The prostaglandins formed in vessel walls react directly on the systemic arterial pressure largely by decreasing peripheral vascular resistance. The prostaglandin released from platelets is a vasoconstrictor. The other important agents for dilating the systemic arterioles are β stimulators and the smooth muscle dilators such as nitroglycerin and nitroprusside and histamine one stimulators.

VEINS

The small veins have a large amount of smooth muscle, are richly innervated, and have the ability to control capillary flow. Thus, they are particularly important in determining capillary hydrostatic pressure. The balance between capillary pressure and plasma colloid osmotic pressure, in large measure, controls the flux of fluid between the vascular and extracellular fluid compartments. Any rise in postcapillary pressure or resistance tends to raise capillary pressure and shift fluid into the interstitial pressures. Similarly, a fall in postcapillary resistance favors the movement of fluid from the interstitial space into the blood (Pappenheimer and Soto-Rivera, 1948).

Capacitance vessels (capillaries, venules, and veins) are important because they contain 60% of total blood volume. If they were maximally dilated, they could contain greater than the normal circulating volume. Thus, venous vasomotor status is a very important determinant of cardiac output due to its substantial influence on return of blood to the heart or preload.

The factors which affect tone of the veins are shown in Table 13.2. In intact man, variations in PO_2 probably play little role in the control of venomotor tone. It is significant that the veins remain responsive in the presence of ischemia and anoxia after the arterioles have lost tone and become dilated (Vanhoutte and Janssess, 1978). This tends to increase microvascular pressure in the postarterial bed and promote the development of edema.

Table 13.1
Arterioles

Constrict	Dilate
Catecholamines	Histamine, bradykinin
Renin-angiotensin	K^+, H^+
Vasopressin	PGI_2, PGE_1
PGA_1-PGF	Lactic acid, adenosine
Correction hypoxia	Hypoxia, hypercapnea

Table 13.2
Veins

Constrict	Dilate
Catecholamines	Histamine
Renin-angiotensin	PGI_2
Serotonin	PGE_1
Bradykinin	Hypoxia, late
PGA_2-PGF_{2a}	

Table 13.3
Capillaries

Dilate	Obstruct
Histamine	Mechanical
Serotonin	Edema
Gravity	Cell aggregates
Venous hypertension	Viscosity

The major role of the veins is to adjust the capacity of the vascular system to ensure appropriate return to the heart. This also forms a major determinant of capillary pressure. Veins can behave as a passive reservoir or react strongly due to their sympathetically innervated muscle. The muscular capacitance vessels under sympathetic control act as an active blood mobilization system, whereas cutaneous veins function more in thermoregulation. Thus, the local effect of temperature is of great importance for the cutaneous veins.

The metabolic regulatory factors, such as anoxia and acidosis, have a lesser effect on venous function in contrast to their very marked effect on the precapillary level. Many neurohumoral substances—histamine, ADP, and acetylcholine—modulate the function of adrenergic nerves and smooth muscle cells in the vein. Frequently used therapeutic agents, such as nitrates or digitalis, can dilate the veins and anesthetics like halothane reduce cardiovascular function by lowering venous return.

CAPILLARIES

The major factors that affect flow through the capillaries are shown in Table 13.3. The capillaries have no intrinsic constrictor mechanism of their own and are thus much more susceptible to extrinsic influences.

PULMONARY RESISTANCE

The pulmonary vascular system, in many respects, responds quite differently from the systemic vasculature (Bergofsky, 1974). Most notable is the response to hypoxia—whether alveolar, arterial, or cellular—which is a rise in pulmonary arteriolar tone (Berry et al., 1965). This has the beneficial effect of reducing blood flow to poorly ventilated areas of the lung, which reduces ventilation perfusion inequities. In sharp contrast, the peripheral arteriolar system is dilated by hypoxia, which increases flow to the ischemic area. Acidosis—whether respiratory or metabolic, or due to increased hydrogen ions such as in aspirated gastric acids—similarly causes increased arteriolar resistance in the lung. Various drugs that increase pulmonary vascular resistance are shown in Table 13.4. In addition, the effect of these agents may be enhanced by β blockade and reduced by α blockade (Porcelli and Bergofsky, 1973). The effects of hypoxia and hypercapneic acidosis are similarly increased by β blockade and reduced by α blockade. α and β blockade depress and enhance, respectively, the vasoconstrictor responses to angiotensin, histamine, epinephrine, and norepinephrine but do not affect the response to serotonin. Various drugs which cause pulmonary vasodilation are shown in Table 13.5.

Physical factors likewise play a significant role in pulmonary vascular resistance. Atelectasis drastically increases resistance by collapsing the capillaries and causing local hypoxia. Overdistension compresses the low pressure capillary bed. With rising alveolar pressures, the pulmonary arterial pressure must rise synchronously to maintain flow. The optimal spatial configuration and lowest resistance coincide with the inflation level of the normal functional residual capacity (Fig. 13.1).

In hypovolemia, systemic resistance may double, but pulmonary resistance may rise manyfold (Fig. 13.2). With restoration of intravascular volume, this response is often aggravated, as the peripheral and pulmonary vasoconstriction is not reversed as quickly as the volume is restored. The overpowering systemic vasoconstriction forces the blood into the lesser circuit, even to produce pulmonary edema.

The prostaglandins, a group of 20 carbon fatty acids and their metabolites, are widely distributed throughout the body and are known to contribute to the regulation of circulation in virtually every organ system in the body. This regulatory function is unusual because the individual organ itself often synthesizes and controls the manner in which its prostaglandins influence function locally. In general, the prostaglandins with two double bonds, such as PGA_2 and PGE_2, tend to cause vasoconstriction, whereas those with a single bond, particularly PGE_1 and the prostacyclines (PGI_2), produce vasodilation, espe-

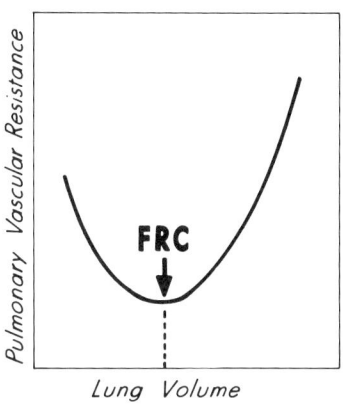

Figure 13.1. Graph showing relationship of pulmonary vascular resistance to lung volume. Note that resistance rises both with progressive atelectasis and with increasing inflation of the lung. Most of the resistance measured here occurs in the alveolar capillaries.

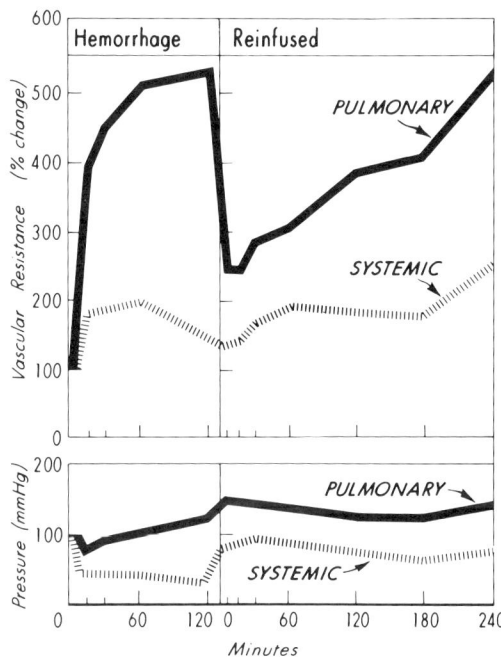

Figure 13.2. Graph comparing systemic and pulmonary pressures and resistance during hemorrhage and reinfusion. Note the much greater increase in resistance in the lung both during hypothermia and after restoration of blood volume.

Table 13.4
Drugs Which Cause Pulmonary Vasodilation

Aminophylline	Nitroprusside
Chlorpromazine	Phentolamine
Dilantin	PGE_1
Isoproterenol	PGA_1
Minipres	PGI_2 (Prostacyclin)
Morphine	Tolazoline
Nitroglycerine	

Table 13.5
Drugs Which Increase PVR

Cyclopropane	Procaine
Dinitrophenol	Propranolol
Dopamine	Prostaglandins
Histamine	Serotonin
Meperidine	Tetracaine
Norepinephrine	Thromboxane
Potassium cyanide	Tyramine

cially in the pulmonary system (Hyman et al., 1978). These agents are not available for clinical use at this time. They can, however, be regulated within the body by the utilization of aspirin and indomethacin and other potent nonsteroidal anti-inflammatory agents which prevent conversion of fatty acid moieties to prostaglandins (Vane, 1971).

One of the key responses to shock in the dog is postcapillary or small vein constriction in the lung, even during the shock phase. This is augmented as interstitial edema and capillary congestion further restrict capillary blood flow (Murakami et al., 1970). Pulmonary reimplantation was found experimentally to be one of the few effective methods for preventing the congestive atelectasis in the lung secondary to hemorrhagic shock, again suggesting that this entity is, in part, neurally controlled (Sugg et al., 1968a and b). The work of Bredenberg et al. (1980) most recently demonstrated that this pulmonary venous constriction in response to hypovolemia alone does not occur in the baboon, suggesting that this probably does not occur in man. It is very possible, however, that secondary factors, such as trauma with the release of serotonin, prostaglandins, and other venoactive agents, may produce venoconstriction. Other factors increasing capillary permeability in trauma and shock are bacteremia, endotoxin, histamine, complement, and inhaled irritants. Moss et al. (1971) demonstrated that cerebral hypoxia can produce a full blown picture of congestive atelectasis in primates and that this is prevented in the reimplanted lung. These findings likewise suggest a cerebral factor which is mediated through the sympathetic system.

CAPILLARY FACTORS CONTROLLING FLUID FLUX

Fluid flux across the capillary membrane, whether systemic or pulmonary, is related to the Starling equation as modified by Kedem and Katchalsky (1961):

$$J_v = Kfc[(P_c - P_t) - \sigma_c(\pi_p - \pi_t)].$$

where J_v = net volume flow (ml/min/100 g of tissue); Kfc = capillary filtration coefficient (ml/min/100 g/mm Hg driving pressure); P_c = capillary hydrostatic pressure (mm Hg); P_t interstitial hydrostatic pressure (mm Hg); σ_c = reflection coefficient of plasma protein ($\sigma_c = 1$ if the membrane is impermeable to the molecule, and $\sigma_c = 0$ if the molecule crosses the membrane as easily as water); π_p = colloid osmotic pressure of the plasma colloids; π_t = the colloid osmotic pressures of the tissues (mm Hg). π is best described by a cubic equation for plasma proteins, i.e., π_p (mm Hg) = 2.8c prot + 0.16 c^2 prot + 0.09c^3 prot.

The reflection coefficient refers to the permeability of the capillaries to protein varying in different organs and in response to different pathologic changes. In the lung, an increase in capillary permeability to larger molecules occurs not only in inflammatory processes but also at high capillary pressures due to the stretched pore phenomenon. A high capillary pressure or a low oncotic pressure favors the egress of fluid from the capillary bed.

In clinical practice, it is unusual for accumulations of peripheral edema to have any very significant effect on tissue survival. On the other hand, relatively small amounts of pulmonary edema can be deleterious.

SAFETY FACTORS

As a result of any imbalance which allows fluid filtration into the interstitium, there is an increase in tissue pressure and lymph flow and decreased interstitial colloid oncotic pressure. The lymph drainage will remove interstitial proteins, decreasing the oncotic effect above the simple dilution effect. Lung lymph flow may increase 20 times the normal to help prevent edema, and this can provide approximately a -7 mm Hg safety factor against edema. By adding the individual safety factors, one can estimate that capillary filtration forces must be increased by 18 or 19 mm Hg before gross edema occurs (Drake and Taylor, 1975; Vergilio et al., 1979).

Acute hypoproteinemia, as is seen after resuscitation with crystalloid solutions, can cause a one-third to one-half reduction in plasma oncotic pressure. All tissues respond to any sudden decrease in plasma oncotic pressure by accumulating fluid in the interstitial spaces. The greatest percentage increase has been found in the lung which may require up to 50 hr to return to normal (Granger et al., 1978).

Intravascular volume can be supported with colloid-free electrolyte solution, but replacement of approximately four to five times the blood volume is required from the beginning of blood loss. This generalized overexpansion of the body's extracellular space and decreased oncotic pressure results in an increase in the interstitial volume of the pulmonary parenchyma (Granger et al., 1978). It is not surprising that acute respiratory distress is frequent in patients in hemorrhagic or burn shock who have lost large quantities of intravascular colloids and have had their intravascular volume maintained with crystalloid (Doty et al., 1978; Labandter et al., 1979).

Experience with burns shows generalized edema of all tissues including the lungs in patients resuscitated using only electrolyte solutions. Resuscitation with hypertonic saline solution with albumin requires roughly 1.8 ml/kg/1% body surface burn as compared to 4 ml of lactated Ringer's solution. The former produces no demonstrable edema of unburned tissue, intestine, or lung even in the patient with respiratory burns. Thus, the theorized generalized capillary permeability of burns is primarily a washout phenomenon of the massive noncolloid therapy. This is supported by the studies of Jelenko et al. (1978, 1979a and b) showing early, normal flux of ^{131}I albumin in burn patients treated with a hypertonic saline albumin solution. Interestingly, the calculated total amount of sodium given, to full resuscitation, is the same by both methods.

This concept is supported, at least by experimental studies, demonstrating that there is increased vascular permeability as shown by increased water content and protein leakage only in the area of the thermal burn—not in distant areas. Segments of skin in burned rats showed water content to be maximal at 3 hr postburn with no increase elsewhere (Bruhar et al., 1978). Similarly, albumin leakage was maximal in the burned skin at 30 min but disappeared by 12 hr postinjury, with no albumin extravasation in nonburned areas. There was never an increase in water content or albumin leakage in tissues or organs not directly injured by burn. Similar clinical studies in burns show no increase in lung water when lesser volumes of fluid containing albumin are used (Morgan et al., 1978). Overall, the most important determinant of flux of water in pulmonary interstitial tissues probably relates to the differential pressure between the colloid oncotic pressure and the pulmonary microvascular pressure. So long as the oncotic pressure is more than 8 mm above the microvascular capillary pressure there is minimal chance of edema. Between 3 and 8 mm Hg it is possible; below 3 mm Hg it is quite probable that pulmonary edema will occur in response to other factors.

PRINCIPLES OF MICROCIRCULATORY REGULATION

In response to fluid loss in traumatic shock, hemorrhage, burns, and other forms of hypovolemic shock, systemic and pulmonary vasculature respond with increased tone and markedly increased resistance at the arteriolar and possibly the venous level. Response to fluid replacement is not always accompanied with appropriate reduction in vascular resistance, which leads to increasing local edema. Accordingly, along with restoration of intravascular volume, which preferably should be done with a colloid solution that will remain within the vascular tree, one must take cognizance of vascular resistance—both in the systemic and pulmonary circuits—and reduce it to normal or even subnormal. Obviously these must be done simultaneously. Vascular resistance can be reduced, e.g., by an infusion of nitroglycerin or nitroprusside. This should be accompanied by monitoring of the cardiac output, central venous pressure, pulmonary systolic and diastolic pressures, and the pulmonary arterial wedge pressure. In the presence of an elevated left atrial pressure (pulmonary arterial wedge pressure) which may significantly increase overall pulmonary vascular resistance, it is important to improve cardiac function by inotropic agents such as dopamine or a dilute adrenalin solution. At the same time, the afterload of the heart may need to be reduced. This is usually accomplished by the same infusion of nitroglycerin and nitroprusside or the use of chlorpromazine (Thorazine).

Thus, it is essential to take cognizance of the vascular tone in the pulmonary and systemic circulations, to increase vascular volume compatible with the pressure and tone of the vessels, and to maintain these in equilibrium as the diminished volume, diminished cardiac output, and increased vascular tone are returned to normal.

References

Berry, W., McLaughlin, J., Clark, W., and Morrow, A.: The effects of acute hypoxia on pressure, flow, and resistance in the pulmonary vascular bed. Surgery 58:404, 1965.
Bergofsky, E.H.: Mechanisms underlining vasomotor regulation of regional pulmonary blood flow in normal and diseased states. Am. J. Med. 57:378, 1974.
Bredenberg, C., Taylor, G., and Webb, W.: Thrombocytopenia altering the pulmonary hemodynamic response to intravenous endotoxin. ACS Surgical Forum 28:186, 1977.
Bredenberg, C.E., Nomoto, S., and Webb, W.R.: Pulmonary and systemic hemodynamics during hemorrhagic shock in baboons. Ann. Surg. 192(1):86, 1980.
Bruhar, B.H., Carvajal, H.F., and Liners, H.A.: Burn edema and protein leakage in the rat: 1. Relationship to time of injury. Microvasc. Res. 15:221, 1978.
Doty, D.B., Hofnagel, H.V., Mosley, R.V.: The distribution of body fluid following hemorrhage and resuscitation in combat casualities. Surg. Gynecol. Obstet. 130:453, 1978.
Drake, R.E., and Taylor, A.E.: The relative importance of net capillary filtration pressure, tissue pressure and tissue fluid colloid osmotic pressure in opposing pulmonary edema. Physiologist 18:197, 1975.
Granger, D.N., Gabel, J.C., Drake, R.E., et al.: Physiologic basis for the clinical use of albumin solutions. Surg. Gynecol. Obstet. 146:96, 1978.
Hyman, A.L., Spannhake, F.W., and Kadowitz, P.J.: Prostaglandins and the lung. Am. Rev. Resp. Dis. 117:111, 1978.
Jelenko, C., Wheeler, M.L., Callaway, B.D., et al.: Studies in shock and resuscitation II: Volume repletion with minimal edema using the "HALFD" method. JACEP 7:326, 1978.
Jelenko, C., Williams, J.B., Wheeler, M.L., et al.: Studies in shock and resuscitation I: Use of a hypertonic albumin-containing fluid demand regimen (HALFD) in resuscitation. J. Crit. Care Med. 7:57, 1979a.
Jelenko, C., Solenberger, R.I., Wheeler, M.L., et al.: Studies in shock and resuscitation III: Accurate refractometric COP determinations in hypovolemia treated with HALFD. JACEP 8:253, July, 1979b.
Kedem, O., and Katchalsky, A.: A physical interpretation of the phenomenological coefficients of membrane permeability. J. Gen. Physiol. 45:143, 1961.
Labandter, H.P., Wax, S.D., and Webb, W.R.: Hypertonic albuminated (HAL) solution burn resuscitation study. Presented at the American Burn Association Meeting, March, 1979.
Morgan, A., Knight, B., and O'Connor, N.: Lung water changes after thermal burns. Ann. Surg. 187:288, 1978.
Moss, G., Staunton, C., and Stein, A.: Cerebral hypoxia as the primary event in the pathogenesis of the "Shock Lung Syndrome." Surg. Forum 22:211, 1971.
Murakami, T., Wax, S., and Webb, W.: Pulmonary microcirculation in hemorrhagic shock. Surg. Forum 21:25, 1970.
Pappenheimer, J.R., and Soto-Rivera, A.: Effective osmotic pressure of the plasma proteins and other quantities associated with the capillary circulation in the hindlimbs of cats and dogs. Am. J. Physiol. 152:471, 1948.
Porcelli, R.J., and Bergofsky, E.H.: Adrenergic receptors in pulmonary vasoconstrictor responses to gases and humoral agents. J. Appl. Physiol. 34:483, 1973.
Sapro, D., and Fulton, G.P. (Eds.): *Microcirculation as Related to Shock*. Academic Press, New York, 1968.
Stevens, K.M.: Anoxemia as the cause of death in shock. Med. Hypotheses 5:699, 1979.
Sugg, W., Webb, W., and Ecker, R.: Prevention of lesions of the lung secondary to hemorrhagic shock. Surg. Gynecol. Obstet. 127:1005, 1968a.
Sugg, W., Webb, W., Nakae, S., Theodorides, T., et al.: Congestive atelectasis an experimental study. Ann. Surg. 168:234, 1968b.
Vane, J.R.: Inhibition of prostaglandin synthesis as a mechanism of action for aspirin-like drugs. Nature: New Biology 231:232, 1971.
Vanhoutte, P.M., and Janssess, W.J.: Local control of venous function. Microvasc. Res. 16:196, 1978.
Vergilo, R.W., Rice, C.L., Smith, D.C., et al.: Crystalloid vs. colloid resuscitation: Is one better? Surgery 85:129, 1979.

CHAPTER 14

Pathology and Pathophysiology of Disseminated Intravascular Coagulation

ROBERT M. HARDAWAY

Disseminated intravascular coagulation (DIC) may occur in a wide variety of clinical conditions. It is a relatively common phenomenon but often not diagnosed (Hardaway, 1961, 1966; Hardaway and McKay, 1959, 1963). It is defined as an acute, transient coagulation occurring in the flowing blood throughout the vascular tree and which may obstruct the microcirculation. It may or may not result in an accumulation of fibrin but does involve the transformation of fibrinogen into fibrin. It includes the agglutination of platelets and red cells and the sticking of leukocytes.

Coagulation and clot lysis are normally, continuously, and simultaneously going on within the vascular tree. The actual lining of the endothelial layer of the blood vessels may consist of a layer of fibrin, which helps to seal the vessel wall. Electron microscopy has shown fibrin fibrils on the endothelial surface. The implication of this observation is that the blood remains fluid normally in spite of a small but dynamic and continuous formation of fibrin inside the vascular tree. This hypothesis assumes that fibrinogen, which has a half-life under normal conditions of approximately 6 days, disappears from the blood because of its conversion to fibrin by the highly active blood clotting system. The fibrin then formed is removed by the fibrinolytic enzyme plasmin (fibrinolysin) or by the reticuloendothelial system (RES). The speed of fibrin accumulation will depend on the concentration of thrombin, the speed of fibrin dissolution on the concentration of fibrinolysin, and the integrity of the RES. If fibrin is not removed with the same speed as it is formed, an accumulation will occur. It can be seen that changes in this equilibrium may result in the accumulation of fibrin. A great many factors are known to shift this equilibrium toward more intravascular coagulation. Changes in this equilibrium result in DIC.

There has been some controversy as to the nomenclature of the phenomenon of DIC. Some prefer the term "consumption coagulopathy." Certainly, clotting factors are consumed in DIC but much more is involved, especially local infarction of tissues and organ failure. This name is not broad enough. Another term, reflecting the first recognition of the phenomenon, is "afibrinogenemia." This is quite inappropriate as afibrinogenemia is not common in DIC. In fact, it is the least likely of all coagulation factors to be depleted in DIC and is often above normal due to its stimulation by stress.

DIC may occur in a wide spectrum of clinical settings. Whenever DIC occurs, it greatly increases the seriousness and complications in whatever setting it takes place. For DIC to occur, there must be some thromboplastic substance which gains access to the circulating blood. There are a wide variety of substances which are known to initiate DIC. However, the mere availability of thromboplastic substances in the blood does not alone produce a continuing and clinically significant intravascular clotting. Other factors are involved in producing this, the most important is speed of blood flow in the capillaries. Slow flow promotes DIC. Other factors are also involved.

FACTORS PROMOTING DIC

Factors Related to Deficient Capillary Flow (Shock)

This is discussed first because it is essential to the initiation of DIC (Fig. 14.1). It is difficult to produce DIC without a deficient capillary flow. Shock may be due to hypovolemia, sepsis, heart failure, trauma, and many other conditions. Decreased capillary flow may be brought about by the following:

1. Decreased cardiac output as a result of hypovolemia, failure of the myocardium, increased pulmonary vascular resistance due to arteriolar constriction or obstruction.
2. Systemic arteriolar constriction secondary to sympathetic stimulation and a high catecholamine level. This decreases flow to the capillaries.
3. Opening of arteriovenous shunts also caused by sympathetic stimulation. This bypasses the capillaries and shunts blood directly into the veins.
4. Low arterial blood pressure from any cause and usually associated with the above named factors.
5. Opening of all capillaries at once. Normally, only

25% of the capillaries are open; in shock all may be open. This causes slowing of flow in all capillaries.

6. Viscosity of blood. Blood, unlike water, is not a Newtonian fluid. Its viscosity varies with its speed of flow. The slower it flows, the greater its viscosity. Whole blood may exhibit viscosities in the order of 100- to 1000-fold higher than water at near zero flow velocities. At high flow velocities, it might show a viscosity of less than

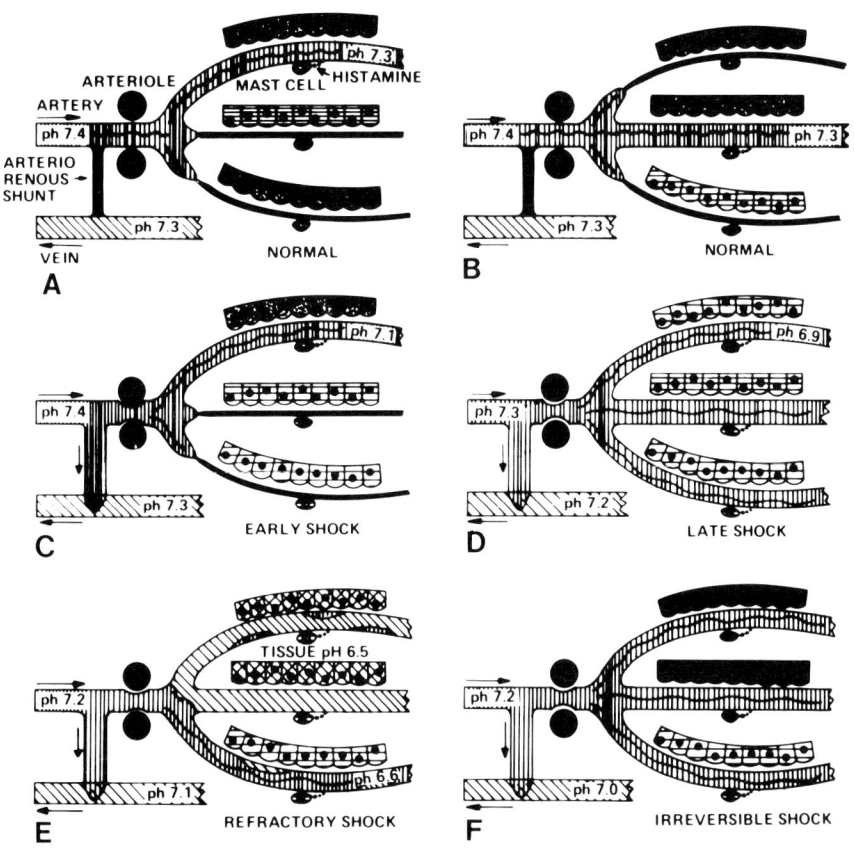

Figure 14.1. Stages in the development of irreversible shock. Diagram represents a small artery ending in an arteriole with sphincter-like action. Arteriole feeds three capillaries, each nourishing a group of cells. A, normal condition. Arteriole is fairly widely opened. Only one capillary is being perfused while the others rest. Capillaries open in rotation on demand of cells adjacent to them. Histamine secreted by mast cells along the capillaries cause capillary sphincters to open. Constant perfusion is not necessary. Blood flow through the capillaries is rapid; pH drop along the capillaries is minimal. Cells of middle capillary are becoming slightly anoxic. Arteriovenous shunt is closed. B, normal condition. Center cells have become slightly anoxic and mast cells have secreted histamine causing the central capillary to open. Upper capillary is now closed, as mast cells have stopped secreting histamine. Arteriole is fairly widely opened. C, shock, phase I (early reversible). Elevated catecholamines have caused vasoconstriction. The arteriovenous shunt has opened as a part of the catecholamine action. There may be a loss of arterial blood pressure due to poor venous return to the heart. All of these cause a slow capillary flow in the upper capillary. D, phase II shock (late reversible). Due to the long time required for adequate perfusion by the cells, because of the slow capillary flow, all capillaries are now open. The result is an expansion of the capacity of the vascular tree. Capillary flow is extremely slow, and pH fall along the capillary is marked due to anaerobic metabolism with lactic acid production. This stage is reversible by adequate volume administration. Hemorrhagic shock is always in this stage. E, phase III shock (refractory). Stage of disseminated intravascular coagulation (DIC). Stagnant acid blood in presence of sepsis or tissue injury has begun to coagulate, causing sticking of red cells—occluding the upper two capillaries. This stops perfusion in these capillaries completely. Cells nourished by these two capillaries are dying. Blood through the lower capillary is sluggish. Circulating blood is incoagulable. Lysis of clotted blood in upper capillary has already started due to endogenous fibrinolysin. F, phase IV (irreversible shock). Cells nourished by the upper two capillaries have died, producing focal tissue necrosis. Capillary clots have lysed, and circulation has been restored. However, large areas of necrosis are producing multiple organ failure, which results in death of organism.

twice that of water. Also, viscosity varies with blood composition. A high hematocrit or a high protein concentration causes a high viscosity. A high level of fibrinogen in blood predisposes the blood to DIC (Hardaway, 1980). The higher the viscosity, the slower the flow. This creates a vicious circle.

Factors Related to Hypercoagulability

This may be difficult to document but is a very real condition. Some blood coagulates faster and easier than other.

1. Acidosis may cause hypercoagulability. In fact, fully heparinized blood which is acidified to pH 7.2 will clot. If acidified to pH 6.8 it will clot very quickly. If an animal is bled to shock levels, the blood becomes more coagulable as acidosis increases. This was first noted by Hewson in the 18th century.

2. High level of clotting factors. Blood of pregnant women is high in fibrinogen and other clotting factors. Pregnant women are more susceptible to clotting than normal women. The two factors are likely related. Dogs with high fibrinogen levels are more susceptible to DIC than are normal ones. This is probably related to blood viscosity.

3. Platelet adhesiveness may increase in hemorrhagic shock, septic shock, and pregnancy. Clumping of platelets may help initiate DIC. Heparin causes platelet clumping.

4. Catecholamines. The intravenous administration of epinephrine decreases the clotting time in animals. Stimulation of splanchnic nerves does the same thing. Shock or other stress produces an elevated catecholamine level.

5. Steroids cause an increase in fibrinogen and other clotting factors as in pregnancy. The Swartzman reaction (an episode of DIC) can be produced with one injection of endotoxin in rabbits if the animal is pregnant, whereas two injections are otherwise required.

6. Fibrinolysin inhibition or absence. The administration of epsilon amino caproic acid (EACA) predisposes to DIC by inhibiting the production of fibrinolysin, which is the body's protection against the fibrin produced by DIC. A spontaneous lack of fibrinolytic activity, also, predisposes to especially marked DIC.

Factors Initiating Coagulation

1. Hemolysis of red cells liberates a thromboplastic substance into the blood. It may be a red cell thromboplastin or, more likely, the red cell stroma may act as particulate matter which is strongly thromboplastic. Hemolysis in the presence of shock produces DIC. Hemolysis alone produces only a temporary incoagulability which is quickly reversed spontaneously.

2. Bacterial toxins, both endotoxins and exotoxins, are strongly thromboplastic. Coagulase acts like thrombin but is not affected by heparin. Coagulase positive staphylococci cause immediate coagulation. Endotoxins act on platelets to cause immediate clumping and disappearance of platelets from the circulation within seconds. They also deplete all the clotting factors, and produce the Swartzman reaction in rabbits, which is DIC.

3. Amniotic fluid, acting by its cellular debris, is a strong thromboplastic agent producing DIC with incoagulability and shock. If amniotic fluid is filtered before injection into animals, it produces no effect.

4. Tissue juices, as liberated by tissue injury, are thromboplastic. This may initiate DIC in the presence of hypovolemic shock.

5. Malignant cells gaining access to the blood stream cause coagulation either locally or disseminated.

6. Antigen antibody complexes may initiate coagulation.

7. Ischemic tissue is thromboplastic when it gains access to the blood stream. This may occur in malignancy or dead fetus syndrome.

8. Anaphylaxis is a typical antigen-antibody reaction and produces DIC. The blood becomes incoagulable in anaphylactic shock.

9. Injection of thrombin or thromboplastin into animals intravenously produces a temporary and self-limiting DIC. If accompanied by hemorrhagic shock, it produces a fatal DIC.

10. Trypsin when artificially injected or absorbed from a pancreatitis is strongly thromboplastic. Its action is similar to thrombin, that is, by splitting fibrinogen to form monomer fibrin.

11. Any particulate matter from talcum powder to hemolyzed red cells stimulates coagulation. Amniotic fluid and meconium act in this way.

12. Snake venoms of the pit viper type cause intravascular coagulation and an incoagulability.

13. Thermal burns cause local thrombosis of microvessels and local necrosis. If widespread, this may produce DIC.

14. Heat stroke produces DIC, possibly by hemolysis and endothelial damage.

15. Contact of blood with foreign surfaces as in extracorporeal circulation initiates coagulation and DIC. It is particularly marked if there is capillary stagnation, as is often the case.

16. Damage to the RES. The RES removes fibrin from the circulation. If the system is occluded with an accumulation of fibrin or other material, it can no longer remove fibrin, and a mild DIC will become fulminating. The Swartzman reaction is an example of this. If the RES is occluded by DIC, it is also impaired in its function to combat bacterial infection. Thus, DIC may predispose to serious sepsis and vice versa.

Factors Related to the Vascular Wall

Injury to the intima causes the accumulation of platelets and subsequently the formation of fibrin. If intimal injury is widespread, as may be the case in a number of viral or rickettsial diseases, DIC may result.

Vicious Circles

All of the above factors may stimulate each other to form vicious circles (see diagram).

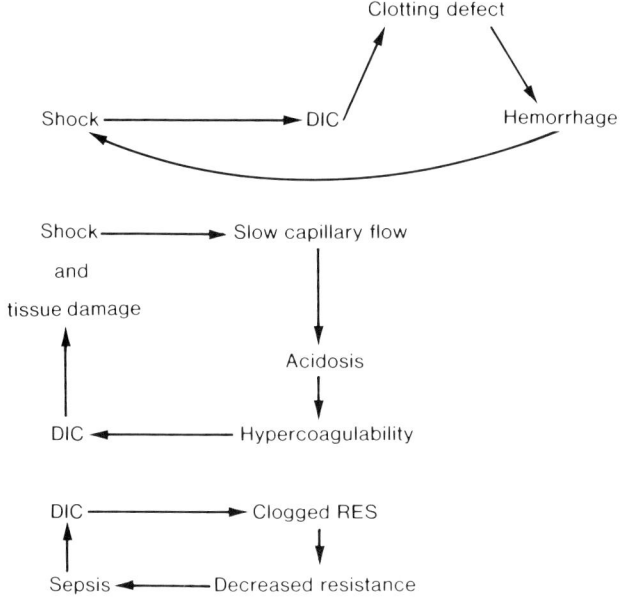

EFFECTS OF DIC

These may be categorized under four headings.

Shock

Shock is both a cause and effect of DIC, noted by a fall in arterial pressure and urine output. It is a slowing or halting of capillary perfusion and may be due to hypovolemia, sepsis, heart failure, or other causes. DIC produces shock by occluding capillaries and causing arteriolar constriction.

Rapid Development of a Coagulation Defect

The coagulation changes of DIC affect every element of coagulation. These changes may be categorized under the following headings:
1. A consumption coagulopathy consisting of Platelet agglutination and thrombocytopenia and Depletion of all clotting factors I through XIII (Table 14.1);
2. Activation of profibrinolysin to fibrinolysin; and
3. Development of anticoagulants:
   a. fibrinogen breakdown products;

Table 14.1
Clotting Factor Depletions Noted in 29 Consecutive Patients in Severe Septic or Traumatic Shock[a]

Patient	Fibrinogen	Platelets	Patient[b]		Control[b]		Factor Assays						
			PT	PTT	PT	PTT	II	V	VIII	IX	X	XI	XII
	mg/100 ml									%				
1	238	16,500	19.0	60.4	13.2	38.4							
2	228	31,000	16.2	72.8	12.5	37.6	46	59	100	57	54		
3	347	111,000	15.6	49.4	12.5	41.6							
4	359	102,000	18.0	215.8	13.2	42.5	45	66	48	2	17		95
5	542	265,000	14.5	120.5	13.0	55.0							
6	318	24,000	15.8	255.0	12.3	43.0	50	32	10	37			77
7	400	99,500	15.8	75.0	13.4	47.4	100	86	59	56			48
8	235	97,500	17.9	71.6	13.9	44.3							
9	280	16,500	19.3	61.9	14.5	48.2							
10	290	154,000	120.0	180.0	14.9	42.0							
11	650	101,500	25.4	93.4	13.5	48.3	100	63	35			26	15
12	320	8,000	22.0	86.2	12.5	41.0							
13	355	8,000	19.0	72.6	13.0	44.3	45	35	67			23	90
14	160	29,000	16.2	132.0	13.6	41.6							
15	165	3,000	37.0	263.4	13.3	46.2	23	5	3			6	18
16	150	57,000	17.8	277.0	14.3	55.9							
17	355	116,000	15.2	49.0	13.7	44.7							
18	184	13,000	26.4	207.0	13.3	44.9	6	12	54			23	29
19	355	110,000	15.2	49.0	14.5	44.8							
20	184	12,500	26.4	207.0	13.5	46.8	6	12	54			23	29
21	50	18,000	33.0	240.0	14.1	40.5							
22	605	83,000	14.9	50.5	14.3	46.5							
23	367	3,500	16.0	116.9	13.1	48.2							
24	240	15,000	52.5	107.4	12.9	35.7							
25	525	29,500	16.6	76.6	14.6	48.5							
26	325	140,000	14.4	44.9	14.2	54.7							
27	465	31,000	22.2	86.6	12.8	47.1							
28	436	33,500	17.4	52.0	12.7	47.3							
29	310	12,000	30.6	94.2	14.5	55.5							
Average	305	59,000	24.5	119	13.5	43.9	46	41	48	38	35	20	50

[a] Fibrinogen was the only factor not usually depleted.
[b] PT, prothrombin time; PTT, partial thromboplastin time.

b. activation of heparin-like substance; and
c. fibrin breakdown products.

If endotoxin is given intravenously to a dog, the circulating platelets completely disappear within seconds. This is due to their instant agglutination and their being filtered out in the microcirculation, primarily in the lungs. This mechanism accounts for the typical thrombocytopenia observed in DIC, particularly, as seen in septic shock.

Depletion of all of the known clotting factors is brought about by their being used in the clotting process, leaving the remaining unclotted blood deficient. The clotting takes place primarily in the capillaries and venules where flow is slowest, leaving the remaining unclotted and unclottable blood to circulate in the major vessels. The amount of depletion of each factor varies. The only factor which seems less susceptible to depletion is fibrinogen. Although fibrinogen was the first factor to be recognized as being depleted, it is in fact less depleted than any other in DIC and is often normal or high. This is due to its remarkably high manufacture rate, which is greatly increased by any stress including injury, shock, hemorrhage, or sepsis (Fig. 14.2).

Activation of endogenous profibrinolysin to fibrinolysin may be viewed as the body's defense mechanism to DIC. The extent of this process varies greatly with individuals. In some, very little activation takes place. These individuals are prone to fatality from DIC as the removal of fibrin from the circulation is then dependent mostly on the RES. In others, a great deal of fibrinolysin digests the fibrin and, in high concentration, also the fibrinogen, with the result that fibrinogen is destroyed, and there may be a fulminating bleeding tendency and fatal bleeding.

The appearance of endogenous anticoagulants may also be considered a protective response. There is some evidence that heparin or a heparin-like substance appears or perhaps increases over the normal level. In addition, the breakdown products of fibrin and fibrinogen are anticoagulant in nature. The anticoagulant effect of these substances may be negated, however, as a protective action against further DIC, because heparin is inactivated in low pH (Fig. 14.3).

Although arterial pH may be perfectly normal, in the presence of shock of even a mild degree with maintenance of a normal arterial pressure, pH of tissues and capillary blood may fall to low levels (pH 6.8 or less). At a pH of 7.2, heparin action is impaired and is totally absent below 7.0.

Microinfarction of Tissues

This very important effect of DIC is frequently lost sight of in the preoccupation of the physician with a clotting defect. Platelet clumping and the appearance of fibrin fibers, particularly as a coating on red cells, causes the formation of red cell and fibrin thrombi, which are most prominent in the capillaries, and other small vessels which often become completely occluded. If fibrinolysin is activated quickly and in a sufficient quantity, these microclots are quickly dissolved. They are almost always dissolved eventually, and thus are not usually seen at postmortem examination. In fact, postmortem blood is usually liquid due to fibrinolytic activity. However, if the microclots remain in place for a half hour or more, they may cause microinfarction in such vital organs as the liver, kidneys, gut, pancreas, and lungs (Figs. 14.4–14.6). If enough of this microinfarction takes place, organ function is progressively impaired and may cause organ failure of the kidney, liver, lungs, and other functions. Pulmonary failure, renal failure, liver failure, heart failure, etc., may result. A healthy organ can be as much as three fourths destroyed without evidence of organ failure because of physiological safety margins. However, old or diseased organs may fail with even a modest amount of cellular necrosis. The cellular damage may be assessed by means of enzyme determination (Figs. 14.7 and 14.8). The clinical syndromes of respiratory distress syndrome, renal failure, liver failure, skin lesions of gangrene and purpura fulminans, pseudomembranous enterocolitis, hemorrhagic pancreatitis, amniotic fluid embolism, heat stroke, anaphylactic shock, snake bite and many bacterial, viral, and rickettsial diseases are associated with DIC. Incompatible transfusion reaction, malaria, favism, sickle cell anemia, extracorporal circulation, and septicemia cause DIC.

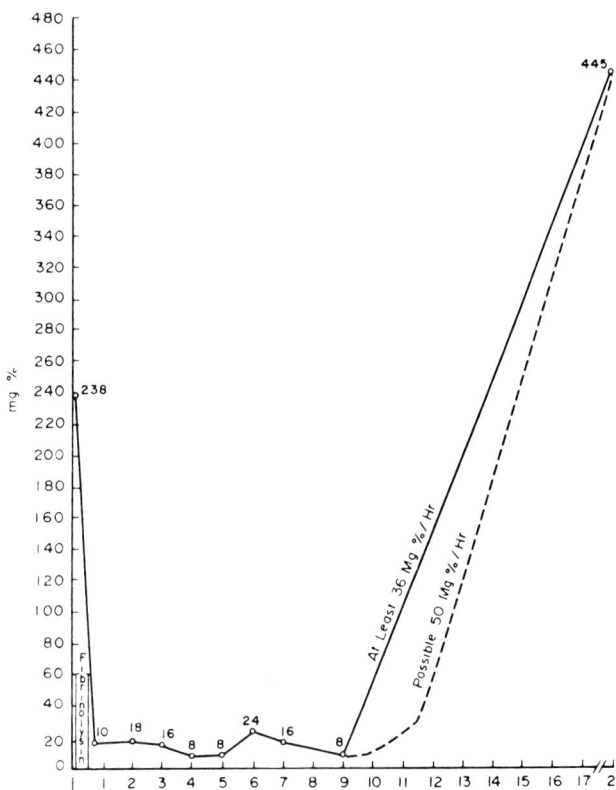

Figure 14.2. Fibrinogen in dogs was destroyed by an infusion of fibrinolysin. Note the rapid spontaneous recovery rate of fibrinogen from 8 to 445 mg/100 ml in 12 hr.

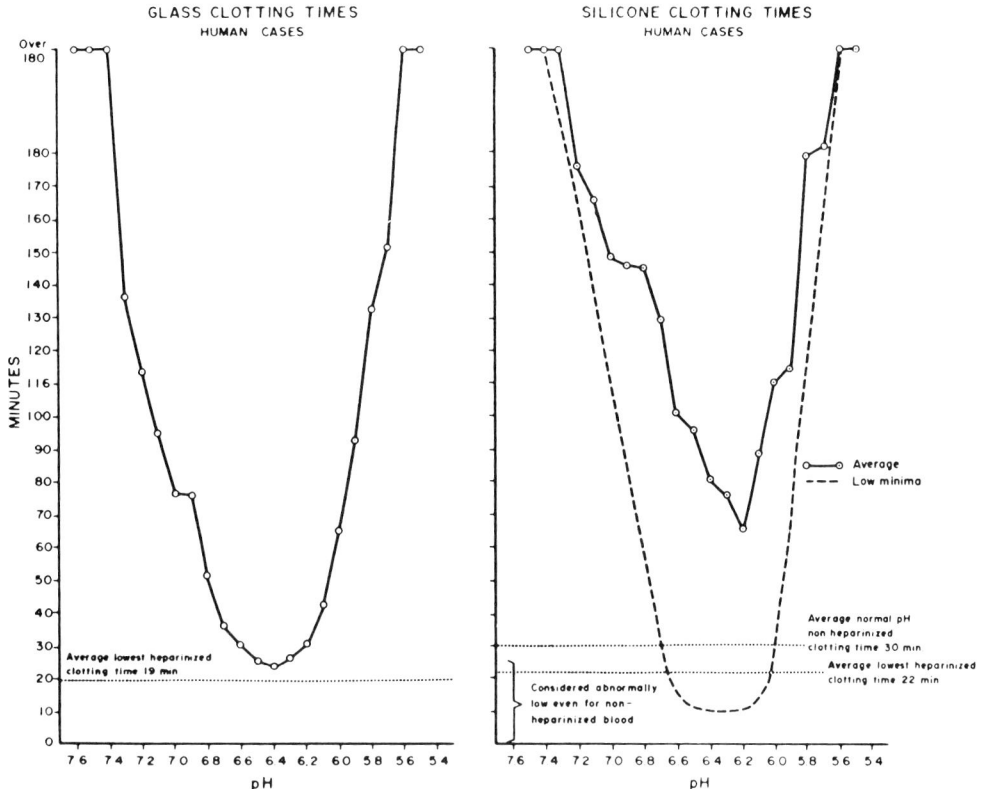

Figure 14.3. Human blood was anticoagulated with heparin and then subjected to various pH levels. Below pH 7.2, the heparin was ineffective.

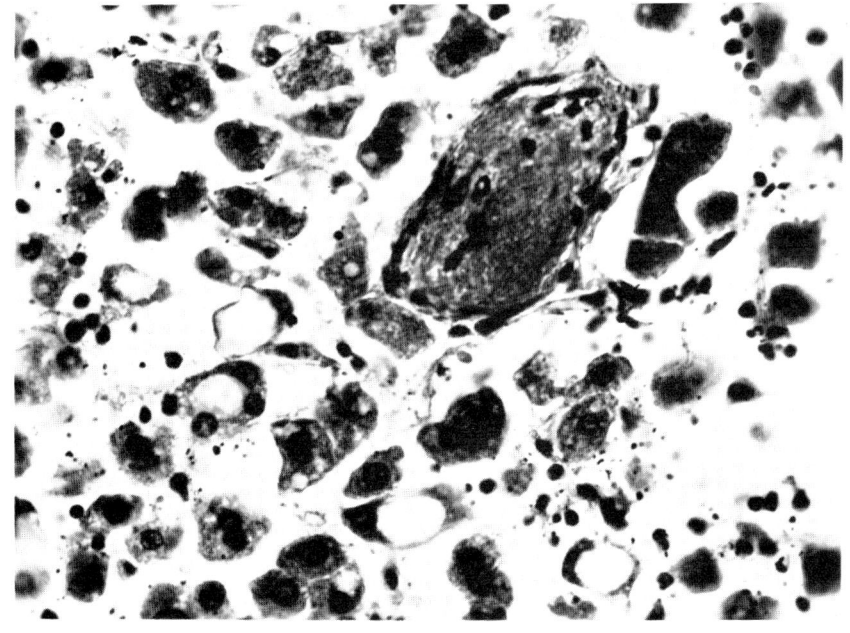

Figure 14.4. Liver of patient dying of septic shock. Note that thrombus in central vein is surrounded by an area of necrosis of liver cells.

Effects on the Body's Defenses

Bacterial toxins can initiate DIC, but DIC can also contribute to sepsis. In a study of patients with proven DIC secondary to severe disease or injury but not due to sepsis, almost all developed sepsis within a few days and most of them died of the combined sepsis and DIC (Effeney et al., 1978). In order to produce the Swartzman reaction (a DIC syndrome) in rabbits, it is necessary to give two separate injections of endotoxin. The first cause a limited DIC which produces fibrin that is removed largely by the RES becoming clogged with the fibrin. A

Figure 14.5. Section of lung of patient dying of severe shock and respiratory failure. Note congestion, edema, hemorrhage, and intravascular thrombi.

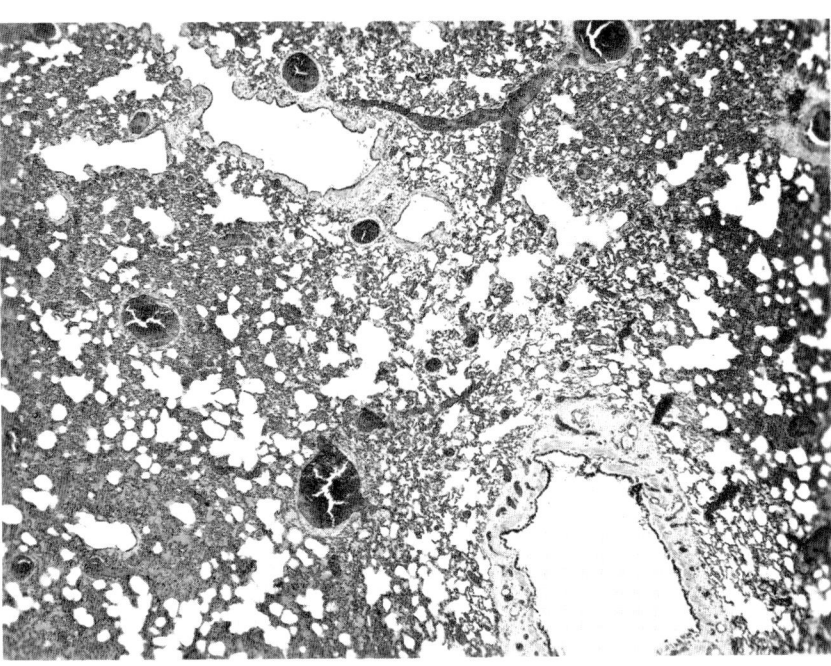

Figure 14.6. Section of kidney of patient dying of severe septic shock. Note thrombus in glomeruli and tubular necrosis.

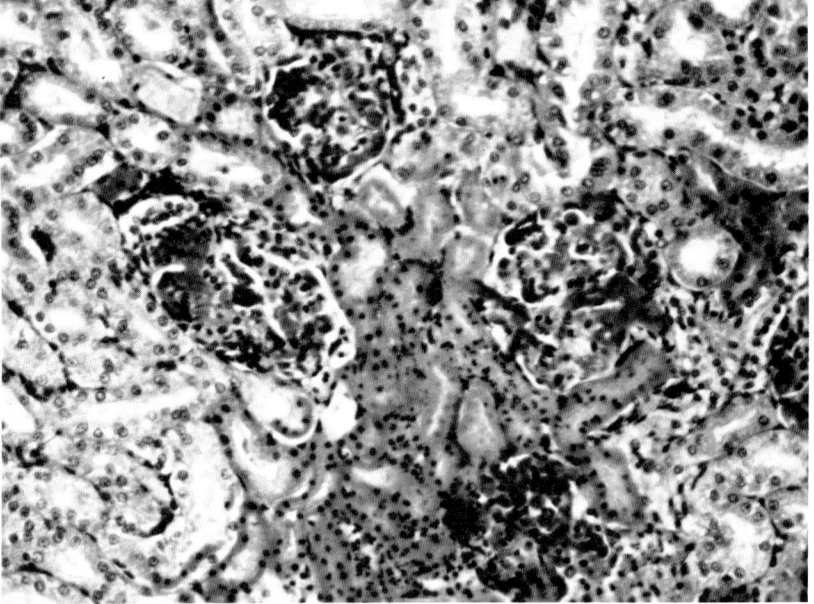

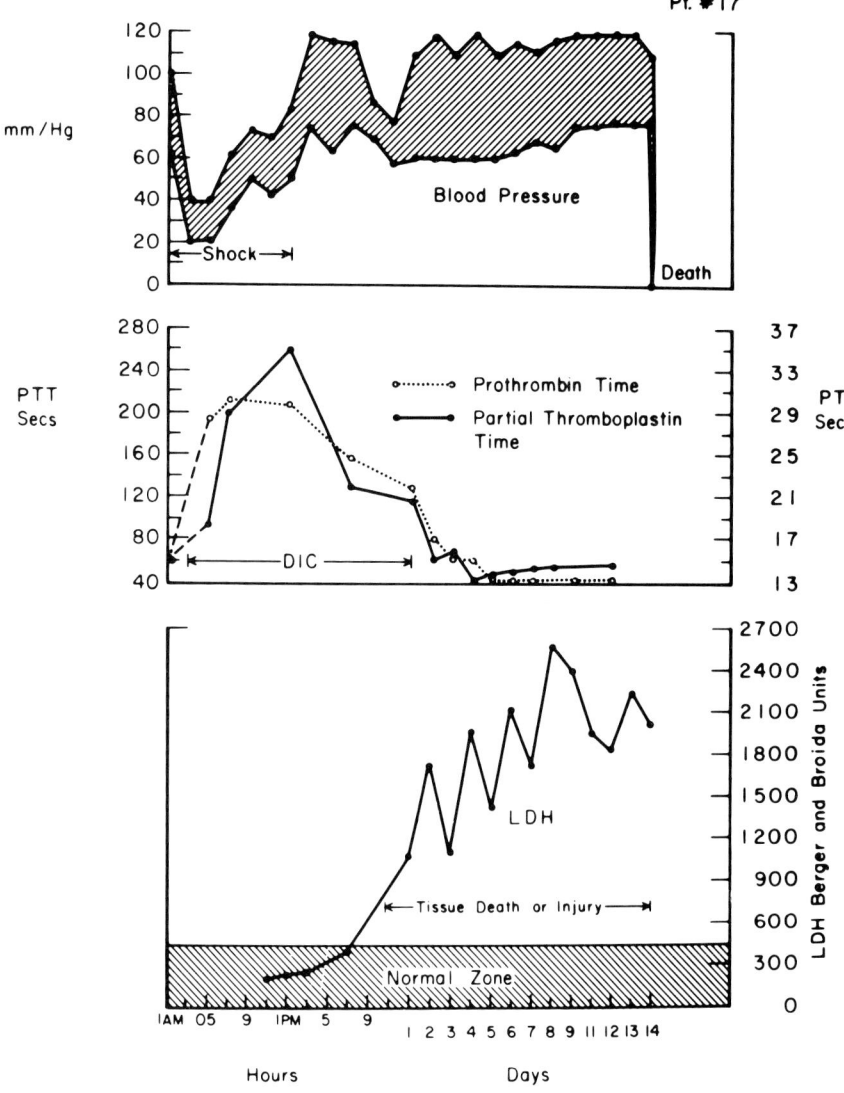

Figure 14.7. Arterial pressure, prothrombin times (PT), partial thromboplastin times (PTT), and LDH of patient dying of severe septic shock. Note rise in PT and PTT denoting onset of DIC. Although treatment resulted in recovery of arterial pressure, resolution of DIC, and clotting defect tissue damage was so severe the patient died with a rising LDH level.

subsequent episode of DIC is fatal because the RES is rendered incapable of removing more fibrin. Clinically, this also may be the case. A mild bacteremia, which normally might be harmless and readily coped with by the body's defenses, may after DIC become a fulminating septicemia.

SYNDROMES OF DIC

Table 14.2 lists a large number of clinical syndromes which may be due to, or complicated by DIC.

DIAGNOSIS

DIC should be suspected in a clinical situation such as sepsis, shock, hemolysis, dead foetus, cancer, or massive trauma. DIC is a relatively common phenomenon and often is not diagnosed unless it is specifically looked for. It becomes obvious if it is marked and produces the classic effects, but the physician must actively seek out chronic, low grade, or mild DIC and call for appropriate diagnostic tests. The bleeding tendency may not be evident unless there is a wound, which may be as small as the needle hole for medication. If there is a larger wound, bleeding may be massive and even fatal. The clotting defect may not be obvious clinically and, in fact, may be revealed only by laboratory tests. These should include prothrombin time, partial thromboplastin time, and platelet count. Factor assays are not necessary, but if done, they usually show deficiencies in all factors. Determination of fibrin split products are highly suggestive of DIC. Fibrinogen level may be high, normal, or low. The level of fibrinogen sheds little light on its speed of consumption. Perhaps the most sensitive index of fibrinogen conversion to fibrin and the presence of DIC is the ^{125}I fibrinogen decay rate (Blaisdell and Braziano, 1978). The rate of fibrinogen catabolism must be increased 300–500% before other tests for DIC become positive. Normally, fibrinogen has a half-life of about 6 days.

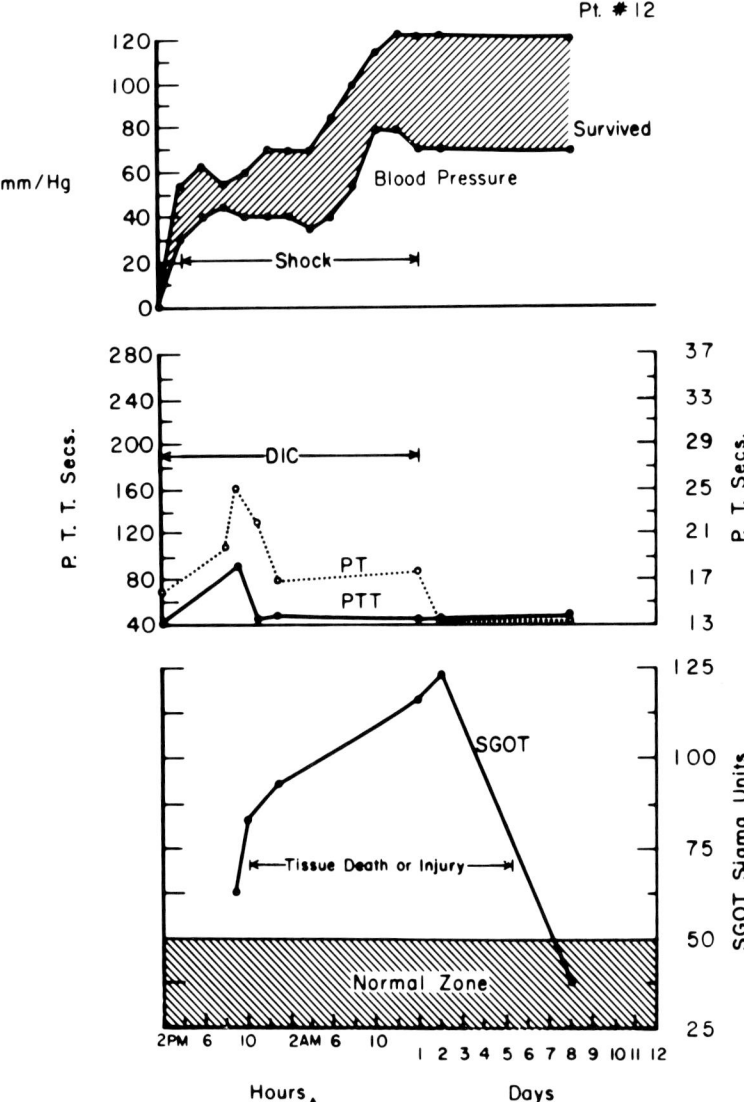

Figure 14.8. Arterial pressure, prothrombin times (PT), partial thromboplastin times (PTT), and SGOT of patient recovering from septic shock with the aid of a vasodilator. Note rise in PT and PTT, indicating onset and resolution of DIC and in SGOT, with onset of DIC and recovery following resolution of shock.

TREATMENT

Treatment of DIC is difficult and the methods controversial. Most important is the removal of the conditions that produced DIC. These include treatment of infection by antibiotics and drainage of abscesses, treatment of shock by intravenous fluids and other shock therapy, removal of cancer, removal of dead tissue, etc.

It would seem at first thought that if clotting is a problem, an anticoagulant such as heparin would be specific and effective treatment. However, this is not the case for a number of reasons. DIC is always characterized by a clotting defect even though it may not be clinically evident. Heparin may aggravate or initiate clinical bleeding; it has no effect on microthrombi already present, and it does not prevent platelet agglutination, which may well be the first step in DIC. In fact, heparin may cause platelet agglutination. Heparin is inactive in a pH of less than 7.2. Whereas arterial pH is usually above this, even in severe septic shock, the capillary pH is often below. It is in the capillary bed, where the blood flow is normally the slowest, that DIC is most apt to take place. Heparin does not affect the clotting effect of coagulase. For these reasons, heparin is not the primary treatment of DIC, although it may be useful in certain circumstances. DIC may have as its most prominent effect a severe bleeding tendency due primarily to an excessive activation of profibrinolysin to fibrinolysin with dissolution of any fibrin formed. This can be directly countered with Epsilon Amino Caproic Acid (EACA). However, this stops the body's attempts to counter the DIC, and widespread intravascular clotting of major as well as microvessels may result. This may be prevented by giving heparin along with the EACA. If DIC is prolonged over several days as indicated by a continued clotting defect, but not a major

Table 14.2
Clinical Syndrome Due to or Complicated by DIC

1. Shock, septic or traumatic
2. Adult respiratory distress syndrome
3. Acute renal failure
4. Hemolytic syndromes:
   Hemolytic transfusion reaction
   Malaria
   Paroxysmal nocturnal hemoglobinuria
   Favism
   Paroxysmal cold hemoglobinuria
   Sickle cell disease
   Injection of hypotonic solution
   Trauma
   Hemolytic uremic syndrome
   Thrombohemolytic thrombocytopenic purpura
5. Syndromes of late pregnancy:
   Eclampsia
   Premature separation of placenta
   Defibrination syndrome
   Amniotic fluid embolism (particulate matter)
   Hydatidiform mole
   Acute renal failure
   Sepsis
   Venous thrombosis
   Acute necrosis of liver
6. Extracorporeal circulation with bleeding
7. Clotting abnormalities due to cancer
8. Snake bite
9. Pseudomembranous enterocolitis
10. Hemorrhagic gastritis
11. Hemorrhagic enterocolitis
12. Acute necrosis of pancreas (includes clotting effect of trypsin)
13. Fat embolism
14. Heat stroke
15. Epidemic hemorrhagic fever ⎫ Endothelial damage
16. Rocky Mountain spotted fever ⎭
17. Swartzman reaction
18. Acute adrenal necrosis (Waterhouse-Friderichsen syndrome)

bleeding problem, heparin may be helpful. It may be given by an initial dose of 10,000 units followed by an infusion of 1000 units an hour to maintain clotting time twice the normal.

The best and safest treatment of DIC is to increase capillary flow, i.e., treat shock (Hardaway, 1968). This is a many faceted program and involves many factors. Intravenous fluid administration with Ringer lactate or other appropriate fluids should be pushed as much as possible using urine output, blood pressure, central venous pressure (CVP), and, in many cases, pulmonary artery pressure as guide lines. If arterial pressure and urine output do not respond adequately and CVP arises above 12 cm H_2O or pulmonary artery pressure rises, a vasodilator may be given (Fig. 14.9). These may include sodium nitroprusside (0.5 to 3 mcg/kg/min intravenously), phentolamine (5 mg/min intravenously), or phenoxybenzamine (1 mg/kg intravenously in 200 ml saline). They must be given only if there is a relative hypervolemia and a CVP of over 12. Careful monitoring of arterial pressure is necessary. If it falls, stop the drug. Usually, arterial pressure rises and cardiac output increases due to the opening up of constricted arterioles of the lungs and systemic circulation. Dopamine stimulates the heart and selectively dilates visceral arterioles, which is helpful (2–5 µg/kg/min). Steroids (methylprednisolone 35 mg/kg in 50 ml saline) may be helpful, but this is not documented.

Because microthrombi occlude the microcirculation and cause focal tissue necrosis and organ failure, it may be possible to help the body lyse these thrombi by augmenting the body's own fibrinolysin. Fibrinolysin has been shown to significantly protect dogs from DIC (Hardaway and Burns, 1963; Hardaway and Johnson, 1963; Hardaway and Drake, 1963). It has been tried in human DIC and seemed to be most effective (Hardaway, 1978) (Fig. 14.10). However, further research is needed to demonstrate its usefulness. It theroretically may increase the chances of a major hemorrhage, hence it should not be used if bleeding is a problem.

It is not usually necessary to treat the coagulation defect for two reasons. First, there may be no clinical bleeding; and second, the defect usually repairs itself rapidly as capillary perfusion improves (Figs. 14.7 and

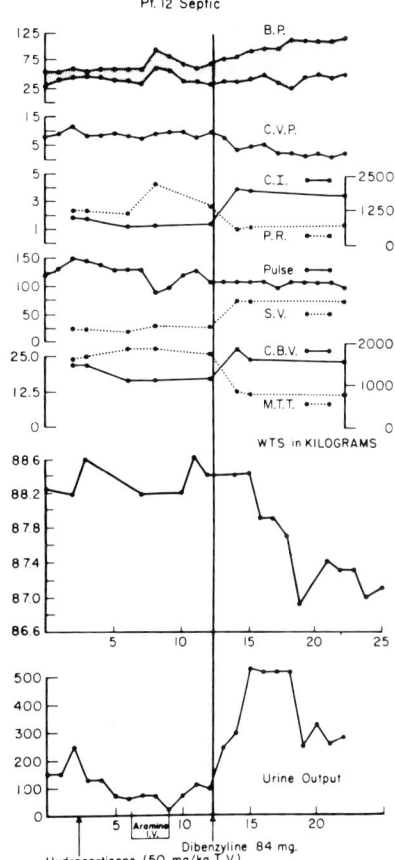

Figure 14.9. Patient in severe septic shock treated with three drugs. Steroids had no demonstrable effect. A pure vasoconstrictor resulted in a rise in arterial pressure but a decrease in capillary perfusion, as indicated by the fall in urinary output. A vasodilator resulted in a rise in arterial pressure, cardiac index, a fall in peripheral resistance and mean transit time, and a diuresis with recovery.

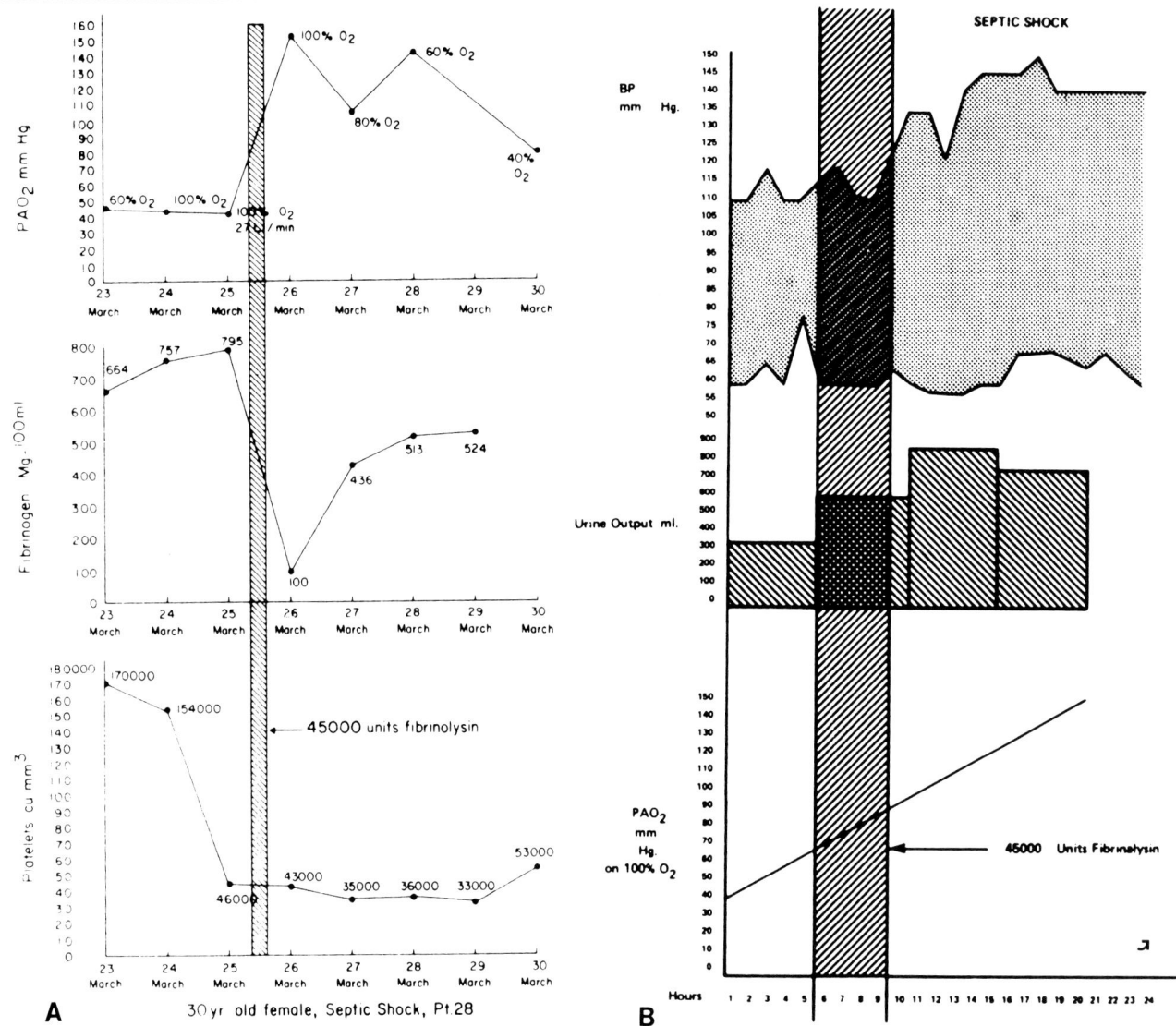

Figure 14.10. A and B, patient in severe septic shock who had adult respiratory distress syndrome. Patient's PaO$_2$ had been 40 torr for 3 days even with 100% oxygen on a respirator and appeared moribund. Administration of 45,000 units of fibrinolysin was followed by a rise in PaO$_2$ to 150 torr and rises in arterial pressure and urine output. The patient recovered rapidly; fibrinogen dropped markedly but not enough to cause a hemorrhage.

14.8). This is due to the rapid manufacture of all clotting factors when DIC is halted. However, if bleeding is severe, treatment may be required. Fresh whole blood given rapidly is best because it supplies all clotting factors, and all are probably deficient. It must be given rapidly to build up an effective level in the face of rapid utilization. Specific clotting factor replacement, except perhaps for platelets, is usually not necessary and is difficult to define. Fibrinogen may occasionally be required if it is very low, but this is rare.

References

Blaisdell, F.W., and Graziano, C.J.: Assessment of clotting by the determination of fibrinogen catabolism. Am. J. Surg. 135:436–443, 1978.

Effeney, D.J., Blaisdell, F.W., McIntyre, K.E., and Graziano, C.J.: The relationship between sepsis and disseminated intravascular coagulation. J. Trauma 18:689–695, 1978.

Hardaway, R.M.: Disseminated intravascular syndromes. Arch. Surg. 83:842–850, 1961.

Hardaway, R.M.: *Syndromes of Disseminated Intravascular Coagulation*. Charles C Thomas, Springfield, IL, 1966.

Hardaway, R.M.: *Clinical Management of Shock*. Charles C Thomas, Springfield, IL, 1968.

Hardaway, R.M.: Acute respiratory distress syndrome and disseminated intravascular coagulation. South. Med. J. 71: 596–598, 1978.

Hardaway R.M.: Influence of fibrinogen levels on mortality from hemorrhagic and traumatic shock. J. Trauma 20:417–419, 1980.

Hardaway, R.M., and Burns, J.W.: Mechanism of action of fibrinolysin in the prevention of irreversible hemorrhagic shock. Ann. Surg. *157*:305–309, 1963.

Hardaway, R.M., and Drake, D.C.: Prevention of irreversible hemorrhagic shock with fibrinolysin. Ann. Surg. *157*:39–47, 1963.

Hardaway, R.M., and Johnson, D.G.: Influence of fibrinolysin on shock. J.A.M.A., *183*:597–599, 1963.

Hardaway, R.M., and McKay, D.G.: Disseminated intravascular coagulation. A cause of shock. Ann. Surg. *159*:462–470, 1959.

Hardaway, R.M., and McKay, D.G.: The syndromes of disseminated intravascular coagulation. Rev. Surg. *20*:297–328, 1963.

Hewson, W.: In *Works of William Hewson SRS*, edited by G. Gulliver. Sydenham Society, London, 1846.

Section 2

Shock and Related Phenomena

PART 1

GENERAL CONSIDERATIONS

EDITORS' SUMMARY

In the first chapter of this section, Chaudry and Baue give an extensive and excellent overview of the pathophysiology of hemorrhagic shock. They stress that shock in all of its types and ramifications results from prolonged deficiency of blood flow resulting in cell hypoxia and ischemia. Most of the important factors occurring in hemorrhagic shock are discussed and the authors present a detailed hypothesis which is largely based on the idea that energy deficits are followed by ion shifts and, therefore, applies the concepts of general cell injury presented in Chapter 1. Clearly then, work from several large laboratories seems to have established the importance of cell energy deficiency and ion shifts. In their review, this hypothesis is also stressed and their views and experimental treatments are reflected in their extensive studies on the utilization of ATP in treatment. These authors and others have obtained considerable experimental evidence of the beneficial effects of ATP and magnesium in shock and related phenomena such as acute renal failure. The mechanism of protection, however, is still not understood as it is not known presently whether the administered ATP is used directly or whether it exerts some other effect, e.g., chelation of calcium. Clearly, changes in membrane permeability in damaged cells may permit the entry of ATP; this complicates the analysis. Much more work in this direction would seem to be desirable since, if the key action of ATP-MgCl$_2$ could be found, perhaps even more effective interventions with a similar action could be devised.

In this context, one wonders why, even if normal hemodynamics and circulating deficits are normalized, the body frequently fails to re-establish its own homeostasis. In our view, the answer lies in the fact that irreversible dysfunction or failure of the injured cell precludes such re-establishment. The ultimate answer, therefore, should result from an understanding of the injured cell and in the development of new concepts regarding the development of interventions designed to prevent or reverse irreversible cell injury by replacement therapy using substrates, enzyme systems, or other therapies which modulate deleterious substances, some of which may even be new to the body. If this fails, another possibility is organ transplantation or replacement. Some metabolic interventions might have to continue for a lifetime; however, if a vital organ becomes irretrievable prior to the institution of therapy, much more development in the field of organ replacement or artificial organs may be necessary to complement cell restitution to promote recovery.

In his chapter, Hinshaw extensively reviews the subject of septic shock. Septic shock remains an extremely important and frequently lethal human condition associated with a variety of primary disease states and, indeed, in most trauma units and general hospitals constitutes a major immediate cause of death. The major cell and tissue factors that initiate the syndrome still elude exact description. The progress that he reports in the baboon model is encouraging and clearly suggests that both bacterial killing and some "membrane" effect on host cells may be implicated. As discussed elsewhere in this volume, especially in Section 1, Part 1, at the cell level some effects of septic and hemorrhagic shock are rather similar; however, it would appear that in septic shock there is an additional major component involving cell membrane damage which further compromises the energy-depleted cell by modifying ion permeability at a time when ion pumping mechanisms are markedly inadequate.

Dr. Siegel and his group have innovated the utilization of a new type of graphic representation of metabolic changes during the progression of shock and related phenomena. Further development of this technique through the use of mathematical models and computer technology could well result in a better and more immediate visualization by the clinician of the immediate status of patients and their response to therapy. This type of charting may well represent a major advance in the presentation of data to the clinician, because at a glance, the patterns depicted in the charts can reveal deviations from the norm, whereas examination of the usual laboratory tables and computer printouts would take many hours to achieve the same goal.

Siegel et al. also consider the human response to sepsis. In the presence of sepsis, the normal catabolic response to trauma is altered in such a way that again the normal pattern of oxidative metabolism shifts toward gluconeogenesis and ketone body formation; in addition, other amino acids liberated from catabolic muscle appear to be diverted away from oxidative metabolism to increased urea formation. The authors also stress that aromatic amino acids which are known to be precursors of catecholamine synthesis may be converted into incompletely metabolized products capable of exerting vasoactive stimuli. Again, characteristic patterns occur which the authors have followed through the use of cluster techniques; these have greatly assisted our conceptualization of the process. Once again, critical blocks in oxidative metabolism, we believe involving membrane deficits in the inner mitochondrial membrane, have to be relieved if effective metabolism of glucose and fatty acids is to be increased and to modify the catabolic process. The question of whether alternate substrates can be utilized needs further exploration; certainly Drs. Chaudry and Baue's results of infusing ATP appear promising, though as mentioned above, the mechanism of action is not known. The role of the liver as an important facet needs to be stressed, and probably further efforts should be directed specifically toward the liver in terms of modifying this response.

Cerra et al. give us a masterful review of their concept of multiple systems organ failure, which is clearly a very important one in patients who survive the initial injury period. Multiple systems organ failure infection is a leading cause of death following traumatic insult. Understanding and effective treatment will require many advances. The syndrome is usually heralded by fever, hypoalbuminemia, cardiopulmonary failure, hyperbilirubinemia, and other evidence of altered liver function. In our experience, this usually is associated with sepsis, but it need not be. At the cellular level, biopsies and autopsies of patients in our unit show extensive cellular alterations of the type mentioned in Chapter 1 with marked mitochondrial swelling, cell death, and numerous autophagic vacuoles. These changes are very marked in the liver. The role of the liver in the syndrome has been stressed in our publications and is mentioned elsewhere in this volume. It is perhaps significant that Cerra et al. point out that patients who have primary liver disease have a lower survival rate than those who do not. The entire syndrome doubtlessly relates to altered hormonal control during the stress state, which is discussed in more detail by Bessman and Renner in Chapter 3. Multiple abnormalities also occur in plasma levels of glucose, lipid, and amino acids, and frequently characteristic profiles occur as plotted, using their cluster techniques. The patient is in a hypercatabolic state as discussed by Bessman and is "set" for gluconeogenesis with marked protein catabolism and release of amino acids. This makes therapy very difficult because at the present time we do not have adequate means to control this regulation and reset the hormonal modulation to normal. Although all of the factors responsible for initiating this disastrous sequence of events are not known, the authors stress the importance of mitochondrial defects, which certainly is compatible with results from other laboratories and from results with experimental animals, as discussed extensively in the chapters by Kahng, Ozawa, Mela, and Carafoli.

Caplan has provided an excellent overall description of the pathophysiology of carbon monoxide and cyanide. These are prototypes of inhibitors of energy metabolism that emanate from the environment. The frequent lack of correlation of severity of symptoms with the carboxyhemoglobin level points to the principal mechanism of toxicity, namely, the interaction with the cytochromes (Goldbaum, 1975).

In the treatment of carbon monoxide poisoning, the 5–10% CO_2 mixed with O_2 is not used at the present time. In our program, we agree that the addition of respiratory acidosis on a metabolic acidosis is unsound.

The figures of 250 min of air and 40 min of pure oxygen breathing as being the half-life times in these two environments is at variance with Peterson and Stewart (1970), where the carbon monoxide in air half-life is 320 min and on 100% oxygen at two and three atmospheres (ATA) is 80 and 23 min. It now appears that the half-life on 100% oxygen is far longer than has been stated. This is also evident in the clinical treatment protocols being followed by hyperbaric units elsewhere.

The proposed protocol for hyperbaric oxygen therapy varies. Kindwall (1975) gave a protocol of three ATA (66 ft sea water) for 46 min with an ascent to two ATA (33 ft sea water) until the patient is conscious, with an exposure of 100% oxygen interrupted with air breaks for up to 2 hr, the more commonly used procedure.

The major delayed effects of carbon monoxide poisoning are in the central nervous system and the myocardium (Garland and Pearce, 1967). Smith and Brandon (1973) have shown a 33% personality deterioration and a 43% memory impairment over a 3-year follow-up in survivors of severe (comatosed) carbon monoxide poisoning.

In the laboratory, the diagnosis of carbon monoxide poisoning, with breath testing using alveolar CO levels, has been utilized as a screening device. Stewart et al. (1976) have shown a fairly good correlation between alveolar carbon monoxide levels and the actual carboxyhemoglobin level.

In the treatment of cyanide poisoning, hyperbaric oxygenation has been effectively used in both the experimental situation (Skene et al., 1966) and in the clinical situation (Trapp, 1980).

The implications of carbon monoxide and cyanide in fire casualities is an extremely important one in the clinical realm, as the contamination with other gases in smoke inhalation has not been widely appreciated. The use of hyperbaric oxygen in smoke inhalation victims thus becomes an extremely effective method of treating both toxicants (carbon monoxide and cyanide).

Finally, in reviewing this section and the other sections of the book, it is quite apparent that what is needed in this field is to begin to develop methods and techniques to extrapolate animal data to man. We still have little information on the relationship between animal models and human organ failure in shock or other related phenomena. In spite of detailed experimental data on animal models, these can only be validated by parallel studies in man in which the animal studies are compared with human data derived from the clinical arena. It is our view that the clinician and the basic scientist need not be in the same geographic locale to accomplish this collaboration, and it is one of our main ideals and one of the

References

Garland, H., and Pearce, J.: Neurological complications of carbon monoxide poisoning. Q. J. Med., New Series XXXVI *144:*445–455, 1967.

Goldbaum, L.R., Ramirez, R.G., and Absalon, K.B.: What is the mechanism of carbon monoxide toxicity? Aviat. Space Environ. Med. *46:*1289–1291, 1975.

Kindwall, E.P.: Carbon monoxide poisoning treated with hyperbaric oxygen. Resp. Ther. *5:*29–33, 1975.

Peterson, J.E., and Stewart, R.D.: Absorption and elimination of carbon monoxide by inactive young men. Arch. Environ. Health *21:*165–175, 1970.

Skene, W.G., Norman, J.N., and Smith, G.: Effects of hyperbaric oxygen on cyanide poisoning. *Proceedings of the Third International Congress on Hyperbaric Oxygen*, edited by I.W. Brown, Jr. and B.G. Cox, pp. 705–710. National Academy of Sciences, Washington, DC, 1966.

Smith, J.S., and Brandon, S.: Morbidity from acute carbon monoxide poisoning at three year follow up. Br. Med. J. *1:* 318–321, 1973.

Stewart, R.D., Stewart, R.S., Staman, W., et al.: Rapid estimation of carboxyhemoglobin level in fire fighters. J.A.M.A. *4:*390-392, 1976.

Trapp, W.: Massive cyanide poisoning with recovery; a boxing day story. Can. Med. J. *102:*517, 1970.

CHAPTER 15

Overview of Hemorrhagic Shock

IRSHAD H. CHAUDRY

ARTHUR E. BAUE

Shock as been recognized for over 100 years; however, a clear definition and dissection of this complex and devastating state has emerged slowly. In the 19th century, Samuel Gross (1872) described shock as a "manifestation of a rude unhinging of the machinery of life." Although this definition of shock is accurate, it is obviously far from precise. Wiggers, in 1942, offered the definition of shock as "a syndrome resulting from a depression of many functions, but in which reduction of the effective circulating blood volume is of basic importance, and in which impairment of the circulation steadily progresses until it eventuates in a state of irreversible circulatory failure." More recently, Simeone (1964) stated that shock may be defined as a "clinical condition characterized by signs and symptoms which arise when the cardiac output is insufficient to fill the arterial tree with blood under sufficient pressure to provide organs and tissues with adequate blood flow." A more precise and current definition of shock to include all of the above alterations is "inadequate blood flow to vital organs or the inability of the body cell mass to metabolize nutrients normally" (MacLean, 1977). Thus, it is clear that shock and all of its ramifications result from a prolonged deficiency of the flow of blood. This inadequate circulation with diminished blood flow to tissues results in cell hypoxia and its sequelae. Hemorrhagic or hypovolemic shock is due to an inadequate circulating blood volume. A review of this area must begin then with consideration of how blood volume is controlled.

BLOOD VOLUME AND ITS CONTROL

A decreased circulating blood volume is the result of hemorrhagic shock. When such a decrease exceeds the ability of the individual to compensate for the loss, either because of the rapidity of the blood loss or continued slow loss, the circulation begins to fall and shock is present. Blood volume is defined as the sum of the volume of cells and plasma inside the circulatory system. However, all components of blood, even the formed elements, are to some degree present outside of blood vessels in the lymph and interstitial or extracellular fluid. In addition, the intravascular fluid is in equilibrium with the extracellular fluid and a dynamic equilibrium is present with intracellular fluid. Thus, disorders of total body hydration seriously affect vascular volume. Normal blood volume is best described in functional terms, rather than by a measurement of volume by dilution and reference to standards tables and is the amount of blood that provides an adequate filling pressure for the heart. The essential role of the blood volume is transport, but the system must be adequately filled in order to ensure the maintenance of adequate venous return and volume flow of blood. An adequate functional blood volume, therefore, is one that provides a normal or adequate circulation if the heart and peripheral circulation system are normal.

A low atrial pressure indicates a less than adequate circulating volume. Even if the patient's arterial circulation in this circumstance was normal, he would have no reserve if circulatory demands increased. Normal atrial pressures with an adequate arterial circulation indicate an adequate blood volume. However, circulating blood volume may be low and the arterial circulation diminished, but atrial pressure may remain normal by compensating mechanisms.

Maintenance of blood volume obviously requires the maintenance of total body water and extracellular fluid volume by the mechanisms of antidiuretic hormone and aldosterone secretion, volume of urine production, saliva production and thirst, red cell population, and mobilization of plasma proteins, particularly from the liver. Maintenance of an adequate volume within the circulatory system is dependent primarily on two mechanisms: the ability of extracellular fluid to provide volume to the circulation in the capillary bed according to the Starling equilibrium (capillary refilling) and the ability of the vascular system to decrease its volume by constriction of capacitance vessels, particularly in the splanchnic bed. The shift in the balance of the capillary circulation between filtration and reabsorption is much more sensitive to changes in venous pressure than it is to changes in arterial pressure. The recent work of Gann and Perkle (1975) indicates that intracellular water contributes to vascular refilling after a loss by a hormonal effect and an extracellular hyperosmolar phenomenon.

Hemodynamic Disturbances in Shock

A common feature of shock is substantially decreased tissue perfusion through the vessels of the microcirculation. Reduced cardiac output due to loss of blood from the intravascular compartment is the most prominent cause of inadequate perfusion. The proportion of cardiac output available to individual organs under normal conditions is dependent upon the perfusion pressure and the degree of smooth muscle tone in the supplying vessels. This is usually considerable and is due to the activity of sympathetic vasoconstrictor fibers to the arterioles, venules, and veins. Tissues, such as the skin and to a certain extent skeletal muscle, have passive pressure-flow relationships. On the other hand, steady state pressure-flow relationship in the renal, cerebral, and coronary vascular beds are almost horizontal, until a pressure of about 50 mm Hg is reached, when flow decreases precipitously. This remarkable ability of an organ to maintain flow despite changes in perfusion pressure is termed autoregulation. Autoregulation occurs in the absence of the motor nerves and is an intrinsic property of the vascular smooth muscle of the organ concerned. Autoregulation, basically, is a protective mechanism by which the body attempts to compensate for a reduced perfusion pressure to vital organs. However, reduction in tissue blood flow in response to a reduced systemic arterial blood pressure (to levels approximately 50% of normal) will obviously be much more marked in tissues and organs that do not exhibit vascular autoregulation.

Another compensatory mechanism available to the body during hemorrhage is increased sympathoadrenal discharge. This release not only increases myocardial contractility but also leads to constriction of the arterioles and of the capacitance vessels. This is an attempt to restore blood pressure towards normal by increasing peripheral resistance and by maintaining venous return to the heart through decreased volume of blood in the venous capacitance system.

Hypotension produces a variable effect in the microcirculation which depends on the dominance of the constrictor influences at each end of the capillary. When the pressure at the arteriole falls, transmural capillary pressure is reduced and there is a net movement of extracellular fluid into the capillary in order to restore blood volume. If, however, venoconstriction is predominant, plasma is lost from the vascular space and hemoconcentration occurs. These responses to severe blood loss are essential for immediate survival. However, prolonged diversion of blood flow from liver, kidney, gastrointestinal tract, and muscle masses are devastating in the long run. Fluid loss is also accelerated by circulating vasoactive substances, such as histamine and plasma kinins, which increase capillary permeability. Other factors which influence blood viscosity are the fibrinogen level and the hematocrit, both of which may be raised in the early stages of shock. These changes in the blood lead to widespread aggregation of red cells and platelets. Platelet aggregation can be induced by substances such as norepinephrine, thrombin, particulate matter, and ADP. Although platelet aggregation may be helpful to the organism for phagocytosis of foreign material, platelet aggregation may obstruct blood flow under conditions of decreased tissue perfusion, and this may result in infarction of the tissue supplied by the obstructed vessel.

The stabilizing reflexes act to restore blood pressure in shock by reducing the capacity of the vascular system. Moreover, other equally effective homeostatic responses are designed to conserve and expand plasma volume. Sodium and water are conserved by the kidney, under the influence of antidiuretic hormones and aldosterones, respectively. If, however, homeostasis is not restored, the injury becomes overwhelming and circulation is redirected in the vital areas of heart, brain, and lungs, at the expense of the remaining tissues and organs.

Compensation for Hypovolemia

The compensation for blood loss has been studied extensively in man by Moore (1965). The loss of 500–1000 ml of blood by slow venous hemorrhage, which does not produce shock in normal man, is followed by a net movement of water, salt, and protein into the plasma. This refilling of plasma from the capillary bed, produced in good part by decreased venous pressure, is rapid at first (as high as 2.0 ml/min) and decreases with time, with plasma volume restored to normal in 20–40 hr. The studies of Perkle and Gann (1976) have suggested that mild hemorrhage leads to an increase in extracellular osmolarity mediated in part by increased cortisol concentrations. As a result of this, there is a shift of intracellular fluid to the interstitium, causing interstitial pressure to increase. The increased interstitial pressure accelerates lymphatic movement of interstitial protein to the vascular system, and this results in a re-equilibration of extracellular fluid toward the plasma. This, then completes the restitution of blood volume.

There is also increased secretion of renin, aldosterone, antidiuretic hormone, and erythropoietin and renal conservation of sodium and water (Skillman et al., 1967a). Cortisol secretion does not seem to increase initially. Interstitial fluid is decreased and is restored only by ingestion or injection. Albumin enters the circulation rapidly at rates initially of up to 4.0 g/hr (Skillman et al., 1967b). A rapid arterial bleed produces even higher initial rates of capillary refilling, so long as shock is not produced. Then adrenal release of epinephrine and adrenal and sympathetic nervous system release of norepinephrine are increased, as is cortisol secretion.

VASOACTIVE AGENTS IN SHOCK

During shock a variety of vasoactive agents are released.

1. Norepinephrine and Epinephrine. Following hemorrhage there is a significant release of epinephrine and norepinephrine. The initial release of norepinephrine may be from the granulated vesicles of the postganglionic sympathetic fibers. The release of both epinephrine and norepinephrine from the adrenal medulla occurs at a later stage. Plasma catecholamine levels increase as high as 200 times normal in experimental hemorrhagic shock (Jakschik et al., 1974a).

2. Prostaglandins. The prostaglandins are unsaturated fatty acid derived compounds, synthesized in the body by cellular microsomes from essential fatty acids. The variety and magnitude of effects which prostaglandins evolve are striking. For the most part, the vascular effects of prostaglandin may be summarized by the statement that PGE_2 and PGI_2 are vasodilators and $PGF_{2\alpha}$ and TxA_2 are vasoconstrictors. The circulatory insult of hemorrhagic hypotension is precisely the circumstance in which one might expect to find increased prostaglandin synthesis. This is due to the fact that the microcirculation is affected during hemorrhage and cells are subjected to hypoxia, which is a potent stimulant of prostaglandin synthesis (Markelonius and Garbus, 1975). The decreased blood flow to organs and tissues, which leads to altered cell function throughout the organism, might lead specifically to a depression of cell membrane transport and metabolism of prostaglandins by the endothelium in the lung. This, in turn, might subject the organism to further increased prostaglandin levels. It has been shown by a number of investigators (Flynn et al., 1975; Frolich, 1977; Jakschik et al., 1974b; Johnston and Selkurt, 1976) that PGE_2 levels increase during hemorrhagic shock. The possibility has been raised that part of the elevated arterial PGE_2 levels might be the result of diminished pulmonary metabolism of circulating PGE. The in vivo studies of a number of investigators (Blasingham and Selkurt, 1976; Fletcher and Ramwell, 1977; Jakschik et al., 1974a) are consistent with this view. These investigators, however, could not distinguish decreased metabolism from increased pulmonary synthesis and release of PGE during hemorrhage.

The experimental use of prostaglandin synthesis blockade by aspirin, indomethacin, and meclofcmate, both as therapeutic intervention and as a pharmacologic tool, has attracted many investigators (Jakschik et al., 1974a; Johnston and Selkurt, 1976; Leffler and Passmore, 1977). The studies of Leffler and Passmore (1977) and Carlson et al. (1979) suggest a protective role for prostaglandins in hemorrhagic shock. A number of other reports have documented (by prostaglandin synthesis blockade) the importance of prostaglandin in the renal blood during hemorrhagic hypotension (Bell et al., 1975; Data et al., 1976; Tyssebough and Kirkebo, 1977). The above mentioned studies suggest that prostaglandin synthesis is increased in the renal bed. The increased synthesis may, perhaps, be to counteract the effects of the renal sympathetics and circulating angiotensin, thereby maintaining renal blood flow. Thus, it appears that renal prostaglandins exert a protective vasodilatory effect during hemorrhagic hypotension. The work of Gerkes and Shand (1975) on hepatic autoregulation is analogous to the studies on the renal bed described above and suggests that prostaglandins play a role in vasodilatation in the hepatic bed. Studies of infusion of prostaglandins E and F during hemorrhage indicate that each of these may have salutary effects (Glenn, 1972; Machido et al., 1973, 1976; Priano et al., 1974; Whitten et al., 1979). Our recent studies, however, have shown that infusion of PGE_2 alone following hemorrhage failed to have any beneficial effects on the survival of animals (Carlson et al., 1979). Thus, infusion of PGE_2 with another PG may be necessary to provide beneficial effects. Moreover, it should be noted that prostaglandin infusions were given intravenously in most of the studies (Glenn, 1972; Machido et al., 1973, 1976; Priano et al., 1974; Whitten et al., 1979). Since prostaglandin E and F are rapidly inactivated by the pulmonary vessel bed in normal circumstances, there is cause for concern that infused prostaglandin would be largely metabolized in one passage through the lung. Since the metabolism of primary prostaglandins is apparently diminished during shock, the amount of prostaglandin reaching the tissues in these studies remains, therefore, unknown. Thus, it could be concluded that arterial PGE levels are elevated during hemorrhage and that, associated with this increase, is an equivocal decrease in the ability of the pulmonary bed to inactivate circulating PGE. The effect of PG synthesis blockade appears to be deleterious to autoregulation, and there is conflicting opinion whether or not prostaglandin infusion during hemorrhage is beneficial.

3. Angiotensin and Vasopressin. A number of studies have indicated that vasopressin secretion and angiotensin formation increases following hemorrhage and that they play major roles in the intestinal and splenic vasoconstriction (Beleslin et al., 1967; Cohen et al., 1970; Rocha and Rosenberg, 1969; Scornik and Paladini, 1964; Weinstein et al., 1960). The sympathetic nerves and adrenal medullary secretions may also contribute to splenic vasoconstriction, but they appear not to be important in the intestinal vasoconstriction. Moreover, the above mentioned studies indicated that the response of the intestinal splenic and hepatic arterial resistance vessels to intravenous infusion of vasopressin and angiotensin were consistent with the postulated roles for these peptides in the splanchnic response to hemorrhage.

Changes in Microcirculation

Substantial evidence is present in the literature which indicates that hemorrhage results in a maldistribution of blood through the microvascular network of skeletal muscle and this results in an altered diffusional transport (Appelgren, 1972; Haglund, 1973; Nickerson, 1970). It has also been shown that microrheological changes accelerate these trends (Chien, 1969; Dintenfass, 1968; Goldstone et al., 1970; Lofstrom, 1966; Schmid-Schoendien and Wells, 1971) and there is a loss of myogenic adjustments in the intestine (Folkow et al., 1963). Nutritional shunting is also present, which suggests an inability of the terminal vascular bed to regulate the systemic distribution of blood in tissues such as the intestines (Appelgren, 1972; Beachstrom et al., 1970; Haglund, 1973; Renkin, 1968). The presence of microcirculatory dysfunction, with the development of irreversibility, is confirmed by direct intravital microscopy (Zweifach, 1958).

If 20–25% of the blood volume is lost, this results in a persistent hypotension and underperfusion of parenchymal tissues and, with time, the syndrome becomes increasingly refractory to blood replacement. The changeover from a reversible situation to an irreversible (which no longer is helped by conventional fluid replacement) is probably the net result of several contributing factors. The failure in microcirculation can occur in a number of different levels, and it will be useful to deal separately with the transport and exchange functions. There are two types of changes encountered at the transport level: a suppression of autoregulation and spontaneous vasomotion (Hinshaw, 1971). There is also a diminished activity of the vascular smooth muscles (Zweifach, 1965). The above phenomena are probably interrelated. Because of an imbalance of pressure and osmotic forces, the net flux of fluid is shifted toward absorption at the exchange level. This results in an initial hemodilution. Subsequently however, the balance shifts the opposite way and results in a secondary loss in fluid.

During hemorrhage, the peripheral vascular bed and splanchnic tissue show that larger arterioles (50–75 μ) remain constricted throughout the oligemic phase (Zweifach and Fronek, 1975). Following the onset of hemorrhage, the microvascular bed develops an intense ischemia, due to precapillary vasoconstriction, which is intermittently relieved at short intervals and allows flow through the capillary network. The progression of hemorrhagic shock syndrome towards irreversibility, within the microcirculation proper, is characterized by features such as: 1) the gradual suppression of spontaneous vasomotion in the precapillary vessels (Zweifach, 1958); 2) a blunted response to constrictor stimuli, such as norepinephrine (Zweifach, 1965); and 3) an inability to maintain capillary pressure within a range compatible with a balanced fluid exchange (Zweifach and Intaglietta, 1968). During shock, the changes in precapillary activity do not increase tissue blood flow significantly because of the sustained arteriolar vasoconstriction. The blood pressure in the capillary bed proper, following hemorrhage, is initially maintained at near normal levels, but then tends to fall (Zweifach, 1971; Zweifach and Intaglietta, 1968). During the later stages of hemorrhagic shock, the terminal vascular bed behaves more as a passive structure and no longer exhibits active adjustments to circulatory disturbances.

HORMONAL ALTERATIONS DURING SHOCK

Circulatory failure produces complex nervous and humoral adjustments that result in a rapid increase in blood glucose level (Frank et al., 1955; Hume, 1957; Seligman et al., 1947; Watts, 1956). As hypovolemia continues, the progressive rise in the glucose level changes to decline (Drucker et al., 1958; Engel, 1952), at least in experimental animals in shock. In man, severe injury and shock are associated with hyperglycemia and an abnormality of glucose tolerance that persists after the injury (Allison et al., 1968; Howard, 1955; Rhoads and Howard, 1963). Insulin is under the dual influence of catecholamines and nutrients. Norepinephrine is released from the sympathetic nerve endings during hemorrhage, and it inhibits insulin release, leading to low absolute levels of circulating insulin. Hiebert et al. (1973) have calculated the insulin secretory rate in monkeys during shock by measuring portal vein flow and the insulin concentration in portal and arterial blood. They found a large and progressive decrease in insulin secretory rate with shock, in spite of an increase in arterial concentrations of insulin in late shock. The low levels of insulin in early stages of shock result in increased amino acid efflux from peripheral skeletal muscle.

Glucagon secretion is also under the influence of

catecholamines and nutrients, and stress induces a rapid increase in glucagon secretion also. The precise effects on muscle of these elevated levels of glucagon remain unknown. However, glucagon stimulates free fatty acids and glycerol production from adipose tissues in conditions of relatively low insulin levels. Glucagon's main site of action is on the liver, where it stimulates gluconeogenesis. Thus, high glucagon concentrations, acting in conjunction with relatively low insulin concentration, ensure a steady supply of glucose, free fatty acids, and ketones during hemorrhage, at the expense of body protein. This loss is reflected in high urine nitrogen excretion (Meguid and Egdahl, 1977). Thus, hemorrhage is usually followed by a period of metabolic instability, the manifestations of which include insulin resistance and protein breakdown with conversion of the released amino acids to glucose and urea (Chaudry et al., 1974a; Olsen and Nuetzell, 1950; Ryan et al., 1977). This process is believed to provide important substrates to support the repair activities necessary for survival and recovery. The changes in metabolism occur in association with increased plasma levels of various catabolic hormones, including the adrenal catecholamine and steroids (Campbell et al., 1954; Gann and Egdahl, 1965; Jaatella, 1972). However, recent studies of Ryan et al. (1977) have shown that hemorrhagic shock was followed by insulin resistance and abnormality of glucose and amino acid metabolism by skeletal muscles, but these abnormalities were not dependent on the concurrent changes in plasma levels of adrenal steroids or catecholamine. The factors responsible for the posttraumatic abnormalities of tissue metabolism are, therefore, still unresolved.

Carbohydrate Metabolism

Claude Bernard (1877) observed that early in hemorrhagic shock the blood sugar level became elevated and remained elevated until the terminal stages. The hyperglycemic feature of hemorrhagic shock has since been confirmed by other investigators (Hift and Strawitz, 1961), and in man the hyperglycemic response seems to correlate with the degree of hemorrhage. Although earlier studies (Drucker and DeKiewiet, 1964) suggested that glucose uptake by tissues from animals subjected to severe shock was increased, more recent studies failed to support this notion (Chaudry et al., 1975a). In the early phases of shock, increased glycogeno lysis has been found both in skeletal muscle and liver of animals (Heath, 1971; Stoner, 1958). Cardiac muscle glycogen increases marginally in the early stages of shock and it decreases at the terminal phases of shock. The glycogen level of the brain also falls towards the terminal phases of shock (Stoner, 1958). In contrast to increased glycogenolysis, the rate of oxidation of carbohydrate is decreased after shock (Heath and Corney, 1973).

Gluconeogenesis in man and other nonruminants comprises the synthesis of glucose and glycogen from lactate, pyruvate, glycerol, and certain amino acids. The liver is the major site of gluconeogenesis, with the kidney becoming an important site of gluconeogenesis during stress conditions. It would appear that the hyperglycemia which is observed in the early stages of shock results from the increased glycogenolysis. In the later stages of shock, there is indirect evidence for increased gluconeogenesis (Kinney et al., 1970). However, more recent studies indicate that gluconeogenesis was not altered during late hemorrhagic shock (Chaudry et al., 1978).

Protein Metabolism

The response of the serum proteins in the early stages of shock is complex because the synthesis rates of some may be increased and that of others decreased, while the catabolic rates of others, e.g., transferrin, may be increased (Gordon, 1970). Thus, although the supply of amino acid influences protein synthesis in a complex fashion (Munro, 1970), the control of the response to early shock is unlikely to be determined by measurement of tissue amino acid levels. Few attempts have been made to assess directly total body protein synthesis after shock. The general conclusion, however, is that protein catabolism is increased, at least in the late stages of shock (Heath and Corney, 1973). Early after injury, liver polysome aggregation and incorporation of amino acids into polysome protein increases. Subsequently, however, there is reduced incorporation of proteins and polysome disaggregation (Khan et al., 1974). These observations are consistent with increased protein synthesis in liver in the early phases of shock and a decrease in the later phases of shock (Randall et al., 1974).

Fat Metabolism

The studies of Shoemaker et al. (1973) indicated that in the early stages of hemorrhage there was a net increase in the release of triglycerides from the liver and increased uptake of free fatty acids, phospholipids, and cholesterol. This effect was of short duration, and the values returned to control levels in the middle stages of hemorrhage. In the late stages of hemorrhage, free fatty acids and phospholipids were released. Furthermore, they showed that nonhepatic splanchnic tissue responded to hemorrhage with an increased output of free fatty acids, triglycerides, and phospholipids, which decreased in the late stages of hypovolemia. Increased glycerol concentrations during hemorrhage were also found by Kovach (1972) and by Spitzer et al. (1973). Thus, it appears that there is a relation between carbohydrates and fat metabolism via pyruvate, acetyl CoA, and glycerol.

Alterations in Cyclic Adenosine Monophosphate Levels

Since the original discovery of cyclic adenosine monophosphate as an intracellular mediator or a second messenger for hormone action, a large number of metabolic regulatory systems have been implicated as acting through this nucleotide by several groups (Butcher et al., 1968; Robinson et al., 1967; Sutherland and Robinson, 1969). It has been suggested that if the effectiveness of cyclic adenosine monophosphate system is decreased, a loss of control of certain vital cellular activities could result. Various hormones affect the levels of cyclic adenosine monophosphate. The levels of hormones such as catecholamines, adrenocorticotropin, cortisol, thyroxin, and insulin have been found to be altered during shock. Some of the metabolic processes controlled by the aforementioned hormones and biogenic amines appear to be defective during shock, as suggested by a number of investigators (Drucker et al., 1958; Lillihei et al., 1964; Shires and Carrico, 1966; Shoemaker and Rall, 1967). The studies of Rutenberg et al. (1971) and Chaudry and Baue (1977) have indicated that there are indeed significant reductions in cyclic adenosine monophosphate levels during hemorrhagic shock.

Alterations in Calcium Concentration

Substantial evidence now indicates that during shock or low flow conditions, there is a significant fall in the serum calcium levels, and it is assumed that the fall in serum calcium is associated with an increase in intracellular calcium levels (Trump et al., 1971). The increased intracellular calcium levels may be due to a defect or a decrease in the activity of the calcium ATPase, which requires ATP for its operation. Calcification of mitochondria is commonly observed in injured cells in vivo. Calcification is also observed in cells at the edges of infarcts and probably in ischemic cells after reflow of blood even if the cells are necrotic. In normal cells, the mitochondria probably do not see calcium in sufficient quantities to accumulate this cation. However, following injury that results in direct damage to the integrity of the cell membrane or indirectly affects the membrane through the loss of ATP production and secondary leak, calcium influx into the cell occurs (Trump et al., 1971). This is reflected by rapid mitochondrial calcium accumulation which promotes mitochondrial swelling and competes with oxidative phosphorylation. Thus, influx of calcium may well be a late manifestation of cell swelling, resulting in inhibition of mitochondrial production of ATP. In addition, it has been suggested that increased mitochondrial calcium levels prevent the translocation of ATP from the mitochondria. A more detailed description of alterations in calcium during adverse circulatory conditions is provided in Chapter 1.

Lysosomal Enzymes

Lysosomes are widely distributed in various tissues including the brain, spleen, thyroid, and lymph nodes. The highest concentrations of lysosomes are found in the liver, kidney, and spleen. As many as 12 different acid hydrolyases have been identified. However, the distribution and absolute concentration varies. Janoff (1964) suggested that lysosomal enzymes are released not only from dead cells undergoing autolysis but also prior to cell death, as a result of cellular anoxia, ischemia, and acidosis (Slater, 1969). Lefer and Glenn (1973) found that the total tissue lysosomal activity of the pancreas and liver was markedly reduced in postoligemia and splanchnic ischemic shock, whereas the spleen and intestines were moderately influenced and the heart was not significantly involved. Significant increases in the plasma level of these enzymes have been reported in hemorrhagic shock (Glenn and Lefer, 1970; Lefer, 1978; Lefer and Bareholz, 1972). However, the release of measurable quantities of lysosomal enzymes in shock has been questioned by Schumer and associates (1969).

It appears, therefore, that in the late stages of hemorrhagic shock, i.e., in the irreversible phases, further deterioration continues and eventually the intracellular organelles, lysosomes, break down and leak (Lefer and Barenholz, 1972). The lysosomes contain hydrolytic enzymes, which may be involved in further damage inside the cell. Eventually the cell is destroyed, and as this happens, other toxic factors (Lefer, 1978) may be released which may make this a vicious cycle, altering adjoining cells and other tissues and organs.

Reticuloendothelial System

A number of studies have documented a relationship between the reticuloendothelial system (RES) phagocytic activity and survival following shock (Altura and Hershey, 1968; Fine et al., 1959; Kaplan and Saba, 1976; Zweifach et al., 1957). Moreover, it has been shown that prior stimulation of the RES enhances resistance to experimental shock and prior depression of the RES attenuates such resistance (Altura and Hershey, 1968; Fine et al., 1959; Kaplan and Saba, 1976; Zweifach et al., 1957). Shock also induces a state of RES depression which is directly proportional to the severity of the shock state (Altura and Hershey, 1968; Kaplan and Saba, 1976; Kaplan et al., 1976). It has also been shown that animals that survive shock manifest only transient reticuloendothelial depression, with subsequent recovery, and that animals that eventually succumb to identical insults are characterized by a persistent and progressive reticuloendothelial depression (Altura and Hershey, 1972).

It has been reported that reticuloendothelial dysfunction following shock is at least in part mediated by a deficiency in circulating opsonic activity (Kaplan and Saba, 1976). The phagocytic depression which occurs in hemorrhagic shock in animals has been functionally associated with such humoral opsonic dysfunction (Loegering and Saba, 1976). It is encouraging to note that recent studies have indicated that administration of preparations rich in α_2-SB-opsonic glycoprotein (cryoprecipitate) restores circulating opsonic activity after injury (Saba, 1978).

Metabolic Alterations

Various metabolic alterations take place during shock. As mentioned above, there may be hyperglycemia initially, due probably to increased hepatic glycogen breakdown from epinephrine secretions. This can produce initial relative hyperkalemia and eventual glycogen depletion. Hypoglycemia may occur in terminal stages. With decreased oxygen available to tissues, there is a shift to anaerobic metabolism, with an increase in lactate production and metabolic acidosis. Free fatty acids increase (Skillman et al., 1970). Insulin secretion is decreased. Shires and his colleagues have suggested that there is a decrease in functional extracellular fluid volume with prolonged oligemic shock (Shires et al., 1973).

Ultrastructural Changes

The studies of Holden and his group (1965) described the cell's swelling, mitochondrial swelling, and the endoplasmic reticulum swelling during hemorrhagic shock in the rat. More recently, George et al. (1978) have shown that marked structural changes in various tissues persisted for a prolonged time after shock. Trump (1974) studied the progressive changes seen in various cells of patients with shock. He found that virtually all of the acute responses of cells to injury such as shock involved alterations of the membrane systems. Early changes that he described after injury including clumping of nuclear chromatin, dilation of endoplasmic reticulum, and swelling of the cell sap. These changes, therefore, can, be correlated with increased cellular sodium, decreased potassium, and increased water.

Disturbances in Cellular Energy Metabolism

Numerous studies have indicated that there is a decrease in circulating plasma volume during the late oligemic and irreversible post-transfusion phase (Abel and Wolf, 1973; Chien et al., 1973; Lillihei et al., 1963). A common feature of all forms of shock is thought to be an inadequate circulation with diminution of blood flow to tissues, thereby resulting in tissue hypoxia. As a result of this decreased availability of oxygen to tissues in shock, an increased demand may be placed on the high energy phosphate compounds, such as ATP and creatine phosphate, eventually resulting in a decreased level of these compounds (Chaudry et al., 1974b, 1976a; Crowell and Smith, 1964; Cunningham and Keaveny, 1977; Kovach and Funyo, 1960; LePage, 1946; McShan et al., 1945). The results also indicate that during hemorrhagic shock, NAD levels decreased and NADH levels increased in various tissues (Chaudry et al., 1976b; Loiselle and Denstedt, 1964). The ratio of NAD and NADH also decreased significantly in tissues of animals in shock.

It is also well known that circulating lactate and pyruvate levels increase in shock (Huckabee, 1961a and b; Paretz et al., 1965; Spitzer et al., 1972; Weil and Shubin, 1972), and greatly increased lactic acid has been correlated with reduced survival (Huckabee, 1961b; Paretz et al., 1965). Lactic acid accumulates within the cell (Chaudry et al., 1973) as a result of an inability of pyruvate, in the absence of adequate oxygen, to pursue its normal pathway via coenzyme A into the Krebs citric acid cycle. This block in the glycolytic pathway leads to a tendency for glucose to leave the cell, and this also results in reduced formation of ATP (Schumer, 1968). The inability of the cell to form ATP leads to an accumulation of phosphates within the cell and later in the blood. With the fall in energy available to the cell, its vital functions deteriorate. Anaerobic glycolysis obviously occurs in shock or low flow conditions and, thus, the Krebs cycle contributes very little to energy production. Despite the return to normal blood volume, most of the derangements of the metabolic process persist in the irreversible state, which indicates persistent ischemia of peripheral tissue or the failure of cells to utilize oxygen efficiently even when oxygen is available (Baue and Sayeed, 1970; Mela et al., 1971).

CELL AND ORGAN FUNCTION IN SHOCK

Alterations in cell function are early features of the shock syndrome but for obvious reasons are less readily recognized than the hemodynamic and respiratory disturbances. Carbohydrate metabolism is impaired at an early stage of shock with an accumulation within the cells of lactic acid, resulting from an inability of pyruvate, in the absence of adequate oxygen, to pursue its normal pathways into the citric acid cycle. Glycogen breakdown also occurs, and this results in hyperglycemia. The ensuing hyperglycemia is relatively resistant to the administration of insulin. As a result of this, increased glycogenolysis occurs in an attempt to maintain normal intracellular levels of glucose. The failure of carbohydrate metabolism to proceed to completion results in reduced formation of ATP. The decreased ability of the cell to form ATP leads to an accumulation of phosphates within the cell, and later in the blood. The failure of the sodium pump (perhaps due to decreased ATP levels) leads to an extrusion of intracellular potassium and swelling of the cytoplasm and the intracellular organelles, as a result of sodium and water influx into the cell. It is, therefore, clear that metabolic problems and alterations in cell function occur during shock.

Changes in the various organ systems occur as organs and capillary blood flow decrease. In the kidney there is vasoconstriction with decreased renal blood flow and an intrarenal distribution of flow from the cortex, favoring the medulla, decreasing glomerular filtration rate and oliguria. There is also decreased medullary sodium, with loss of the medullary hypoosmolar zone and countercurrent concentrating system. Eventually, tubular necrosis and acute renal failure may occur if the insult persists. This is augmented by pigment excretion of myoglobin and hemoglobin, followed by total renal shutdown with azotemia, hyperkalemia, and acidosis.

In the heart, there is decreased coronary flow which may contribute to a further decrease in cardiac output. The coronary circulation, however, has the capacity of autoregulation and dilates as cardiac output decreases. Electrocardiographic changes and myocardial ischemia may also be seen. In the liver, there is decreased ability to break down lactate and, probably, to detoxify other substances. Unidentified depressor substances may appear. The liver's synthetic activities, particularly production of albumin, are decreased. In the brain, the sensorium and electroencephalographic activity may be depressed if circulatory failure and hypotension are severe. The effects on other vital centers are not well understood. Hyperventilation occurs, probably from decreased central nervous system blood flow, which may initially produce respiratory alkalosis and further decrease cerebral blood flow by a fall in arteriole PCO_2. Later, hyperventilation occurs, owing to metabolic acidosis from increased lactate production. Decreased blood flow in the lungs may contribute to hypoxia and carbon dioxide retention. Much has been written recently about so called "shock lung;" however, a number of studies have shown that little permanent pulmonary dysfunction results from hemorrhagic hypotension (Fulton and Fischer, 1974; Kallos et al., 1973; Moss et al., 1971). Despite findings of arterial desaturation in wounded men in Viet Nam (Martin et al., 1969), it is unlikely that hemorrhage without resuscitation results in overt pulmonary distress (Meyers and Baue, 1973).

It, therefore, seems that oligemic shock per se, does not alter the lungs greatly. However, it certainly could set the stage for making the individual and the lungs more susceptible to further insult.

Bounous et al. (1964) demonstrated that when hemorrhagic hypotension progressed beyond a certain point in dogs, reinfusion of oxygenated blood could restore normal blood flow and near normal oxygen consumption in the liver and limbs, but not in the intestine. They further reported that metabolism of the mucosal cells was decreased and this impaired the energy-dependent defense mechanism which protects the epithelial cells of the mucosa from *Proteus* and toxins. Although extensive destruction of the mucosal layer of the gastrointestinal tract characterizes all forms of shock in dogs, it is exceptionally rare in man. Thus, comparisons based on canine shock models to human are difficult.

HYPOTHESIS ON PROGRESSIVE CELL DETERIORATION WITH ISCHEMIA

Using work over the years from a number of laboratories including our own, we have developed an hypothesis about progressive cell injury with insults such as shock and other forms of trauma (Baue et al., 1974). The initial change in the cell population during shock seems to occur at the cell membrane. The membrane potential decreases (perhaps due to catecholamines or other circulating factors), sodium enters, and potassium leaves the cell. The sodium-potassium ATPase system is activated, ATP is used, the mitochondria are stimulated, and cyclic AMP decreases, which may alter effects of various hormones. ATP further decreases, more sodium gets into the cell, the cell swells, mitochondria swell, and endoplasmic reticulum swells. The above alterations lead to decreased metabolic capability and, eventually, lysosomes leak and there is cell destruction. This, then may be a cycle of deterioration by which one cell and its products can damage adjoining cells.

Evidence for the Hypothesis. Potential difference measurements across the cell membrane were conducted by Shires et al. (1973) and Haljamae et al. (1979). They found that with prolonged and severe hemorrhagic shock the resting trasmembrane potential of the muscle cell decreases. With this change in potential difference, they predicted according to chloride space and the Nerst equation that sodium and water entered the cell and potassium came out. Catecholamines are released during shock (Jakschik et al., 1974b; Ryan et al., 1977), and they also affect membrane potential and function. Shires et al. (1973) and Haljamae et al. (1979) also sampled the interstitial fluid around muscle from animals in shock and found that potassium values were 15–18 mEq/liter after 120 min of shock. This also indicated that with severe prolonged shock, potassium leaves the cell as membrane potential decreases. Studies from our laboratory have shown that the capacity of liver cells to transport sodium and potassium was significantly decreased in prolonged hemorrhagic shock (Sayeed and Baue, 1973). In late shock, the liver cells lose the capability to extrude sodium and maintain intracellular potassium concentrations. These cells seem, therefore, to lose potassium and take up sodium and probably water along with it. As membrane potential and transport capability are altered, the enzyme sodium-potasssium ATPase, which is responsible for sodium and potassium transport, was found to have greatly increased activity, probably in response to increased sodium getting into the cell (Wurth et al., 1973). As this happens, the high energy phosphate compound adenosine triphosphate (ATP) is utilized in increasing amounts. Mitochondria are stimulated to increase ATP production, further sodium gets into the cell and also into the mitochondria, and potassium is lost. ATP levels within the cell begin to decrease. Evidence showing that ATP levels, in various tissues and organs, decrease shock came from the studies of our laboratory (Chaudry et al., 1974b, 1976a) as well as from a number of other investigators (Crowell and Smith, 1964; Cunningham and Keaveny, 1977; Kovach and Funyo, 1960; LePage, 1946; McShan et al., 1945). In studies by Rutenbug et al. (1971) as well as in studies from our own laboratory (Chaudry and Baue, 1977), cellular cyclic AMP levels have been shown to decrease during hemorrhagic shock. Decreased levels of cyclic AMP may produce alterations in the effects of various hormones such as insulin, glucagon, catecholamines, and perhaps, corticosteroids (Campbell et al., 1954; Gann and Egdahl, 1965; Ryan et al., 1977). As the sequence of cell injury with decreased blood flow continues, the cell tends to swell, the mitochondria swell, and the endoplasmic reticulum swells. The work of Holden and his group (1965) describes the cells swelling, mitochondrial swelling, and endoplasmic reticulum swelling during hemorrhagic shock in the rat. Studies from our laboratory have also confirmed these alterations. More recently, George et al. (1978) have shown that marked structural changes in tissues persisted for a prolonged period of time after shock. Trump (1974) studied the progressive changes seen in various cells of patients with shock. He found that virtually all of the acute responses of cells to injury, such as shock, involved alterations of the membrane systems. Early changes, which he described after injury, include clumping of nuclear chromatin, dilitation of the endoplasmic reticulum, and swelling of the cell sap. These changes can therefore be correlated with increased cellular sodium, decreased potassium, and increased water. As a result, the metabolic capability of the cell is further decreased and less ATP is produced because of the shift to anaerobic glycolysis. This leads, therefore, to increased lactic acid production (Chaudry et al., 1973). Further deterioration continues, and eventually, the intracellular organelles, called lysosomes, begin to break down and leak (Glenn and Lefer, 1970). The lysosomes contain hydrolytic enzymes, and these may be involved in further damage inside the cell. Eventually the cell is destroyed and, as this happens, other toxic factors (Lefer, 1978) may be released which may make this a vicious cycle, altering adjoining cells and other tissues and organs. By examining liver mitochondrial function, it was found that there is a progressive decrease in the capability of liver mitochondria to utilize α-ketoglutarate (Mela et al., 1971; Sayeed and Baue, 1971) and therefore to produce high energy phosphate compounds during shock. We have also found decreased protein synthesis in the liver and resistance of muscle membrane to the effects of insulin in promoting glucose uptake by the muscle (Chaudry et al., 1974a; Randall et al., 1974). Blood glucose levels have been reported to increase during the early phases of hypovolemic shock (Bauer et al., 1969; Garcia-Barreno and Balibrea, 1978; Printen et al., 1974). The above mentioned progressive and interrelated effects on cell function will continue in any organ where blood flow is decreased and forms a cycle of alterations progressing to cell and organ death.

TREATMENT PROGRAMS

Preservation of Cell Damage Before the Insult (Before Ischemia)

It is generally accepted that a cell, an organ, or the entire individual will tolerate an episode of ischemia or shock better if organ and cell function is normal before and there are adequate nutrients stored within the cell.

It has been reported that intravenous infusion of inosine 20 min before renal ischemia afforded significant production of the kidneys and significantly improved the survival of animals (Fernando et al., 1976). It has also been shown that kidneys perfused with inosine maintained higher purine nucleotide levels during ischemia and rapidly resynthesized ATP when blood flow was restored in vivo (Fernando et al., 1976). These investigators suggested that inosine provided the pool of ATP precursors and suggested that the resulting high ATP concentration would facilitate the energy-requiring processes of osmotic regulation, tubular function, urine concentration and tissue regeneration in the postischemic period. These are promising results for protection against ischemia and possibly against hemorrhagic shock.

Allopurinal inhibits the enzyme xanthine oxidase. It has been suggested that such an agent may prevent the irreversible conversion of xanthine to uric acid and thus preserve high energy nucleotides of tissues during hemorrhagic shock. The studies of Crowell et al. (1969) have shown that pretreatment of animals with allopurinol significantly improved the survival of animals following hemorrhagic shock. Similar results have been obtained by Baker (1972). Since the salvage pathways normally contribute far more to purine nucleotide synthesis than the de novo pathways and also requires considerably less energy (Murray, 1971), the high plasma levels of uric acid and allantoin formed during hypotension can be expected to severely limit the ability of cells and tissues to restore normal ATP and total adenine nucleotide concentrations following reinfusion. Thus, it could be concluded on the basis of these studies that one aspect of irreversibility in hemorrhagic shock or organ ischemia is probably related to loss of purine base for the restoration of cellular ATP and that allopurinol prevents this loss of purine nucleotides. In other organs such as the heart, ischemia is better tolerated if glycogen levels are built up before the insult.

Treatment of Hemorrhagic Shock

The cornerstone of treatment of cellular and metabolic defects produced by shock is the restoration of circulation. Fluids or blood is given first to provide or maintain an adequate vascular volume. This is often sufficient to correct the problem. If not, then an inotropic agent is used to increase cardiac output and improve blood flow. Along with this, various adjunctive agents and approaches may be used such as steroids and buffering agents (Baue, 1968). However, the discussion now will only include the use of substrates and energy as adjunctive measures, specifically for treating cell injury in shock.

As mentioned above, alterations in cell function are early features of the shock syndrome. Carbohydrate metabolism is impaired in the early stage of shock, and the failure of carbohydrate metabolism to proceed to completion results in reduced formation of ATP. The decreased ability of the cell to form ATP leads to an accumulation of phosphates within the cell and later in the blood. The failure of the sodium pump leads to an inability to maintain intracellular potassium and swelling of the cytoplasm and the intracellular organelles as a result of sodium and water influx into the cell. It is, therefore, clear that metabolic problems and alterations in cell function occur during shock. In view of this, an exciting area of clinical and animal research for the treatment of shock now and in the future is that of correction of the various metabolic problems and alterations in cell functions described previously. If a depressed circulation, such as with hypovolemic shock, alters cell function by decreasing cell membrane capability and decreasing energy capability within the cell, then this can be considered a form of energy crisis for the cell and various organ systems (Baue, 1974). Thus, attempts are being made to provide for these needs by:

1. Providing substrates or compounds which provide for energy production in the cell under adverse circulatory conditions. These include the use of hypertonic glucose and other approaches.

2. Utilizing solutions which provide protection or help for the cell membrane and its functions. These include the so called polarizing solutions containing glucose-insulin-potassium.

3. Providing energy directly by the utilization of the high energy phosphate compound ATP.

Although a high priority is given to the re-establishment of adequate tissue perfusion, the metabolic problems and disturbed cell function which follow shock present potential points for therapeutic intervention.

GLUCOSE

Glucose has been given to provide added energy in hemorrhagic shock (McNamara et al., 1970; Moffatt et al., 1968; Stremple et al., 1976). Administration of hypertonic glucose significantly improves hemodynamics in critically ill patients (Pindyck et al., 1974) and in experimental animals (Baue et al., 1967). The above investigators (Pindyck et al., 1974) propose that exogenous glucose prolongs survival by providing energy substrate. This is in agreement with the hypothesis that increased ATP synthesis resulting from stimulation of glycolysis plays an important role in the adaptation to acute hemorrhage. However, the proposal that exogenous glucose prolongs survival by providing energy does not appear to be true in view of the studies of Stoner et al. (1960). These investigators showed that oxidation of [^{14}C]glucose to $^{14}CO_2$ was decreased by 48% in the shocked rat as compared to control animals. Decreased CO_2 production from [^{14}C]glucose in dogs subjected to hemorrhagic hypotension was also reported by Gump et al. (1973). The studies of Stremple (1974) have shown that rapid and transient increase in blood pressure following adminstration of hypertonic glucose is not mediated by an increased absolute content or tissue uptake of glucose in the myocardium. The above studies (Gump et al., 1973; Stoner et al., 1960; Stremple, 1974),therefore, suggest that the beneficial effects of glucose seen by other investigators (McNamara et al., 1970; Moffatt et al., 1968) were not through provision of energy, since oxidation of glucose to CO_2 is decreased during shock. Thus, the above mentioned studies raise serious questions concerning the efficacy of glucose administration in hemorrhagic shock.

GLUCOSE-INSULIN-POTASSIUM

The addition of pharmacological doses of insulin with potassium to an infusion of hypertonic glucose has been reported to overcome the relative state of hypoinsulinemia of trauma, improving survival rates after hemorrhagic shock (Whitten and Egdahl, 1976). The mechanism of actions proposed for glucose-insulin-potassium include the stabilization of cell membranes, increased osmolarity and an increased inotropic effect. For this reason, these solutions have been called polarizing solutions. The question which remains to be answered, however, is whether treatment with glucose-insulin-potassium is really effective.

CYCLIC AMP AND NICOTINAMIDE

Administration of cyclic AMP after hemorrhagic shock was also attempted. However, the cardiovascular effects of cyclic AMP in animals during shock are inconsistent. Some investigators have reported the effects to be absent (MacRae et al., 1975), small and variable (Henion et al., 1962), or dramatic (Levine et al., 1968). Injection of nicotinamide into rats has been shown to increase the hepatic nicotinamide adenine dinucleotide (NAD) concentration (Lagunas et al., 1970). A number of studies have shown that the activity of many metabolic pathways is dependent on the ratio of oxidized to reduced nicotinamide adenine dinucleotide (Flatt and Ball, 1966; Williamson et al., 1967). Also the injection of nicotinamide provides the means of increasing tissue NAD levels and the NAD/NADH ratio without the necessity of supplying a metabolite. Therefore, it seemed of interest to study the effects of nicotinamide infusion on the survival of animals following shock. While nicotinamide administration may have a beneficial effect in endotoxin shock (Fulton, 1974), it was not found to be of any benefit in hemorrhagic shock (Chaudry et al., 1976b).

KREBS CYCLE INTERMEDIATES

Some efforts have been exerted to identify the metabolic intermediates which if given in large amounts might reverse some of the biochemical deteriorations which occur during shock. Chick et al. (1968) reported that administration of Krebs cycle intermediates (fumarate or a combination of oxaloacetate plus α-ketoglutarate) increased 24 hr survival in rabbits, and they postulated that increased survival was due to stimulation of ATP synthesis. However, measurement of tissue ATP levels was not performed in their studies. It has also been reported that Krebs cycle intermediates produced vasodilitation in the perfused kidney or forelimb of the dog (Frohlich, 1965). Thus, it is conceivable that these agents increased survival in shock through vasodilatation rather than stimulation of ATP synthesis. Conversely, Rush (1971) subsequently reported that infusion of succinate, α-ketoglutarate, and glucose-6-phosphate were given without success.

ADENOSINE AND CREATINE PHOSPHATE

It has recently been reported that administration of more than 6.7 mg adeosine/100 g body wt enhanced recovery of the energy charge and adenine nucleotide levels following shock (Ida et al., 1978). Although these investigators reported that higher concentrations of adenosine restored liver adenine nucleotide and energy charge, the effect of this on the survival of animals following shock was not determined. Moreover, adenosine is known to be a potent vasodilator; in view of the high concentrations of adeonsine used, it is quite possible that the restoration in hepatic nucleotide levels was due to improved blood flow.

The studies of Boonsong et al. (1974) showed that hepatic ATP levels decreased during hemorrhage shock. However, infusion of creatine phosphate following shock significantly increased the hepatic ATP levels. These investigators did not measure the survival of animals following treatment. However, they concluded that high energy phosphate compounds might have therapeutic value in hemorrhagic shock.

ATP

If infused ATP could be used by the cell, it would be of tremendous benefit since it would save time for resynthesis of ATP, which may be a rate-limiting factor during adverse circulatory conditions. Moreover, it seems logical that the most direct approach for raising or restoring tissue ATP levels would be to infuse ATP rather than administer agents which would synthesize ATP. This approach was used by Tallat and associates (1964), who showed that ATP infusion before or during shock proved beneficial for the survival of animals. Sharma and Eiseman (1966) showed that ATP was protective if given prior to hemorrhage, but that it was not protective if it was administered following severe hemorrhagic shock. Our studies extended the observation of the above investigators and showed that administration of ATP-$MgCl_2$ (25 μmoles each) before, during, or even after a period of severe shock had a beneficial effect on the survival of animals (Chaudry et al., 1974c). The essential difference between our studies (Chaudry et al., 1974c) and those of the others (Sharma and Eiseman, 1966; Tallat et al., 1964) is that we gave $MgCl_2$ along with ATP. ATP is a biologically complex agent (Ohnishi and Ebashi, 1963; Sanui and Page, 1967) and when given alone may chelate divalent cations from the vascular system and produce a different hemodynamic effect. Such undesirable effects may be eliminated by giving equimolar amounts of $MgCl_2$. Moreover, it has been shown that Mg^{2+} in vitro and in vivo inhibits the deamination and dephosphorylation of ATP by tissues (Green and Stoner, 1950). Thus, by giving ATP along with $MgCl_2$, higher concentrations of ATP could be available to tissues as compared to when ATP is given alone. Our observations of the beneficial effects of ATP-$MgCl_2$ following hemorrhagic shock have now been confirmed by DiStazio et al. (1980) and by Kraven et al. (1979a).

MECHANISM OF THE BENEFICIAL EFFECT OF ATP-$MgCl_2$

Although the above mentioned studies indicate that administration of ATP-$MgCl_2$ following hemorrhagic shock beneficially affects survival, the precise mechanism by which this occurs remains to be determined. The administration of ATP could produce vasodilitation (Green and Stoner, 1950) and other hemodynamic effects or provide ATP directly to tissues in which ATP levels were lowered or both. The possibility that ATP in these studies in combination with $MgCl_2$ produce beneficial effects through vasodilitation alone does not seem to be a major factor since agents such as ADP and AMP, which are more potent vasodilators, had no beneficial effects (Chaudry et al., 1974c). Another possible explanation is that ATP-$MgCl_2$ has a beneficial effect on the circulation, on microcirculatory blood flow, or on regional perfusion which was not provided by returning blood or blood plus Ringer's lactate (Chaudry et al., 1974c).

The possibility that the beneficial effects of ATP-$MgCl_2$ following hemorrhagic shock are through provision of energy is much more attractive, but also very controversial. Although it has been a popular belief that ATP does not cross the cell membrane (Glynn, 1968), a number of experimental observations now provide clear evidence which contradict this concept (Chaudry and Gould, 1970; Clemens and Forrester, 1979; Forrester, 1972; Maxild, 1978; Pant et al., 1979; Williams et al., 1979). The evidence provided by the above investigators strongly suggests that the release and uptake of ATP by tissues and organs is a physiological process.

Previous studies from our laboratory have shown that ATP levels decreased significantly during shock and that following ATP-$MgCl_2$ infusion, ATP levels in various tissues were restored (Chaudry et al., 1974d). Similar results have been obtained recently by Kraven et al., (1979a). Moreover, our studies have shown that ATP uptake by liver, kidney, and muscle of animals in shock was two and one-half times greater than the corresponding uptake by control tissues (Chaudry et al., 1975b, 1977a). The experiments of Ely (1944) and Sharma and Eiseman (1966) have shown that administration of ATP is selectively taken up by the liver, spleen, heart, and kidney. Kraven et al. (1979b) recently measured tissue lactate production during shock and showed that infusion of ATP-$MgCl_2$ following shock significantly reduced tissue lactate levels. Inhibition of lactate production is a well known effect of ATP and is a manifestation of the Crabtree effect. The Crabtree effect has been utilized to demonstrate permeability of cancer cells to adenine nucleotides (Gosalvez et al., 1978). Since the significant presence of the Crabtree effect in tissue cells of animals in shock was demonstrated by Kraven et al. (1979b), their results therefore demonstrate that such cells are indeed permeable to ATP. Relating all of these findings to our observations (Chaudry et al., 1974c) as well as the observations of other investigators who found beneficial effects of ATP-$MgCl_2$ following hemorrhagic shock (DiStazio et al., 1980; Kraven et al., 1979a), it may be concluded that the beneficial effects of ATP-$MgCl_2$ infusion to animals in shock could be through direct provision of energy to cells in which ATP levels were lowered. It is also possible that infused ATP-$MgCl_2$ has a "priming" effect on the resynthesis of cellular adenine nucleotides. Moreover, infused ATP could be switching the prevailing anaerobiosis to aerobic cycle during shock.

The idea that ATP may have some specific salutary effects in shock is controversial because: 1) ATP is thought to be rapidly broken down or degraded when given into the blood, 2) ATP has been thought not to be able to cross the cell membranes, and 3) ATP has profound hemodynamic effects. However, our studies as well as the studies of a number of investigators have now provided evidence that ATP does have salutary effects following adverse circulatory conditions.

RATIONALE FOR THE USE OF ATP IN THE TREATMENT OF SHOCK

The vital role of ATP in membrane function, carbohydrate metabolism, and tissue respiration (Long, 1943) as an energy supplier for various intracellular reactions and in muscle contractions is well recognized (Dreizen and Gersham, 1970; Green and Stoner, 1950). In an aerobic organism, the production of ATP occurs by two different types of phosphorylation process. One of these processes consists in the substrate phosphorylation encountered in glycolysis and the other is the oxidative phosphorylation associated with the electron transport mechanism. The latter process accounts for over 90% of all ATP generated from ADP, at the expense of energy liberated during metabolism of fuel substrates. Thus, it is clear that in order for ATP levels to be maintained, oxidative phosphorylation must continue. This, however, is not the case during low flow conditions since oxygen delivery as well as substrate delivery to tissues is decreased. Moreover, since glycolysis cannot match ATP production, in relation to its utilization during shock, the cellular adenine nucleotide levels are eventually lowered. The available evidence indicates that during shock the decrease in ATP concentration is accompanied by a decrease in total adenine nucleotide with an irreversible loss of adenine from the cells (Baker, 1972; Crowell et al., 1969). Thus, shock is associated with activation of ATP degradation, probably through AMP deaminase and ultimate hydrolysis of IMP to hypoxanthine, which would be oxidized by xanthine oxidase to uric acid. It would be anticipated from the key role that ATP plays in the cell economy that any significant drop in ATP concentration may have many metabolic consequences.

It has been reported that when the hepatic ATP levels reach approximately 35% of control values, the mitochondria begin to show changes in the control of the generation of energy via respiration (Vogt and Farber, 1970). Liver ATP levels do decrease more than 35% during shock (Chaudry et al., 1974b) and functional (Baue et al., 1974) as well as morphological (George et al., 1978; Holden et al., 1965; Trump, 1974) alterations have been demonstrated during such conditions. Thus, energy is required for structural as well as functional purposes of the cell, and both of the above processes are affected during shock. Because of the above mentioned reasons, it is crucial to try to maintain cellular ATP levels during shock by provision of substrates or energy so the cell can continue to function and, therefore, prevent irreversible cellular damage.

SUMMARY

Simple hypovolemic shock brings about progressive and profound alterations in cellular and, therefore, organ function. We have developed a hypothesis about the progressive cell injury which occurs with shock based on the work from our laboratory, as well as on the work of others. This hypothesis is as follows: With decreased circulation, initial changes take place in the cell and in the function of the cell membrane in the various organs. Membrane potential of the cell decreases and with this decrease in membrane potential, sodium tends to enter the cells while potassium leaves cells. As this occurs, sodium potassium ATPase is activated. ATP is utilized, mitochondria are stimulated, and oxygen availability decreases along the way. Energy levels decrease, cyclic AMP levels decrease, and nuclear function is also depressed. Further, sodium and, perhaps, water enter the cells, potassium leaves the cells, and the cells tend to swell. Water also enters the mitochondria, which appear rounded and swollen. The endoplasmic reticulum seems to have increased hydration. Further membrane changes occur. Tissue responses to insulin decrease. The effect of glucagon, catecholamines, and corticosteroids on the cell are altered. Metabolic capability further decreases, with less availability of utilizable substrate for mitochondria, and uncoupling of mitochondrial energy production takes place. Protein synthesis is also altered. As this sequence of events continues and intensifies, the lysosomes begin to leak and eventually break down. As this occurs, further intracellular disruption develops, the mitochondria are disrupted, and the particular cell is finally destroyed. Based on this information, attempts have been made to directly support and maintain cell function during low flow conditions. The first approach, of course, must be to replace lost volume and increase blood flow generally and to each organ. Oxygen can be provided. Other measures may be in order. We must now also consider how to support cells and reverse the insult on a cellular level. One approach to maintain cellular function during adverse circulatory conditions is to provide substrates, precursors of ATP synthesis, or ATP itself directly.

Additional beneficial effects on cellular functions and survival can be achieved by increasing cellular energy levels. Substrates and energy factors may produce beneficial effects by improving microcirculatory blood flow, by improving membrane function, or by helping other aspects of cell function. In addition, cellular energy levels seem to be increased even after the insult by infusion of ATP complexed with $MgCl_2$. Other approaches to aiding the cell may also be in order.

Acknowledgments. Supported by USPHS Grant 5 RO1 HL 19673 04 and U. S. Army Contract DAMD-17-76-C-6026. The authors express their thanks to Ms. Terrill S. Moorehouse, Ms. Paula Smus, and Ms. Irene Sobochinski for their skill and assistance in typing this chapter.

References

Abel, F.L., and Wolf, M.B.: Increased capillary permeability of 125 labelled albumin during experimental hemorrhagic shock. Trans. N.Y. Acad. Sci. *35:*243, 1973.

Allison, S.P., Hinton, P., and Chamberlain, M.J.: Intravenous glucose tolerance, insulin and free fatty acid levels in burn patients. Lancet *2:*1113, 1968.

Altura, B.M., and Hershey, S.B.: RES phagocytic function in trauma and adaptation to experimental shock. Am. J. Physiol. *215:*1414, 1968.

Altura, B.M., and Hershey, S.B.: Sequential changes in reticuloendothelial system function after acute hemorrhage. Proc. Soc. Exp. Biol. Med. *139:*935, 1972.

Appelgren, L.: Perfusion and diffusion in shock. Acta Physiol. Scand. (Suppl.) *378:*1, 1972.

Baker, C.H.: Protection against irreversible hemorrhagic shock by allopurinol. Proc. Soc. Exp. Biol. Med. *141:*694, 1972.

Baue, A.E.: Recent developments in the study and treatment of shock. Surg. Gynecol. Obstet. *127*:849, 1968.

Baue, A.E.: The energy crisis in surgical patients. Arch. Surg. *109*:349, 1974.

Baue, A.E., and Sayeed, M.M.: Alterations in the functional capacity of mitochondria in hemorrhagic shock. Surgery *68*:40, 1970.

Baue, A.E., Tragus, E., and Parkins, W.: A comparison of isotonic and hypertonic solutions on blood flow and oxygen consumption in the initial treatment of hemorrhagic shock. J. Trauma *7*:743, 1967.

Baue, A.E., Sayeed, M.M., Chaudry, I.H., and Wurth, M.A.: Cellular alterations with shock and ischemia. Angiology *25*:31, 1974.

Bauer, W.A., Vigas, S.M., Haist, R.E., and Drucker, W.R.: Insulin response during hypovolemic shock. Surgery *66*:80, 1969.

Beachstrom, P., Folkow, B., Kovach, A.G.B., et al.: Evidence of plugging in the microcirculation following acute hemorrhage. *Sixth European Conference on Microcirculation*, p. 16. Allborg, 1970.

Beleslin, D., Biset, G.W., Halder, J., and Polak, R.L.: The release of vasopressin without oxytocin in response to hemorrhage. Proc. R. Soc. Lond. [Biol.] *166*:443, 1967.

Bell, R.D., Sinclair, R.J., and Perry, W.L.: The effects of indomethacin on autoregulation and the renal response to hemorrhage. Circ. Shock *2*:57, 1975.

Bernard, C.: *Leçons sur le Diabete*, p. 410. Librairie J.B. Bailliere et fils, Paris, 1877.

Blasingham, C., and Selkurt, E.E.: Changes in metabolism of prostaglandin E by the dog lung during hemorrhagic shock. Fed. Proc. *35*:608, 1976.

Boonsong, C., Moussali, S., Frowell, J.G., Blackwood, J.M., and Rush, B.F.: Induction of aerobic metabolism by phosphocreatine following hemorrhagic shock. Surg. Forum *25*:7, 1974.

Bounous, G., Scholefield, P.G., Hampson, L.G., and Gurd, F.N.: Phosphate metabolism in intestine during hemorrhagic shock. J. Trauma *4*:424, 1964.

Butcher, R.W., Robinson, G.A., Hardmann, J.G., and Sutherland, E.W.: The role of cyclic AMP in hormone actions. In *Advances in Enzyme Regulation*, edited by G. Weber, p. 357. Pergamon Press, New York, 1968.

Campbell, R.M., Sharp, G., Boyne, A.W., and Cuthbertson, D.G.: Cortisone and metabolic response to injuries. Br. J. Exp. Pathol. *35*:566, 1954.

Carlson, R.D., Chaudry, I.H., and Baue, A.E.: Prostaglandin (PG) metabolism, synthesis and blockade in hemorrhage and sepsis. Surg. Forum *30*:476, 1979.

Chaudry, I.H., and Baue, A.E.: Depletion and replenishment of cellular cyclic adenosine monophosphate in hemorrhagic shock. Surgery *145*:877, 1977.

Chaudry, I.H., and Gould, M.K.: Evidence for the uptake of ATP by rat soleus muscle in vitro. Biochim. Biophys. Acta *196*:320, 1970.

Chaudry, I.H., Sayeed, M.M., and Baue, A.E.: The effect of low ATP on glucose uptake in soleus muscle during hemorrhagic shock. Proc. Soc. Biol. Med. *144*:321, 1973.

Chaudry, I.H., Sayeed, M.M., and Baue, A.E.: Insulin resistance in experimental shock. Arch. Surg. *109*:412, 1974a.

Chaudry, I.H., Sayeed, M.M., and Baue, A.E.: Effect of hemorrhagic shock on tissue adenine nucleotides in conscious rats. Can. J. Physiol. Pharmacol. *52*:131, 1974b.

Chaudry, I.H., Sayeed, M.M., and Baue, A.E.: Effect of adenosine triphosphate-magnesium chloride administration in shock. Surgery *75*:220, 1974c.

Chaudry, I.H., Sayeed, M.M., and Baue, A.E.: Depletion and restoration of tissue ATP in hemorrhagic shock. Arch. Surg. *108*:28, 1974d.

Chaudry, I.H., Sayeed, M.M., and Baue, A.E.: The effect of insulin on glucose uptake in soleus muscle during hemorrhagic shock. Can. J. Physiol. Pharmacol. *53*:67, 1975a.

Chaudry, I.H., Sayeed, M.M., and Baue, A.E.: Evidence for enhanced uptake of adenosine triphosphate by muscles of animals in shock. Surgery *77*:833, 1975b.

Chaudry, I.H., Sayeed, M.M., and Baue, A.E.: Alterations in high energy phosphates in hemorrhagic shock as related to tissue and organ function. Surgery *79*:66, 1976a.

Chaudry, I.H., Sayeed, M.M., and Baue, A.E.: Failure of nicotinamide in the treatment of hemorrhagic shock. J. Surg. Res. *21*:27, 1976b.

Chaudry, I.H., Sayeed, M.M., and Baue, A.E.: Evidence for enhanced uptake of ATP by liver and kidney in hemorrhagic shock. Am. J. Physiol. *233*:R33, 1977.

Chaudry, I.H., Adzick, N.S., and Baue, A.E.: Glucocorticoid effects on gluconeogenesis during hemorrhagic shock. J. Surg. Res. *24*:26, 1978.

Chick, W.L., Weiner, R., Cascarano, J., and Zweifach, B.W.: Influence of Krebs cycle intermediates on survival in hemorrhagic shock. Am. J. Physiol. *215*:1107, 1968.

Chien, S.: Blood rheology and its relation to flow resistance and transcapillary exchange with special reference to shock. Adv. Microcirc. *2*:89, 1969.

Chien, S., Dellenback, R.J., and Usami, S.: Blood volume, hemodynamic and metabolic changes in hemorrhagic shock in the normal and splenectomized dogs. Am. J. Physiol. *225*:866, 1973.

Clemens, M.G., and Forrester, T.: Release of ATP from hypoxic isolating working rat heart. Fed. Proc. *28*:1037, 1979.

Cohen, M.M., Sitar, D.S., MacNeal, J.R., and Greenway, C.V.: Vasopressin and angiotensin on resistance vessels of spleen, intestine and liver. Am. J. Physiol. *218*:1704, 1970.

Crowell, J.W., and Smith, E.E.: Oxygen deficit and irreversible hemorrhagic shock. Am. J. Physiol. *206*:313, 1964.

Crowell, J.W., Jones, T.E., and Smith, E.E.: Effect of allopurinol on hemorrhagic shock. Am. J. Physiol. *216*:744, 1969.

Cunningham, S.K., and Keaveny, T.M.: Splanchnic organ adenine nucleotides and their metabolites in hemorrhagic shock. Ir. J. Med. Sci. *146*:136, 1977.

Data, J.L., Chang, L.C.T., and Nies, A.S.: Alterations of renal vascular response to hemorrhage by inhibition of prostaglandin synthesis. Am. J. Physiol. *230*:940, 1976.

Dintenfass, L.: Blood viscosity, internal fluidity of the red cell, dynamic coagulation and the critical capillary radius as factors in the physiology and pathology of circulation and microcirculation. Med. J. Aust. *1*:688, 1968.

DiStazio, J., Maley, W., Thompson, B., et al.: Effects of ATP-$MgCl_2$ administration during hemorrhagic shock on cardiovascular function, metabolism and survival. Adv. Shock Res. *3*:153, 1980.

Dreizen, P., and Gersham, L.C.: Molecular basis of muscle contraction. Myosin. Trans. N.Y. Acad. Sci. *32*:170, 1970.

Drucker, W.R., and DeKiewiet, J.C.: Glucose uptake by diaphragms from rats subjected to hemorrhagic shock. Am. J. Physiol. *206*:317, 1964.

Drucker, W.R., Kaye, M., Kendrick, R., et al.: Metabolic aspects of hemorrhagic shock. 1. Changes in intermediary metabolism during hemorrhage and depletion of blood. Surg. Forum *9*:49, 1958.

Ely, J.O.: Distribution in the heart of injected radioactive "muscle shock factor" of Green. J. Franklin Inst. *238*:378, 1944.

Engel, F.L.: The significance of the metabolic changes during shock. Ann. N.Y. Acad. Sci. *55:*381, 1952.

Fernando, A.R., Armstrong, D.M.G., Griffiths, J.R., et al.: Enhanced preservation of ischemic kidney with inosine. Lancet *13:*555, 1976.

Fine, J., Rutenberg, S., and Schweinberg, F.B.: The role of RES in hemorrhagic shock. J. Exp. Med. *110:*547, 1959.

Flatt, J.T., and Ball, E.G.: Studies on the metabolism of adipose tissues. XVIII. An evaluation of the major pathways of glucose catabolism as influenced by acetate in the presence of insulin. J. Biol. Chem. *241:*2868, 1966.

Fletcher, J.R., and Ramwell, P.W.: Altered lung metabolism of prostaglandins during hemorrhagic and endotoxin shock. Surg. Forum *28:*184, 1977.

Flynn, J.T., Appert, H.E., and Howard, J.M.: Arterial prostaglandin A_1, E_2 and $F_{2\alpha}$ concentration during hemorrhagic shock in the dog. Circ. Shock *2:*155, 1975.

Folkow, B., Lundgren, O., and Wallentin, I.: Studies on the relationship between flow resistance capillary filtration coefficient and regional blood volume in the intestine of the cat. Acta Physiol. Scand. *57:*270, 1963.

Forrester, T.: An estimation of adenosine triphosphate release into the venous effluent from exercising human forearm muscle. J. Physiol. (Lond.) *224:*611, 1972.

Frank, H.A., Frank, E.D., Korman, H., Macchi, I.A., and Hechter, O.: Corticosteroid output and adrenal blood flow during hemorrhagic shock in the dog. Am. J. Physiol. *182:*24, 1955.

Frohlich, E.D.: Vascular effects of Krebs intermediate metabolites. Am. J. Physiol. *208:*149, 1965.

Frolich, J.C.: Gas chromatography—mass spectrometry of prostaglandins. In *The Prostaglandins,* edited by P.W. Ramwell, vol. 3, p. 1. Plenum Press, New York, 1977.

Fulton, R.L.: Prevention of endotoxic death with nicotinamide and adenosine triphosphate. Surg. Forum *25:*17, 1974.

Fulton, R.S., and Fischer, R.P.: Pulmonary changes due to hemorrhagic shock resuscitation with isotonic and hypotonic saline. Surgery *75:*881, 1974.

Gann, D.S., and Egdahl, R.H.: Responses of adrenal corticosteroid secretion to hypotension and hypovolemia. J. Clin. Invest. *44:*1, 1965.

Gann, D.S., and Perkle, J.C.: Role of cortisol in the restitution of blood volume after hemorrhage. Am. J. Surg. *130:*565, 1975.

Garcia-Barreno, P., and Balibrea, J.L.: Metabolic response in shock. Surg. Gynecol. Obstet. *146:*186, 1978.

George, B.C., Ryan, N.T., Ullrick, W.C., and Egdahl, R.H.: Persisting structural abnormalities in liver, kidney, and muscle tissues in hemorrhagic shock. Arch. Surg. *113:*239, 1978.

Gerkes, J.F., and Shand, D.J.: Inhibition by indomethacin of hepatic arterial autoregulation in hemorrhage in the dog. Pharmacologist *17:*221, 1975.

Glenn, T.M.: Alteration of the course of feline post-oligemic shock by prostaglandin infusion. Fed. Proc. *31:*545, 1972.

Glenn, T.M., and Lefer, A.M.: Significance of splanchnic proteases in production of a toxic factor in hemorrhagic shock. Circ. Res. *27:*783, 1970.

Glynn, I.M.: Membrane adenosine triphosphate and cation transport. Br. Med. Bull. *24:*165, 1968.

Goldstone, J., Schmid-Schoendien, H., and Wells, R.E.: The rheology of red blood cell aggregates. Microvasc. Res. *3:*273, 1970.

Gordon, A.H.: The effects of trauma and partial hepatectomy on the rates of synthesis of plasma protein by the liver. In *Plasma Protein Metabolism,* edited by M.A. Rothschild and T. Waldmann, p. 351. Academic Press, New York, 1970.

Gosalvez, M., Garcia-Suarez, S., and Lopez-Alarcon, L.: Metabolic control of glycolysis in normal and tumor permeabilized cells. Cancer Res. *38:*140, 1978.

Green, H.N., and Stoner, H.B.: *Biological Actions of Adenine Nucleotide.* H. K. Lewis & Co. Ltd., London, 1950.

Gross, S.G.: *System of Surgery: Pathological Diagnostic, Therapeutique, and Operative.* Lea & Febiger, Philadelphia, 1872.

Gump, F.E., Long, C.F., Wong, M., and Kinney, J.M.: Exogenous glucose as an energy substrate in experimental hemorrhagic shock. Surg. Gynecol. Obstet. *136:*611, 1973.

Haglund, U.: Vascular reaction in the small intestine of the cat during hemorrhage. Acta Physiol. Scand. *89:*129, 1973.

Haljamae, H., Amundson, B., Bagge, U., Jennische, E., and Branemark, P.I.: Pathophysiology of shock. Pathol. Res. Pract. *165:*200, 1979.

Heath, D.F.: Liver metabolism after injury. Adv. Exp. Biol. Med. *33:*271, 1971.

Heath, D.F., and Corney, P.L.: The effects of starvation, environmental temperature and injury on the rate of disposal of glucose by the rat. Biochem. J. *136:*519, 1973.

Henion, W.F., Sutherland, E.W., and Posternak, T.H.: Effects of derivatives of adenosine 3'-5'-monophosphate in liver slices and intact animals. Biochim. Biophys. Acta *65:*558, 1962.

Hiebert, J.M., McCormick, J.M., and Egdahl, R.H.: Direct measurement of insulin secretory rates: Studies in shocked primates and post-operative patients. Ann. Surg. *176:*296, 1973.

Hift, H., and Strawitz, J.G.: Irreversible hemorrhagic shock in dogs: Problem of onset of irreversibility. Am. J. Physiol. *200:*269, 1961.

Hinshaw, L.B.: Autoregulation in normal and pathological states including shock and ischemia. Circ. Res. (Suppl. 1) *28:*46, 1971.

Holden, W.D., DePalma, R.G., Drucker, W.R., and McKalan, A.: Ultrastructural changes in hemorrhagic shock. Electron microscopic study of liver, kidney and striated muscle cells in rats. Ann. Surg. *162:*517, 1965.

Howard, J.M.: Studies on the absorption and metabolism of glucose following injury—the systematic response to injury. Ann. Surg. *141:*321, 1955.

Huckabee, W.E.: Abnormal resting blood lactate. 1. The significance of hyperlactemia in hospitalized patients. Am. J. Med. *30:*833, 1961a.

Huckabee, W.E.: Abnormal resting blood lactate. 2. Lactic acidosis. Am. J. Med. *30:*840, 1961b.

Hume, D.M.: The secretion of epinephrine, norepinephrine, and corticosteroids in the adrenal venous blood of the dog following single and repeated trauma. Surg. Forum *8:*111, 1957.

Ida, T., Ukikusa, M., Yamamoto, M., et al.: Stimulatory effects of adenosine on hepatic adenine nucleotide and energy charge levels in shocked rats. Circ. Shock *5:*383, 1978.

Jaatella, A.: Effect of traumatic shock on plasma catecholamine levels in man. Ann. Clin. Res. *4:*204, 1972.

Jakschik, B.A., Kourik, J.L., and Needleman, P.: Prostaglandin metabolism and release by the lung during hemorrhage. Pharmacologist *16:*197, 1974a.

Jakschik, B.A., Marshall, G.R., Kourik, J.L., and Needleman, P.: Profile of circulating vasoactive substances in hemorrhagic shock and their pharmacologic manipulation. J. Clin. Invest. *54:*842, 1974b.

Janoff, A.: Alterations in lysosomes (intracellular enzymes) during shock: Effects of precondition (tolerance) and protective drugs. In *Shock,* edited by S.G. Hershey. Little, Brown, Boston, 1964.

Johnston, P.A., and Selkurt, E.E.: Effect of hemorrhagic shock on release of prostaglandin E. Am. J. Physiol. *230:*831, 1976.

Kallos, T., Wyche, M.Q., and Marshall, B.E.: Effects of hemorrhagic shock on pulmonary diffusion and capillary blood volume of the dog. J. Trauma *13:*218, 1973.

Kaplan, J.E., and Saba, T.M.: Humoral deficiency in reticuloendothelial depression after traumatic shock. Am. J. Physiol. *230:*7, 1976.

Kaplan, J.E., Saba, T.M., and Cho, E.: Serological modifications of reticuloendothelial capacity and altered resistance to traumatic shock. Circ. Shock *2:*203, 1976.

Khan, S.N., Tilstone, W.J., Fleck, A., and Broom, I.: Protein synthesis in the rat liver after fracture of the femur. Proc. Nutr. Soc. *33:*93A, 1974.

Kinney, J. M., Duke, J.H., Jr., Long, C.L., and Gump, F.E.: Tissue fuel and weight loss after injury. J. Clin. Pathol. (Suppl. 4) *23:*65, 1970.

Kovach, A.G.B.: Metabolic changes in hemorrhagic shock. Adv. Exp. Biol. Med. *23:*275, 1972.

Kovach, A.G.B., and Funyo, A.: Metabolic responses to injury in cerebral tissue. In *The Biochemical Response to Injury*, edited by H.B. Stoner and B.J. Threlfall, p. 129. Oxford Press, Blackford, 1960.

Kraven, T., Rush, B.F., Gosh, A., et al.: Correlation of survival and metabolic response produced by ATP-$MgCl_2$ in hemorrhagic shock. Circ. Shock *6:*186, 1979a.

Kraven, T., Rush, B.F., Slotman, G.J., and Adams-Griffin, M.: Permeability of the shocked cell to ATP-$MgCl_2$. Surg. Forum *30:*7, 1979b.

Lagunas, R., McLean, P., and Greenbaum, A.L.: The effect of raising the NAD content on the pathways of carbohydrate metabolism and lipogenesis in rat liver. Eur. J. Biochem. *15:*179, 1970.

Lefer, A.M.: Properties of a cardio-inhibitory factors produced in shock. Fed. Proc. *37:*2734, 1978.

Lefer, A.M., and Barenholz, Y.: Pancreatic hydrolyases and the formation of the myocardial depressant factor in shock. Am. J. Physiol. *223:*1103, 1972.

Lefer, A.M., and Glenn, T.M.: The lysosomal protease-myocardial depressant factor system in circulatory shock. In *Neurohumoral and Metabolic Aspects of Injury*, edited by H.B. Stoner and J.J. Spitzer, p. 367. Plenum Press, New York, 1973.

Leffler, C.W., and Passmore, J.C.: Effects of indomethacin on hemodynamics of dogs in refractory hemorrhagic shock. J. Surg. Res. *23:*392, 1977.

LePage, G.A.: Biological energy transformation during shock as shown by tissue analysis. Am. J. Physiol. *146:*267, 1946.

Levine, R.A., Dixon, L.M., and Franklin, R.B.: Effects of exogenous adenosine 3'-5'-monophosphate in man: Cardiovascular responses. Clin. Pharmacol. Ther. *9:*168, 1968.

Lillihei, R.C., Johnson, D.J., and Hardway, R.M.: The nature of irreversible shock: Experimental and clinical observations. Ann. Surg. *160:*1682, 1963.

Lillihei, R.C., Longerbean, J.K., Bloch, H.H., and Mannix, W.D.: The nature of irreversible shock: Experimental and clinical observations. Ann. Surg. *160:*682, 1964.

Loegering, D.J., and Saba, T.M.: Hepatic Kupffer cell dysfunction during hemorrhagic shock. Circ. Shock *3:*107, 1976.

Lofstrom, B.: Changes in the flow properties of blood related to nutritive blood flow. Acta Anaesthesiol. Scand. (Suppl.) *25:*305, 1966.

Loiselle, J.M., and Denstedt, O.F.: Biochemical changes during acute physiological failure in the rat. II. The behavior of adenine and pyridine nucleotides of the liver during shock. Can. J. Biochem. *42:*21, 1964.

Long, C.: The *in vitro* oxidation of pyruvic and ketobutric acids by ground preparation of pigeon brains: The effect of inorganic phosphate and adenine nucleotide. Biochem. J. *37:*215, 1943.

Machido, G.W., Brown, C.S., Lavigne, J.E., and Rush, B.F.: Prostaglandin E_1 as therapeutic agent in hemorrhagic shock. Surg. Forum *24:*12, 1973.

Machido, G.W., Brown, C.S., Lavigne, J.E., and Rush, B.F.: Beneficial effects of prostaglandin E_1 in experimental hemorrhagic shock. Surg. Gynecol. Obstet. *143:*433, 1976.

MacLean, L.D.: Shock: Causes and management of circulatory collapse. In *Davis-Christopher's Textbook of Surgery*, edited by D.C. Sabiston, p. 65. W.B. Saunders, Philadelphia, 1977.

MacRae, M.L., Chiu, C.J., and Hinchey, E.J.: Effects of exogenous cyclic adenosine monophosphate in hemorrhagic shock. Surgery *78:*254, 1975.

Markelonis, G., and Garbus, J.: Alterations of intracellular oxidative metabolism as stimuli evoking prostaglandin biosynthesis. Prostaglandins *20:*1087, 1975.

Martin, A.M., Simmons, R.L., and Heistercamp, C.A.: Respiratory insufficiency in combat casualties. 1. Pathologic changes in the lung of patients dying of wounds. Ann. Surg. *170:*30, 1969.

Maxild, J.: Effect of externally added ATP and related compounds on active transport of P-aminohippurate and metabolism in cortical slices of the rabbit kidney. Arch. Int. Physiol. Biochim. *86:*509, 1978.

McNamara, G.G., Mills, D., and Aby, G.B.: Effect of hypertonic glucose on hemorrhagic shock in rabbits. Ann. Thorac. Surg. *9:*116, 1970.

McShan, W.H., Potter, V.R., Goldman, M.A., Shipley, E.G., and Meyer, R.K.: Biological energy transformations during shock as shown by blood chemistry. Am. J. Physiol. *145:*93, 1945.

Meguid, M.M., and Egdahl, R.H.: Neuroendocrine response to operation. In *Textbook of Surgery*, edited by J.D. Hardy, p. 10. J.B. Lippincott, Philadelphia, 1977.

Mela, L., Bacalzo, L.V., Jr., and Miller, L.D.: Defective oxidative metabolism of rat liver mitochondria in hemorrhagic or endotoxin shock. Am. J. Physiol. *220:*571, 1971.

Meyers, J.R., and Baue, A.E.: Does hemorrhagic shock damage the lung? J. Trauma *13:*509, 1973.

Moffatt, J.G., King, J.A.C., and Drucker, W.R.: Tolerance to prolonged hypovolemic shock: Effect of infusion of an energy substrate. Surg. Forum *19:*5, 1968.

Moore, F.D.: The effects of hemorrhage on body composition. N. Engl. J. Med. *273:*567, 1965.

Moss, G.S., Siegel, D.C., Cochin, A., and Fresquez, V.: Effects of saline and colloid solutions on pulmonary function in hemorrhagic shock. Surg. Gynecol. Obstet. *133:*53, 1971.

Munro, H.N.: A general survey of mechanisms regulating protein metabolism in mammals. In *Mammalian Protein Metabolism*, edited by H.N. Munro, vol. 4, p. 3. Academic Press, New York, 1970.

Murray, A.W.: The biological significance of purine salvage. Annu. Rev. Biochem. *40:*811, 1971.

Nickerson, M.: Vascular adjustments during the development of shock. Can. Med. Assoc. J. *103:*853, 1970.

Ohnishi, T., and Ebashi, S.: Spectrophotometrical measurements of instantaneous calcium binding of the releasing factor of muscle. J. Biochem. (Tokyo) *54:*506, 1963.

Olsen, N.S., and Nuetzell, J.A.: Resistance to small doses of insulin in various clinical situations. J. Clin. Invest. *29:*862, 1950.

Pant, H.C., Terakawa, S., Yoshioki, T., Tasaki, I., and Gainer, H.: Evidence for the utilization of extracellular [α-^{32}P]ATP for the phosphorylation of intercellular proteins in the squid giant axon. Biochim. Biophys. Acta *582:*197, 1979.

Paretz, D.I., Scott, H.M., Duff, J., Dosseter, J.B., MacLean, L.D., and McGregor, M.: The significance of lactic acidemia in the shock syndrome. Ann. N.Y. Acad. Sci. *119:*1133, 1965.

Perkle, J.C., and Gann, D.S.: Restitution of blood volume after hemorrhage: Role of the adrenal cortex. Am. J. Physiol. *230:* 1683, 1976.

Pindyck, F., Drucker, W.R., Brown, R.S., and Shoemaker, W.C.: Cardiorespiratory effects of hypertonic glucose in the critically ill patient. Surgery *75:*11, 1974.

Priano, S.L., Miller, T.H., and Traber, D.L.: Views of prostaglandin E_1 in the treatment of experimental hypovolemic shock. Circ. Shock *1:*221, 1974.

Printen, K.J., Keefe, W.E., Foster, E., and Brown, W.: Fluxes in serum glucose and fatty acids in early endotoxemia and hemorrhage. Surg. Gynecol. Obstet. *138:*686, 1974.

Randall, G.R., Sayeed, M.M., Chaudry, I.H., and Baue, A.E.: Protein synthesis by rat liver slices in hemorrhagic shock. Fed. Proc. *33:*318, 1974.

Renkin, E.M.: Neurogenic factors in microcirculatory low flow states. In *Microcirculation as Related to Shock*, edited by D. Shepro and G. Fulton, p. 139. Academic Press, New York, 1968.

Rhoads, J.E., and Howard, J.M.: Carbohydrate metabolism. In *Chemistry of Trauma*, p. 113. Charles C Thomas, Springfield, IL, 1963.

Robinson, G.A., Butcher, R.W., and Sutherland, E.W.: Adenyl cyclase as an adrenergic receptor. Ann. N.Y. Acad. Sci. *319:* 703, 1967.

Rocha, S.E., Jr., and Rosenberg, M.: The release of vasopressin in response to hemorrhage and its role in the mechanism of blood pressure regulation. J. Physiol. (Lond.) *202:*535, 1969.

Rush, B.F.: Irreversibility of the post-transfusion phase of hemorrhagic shock. Adv. Exp. Med. Biol. *23:*215, 1971.

Rutenberg, A.M., Bell, M.L., Butcher, R.W., Polgar, P., Dorn, B.D., and Egdahl, R.H.: Adenosine-3'-5'-monophosphate levels in hemorrhagic shock. Ann. Surg. *174:*461, 1971.

Ryan, N.T., George, B.C., Harlowe, T.L., Hiebert, J.M., and Egdahl, R.H.: Endocrine activation and altered muscle metabolism after hemorrhagic shock. Am. J. Physiol. *233:*E439, 1977.

Saba, T.M.: Prevention of hepatic reticuloendothelial host-defense failure after surgery by intravenous opsonic glycoprotein therapy. Ann. Surg. *188:*142, 1978.

Sanui, H., and Page, M.: Effect of ATP, EDTA and EGTA on the simultaneous binding of sodium, potassium, magnesium and calcium by rat liver microsomes. J. Cell. Physiol. *69:*11, 1967.

Sayeed, M.M., and Baue, A.E.: Mitochondrial metabolism of succinate, beta-hydroxybutyrate and alpha-ketoglutarate in hemorrhagic shock. Am. J. Physiol. *205:*1275, 1971.

Sayeed, M.M., and Baue, A.E.: Na-K transport in rat liver slices in hemorrhagic shock. Am. J. Physiol. *224:*1265, 1973.

Schmid-Schoendien, H., and Wells, R.E.: Rheological properties of human erythrocytes and their influence upon the anomalous viscosity of blood. Ergeb. Physiol. Biol. Chem. Exp. Pharmakol. *63:*146, 1971.

Schumer, W.: Localization of the energy pathway block in shock. Surgery *64:*55, 1968.

Schumer, W., Kapica, S.K., and Teng, T.L.: Validity of the lysosomal theory in oligemic shock. Arch. Surg. *99:*325, 1969.

Scornik, O.A., and Paladini, A.C.: Angiotensin blood levels in hemorrhagic hypotension and other related conditions. Am. J. Physiol. *206:*553, 1964.

Seligman, A.M., Frank, H.A., Alexander, B., and Fine, J.: Traumatic shock. XV. Carbohydrate metabolism in hemorrhagic shock in the dog. J. Clin. Invest. *26:*536, 1947.

Sharma, G.P., and Eiseman, B.: Protective effect of ATP in experimental hemorrhagic shock. Surgery *59:*66, 1966.

Shires, T., and Carrico, C.J.: Current status of shock problems. In *Current Problems in Surgery*. Year Book Medical Publishers, Chicago, 1966.

Shires, G.T., Carrico, C.J., and Canizaro, P.C.: *Shock*, vol. 13, ch. 2. W.B. Saunders, Philadelphia, 1973.

Shoemaker, E.W., and Rall, T.W.: *Shock: Chemistry, Physiology, and Therapy*. Charles C Thomas, Springfield, IL, 1967.

Shoemaker, W.C., Stahr, L.J., Kim, S.I., and Elwyn, D.H.: Sequential circulatory and metabolic changes in the liver and whole body during hemorrhagic shock. Adv. Exp. Med. Biol. *33:*293, 1973.

Simeone, F.A.: Shock. In *Christopher's Textbook of Surgery*, p. 58. W.B. Saunders, Philadelphia, 1964.

Skillman, J.J., Lawler, D.P., Hickler, R.B., Lyons, J.H., Olson, J.E., Ball, M.R., and Moore, F.D.: Hemorrhage in normal man: Effect on renin, cortisol, aldosterone, and urine composition. Ann. Surg. *166:*865, 1967a.

Skillman, J.J., Awwad, H.K., and Moore, F.D.: Plasma protein kinetics of the early transcapillary refill after hemorrhage in man. Surg. Gynecol. Obstet. *125:*983, 1967b.

Skillman, J.J., Hedley-White, J., and Pallotta, J.A.: Hormonal fuel and respiratory relationships after acute blood loss in man. Surg. Forum *21:*23, 1970.

Slater, T.F.: Lysosomes in experimentally induced tissue injury. In *Lysosomes in Biology and Pathology*, edited by J.T. Dingel and H.B. Fell, p. 469. Elsevier, New York, 1969.

Spitzer, J.J., Spitzer, J.A., Wang, J.T., and Scott, J.C.: Myocardial metabolism during acute hemorrhage or endotoxin shock. Adv. Exp. Med. Biol. *23:*267, 1972.

Spitzer, J.J., Weiner, R., and Wolf, E.H.: Non-esterified fatty acid (FFA) metabolism following severe hemorrhage in the conscious dog. Adv. Exp. Med. Biol. *33:*221, 1973.

Stoner, H.B.: Studies on the mechanism of shock. The quantitative aspects of glycogen metabolism after limb ischaemia in the rat. Br. J. Exp. Pathol. *39:*635, 1958.

Stoner, H.B., Heath, D.F., and Collins, O.M.: The metabolism of ^{14}C-glucose, ^{14}C-fructose and 2-^{14}C-pyruvate after limb ischemia in the rat. Biochem. J. *76:*135, 1960.

Stremple, J.F.: Rapid hypertonic glucose infusion: Organ localization of label after ^{14}C-glucose during hemorrhagic shock. J. Surg. Res. *17:*90, 1974.

Stremple, J.F., Thomas, H., Sakach, V., and Trelka, D.: Myocardial utilization of hypertonic glucose during hemorrhagic shock. Surgery *80:*4, 1976.

Sutherland, E.W., and Robinson, G.A.: The role of cyclic adenosine monophosphate in control of carbohydrate metabolism. Diabetes *18:*797, 1969.

Tallat, S.M., Massion, W.H., and Schilling, J.A.: Effects of adenosine triphosphate administration in irreversible hemorrhagic shock. Surgery *55:*813, 1964.

Trump, B.F.: The role of cellular membrane systems in shock. In *The Cell in Shock*, p. 16. The Upjohn Co., Kalamazoo, 1974.

Trump, B.F., Crocker, B.P., and Mergner, W.J.: The role of energy metabolism, ion and water shifts in the pathogenesis of cell injury. In *Cell Membranes, Biological and Pathological Aspects*, edited by G.W. Richter and D.G. Scarpelli, p. 84. Williams & Wilkins, Baltimore, 1971.

Tyssebough, I., and Kirkebo, A.: The effect of indomethacin on renal blood flow distribution during hemorrhagic shock in dogs. Acta Physiol. Scand. *101:*15, 1977.

Vogt, M.T., and Farber, E.: The effects of ethionine treatment on the metabolism of liver mitochondria. Arch. Biochem. Biophys. *141:*162, 1970.
Watts, D.T.: Arterial blood epinephrine levels during hemorrhagic hypotension in dogs. Am. J. Physiol. *184:*271, 1956.
Weil, M.H., and Shubin, H.: Proposed reclassification of shock states with special references to distributive effects. Adv. Exp. Med. Biol. *23:*13, 1972.
Weinstein, H., Berne, R.M., and Sachs, H.: Vasopressin in blood: Effect of hemorrhage. Endocrinology *66:*712, 1960.
Whitten, R.H., and Egdahl, R.H.: High dose glucose-insulin-potassium in treatment of irreversible hemorrhagic shock. Surg. Forum *27:*60, 1976.
Whitten, R.H., Ryan, N.T., and Egdahl, R.H.: PGE$_2$ in treatment of "irreversible" hemorrhagic shock. Surg. Forum *30:* 473, 1979.
Wiggers, C.J.: Present status of shock problem. Physiol. Rev. *22:*74, 1942.
Williams, D., Reibel, D., and Rovetto, J.J.: ATP induced increase in ATP content in cultured myocardial cells. Fed. Proc. *38:*1389, 1979.
Williamson, D.H., Lind, P., and Krebs, H.A.: The redox state of free nicotinamide-adenine dinucleotide in the cytoplasm and mitochondria of rat liver. Biochem. J. *103:*514, 1967.
Wurth, M.A., Sayeed, M.M., and Baue, A.E.: Na-K-ATPase activity in the liver with hemorrhagic shock. Proc. Soc. Exp. Biol. Med. *139:*1238, 1973.
Zweifach, B.W.: Etiology of the shock syndrome. Heart Bull. *14:*21, 1965.
Zweifach, B.W.: Local regulation of capillary pressure. Circ. Res. (Suppl. 1) *28:*129, 1971.
Zweifach, B.W., and Fronek, A.: The interplay of central and peripheral factors in irreversible hemorrhagic shock. Prog. Cardiovasc. Dis. *18:*147, 1975.
Zweifach, B.W., and Intraglietta, M.: Fluid exchange across capillaries during hemorrhagic hypotension. Fed. Proc. *27:* 512, 1968.
Zweifach, B.W., Banacerras, B., and Thomas, L.: Relationship between the vascular manifestation of shock produced by endotoxin, trauma, and hemorrhage. 2. The possible role of the RES in resistance to each type of shock. J. Exp. Med. *106:*403, 1957.
Zweifach, B.W.: Microcirculatory derangements as a basis for the lethal manifestation of experimental shock. Br. J. Anesth. *30:*446, 1958.

CHAPTER 16

Overview of Endotoxin Shock

LERNER B. HINSHAW

Endotoxin shock is a pathophysiologic phenomenon resulting from the release of endotoxin from gram-negative organisms (Berry, 1977) or following the exogenous administration of endotoxin experimentally (Weil et al., 1956; MacLean and Weil, 1956; MacLean et al., 1956; Visscher, 1958). Endotoxins are lipopolysaccharide protein lipid complexes (Morrison and Ulevitch, 1978) which are released from cell membranes of killed bacteria. The term, "endotoxin shock," is usually considered to be similar or equal to "endotoxic shock," "gram-negative shock," "septic shock," and "septicemic shock," and has been associated generally with the terms, "bacterial shock," "bacteremic shock," "septicemia," and "bacteremia." Concerns for definitions of endotoxin shock and questions regarding the relevance of experimental animal models in terms of their application to man have been expressed by Waisbren (1964), Powrie and Norman (1976), Sibbald (1976), and Weil (1977).

History

Brill and Libman described the first cases of gram-negative bacteremia in 1899. The first indication that endotoxin participates in the genesis of shock arose from the clinical observations of Spink et al. (1948): following the use of an antibiotic in bacteremic patients, they documented the elicitation of shock, including the presence of fever, systemic hypotension, and tachycardia. Waisbren (1951) was the first to point out that a specific "shock-like picture" could be seen in some patients with bacteremia, which included systemic hypotension, cold and clammy skin, and lethargy. During the same period,

Borden and Hall (1951) and Braude et al. (1953) observed severe shock in patients transfused with blood contaminated with gram-negative organisms. Studdiford and Douglas (1956) first drew attention to the precipitation of shock associated with septic abortion.

The Genesis of Endotoxin Shock and Its Relation to "Septic Shock" in Man

Spink et al. (1948) and Borden and Hall (1951) presumed that shock in humans is caused by the release of endotoxin. Spink (1972) pointed out that endotoxin alone can cause shock in man but that living, invasive gram-negative bacterial cells may conceivably contribute other toxic factors in patients. It has also been suggested that the combination of live organisms and endotoxin may elicit an accelerated Schwartzman phenomenon or an acute allergic reaction, either of which may lead to shock (Waisbren, 1964). It is generally believed that endotoxin is the chief factor which precipitates the shock state (Cavanagh et al., 1977). In an extensive review on the molecular aspects of endotoxins, Nowotny (1969) pointed out that the presence of certain functional groups and structural arrangements of the endotoxin moiety determine its toxic effects in man and animals.

Regardless of possible distinctions between the modes of action of live organisms or endotoxins, gram-negative organisms account for the majority of the cases of septic shock in man (Murdoch et al., 1968). The most common are *Escherichia coli, Aerobacter aerogenis, Proteus mirabilis* or *vulgaris*, and *Pseudomonas aeroginosa*, according to Cavanagh et al. (1977), and according to Weil (1977), *Escherichia coli, Klebsiella-Enterobacter-Serratia* group, *Proteus* species, *Pseudomonas* species, *Bacteroides* species, and *Salmonella* species. The underlying pathophysiological process of septic or endotoxic shock appears to have an immunological basis involving the release of vasoactive substances and neurohumoral agents and the precipitation of coagulation abnormalities (Spink et al., 1964; McKay et al., 1959; Cavanagh et al., 1977; Lees, 1976).

The Medical Significance of Septic and Endotoxic Shock

There is a critical need for research in clinical septic shock. The serious nature of septic shock in man has been underscored recently by McCabe (1974), who points out that since the time of Waisbren's report of 29 cases of bacteremia (Waisbren, 1951), the numbers of cases and deaths from gram-negative bacteremia have increased progressively each year. He estimates that as many as 330,000 bacteremias, with 132,000 deaths, may occur each year (McCabe, 1974).

There is a serious need for research regarding the basic mechanisms responsible for the drastic effects of endotoxins and live organisms on host systems. Endotoxin and bacterial organisms are known to exert profound multiple biologic effects on living organisms. In 1974, Thomas commented that, "Our arsenals for fighting off bacteria are so powerful and involve so many different defense mechanisms, that we are in more danger from them than from the invaders." He further stated that "these (endotoxin) macromolecules are read by our tissues as the very worst of bad news. When we sense lipopolysaccharide (endotoxin), we are likely to turn on every defense at our disposal." Morrison and Ulevitch (1978), in their extensive review on the effects of bacterial endotoxins on host mediation systems, concluded that endotoxins have significant effects on coagulation and complement, on platelets, polymorphonuclear leukocytes and endothelial cells, especially on macrophages and monocytes, and, perhaps to a lesser extent, mast cells. These effects have been demonstrated to be the result of both indirect and direct endotoxin mediator interactions. Two major areas of basic research are sorely in need of increased support: 1) the contributions of the interactions of various host mediation systems during the pathophysiologic effects of endotoxins; and 2) identification of the critical molecular parameters which regulate the interactions between endotoxins and plasma proteins and mediator cell membranes (Morrison and Ulevitch, 1978).

General Description of Endotoxin Shock and Its Classification

The four general forms of shock, according to the most recent classification, are hypovolemic, cardiogenic, distributive, and obstructive shock (Weil, 1972). Endotoxin shock has been placed in the category of "distributive shock" by Weil, who terms it "bacterial shock." As such, it possesses a defect in blood volume distribution inasmuch as alterations in capacitance account for sequestion of blood in the venous circuit. It is expressed in two forms: 1) high or normal vascular resistance, and 2) low vascular resistance, both forms ultimately encompassing perfusion and ventilation defects and, in some instances, cardiac depression.

Patients with the "low vascular resistance" form of sepsis, if adequately hydrated, tend to possess a warm, flushed, dry skin and usually have a normal or increased cardiac output (Wilson, 1976). In contrast, septic patients with the "high vascular resistance" form have low cardiac outputs and almost invariably have prolonged shock with hypovolemia or cardiac failure (Wilson, 1976). In both of these forms of shock, as cardiac output falls, there are substantial increases in mortality (Weil, 1977).

Experimental Shock Models Developed to Study the Mechanisms of Human Septic Shock

Many questions have arisen concerning the adequacy of animal shock models in regard to their application in human septic shock. Waisbren (1964) pointed out dissimilarities between the responses of dogs to endotoxin and man administered endotoxin in the form of killed typhoid organisms. He concluded:

In the last analysis, the true explanation of the pathophysiology of gram-negative shock will come from more intensive studies of patients while they are suffering from the condition and, perhaps more practically, from intensive study of an animal model that more closely simulates the clinical condition in man. ... These further studies ... may prove that endotoxin has a role in gram-negative shock, but at this time the equation of endotoxin and gram-negative shock seems unwarranted.

Weil (1977) commented that "the extent to which the reactions to endotoxin in experimental animals serves as an applicable model of bacterial shock in patients is controversial."

In order to develop more realistic animal models, recent emphasis has been placed on the administration of live organisms rather than endotoxin, and results from these two means of eliciting experimental septic shock have been compared in both canine and primate species (Hinshaw, 1972). Use of live *E. coli* organisms in contrast to endotoxin elicits a "warm phase" of shock, including elevation of regional blood flow, and possesses the more clinically relevant characteristic of a slow release of endotoxin within the circulation following destruction of *E. coli* (Hinshaw, 1972).

Other models include: 1) the canine "septic leg" procedure of Thal (1972); 2) the injection of live *E. coli* into the canine gallbladder following division of the cystic artery and duct (Perbellini et al., 1978); 3) the placing of human fecal material within gelatin capsules which are placed within the peritoneal cavity of the rat (Nichols et al., 1978); 4) the performing of an appendectomy in dogs without closure of the appendiceal stump allowing cecal contents to flow into the peritoneal cavity (Stone et al., 1979); and 5) cecal ligation in dogs (Richardson et al., 1979)—to cite a few experimental procedures developed to better simulate clinical septic shock. All of the aforementioned methods possess their advocates who characteristically draw attention to certain particular responses of their animal model which seem to more closely simulate the clinical entity. It is probably true that each procedure will bear its own unique contribution to our understanding of the mechanisms of septic shock.

Problems of Obtaining Control Clinical Findings in Untreated Septic Shock

In attempts to summarize the most current understanding of septic shock in man, the quotation by Udhoji is most pertinent: "There are formidable limitations in studying bacterial shock in patients rather than in experimental animals, for example, the (human) subjects are sick persons who have had infections for a variable period of time, and previous treatment is a factor which is entirely uncontrolled" (Udhoji et al., 1963). From the basic scientist's point of view, it seems particularly difficult to interpret control or baseline values, especially hemodynamic parameters, since treatment may have been instituted before any measurements are taken (Clowes et al., 1966; MacLean et al., 1967; Shoemaker et al., 1970; Dietzman et al., 1971; Wilson et al., 1972; Siegel et al., 1972; Wilson, 1976; Cerra et al., 1978). Clowes et al. (1966) reported that when baseline circulatory and metabolic parameters were recorded in patients with extensive peritonitis, each had already received one or more liters of fluid. Cerra et al. (1978) have stated that baseline cardiac output measurements in septic shock patients were recorded only following fluid resuscitation. Therefore, one has to consider fluid administration as a significant additive factor in eliciting the "high cardiac output phenomenon" of septic shock. One difficulty in understanding the mechanism of septic or endotoxic shock by studying the responses of patients is, therefore, the multiple effects of therapy, particularly because of those procedures instituted early, prior to the attainment of baseline values. There is a need for well controlled animal studies in this form of shock, patterned closely after the clinical entity which will reveal the underlying mechanisms of shock or impending shock in the untreated subject, as well as identifying the responses to experimentally controlled therapeutic procedures. Thus, animal and man become useful adjunctive partners in the conquering of this form of shock by vigorous cross fertilization of findings between species achieved through well designed and executed studies.

Objective of This Overview

A literal explosion of publications on endotoxic and septic shock has occurred during the last two decades, incorporating studies ranging the entire gamut, from subcellular aspects to treatment of patients. Such an all encompassing inquiry into the mechanisms and treatment of this form of shock creates serious difficulty with attempts to address reports in the published literature. The primary purpose of this overview is merely to summarize some aspects of inquiry while emphasizing others which are deemed by the author to be more directly related to clinical application.

Published reviews, symposia, and texts pertaining to endotoxic and septic shock are referred to in this overview; included are several important publications providing detailed information pertaining to specialized fields of inquiry. To cite a few, there are those by Thomas (1954), early history; Bennett and Cluff (1957), pyrogenic aspects; Gilbert (1960), physiology and hemodynamics; Spink (1962), clinical; Raskova and Vanecek (1964), pharmacology; Zweifach and Janoff (1965), physiology; Nowotny (1969), chemistry; Halinen (1976), nervous system; Utili et al. (1977), liver; Berry (1977), metabolism; and Morrison and Ulevitch (1978), cellular and subcellular aspects.

Several detailed books or published symposia are: Landy and Braun (1964), *Bacterial Endotoxins*; Mills and Moyer (1965), *Shock and Hypotension: Pathogenesis and Treatment*; Shoemaker (1967), *Shock*; Weil and Shubin (1967), *Diagnosis and Treatment of Shock*; Shepro and Fulton (1968); *Microcirculation as Related to Shock*; Thal et al. (1971), *Shock*, Kadis et al. (1971), *Bacterial Endotoxins: A Comprehensive Treatise*; Hershey et al. (1971), *Septic Shock in Man*; Hinshaw and Cox (1972), *The Fundamental Mechanisms of Shock*; Forscher et al. (1972), *Shock in Low- and High-Flow States*; Kovach et al. (1973), *Neurohumoral and Metabolic Aspects of Injury*;

Urbaschek et al. (1975), *Gram-Negative Bacterial Infections and Mode of Endotoxin Actions*; Cavanagh et al. (1977), *Septic Shock in Obstetrics and Gynecology*; Weil and Henning (1978), *Handbook of Critical Care Medicine*; and Jeljaszewicz and Wadstrom (1978), *Bacterial Toxins and Cell Membranes*.

CHARACTERIZATION OF RESPONSES IN ENDOTOXIC AND SEPTIC SHOCK IN MAN AND ANIMALS

Hemodynamic Responses

Abnormal hemodynamic responses comprise a primary hallmark of endotoxic or septic shock. They are of great complexity and variability and differ between the species and vary according to the severity, sequential time periods, and duration of shock. In animal models, and in humans, at least four sequential phases of shock have been recognized: 1) preshock period, lasting minutes to a few hours, characterized by a moderate decrease in mean systemic pressure, tachycardia, tachypnea, fever, restlessness, and irritation; 2) a period of slowly or rapidly developing systemic hypotension, decreased venous return, and depressed cardiac output; 3) a compensatory period precipitated by the presence of systemic hypotension, involving neurohumoral and autonomic reflex activations; followed by 4) a period of improvement if survival is to be attained, or progressive circulatory deterioration with sequentially developing multiple organ failure, terminating in irreversible shock and death. No organ system or biologic function appears to escape the ravages of lethal endotoxic or septic shock.

The hemodynamic responses to gram-negative organisms or endotoxin include several diverse physiologic alterations. The pathologic implementation of these alterations is believed to lead to inadequate perfusion of vital organs, resulting in the inability of body cells to maintain a steady state metabolic status. Weil (1977) has developed the concept that the primary underlying defect in the state of shock caused by bacterial infections is a blood volume *distributive defect*. According to this view, blood is redistributed within the vascular bed in a fashion which results in a lowered cardiac output and subsequent organ malperfusion. Weil describes five primary components of the cardiovascular system which contribute to an understanding of this process. One component is the *heart*, which serves as the power source for circulation. A second component is the *blood*, consisting of an adequate volume for body perfusion. The three remaining components are the *arteries and arterioles* (the resistance unit), the *capillaries* (a passive circuit), and the *veins* (a variable capacitance bed normally containing approximately 80% of the total blood volume).

According to Weil's classification, pure uncomplicated septic shock has the underlying problem of the blood being in the wrong places due to maldistribution. This interesting concept paves the way for a clearer understanding of how the other forms of shock (Weil, 1977)—hypovolemic, cardiogenic, and obstructive shock—may be additionally involved in septic shock, complicate our understanding of the underlying mechanisms of the shock state, and confound attempts at therapy.

Distributive shock (septic shock) is further subdivided into "high or normal resistance" or "low resistance" forms (Weil, 1977). The low resistance form of shock is usually associated with normal or increased cardiac output during the early ("warm shock") phase, and the high resistance form ("cold phase") is lowered cardiac output, decreased blood volume, and elevated pulmonary and systemic vascular resistances (Udjohi and Weil, 1965; Clowes et al., 1966; MacLean et al., 1967; Siegel et al., 1967; Wilson, 1976; Weil, 1977; Cerra et al., 1978).

The hyperdynamic (high flow) and hypodynamic (low flow) states represent in general the difference between survival (the former state) and nonsurvival (the latter state), since increased mortality and decreased cardiac output are clearly related (Weil, 1977). Suggested mechanisms accounting for the hyperdynamic and hypodynamic states are shown in Fig. 16.1. This diagram portrays the concept that the state of elevated cardiac output is consistent with survival (which is supported by clinical findings) but that there may be a progression from this early condition to the hypodynamic state, which possesses ominous lethal overtones. It should be pointed out that as diminished tissue perfusion in shock becomes a sustained feature, positive feedback pathways set up "vicious circles," resulting in an enhanced rate of progressive deterioration (see "+," Fig. 16.1).

A key feature of this form of shock is the maldistribution of blood volume, hence its identification as a "distributive" form of shock. In large measure, the hypovolemic feature of the low flow state is primarily related to a distribution abnormality, blood being translocated to the venous system, including both hepatosplanchnic and peripheral vascular regions (Gilbert, 1960; Hinshaw et al., 1970; Hinshaw, 1971; Blattberg and Levy, 1971; Weil, 1977; Guntheroth and Kawabori, 1977). Therapeutically, this defect may be overridden by fluid administration, or the distributive defect may be corrected by infusion of methylprednisolone sodium succinate (Hinshaw et al., 1967, 1979a). In the latter instance, exogenous fluid administration is not required since the steroid apparently corrects the distributive defect by intravascular shifts of blood volumes to the normal anatomical sites (Hinshaw et al., 1967, 1979a), which results in restored blood flow.

The role of the heart in endotoxic and septic shock has received renewed interest. Although earlier observations failed to document the development of myocardial dysfunction during the 1st hr of endotoxin shock, several reports provide evidence that the heart is depressed during later phases of shock in animals given endotoxin or *E. coli* (Hinshaw, 1974, 1979; Hinshaw et al., 1979c) and in patients with septic shock (Bell and Thal, 1970; Siegel et al., 1967; Clowes et al., 1970). Our current understanding regarding the causes of myocardial dysfunction in experimental septic shock is as fol-

Endotoxin Shock

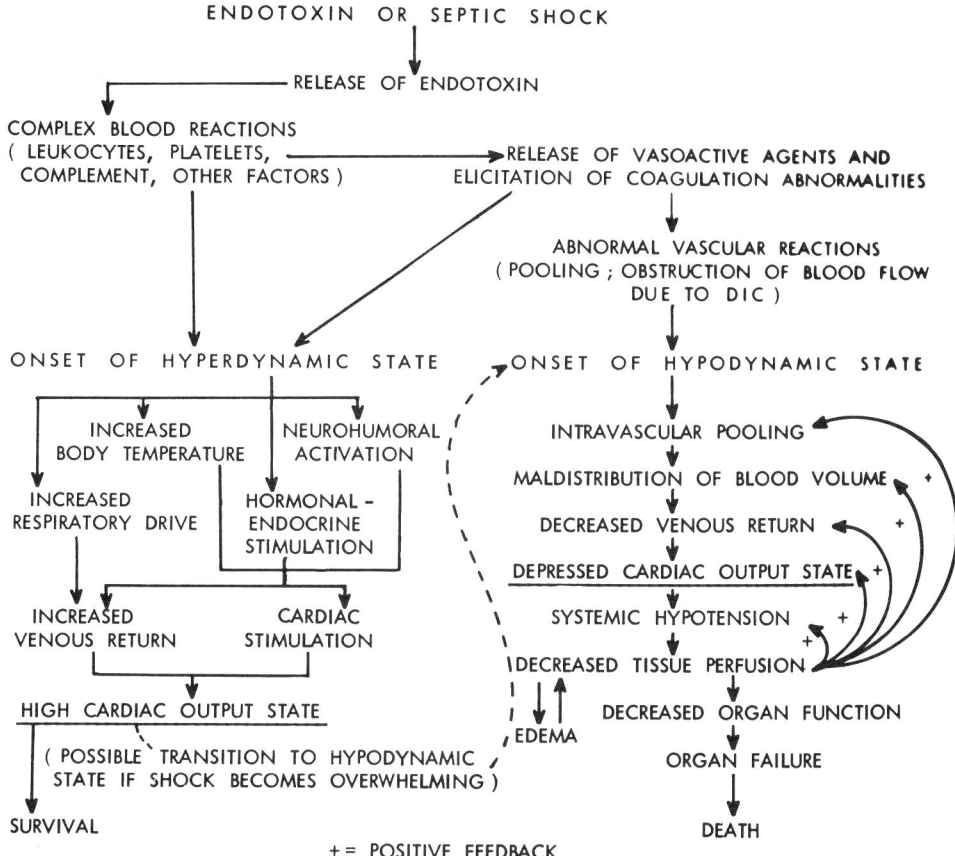

Figure 16.1. Suggested mechanisms for elicitation of hyperdynamic and hypodynamic states of endotoxic or septic shock.

lows: 1) coronary hypoperfusion and depressed responses to beta-adrenergic stimuli are prime factors in the elicitation of cardiac dysfunction; and 2) intracardiac disturbances perform a major role but their causes are obscure. Associated in this latter category are development of edema in the myocardium, occurring in both the contractile elements and mitochondria; ionic imbalances of potassium and probably calcium; and elevations of left ventricular end-diastolic pressure and depressions of negative dP/dt_{max}, cardiac power, and efficiency. The interactions and additive effects of these factors are responsible for the development of myocardial dysfunction in endotoxin shock (Hinshaw, 1979).

Since substantial evidence has been produced for a crucial and prominent role of the myocardium in the development of irreversible endotoxic (septic) shock in animals and in man himself, consideration should be provided for possible therapeutic support of the heart in septic shock.

Pathologic Manifestations and Coagulation Abnormalities

A major problem in endotoxin shock research has been the observation of species differences in morphologic findings. Powrie and Norman (1976) have expressed concern that the use of experimental animals such as the dog is frought with danger inasmuch as infusions of endotoxin in this species produce primary lung and gut lesions, whereas in primates the gut lesions may be much smaller and the liver and kidneys more affected.

During the Oklahoma Shock Tour (Shock Tour Symposium, 1966), 159 mongrel dogs were given $E.\ coli\ LD_{80}$ endotoxin. Of this number, 39 were given endotoxin alone and 120 received various therapeutic procedures 15 min after the intravenous injection of endotoxin. Examination of the gross and microscopic data simultaneously carried out by three pathologists from different medical centers (Drs. J. G. Brunson, D. M. Schultz, and D. M. Angevine) revealed a more or less consistent chronologic patern of development of the lesions in the untreated animals: the earliest detectable lesions were observed in the heart, liver, and gallbladder, which consisted of myocardial hemorrhages, marked hepatic congestion, and edema and hemorrhage in the gallbladder. During the next 5–12 hr after endotoxin administration, the cardiac, hepatic, and gallbladder lesions increased in severity and were characterized by frank areas of hepatic necrosis and profound gallbladder edema. Additionally, during this period, hemorrhagic lesions of the small bowel and the adrenal gland began to appear, and pulmonary congestion, edema, and hemorrhages developed. The pulmonary, liver, gallbladder, small bowel, and adrenal lesions increased in severity during the second 12-hr postendotoxin period, associated also with hemorrhages in the wall and lumen of the large bowel. In contrast, cardiac changes were minimal during this period. Following the 24th hr in a smaller group of still surviving dogs, pulmonary and small and large bowel changes persisted or increased in severity, while there was a pronounced decrease in the incidence and severity of changes in other organs.

Occlusive vascular lesions were rarely observed, while most lesions were characterized by edema and hemorrhage. In the liver there was early marked central lobular congestion and hemorrhage that eventually involved all portions of the lobules, which then greatly decreased and was associated with ischemic areas of necrosis. In some animals, bloody ascitic fluid was noted. The adrenal gland showed a persistent hemorrhagic lesion which involved the outer medulla and inner cortex. Eighty-eight percent of the control group of dogs died within the first 24 hr after endotoxin administration.

One initiating mechanism accounting for the pathologic changes observed in dogs, especially the gastrointestinal lesions, may be intravascular coagulation or disseminated intravascular coagulation (DIC), as reported by Hardaway (1962) and Kondo et al. (1978). Hardaway and McKay (1959) have stated that rather than DIC accompanying gram-negative bacteremic shock, their observations point to the probability that intravascular coagulation may be a cause of shock.

Colman et al. (1979) have defined DIC as a pathologic syndrome resulting from the formation of thrombin, subsequent activation and consumption of certain coagulant proteins, and production of fibrin thrombi. Others have reported that in man bloodstream infections due to endotoxin-producing gram-negative bacteria prevail as a cause of DIC (Corrigan et al., 1968; Levine et al., 1972; Robboy et al., 1972). Corrigan and Jordan (1970) have found that DIC and shock-complicating bacteremic episodes contribute substantially to mortality.

According to Colman et al. (1972), the clinical criteria for DIC include bleeding tendency with or without hypotension. The laboratory criteria for detection of DIC include thrombocytopenia, prolongation of prothrombin and partial thromboplastin times, reduced factor V and VIII activity levels, hypofibrinogenemia, and evidence of enhanced fibrinolysis manifested by increased amounts of degradation products of fibrinogen and fibrin (FDP, fibrin breakdown products, fibrinogen-related antigen) (Colman et al., 1979). There are two distinct modes of presentation of DIC: acute and chronic. Acute DIC develops rapidly over a period of a few hours to days. The patient often presents with a multisite bleeding diathesis that can range from oozing to catastrophic life-threatening hemorrhage (Colman et al., 1979). The mortality associated with acute DIC is high, ranging from 54 to 67% (Siegal et al., 1978; Minna et al., 1974). Siegal et al. (1978) found the mortality directly related to age, the number of clinical manifestations of DIC, and the severity of the laboratory manifestations.

Patients with DIC often have signs and symptoms of dysfunction of multiple organs. Some situations where organ dysfunction appears related to DIC or is out of proportion to other features of the illness include the adult respiratory distress syndrome or shock lung (Bone et al., 1976) and renal insufficiency and oliguria associated with gram-negative septicemia (Preston et al., 1973). The spectrum of pathologic findings in DIC includes fibrin thrombi, major vessel thrombosis, small vessel thrombosis, hemorrhage, and complications thereof (Robboy et al., 1972). The pathologic hallmark of DIC is the fibrin thrombi. Fibrin thrombi are observed more frequently in the kidney (68%) than in any other organ and involve 2–10% of the glomeruli (Robboy et al., 1972).

McGovern (1971, 1972) reported postmortem findings in patients in shock or from whom positive blood cultures were obtained. He stated that the pathology of shock in man centers upon intravascular fibrin formation, hemorrhages, and necrosis of tissues. These kinds of pathologic lesions are similar to the microscopic data gathered by Drs. Brunson, Schulz, and Angevine at the Shock Tour in shocked dogs (Shock Tour Symposium, 1966). McGovern (1971) reported that in the first 18 hr in the lung, there were petechial hemorrhages, microthrombi, scattered foci of congestion and edema, and atelectasis of the dependent portion of the lower and middle lobes. After 72 hr the cut surface of the lung resembled liver in consistency while, microscopically, hyaline membranes were found in addition to hemorrhages. Fibrin thrombi, hemorrhage, and tissue necrosis were seen in the intestines, kidneys, and adrenals. He further stated that in acute ischemic enterocolitis, which is characteristic of the shock syndrome, the first lesion is the formation of fibrin thrombin in capillaries and venules of the mucosa and submucosa, which is almost always accompanied by hemorrhages. This mechanism of pathogenesis of gut lesions in shock patients corroborates the findings in dogs of Hardaway et al. (1962) and Kondo et al. (1978).

McGovern (1971) stated that zonal necrosis of the liver was the most common histologic manifestation of shock encountered at autopsy. Remmele and Harms (1968) also reported that the hepatic sinusoids were the most common site for demonstration of fibrin thrombi in shock but thrombi were seldom seen at this site unless death occurred within 3 days of the onset of shock. Colman et al. (1979) stated that enhanced fibrinolysis is probably responsible for the disappearance of fibrin thrombi in advanced cases of DIC, making difficult their detection at autopsy.

McGovern (1971) further demonstrated that shock in the adrenal gland manifests itself by hemorrhage, fibrin thrombi, and necrosis. These findings are strongly supported by recent studies from our laboratory in *E. coli*-shocked (LD_{100}) baboons in which microscopic examination of adrenal tissue without prior knowledge of treatment revealed that all fully treated animals (methylprednisolone sodium succinate plus gentamicin sulfate) showed only congestion of cortical vessels or normal morphology, whereas untreated shocked baboons revealed massive hemorrhage and necrosis of both zonae fasiculata and glomerulosa of the adrenals (Hinshaw et al., 1980).

Coalson et al. (1979) described the following morphologic changes in baboons receiving LD_{100} E. coli organism infusions: the acute lung lesion previously observed in baboons dying within 6 hr was not observed in this prolonged shock model (24 hr). Fibrin thrombi and hepatocyte damage were observed in the liver and were associated with increases in LDH, FLDH, and hypoglycemia. Glomerular fibrin thrombi and tubular epithelial changes of cytoplasmic vacuolization and brush border loss were present in the kidney and increases in BUN levels were noted. Hinshaw et al. (1980) reported the presence of severe adrenal hemorrhage in the baboon receiving LD_{100} E. coli; however, no pathologic changes were observed in the intestines. Coalson et al. (1978a) reported a striking similarity between the pathologic findings in tissues obtained from septic patients and those from live E. coli-infused baboons. Similar findings were observed after endotoxin administration in baboons except that renal fibrin thrombi were absent (Coalson et al., 1978b). Finally, McGovern (1971) concluded that the most persistent lesions in the shock patient were microthrombosis of the vasculature, hemorrhage, and tissue necrosis. He observed that a chief characteristic of gram-negative septicemia was the prominent incidence of pulmonary hemorrhage.

The histologic abnormalities of pulmonary edema and intraalveolar hemorrhage account for the precipitation of the "adult respiratory distress syndrome" or "shock lung" described by Clowes et al. (1974) in this form of shock. It is not known to what extent therapeutic interventions, including fluid administration, may have enhanced the degree of pulmonary pathology, inasmuch as it is absent in baboons dying from E. coli shock and not receiving therapy (Hinshaw et al., 1980).

In a recent report, Hardaway (1978) also asks the pertinent question, "Why do some patients in shock develop DIC and respiratory failure while others do not?" He states that shock is characterized by deficient capillary perfusion and that a mere slowing of blood in capillaries will not initiate coagulation but only predisposes to it. In the presence of a slow capillary flow, a thromboplastic substance such as bacterial toxins or tissue juices (crushed tissue) entering the bloodstream initiates DIC, which may produce lesions in the lungs—a prime target.

In view of these data, it seems reasonable to hypothesize that disseminated intravascular coagulation and the deposition of fibrin thrombi in virtually every organ system could contribute to the many pathophysiologic derangements characteristic of septic or endotoxic shock.

Metabolic-Endocrinologic Interactions and Participation of Vasoactive Agents

To date, research and clinical observations clearly implicate the development of a serious energy supply deficit in septic shock, and glucose metabolism appears to occupy a central position in the pathogenesis of the shock state. Septic or endotoxic shock exerts a major impact on metabolic requirements, and metabolic-endocrinologic derangements may represent the primary kinds of defects in this form of shock. In fact, the balance of findings in recent times has shifted increasingly to a major concern of energy deficits in the septic shock

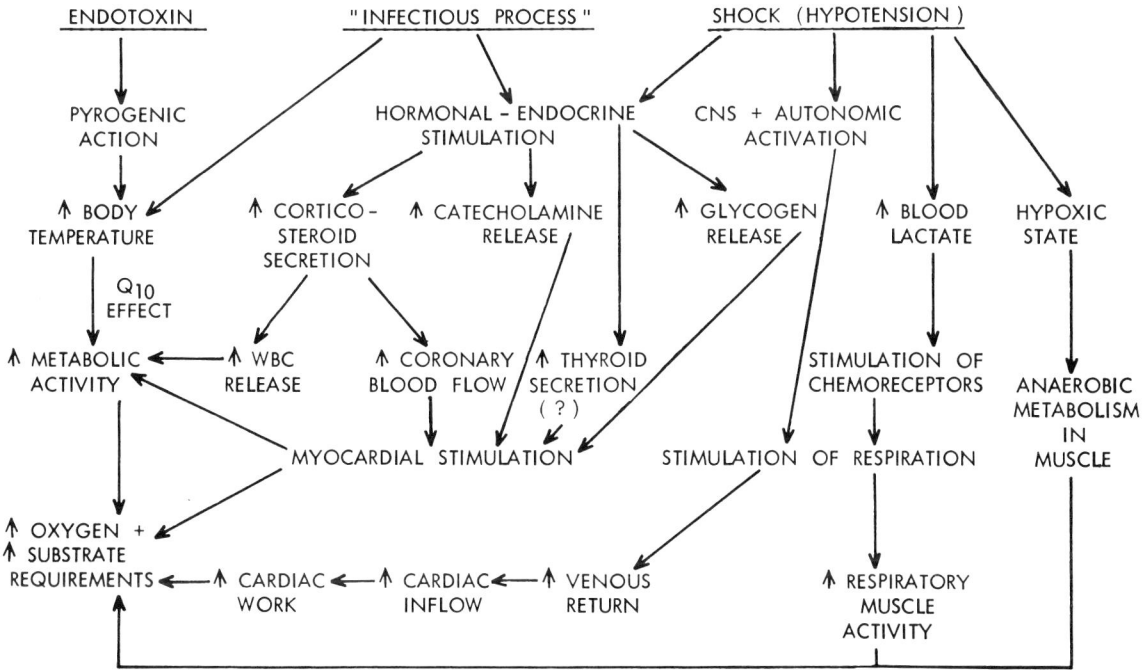

Figure 16.2. Suggested factors causing increased metabolic demand in septic shock.

patient. Figure 16.2 illustrates some possible mechanisms which may account for the increased metabolic requirements. An initial action in the early phase of shock ("warm shock") is related to driving forces causing an increase in metabolic rate, by virtue of an increase in body temperature. In addition, hormonal-endocrinologic activation, occurring early in shock and more significantly in the hypotensive low flow state ("cold shock"), appears to set into motion a diverse set of influences which result in markedly elevated metabolic requirements. For example, catecholamine and glucagon release stimulate the myocardium; increased secretions of adrenal and possibly thyroid glands drive the heart or metabolism in general; neural and chemoreceptor involvements stimulate the muscles of respiration; and adrenocorticosteroid secretion stimulates the outpouring of leukocytes from bone marrow. These forces all contribute to the already increased drain on the total energy availability.

The reasons for the underlying alterations in energy requirements and utilization of tissue fuel associated with septic shock are not readily explained (Kinney, 1972). Caloric expenditures in the early phase of human septic shock are markedly in excess of those predicted from body temperature elevations alone (Q_{10} effect). Kinney discusses several other mechanisms which may explain the energy deficit: uncoupling of oxidation and phosphorylation, which is a possibility but remains unproven; and the indication that the septic state is accompanied by an increased turnover rate of glucose in the blood, with an acceleration of glucose oxidation. Kinney further pointed out that increases in caloric expenditure are only partly related to gluconeogenesis, and approximately half of the increase in expenditure must be sought in other viscera or peripheral tissues. Hinshaw et al. (1978a) have reported that part of the glucose "sink" lies within the phagocytes, whose increased numbers and elevated glucose requirements are apparent in endotoxin shock. Raymond and associates (1979) have identified a glucose "sink" in endotoxin shock, namely, the skeletal muscle bed during the condition of hypoxia.

The development of hypoglycemia and the depletion of the reserves of liver glycogen were the first metabolic effects of endotoxin reported in the literature (Berry, 1977). A most significant development has been the recognition of impaired liver function in endotoxin shock and the resultant depression of hepatic gluconeogenesis (Berry, 1977; Utili et al., 1977; Schuler et al., 1976). Both hyperglycemia and hypoglycemia have been observed in animals and man (Cavanagh et al., 1977; Hinshaw et al., 1975; Hinshaw, 1976; Filkins, 1978); however, these variations are probably related to the stage of shock in which observations are made and to species differences (Cavanagh et al., 1977).

Recently, Filkins (1978) described a temporal course of changes in plasma glucose, gluconeogenesis, and glucose oxidation incident to low dose (LD_{20}) and high dose (LD_{95}) endotoxin administration in rats. Either low dose or early high dose endotoxin injection is associated with hyperglycemia, hepatic glycogen depletion (fed state), increased gluconeogenesis (fasted state), and increased glucose oxidation. Late or high dose administration is characterized by depressed gluconeogenesis, maintained enhancement of glucose oxidation, and a progressive, profound hypoglycemia (Filkins, 1978). The ultimate net effect of endotoxin in bringing about a profound hypoglycemia is due to the increased rate of glucose uptake by leukocytes and skeletal muscle in severe shock, together with inhibition of hepatic gluconeogenesis and depletion of high energy adenine nucleotides (Schuler et al., 1976). Hypoglycemia and death in LD_{70} endotoxin shock are prevented by hypertonic glucose administration (Hinshaw et al., 1974a); in LD_{100} endotoxin shock, by steroid infusion (White et al., 1978); and in live *E. coli* shock, by repeated maintenance doses of steroid and antibiotic (Hinshaw et al., 1979a).

Both animals and man subjected to septic shock reveal a bizarre metabolic endocrine abnormality termed "pseudodiabetes": in this condition, plasma insulin concentrations are abnormally low, while glucose concentrations are high, normal, or low (Clowes et al., 1974, 1978; Hinshaw et al., 1975). Recent literature has ascribed the elicitation of low insulin concentrations to intensely increased catecholamine activity and impaired vascular perfusion of the pancreas. Also, the already depressed glucose uptake by tissues is lowered even further because of the presence of peripheral insulin resistance (ineffectiveness of insulin) (Clowes et al., 1974, 1978; Gump et al., 1974; Hinshaw et al., 1975; Hinshaw, 1976). Clowes et al. (1974) reported abnormal insulin levels and an ineffectiveness of insulin for the transport of glucose during low cardiac output septic shock and increased insulin resistance in the high cardiac output state (Clowes et al., 1978). In human septic shock, infusions of insulin together with glucose and potassium have produced an elevation in cardiac output (Clowes et al., 1974) and improved myocardial performance (Weisul et al., 1975).

Defects in aerobic metabolism in human septic shock are readily apparent. Shoemaker and others (1970) described a deficit in oxygen transport relative to the total needs of the patient in the state of hyperthermic, hypermetabolic septic shock. Duff et al. (1972) identified an increased oxygen need in the hypermetabolic state and also noted a possible impaired ability of tissues to extract oxygen. Irreversible damage of mitochondria caused by low blood flow may destroy the oxidative metabolic machinery in vital organs (Mela, 1979).

The endogeneous adrenocortical hormone, cortisol, is notably elevated in septic shock in baboons (Hinshaw et al., 1978b) and in man (Sibbald, 1976; Sibbald et al., 1977). Infusion of exogenous corticosteroid is without effect when given alone to baboons in *E. coli* shock (Hinshaw et al., 1978b) but is extremely effective when infused together with an antibiotic (Hinshaw et al., 1979a). Sibbald et al. (1977) have described a condition of adrenocortical insufficiency in septic patients. The need for additional steroid is well documented in the experimental literature, but the mechanisms of its various beneficial actions are complex and not well delineated.

It is probable that a great variety of vasoactive agents, including histamine, serotonin, kinins, and others, are released following endotoxin administration. Their roles are not well understood although the kinds and quantities of such agents must be of critical significance in the pathogenesis of shock, since they exert profound effects on regional blood flow and vascular resistance and may alter microvascular pressure and capillary permeability (Hinshaw, 1971; Berry, 1977; Altura and Halevy, 1977).

Alterations in Host Defense

In the 1890s, Metchnikoff deduced that phagocytic cells protected animals from assault by microorganisms and championed the cause of phagocytosis as the basis of survival against infections (Metchnikoff, 1893). Recent reports emphasize the importance of host defense in the prevention or resolution of infections and sepsis in experimental animals and man, but each seems concerned with the separate components of host defense [humoral (immunoglobulin) system, cellular-phagocytic (neutrophil and macrophage) system and cell-mediated (T-lymphocyte) immunity]. Alexander (1974) discusses host defense in terms of phagocytic cells, opsonins, and vascular response.

PHAGOCYTIC CELLS

Cline (1975) points out that the neutrophilic granulocytes constitute one of the body's most important defense systems against microbial pathogens because of their active motility, phagocytic activity, and complex microbicidal systems. In fact, Stossel (1972) has called the neutrophil the host's "first line of defense."

Recent reports from our laboratory demonstrate that increased numbers of leukocytes (neutrophils) play a key role in increasing survival rate in dogs given injections of either live *E. coli* or endotoxin. In vitro studies reveal an acceleration of glucose uptake by leukocytes in the presence of live *E. coli* or endotoxin (Hinshaw et al., 1977a and b). An increase in the neutrophil's basal metabolic activity, as well as the effect of increased numbers of cells, have been implicated as the primary factors accounting for the elevated glucose uptake and increased survival of animals (Hinshaw et al., 1977a and b; White et al., 1977; Archer et al., 1978).

Hollingsworth and Beeson (1955) found that if irradiated rats are transfused with leukocytes, injections of *E. coli* are cleared normally despite the fact that the transferred leukocytes have disappeared from the blood. Recent reports have described beneficial effects of transfused white blood cells as a treatment for septicemia in neutropenic dogs (Epstein et al., 1974) and patients (Graw et al., 1972).

Abnormalities in neutrophil function apparently predispose the patient to sepsis. Alexander (1974) has shown that quantitative burn wound cultures and incidence of sepsis in patients are related to abnormal neutrophil function. High caloric and high protein enteric alimentation were found to reverse in part abnormal neutrophil function and reduce the incidence of sepsis. Hellum and Solberg (1977; Solberg and Hellum, 1972) have shown defects in neutrophil granulocyte function caused by bacterial infections and suggest that these defects may contribute to mortality.

OPSONINS

Several investigations have been concerned with the importance of "humoral" factors in determining the outcome of sepsis or septic shock (Alexander, 1974; Saba, 1975, 1978; Kaplan and Saba, 1976; Scovill et al., 1976; Meakins, 1976; Kaplan et al., 1977; Saba et al., 1978). These reports emphasize that when humoral factors or opsonins are depleted, phagocytic cells (neutrophils and macrophages) may not "recognize" the microorganisms and therefore may not ingest them. Stossel (1974) states that antibodies of the IgG class and activated C3 of the complement proteins are the most important opsonins of serum. Alexander (1974) found that when burned patients were vaccinated with a vaccine to *Pseudomonas aeruginosa*, they survived for 5 days without incidence of *Pseudomonas* septicemia. In a consecutive group of similar but nonvaccinated patients, death from *Pseudomonas* sepsis occurred in 15%. However, with the availability of a hyperimmune anti-*Pseudomonas* gamma globulin to treat bacteremia after vaccine failure, death from *Pseudomonas* infections did not occur. This observation may be related to the ability of immune antibodies to opsonize bacteria in the absence of complement (Alexander, 1974).

The opsonic factor of prime importance during an infection with *E. coli* apparently is C3, which has been activated in the alternate complement or properdin pathway (Alexander, 1974). Serum obtained from patients showed reduced opsonic activity for *Pseudomonas* and *E. coli* for 4–28 days postburn (Bjornson and Alexander, 1974). These opsonic alterations both preceded and followed the onset of septic episodes, suggesting that they contributed to the pathogenesis of sepsis but could also occur as its consequence. Further, opsonins supporting phagocytosis of *E. coli* were consumed during infection with *E. coli* (Alexander, 1974).

These findings provide strong support for the hypothesis that consumption of opsonic proteins can occur during active infection. Alexander (1974) has named this condition, "consumptive opsoninopathy," a state which may be corrected by administration of plasma or blood containing a full component of normal serum proteins.

Saba (1975) states that resistance to septicemia involves both nonspecific and specific factors; however, his studies have emphasized the function of the reticuloendothelial system (RES) as a determinant of survival after severe trauma and shock. Saba and others also support the view of a "consumptive opsoninopathy" being of prime importance since phagocytic depression in man and experimental animals following surgery, hemorrhage, or multiple trauma appears to be due to consumption of an opsonic α_2 surface binding glycoprotein (α_2-SB-glycoprotein) (Saba, 1975, 1978; Kaplan and Saba, 1976; Scovill et al., 1976; Blumenstock et al., 1976, 1977; Kaplan et al., 1977; Saba et al., 1978).

The decrease of this protein in the serum contributes to the observed RES phagocytic depression. Reticuloendothelial (RE) cells in the liver and spleen remove bacteria, microaggregates of fibrin, injured platelets, denatured protein, and immune complexes from the blood and thus serve as a clearance mechanism to protect the pulmonary and systemic vascular beds from microembolization and injury (Saba, 1975).

Saba et al. (1978) intravenously infused fresh plasma cryoprecipitate containing fibronectin or opsonic α2-SB-glycoprotein into three severely ill, septic surgical and trauma patients with marked opsonic deficiency and RES failure and tested for augmented systemic defense against persistent septicemia and associated pulmonary insufficiency. Within 3 days after therapy, the serum concentration of this protein gradually rose concurrent with patient stabilization and reversal of the febrile and septic state.

THE VASCULAR RESPONSE

In considering the vascular response as a component of host defense, Alexander (1974) stated that decreased perfusion of tissues or blockage of the development of the inflammatory lesion will result in an inadequate delivery of phagocytic cells and opsonins and an increased susceptibility to infection. Therefore, conditions such as shock or disseminated intravascular coagulation may contribute significantly to surgical infection.

CELL-MEDIATED IMMUNITY

Neither the phagocytic nor the humoral components of the host defense system encompass the cell-mediated immunity component as discussed by Meakins (1976). He states that the only measure of immunologic activity in patients which correlates with morbidity and mortality from sepsis is skin reactivity. The presence of anergy, defined as the failure to react to any five standard skin test antigens, indicated the gravest prognosis and highest incidence of sepsis. Although the relative role of anergy or failure of delayed hypersensitivity has not been completely resolved, Meakins et al. (1979) suggest that it is important to restore patients to a better immune status using surgery itself, immunorestorative drugs, or adequate alimentation.

THERAPEUTIC ASPECTS: NONHUMAN PRIMATE

There has been a recent acceleration of interest in the combined use of steroids and antibiotics in the treatment of experimental and clinical septic shock (Schumer, 1976; Pitcairn et al., 1975; Greisman et al., 1979; Balis et al., 1979; Hinshaw et al., 1978b, 1979a and b, 1980. Recent findings have clearly shown that dogs subjected to 100% lethal intravenous infusion of *E. coli* are completely protected against the characteristic pathophysiologic and lethal actions of the *E. coli* by multiple sustaining infusions of both methylprednisolone sodium succinate and gentamicin sulfate (Hinshaw et al., 1979a). Either agent, administered by itself without the other, offered no protection to the animal.

As a follow-up study to this successful treatment regimen in canine *E. coli* shock, experiments were conducted on adult baboons (Hinshaw et al., 1979b, 1980). Table 16.1 outlines the treatment regimen. Three groups of animals were studied: *Group A*, *E. coli* alone; *Group B*, *E. coli* plus infusions of both methylprednisolone sodium succinate (total of 75 mg/kg in 12 hr) and gentamicin sulfate (total of 18 mg/kg in 10 hr); and *Group C*, *E. coli* plus gentamicin sulfate (total of 18 mg/kg in 10 hr). Animals were monitored during a 12-hr period and observed up to 28 days or until death intervened. Results from these studies showed that systemic hypotension occurred in all groups within 2 hr of *E. coli* infusion. Subsequent hypotension, hypoglycemia, hypoinsulinemia, neutropenia, anuria, and death were prevented, however, in all fully treated baboons (Group B), while all animals of Groups A and C died within 42 hr.

Table 16.1
Treatment Regimen in Baboons Subjected to *E. coli*-Induced Shock[a]

Group Agent Administered	Dosage, *E. coli*/kg[b]	Time After Onset of *E. coli* Infusion	Duration and Route of Administration
A. *E. coli* organisms	2.1 (±0.1) × 10^{10}	Zero time (0)	0–120 min, IV
B. *E. coli* organisms	2.6 (±0.4) × 10^{10}	Zero time (0)	0–120 min, IV
Methylprednisolone[c]	30 mg/kg	+30 min	15 min, IV
Gentamicin[d]	9 mg/kg	+130 min	60 min, IV
Methylprednisolone	15 mg/kg	+150 min	120 min, IV
Gentamicin	4.5 mg/kg	+365 min	30 min, IV
Methylprednisolone	15 mg/kg	+365 min	120 min, IV
Gentamicin	4.5 mg/kg	+9 hr	30 min, IV
Methylprednisolone	15 mg/kg	+10 hr	120 min, IV
Gentamicin	4.5 mg/kg	+12 hr	IM
Gentamicin	4.5 mg/kg	Twice daily, 3 days	IM
C. Same procedure as group B [2.9 (±0.6) × 10^{10} *E. coli*], but no methylprednisolone administered			

[a] Saline infusions are substituted for drugs, when latter are not administered. (Hinshaw et al., 1980.)
[b] All groups, volume infused, 2.1 ml/kg.
[c] Methylprednisolone sodium succinate.
[d] Gentamicin sulfate.

Survival times of the three groups of baboons are shown in Table 16.2. Surviving animals of Group B—those receiving both steroid and antibiotic—showed remarkable recovery, drinking and moving about within 24 hr following onset of LD_{100} *E. coli* infusions. Return to normal health was evident within 3 days when all fully treated baboons demonstrated normal behavior and eating habits together with their characteristic responsiveness, alertness and aggressiveness, absence of diarrhea, and presence of urine flow. Surviving animals (Group B) were sacrificed between 7 and 28 days for tissue evaluation by light and electron microscopy, and the only histologic finding of note was a mild degree of adrenal congestion. These treatment studies, conducted on baboons, prove that implementation of vigorous post-treatment therapy with both methylprednisolone sodium succinate and gentamicin sulfate is strikingly effective in assuring permanent survival of animals subjected to massively lethal *E. coli* shock.

Recent studies demonstrate the effectiveness of the above described treatment when the onset of therapy is begun only after LD_{100} (100% lethal) *E. coli* organisms have been infused in baboons. Figure 16.3 portrays the responses of an adult baboon following a lethal (LD_{100}) infusion of live *E. coli* organisms. Systemic hypotension, tachycardia, fever, hypoglycemia, lactacidemia, and hypocarbia were early occurrences which are the typical nonhuman primate responses to lethal *E. coli* administration. Death occurred in 4 hr following the 12th-hr recording of relatively normal mean arterial pressure, pH, and PO_2, decreased PCO_2 and blood glucose concentrations, and elevated heart rates and lactic acid concentrations. The animal was totally anuric, and there was massive diarrhea from the 6th to 12th hr. No treatment was given the baboon other than continuous infusions of saline approximately equal to the rate of insensible loss. Figure 16.4 provides data in an experiment similar to that shown in Figure 16.3 except that the baboon was treated with intermittent infusions of steroid and antibiotic as shown in the figure and in the manner outlined in Table 16.1. Following infusion of organisms, blood glucose concentration increased, lactic acid concentration rose but leveled, heart rate elevations were modest, pH and PO_2 were normal, while PCO_2 was minimally depressed. Body temperature returned to con-

Table 16.2
Survival Data in Baboons Receiving *E. coli* Organisms and Treated with Methylprednisolone Sodium Succinate and Gentamicin Sulfate[a]

Group	Description of Group	Baboon No.	Survival Time
A	*E. coli* alone	1	10.5 hr
		4	3 hr
		7	5 hr
		10	32 hr
		13	42 hr
B	*E. coli* plus methylprednisolone sodium succinate + gentamicin sulfate	2	7 days[b]
		6	9 days[b]
		8	15 days[b]
		11	28 days[b]
		14	16 days[b]
C	*E. coli* plus gentamicin sulfate	3	29 hr
		9	17 hr
		12	15 hr
		15	35 hr

[a] Hinshaw et al., 1980.
[b] Euthanized.

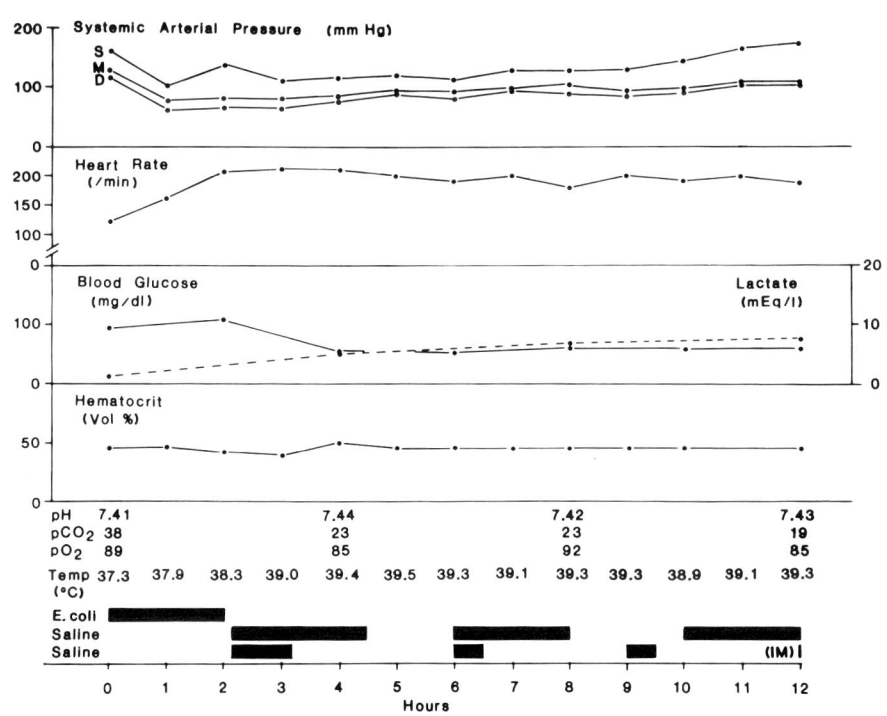

Figure 16.3. Responses of baboon to 2-hr infusion of LD_{100} *E. coli* (2.3×10^{10} organisms per kg body weight). No treatment was administered and animal died in 16 hr.

trol, continuous urine flow was observed, and diarrhea was absent during the 12-hr observation period. These changes were of significant magnitude to be readily contrasted with the nontreated baboon shown in Figure 16.3 and reflect the benefits accrued from early vigorous treatment with steroid and antibiotic. This baboon was a permanent survivor; however, since the steroid therapy was not begun until all of the organisms were administered, the recovery of the animal was slower than observed in our above report. Figure 16.5 presents data

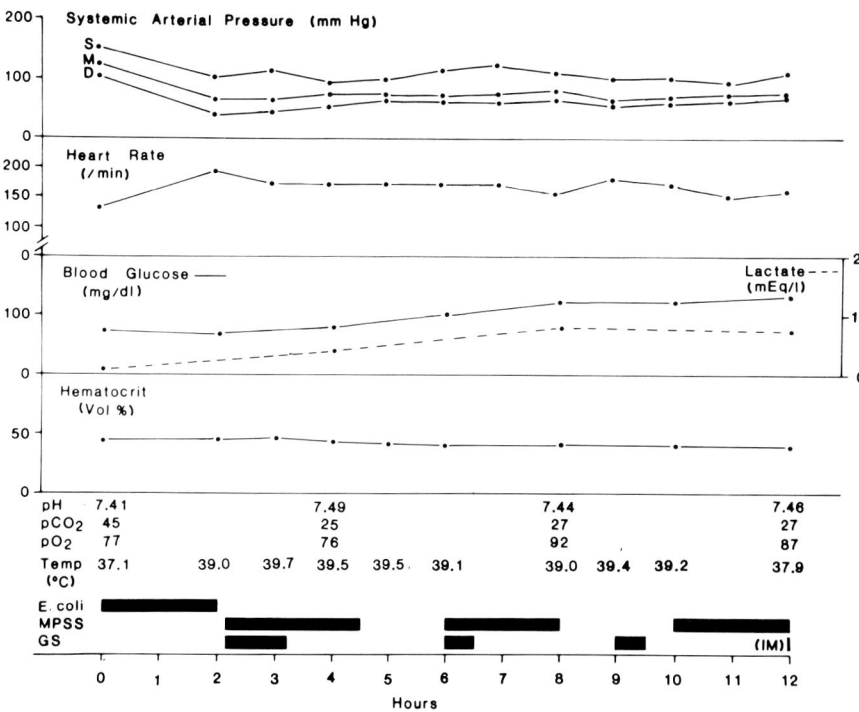

Figure 16.4. Responses of baboon to 2-hr infusion of LD_{100} E. coli (2.7×10^{10} organisms per kg body weight). Treatment with methylprednisolone sodium succinate (MPSS) and gentamicin sulfate (GS) begun *after* all organisms had been infused (see lower frame of figure). Animal was a permanent survivor.

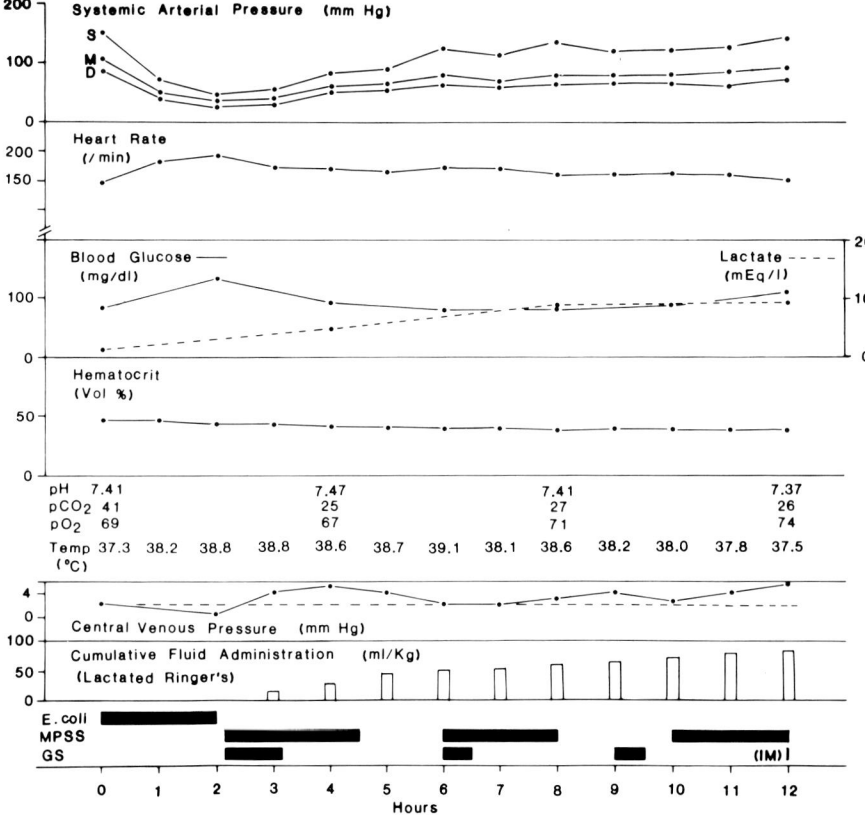

Figure 16.5. Responses of baboon to 2-hr infusion of LD_{100} E. coli (3.2×10^{10} organisms per kg body weight). Treatment with methylprednisolone sodium succinate (MPSS) and gentamicin sulfate (GS) begun *after* all organisms had been infused (see lower frame of figure). Animal was a permanent survivor.

from a baboon treated exactly as the animal depicted in Figure 16.4, except that fluid administration, exceeding that replacing insensible loss, was provided as shown in the next to the bottom frame. Additional fluid was provided inasmuch as the baboon experienced a mean systemic pressure during the 2nd hr of *E. coli* infusion averaging only 35 mm Hg and remained severely hypotensive until the end of the 3rd hr following the onset of *E. coli* infusion. This baboon demonstrated a remarkable response to steroid-antibiotic therapy: systemic hypotension disappeared, heart rate returned to normal, blood glucose concentration remained in the normal range, body temperature returned to control, and pH, PO_2, and PCO_2 were sustained with acceptable values. This baboon, in contrast to nontreated controls receiving *E. coli* only, exhibited no diarrhea, and urine flow was extensive during the 6-12 hr period. The animal was a permanent survivor and, following a slower recovery than animals treated with steroid at an earlier period, demonstrated behavior characteristics and health status consistent with complete recovery from shock.

Results from these studies demonstrate the remarkable effectiveness of methylprednisolone sodium succinate and gentamicin sulfate therapy even when the therapy is begun only after massive organism infusion greater than 2×10^{10} organisms per kg body weight. Findings suggest that the large doses of steroid used during treatment do not depress phagocytic activity (Hinshaw et al., 1978b) or delay time of recovery of the animal during treatment following administration of *E. coli* (Hinshaw et al., 1979a, 1980). The present observations in primates indicate that the high initial doses of antibiotic after *E. coli* are not detrimental to the animal (Hinshaw et al., 1980).

Several mechanisms have been proposed to explain the beneficial actions of steroids in shock: they exert beneficial hemodynamic effects during shock including elevating the cardiac output (Sambhi et al., 1965); they augment venous return by diminishing peripheral pooling (Hinshaw et al., 1967); increase coronary blood flow (Hinshaw et al., 1974b); and elevate regional blood flow (Hinshaw et al., 1967; Vaughn et al., 1967; Sullivan and Cavanagh, 1966). Steroids have been reported to stimulate hepatic gluconeogenesis (Berry, 1971; Holtzman et al., 1974), support liver carbohydrate metabolism (Schuler et al., 1976), stabilize hepatic lysosomal membranes (Galvin et al., 1978), and inhibit the development of disseminated intravascular coagulation (Balis et al., 1978). These beneficial actions have undoubtedly accounted for the improved survival rates of septic shock patients (Schumer, 1976). The nature of the protective linkage between steroid and antibiotic which so effectively promotes survival in animal shock studies remains elusive and must await further investigation.

References

Alexander, J.W.: Emerging concepts in control of surgical infections. Surgery 75:934, 1974.
Altura, B.M., and Halevy, S.: Circulatory shock, histamine, and antihistamines: therapeutic aspects. In *Handbuch der Experimentellen Pharmakalogie*, edited by G. V. R. Born, O. Eichler, A. Farah, H. Herken, and A. D. Welch, p. 575. Springer-Verlag, Berlin, 1977.
Archer, L.T., White, G.L., Coalson, J.J., Beller, B.K., Elmore, O., and Hinshaw, L.B.: Preserved liver function and leukocyte response in superlethal endotoxic shock. Circ. Shock 5: 279, 1978.
Balis, J.U., Rappaport, E.S., Gerber, L., Fareed, J., Buddingh, F., and Messmore, H.L.: A primate model for prolonged endotoxin shock. Blood-vascular reactions and effects of glucocorticoid treatment. Lab. Invest. 38:511, 1978.
Balis, J.U., Peterson, J.F., Shelley, S.A., Larson, C.H., Fareed, J., and Gerber, L.I.: Glucocorticoid and antibiotic effects on hepatic microcirculation and associated host responses in lethal gram-negative bacteremia. Lab. Invest. 40:55, 1979.
Bell, H., and Thal, A.: The peculiar hemodynamics of septic shock. Postgrad. Med. 48:106, 1970.
Bennett, I.L., Jr., and Cluff, L.E.: Bacterial pyrogens. Pharmacol. Rev. 9:427, 1957.
Berry, L.J.: Metabolic effects of bacterial endotoxins. In *Microbial Toxins*, edited by S. Kadis, G. Weinbaum, and S. J. Ajl, p. 165. Academic Press, New York, 1971.
Berry, L.J.: Bacterial toxins. CRC Crit. Rev. Toxicol. 5:239, 1977.
Bjornson, A.B., and Alexander, J.W.: Alterations of serum opsonins in patients with severe thermal injury. J. Lab. Clin. Med. 83:372, 1974.
Blattberg, G., and Levy, M.N.: Sites of extrahepatic pooling in early response to endotoxin. Am. J. Physiol. 220:1267, 1971.
Blumenstock, F.A., Saba, T.M., Weber, P.B., and Cho, E.: Purification and biochemical characterization of a macrophage stimulating alpha-2 globulin opsonic protein. J. Reticuloendothel. Soc. 19:157, 1976.
Blumenstock, F.A., Weber, P.B., Saba, T.M., and Laffin, R.: Electroimmunoassay of alpha-2-opsonic protein levels during reticuloendothelial blockade. Am. J. Physiol. 232:80, 1977.
Bone, R.C., Francis, P.B., and Pierce, A.K.: Intravascular coagulation associated with the adult respiratory distress syndrome. Am. J. Med. 61:585, 1976.
Borden, C.W., and Hall, W.H.: Fatal transfusion reactions from massive bacterial contamination of blood. N. Engl. J. Med. 245:760, 1951.
Braude, A.I., Williams, D., Siemienski, J., and Murphy, R.: Shock-like state due to transfusion of blood contaminated with gram-negative bacilli. Successful treatment with antibiotics and arterenol. Arch. Intern. Med. 92:75, 1953.
Brill, N.E., and Libman, E.: Pyocaneus bacilliaemia. Am. J. Med. Sci. 118:153, 1899.
Cavanagh, D., Rao, P.S., and Comas, M.R.: *Septic Shock in Obstetrics and Gynecology. In Major Problems in Obstetrics and Gynecology*, vol. 11, 135 pp. W. B. Saunders, Philadelphia, 1977.
Cerra, F.B., Hassett, J., and Siegel, J.H.: Vasodilator therapy in clinical sepsis with low output syndrome. J. Surg. Res. 25: 180, 1978.
Cline, M.J.: *The White Cell*, 564 pp. Harvard University Press, Cambridge, MA, 1975.
Clowes, G.H.A., Vucinic, M., and Weidner, M.G.: Circulatory and metabolic alterations associated with survival or death in peritonitis. Ann. Surg. 163:866, 1966.
Clowes, G.H.A., Farrington, G.H., Zieschneid, W., Cossette, G.R., and Saravis, C.: Circulating factors in the etiology of pulmonary insufficiency and right heart failure accompanying severe sepsis (peritonitis). Ann. Surg. 171:663, 1970.
Clowes, G.H.A., O'Donnell, T.F., Ryan, N.T., and Blackburn,

G.L.: Energy metabolism in sepsis: treatment based on different patterns in shock and high output stage. Ann. Surg. *179*:684, 1974.

Clowes, G.H.A., Martin, H., Waiji, S., Hirsch, E., Gazitua, R., and Goodfellow, R.: Blood insulin responses to blood glucose levels in high output sepsis and septic shock. Am J. Surg. *135*:577, 1978.

Coalson, J.J., Benjamin, B.A., Archer, L.T., Beller, B.K., Spaet, R.H., and Hinshaw, L.B.: A pathologic study of *Escherichia coli* shock in the baboon and the response to adrenocorticosteroid treatment. Surg. Gynecol. Obstet. *147*:726, 1978a.

Coalson, J.J., Benjamin, B., Archer, L.T., Beller, B., Gilliam, C.L., Taylor, F.B., Jr., and Hinshaw, L.B.: Prolonged shock in the baboon subjected to infusion of *E. coli* endotoxin. Circ. Shock *5*:423, 1978b.

Coalson, J.J., Archer, L.T., Benjamin, B.A., Beller-Todd, B.K., and Hinshaw, L.B.: A morphologic study of live *Escherichia coli* organism shock in baboons. Exp. Mol. Pathol. *31*:10, 1979.

Colman, R.W., Robboy, S.J., and Minna, J.D.: Disseminated intravascular coagulation (DIC): an approach. Am. J. Med. *52*:679, 1972.

Colman, R.W., Robboy, S.J., and Minna, J.D.: Disseminated intravascular coagulation: a reappraisal. Annu. Rev. Med. *30*:359, 1979.

Corrigan, J.J., Jr., and Jordan, C.M.: Heparin therapy in septicemia with disseminated intravascular coagulation. N. Engl. J. Med. *283*:778, 1970.

Corrigan, J.J., Ray, W.L., and May, N.: Changes in the blood coagulation system associated with septicemia. N. Engl. J. Med. *279*:851, 1968.

Dietzman, R.H., Motsay, G., and Lillehei, R.C.: The use of corticosteroids in the treatment of septic shock. In *Septic Shock in Man*, edited by S. G. Hershey, L. R. M. Del Guercio, and R. McConn, p. 231. Little, Brown, Boston, 1971.

Duff, J.H., Wright, C.J., McLean, A.P.H., and MacLean, L.D.: Oxygen consumption in septic shock. In *Shock in Low- and High-Flow States*, edited by B. K. Forscher, R. C. Lellehei, and S. S. Stubbs, p. 235. Excerpta Medica, Amsterdam, 1972.

Epstein, R.B., Waxman, F.J., Bennett, B.T., and Andersen, B.R.: *Pseudomonas* septicemia in neutropenic dogs. I. Treatment with granulocyte transfusions. Transfusion *14*:51, 1974.

Filkins, J.P.: Phases of glucose dyshomeostasis in endotoxicosis. Circ. Shock *5*:347, 1978.

Forscher, B.K., Lillehei, R.C., and Stubbs, S.S.: *Shock in Low- and High-Flow States*, 314 pp. Excerpta Medica, Amsterdam, 1972.

Galvin, M.J., Shupe, K., and Lefer, A.M.: Anti-endotoxin actions of methylprednisolone in the isolated perfused cat liver. Pharmacology *17*:181, 1978.

Gilbert, R.P.: Mechanisms of the hemodynamic effects of endotoxin. Physiol. Rev. *40*:245, 1960.

Graw, R.G., Jr., Herzig, G., Perry, S., and Henderson, E.S.: Normal granulocyte transfusion therapy. Treatment of septicemia due to gram-negative bacteria. N. Engl. J. Med. *287*:367, 1972.

Greisman, S.E., DuBuy, J.B., and Woodward, C.L.: Experimental gram-negative bacterial sepsis: prevention of mortality not preventable by antibiotic alone. Infect. Immun. *25*:538, 1979.

Gump, F.E., Long, C., Killian, P., and Kinney, J.M.: Studies of glucose intolerance in septic injured patients. J. Trauma *14*:378, 1974.

Guntheroth, W.G., and Kawabori, I.: The contribution of splanchnic pooling to endotoxin shock in the dog. Circ. Res. *41*:467, 1977.

Halinen, M.: Review on endotoxin shock. Acta Physiol. Scand. (Suppl. 439):1, 1976.

Hardaway, R.M.: The role of intravascular clotting in the etiology of shock. Ann. Surg. *155*:325, 1962.

Hardaway, R.M.: Acute respiratory distress syndrome and disseminated intravascular coagulation. South. Med. J. *71*:596, 1978.

Hardaway, R.M., and McKay, D.G.: Disseminated intravascular coagulation: a cause of shock. Ann. Surg. *149*:462, 1959.

Hellum, K.B., and Solberg, C.O.: Granulocyte function in bacterial infections in man. Acta Pathol. Microbiol. Scand. [C] *85*:1, 1977.

Hershey, S.G., Del Guercio, L.R.M., and McConn, R.: *Septic Shock in Man*, 313 pp. Little, Brown, Boston, 1971.

Hinshaw, L.B.: Release of vasoactive agents and the vascular effects of endotoxin. In *Microbial Toxins*, edited by S. Kadis, G. Weinbaum, and S. J. Ajl, vol. 5, p. 209. Academic Press, New York, 1971.

Hinshaw, L.B.: Comparison of responses of canine and primate species to bacteria and bacterial endotoxin. In *Shock in Low- and High-Flow States*, edited by B. K. Forscher, R. C. Lellehei, and S. S. Stubbs, p. 245. Excerpta Medica, Amsterdam, 1972.

Hinshaw, L.B.: Role of the heart in the pathogenesis of endotoxin shock: a review of the clinical findings and observations on animal species. J. Surg. Res. *17*:134, 1974.

Hinshaw, L.B.: The role of glucose in endotoxin shock. Circ. Shock *3*:1, 1976.

Hinshaw, L.B.: Myocardial function in endotoxin shock. Circ. Shock (Suppl. 1):43, 1979.

Hinshaw, L.B., and Cox, G.B.: *The Fundamental Mechanisms of Shock*, 449 pp. Plenum Press, New York, 1972.

Hinshaw, L.B., Solomon, L.A., Freeny, P.C., and Reins, D.A.: Hemodynamic and survival effects of methylprednisolone in endotoxin shock. Arch. Surg. *94*:61, 1967.

Hinshaw, L.B., Shanbour, L.L., Greenfield, L.J., and Coalson, J.J.: Mechanism of decreased venous return in subhuman primate administered endotoxin. Arch. Surg. *100*:600, 1970.

Hinshaw, L.B., Peyton, M.D., Archer, L.T., Black, M.R., Coalson, J.J., and Greenfield, L.J.: Prevention of death in endotoxin shock by glucose administration. Surg. Gynecol. Obstet. *139*:851, 1974a.

Hinshaw, L.B., Archer, L.T., Black, M.R., and Greenfield, L.J.: Effects of methylprednisolone sodium succinate on myocardial performance, hemodynamics and metabolism in normal and failing hearts. In *Steroids and Shock*, edited by T. M. Glenn, p. 253. University Park Press, Baltimore, 1974b.

Hinshaw, L.B., Benjamin, B., Coalson, J.J., Elkins, R.C., Taylor, F.B., Jr., Price, J.T., Smith, C.W., and Greenfield, L.J.: Hypoglycemia in lethal septic shock in subhuman primates. Circ. Shock *2*:197, 1975.

Hinshaw, L.B., Archer, L.T., Beller, B.K., White, G.L., Schroeder, T.M., and Holmes, D.D.: Glucose utilization and the role of blood in endotoxin shock. Am. J. Physiol. *233*:E71, 1977a.

Hinshaw, L.B., Beller, B.K., Archer, L.T., and White, G.L.: Associated leukocyte responses in the lethal aspects of *E. coli* shock. Proc. Soc. Exp. Biol. Med. *155*:179, 1977b.

Hinshaw, L.B., Beller, B.K., Majde, J.A., Archer, L.T., and White, G.L.: In vitro effects of methylprednisolone sodium succinate and *E. coli.* organisms on neutrophils in baboon blood. Circ. Shock *5:* 271, 1978a.

Hinshaw, L.B., Coalson, J.J., Benjamin, B.A., Archer, L.T., Beller, B.K., Kling, O.R., Hasser, E.M., and Phillips, R.W.: *Escherichia coli* shock in the baboon and the response to adrenocorticosteroid treatment. Surg. Gynecol. Obstet. *147:* 545, 1978b.

Hinshaw, L.B., Beller, B.K., Archer, L.T., Fluornoy, D.J., White, G.L., and Phillips, R.W.: Recovery from lethal *Escherichia coli* shock in dogs. Surg. Gynecol. Obstet. *149:*545, 1979a.

Hinshaw, L.B., Archer, L.T., Beller-Todd, B., Flournoy, D.J., Passey, R., Benjamin, B., White, G.L., and Coalson, J.J.: Is antibiotic/steroid post-treatment capable of preventing death in *E. coli* LD$_{100}$ shocked baboons? Fed. Proc. *38:*1192, 1979b.

Hinshaw, L.B., Benjamin, B., Archer, L.T., and Peyton, M.D.: The heart and endotoxin shock. In *Factors Contributing to Cardiovascular Function.* Tex. Rep. Biol. Med., *39:*173, 1979c.

Hinshaw, L.B., Archer, L.T., Beller-Todd, B.K., Coalson, J.J., Flournoy, D.J., Passey, R., Benjamin, B., and White, G.L.: Survival of primates in LD$_{100}$ septic shock following steroid/antibiotic therapy. J. Surg. Res. *28:*151, 1980.

Hollingsworth, J.W., and Beeson, P.B.: Experimental bacteremia in normal and irradiated rats. Yale J. Biol. Med. *29:*56, 1955.

Holtzman, S., Schuler, J.J., Earnest, W., Erve, P.R., and Schumer, W.: Carbohydrate metabolism during endotoxemia. Circ. Shock *1:*99, 1974.

Jeljaszewicz, J., and Wadstrom, T.: *Bacterial Toxins and Cell Membranes,* 432 pp. Academic Press, New York, 1978.

Kadis, S., Weinbaum, G., and Samuel, J.A.: *Bacterial Endotoxins: Comprehensive Treatise,* vol. 5, 507 pp. Academic Press, New York, 1971.

Kaplan, J.E., and Saba, T.M.: Humoral deficiency and reticuloendothelial depression after traumatic shock. Am. J. Physiol. *230:*7, 1976.

Kaplan, J.E., Scovill, W.A., Bernard, H., Saba, T.M., and Gray, V.: Reticuloendothelial phagocytic response to bacterial challenge after traumatic shock. Circ. Shock *4:*1, 1977.

Kinney, J.M.: Energy expenditure and tissue fuel in the septic patient. In *Shock in Low- and High-Flow States,* edited by B. K. Forscher, R. C. Lillehei, and S. S. Stubbs, p. 145. Excerpta Medica, Amsterdam, 1972.

Kondo, M., Yoshikawa, T., Takemura, S., Yokoe, N., Kawai, K., and Masuda, M.: Hemorrhagic necrosis of the intestinal mucosa associated with disseminated intravascular coagulation. Digestion *17:*38, 1978.

Kovach, A.G.B., Stoner, H.B., and Spitzer, J.J.: *Neurohumoral and Metabolic Aspects of Injury.* Plenum Press, New York, 1973.

Landy, M., and Braun, W.: *Bacterial Endotoxins* (symposium), 691 pp. Quinn & Boden, Rahway, NJ, 1964.

Lees, N.W.: The diagnosis and treatment of endotoxic shock. Anaesthesia *31:*897, 1976.

Levine, J., Poore, T.E., Young, N.S., Margolis, S., Zauber, N.P., Townes, A.S., and Bell, W.R.: Gram-negative sepsis: detection of endotoxemia with the Limulus test. Ann. Intern. Med. *76:*1, 1972.

MacLean, L.D., and Weil, M.H.: Hypotension (shock) in dogs produced by *Escherichia coli* endotoxin. Circ. Res. *4:*546, 1956.

MacLean, L.D., Weil, M.H., Spink, W.W., and Visscher, M.B.: Canine intestinal and liver weight changes induced by *E. coli* endotoxin. Proc. Soc. Exp. Biol. Med. *92:*602, 1956.

MacLean, L.D., Mulligan, W.G., McLean, A.P.H., and Duff, J.H.: Patterns of septic shock in man—a detailed study of 56 patients. Ann. Surg. *166:*543, 1967.

McCabe, W.R.: Gram-negative bacteremia. Adv. Intern. Med. *19:*135, 1974.

McGovern, V.J.: Shock. In *Pathology Annual,* edited by S. Sommers, vol. 6, p. 279. Appleton-Century-Crofts, New York, 1971.

McGovern, V.J.: The pathophysiology of gram-negative septicaemia. Pathology *4:*265, 1972.

McKay, D.G., Jewett, J.F., and Reid, D.E.: Endotoxin shock and the generalized Shwartzman reaction in pregnancy. Am. J. Obstet. Gynecol. *78:*546, 1959.

Meakins, J.L.: Pathophysiologic determinants and prediction of sepsis. Surg. Clin. North Am. *56:*847, 1976.

Meakins, J.L., Christou, N.V., Shizgal, H.M., and MacLean, L.D.: Therapeutic approaches to anergy in surgical patients: surgery and levamisole. Ann. Surg. *190:*286, 1979.

Mela, L.: Reversibility of mitochondrial metabolic response to circulatory shock and tissue ischemia. Circ. Shock (Suppl. 1):61, 1979.

Metchnikoff, E.: *Lectures on the Comparative Pathology of Inflammation.* Kegan Paul, London, 1893.

Mills, L.C., and Moyer, J.H.: *Shock and Hypotension: Pathogenesis and Treatment. Twelfth Hahnemann Symposium,* 718 pp. Grune & Stratton, New York, 1965.

Minna, J.D., Robboy, S.J., and Colman, R.W.: Conditions initiating or predisposing patients to DIC. In *Disseminated Intravascular Coagulation in Man,* p. 26. Charles C Thomas, Springfield, IL, 1974.

Morrison, D.C., and Ulevitch, R.J.: The effects of bacterial endotoxins on host mediation systems. Am. J. Pathol. *93:* 526, 1978.

Murdoch, J.C.McC., Speirs, C.F., and Pullen, H.: The bacteraemic shock syndrome. Br. J. Hosp. Med. *1:*346, 1968.

Nichols, R.L., Smith, J.W., and Balthazar, E.R.: Peritonitis and intraabdominal abscess: an experimental model for the evaluation of human diseases. J. Surg. Res. *25:*129, 1978.

Nowotny, A.: Molecular aspects of endotoxic reactions. Bacteriol. Rev. *33:*72, 1969.

Perbellini, A., Shatney, C.H., MacCarter, D.J., and Lillehei, R.C.: A new model for the study of septic shock. Surg. Gynecol. Obstet. *147:*68, 1978.

Pitcairn, M., Schuler, J., Erve, P.R., Holtzman, S., and Schumer, W.: Glucocorticoid and antibiotic effect on experimental gram-negative bacteremic shock. Arch. Surg. *110:*1012, 1975.

Powrie, S., and Norman, J.: Septicaemia. Br. J. Anaesth. *49:* 41, 1976.

Preston, F.E., Malia, R.G., Sworn, M.J., and Blackburn, E.K.: Intravascular coagulation and *E. coli* septicemia. J. Clin. Pathol. *26:*120, 1973.

Raskova, H., and Vanecek, J.: Pharmacology of bacterial toxins. Pharmacol. Rev. *16:*1, 1964.

Raymond, R.M., Harkema, J.M., and Emerson, T.E., Jr.: Mechanisms of increased glucose uptake by gracilis muscle during endotoxin shock in the dog. Physiologist *22:*105, 1979.

Remmele, W., and Harms, D.: Zur pathologischen anatomie des kreislaufschocks beim meuschen. Klin. Wochenschr. *46:* 352, 1968.

Richardson, J.D., Fry, D.E., Arsdall, L.V., and Flint, L.M., Jr.:

Delayed pulmonary clearance of gram-negative bacteria: the role of intraperitoneal sepsis. J. Surg. Res. 26:499, 1979.

Robboy, S.J., Colman, R.W., and Minna, J.D.: Pathology of disseminated intravascular coagulation (DIC): analysis of 26 cases. Hum. Pathol. 3:327, 1972.

Saba, T.M.: Reticuloendothelial systemic host defense after surgery and traumatic shock. Circ. Shock 2:91, 1975.

Saba, T.M.: Prevention of liver reticuloendothelial systemic host defense failure after surgery by intravenous opsonic glycoprotein therapy. Ann. Surg. 188:142, 1978.

Saba, T.M., Blumenstock, F.A., Scovill, W.A., and Bernard, H.: Cryoprecipitate reversal of opsonic α2-surface binding glycoprotein deficiency in septic surgical and trauma patients. Science 201:622, 1978.

Sambhi, M.P., Weil, M.H., and Udhoji, U.H.: Acute pharmacodynamic effects of glucocorticoids: cardiac output and related hemodynamic changes in normal subjects and patients in shock. Circulation 31:523, 1965.

Schuler, J.J., Erve, P.R., and Schumer, W.: Glucocorticoid effect on hepatic carbohydrate metabolism in the endotoxin-shocked monkey. Ann. Surg. 183:345, 1976.

Schumer, W.: Steroid in the treatment of clinical septic shock. Ann. Surg. 184:333, 1976.

Scovill, W.A., Saba, T.M., Kaplan, J.E., Bernard, H., and Powers, S.R.: Deficits in reticuloendothelial humoral mechanisms after trauma. J. Trauma 17:898, 1976.

Shepro, D., and Fulton, G.P.: *Microcirculation as Related to Shock*, 276 pp. Academic Press, New York, 1968.

Shock Tour Symposium: Mechanisms and Therapy of Endotoxin Shock. J. Okla. State Med. Assoc. 59:407, 1966.

Shoemaker, W.C.: *Shock*, 306 pp. Charles C Thomas, Springfield, IL, 1967.

Shoemaker, W.C., Printen, K.J., Carey, J.C., Reinhard, J.M., and Kark, A.E.: Use of sequential physiologic measurements for evaluation and therapy of uncomplicated septic shock. Surg. Gynecol. Obstet. 131:245, 1970.

Sibbald, W.J.: Bacteremia and endotoxemia: a discussion of their roles in the pathophysiology of gram-negative sepsis. Heart Lung 5:765, 1976.

Sibbald, W.J., Short, A., Cohen, M.P., and Wilson, R.F.: Variations in adrenocortical responsiveness during severe bacterial infections. Ann. Surg. 186:29, 1977.

Siegal, T., Seligsohn, U., Aghai, E., and Kodan, M.: Clinical and laboratory aspects of disseminated intravascular coagulation (DIC): a study of 118 cases. Thromb. Haemost. 39:122, 1978.

Siegel, J.H., Greenspan, M., and Del Guercio, L.R.M.: Abnormal vascular tone, defective oxygen transport and myocardial failure in human septic shock. Ann. Surg. 163:504, 1967.

Siegel, J.H., Farrell, E.J., Goldwyn, R.M., and Friedman, H.P.: Myocardial function in human septic shock states. In *Shock in Low- and High-Flow States*, edited by B. K. Forscher, R. C. Lillehei, and S. S. Stubbs, p. 250. Excerpta Medica, Amsterdam, 1972.

Solberg, C.O., and Hellum, K.B.: Neutrophil granulocyte function in bacterial infections. Lancet 2:727, 1972.

Spink, W.W.: Endotoxin shock. Ann. Int. Med. 57:538, 1962.

Spink, W.W.: The role of endotoxin in shock. In *Shock in Low- and High-Flow States*, edited by B. K. Forscher, R. C. Lillehei, and S. S. Stubbs, p. 226. Excerpta Medica, Amsterdam, 1972.

Spink, W.W., Braude, A.I., Castaneda, M.R., and Groytea, R.S.: Aureomycin therapy in human brucellosis due to *Brucella melitensis*. J.A.M.A. 138:1145, 1948.

Spink, W.W., Davis, R.B., Potter, R., and Chartrand, S.: The initial stage of canine endotoxin shock as an expression of anaphylactic shock: studies on complement titres and plasma histamine concentrations. J. Clin. Invest. 43:696, 1964.

Stone, A.M., Stein, T., LaFortune, J., and Wise, L.: Effect of steroids on the renovascular changes of sepsis. J. Surg. Res. 26:565, 1979.

Stossel, T.P.: Phagocytosis: the department of defense. N. Engl. J. Med. 286:776, 1972.

Stossel, T.P.: Phagocytosis. N. Engl. J. Med. 290:717, 1974.

Studdiford, W.E., and Douglas, G.W.: Placental bacteremia: a significant finding in septic abortion accompanied by vascular collapse. Am. J. Obstet. Gynecol. 71:842, 1956.

Sullivan, T.J., III, and Cavanagh, D.: Corticosteroids in endotoxin shock. Effect on renal vasomotion. Arch. Surg. 92:732, 1966.

Thal, A.P.: The cardiovascular response to sepsis. In *Shock in Low- and High-Flow States*, edited by B. K. Forscher, R. C. Lillehei, and S. S. Stubbs, p. 240. Excerpta Medica, Amsterdam, 1972.

Thal, A.P., Brown, E.B., Jr., Hermreck, A.S., and Bell, H.H.: *Shock*, 304 pp. Year Book Medical Publishers, Chicago, 1971.

Thomas, L.: The physiological disturbances produced by endotoxins. Annu. Rev. Physiol. 16:467, 1954.

Thomas, L.: *The Lives of a Cell: Notes of a Biology Watcher*, p. 78. Viking Press, New York, 1974.

Udhoji, V.N., and Weil, M.H.: Hemodynamic and metabolic studies on shock associated with bacteremia. Ann. Int. Med. 62:966, 1965.

Udhoji, V.N., Weil, M.H., Sambhi, M.P., and Rosoff, L.: Hemodynamic studies on clinical shock associated with infection. Am. J. Med. 34:461, 1963.

Urbaschek, B., Urbaschek, R., and Neter, E.: *Gram-Negative Bacterial Infections and Mode of Endotoxin Actions*, 524 pp. Springer-Verlag, New York, 1975.

Utili, R., Abernathy, C.O., and Zimmerman, H.J.: Minireview: endotoxin effects on the liver. Life Sci. 20:553, 1977.

Vaughn, D.T., Kirschbaum, T., Bersentes, T., and Assali, N.S.: Effects of corticosteroid hormones on regional circulation in endotoxin shock. Proc. Soc. Exp. Biol. Med. 124:760, 1967.

Visscher, M.B.: Shock with particular reference to endotoxin shock. Postgrad. Med. 23:545, 1958.

Waisbren, B.A.: Bacteremia due to gram-negative bacilli other than the *salmonella*. A clinical and therapeutic study. Arch. Int. Med. 88:467, 1951.

Waisbren, B.A.: Gram-negative shock and endotoxin shock. Am. J. Med. 36:819, 1964.

Weil, M.H.: Proposed classification of shock states, with special reference to distributive defects. In *The Fundamental Mechanisms of Shock*, edited by L. B. Hinshaw and B. G. Cox, p. 13. Plenum Press, New York, 1972.

Weil, M.H.: Current understanding of mechanisms and treatment of circulatory shock caused by bacterial infections. Ann. Clin. Res. 9:181, 1977.

Weil, M.H., and Henning, R.J.: *Handbook of Critical Care Medicine*, 559 pp. Symposia Specialists, Miami, 1978.

Weil, M.H., and Shubin, H.: *Diagnosis and Treatment of Shock*, 391 pp. Williams & Wilkins, Baltimore, 1967.

Weil, M.H., MacLean, L.D., Visscher, M.B., and Spink, W.W.: Studies on the circulatory changes in the dog produced by endotoxin from gram-negative microorganisms. J. Clin. Invest. 35:1191, 1956.

Weisul, J.P., O'Donnell, T.F., Stone, M.A., and Clowes, G.H.A., Jr.: Myocardial performance in clinical septic shock: effects of isoproterenol and glucose potassium insulin. J. Surg. Res. 18:357, 1975.

White, G.L., Archer, L.T., Beller, B.K., Holmes, D.D., and

Hinshaw, L.B.: Leukocyte response and hypoglycemia in superlethal endotoxic shock. Circ. Shock 4:231, 1977.
White, G.L., Archer, L.T., Beller, B.K., and Hinshaw, L.B.: Increased survival with methylprednisolone treatment in canine endotoxin shock. J. Surg. Res. 25:357, 1978.
Wilson, R.F.: The diagnosis and management of severe sepsis and septic shock. Heart Lung 5:422, 1976.
Wilson, R.F., Mohammed, A., Verandhen, A., McCarthy, B., Pitt, J., Hayes, D., Percinel, A., and Leblank, L.P.: Effects of vasoactive agents in clinical shock. In *Shock in Low- and High-Flow States*, edited by B. K. Forscher, R. C. Lillehei, and S. S. Stubbs, p. 269. Excerpta Medica, Amsterdam, 1972.
Zweifach, B.W., and Janoff, A.: Bacterial endotoxemia. Annu. Rev. Med. *16*:201, 1965.

CHAPTER 17

Human Response to Sepsis: A Physiologic Manifestation of Disordered Metabolic Control

JOHN H. SIEGEL
FRANK B. CERRA
JOHN R. BORDER
BILL COLEMAN
RAPIER H. MCMENAMY

The establishment of an invasive septic process initiates a state of disordered metabolic control in the host which alters the normal adaptive mechanisms to traumatic injury. As a consequence, the normal catabolic response to trauma is altered in such a way as to cause diversion of the normal pattern of glucose and gluconeogenic amino acid metabolism away from oxidative energy engendering aerobic metabolic pathways towards increased gluconeogenesis and fatty acid formation. In addition, other amino acids liberated from catabolic muscle appear also to be diverted from oxidative metabolism and protein synthesis to increased urea formation. In particular, the aromatic amino acids which are precursors of catecholamine synthesis may be converted into incompletely metabolized by-products which are capable of vasoactive stimuli as false neurotransmitters. There also appears to be impairment in the utilization of triglycerides and free fatty acids with pathologic hypertriglyceridemia and an apparent reduction in oxidative fat metabolism. This state of metabolic insufficiency is reflected in the adaptive pattern of cardiorespiratory vascular and physiologic compensation, which can be quantitatively measured at the bedside. The magnitude of the resultant pathophysiologic compensation and its rate and direction of change can be quantified by the use of physiologic state trajectories, which also reflect the magnitude of the underlying metabolic derangements. The tightness of the correlation between the physiologic and metabolic abnormalities in severe human sepsis suggests that the fundamental mechanisms of physiologic compensation are directly mediated by the categoric necessity of responding to the abnormal metabolic process. Because of the linkage, the pattern of physiologic abnormalities provides the key to clinical classification and staging. It also becomes an organizing principle by which one can understand and explore the altered biochemical control mechanisms of intermediary metabolism in the critically ill septic patient.

For many years, the understanding of the nature and magnitude of the physiologic response to sepsis in man was obscured by reliance on an animal model of endotoxin shock as the prototype for the human septic response. However, when clinical investigators began to adapt the techniques of cardiac catheterization with quantitative measurement of cardiac output and other cardiorespiratory physiologic parameters to the study of the critically ill at the bedside, it became apparent that the initial physiologic response to severe human septic illness was considerably different from the canine response to the intravenous injection of a lethal or sublethal quantity of bacterial endotoxin. Rather than there being a profound hypotension induced by a fall in cardiac output and visceral venous pooling of blood as seen in the dog, the initial response to human sepsis is a hyperdynamic state characterized by an increasing cardiac output and a fall in peripheral arterial vascular resistance (Weil et al., 1964; MacLean et al., 1967; Clowes et al., 1966). Careful analysis of this response demonstrated that the decrease in vascular tone, which reflects the pressure:flow relationship of the body, was disproportionate to the increase in cardiac output (Siegel et al., 1967). As a consequence, the critically ill septic patient was found to have a lower vascular resistance for the same body flow when compared to patients studied after traumatic injury. It was also noted that this response was different from that seen in patients in hypovolemic and cardiogenic shock states, where the vascular tone relationship was increased as compared to normal.

The critical observation, which suggested that the septic process was fundamentally different than that seen in response to nonseptic, traumatic, or surgical injury, was that after hypovolemia was corrected, most nonseptic patients increased cardiac outputs and oxygen consumption. In the most seriously ill hyperdynamic septic patients, the decrease in vascular tone relationships was accompanied by a fall in oxygen consumption and metabolic acidosis (Siegel et al., 1967, 1973). Further examination of this process demonstrated that the septic decrease in oxygen uptake was due to a failure of extraction rather than to a failure of delivery of oxygen to the peripheral tissues, as seen in hypovolemic and cardiogenic shock. Initially, the very close correlation between decreasing vascular tone and the rising mixed venous oxygen content, which produced the fall in oxygen consumption, was interpreted as being compatible with a pathophysiologic arteriovenous shunt, in which capillary beds were bypassed by the opening of pathologic vasculature, possibly in the area of inflammation (Siegel et al., 1967). While it became clear that there was some precapillary shunting through skin and areas of granulating tissue, it was also found that there was an increase in microvascular flow in capillary beds remote from the primary septic process. Xenon washout studies in septic human skeletal muscles demonstrated an increased rather than decreased capillary flow (Wright et al., 1971).

As more septic patients were studied throughout the course of their process of recovery or death from sepsis, it became clear that the nature of the septic process was not that of a steady state with a predetermined outcome but that patients manifesting a high level of oxygen consumption could make a transition into the state of low oxygen consumption and that considerable oscillation between the states could occur (Siegel, 1976b). These transitions appear to be functions of the successful or unsuccessful modalities of surgical drainage and antibiotic therapy. Deterioration of the septic process characteristically shows as an important component a fall in oxygen consumption during a period when cardiovascular function remains increased. This decrease in oxygen consumption is the earliest predictor of an increased chance of physiologic decompensation and death. It became clear that a characterization of the process of pathophysiologic adaptation in the septic patient and its time course of evolution would be critical factors in understanding the fundamental biochemical abnormalities, and in providing a meaningful classification system whereby the severity of sepsis could be compared in the same patient at different times and between different patients.

PHYSIOLOGIC STATE CLASSIFICATIONS AS AN INDEX OF THE CARDIOVASCULAR ADAPTIVE RESPONSE TO SEPSIS AND INJURY

In order to develop a classification system by which a physiologic pattern and pathologic process could be quantified, it was necessary to develop a frame of reference by which abnormal pathophysiologic patterns could be discriminated from normal adaptive stress responses to injury and to define a scale by which a change in the pattern of response could be quantified from one time period to the next. To this end, the principles of statistical pattern recognition were applied to a set of physiologic data obtained from patients with various forms of critical illness including shock, sepsis, traumatic injury, and cardiogenic decompensation (Siegel et al., 1972b; Friedman et al., 1975). After considerable preliminary analysis, a baseline set of 11 physiologic measurements which were obtained simultaneously in time at each stage of the patient's adaptive response to injury or sepsis were studied. In the initial analysis of the data (Siegel et al., 1972b), 695 sets of these 11 simultaneously obtained physiologic variables from 157 patients were analyzed. In some patients, the measurement sets were obtained in a control period preoperatively before major surgical operations; at a time when no evidence of stress response, sepsis, liver disease, or cardiogenic decompensation existed. In other instances, the patients evaluated manifested severe hypovolemic, cardiogenic, or septic shock states.

The multivariable data set of physiologic data included the determination of cardiac output by the indicator dilution technique, using indocyanine green dye injected in the right atrium and sampled in the arterial system for computation of the cardiac index (CI). In addition, two other important parameters of cardiac function were obtained from the indicator dilution curve, as observed in its transit across the central circulation. These were the pulmonary dispersive time (td), which has been shown to be primarily a measure of the mean transit time of dye containing blood across the pulmonary vascular bed, and the cardiac washout or mixing time (tm) (Siegel et al., 1972a). From the td in seconds times the

CI in liters/second, one can obtain a measure of pulmonary dispersive blood volume (DV/m^2) corrected for body surface area ($td \times CI = DV/m^2$). This has been shown experimentally to be within 10% of the pulmonary blood volume, as obtained from injection of dye in the pulmonary artery with sampling in the left atrium (Siegel et al., 1972a; Siegel, 1976a). The tm is the time constant of washout of dye containing blood from the left ventricle. It has been shown to be a function of the cardiac ejection fraction and as such to directionally reflect the factors which increase the myocardial force velocity relationship by reducing the duration of contractile active state (Siegel et al., 1972a; Siegel, 1976a). From this time constant of washout, it is possible to compute a minute cardiac ejection fraction (EFx) (Siegel et al., 1979c). This ejection fraction is analogous to, but is not identical with, the angiographic ejection fraction. It represents rather the proportion of blood volume contained in the heart during 1 min of cardiac output, which is involved in the ejection fraction function. It is in fact the mean of all the beat ejection fractions studied during the washout period. It has the advantage of being obtainable at the bedside by standard indicator dilution techniques, without use of x-ray, radioactive clearances, or expensive nuclear image equipment being necessary. This EFx, as any measure of ejection fraction, is influenced both by the intrinsic contractile dynamics of the myocardium as well as by the afterload effects of the total peripheral resistance (TPR) (Siegel, 1976a; Siegel et al., 1979c). It therefore represents a point on the myocardial force-velocity relationship. However, from the determination of the stroke volume (SV) and the EFx, an estimate of the effective mean left ventricular end-diastolic volume (LVEDV) can be obtained (LVEDV = SV/EFx).

In addition to these parameters obtained from the indicator dilution curve, simultaneous measurement of the mean heart rate (HR), mean arterial pressure (MAP), right atrial mean pressure (RAP), systolic ejection time (ET), arterial and mixed venous (PO_2, PCO_2), and hemoglobin concentrations and saturations were obtained. In addition, the P_{50} of the blood was determined from the mixed venous sample by an adaptation of the Kellman technique (Farrell and Siegel, 1976). From these data, the arteriovenous oxygen difference (A-VO_2Dif) could be directly calculated. In addition the oxygen consumption index (O_2CI) was computed as the product of CI times the A-VO_2Dif. The TPR, SV, and cardiac minute work were computed by standard formulas (Siegel, 1976a). A respiratory index (RI) (Siegel et al., 1973) was obtained which estimated the effective AaO_2/PaO_2 gradient by adjustment of the PIO_2 by barometric pressure, pH and body temperature, and $PaCO_2$ (as an estimate of $PACO_2$).

From the primary data, an 11 variable physiologic frame of reference was developed which could permit the delineation of the normal state of compensation for the older aged high risk patient who did not have shock, acute myocardial decompensation, sepsis, or liver disease. In defining this state (Fig. 17.1), the 11 variables used were the CI, HR, MAP, RAP, systolic ET, pulmonary td, cardiac tm, A-VO_2Dif, and mixed venous PO_2 (VPO_2), PCO_2 ($VPCO_2$), and pH (VpH); these variables were used as the normal frame of reference by which the variables of other types of patients in different states

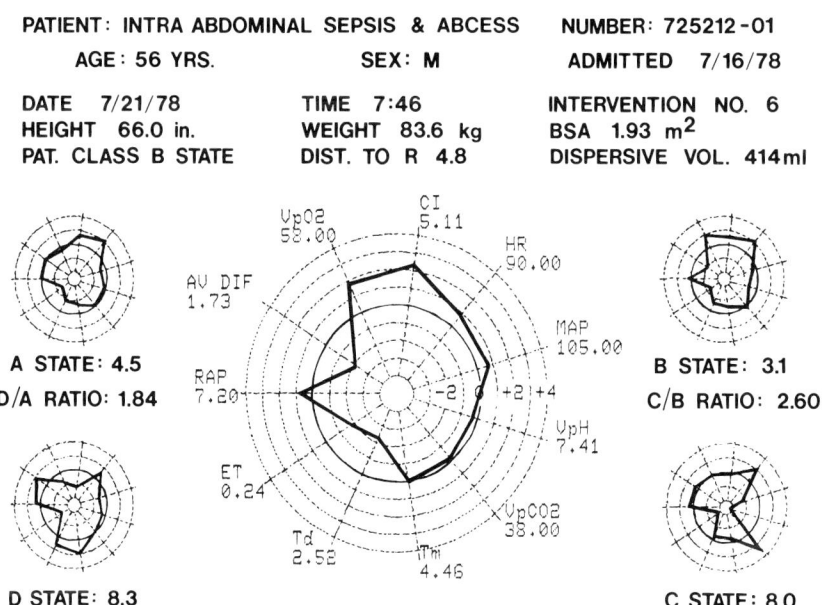

Figure. 17.1. Circle diagram of physiologic state. At corners are shown the prototype patterns for the A, B, C, and D states. In the large circle in the center is the physiologic pattern manifested by a 56-year-old man with intra-abdominal sepsis and abscess. The perfect circle in the center = 0 SD to reference control R state. Each *dotted line* represents 1 SD from R, either increased or decreased. Adjacent to each state is the state distance in normalized units from that prototype. Patient is closest to a B state (3.1) and therefore is classified as B. The real values of physiologic variables are given together with variable name on each ray. (Reprinted with permission from J. H. Siegel, F. B. Cerra, B. Coleman, I. Giovannini, M. Shetye, J. R. Border, and R. N. McMenamy: Surgery 86:163, 1979.)

could be compared by virtue of their standard deviation, positive or negative from the normal reference R state (0 SD = *dark circle* in Fig. 17.1). When compared to this reference control group (R state), it was noted that the entire spectrum of clinical severity in patients with trauma, sepsis, and cardiogenic shock could be viewed in terms of four pathophysiologic states A, B, C, and D. These states were derived by a technique of clustering all of the individual physiologic pattern data obtained from each of the 695 original data sets (Siegel et al., 1972b). The original groupings have been confirmed by additional studies of more than 1000 patients. The critical mathematic technique used in deriving these prototype states, which are seen in the four corners of Fig. 17.1, is the technique of clustering (Friedman et al., 1975). While this technique is rather complex from a statistical point of view, it is simple in concept. It is basically the logical principle used in grouping together individuals as being of the same family, and different from other family groupings, on the basis of their pattern of physical resemblance. In this statistical technique, the individual multivariable patterns are grouped in terms of similarity of pattern, and from these groupings a mean pattern which characterizes the nature of the adaptive response can be defined.

The A state is a normal stress response pattern. It is seen after injury or a major surgical procedure and also is the pattern found in compensated sepsis. This pattern is characterized by an increase in heart rate and CI, an improvement in the contractility as evidenced by a reduced tm, and an increased EFx. It also manifests an increase in oxygen consumption without any evidence of metabolic abnormality. This is seen in the fact that while the CI rises the A-V$\bar{O}_2$Dif remains normal or increases slightly; consequently O_2CI, which is the product of A-V$\bar{O}_2$Dif times flow, increases, while VpH, P$\bar{v}CO_2$, and P$\bar{v}O_2$ remain normal.

The *B* and *C* states represent increasing stages of severity characteristic of the deteriorating septic process. In the B state, a hyperdynamic cardiovascular pattern, reflected in the increase in cardiac output, the reduction in tm, the increase in cardiac EFx, and the shortened systolic ET, appears to fail to supply peripheral metabolic needs adequately. There is a reduced oxygen consumption, which is a function of the reduced extraction of oxygen (narrow A-V$\bar{O}_2$Dif), and this extraction is accompanied by a metabolic acidosis. On occasion, the magnitude of the acidosis may be concealed by a compensatory alkalosis as CO_2 is reduced by hyperventilation, but the metabolic acidosis is *always* present. In the C state, respiratory decompensation is superimposed on the unbalanced metabolic processes seen in the B state level of decompensation. Consequently, a profound metabolic and respiratory acidosis occurs. The C state is characteristic of profound septic shock with hypotension in spite of a normal or increased cardiac output. It is marked by a profound reduction in arterial vascular tone to a magnitude even greater than that seen in the B state. It is occasionally seen in acute postoperative or posttraumatic respiratory distress syndrome as a terminal phenomenon.

In contrast to the metabolic B and respiratory failure C states, the cardiogenic or the D state demonstrates a pattern of primary myocardial rather than primary peripheral failure. In this cardiogenic state, there is a decline in myocardial contractility manifested by a prolonged tm with a reduced EFx. Consequently, there is a fall in cardiac output and a widening of the A-V$\bar{O}_2$Dif as the peripheral tissues attempt to compensate for the oxygen delivery failure by increasing oxygen extraction. The pulmonary blood volume (DV/m^2) rises as a function of the cardiac failure and as a result the mean td is prolonged. Varying degrees of hypotension and acidosis may occur in this state as a function of the magnitude of the oxygen delivery and extraction failure. This D state pattern is the characteristic hemodynamic response seen in acute myocardial infarction (Siegel et al., 1972b) and is also the most common pattern seen in the immediate postoperative period following coronary artery bypass grafting (CABG), usually evolving into an A state in a few hours as the transient myocardial depression following surgery is resolved into a normal stress response (Siegel et al., 1975; Raza et al., 1977).

While these prototype R, A, B, C and D patterns provide understanding as to the nature of human adaptive responses to stress, their most important value with regard to the classification of an individual patient is that they can be considered as a grid point in a physiologic hyperspace in which the real patient moves as his degree of recovery or compensation to a physiologic stress occurs (Siegel et al., 1979b). Since the principle behind the classification technique is to transform all of the individual physiologic variables into a common unit, *the standard deviation of that variable from the control state*, it becomes possible to quantify the specific multivariable physiologic state of an individual real patient in terms of a "distance" at a given moment in time from each of the points represented by the prototype (R, A, B, C, or D) mean states. The nature and degree of the individual patient's physiologic inadequacy can thus be quantified at a given moment in time from his absolute distance from a given state or from a distance ratio between various states (Siegel, 1976b; Siegel et al., 1979b). This is also demonstrated in Figure 17.1 which shows the computer printout from a severely ill septic patient studied following a traumatic injury resulting in localized bowel perforation with intraabdominal abscess formation. It can be seen that this patient manifests a B state pathophysiologic pattern. By comparing the patient's individual pattern to each of the four prototype state patterns (A, B, C, and D) and the reference R state (perfect *dark circle* on all patterns), it is possible to derive a quantitative physiologic distance from each state and some important state distance ratios. While it is evident that at a given particular moment in a patient's physiologic course he has some quantifiable relationship to all of the prototype states; however, for simple classification purposes the patient is designated by the closest state distance as being either the A, B, C, D, or R state at a given study time.

INTERPRETATION OF CARDIOVASCULAR AND CARDIOPULMONARY RELATIONS IN THE LIGHT OF THE PATIENT'S PHYSIOLOGIC STATE

The recognition that a patient is in a particular physiologic state has considerable implications for understanding the specific cardiovascular interrelationships seen in patients with septic and nonseptic forms of critical illness. This is shown in Figure 17.2, which demonstrates the relationship between the CI level as a function of the cardiac EFx and the DV/m^2. This figure demonstrates a total of 374 observations from 151 critically ill patients (202 septic and 172 cardiogenic or hypovolemic nonseptic). None of these patients were in the original group of 157 used for the derivation of the original state classifications (Siegel et al., 1979c). This figure demonstrates clearly that critically ill patients *do* obey the basic cardiovascular interrelationships described by the Starling-Sarnoff law of the heart. This can be seen in the fact that at a given level of EFx, the CI can be increased by an increase in the DV/m^2, which acts as the filling reservoir of the left heart. This increase in output as a function of the increased filling volume of the heart is the classic Frank-Starling mechanism. Conversely, at a given pulmonary reservoir and therefore left atrial filling volume (DV/m^2), the CI can also be increased by interventions which change the basic inotropic force of contraction, thus moving the patient from one Starling curve to an improved one, the inotropic mechanism. This occurs in the critically ill patient because the ordinary mechanisms for reflex control of the circulation, which achieve a sympathetic balance in normal individuals, are obviously already operating at the maximum stress response level. The importance of recognizing that these mechanisms are important can be seen by observing that a different mechanism for circulatory support would be utilized in a patient with a low CI and a low ejection fraction who was already operating at high DV/m^2, compared to that which should be used in a similar patient with a low CI who had a high ejection fraction but a low DV/m^2. In the former instance since filling volume was already at maximum, the use of cardiac inotropic agents such as isoproterenol or dopamine would be the therapeutic choice. In the latter, however, where cardiac inotropic

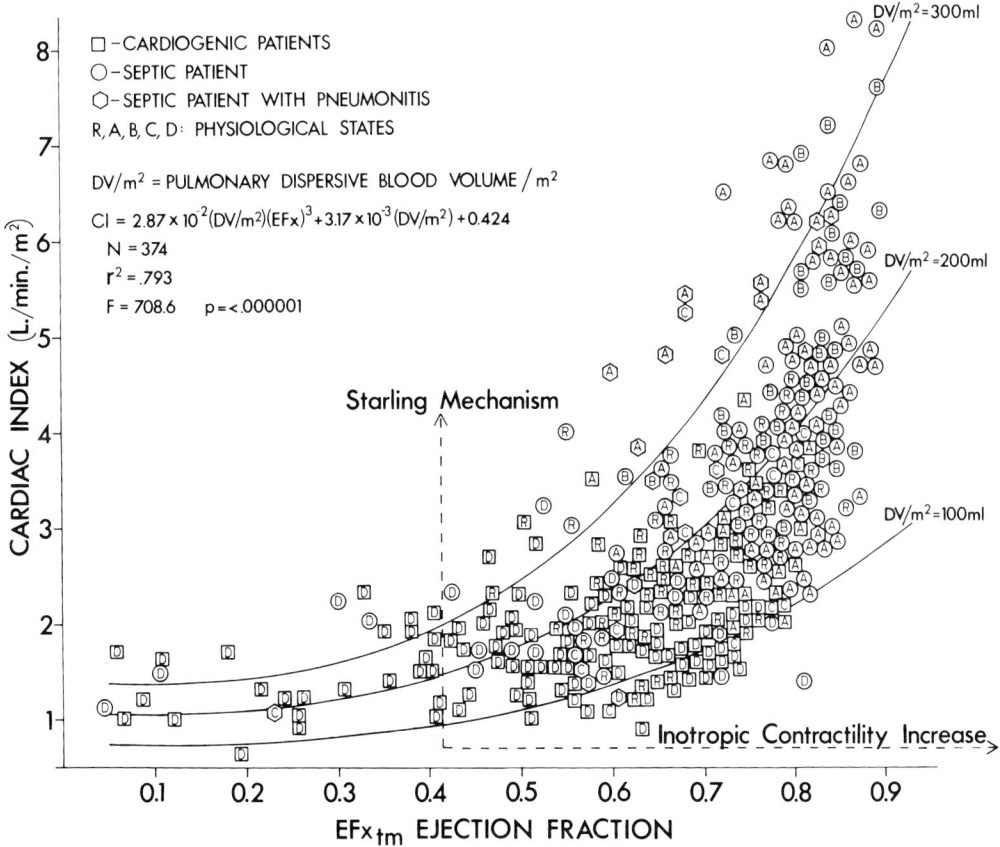

Figure 17.2. Relationship between (CI) and ejection fraction (EFx) computed from the cardiac mixing time (tm). The mean lines of constant pulmonary dispersive volume (DV/m^2) as shown in the regression equation. Labeled by physiologic state. (Reprinted with permission from J. H. Siegel, F. B. Cerra, B. Coleman, I. Giovannini, M. Shetye, J. R. Border, and R. H. McMenamy: Surgery 86:163, 1979.)

action was already high, as evidenced by an increased EFx, the low cardiac output would be clearly on the basis of a low reservoir volume. Therefore, infusion of colloid or blood volume would be the modality best suited to increase the cardiac output by increasing the filling volume of the already maximally stimulated heart.

Within this framework, it is also clear that in general there is a different distribution of patients with sepsis (*circles*) and those with nonseptic cardiogenic or hypovolemic states (*squares*). The septic A and B state, patients can be seen to have high CI and large ejection fractions over the entire range of pulmonary dispersive volume. In contrast, the cardiogenic or hypovolemic patients are seen to be primarily in a D state and have in general lower ejection fractions regardless of whether the filling volume is increased, normal, or decreased. It can also be seen that there are some septic patients who are in a D or cardiogenic state, and these patients' behavior in terms of cardiac adaptive mechanisms is similar to that found in other cardiogenic patients. The importance of this will be discussed later. However, the most important aspect is the fact that the patients with the highest cardiac indices and the greatest levels of contractility are primarily septic in the B state, or a few A state patients who are near to a B state transformation. This has considerable significance since it is evident from the previous state patterns that the B state patients are those with the lowest vascular resistance and the most reduced oxygen consumption, suggesting that metabolic factors may play some role in the final level of adaptation of the cardiovascular response.

This is made even more clear when one considers the relationship between cardiac output and TPR (Fig. 17.3). Also, shown are lines of constant cardiac minute work. The normal older patient in a controlled nonseptic, nonstress state will have a CI between 5 and 6 liters/min, a range of total peripheral resistance between 1200 and 1500 dyne-sec-cm^{-5}, and a level of cardiac work at approximately 6 kg-m/min. Compared with these patients, it can be seen that the septic patients (*circles*) in the A or B hyperdynamic states have considerably higher CI performed at substantially lower levels of TPR. In contrast, the patients with cardiogenic syndromes (D state), whether they are septic (*circles*) or cardiogenic (*squares*), are seen to have low levels of cardiac output performed at relatively high levels of TPR. In general,

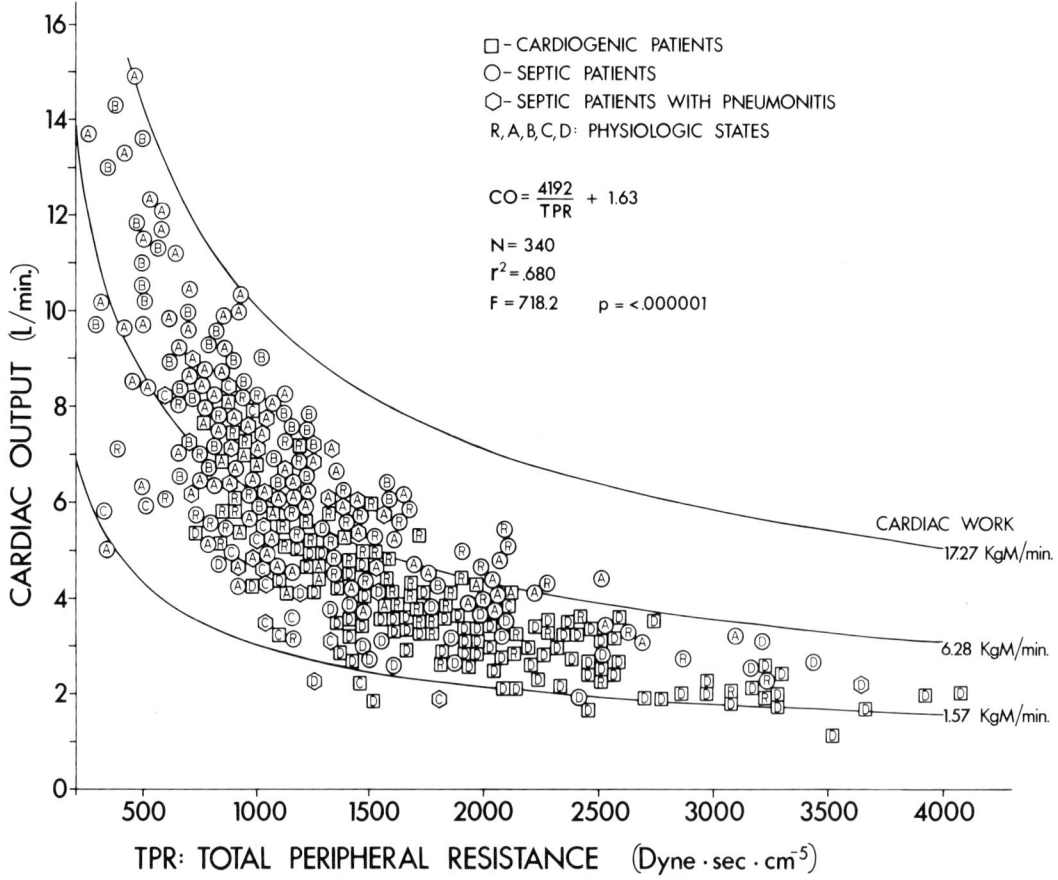

Figure 17.3. Relationship between cardiac output and total peripheral resistance (TPR) labeled by physiologic state classification. Lines of constant cardiac work in kilograms per minute are shown. (Reprinted with permission from J. H. Siegel, F. B. Cerra, B. Coleman, I. Giovannini, M. Shetye, J. R. Border, and R. H. McMenamy: Surgery 86: 163, 1979.)

they do less work than normal, but this work is primarily *pressure* work done at high resistance. This figure demonstrates clearly why it is in the interest of the patient with a D state cardiogenic syndrome to utilize an afterload unloading agent such as nitroglycerine paste, intravenous nitroglycerine, or nitroprusside, since by this means one may increase the body flow by reducing TPR without increasing the level of cardiac minute work and therefore cardiac oxygen consumption.

When one considers cardiac work as a critical aspect of the septic process, with regard to the metabolic needs of the septic patient, it is of critical interest to note that the hyperdynamic A and B state septic patients who have the highest cardiac output and the lowest TPR are also those patients performing the largest amount of cardiac minute work. Indeed, in the B state patients and in those A state patients close to a B state transformation, the cardiac work ranges between 10 and 17 kg-m/min. This is an especially significant figure, since the maximum cardiac work that can be achieved under ordinary circumstances ranges between 20 and 30 kg-m/min and is generally performed for only short periods of time such as in maximal exercise. However, these desperately ill septic patients are operating at high levels of cardiac minute work not for just a few minutes, but for days or weeks. The cost of this work in terms of myocardial energetic needs is enormous and demonstrates the great dependence of the cardiac performance of the septic patient on an adequate level of myocardial metabolism. As is shown in the next figure (Fig. 17.4), the enormous myocardial requirement for energetics in order to maintain the hyperdynamic state often induces a metabolic myocardial depression type of cardiac failure. That this is not an uncommon phenomena can be seen in the significant number of D state septic patients shown in Figures 17.2 and 17.3.

As will be shown later, the myocardial failure of sepsis may be due to the progressive sequence of metabolic abnormalities seen as the septic state transitions from the A to B state. These tend to restrict the availability or utilization of metabolic fuels by oxidative metabolism. This is well shown in Figure 17.4, which demonstrates sequential physiologic patterns from a critically ill patient who was studied following vascular occlusion of distal arteries to the small bowel resulting in infarction and necrosis. After resection, he developed peritonitis, sepsis, and a wide range of complications related to the septic process. The three studies in Figure 17.4 demon-

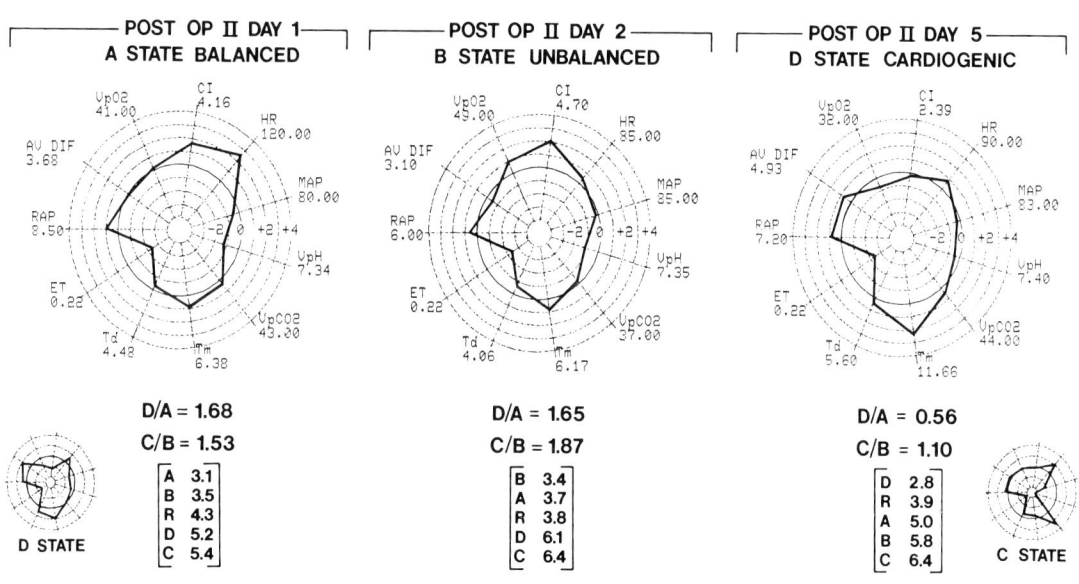

Figure 17.4. State transitions in severe sepsis. Changing physiologic patterns together with their state distances and state distance ratios are shown for a 62-year-old man with bowel infarctions and resection who developed peritonitis and sepsis followed by wound dehiscence. He had a closure of dehiscence, ileostomy, colostomy, and tracheostomy as a second operation procedure (Op II). The state transitions following his second operation from an A-balanced physiologic state to a B state of metabolic imbalance, followed by comparison of the patient's states with the prototypes of the A, B, C, and D states. (Reprinted with permission from J. H. Siegel, F. B. Cerra, B. Coleman, I. Giovannini, M. Shetye, J. R. Border, and R. H. McMenamy: Surgery 86: 163, 1979.)

strate serial aspects of the time course showing a typical progression into a D state of cardiogenic decompensation. As can be seen, the patient transitioned from an A state of balanced stress response to a B state unbalanced pattern with narrowing of the A-VO$_2$Dif and evidence of metabolic decompensation with production of metabolic acidosis. Following this metabolic decompensation, the patient transitioned to a D state myocardial decompensation demonstrating reduction in EFx (producing a prolongation in tm and a fall in CI). This is a classic sequence of state transitions in the septic patient, and it demonstrates the extreme vulnerability of the hyperdynamic septic patient who manifests a B state metabolic imbalance to develop myocardial failure. This emphasizes particularly well the need for the early recognition of even minimal levels of myocardial decompensation and the prophylactic use of cardiac inotropic agents to prevent acute metabolic myocardial failure in the septic patient.

The abnormal cardiovascular physiologic abnormalities seen in the septic A and B states and their differences compared to the abnormalities found in the state of cardiogenic decompensation (D state) have their analog in the cardiopulmonary interrelationships found in the septic patient (Siegel et al., 1979c). This is seen in Figure 17.5, which demonstrates the relationship between abnormalities in the ventilation/perfusion ($\dot{V}_A/\dot{Q}_T$) ratio as a function of the alterations in pulmonary shunt ($\dot{Q}_S/$

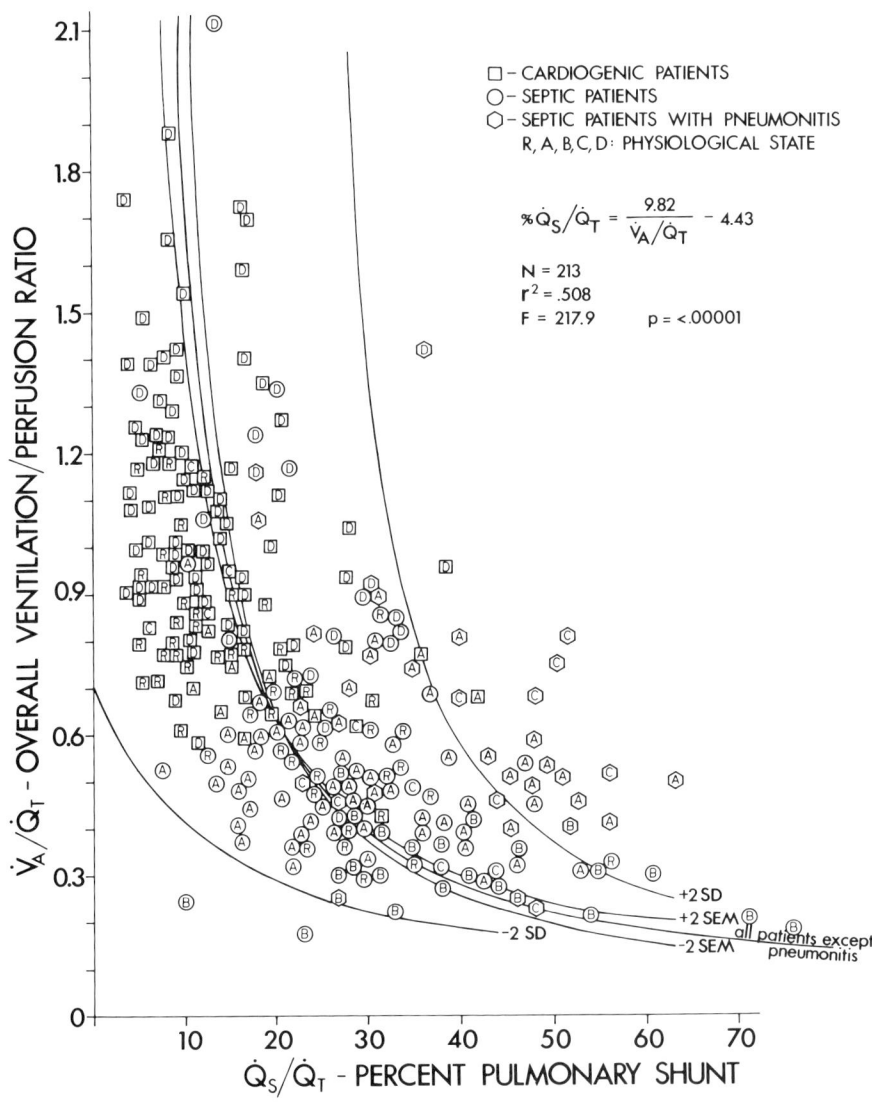

Figure 17.5. Relationship between overall ventilation/perfusion ratio ($\dot{V}_A/\dot{Q}_T$) and percentage of pulmonary shunt ($\dot{Q}_S/\dot{Q}_T$) labeled by physiologic state. Shown are the mean, ±2 SEM, and ±2 SD lines for the regression for all patients, excluding those with pneumonitis. Septic patients with pneumonitis are shown by a hexagonal symbol and generally lie more than 2 SD above the nonpneumonitis regression mean. (Reprinted with permission from J. H. Siegel, F. B. Cerra, B. Coleman, I. Giovannini, M. Shetye, J. R. Border, and R. H. McMenamy: Surgery 86: 163, 1979.)

$\dot{Q}_T$). In this figure, it can be seen that in septic patients without pneumonitis, the A and B state patients who have the lowest $\dot{V}_A/\dot{Q}_T$ also have the highest percentage of shunt ($\dot{Q}_S/\dot{Q}_T$) (Siegel et al., 1979c). It has also been shown that the marked disparity in $\dot{V}_A/\dot{Q}_T$ seen in the septic patient is correlated with the major increase in the ratio of respiratory dead space to tidal ventilation (V_D/V_T), which suggests a major maldistribution of perfusion in spite of the increased cardiac output and increased pulmonary blood flow seen in the A and B state septic patients. This pathologic relationship is most marked in the patients with the unbalanced metabolic B state who show the most significant reductions in TPR and who have the highest EFx due to a reduction in afterload. In these patients, there is also evidence that there is a marked shift of the Starling curve to the left such that there is a smaller left ventricular end-diastolic volume (LVEDV) per increase in cardiac output (Siegel et al., 1979c).

These factors suggest that the peripheral vascular abnormalities, which are the primary pathophysiologic lesions of the septic (Siegel et al., 1967; Maclean et al., 1967), may induce the abnormal pulmonary ventilation/perfusion maldistribution by diverting a higher percentage of the increased pulmonary blood flow to dependent lung segments. This would occur because of the major passive dependence of blood flow through the pulmonary bed on the difference in pressure between pulmonary inflow and left atrial (LAP) and left ventricular end-diastolic (LVEDP) pressure on the outflow side of the pulmonary vascular run off. The marked reduction in vascular resistance, which is the characteristic feature of the peripheral abnormality in sepsis, is most abnormal in the B state. Therefore, by reducing the afterload and permitting the large cardiac ejection fraction, which reduces LVEDV and thus LVEDP and LAP, the perfused segments of lung and consequently the area of optimum $\dot{V}_A/\dot{Q}_T$ would decrease markedly. These pulmonary perfusion abnormalities seen in sepsis are in marked contrast to the $\dot{V}_A/\dot{Q}_T$ and $\dot{Q}_S/\dot{Q}_T$ abnormalities in patients with cardiogenic failure, in whom $\dot{V}_A/\dot{Q}_T$ levels are actually increased over normal (normal = 0.8) (Fig. 17.5). The degree of $\dot{Q}_S/\dot{Q}_T$ is largely a function of alveolar collapse and edema due to the high level of LAP, with increased pulmonary interstitial edema and in some instances pulmonary edema. These markedly different pathophysiologic pictures demonstrate clearly how the physiologic state and its pattern of adaptation to stress are totally different in different forms of human critical illness and shock and that the state classification provides a means of summarizing and characterizing these abnormalities in a concise and practical way.

PHYSIOLOGIC TRAJECTORY AND ITS VALUE AS A MEANS OF CLASSIFYING THE MAGNITUDE OF METABOLIC ABNORMALITIES IN SEPSIS

A key corollary to the concept of physiologic state classification as a pattern of adaptation to stress is the understanding that changes in this state may occur over a period of time as the patient's condition improves or deteriorates. This is shown in Figure 17.4 in which the changing physiologic patterns reflect the nature of the physiologic adaptive responses to septic stress. From observing this figure, it is also clear that no individual patient's pattern of adaptation is exactly like any of the mean prototype states shown in the four corners. However, the value of the prototype states, which have been derived from the cluster analysis of large numbers of critically ill patients, is that they provide known reference points in a physiologic space by which an individual patient's similarity or dissimilarity to each state can be stated in terms of a relative Euclidean "distance" from each of these five states (Friedman et al., 1975; Siegel et al., 1979b). Using these physiologic state distances as a kind of coordinate system whereby a patient's physiologic position can be determined, it is possible to track the vector change, in a quantitative way, from one moment to the next. Thus, a patient's exact physiologic position can be determined, and his course of recovery or nonrecovery can be analyzed and correlated with other physiologic and metabolic measurements. It is also possible to follow the time course of a number of patients in similar clinical conditions or types of surgical operations and thereby determine whether they are following acceptable or unacceptable recovery trajectories. By this means, one may determine whether deviation from a particular type of recovery trajectory is associated with success or failure of the therapy. If one considers Figures 17.1 and 17.4, it is possible to determine that the similarity a patient has at any given time to the prototype A state of normal stress response as compared to that of the prototype D state of cardiogenic compensation, the D/A ratio, is a measure of cardiovascular adequacy. Similarly, the relationship between the B state of metabolic insufficiency and the C state of respiratory insufficiency, the C/B ratio, provides an indication of the relative adequacy of the patient's metabolic and respiratory function. Considering these two ratios together, a useful way of describing and plotting a recovery trajectory is shown in Figure 17.6. Patients with a close similarity to a normal stress response therefore have a high D/A ratio, whereas those with cardiogenic decompensation have a low D/A ratio. Also, patients with a large degree of respiratory insufficiency would have a low C/B ratio, whereas those with a major degree of metabolic insufficiency characterized by decreasing oxygen consumption and metabolic acidosis would demonstrate a high C/B ratio.

In this analysis, it has also been possible to determine the definite areas of acceptable and unacceptable recovery for various types of surgical patients undergoing elective procedures. These regions are shown in the outlined boxes in Figure 17.6. Two very different types of surgical response patterns have been identified. In coronary bypass patients, used as the prototype for patients in myocardial dysfunction, when studied prior to surgery (CABG-P) were found to have D/A ratios and C/B ratios that were both greater than 1.0. The ±1

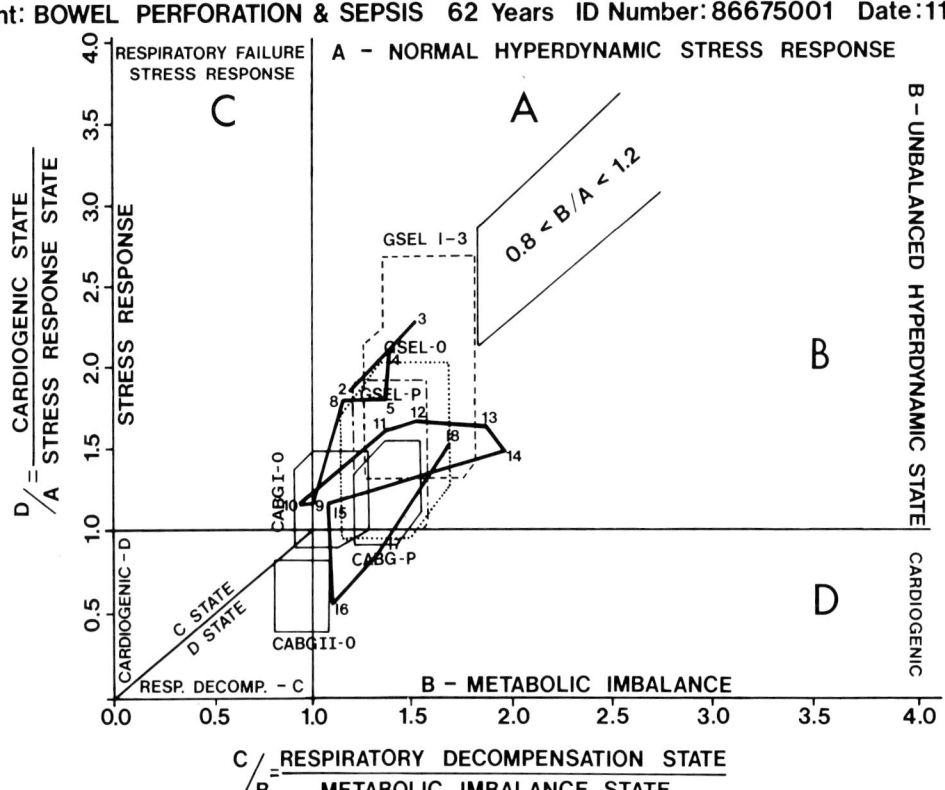

Figure 17.6. Physiologic state trajectory plot for the patient in Fig. 17.4. This figure shows the cardiovascular related D/A ratio as a function of the respiratory: metabolic C/B ratio. Envelopes of recovery for coronary bypass patients (CABG) and routine major nonseptic general surgery patients (GSEL) are outlined in this physiologic space. The ±1 SD region of the postoperative day trajectories for GSEL patients are shown. The areas occupied by patients whose state classification are, respectively, A, B, C, or D are shown outside of the physiologic recovery envelope of the GSEL patients. (Reprinted with permission from J. H. Siegel, F. B. Cerra, B. Coleman, I. Giovannini, M. Shetye, J. R. Border, and R. H. McMenamy: Surgery 86: 163, 1979.)

standard deviation (SD) box for CABG-P is shown in Figure 17.6 for these patients. Immediately after surgery (day 0), three types of recovery patterns were identified (Siegel et al., 1975; Raza et al., 1977). Patients who did well, type I (CABG-I-0), showed a negligible fall in the D/A ratio but demonstrated a slight movement toward a moderate degree of respiratory insufficiency (decrease in the C/B ratio). The ±1 SD region of the CABG-I-0 group is shown in Figure 17.6. Within 12–18 hr, the type I CABG patient returned to the preoperative level (CABG-P). In the type II cardiogenic recovery (CABG-II), which is the minimum acceptable recovery for coronary bypass patients, there was a fall in cardiovascular compensation in the immediate (day 0) postoperative period, as evidenced by a decreased D/A ratio. At the same time, there was evidence of a significant degree of respiratory insufficiency, and the C/B ratio also fell. The ±1 SD for these patients is shown in the CABG-II-0 area in Figure 17.6. Type II cardiogenic patients showed the relatively rapid return of cardiovascular adequacy with a physiologic recovery trajectory that returned to the preoperative region (CABG-P) within an 18–24 hr period. However, patients who subsequently had a poor clinical course, the cardiogenic type III recovery trajectory, failed to return to the CABG-P region and tended to have an oscillatory course that kept them in the region of myocardial depression (CABG-II-0) for longer than 18–24 hr. These patients either had a difficult postoperative recovery with a very slow return to the preoperative level or they failed to recover and died in or near the CABG-II-0 region with both D/A and C/B ratios usually less than 1.0 (Siegel et al., 1975). This type of recovery is also found in patients with myocardial depression or failure due to other causes such as acute myocardial infarction (Siegel et al., 1972b), myocardiopathy, or toxic myocardial depression. It is also seen in the metabolic myocardial failure of sepsis (Siegel et al., 1967, 1979a).

In contrast, general surgical (GSEL) patients manifest a very different type of recovery trajectory. Preoperatively (GSEL-P), these patients are seen to have some overlap with the CABG-P patients, reflecting the fact that some general surgical patients have mild degrees of occult myocardial insufficiency. However, generally they fall into a broader region with higher preoperative D/A ratios. There is no significant difference from the CABG-

P in the level of respiratory and metabolic compensation, the C/B ratio. The region of ±1 SD in preoperative GSEL patients is shown (GSEL-P). Following the stress of major surgical therapy, the general surgical patient has a trajectory which is in a very different direction from the coronary bypass patient. There is a progressive increase in the D/A ratio from the immediate postoperative study (GSEL-0) through the first 3 days after operation (GSEL-1-3). This reflects a heightened stress response as the patient moves closer to an A state prototype. There is also a moderate increase in the C/B ratio as the patient demonstrates a mild metabolic insufficiency. This is rapidly corrected, and by the 3rd day after operation the well compensated general surgical patient has already returned toward the preoperative level. In some cases, definitive recovery may take up to 5 days, but the patient's physiologic recovery seldom moves outside of the ±1 SD envelope of the general surgical (GSEL) trajectory.

The advantage of using this type of graphic representation of the physiologic response envelope for different types of surgical recoveries is that it is possible to evaluate an individual patient with regard to his deviation from the ±1 SD course of previously studied patients. In other words, the entire time course of a patient can be evaluated with regard to the degree to which his or her trajectory remains in the envelope of acceptable recovery. Figure 17.6, using this type of course analysis to follow the major metabolic and cardiogenic decompensations shown in the septic patient whose individual physiologic patterns were shown in Figure 17.4, clearly demonstrates that during the initial septic period the patient's course was marked by an adequate stress response. From studies 2–8 the patient moved within the envelope of the normal GSEL recovery; however, by the ninth study he began to demonstrate evidence of mild respiratory insufficiency with a fall of C/B ratio, even though there were adequate cardiovascular dynamics (D/A ratio). This was treated with aggressive ventilatory support (studies 9 and 10), and following the correction of respiratory insufficiency it was noted that the patient began to have evidence of increasing metabolic insufficiency, indicated by a rising C/B ratio. This pathophysiologic course carried him through the normal GSEL region into the area of unmodified B state (studies 13 and 14); this transition is shown in its prototype patterns (the A and B state studies) in Figure 17.4. After the severe metabolic insufficiency response seen in studies 13 and 14, when falling oxygen consumption and marked reduction in vascular tone had been ameliorated through surgical drainage, antibiotics, and host response, the patient returned through the GSEL envelope. However, as was noted earlier, following this metabolic insufficiency response, the patient manifested a sudden myocardial depression, and his trajectory fell into the region of CABG-II-0, evidencing a picture similar to the myocardial depression seen in patients with nonseptic cardiogenic syndrome (study 16). This specific physiologic pattern is seen in the D study in Figure 17.4. Through the aggressive use of cardiogenic support (digoxin and isoproterenol) and a vasodilating agent (nitroglycerine paste), it was possible to effect a return to a normal stress response over the 17th and 18th studies. This time course trajectory demonstrates that significant cardiovascular and metabolic interactions can be summarized in a fashion which provides quantitative information regarding the specific nature of the physiologic accommodations to a septic stress.

PHYSIOLOGIC STATE AS A QUANTITATIVE CORRELATE OF THE NATURE AND MAGNITUDE OF METABOLIC INSUFFICIENCY IN SEPSIS

The most important aspect of the study of physiologic trajectories has been the understanding that the physiologic state can be used as the organizing principle and the physiologic correlate of the magnitude and nature of metabolic inadequacy in the critically ill septic patient (Siegel et al., 1979a and b). These relationships are demonstrated in Figure 17.7, which shows the pattern of abnormalities in branched chain amino acids, glucose metabolites, glucose regulating hormones, fat metabolites, aromatic amino acids, and the amino acids involved in urea synthesis as well as the parameters of cardiovascular function and the D/A and C/B ratios from 136 observations in 49 patients representing three different clinical groups. These three groups were patients with major nonseptic traumatic injury and septic patients in the A or B states of metabolic adequacy. The mean values from these groups are compared with regard to the magnitude of their standard deviational differences with the mean of a group of control elective general surgical patients in the R state of compensation (perfect *circle*) at 0 SD. A physiologically important alteration can be assumed for a change of $> \pm 1$ SD from the control. It is clearly evident that very major differences exist within the pattern of cardiovascular compensation and the circulating concentrations of the various hormones and metabolic products when one compares the nonseptic traumatized patient with the septic patients in the A or B states of physiologic compensation. More importantly there appears to be a progressive magnitude of abnormality as the patient moves from A to B state in the septic process.

It can be seen that all three groups have certain similarities in the adaptive response of the cardiovascular system. They all demonstrate an increased D/A ratio, which is mostly increased in the septic B state patient. All have an increase in CI, which is most prominent in the traumatized patient. All show an increase in EFx, a reduction in pulmonary mean td, and a fall in TPR. The important differences in the cardiovascular functional area between the septic and nonseptic patients lie in the decrease in mixed venous pH (VpH) and the narrow A-VO_2 in the B state septic patient. Both of these means are approximately 1 SD less than control in the septic B patients and at normal levels in the trauma patients. However, the most important physiologic difference is in the O_2CI. Whereas trauma patients have an oxygen

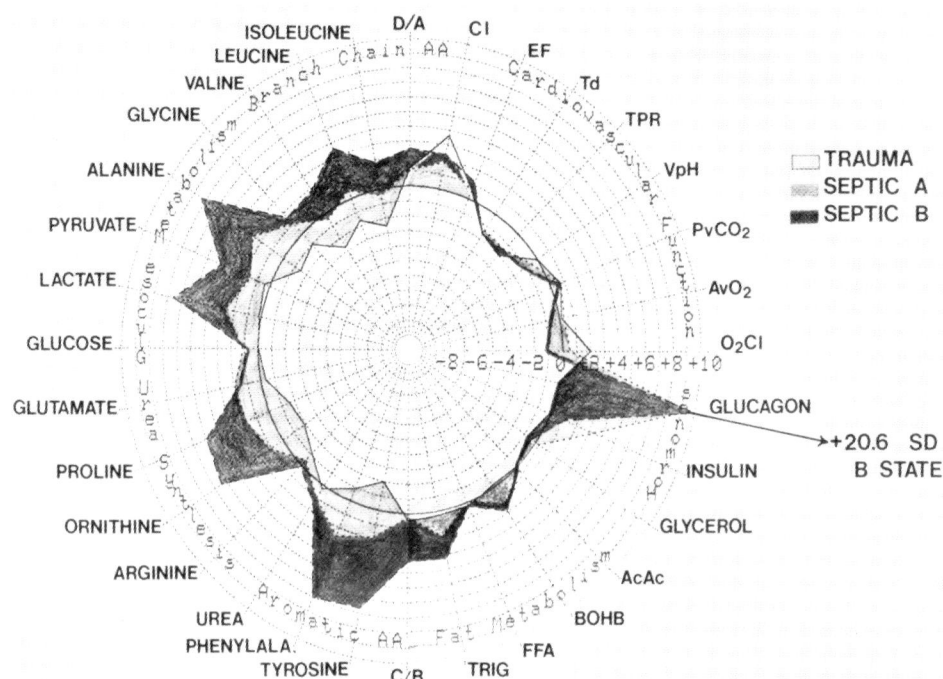

Figure 17.7. Physiologic and metabolic circle diagram for patients with nonseptic major trauma and for patients in septic A and B states. The perfect circle at 0 SD represents the mean values for a control group of general surgical patients in the R state of physiologic compensation. All other mean lines are normalized by the SD of the control group. The mean value for the trauma patients is shown by the *light gray shading*, mean value for the septic A patients by the *intermediate gray*, and mean value for the septic B patients by the *black*. Data are grouped in terms of appropriate physiologic-metabolic functional interrelations. (Reprinted with permission from J. H. Siegel, F. B. Cerra, B. Coleman, I. Giovannini, M. Shetye, J. R. Border, and R. H. McMenamy: Surgery *86:* 163, 1979.)

consumption which is approximately 2 SD *above* normal and the septic A state patients show an oxygen consumption which is only slightly increased over normal, the septic B state patients show a markedly *reduced* oxygen consumption. This is 1 SD less than the control R state and more than 3 SD less than the mean of the trauma patients. If it can be assumed that the normal response to nonseptic trauma is the basic adaptive mechanism, then this reduction in O_2CI reflects a very severe impairment of oxidative metabolism at a time of major metabolic and physiologic stress.

This difference in oxidative metabolism becomes even more significant when viewed in the light of the pattern of plasma concentrations of circulating metabolic substrates. Again, considering that the nonseptic trauma response is truly the basal adaptive response to injury, it can be seen that the levels of branched chain amino acids valine, leucine, and isoleucine are between 1 and 3 SD below normal, suggesting an improved utilization of these essential amino acids if the circulating levels reflect equilibration with the rate of utilization. The level of the carrier amino acids glycine and alanine, which are major precursors of the gluconeogenic response, are also reduced, suggesting an increased utilization of these amino acids, since they are known to be released from muscles in patients following traumatic injury (Cerra et al., 1979a;

Marchuck et al., 1977; O'Donnell et al., 1976; Woolf et al., 1979). The levels of pyruvate, lactate and glucose seem to be approximately at the level of control general surgical patients, which again suggests that there may be increased utilization of muscle released gluconeogenic amino acids in traumatized patients, but that these are oxidatively metabolized and may therefore contribute to the increased O_2CI found in the trauma group. In a similar fashion, the amino acids used as markers of urea synthesis, glutamate, proline, ornithine, and arginine also show somewhat lower levels than does the control, whereas urea levels are essentially normal. The levels of the aromatic amino acids phenylalanine and tyrosine are also reduced as compared to control levels, perhaps reflecting a generally improved metabolism of all amino acids released from muscle catabolism in trauma. The C/B ratio is normal, and the levels of fat intermediates triglycerides, free fatty acids (FFA), β-hydroxybutyrate, acetoacetate (AcAc), and glycerol, which is also a gluconeogenic precursor, are all at normal levels. The most important aspects of the traumatic response are that there are no significant increases over R state general surgical controls in either insulin or glucagon, perhaps reflecting a normal balance between anabolic and catabolic stimuli in the post-traumatic patient.

Considering the trauma response as the normal prototype of stress adaptation, the progressive alterations in the septic patient as the physiologic state progresses from a balanced stress response (septic A state) to an unbalanced metabolic response (septic B state) reflect a deteriorating pattern of oxidative fuel utilization. As the A to B state transition occurs, marked by a progressive rise in C/B ratio and a progressive fall in O_2CI, it can be seen that there is a gradual increase of the circulating levels of branch chain amino acids when compared to the posttraumatic cases. While the levels of branched chain amino acids in A state patients appear to be normal, they are more than 2 SD increased when one compares them to the traumatized patients. The septic B state patients represent a 4–5 SD increase compared to the levels seen in nonseptic traumatic injury. There are also significant increases over the trauma patient in the carrier amino acids glycine and alanine, which can serve as gluconeogenic precursors. In common with the increases in the gluconeogenic amino acids, there are progressive rises in pyruvate-lactate and glucose which reflect the increased levels of gluconeogenesis, which appear to be occurring in sepsis (Long et al., 1976). The level of urea precursors, glutamate, proline, ornithine, and arginine also rise progressively as the septic patient deteriorates. These increases are accompanied by increases in circulating levels of urea in patients in whom adequate renal function is maintained. This suggests a marked increase in net urea synthesis, probably from the amino acid ammonia moiety resulting from the increased peripheral tissue production and hepatic utilization of muscle released amino acids, especially alanine (Felig, 1975; Cerra et al., 1979b).

In the area of fat metabolism, there is evidence of increased lipolysis with a progressive rise in triglycerides, even though free fatty acids levels and glycerol levels remain normal or slightly decreased. This suggests that free fatty acids can be taken up and metabolized to some degree in sepsis, and glycerol has been shown to represent an important gluconeogenic precursor in this condition (Long et al., 1976). However, there is evidence of alteration in the redox state of the septic patient since there are progressive rises in β-hydroxybutyrate (BOHB) as the septic conditions worsen from A to B with a maintenance of relatively normal or decreased levels of AcAc so that the BOHB/AcAc ratio progressively rises. The most significant difference between nonseptic traumatized patients and the progressively worsening septic condition lies in the marked increase in glucagon, which rises from approximately 10 SD in the septic A state to more than 20 SD above control in the septic B state. This is also accompanied by increases in insulin, but the glucagon/insulin ratio is progressively increased as the septic deterioration, with a transition from the A to B state (marked by a rising C/B ratio), occurs.

The magnitude of these changes are shown in Figure 17.8 in which the mean values of standard deviational changes seen in Figure 17.7 for circulating amino acids, fat, and glucose precursor levels are shown for the control, nonseptic trauma, and septic A and B state patients. These are arranged in the form of a metabolic map so that the major catabolic interrelationships between the substrates and the level of O_2CI can be demonstrated.

With regard to the specific relationships of interest in the area of gluconeogenic control, the relationship between pyruvate and alanine and pyruvate and lactate are shown in Figure 17.9 for septic versus nonseptic general surgical and trauma patients. As can be seen in this figure, while the levels of lactate and pyruvate are generally higher in the septic patients, especially in the septic B patients or in those septic A patients close to a B state transition, the slope of the relationship between lactate and pyruvate is essentially the same as that seen in the nonseptic patients. This indicates that rather than there being an excess lactate production, the equilibration relationship between lactate and pyruvate remains the same. However, there appear to be increased levels of pyruvate formation in the septic patients when compared to nonseptic trauma patients. One of the reasons for this is suggested by observing the relationship between pyruvate and alanine. Where as in the nonseptic trauma and general surgical patients there is no statistical significant relationship for blood alanine as a precursor of pyruvate, indicating that it may be one of many substrates playing a role in pyruvate synthesis, in the septic patient the change in pyruvate is mainly dependent on the blood concentration level of alanine ($r^2 = 0.749$). In the septic patient, alanine appears to become the major precursor for pyruvate formation and therefore largely determines the pyruvate level. Thus, alanine becomes the major substrate precursor for gluconeogenesis as well as for lactate formation (Long et al., 1976; Siegel et al. 1979a; Kuttner and Spitzer, 1978). It is of great physiologic importance that in spite of the high levels of oxygen delivery, the O_2CI is seen to fall as the A to B state transition occurs. These data suggest that a major impairment may occur in the oxidative utilization of pyruvate with an increased diversion of pyruvate through the Cori cycle to gluconeogenesis (Fig. 17.10), and this may be accelerated by the increased supply of the alanine precursor (Dietze et al., 1976).

METABOLIC FUEL-ENERGY DEFICIT OF SEPSIS

In an attempt to integrate the physiologic and metabolic statistical data (Siegel et al., 1979a), a hypothesis has been developed concerning the nature of the cell and organ metabolic abnormalities which produce the observations seen in the septic patient. It is based on the present observations, the known interrelationships between skeletal muscle and hepatic metabolism (Border et al., 1976; Felig, 1975), and the possible implications of the statistically significant relationships between precursors and by-products of metabolism observed in the septic patient (Siegel et al., 1979a). The hypothesis explaining these interrelationships is shown in Fig. 17.10 for the hyperdynamic B state septic patient.

In this model, the septic process triggers an unknown septic mediator of hormonometabolic effects which stimulates *protein catabolic phenomena* in skeletal muscle as

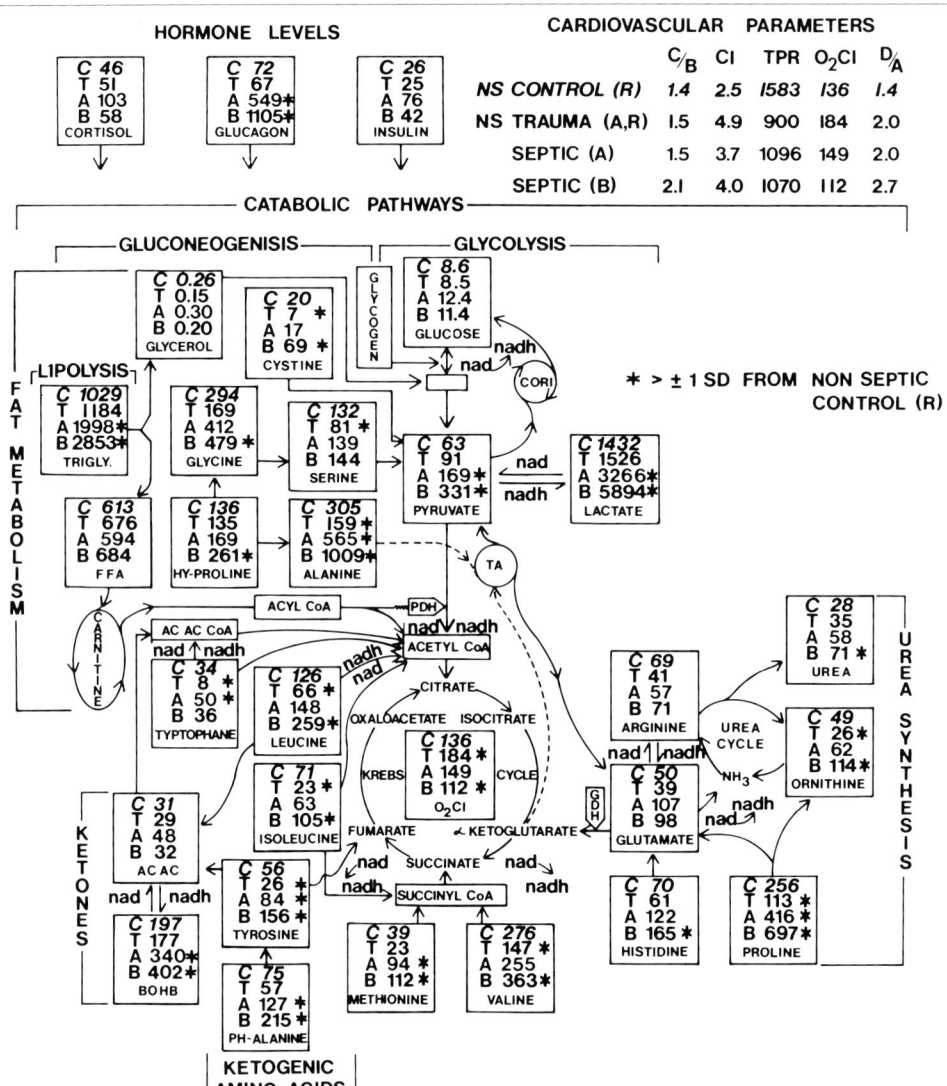

Figure 17.8. Metabolic map of known catabolic pathways in liver for amino acids, fat metabolites, glucose precursors, and precursors of urea synthesis. Values indicate means of physiologic study groups. *C*, nonseptic control general surgical patients in R state; *T*, nonseptic traumatized patients in A or R state; *A*, septic A state patients; *B*, septic B state patients. Cardiovascular parameters for these groups are shown in the right upper corner. (Reprinted with permission from J. H. Siegel, F. B. Cerra, B. Coleman, I. Giovannini, M. Shetye, J. R. Border, and R. H. McMenamy: *Surgery 86*:163, 1979.)

well as the related release of catabolic hormones such as glucagon, corticosteroids, and catecholamines (Wilmore et al., 1973). The exact nature of this septic mediator is unknown but may be related to the immunologic host response to bacterial invasion which occurs through a complement cascade with the formation of various kinins (Schumer et al., 1974). It is possible that the increased levels of kinins may be the initiating stimulus. For example, bradykinin has been shown experimentally to alter the permeability of muscle to glucose entry at high concentrations (Rita McConn, personal communication, 1979) perhaps accounting for an effective insulin resistance. It has also been found to decrease limb oxygen extraction at controlled blood flow (Siegel et al., 1971).

While this septic initiating mechanism is speculation, the net effect is to stimulate a marked protein catabolism in which all of the sequence of amino acids contained in various muscle proteins are broken down. Consequently, branched chain amino acids, proline and other ureagenic and aromatic and sulfur-containing amino acids are all released in concentrations proportionate to their concentration in the muscle proteins (Marchuk et al., 1977; O'Donnell et al., 1976). However, the *muscle* itself is only able to utilize the branched chain amino acids effectively as metabolic substrates (Freund et al., 1978). These branched chain amino acids (BCAA), leucine, isoleucine, and valine, are converted to their respective ketoacids which then can enter the Krebs tricarboxylic acid (TCA)

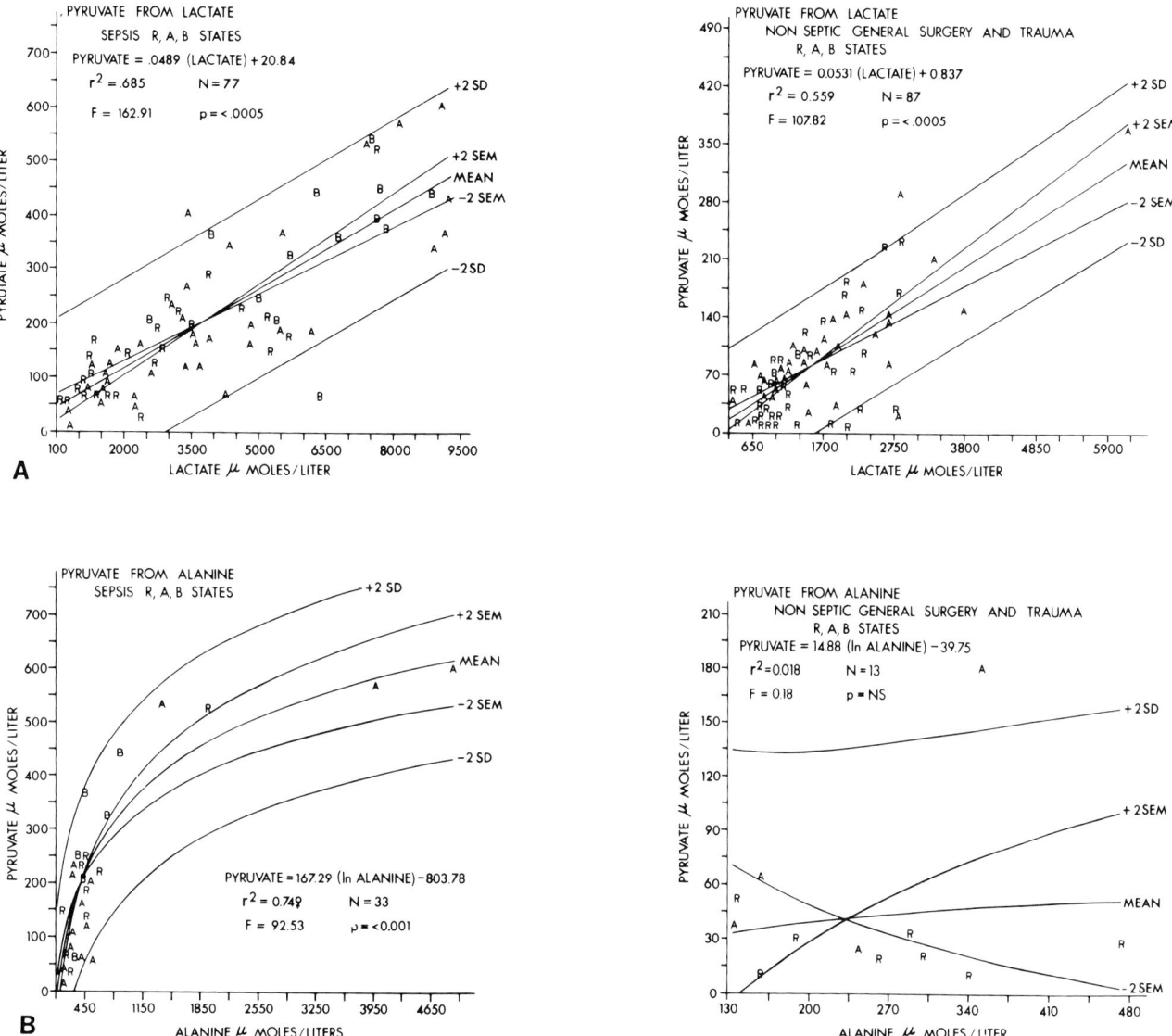

Figure 17.9. A, relationship between pyruvate and lactate concentration in blood for septic and nonseptic general surgical and trauma patients. Labeled by physiological state classifications. B, relationship between pyruvate concentration and alanine concentration in blood for septic and nonseptic general surgical and trauma patients labeled by physiologic state. (Reprinted with permission from J. H. Siegel, F. B. Cerra, B. Coleman, I. Giovannini, M. Shetye, J. R. Border, and R. H. McMenamy: 86:163, 1979.)

cycle for oxidative metabolism. The ammonia nitrogen (NH_3^+) liberated by this process is combined with pyruvate developed from muscle glycogen, or exogenous glucose, via glucose-6 phosphate, to form the carrier amino acids alanine and glycine (Felig, 1975). These carrier amino acids, and especially alanine, which is produced in large quantity in the septic process, are transported through the blood to liver and kidney.

In these visceral organs, alanine is reconverted to pyruvate through a mechanism of transamination where alanine plus α-ketoglutarate yields pyruvate and glutamate (Krebs et al., 1976). Under ordinary circumstances in the nonseptic patient, the major fraction of the pyruvate so produced would then be metabolized oxidatively through acetyl-CoA to the TCA cycle generating ATP as a by-product of the election transport, yielding oxygen consumption and carbon dioxide production. However, in the septic patient, and especially in the B state septic patient, there appears to be an increased *hepatic* diversion of pyruvate to gluconeogenic pathways via the Cori cycle, with increased formation of glucose-6 phosphate and a higher level of equilibration with lactate. In the liver, a significant portion of the glucose-6 phosphate appears to be hydrolyzed, producing a glucose which is emptied into the blood stream and transported to the visceral organs including skeletal muscle and brain (Long et al., 1976). Thus, increased gluconeogenesis may account for the *hyperglycemia* of the septic process.

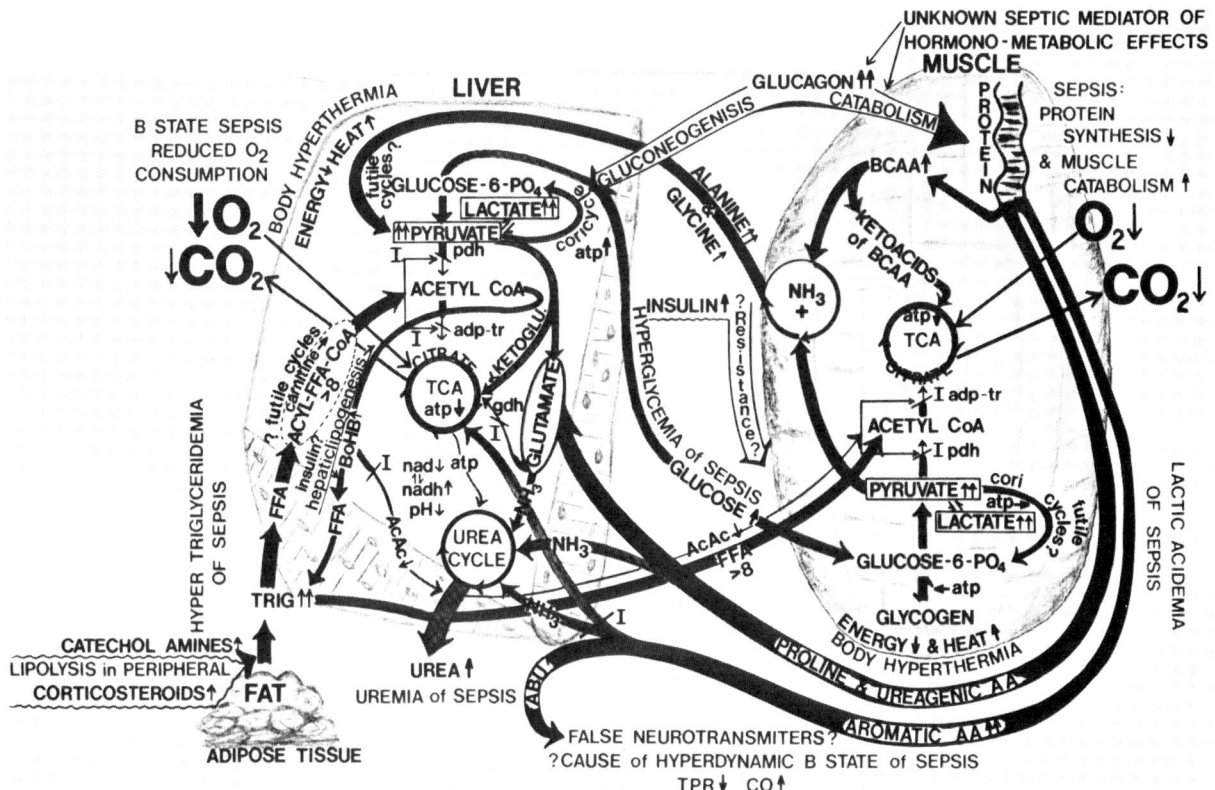

Figure 17.10. Schematic diagram of metabolic fuel-energy deficit in hyperdynamic B state sepsis.

Under conditions of nonseptic stress adaption, the other amino acids liberated by protein catabolism, such as proline and the other ureagenic amino acids, the aromatic amino acids, and sulphur-containing amino acids are also transported through the blood stream from muscle to liver and kidney where oxidative catabolism of the carbon skeleton occurs and the amino acid nitrogen residue is disposed of by urea synthesis (Krebs et al., 1976). However, in the severely ill B state septic patient, there appears to be impairment in some of these mechanisms. Thus, in the case of the proline and related amino acids (Fig. 17.10) (which enter into urea synthesis and oxidative metabolism through the medium of glutamate), while there appears to be an increased urea synthesis through the ornithine, arginine, and citruline cycle, there also appears to be some impairment of glutamate entry into oxidative pathways via glutamate dehydrogenase (GDH) so that the concentration of glutamate increases disproportionately at a time when oxygen consumption is falling (Cerra et al., 1980).

With regard to the aromatic amino acids, especially tyrosine, there appears to be some impairment in catabolism with increased levels of incomplete oxidation products, also α-amino butyric acid increases (Cerra et al., 1979b). In preterminal stage B state sepsis, it seems as though the impairment in the metabolism of aromatic amino acids, especially tyrosine, reaches such a degree that the synthesis of catecholamines is impaired and the levels of epinephrine actually decrease in spite of the enormous stress response (F.B. Cerra et al., unpublished observations, 1979). There is some evidence that the abnormal precursors of catecholamine synthesis and other by-products of incomplete aromatic amino acid catabolism may also form *false neurotransmitters* such as octopamine, which has been shown experimentally to produce reductions in vascular pressure/flow relationships (Nespoli et al., unpublished observations, 1979). This may be the mechanism for the reduction in vascular tone which appears to be the primary hemodynamic lesion of the septic process and becomes most severe in the B state of sepsis (Siegel et al., 1967, 1979b). Nevertheless, the incomplete catabolism of these amino acids does result in increased diversion of amino acid ammonia nitrogen to the urea cycle with an increased urea production, and this is the primary factor behind the *uremia* of sepsis.

At the level of the third major organ of substrate fuel production, adipose tissue, the increased glucagon, corticosteroids and catecholamines result in increased peripheral lipolysis with production of the *hypertriglyceridemia* of sepsis. Since, in spite of the increased plasma levels of triglycerides, free fatty acids and glycerol levels appear not to be increased above levels found in the nonseptic traumatized patient, this suggests that triglyceride breakdown into free fatty acids and glycerol is occurring and that these latter substrates are being utilized, at least to some extent. Carpenter et al. (1979) in studying lipids showed that glycerol does serve as a significant gluconeogenic fuel in the septic patient. An additional factor in the septic hypertriglyceridemia appears to be an increase in hepatic lipogenesis (Pace, 1980). This results from a diversion of citrate and acetyl CoA away from oxidative metabolism and ketogenesis into formation of acyl-free fatty acid-CoA complexes in the cytosol. In general, it appears that the longer chain free fatty acids predominate under the circumstances of septic lipogenesis.

It is possible that in this particular manifestation of the septic process lies the underlying modality for pathophysiologic control of oxidative metabolism by distortion of the normal control mechanisms. While other as yet undescribed mechanisms may play an important role in this process, the known inhibitory and stimulatory actions of long chain free fatty acids (Shrago et al., 1976) through the medium of acyl-free fatty acid-CoA esters, in the presence of the increased levels of alanine and pyruvate and with the gluconeogenic facilitating capability of the elevated circulating glucagon (Chiasson et al., 1974; Wise et al., 1972) could explain much of what is seen in the B state septic process. It is known that long chain acyl-free fatty acid-CoA esters inhibit pyruvate entry into the Krebs cycle by reducing the activity of pyruvate dehydrogenase (PDH) (Shrago et al., 1976). At the same time these esters stimulate pyruvate carboxylase activity (Barritt et al., 1976), the first step in the Cori cycle. Once this enzyme is stimulated, the conversion of pyruvate to glucose through the gluconeogenic pathways becomes dependent on the concentration of pyruvate, which is increased in sepsis. It is of interest in this regard that glucagon has also been shown to enhance gluconeogenesis from alanine (Chiasson et al., 1974; Wise et al., 1972) by stimulating the conversion of pyruvate and oxaloacetate to phosphoenolpyruvate (Tilghman et al., 1976), the second key step in the Cori cycle synthesis of glucose from pyruvate. In addition, the long-chain acyl-free fatty acid-CoA esters have been shown to inhibit adenine nucleotide translocase from the mitochondria, which serves as a regulator for the conversion of acetyl-CoA into acetoacetate, reduced to BOHB, rather than into citrate formation (Shrago et al., 1976). This effect would be constant with the observation that BOHB levels rise in sepsis and become higher as the transition from the septic A to septic B state occurs.

These long chain acyl-free fatty acid-CoA esters also have been implicated in inhibiting the Malate-Aspartate shuttle and the related transport of hydrogen ions across the mitochondrial membrane, which would produce a decrease in the mitochondrial redox potential (Shrago et al., 1976). Also, the increased level of lactate in the presence of lactate dehydrogenase may influence hydrogen ion availability in the cytoplasmic portion of the cell (Williamson et al., 1976). The net result of this would be to produce intracellular and intramitochondrial acidosis and a tendency to saturate the nicotinamide adenine dinucleotide hydrogen acceptor, so that NADH rather than NAD would occur in preponderance (Williamson, 1976). This lack of a hydrogen acceptor in the presence of a reduced redox potential may be responsible for the lack of oxidation of BOHB to AcAc, which is seen in the septic process, and may account for the rising BOHB/AcAc ratio. In addition, since a large number of the critical enzymes in amino acid catabolism are NAD $\rightleftarrows$ NADH or NADP $\rightleftarrows$ NADPH dependent, especially GDH as well as some of the critical enzyme systems for the utilization of leucine, isoleucine, valine, and tryptophane, this may well account for the generalized impairment in amino acid metabolism which occurs late in the B state septic process, where all amino acid levels including branched chain amino acid levels rise as a preterminal event (Cerra et al., 1979a). The net result of all these factors would be to reduce the amount of substrate which enters the TCA cycle. This would be expected to produce a fall in oxygen consumption and CO_2 production, and these seem to occur as the A to B state septic transition develops.

An additional critical consideration in the septic process is the fact that at a time when oxidative metabolism and, therefore, ATP synthesis are declining, two processes which are extremely competitive for ATP, namely urea synthesis and gluconeogenesis (Krebs et al., 1976), are increasing. At the reduced level of oxygen consumption, which occurs in the septic B state patient, it is possible that a major fraction of the already diminished ATP produced is being diverted into these two synthetic cycles, rather than supporting other catabolic metabolic pathways and protein synthesis which are also energy-dependent. Indeed, the synthesis of acute phase proteins and immunologic proteins has been demonstrated to decrease, and skin test hypersensitivity is reduced even to the point of complete anergy in B state sepsis.

Another possible consequence of the increased gluconeogenesis, at a time when pyruvate access to oxidative metabolism through acetyl-CoA is inhibited, is the production of a *futile cycle* in which pyruvate is synthesized to fructose-6 phosphate through the gluconeogenic pathway and then returned by glycolysis to pyruvate without oxidation (Söling and Kleineke, 1976). This process, which is extremely wasteful of ATP, produces increased heat and net reduction in energy and may be related to the *body hyperthermia*, which is characteristically seen in sepsis. Another septic futile cycle may occur from the diversion of acetyl-CoA away from ketogenesis and citrate from oxidation into condensation with malonyl-CoA and FFA formation (Pace, 1980). This is ATP using, and also results in increased *hepatic lipogenesis* with a net diversion of acetyl CoA into resynthesis of free fatty acids and triglycerides rather than fat oxidation. This may account for the histologic fatty degeneration seen in the livers of nonsurviving patients with severe sepsis. This concept is also supported by clinical observations that when death occurs in the B state septic patient, there is evidence of marked muscle catabolism with wasting of all skeletal muscle, at a time when peripheral adipose tissue fat deposits remain prominent, and marked hepatic fat deposition occurs.

QUESTIONS FOR THE FUTURE

The critical questions raised by this hypothesis of septic deterioration are related to the proof by biochemical tracer studies of the interacting mechanisms for this pathophysiologic metabolism and its physiologic correlates. This hypothesis also raises questions of how to maximize utilization of alternative fuels which may bypass the critical blocks in oxidative metabolism so as to restore to normal the energetic generation of ATP. At the peripheral locus, if these blocks to the effective oxidative metabolism of glucose and fatty acids are the critical factors in stimulating skeletal muscle protein catabolism and increased muscle utilization of branched chain amino acids, possibly this muscle catabolic process, which also seems to be the major factor in the increase of gluconeogenic substrates, could be reduced.

At the hepatic level, the question as to why fat sources, especially long chain fatty acids, cannot be utilized effectively in severe sepsis in the face of a pathologic hypertriglyceridemia, thus denying the availability of the major energetic fuel as a source for oxidative metabolism, remains to be elucidated. However, it is possible that a level of effective intracellular energetics and ATP synthens can be achieved by the use of simple alternative fuels. If so, some of the metabolic blocks to hepatic fat oxidation may be overcome, allowing a more effective utilization of circulating free fatty acids and triglycerides. If this hypothesis is correct, an alternative simple fuel would be expected to prevent the hepatic fat deposition and to produce sufficient energy to permit the complete utilization of the ureagenic and aromatic amino acids.

It seems likely that the false neurotransmitters, which can be the by-product of incomplete aromatic amino acid metabolism, may be the major pathophysiologic factors causing the abnormal vascular tone and the reflex mediated hyperdynamic state. Improved utilization of these aromatic amino acids, therefore, may reverse the abnormal physiology, and thus the quantification of the physiologic state would appear to be the best clinical guide to the effective utilization of an alternative fuel and the reversal of this pathologic-metabolic process of metabolic fuel-energy deficit. The investigation of these biochemical regulatory mechanisms and their influence on metabolic energy engendering pathways remain the major objectives of our research investigations.

The concept of organ interaction in the development of the septic syndrome is critical to the understanding of this process. It remains to be demonstrated whether sepsis is always a factor in the development of the multiple organ failure syndrome, discussed in Chapter 18, or whether other types of stimuli can produce this condition. However, this type of septic metabolic failure remains the major cause of death, excluding head injury, in the traumatized patient who survives acute hypovolemia and the acute pulmonary insufficiency of volume replacement therapy long enough to become infected. It is clearly the major cause of death in the severely ill patient who is septic from peritonitis or intraabdominal abscess formation. Unfortunately, no good animal model of the septic metabolic failure syndrome exists, probably because it requires intensive care at a high level in order to prevent death from septic shock or fluid shifts at a much earlier stage in the septic process. Therefore, this process must be studied in humans under conditions of intensive care. The physiologic state classification and its correlation with the underlying metabolic abnormalities still remain the best means of classification of the severity of the septic illness and is the yardstick by which we may gauge the effectiveness of newer metabolic and physiologic therapies.

References

Barritt, J.G., Zander, G.L., and Utter, M.F.: The regulation of pyruvate carboxylase activity in gluconeogenic tissues. In *Gluconeogenesis: Its Regulation in Mammalian Species*, edited by R.W. Hanson and M.A. Mehlman. John Wiley & Sons, New York, 1976.

Border, J.R., Chenier, R., McMenamy, R.H., LaDuca, J., Seibel, R.W., Birkhan, R., and Yu, L.: Multiple systems organ failure: Muscle fuel deficit with visceral protein malnutrition. Surg. Clin. North Am. *56:*1147, 1976.

Carpenter, G.A., Askanazi, J., Elwyn, D.H., and Kinney J.M.: Effects of hypercaloric glucose infusion on lipid metabolism in sepsis. J. Trauma *19:*649, 1979.

Cerra, F.B., Siegel, J.H., Border, J.R., Peters, D.M., and McMenamy, R.H.: The correlation between metabolism and physiology in trauma, general surgery and sepsis. J. Trauma *19:*621, 1979a.

Cerra, F.B., Siegel, J.H., Border, J.R., and McMenamy, R.H.: The hepatic failure of sepsis: Cellular vs. substrate. Surgery *86:*409, 1979b.

Cerra, F.B., Caprioli, J., Siegel, J.H., Border, J.R., and McMenamy, R.H.: Abnormal proline metabolism in human sepsis: evidence of specific metabolic blocks. Ann. Surg., *190:*577, 1980.

Chiasson, J.L., Cook, J., Liljenquist, J.E., and Lacy, W.W.: Glucagon stimulation of gluconeogenesis from alanine in the intact dog. Am. J. Physiol. *227:*19, 1974.

Clowes, G.H.A., Vucinic, M., and Widner, M.G.: Circulatory and metabolic alteration associated with survival or death in peritonitis. Ann. Surg. *16:*866, 1966.

Dietze, G., Wicklmayr, M., and Hepp, K.D.: On gluconeogenesis of human liver. Accelerated hepatic glucose formation induced by increased precursors supply. Diabetologia *12:* 555, 1976.

Farrell, E.J., and Siegel, J.H.: Estimation of blood gas contents from expired air under normal and pathologic conditions. Respir. Physiol. *26:*303, 1976.

Felig, P.: Amino acid metabolism in man. Annu. Rev. Biochem. *44:*933, 1975.

Friedman, H.P., Goldwyn, R.M., and Siegel, J.H.: The use and interpretation of multivariate methods in the classification of stages of serious infectious disease processes in the critically ill. In *Prospectives in Biometrics*, edited by R. Blashoff, p. 81. Academic Press, New York, 1975.

Freund, H.R., Ryan, J.A., Jr., and Fischer, J.E.: Amino acid derangements in patients with sepsis: treatment with branched chain amino acid rich effusions. Ann. Surg. *188:* 423, 1978.

Krebs, H.A., Lund, P., and Stubbs, M.: Interrelations between gluconeogenesis and urea synthesis. In *Gluconeogenesis: Its Regulation in Mammalian Species*, edited by R.W. Hanson and M.A. Mehlman, p. 269. John Wiley & Sons, New York, 1976.

Kuttner, R.E., and Spitzer, J.J.: Gluconeogenesis from alanine in endotoxin treated dogs. J. Surg. Res. *25:*166, 1978.

Long, C.L., Kinney, J.M., and Geiger, J.W.: Nonsuppressibility of gluconeogenesis by glucose in septic patients. Metabolism 25:193, 1976.

MacLean, L.D., Mulligan, W.G., McLean, A.P.H., and Duff, J.M.: Patterns of septic shock in man—a detailed study of 56 patients. Ann. Surg. 166:543, 1967.

Marchuk, J.B., Finley, R.J., Groves, A.C., Wolfe, L.I., Holliday, R.L., and Duff, J.H.: Catabolic hormones and substrate patterns in septic patients. J. Surg. Res. 23:177, 1977.

O'Donnell, T.F., Clowes, G.H.A., Blackburn, G.L., Ryan, N.T., Benotti, P.N., and Miller, J.D.: Proteolysis associated with a deficit of peripheral energy fuel substrate man. Ann. Surg. 80:192, 1976.

Pace, J.G.: Fatty acid metabolism and ketogenesis during a *streptococcus pneumonae* infection in the rat. Dissertation. Graduate School of Arts and Sciences, George Washington University, 1980.

Raza, S.T., Vidne, B.A., Farrell, E.J., Lajos, T.Z., Lee, A.B., Schimert, G., and Siegel, J.H.: Early and longterm effects of direct myocardial revascularization on cardiac function: a prospective study using multivariable physiologic analysis. Ann. Thorac. Surg. 23:99, 1977.

Schumer, W., Erve, P.E., and Miller, B.: Immune response in septic shock. Therapeutic implications. In *Treatment of Shock: Principles and Practice*, edited by L. Nyhus, W. Schumer, p. 141. Lea & Febiger, Philadelphia, 1974.

Shrago, E., Shug, A., and Elson, C.: Regulations of cell metabolism by mitochondrial transport systems. In *Gluconeogenesis: Its Regulation in Mammalian Species*, edited by R.W. Hanson and M.A. Mehlman, p. 221. John Wiley & Sons, New York, 1976.

Siegel, J.H.: Physiologic assessment of cardiac function in the aged and high risk surgical patient. In *The Aged and High Risk Surgical Patient: Medical, Surgical, and Anesthetic Management*, edited by J.H. Siegel and P. Chodoff, p. 23. Grune & Stratton, New York, 1976a.

Siegel, J.H.: Pattern and process in the evolution of and recovery from shock. In *The Aged and High Risk Surgical Patient: Medical, Surgical, and Anesthetic Management*, edited by J.H. Siegel and P. Chodoff, p. 381. Grune & Stratton, New York, 1976b.

Siegel, J.H., Greenspan, M., and DelGuercio, L.R.M.: Abnormal vascular tone, defective oxygen transport and myocardial failure in human septic shock. Ann. Surg. 165:504, 1967.

Siegel, J.H., Goldwyn, R.M., and DelGuercio, L.R.M.: Patterns of cardiovascular response in septic shock. In *Septic Shock in Man*, edited by S.G. Hershey, L.R.M. DelGuercio and R. McConn, p. 173. Little, Brown, Boston, 1971.

Siegel, J.H., Farrell, E.J., and Lewin I.: Quantifying the need for cardiac support in human shock by a functional model of cardiopulmonary vascular dynamics: with special reference to myocardial infarction. J. Surg. Res. 13:166, 1972a.

Siegel, J.H., Farrell, E.J., Goldwyn, R.M., and Friedman, H.P.: The surgical implications of physiologic patterns in myocardial infarction shock. Surgery 72:126, 1972b.

Siegel, J.H., Farrell, E.J., Miller, M., Goldwyn, R.M., and Friedman, H.P.: Cardiorespiratory interactions as determinants of survival and the need for respiratory support in human shock states. J. Trauma 13:602, 1973.

Siegel, J.H., Farrell, E.J., Fichthorn, J., Lajos, T.Z., Lee, A.B., Schimert, G., and Eberhardt, R.C.: The use of multivariable trajectories in identifying normal and abnormal time courses of recovery after coronary bypass surgery. J. Surg. Res. 18:341, 1975.

Siegel, J.H., Cerra, F.B., Coleman, B., Giovannini, I., Shetye, M., Border, J.R., and McMenamy, R.H.: Physiological and metabolic correlations in human sepsis. Surgery 86:163, 1979a.

Siegel, J.H., Cerra, F.B., Peters, D., Moody, E., Brown, D., McMenamy, R.H., and Border, J.R.: The physiologic recovery trajectory as the organizing principle for the quantification of hormonometabolic adaptation to surgical stress and severe sepsis. In *Advances in Shock Research*, edited by W. Schumer, J.J. Spritzer, B.E. Marshal, p. 177. Alan R. Liss, New York, 1979b.

Siegel, J.H., Giovannini, I., and Coleman, B.: Ventilation: perfusion maldistribution secondary to the hyperdynamic cardiovascular state as the major cause of increased pulmonary shunting in human sepsis. J. Trauma. 19:432, 1979c.

Söling, J., and Kleineke, J.: Species dependent regulation of hepatic gluconeogenesis in higher animals. In *Gluconeogenesis: Its Regulation in Mammalian Species*, edited by R.W. Hanson and M.A. Mehlman, p. 449. John Wiley & Sons, New York, 1976.

Tilghman, S.M., Hanson, R.W., and Ballard, F.S.: Hormonal regulation of phosphoenolpyruvate carboxykinase (GTP) in mammalian tissues. In *Gluconeogenesis: Its Regulation in Mammalian Species*, edited by R.W. Hanson and M.A. Mehlman, p. 47. John Wiley & Sons, New York, 1976.

Weil, M.H., Shubin, H., and Biddle, M.: Shock caused by gram-negative microorganisms: Analysis of 169 cases. Ann. Intern. Med. 60:384, 1964.

Williamson, J.R.: Role of anion transport in the regulation of metabolism. In *Gluconeogenesis: Its Regulation in Mammalian Species*, edited by R.W. Hanson and M.A. Mehlman, p. 197. John Wiley & Sons, New York, 1976.

Williamson, J.R., Scheffer, S.W., Ford, C., and Safer, B.: Contribution of tissue acidosis to ischemic injury in the perfused rat heart. Circulation (Suppl. 1) 53:1, 1976.

Wilmore, D.W., Moyland, J.A., Jr., Lundsey, C.A., Falonna, G.R., Unger, R., and Pruitt, B.A., Jr.: Hyperglucagonemia following thermal injury: insulin and glucagon in the postraumatic catabolic state. Surg. Forum 24:97, 1973.

Wilmore, D.W., Mason, A.D., and Pruitt, B.A.: Impaired glucose flow in burned patients with gram-negative sepsis. Surg. Gynecol. Obstet. 143:720, 1976.

Wise, J.K., Hendler, R., and Felig, P.: The glycemic response to alanine: index of glucagon secretion in man. Clin. Res. 20:561, 1972.

Wolfe, R.R., and Burke, J.F.: Effect of glucose infusion on glucose and lactate metabolism in normal and burned guinea pigs. J. Trauma 18:800, 1978.

Wolfe, R.R., Elahi, D., and Spitzer, J.F.: Glucose and lactate kinetics following endotoxin administration in dogs. Am. J. Physiol. 232:E180, 1977.

Woolf, L.I., Groves, A.C., and Duff, J.H.: Amino acid metabolism in dogs with *E. coli* bacteremic shock. Surgery 85:212, 1979.

Wright, C.J., Duff, J.H., McLean, A.P.H., and MacLean, L.D.: Regional capillary blood flow and oxygen uptake in severe sepsis. Surg. Gynecol. Obstet. 132:637, 1971.

CHAPTER 18

Multiple Systems Organ Failure

FRANK B. CERRA
JOHN R. BORDER
RAPIER H. McMENAMY
JOHN H. SIEGEL

CLINICAL SYNDROME

Multiple systems organ failure is a recently recognized clinical syndrome (Border et al., 1976; Eiseman et al., 1977). If myocardial infarction, pulmonary emboli, and irreversible hypovolemia are excluded, multiple systems organ failure is a leading cause of death following traumatic insult. Its recognition is the result of advances in critical care support techniques. With the advent of these techniques of monitoring and a better understanding of cardiopulmonary physiology and its support and manipulation, patients who ordinarily would have expired a few days after a traumatic insult now live for many days to weeks. This phenomenon has resulted in the unmasking of the multiple systems organ failure syndrome.

It is generally agreed that the syndrome is initiated by a severe physiologic insult such as multiple trauma or septicemia with septic shock. The patients are usually easily resuscitated from this insult and then enter into a latent period of "well being." During this interval, the patients seem to be doing well by the usual clinical criteria. After several days, the onset of a cumulative sequence of organ failure occurs. This is usually heralded by the appearance of fever, hypoalbuminemia, and cardiopulmonary failure. The cardiopulmonary failure is initially compensable by exogenous support, e.g., positive pressure ventilation, PEEP, and cardiovascular manipulation by volume loading, inotropic support, or afterload reduction therapy. Hyperbilirubinemia shortly ensues along with an elevation of the other standard clinical tests of liver function (SGOT, SGPT, LDH).

The patient is usually felt to have a source of sepsis and a septic workup ensues. Frequently a septic focus is found and surgical drainage or removal is instituted. In spite of this intervention, the sequence of organ failures continues to progress. Cerebral function deteriorates with the onset of obtundation and coma. Stress ulcers of the gastrointestinal tract with gastrointestinal bleeding are common. The nonhealing of wounds is frequently present as are the development of multiple decubitus ulcers.

Bacteremia eventually appears. Initially it is intermittent and controlled by antibiotics. Eventually the bacteremia becomes persistent in spite of adequate plasma levels of antibiotics to which the cultured organisms are sensitive in vitro. Frequently, polymicrobial bacteremia is present. Anergy to a battery of recall skin test antigens occurs, along with an absolute and relative lymphopenia.

The cardiopulmonary failure worsens and becomes unresponsive to vigorous exogenous support. Large doses of albumin become necessary to maintain an albumin level within the minimal normal range. The hepatic function tests begin to progressively deteriorate; renal insufficiency and eventually frank renal failure become a prominent part of the clinical picture. The terminal event is usually heralded by the onset of a coagulopathy manifested by an elevation of the protime, partial thromboplastin time, and thrombocytopenia. This coagulopathy eventually becomes refractory to exogenous support and death ensues with the onset of hypotension and arrythemia.

Several other clinical observations can be made about the patients who enter into this progressively deteriorating syndrome. Healthy, well nourished patients take longer to die than those who enter it with previously existing malnutrition. Patients with pre-existing liver disease, such as hepatic cirrhosis, have a much shorter time course than those patients who do not have pre-existing liver disease. Exogenous nutritional support with the currently available amino acid formulas seems to prolong the time to death. Progressive muscle wasting occurs with little or no loss in the clinically observed fat mass. At death, the patients have a rather striking reduction of muscle mass; but a preponderance of adipose tissue remains. At postmortem examination, if the patient has been treated properly during his course, no additional abscesses or surgically remediable sepsis is found.

Fever and bacteremia are prominent features of this syndrome and deaths are commonly interpreted as being due to sepsis. Several investigators, however, have noted that approximately one-third of the patients never have bacteremia during the course of their disease under circumstances that are highly suggestive of infection

(Border et al., 1976; Eiseman et al., 1977). Undrained sepsis or surgically remediable sepsis is usually not found at postmortem. The bacteremias in these patients are frequently changing and polymicrobial in nature. As the clinical syndrome evolves and the bacteremia becomes apparent, the onset of anergy to recall skin test antigens together with an absolute and a relative lymphopenia becomes evident.

Causes of fever other than sepsis are present. There are usually multiple sites of phagocytotic stimulation such as wounds, hematomas, or crushed deep muscle or fat. This phagocytic stimulation can cause the release of endogenous pyrogen. Acting through prostaglandin stimulation of hypothalamus, the endogenous pyrogen could easily account for the fever (Beisel and Wannemacher, 1977). Gastrointestinal ulcerations, only a portion of which bleed, could also provide access portals to the blood stream and may therefore result in bacteremia, which is a consequence of the multiple systems organ failure and not a cause of it. The bacteriologic problem is further compounded by the difficulty of cultural identification of anaerobes.

The question then of the association between the systemic septic response and multiple organ failure syndrome, therefore, is presently unanswered. It seems reasonable to say at this point that multiple systems organ failure is frequently associated with clinical settings highly suggestive of sepsis. Whether or not it is always associated with sepsis and whether or not sepsis is a cause or an effect, however, is presently unanswerable.

PHYSIOLOGIC TIME COURSE

The physiologic response to multiple systems organ failure syndrome is somewhat heterogeneous in nature. For this reason, a system must be devised such that one can precisely define where a patient is in the time course of this physiologic response. A detailed discussion of this physiologic assessment and state classification system is presented elsewhere. A brief review is presented here for purposes of continuity in discussing the metabolism and metabolic-physiologic correlations in the multiple systems organ failure syndrome.

The physiologic staging is derived from the indocyanine green indicator dilution curve together with an arteriovenous oxygen saturation difference. (A-VO_2). The variables determined are cardiac output (CO), cardiac index (CI), pulmonary dispersive volume (dv) (a reflection of pulmonary blood volume), cardiac mixing time (tm) (an indication of myocardial contractility), systolic ejection time, right atrial pressure (RAP), total peripheral resistance (TPR), arterial and central venous blood gases, A-VO_2, and oxygen consumption index (O_2CI). The oxygen consumption index is calculated as a product of cardiac index and A-VO_2.

The primary variables are then analyzed according to the method of Siegel (1976; Siegel et al., 1979b) and a physiologic response state determined. In this state classification system, the data is compared to a previously studied group of nonstressed elective preoperative general surgery patients who serve as the reference (R) or control state. Each datum is then normalized by the standard deviation of that variable to this reference control value. In this way, the statistical deviation from the reference control state can be determined in standard deviational units.

By clustering techniques, the data from critically ill patients with a variety of pathologies have resulted in a description of four prototype stress response states (A, B, C, D; Fig. 18.1). The *A* state represents the normal balanced stress response state seen in such situations as compensated sepsis and after a significant insult such as major elective general surgery or trauma. The A state is characterized by a balanced physiologic response consisting of an increased cardiac output and heart rate, a decrease in contractility and mean pulmonary transit time, and a decrease in cardiac ejection time. The vascular tone remains balanced and the A-VO_2 is unchanged or slightly increased. Oxygen consumption is therefore generally increased. The D state represents the opposite extreme of the physiologic spectrum and results in the classic prototypic cardiogenic state consisting of a low cardiac output, high peripheral resistance, wide A-VO_2 difference, and reduced oxygen consumption on a perfusional basis, in the presence of a reduced myocardial contractility.

The B state, however, represents a state of unbalanced vascular tone characterized by a marked elevation of cardiac output with a reduction in total peripheral resistance that is disproportionate to this increase in flow and in the narrowing of the A-VO_2. The result is an absolute reduction in oxygen consumption. As will be seen when the metabolic data are discussed, this does not seem to be on the basis of perfusion-related phenomena. Metabolic acidosis commonly occurs at this point. This state is characteristic of patients with decompensating organ failures. It is associated with increased morbidity and mortality if the metabolic derangement cannot be corrected. The C state represents a continued deterioration of the organ failure syndrome in which the cardiopulmonary failure is no longer responsive to exogenous support and becomes superimposed upon the unbalanced B state, producing a combined metabolic and severe respiratory acidosis. Death inevitably ensues.

Following a physiologic intervention, the data are statistically compared to the five prototypic states and the patient's similarity and dissimilarity to each prototypic state determined in terms of his Euclidian distance from each of these states. Consequently, the existing physiologic state of the patient can be precisely defined and categorized as the state to which the patient has the most resemblance (the closest distance). By taking the ratio of the distance of the patient to the D state relative to the A state, the D/A ratio, a measure of cardiovascular adequacy, is determined. Likewise, the relationship between the B state of metabolic insufficiency and the C state of respiratory insufficiency can be represented in the C/B ratio and provides an indication of the patient's balance of metabolic and respiratory function. Thus, the data can be reduced to state distances and ratio. By

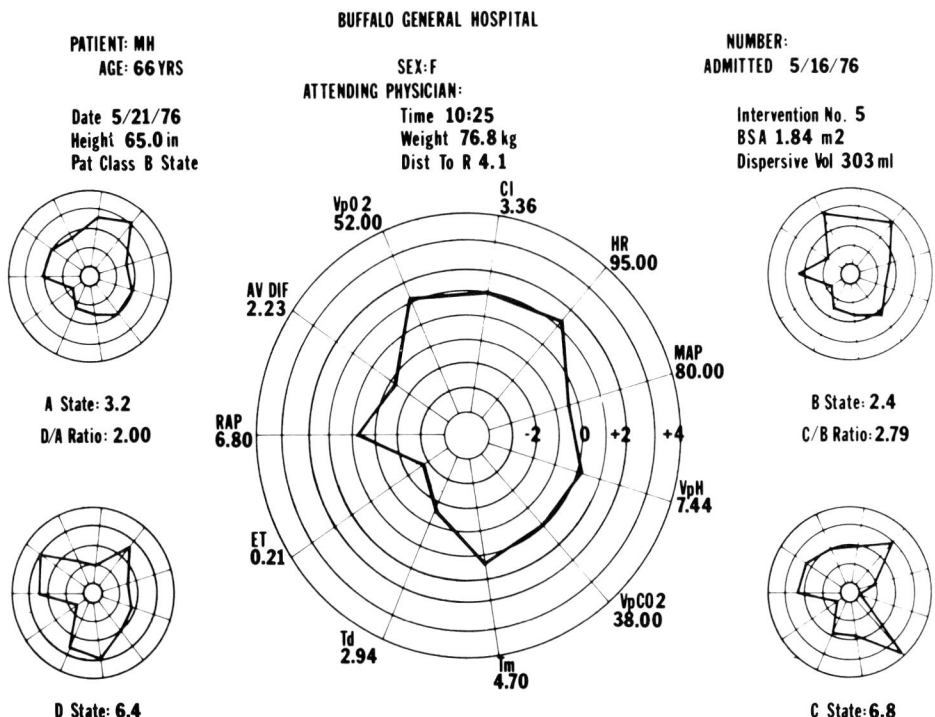

Figure 18.1. Computer printout of a patient's state classification following a physiologic intervention. The standard deviation differences for each variable, along with the absolute values and state distances are illustrated.

plotting the D/A and C/B ratios from multiple interventions relative to one another, it is then possible to plot the patient's trajectory over the time course of his disease. Furthermore, within a given pathologic state, the time course of the patient's physiologic response can be precisely and statistically quantified and compared to known response trajectories from other pathologies (Fig. 18.2).

A given patient with multiple systems organ failure may present in any one of the five prototype states discussed. Over the course of the disease, the patient moves in time from one state to another as the organ failures progress. At some point in this process, myocardial depression occurs and the cardiogenic state becomes superimposed on the other states that the patient was previously in. In patients with pre-existing myocardial disease, this cardiogenic response may be the initial presentation. A patient presenting in an A state can move into a B state when the severity of the metabolic defect becomes severe enough.

In patients without prior cardiopulmonary disease, the recovery from the severe physiologic insult is generally heralded by the onset of the physiologic A state. The cardiac index is increased; the vascular tone remains balanced; peripheral oxygen extraction as manifested in the A-VO$_2$ is normal or high normal; and oxygen consumption index is generally increased. As the organ failures unfold, the patients generally move into the unbalanced B state that is heralded by the onset of the vascular tone abnormality, whereby the peripheral resistance is inappropriately low for the level of cardiac output. The mass flow of oxygen to the periphery is markedly increased, as evidenced by the product of the oxygen content and the cardiac index. Peripheral extraction, as reflected in the A-VO$_2$ difference, progressively falls such that there is a progressive fall in oxygen consumption. This physiologic complex was previously interpreted as indicative of physiologic shunting being present in the periphery. Because of further work on the peripheral flow distribution and the metabolic data that is to be presented, the presence of shunts seems to be only a small component of this phenomena (Cerra et al., 1979a and c; Finley et al., 1975). As will be seen, the major reason for the fall in oxygen consumption seems to be one of nonutilization rather than of delivery to the periphery. As the organ system failure progresses and cardiopulmonary failure ensues, it is no longer compensable by exogenous support; the patient generally moves into a cardiogenic or D state. Even though this is physiologically a low output, high resistance, increased extraction with low oxygen consumption, the metabolic profile remains that of the septic patient. Frequently the patient will proceed directly to the C state with combined acidosis and expire.

The pulmonary failures observed in patients with multiple systems organ failure fall into three basic categories. The first type of pulmonary failure is that which is characterized by hypoxemia, with a widening of an A-a gradient, together with pulmonary hypertension and a normal appearing chest x-ray. This type of pulmonary

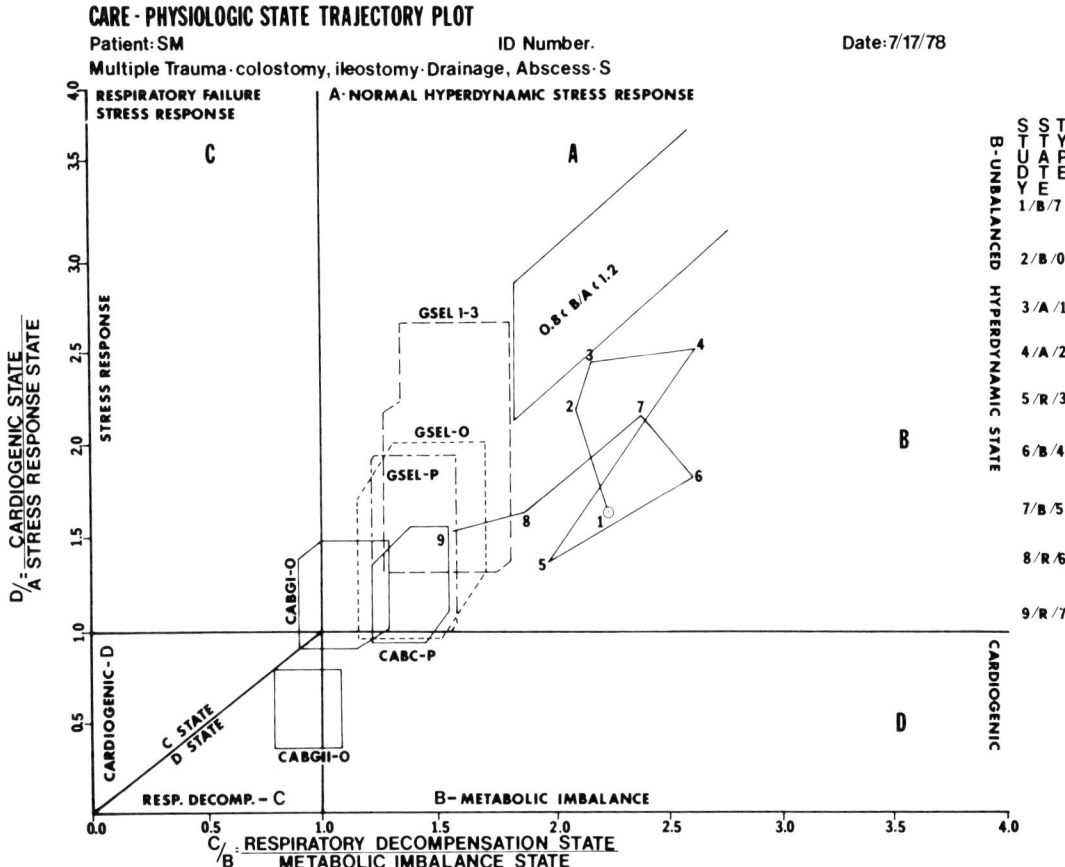

Figure 18.2. Computer printout of a time course trajectory plot of seven daily physiologic interventions in a patient with sepsis and multiple systems organ failure. The reference trajectories for clean general and cardiac surgery serve as a reference for known, normal trajectories. The changing nature of the physiologic response is evident.

failure occurs with the onset of the vascular tone abnormality in multiple system organ failure patients. Work by Siegel et al. (1979a) have indicated that this kind of pulmonary failure is a manifestation of the vascular tone abnormality with the production of a rather large absolute shunt in the pulmonary circuit. This Q_S/Q_T abnormality accounts for the phenomena observed in this type of pulmonary failure.

The second type of pulmonary failure falls in the category of adult respiratory distress syndrome. It is heralded by the onset of a widening A-a gradient together with hypocarbia and hyperventilation in the non-mechanically ventilated patient. In the mechanically ventilated patient, it generally becomes manifest by the onset of an x-ray picture characterized by diffuse interstitial-alveolar infiltrations. Multiple studies with pulmonary artery flotation catheters have indicated that this phenomenon is associated with a marked increase in lung water that is noncardiac in etiology (Chs. 25 and 26). It is frequently associated with hypoalbuminemia systemically. Physiologically, the patients are usually in the unbalanced vascular tone B state. An increased capillary permeability with the presence of perivascular and peribronchiolar edema seems to be a prominent feature (Ch. 25). A significant percentage of these patients go on to pulmonary fibrosis. Recent work by Mittermayer et al. (Ch. 25) has indicated that this pulmonary fibrosis is in response to a factor that is present in the interstitial edema. The etiology of the onset of this respiratory distress syndrome is unknown. Many investigators have indicated a correlation with the activation of complement, prostaglandin formation, and intravascular coagulation systems (Chs. 12 and 26).

The third type of pulmonary failure that occurs is the onset of parenchymatous pneumonias. These are usually multilobed and gram-negative in bacteriology and are often refractory to treatment with the usual combinations of antibiotics.

METABOLIC TIME COURSE

Studies of the metabolism of multiple systems organ failure syndrome have mainly involved sampling of plasma substrate concentrations over time. In addition to the endogenous factors that effect the plasma substrate levels, two major exogenous factors are present. One is the type of nutritional support that the patient is on and the other is the reference standard to which the plasma levels of metabolic substrate are compared. The influence of exogenous nutritonal support is significant and will be discussed in greater detail subsequently. The plasma levels of metabolic substrate in patients with multiple systems organ failure are much different from those observed in overnight fasting man and in trauma hypermetabolic man (Cerra et al., 1979a and b; Clowes et al., 1976) (Figs. 18.3 and 18.4). The patterns of the metabolic substrate changes in multiple systems organ failure patients will therefore vary, depending upon which of these two standards are used as a reference. The reference will be carefully emphasized in the ensuing discussion.

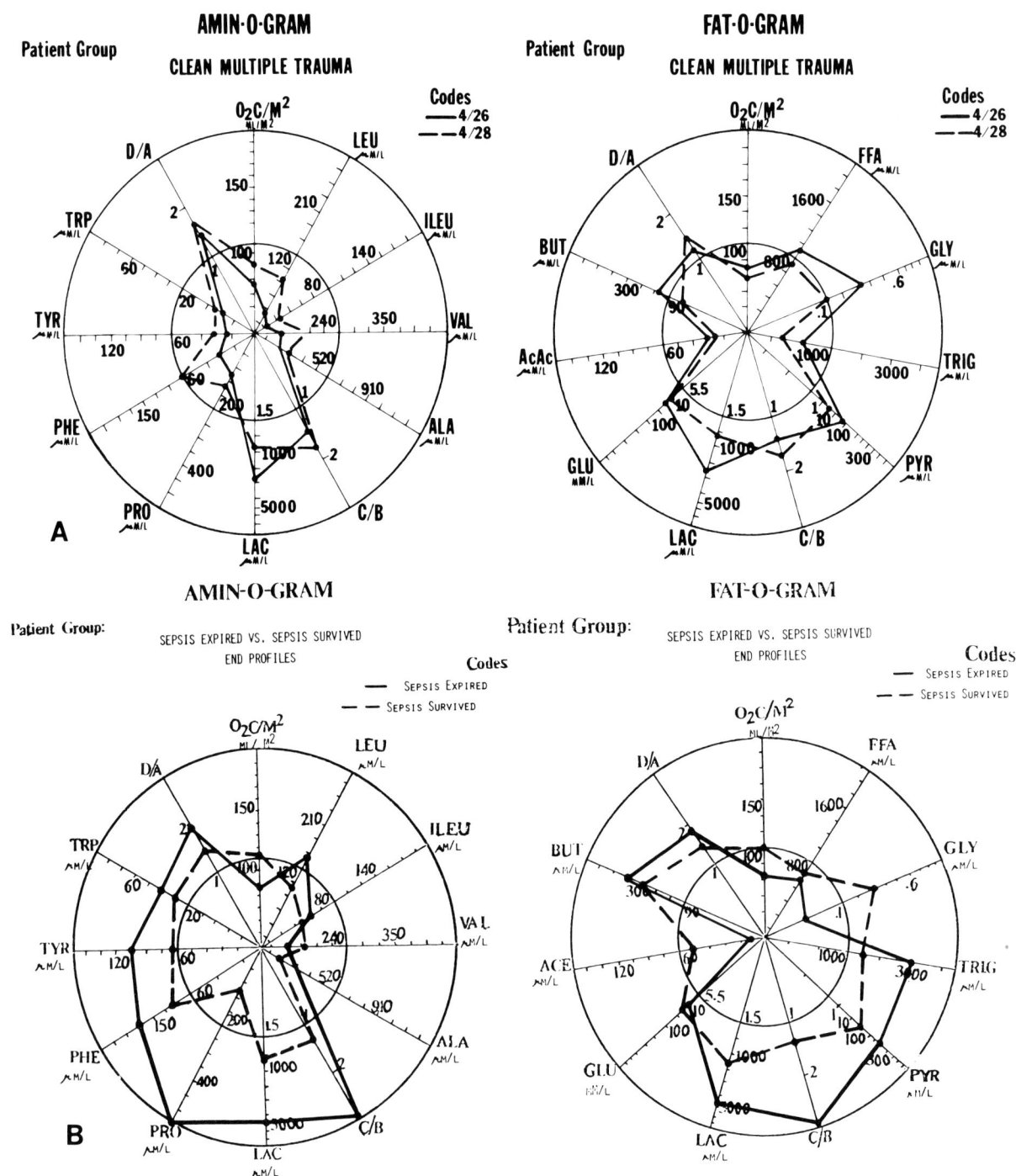

Figure 18.3. Physiologic-metabolic profile patterns of clean, hypermetabolic polytrauma (A) and sepsis multiple organ failure patients (B). The inner circle is the reference values for overnight fasting man. The altered values for each variable relative to this reference standard are apparent.

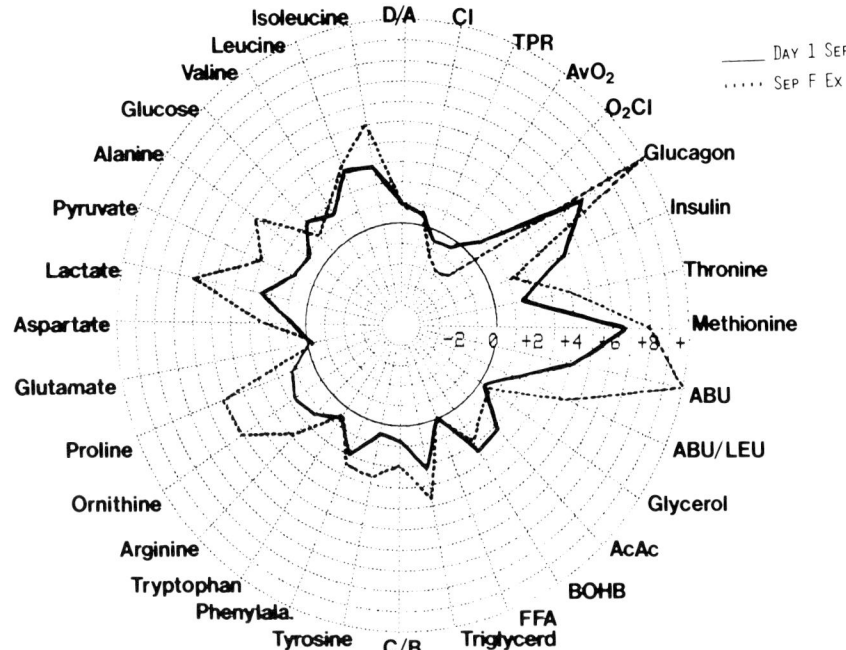

Figure 18.4. Hormonometabolic-physiologic statistical profile plot of patients with sepsis and multiple organ failure early in their time course and within 3 days of death. The dark inner circle is the reference of nonseptic, trauma-hypermetabolic man at the same point in time. Each of the *dotted circles* represents one standard deviational difference from the reference mean. When considered with Fig. 18.3, the importance of stating the reference standard when discussing plasma levels is emphasized. (Reprinted with permission from F. B. Cerra, J. H. Siegel, J. R. Border, et al.: Surgery 86:409, 1979b.)

The metabolic profile patterns to be described are from patients who were supported nutritionally on a commercial amino acid mix (Aminosyn), given with glucose in a ratio of 100 glucose calories per gram of administered protein nitrogen. The protein was administered at a rate of 1 g/kg/24 hr by constant infusion.

Regardless of the reference standard used, the first feature of multiple systems organ failure is the onset of hyperglycemia. This hyperglycemia is in the range of 250–300 mg/100 ml. It has two additional characteristics: it is refractory to the administration of exogenous insulin, and it is sensitive to the administration of exogenous glucose. If higher concentrations of glucose are administered, a hyperosmolar state with very high blood glucose levels ensues. To attempt to control the hyperglycemia with exogenous insulin results in the use of very high quantities of regular insulin, sometimes up to 40 units of regular insulin per hour by continuous infusion. Even with these doses, it is difficult to maintain the blood sugar below the 200 mg/100 ml range. This hyperglycemia is associated in time with elevations of lactate, pyruvate, and alanine. As the multiple systems organ failure syndrome progresses, the lactate, pyruvate, and alanine rise proportionately in a constant relationship with one another. For a given level of lactate, there is a predictable level of pyruvate and alanine. The lactate-pyruvate relationship is also of considerable interest. The initial lactate/pyruvate ratio is normal. As the syndrome progresses, the lactate and pyruvate rise proportionately but the lactate/pyruvate ratio remains constant (Cerra et al., 1979a and c) (Fig. 18.4). Subsequent studies by Kinney et al. have recently shown that this constancy of the lactate/pyruvate ratio, in spite of rising concentrations of both lactate and pyruvate, is also present on intracellular muscle measurements (Liaw et al., 1980). To state it another way, there is no excess of lactate production relative to pyruvate. This observation provides strong supporting evidence that the syndrome does not seem to be resulting from a perfusion related deficit, at least in a total body sense.

Irrespective of the reference chosen, the abnormalities in fat metabolism are significant (Cerra et al., 1979a and b; Wannemacher et al., 1978) (Fig. 18.4). With the onset of multiple systems organ failure syndrome, hypertriglyceridemia becomes a very prominent feature; the triglyceride level progressively rises as the organ degeneration proceeds towards death. Frequently the serum is hyperlipemic. In addition, if exogenous triglyceride loading is done, a markedly prolonged clearance time of the administered triglyceride is noted. The free fatty acid levels are inappropriately high for the level of glucose. Initially there are large amounts of circulating ketone bodies. The β-hydroxybutyrate is initially increased regardless of the reference standard. Relative to trauma-hypermetabolic man, the acetoacetate levels in multiple systems organ failure syndrome are increased (Fig. 18.4). As these organ failures proceed toward death, the acetoacetate level progressively falls while there is a rise in β-hydroxybutyrate level. The β-hydroxybutyrate/acetoacetate ratio, therefore, progressively increases towards death. If measurements on the day of death are reviewed, however, the acetoacetate level is barely detectable and the β-hydroxybutyrate level has fallen precipitously (Fig. 18.5). Glycerol levels are elevated regardless of the reference source and progressively rise as death approaches.

The branched chain amino acid levels are of considerable interest. With the onset of the multiple systems organ failure syndrome, the levels of leucine, isoleucine, and valine are reduced relative to overnight fasting man (Cerra et al., 1979a) (Fig. 18.3). Relative to trauma-hypermetabolic man, at the same point in time as in multiple systems organ failure patients, the levels of the

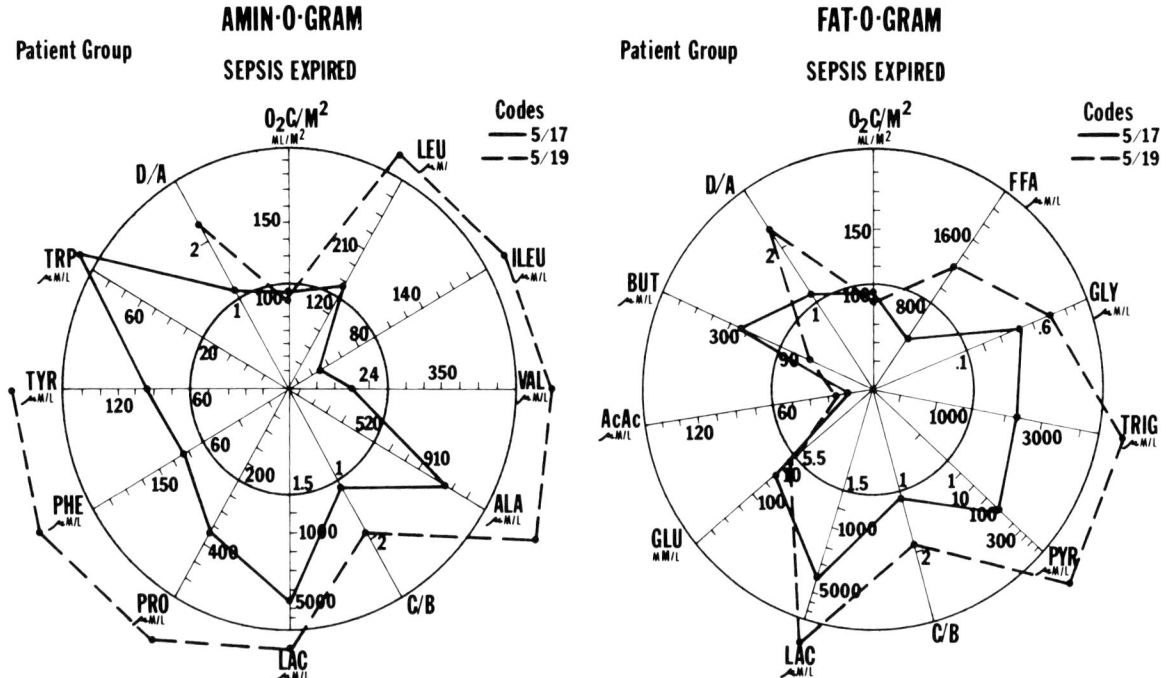

Figure 18.5. Physiologic-metabolic profile illustrating the terminal "blow-out" pattern of substrate levels on the day of death. All substrate levels rise except ketone bodies and glucose. The B state physiologic transition has occurred. The reference inner circle is overnight fasting man.

branch chain amino acids are significantly increased (Cerra et al., 1979b) (Fig. 18.4). The influence of the reference standard therefore becomes quite apparent, and precise definition must be given. As the organ failure syndrome evolves, the branched chain amino acids eventually begin to rise, and when they are seen on the day of death, the leucine, isoleucine, and valine levels are extremely high (Fig. 18.5). In detailed studies of the splanchnic clearance of the amino acids, the hepatic clearance of the branched chain amino acids is reduced (McMenamy et al., 1981). The aromatic amino acids phenylalanine, tyrosine, and tryptophane are elevated in the plasma regardless of the reference standard. These amino acids continue to rise in concentration as the organ failure progresses. This is happening at a time when the splanchnic clearance of these amino acids is increasing (McMenamy et al., 1981).

Amino acids threonine and methionine, as well as aminobutyric acid (ABU), begin to rise with the onset of multiple systems organ failure (Fig. 18.4). As the organ failure progresses, the levels of these three substances continue to rise. The ABU/leucine ratio likewise rises with the ABU rising in excess of leucine. The levels of aspartate, glutamate, proline, ornithine, arginine, and ammonia are also elevated early in the organ failure process and progressively rise as death approaches. Correlated with a rise in these amino acids is a progressive increase in urea excretion in the urine.

The onset of multiple systems organ failure, therefore, is associated with abnormalities in the plasma substrate levels of glucose, fat, and amino acids. In the few patients who survive this syndrome, the plasma substrate levels eventually go back toward that for overnight fasting man (Fig. 18.6). Most of the patients, however, expire. As has been stated, as death approaches the levels of all plasma, substrates tend to rise such that on the day of death, most plasma substrate levels are at very high levels. The exceptions are ketone bodies and glucose, which tend to fall and reach very low plasma levels on the day of death (Fig: 18.5).

This plasma substrate profile is markedly different from that as seen in overnight fasting man or in trauma-hypermetabolic man. It is also markedly different from that which is seen in patients with hepatic cirrhosis who are encephalopathic and either survive or expire (Job et al., 1966). The patients with hepatic cirrhosis do have the abnormalities in amino acid metabolism which are similar to those seen in organ failure syndrome patients. They do not, however, have the abnormalities of glucose, lactate, pyruvate, and fat metabolism that are present in organ failure syndrome patients (Cerra et al., 1979b; Fischer et al., 1974) (Fig. 18.7). When the cirrhotic patient becomes septic, however, he develops a profile pattern which is very similar to those patients with multiple organ failure syndrome and which follows a much more rapid course towards death (Cerra et al., 1979b) (Fig. 18.8).

The exogenous nutritional support that a patient is receiving does have an influence on the plasma substrate levels. If the patient is supported just on intravenous protein in the form of albumin without any exogenous amino acid, profound effects on the amino acid levels

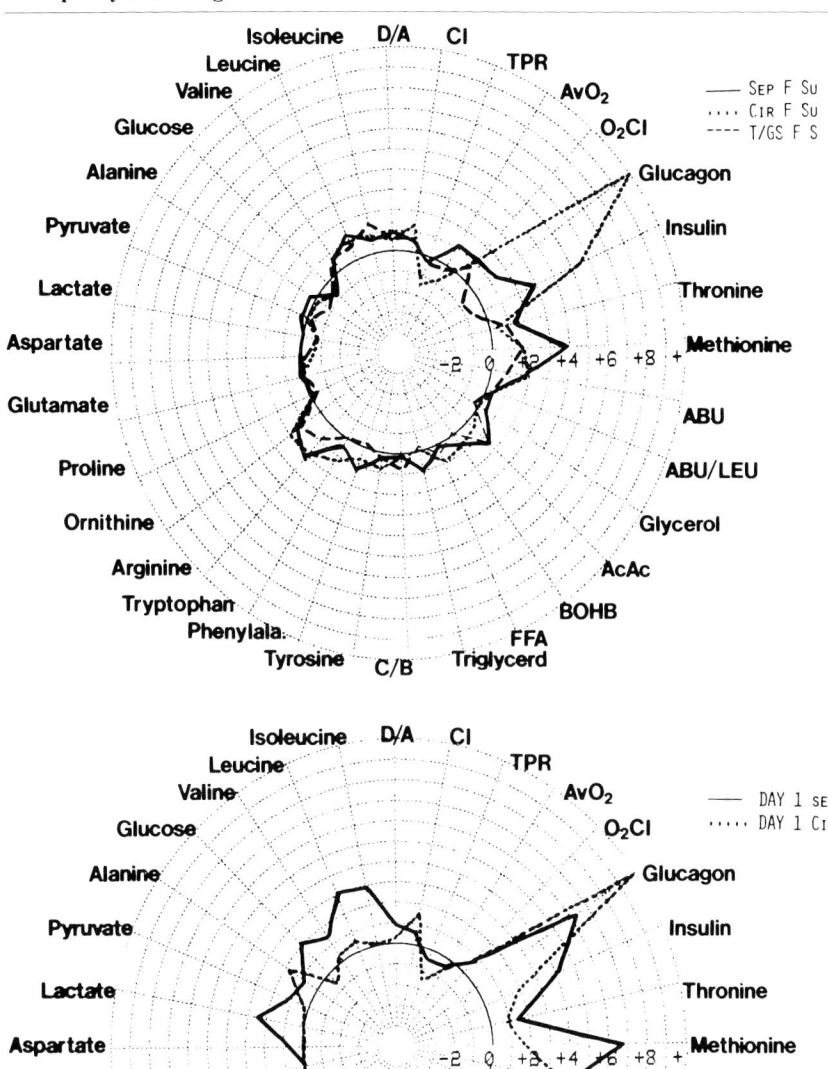

Figure 18.6. Profile patterns for surviving septic (*Sep*), cirrhotic (*Cir*) and nonseptic-noncirrhotic general surgery patients (*T/GS*) 7–10 days after the initial insult. The reference is the same as Fig. 18.4. Substrate levels return toward the reference values. (Reprinted with permission from F. B. Cerra, J. H. Siegel, J. R. Border, et al.: Surgery 86:409, 1979b.)

Figure 18.7. Profile patterns comparing sepsis organ failure patients early in their time course with cirrhotic patients with encephalopathy following protocaval decompression. The reference is the same as Fig. 18.4. The absence of significant abnormalities in the glucose and fat substrates in the cirrhotic group is evident. (Reprinted with permission from F. B. Cerra, J. H. Siegel, J. R. Border, et al.: Surgery 86:409, 1979b.)

occur. These are mainly evident in the branched chains, particularly isoleucine, in which albumin and plasma protein fractions of various kinds are very deficient. The use of this kind of support produces a progressively falling isoleucine/leucine ratio (Moyer et al., 1981a). When exogenous amino acids are used, the effect in survivors and nonsurvivors is much different. In both cases, there is some increase in plasma substrate levels as a function of the amino acid load. The levels most effected are glycine, alanine, lactate, pyruvate, and aromatic amino acids. This phenomena is significant in the range of 75–100 g of intravenous amino acids per day. The effect is more prominent in survivors, with little effect in nonsurvivors (Cerra et al., 1980; Moyer et al., 1981b). In addition, exogenous amino acid support seems to profoundly influence the levels of prealbumin, ceruloplasmin, and retinol binding protein in survivors, whereas there is little effect in nonsurviving patients (Skillman et al., 1976).

As has been pointed out, there is a very tight correlation in time in patients developing the organ failure syndrome between the evolving unbalanced physiology

Figure 18.8. Profile patterns of septic cirrhotic patients with multiple organ failure relative to noncirrhotic, septic organ failure patients. The reference is the same as in Fig. 18.4. When the cirrhotic patient develops sepsis, his profile pattern becomes that of sepsis, and the time course to death is faster. (Reprinted with permission from F. B. Cerra, J. H. Siegel, J. R. Border, et al.: Surgery 86:409, 1979b.)

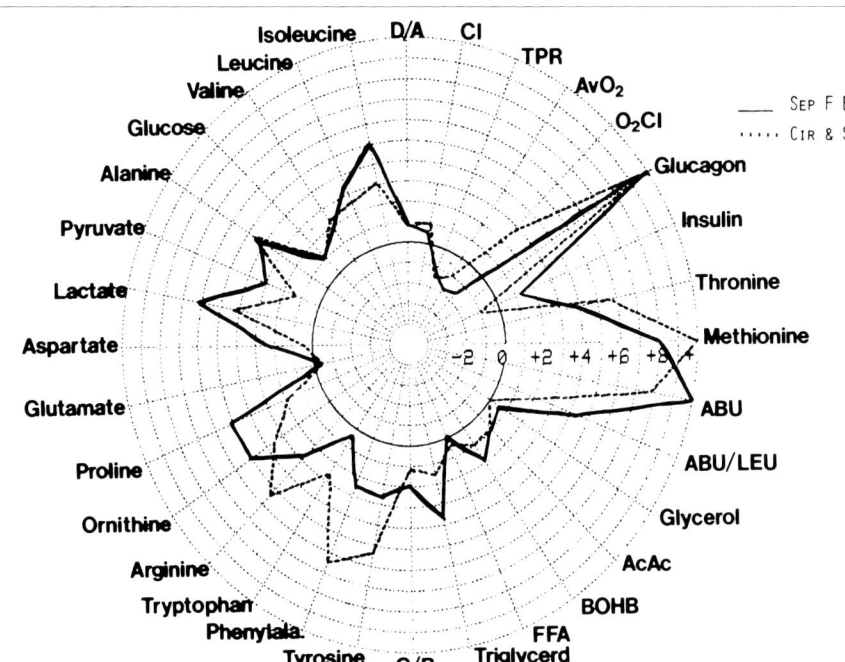

and unbalanced metabolism. This relationship is further pointed out by analyzing two of the amino acids in detail. Proline is an amino acid which is mainly catabolized by liver and which cannot be catabolized by muscle. Proline levels in multiple systems organ failure progressively rise in an exponential fashion as death approaches (Cerra et al., 1979c). As the proline level rises, the total peripheral resistance and oxygen consumption index fall in a very tight linear relationship (Fig. 18.9). This rise in proline level is also associated with progressive rises in the lactate and pyruvate levels, with the constancy of the lactate/pyruvate ratio (Cerra et al., 1979c). In the hepatic degradation pathways of proline, it is converted to an intermediate, which then comes into equilibrium with ornithine or glutamate. The action of glutamate dehydrogenase can convert glutamate into α-ketoglutarate, with entrance into the Krebs cycle and the production of ammonia. The glutamate concentration likewise rises exponentially as death approaches. This is associated with linear rises in proline, ornithine, and ammonia (Fig. 18.10). These changes are again tightly correlated with a progressive fall in total peripheral resistance and oxygen consumption (Cerra et al., 1979c).

Threonine and methionine are likewise catabolized in the liver. Initially they are catabolized to α-ketobutyrate. This intermediate can then be oxidized or converted to aminobutyric acid by the addition of an ammonia molecule. As has been seen, the concentrations of threonine, methionine, aminobutyric acid, and ammonia rise proportionately. It is felt that the ammonia probably facilitates the conversion of α-ketobutyrate into the nonoxidative pathway with the subsequent formation of aminobutyric acid (Cerra et al., 1979b).

Other studies in septic patients have demonstrated an increase in glucose pool size with an increase in mass flow of glucose to the periphery (Long, 1977; Long et al., 1971). This is associated with an increase turnover rate for glucose with the recycling of glucose through the Cori and alanine cycles. Carbon-14 glucose and alanine infusions, however, indicate that although there is a marked increase in the gluconeogenic response, it is not suppressed by the administration of exogenous glucose, a phenomenon not characteristic of the nonseptic state (Long et al., 1976). Animal models have indicated a reduced clearance of exogenous triglycerides with the reduction of postheparin lipolytic activity (Imamura et al., 1975). Recent human studies also suggest that glycerol turnover is increased in the septic process (Kaufmann et al., 1976).

A common feature of the systemic septic response seems to be a marked increase in muscle catabolism with an apparent utilization of branched chain amino acids by muscle as an energy source (Border, 1970; Border et al., 1976; Clowes et al., 1976). This concept is very consistent with the observed levels and phenomena seen in multiple systems organ failure. Studies by Wannemacher and others (1978; Beisel and Wannemacher, 1977) of the septic model do show enhanced muscle clearance of branched chain amino acids increased plasma alanine, reduced hepatic and plasma ketone bodies, hyperglycemia, and hypertriglyceridemia with reduced peripheral clearance of triglycerides and an increase in hepatic liponeogenesis. Studies by Clowes et al. (1976) in an animal model have shown an advanced state of leucine oxidation together with insulin resistance. Their study on septic man using lower extremity clearances also showed reduced fatty acid and ketone body clearance in association with an unchanged glucose clearance and an increased output of lactate and alanine relative to starved man (Ryan et al., 1974).

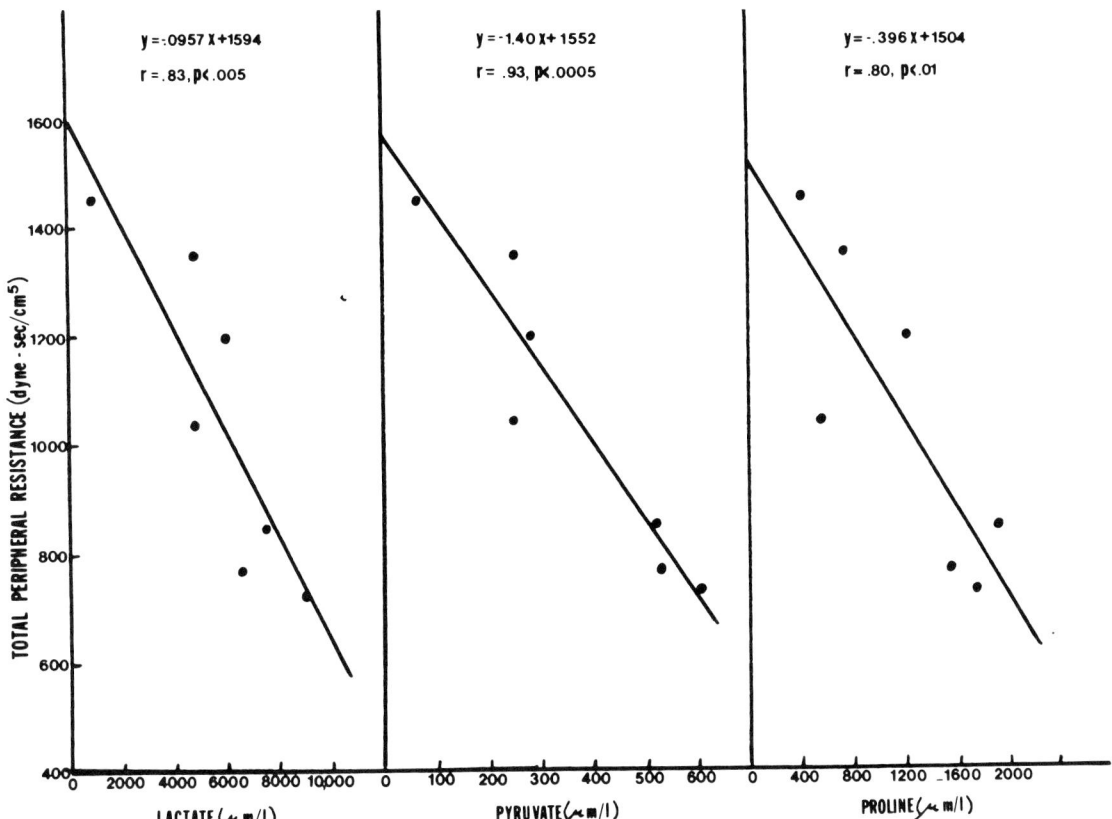

Figure 18.9. Physiologic-metabolic time course correlations in nonsurviving patients with sepsis organ failure syndrome. Total peripheral resistance (TPR) falls as the levels of lactate, pyruvate, and proline rise. The lactate/pyruvate ratio remains constant. The O_2CI relationships are the same. (Reprinted with permission from F. B. Cerra, J. Caprioli, and J. H. Siegel: Annals of Surgery 190:577, 1979c.)

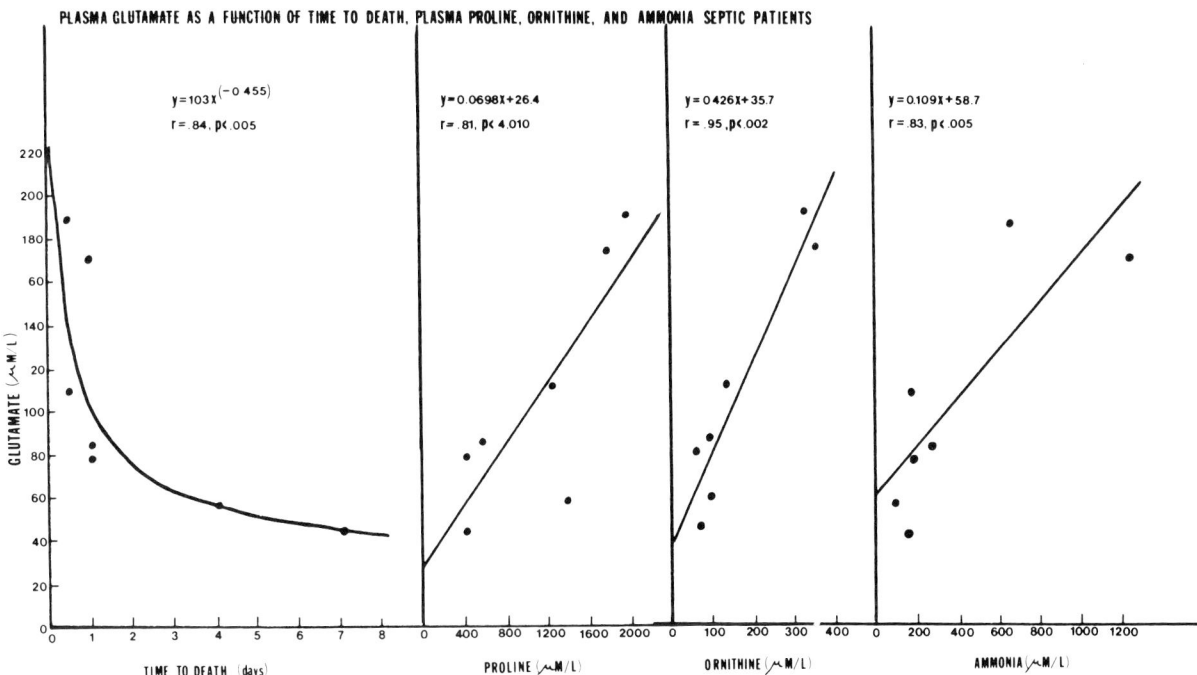

Figure 18.10. Metabolic substrate correlation time course for the components of the glutamate dehydrogenase pathway. As the levels rise, TPR and O_2CI falls (the B state). (Reprinted with permission from F. B. Cerra, J. Caprioli, and J. H. Siegel: Annals of Surgery 190:577, 1979c.)

NEUROHUMORAL TIME COURSE

Data on humans on the neural response to stress is difficult to obtain. A number of studies have shown that the neural reflexes play an important part in the metabolic and physiologic response to stress. Local blocking of an injured area, prior to the onset and release of humoral factors, can control the response to stress (Hume, 1974). Selective hypothalamic stimulation of the rat can produce most of the observed metabolic phenomena of multiple systems organ failure (Bernardis et al., 1975). Although direct measurements of this sympathetic tone in man have not been possible, indirect evidence from changes in heart rate, myocardial contractility, cardiovascular characteristics, and norepinephrine excretion data do indicate that increased sympathetic tone is at play. An active field of investigation is in the influence of this sympathetic tone on the cellular metabolic machinery. Stimulation of glucogenolysis and, indirectly, gluconeogenesis have been demonstrated in the liver.

The glucagon and insulin response in multiple systems organ failure and in other pathologic states has been studied. Early in the course, there is marked elevation in circulating glucagon levels (Fig. 18.4). Insulin levels are generally increased but not to the extent of glucagon, such that there is an increase in the glucagon/insulin ratio (Cerra et al., 1979b). This phenomenon is occurring at the time of the hyperglycemia and elevated free fatty acid levels that were previously discussed. The insulin levels that are present are inappropriately low for the level of existing glucose; the normal inverse relationship between glucose and free fatty acids is absent. As the multiple systems organ failure syndrome progresses, the high glucagon/insulin ratio persists (Cerra et al., 1979b). This characteristic is significantly different than the glucagon and insulin response that is seen in trauma-hypermetabolic man, overnight fasting man, and cirrhotic man (Figs. 18.3 and 18.4). In a cirrhotic patient under stress with encephalopathy, there is a marked elevation of glucagon level with an initial increase in the glucagon/insulin ratio (Fig. 18.11). As the cirrhotic patients following portocaval shunt go on to survival, the insulin levels increase such that there is a progressive decrease in the glucagon/insulin ratio. This phenomenon is occurring in a setting characterized by the absence of hyperglycemia and a rather significant elevation in circulating free fatty acid levels and free fatty acid flux. These marked elevations of glucagon are not characteristic of overnight fasting man or in nonseptic, noncirrhotic trauma-hypermetabolic man (Cerra et al., 1979a).

The cortisol levels in stressed man are elevated relative to overnight fasting man. The cortisol level throughout the time course in stressed man, however, does not discriminate between the presence or absence of sepsis, the presence or absence of cirrhosis, or the presence or absence of the hypermetabolic state (Cerra et al., 1979a).

The excretion of epinephrine, norepinephrine, their meta derivatives, and their conjugated forms are increased with all kinds of stress. To date, no significant differences in the patterns of this catecholamine response have been demonstrated relative to the pathology of the stress state, e.g., multiple systems organ failure versus sepsis versus nonseptic trauma-hypermetabolic man. In patients who expire, the norepinephrine levels generally remain increased, while the epinephrine levels dropped towards zero (Benedict and Graham-Smith, 1978).

Recent attention has been turned toward the thyroid hormone levels in the septic multiple systems organ failure process. These studies have indicated that there is a drop in the levels in T3 and T4 with an increase in reverse T3 during the septic process (Cavalieri, 1977).

Looking at the total picture of the hormone pattern profiles, there is a considerable lack of correlation with the pathologic state. Cirrhotic patients have the glucagon, insulin, and catecholamine changes as described. At the same time, the cirrhotic patients under stress do not demonstrate the abnormalities of glucose, fat, and amino acid metabolism that are seen in the patients with sepsis and the multiple systems organ failure. Nonseptic, noncirrhotic, hypermetabolic man does not have elevations of glucagon and insulin, although they do have elevations of their catecholamine excretions, which are not statistically different from those of cirrhotic patients under stress or patients with sepsis or the multiple systems organ failure. The trauma-hypermetabolic patients, however, do not have the abnormalities of glucose, fat, and amino acid metabolism that are seen in sepsis and multiple systems organ failure syndrome. The patients with sepsis and the organ failure syndrome, on the other hand, have a hormone profile picture that is not unlike the cirrhotic under stress, yet they have the previously described abnormalities of glucose, fat, and amino acid metabolism (Fig. 18.11).

As has been stated, in septic patients who expire, norepinephrine excretion remains high. This phenomenon is compatible with sustained sympathetic activity in critically ill patients. Sympathetic tone is known to be one of the most potent stimuli to glucagon production. There is also a close correlation between catecholamine excretion rate and glucagon levels, indicating a possible relationship between sympathetic tone and the level of glucagon in critically ill patients (Wilmore, 1976; Wilmore et al., 1974). Studies of isolated heart and diaphragm indicate that epinephrine stimulates the utilization of alanine and branched chain amino acids (Buse et al., 1973). Catecholamines have also been shown to increase glucagon and decrease insulin secretion from the islet cells (Gerich et al., 1973). The rat peritonitis model has been shown to induce a hyperinsulin response with a reduction in fat utilization from peripheral fat stores (Ryan et al., 1974).

In cirrhotic patients, insulin has been shown to be a potent stimulator of the uptake of branched chain amino acids by muscle (Munro et al., 1975). Patients with cirrhosis who are undergoing portocaval decompression have skeletal muscle concentrations of leucine, isoleucine, and valine that are low at the time when their serum concentrations are low and the serum concentrations of aromatic amino acids are increased (Job et al., 1967). Hepatic tissue biopsies in these same patients,

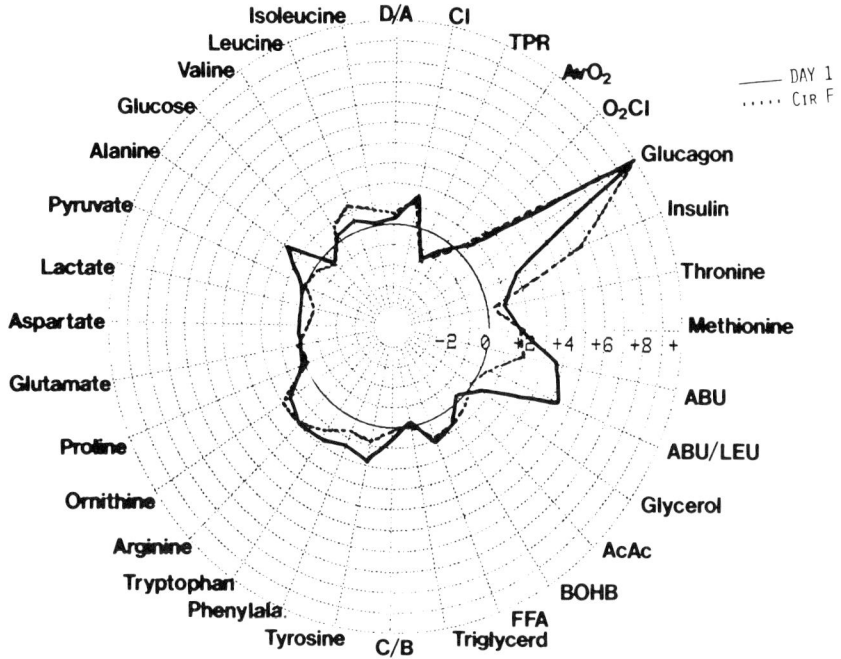

Figure 18.11. Profile time course patterns of cirrhotic patients who survive following portocaval decompression. The reference is the same as Fig. 18.4. The stability of the pattern through their courses is evident. (Reprinted with permission from F. B. Cerra, J. H. Siegel, J. R. Border, et al.: Surgery 86: 409, 1979b.)

however, indicate that the levels of branched chain amino acids in hepatic tissue are the same as those of the control tissue (Job et al., 1967). This is in contradistinction to recently reported skeletal muscle biopsies in patients with sepsis, in which the levels of branched chain amino acids are increased as well as those of aromatic amino acids, at a time when insulin levels are increased and are at a level comparable to those seen in cirrhotic patients (Liaw et al., 1980).

The abnormal amino acid profiles seen in patients with cirrhosis under stress seem to be a function of primary hepatocellular deficiency in the metabolism of aromatic amino acids, together with a normal response of the peripheral metabolic machinery to the modulating hormonal stimulators—mainly, insulin (Cerra et al., 1979b). This does not seem to be true in the patient with sepsis and multiple systems organ failure syndrome, where the hormone patterns are similar to those seen in cirrhotic patients and yet the plasma substrate level profiles are markedly different, with abnormalities in glucose, fat, and amino acid metabolism.

TIME COURSE CORRELATIONS

With the onset of multiple systems organ failure, a characteristic chain of events in physiology, metabolism, and the neurohumoral system comes into play. As the patients proceed toward death, they progressively evolve the unbalanced physiologic state characterized by a total peripheral resistance that is inappropriately low for the level of cardiac output; an increase in cardiac output with a marked increase in the delivery of oxygen and metabolic substrate to the periphery; a progressive reduction in oxygen extraction by the periphery with a subsequent fall in absolute oxygen consumption that becomes refractory to increases in cardiac output (and thus increases oxygen delivery to the periphery) (Fig. 18.4).

The metabolic data indicate that the overall peripheral problem is not one of a maldistribution of flow and oxygenation. An increase in muscle blood flow in sepsis has been demonstrated. Although there may be some local maldistribution, the metabolic characteristics of multiple systems organ failure, such as the constancy of the lactate/pyruvate ratio, indicate that there is an overall matching between perfusion and the cells perfused in the capillary beds.

The metabolic and clinical data indicate that there are progressive abnormalities in substrate levels that occur in time with the development of the physiologic abnormalities (Cerra et al., 1979a and c). The characteristic changes of hyperglycemia, elevation of lactate and pyruvate with a constant lactate/pyruvate ratio, progressive elevations of triglycerides, the progressive increase in the betahydroxybutyrate/acetoacetate ratio, and the amino acid profile characteristics described become progressively more apparent as the unbalanced physiologic state unfolds. The implication of this correlation is that metabolic changes are occurring and are reflected in the changes in physiology. The data indicate a progressive inabilitiy for the utilization of glucose, followed by fat, followed by ketone bodies, and finally of protein as the multiple systems organ failure process unfolds. Early in the course there seems to be a marked increase in the utilization of branched chain amino acids by the periphery. As death approaches, the ability to utilize branched chain for energy production also seems to become inhibited. The clinical correlation of this protein base energy production economy is seen in the rapidly declining muscle mass in these patients at a time when fat mass does not seem to be as rapidly declining. The clinical indicators of reduced protein synthesis are also apparent:

the onset of hypoalbuminemia, anergy, intestinal mucosal ulceration, and the failure of wound healing. The alterations in mentation are quite likely associated with the abnormalities in amino acid profiles that are seen and could be due to processes similar to the false neurotransmitters and alterations in brain catecholamines that have been documented in hepatic encephalopathy (Fischer and Baldessarini, 1971; Munro et al., 1975). This is another way of saying that there is most likely an alteration of the blood-brain barrier in the multiple systems organ failure syndrome. The progression of this syndrome is likewise associated with altered drug metabolism, as has been demonstrated with chloromycetin and cimetidine (Schentag et al., 1979; Slaughter et al., 1979). Much lower doses of these drugs are necessary in this setting.

As was previously discussed, the hormone profile in multiple systems organ failure is such as to be highly suggestive of a reduced influence of the hormonal-metabolic systems on the cellular metabolic machinery. The eventual result of these processes is the failure of energy production and, in most patients, death.

ETIOLOGIC CONSIDERATIONS

In normal man, the regulation of metabolism proceeds through a combination of local factors with modulation, when necessary, by the neurohumoral systems. The end result of this system is a coordinated, modulated, and balanced interorgan flow of substrate in accordance with demand. Thus, the liver produces glucose which is used by the obligate glucose users such as red blood cells, the brain and, to what ever extent possible, by other organs such as muscle. Ketone bodies are produced by the liver, used by the periphery, and become a perferred source of fuel for such organs as muscle. Liver, however, has no capacity to metabolize ketone bodies. Free fatty acids and glycerol are mobilized from adipose tissue, become sources for ketone body formation by the liver, and are a primary fuel for such organs as cardiac muscle and skeletal muscle. The liver has a marked capacity for the catabolism of aromatic- and sulfur-containing amino acids, but takes up branched chain amino acids only in accordance with its needs for protein synthesis and not for energy production. Muscle on the other hand has a marked ability to use branched chain amino acids for protein synthesis and, more importantly in stress states, for use in energy production.

The neuroendocrine modulator serves to increase this interorgan, balanced substrate flow in accordance with existing demand. The substrate flow, however, remains balanced in normal man under stress.

In patients with sepsis and multiple systems organ failure, there appears to be a progressive ineffectiveness of normal, hormonal, modulating mechanisms on the primordial metabolic machinery, with subsequent alterations in substrate flow resulting in the plasma profiles as have been described. To date studies of intracellular substrate have demonstrated that the plasma profiles are reflecting reasonably well what is happening on an intracellular basis (Bergstrom et al., 1976; Liaw et al., 1980). There appears to be a marked increase in gluconeogenesis with an increase in mass flow of glucose to the periphery but an ineffective oxidation of glucose once the periphery is reached. There is subsequent recycling in the form of lactate, pyruvate, and alanine back to the liver with a marked increase in substrate flow to the liver for gluconeogenesis. There seems to be a marked increase in the hepatic production of triglycerides at a time when there is a decreased clearance and probable reduced oxidative utilization of triglyceride and fatty acid in the periphery. The primary energy substrate seems to be protein. This is thought to be a preferential burning of branched chain amino acids for energy production. The one exception to this may be acetoacetate, but data is currently lacking. The source of the branched chain appears to be from muscle itself. When the muscle protein is broken down in preparation for catabolism, the branched chain amino acids cannot be preferentially removed from the actin myosin, but all of the amino acids must be released. The branched chains seem to be preferentially burned in the mitochondria for energy production. Other amino acids seem to be converted to alanine and sent back to the liver for reprocessing. The amino acids that muscle cannot catabolize or interconvert, such as proline, methionine, threonine, and the aromatic amino acids, are released into the blood stream and sent back to the liver for disposition. The result of this phenomenon is a protein-based energy economy, with marked muscle wasting and a progressively unbalanced amino acid pattern that is presented to the liver, which the liver can no longer normalize. In such a setting, hepatic protein synthesis seems to become progressively inefficient (Fig. 18.12).

In addition, this progressive preference for nonoxidative catabolic pathways also appears very early in the liver. This seems to be manifest in the levels of methionine and threonine, together with aminobutyric acid production and the proline catabolic data that was discussed previously in the metabolic section. To this data

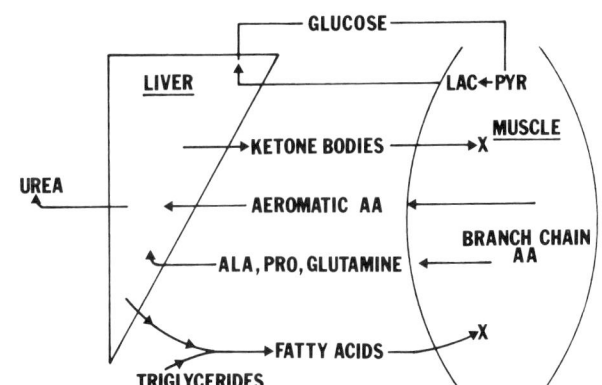

Figure 18.12. Fuel deficit feedbacks. Substrate flow diagram in sepsis multiple organ failure. The effects of the mitochondrial dysfunction and the energy deficit are illustrated.

must be added that of the rising β-hydroxybutyrate/acetoacetate ratio. This is again consistent with the onset of a progressively falling redox state of the mitochondria.

The primary problem in the etiology and pathogenesis of the multiple systems organ failure syndrome, therefore, appears to be mitochondrial in nature. The mitochondrial defect at this point in time can be characterized as one of an energy deficit associated with a progressive fall in redox potential and a progressive preference for nonoxidated pathways of catabolism. Muscle biopsy studies in septic patients have shown a marked reduction in high energy phosphate and high energy phosphate-containing compounds that is consistent with this hypothesis (Finley et al., 1975; Bergstrom et al., 1976). The fall in redox potential appears to be one of an inability to regenerate NAD from NADH with a subsequent progressive failure of the NAD/NADH-dependent systems. One of the most sensitive is the pyruvate hydrogenase system for the conversion of pyruvate to acetyl CoA. The acetyl CoA entrance into the Krebs cycle is, of course, the cornerstone for the entrance of glucose, fat, and ketone bodies into the process of oxidative phosphorylation. This inhibition of pyruvate dehydrogenase on a progressive basis would account for the observed alterations in lactate, pyruvate, and glucose as described. In addition, the high NADH concentrations would, with the reduced redox potential of the mitochondrial, account for the decreased utilization of fatty acids by an inhibition of the "chipping enzyme" and subsequent reduced entry into acetyl CoA. The redox state would also favor the ketone bodies to be present in the form of β-hydroxybutyrate rather than in the utilization form of acetoacetate. There is some indication, however, that acetoacetate may be utilized until very late in the multiple systems organ failure syndrome.

The branched chain amino acids likewise enter through NAD/NADH-dependent systems and become progressively inhibited, such that at the time of death, even these sources of high energy phosphate production become unavailable. Glutamate dehydrogenase also seems to be inhibited very early in the septic process and the process of multiple systems organ failure. This inhibition is indicated from the proline data analysis that was described previously and seems to be primarily a hepatic phenomenon. The progressive rise in intracellular and probably intramitochondrial ammonia would seem to be having some influence on the pathways of preference for catabolism. The aminobutyric acid data are consistent with this concept.

The end result of this process is the progressive inability of substrate entry into the mitochondria for high energy phosphate production. This energy deficit would also serve to account for the seemingly progressive inability of the hormones to modulate the metabolic machinery. Such an energy deficit with a reduction in cytosol ATP would severely inhibit the cyclic AMP system through which most of the hormones were felt to act in their process of modulating metabolism (Ch. 10).

The exact etiology to this progressive mitochondrial dysfunction is currently unknown. This is likewise true for the actual prime mover or prime movers, in that they are currently unidentified. One fact that has become evident is that the processes of multiple systems organ failure are not organism-dependent but seem to be a generalized host phenomenon. These data were obtained by looking at a large number of septicemic patients who were infected with a variety of gram-positive, gram-negative, anaerobic, and fungus organisms (Wiles et al., 1980). A great deal of work has been done on endotoxemia and endotoxic shock (Ch. 16). Although significant derangements of physiology and metabolism have been demonstrated, these derangements are still not what is typically seen in patients with sepsis and the organ failure syndrome. This is not to imply that endotoxin may not be involved in part, although this is yet to be demonstrated in the human model.

Several hypotheses become evident for the derangement in mitochondrial function. It seems likely that this must involve the hydrogen ion shuttle systems across the mitochondrial membrane. There has been a marked increase interest in calcium metabolism and its action as a messenger in cellular function of both a metabolic and contractile nature. Hydrogen ion transport has been shown to be intimately involved with the sodium-calcium pump across the mitochondrial membrane. This energy-dependent mechanism seems to be involved in all tissues but the liver, kidney, lung, and smooth muscle (Carafoli et al., 1976). Certainly a lack of high energy phosphate would inhibit this sodium-calcium pump with a progressively reduced ability for removal of hydrogen ion from the mitochondria. Whether or not this phenomenon would be a primary or secondary change is as yet uncertain.

A second hypothesis for the reduced ability for hydrogen ion transport across the mitochondria is concerned with the malate-aspartate shuttle as proposed by Shargo et al. (1976). An elevation of long chain fatty acid acyl-CoA esters serves to inhibit the malate-asparate shuttle and the subsequent transport of hydrogen ions across the mitochondrial membrane. This would produce the resultant fall in mitochondrial redox potential and the changes that have been previously described. Recent studies have also shown that the plasma carnitine is not deficient in patients with sepsis and the multiple systems organ failure syndrome. The plasma carnitine levels are mainly dependent upon the level of renal function and were no different from the normal control levels. There is some experimental evidence to indicate, however, that intracellular carnitine is deficient in the systemic septic response (Cerra et al., 1981c). This may be reflected in a normal carnitine level, in the sense that it might still be inappropriately low to allow sufficient entry of carnitine into the cytsol. An intracellular deficiency of carnitine would result in an excess of fatty acid acyl-CoA esters and the inhibition of the malate-aspartate shuttle as described.

A great deal of investigation is being done to the role of complement, prostaglandins and coagulation systems in the pathogenesis of the systemic septic response and the multiple systems organ failure syndrome (Chs. 12 and 26). There seems to be activation of all three systems through several common pathways. The results of the activation of these systems can produce many of the physiologic effects and some of the observed metabolic effects that are seen in multiple systems organ failure. In the human model, whether or not the activation of these autocoid systems is occuring as a primary response to an infecting agent or as a secondary response to other primary responses caused by the infecting agent is currently unknown.

THERAPEUTIC CONSIDERATIONS

In the absence of detailed knowledge as to what the prime mover or prime movers are in the etiology and pathogenesis of this syndrome, the treating physician is really left to the control of sepsis and the treatment of symptoms and signs while attempting to provide metabolic support. Much of the treatment regimens of this syndrome are aimed at cardiopulmonary support together with the use of systemic antibiotics and the removal of all septic sources. It is unquestionably true that if all surgically remediable sepsis is not controlled by surgery, mortality from sepsis is very high.

The newer cardiopulmonary support mechanisms are able to provide adequate perfusion and ventilation support throughout most of the time course of this syndrome until the ultimate metabolic failure occurs. The application of vasodilator therapy in those patients who have a prior state of myocardial depression or who develop it as part of the metabolic defect of the multiple systems organ failure syndrome has resulted in the salvage of a group of patients who ordinarily would have expired. In this setting, the mortality was most probably due to the perfusion related deficit rather than the metabolic deficit. A significant percentage of this group still proceeds to expire with the metabolic defect even though the perfusion deficit has been corrected (Cerra et al., 1978).

One recently recognized advance is the early aggressive maintenance of the upright chest and the restoration of normal pulmonary physiology (Sturm et al., 1979). When coupled with techniques of the maintenance of preload and a dry interstitial pulmonary space, this seems to have aborted the onset of this syndrome in patients in whom it would have ordinarily developed. The statistical documentation of this concept is forthcoming. The implications of this phenomenon in terms of etiology are at present unclear.

Broad spectrum antibiotics providing both aerobic and anaerobic coverage become an integral part of the therapy of this syndrome. Eventually, however, the blood is unable to be sterilized as the process proceeds towards death. The changing nature of the bacteremias and septicemias also provide considerable difficulty in the selection of antibiotics. Once the metabolic failure phase of the syndrome has occurred, the presence or absence of antibiotics seems to have little effect on the ultimate outcome.

The newest area of therapy in this syndrome is in the area of metabolic support and manipulation. From the proceeding discussion it becomes evident that there is differential fuel usage as the syndrome progresses towards the ultimate outcome. The branched chain amino acids seem to be in great use early on and throughout the course of the syndrome. There is some indication that acetoacetate is used during the early part of the syndrome with a subsequent inability to use it as death approaches (Cerra et al., 1979a and b.) From the triglyceride data that was discussed, there seems to be little use for the current forms of intravenous triglyceride that are commercially available. Indeed, the use of intravenous triglycerides in this setting has been associated with the aggravation of pulmonary failure.

The commercial amino acid mixes do not seem to be designed for use in this kind of patient. Unfortunately, at this point in time, there is little else with which to provide protein support. It is evident that the use of blood products as metabolic support only contributes to the progression of the syndrome. It is also understood, that during the hypermetabolic phase, there is no known way to contain the hypermetabolism and to stop the tremendous negative nitrogen balance. Evidence is accruing that the use of exogenous amino acids can have a sparing effect on the peripheral protein. Whether or not it can induce a state of positive protein production is currently unknown. The problem with using current commercial amino acid mixes in multiple systems organ failure is that the amino acids seem to be providing a fuel source. As such, because the commercial mixtures are low in branched chain relative to demand and high in those amino acids which are already flowing to the liver at an increased rate from muscle (sulfur and aromatic amino acid), a marked increase in ureagenesis can and does occur. Ideally these patients should be kept on as much intravenous protein as possible. The routine use of Kjedahl nitrogen balance to monitor the efficiency of this utilization is impractical. A reasonable bedside monitor is to use the BUN/creatinine ratio. When the BUN exceeds what is appropriate for the creatinine by 20 mg/100 ml, appropriate or maximized nitrogen utilization has probably occurred. Thus, if the patient's creatinine is 3 and the BUN is 60, continued increase in amino acid load is appropriate. In this same patient, once the BUN has reached 90, maximum tolerable utilizaton has been probably achieved.

It has become evident that excess of caloric support in the form of glucose is frequently detrimental to patients with the systemic septic response and the multiple systems organ failure syndrome. The administration of glucose in excess of demand really seems to aggravate the formation of triglyceride and fatty metamorphosis of the liver (Wannemacher et al., 1978). Consequently, the use of standard intravenous hyperalimentation during the phase of glucose intolerance seems to potentiate the progression of the syndrome (Lowry & Brennan, 1981). The use of insulin drive to control the blood glucose level is usually difficult, and the large amounts of regular insulin that are used seem to potentiate hepatic fatty metamorphosis. The current recommendation for the use of glucose and amino acids in patients with a systemic septic response and the multiple systems organ failure syndrome who are manifesting this kind of glucose intolerance is to provide 100 glucose calories per gram of administered protein nitrogen. This calorie/nitrogen ratio is quite well tolerated and seems to provide what is optimal exogenous support at this point in time. The addition of $ATP-MgCl_2$ with glucose may also be of some benefit (Wilmore et al., 1974).

What is apparent is that the use of branched chain-rich solutions needs to be thoroughly investigated in this syndrome. The use of these solutions for normalization of the aminogram in hepatic failure patients has produced positive clinical results with reversal of encephalopathy and a more rapid and effective reversal of the protein-calorie malnutrition in that setting (Fischer et al., 1976). Some preliminary reports by Freund et al. (1977) in septic patients indicates that it might possibly be true in this setting also. Actual detailed clinical data to date, however, is lacking.

The use of acetoacetate infusions, carnitine-independent fuels, and carnitine infusions in the systemic septic response and the multiple systems organ failure are also other forms of metabolic support and manipulation that are currently in the investigative process. The continued research into the metabolism of this frequently fatal disorder is necessary if the morbidity and mortality is to be reduced.

References

Beisel, W.R., and Wannemacher, R.W.: Metabolic response of the host to infectious disease. In *Nutritional Aspects of Care in the Critically Ill*, edited by J.R. Richards and J.M. Kinney, pp. 135–161. Churchill-Livingstone, New York, 1977.

Benedict, C.R., and Graham-Smith, D.C.: Plasma noradrenalin and adrenalin and dopamine β-hydroxylase activity in patients with shock due to septicemia: Trauma and hemorrhage. Q. J. Med. *57:*1, 1978.

Bergstrom, J., Bostrous, H., and Furst, P., et al.: Preliminary studies of energy rich phosphagens in critically ill patients. Crit. Care Med. *4:*197, 1976.

Bernardis, L.L., Goldman, J.K., and Border, J.R.: Production of weaning rat dorsomedial hypothalamic lesions by cathodal stimulation. Proc. Can. Fed. Biol. Soc. *18:*106, 1975.

Border, J.R.: Metabolic response to short term starvation, sepsis, and trauma. In *Surgery Annual*, edited by L. Cooper. Appleton-Century-Crofts, New York, 1970.

Border, J.R., Chenier, R., and McMenamy, R.H., et al.: Multiple systems organ failure muscle fuel deficit with visceral protein malnutrition. Surg. Clin. North Am. *56:*1147, 1976.

Buse, M.G., Biggers, J.F., and Drier, C., et al.: The effect of epinephrine, glucagon and the nutritional status on the oxidation of branched chain amino acids and pyruvate in isolated hearts and diaphragms of the rat. J. Biol. Chem. *248:*697, 1973.

Carafoli, E., Crompton, M., and Malsronm K., et al.: Mitochondrial calcium transport and the intracellular calcium homeostasis. In *Biochemistry of Membrane Transport*, edited by G. Semenya and E. Carafoli, pp. 535–551. Springer-Verlag, Berlin, 1977.

Cavalieri, R.R.: Impaired peripheral conversion of thyroxine to tricodothyronine. Annu. Rev. Med. *28:*57, 1977.

Cerra, F.B., Hassett, J., and Siegel, J.H.: Use of vasodilator therapy in septic myocardial depression. J. Surg. Res. *25:*180, 1978.

Cerra, F.B., Siegel, J.H., and Border, J.R., et al.: Correlations between metabolic and cardiopulmonary measurements in patients after trauma, general surgery and sepsis. J. Trauma *19:*621, 1979a.

Cerra, F.B., Siegel, J.H., and Border, J.R., et al.: The hepatic failure of sepsis: Cellular vs. substrate. Surgery *86:*409, 1979b.

Cerra, F.B., Caprioli, J., and Siegel, J.H., et al.: Proline metabolism in sepsis, cirrhosis and general surgery: The peripheral energy deficit. Ann. Surg. *190:*577, 1979c.

Cerra, F.B., Siegel, J.H., Coleman, B., et al.: Septic autocannibalism. A failure of exogenous nutritional support. Ann. Surg. *192:*570, 1980.

Cerra, F.B., Aswald, G., and Border, J.R.: Does the plasma carnitine matter in sepsis? J. Trauma, submitted for publication, 1981.

Clowes, G.H.A., O'Donnell, T.F., and Blackburn, G.L., et al.: Energy metabolism and proteolysis in traumatized and septic man. Clin. North Am. *56:*1169, 1976.

Eiseman, B., Beart, R., and Horton, L.: Multiple organ failure. Surg. Gynecol. Obstet. *144:*323, 1977.

Finley, R.H., Duff, J.H., and Holliday, R.L., et al.: Capillary muscle blood flow in human sepsis. Surgery *78:*87, 1975.

Fischer, J.E., and Baldessarini, R.J.: False neurotransmitters and hepatic failure. Lancet *10:*75, 1971.

Fischer, J.E., Yoshimura, N., and Aguirre A., et al.: Plasma amino acids in patients with hepatic encephalopathy. Am. J. Surg. *127:*40, 1974.

Fischer, J.E., Rosen, H.M., and Ebeid, A.M.: The effect of normalization of plasma amino acids on hepatic encephalopathy in man. Surgery *80:*77, 1976.

Freund, H.R., Ryan, J.A., and Fischer, J.E.: Amino acid derangements in patients with sepsis: Treatment with branch chain amino acid rich infusions. Ann. Surg. *83:*657, 1977.

Gerich, J.E., Karam, J.H., and Forsham, P.H.: Stimulation of glucagon secretion by epinephrine in man. J. Clin. Endocrinol. Metab. *37:*479, 1973.

Hirasawa, H., Chaudry, I.H., and Bave, A.E.: Beneficial effect of $ATP-MgCl_2$-glucose administration on survival following sepsis. Surg. Forum *19:*11, 1978.

Hume, D.M.: Endocrine and metabolic response to injury. In *Principles of Surgery*, edited by S.I. Schwartz. McGraw-Hill, New York, 1974.

Imamura, M., Clowes, G.H.A., and Blackburn, G.L., et al. Liver metabolism and glucogenesis in trauma and sepsis. Surgery *77:*868, 1975.

Job, V., Coon, W.W., and Sloan, M.: Altered clearance of free amino acids from plasma of patients with cirrhosis of the liver. J. Surg. Res. *6:*233, 1966.

Job, V., Coon, W.W., and Sloan, M.: Free amino acids in liver, plasma and muscle of patients with cirrhosis of the liver. J. Surg. Res. *7:*41, 1967.

Kaufmann, R.L., Matson, C.F., and Rowberg, A.H., et al.: Defective lipid metabolism during bacterial infection in rhesus monkeys. Metabolism *25:*615, 1976.

Liaw, K.Y., Askanazi, J., and Michelson C.B., et al.: Effect of operative injury and sepsis on high energy phosphate activity and glycolytic activity in muscle and red cells. J. Trauma *20:*755, 1980.

Long, C.L.: Energy balance and carbohydrate metabolism in infection and sepsis. Am. J. Clin. Nutr. *30:*1301, 1977.

Long, C.L., Spencer, J.L., and Kinney, J.M., et al.: Carbohydrate metabolism in man. Effect of elective operations and major inury. J. Appl. Physiol. *13:*110, 1971.

Long, C.L., Kinney, J.L., and Geiger, J.W.: Nonsuppressibility of gluconeogenesis by glucose in septic patients. Metabolism *25:*193, 1976.

Lowry, S.F., and Brennan, M.F.: Abnormal liver function during parenteral nutrition: Correlation with infusion excess. J. Surg. Res., in press, 1981.

McMenamy, R.H., Border, J.R., and Cerra, F.B., et al.: Splanchnic substrate balances and biochemical changes during sepsis. J. Trauma, in press, 1981.

Moyer, E.D., Border, J.R., and Cerra, F.B.: Imbalances in plasma amino acids associated with exogenous albumin in the trauma-septic patient. J. Trauma, submitted for publication, 1981a.

Moyer, E.D., Border, J.R., and Cerra, F.B., et al.: Contrasts in plasma amino acid profiles in trauma-septic patients who survive or die. Effects of intravenous amino acids. J. Trauma, submitted for publication, 1981b.

Munro, H.N., Fernstrum, J.D., and Wurtman, R.J.: Insulin plasma amino acid imbalance and hepatic coma. Lancet *26:* 986, 1975.

Ryan, N.T., Blackburn, G.L., and Clowes, G.H.A.: Differential tissue sensitivity to elevated endogenous insulin levels during experimental peritonitis in rats. Metabolism *23:*1081, 1974.

Schentag, J.J., Cerra, F.B., and Calleri, G., et al.: Pharmacokinetic and clinical studies in patients with cimetidine-associated mental confusion. Lancet *1:*177, 1979

Shrago, E., Shrey, A., and Ellison, C.: Regulation of cell metabolism by mitochondrial transport system. In *Gluconeogenesis: Its Regulations in Mammalian Species*, edited by R.W. Henson and M. A. Mehlman, pp. 221-239. Wiley-Interscience, New York, 1976.

Siegel, J.H.: Pattern and process in the evolution of and recovery from shock. In *The Aged and High Risk Surgical Patient: Medical, Surgical and Anesthetic Management*, edited by J.H. Siegel and P. Chodoff, pp. 381–455. Grune & Stratton, New York, 1976.

Siegel, J.H., Giovannini, I., and Coleman, B.: Ventilation perfusion maldistribution secondary to the hyperdynamic cardiovascular state as the major cause of increased pulmonary shunting in human sepsis. J. Trauma *19:*432, 1979a.

Siegel, J.H., Cerra, F.B., and Peters, D., et al.: The physiologic recovery trajectory as the organizing principle for the quantification of hormonometabolic adaption to surgical stress and severe sepsis (symposium). Adv. Shock Res. *2:*177, 1979b.

Skillman, J.J., Rosenoer, V.M., and Smith, P.C., et al.: Improved albumin synthesis in postoperative patients by amino acid infusion. N. Engl. J. Med. *293:*1037, 1976.

Slaughter, R., Koup, J., and Cerra, F.B.: The pharmacokinetics of chloramphenicol in critically ill patients. Clin. Pharmacol. Ther. *25:*88, 1979.

Sturm, J.A., Trentz, O., and Oestern, H.J., et al.: Cardiopulmonary parameters and prognosis after severe multiple trauma. J. Trauma *19:*305, 1979.

Wannemacher, R.W., Dinterman, R.E., and Hadick, C.L.: Metabolic fuel utilization by skeletal muscle of rhesus monkey during pneumococcal sepsis (abstract). Fed. Proc. *37:* 849, 1978.

Wiles, J., Cerra, F.B., Siegel, J.H., et al.: The systemic septic response: Does the organism matter? Crit. Care Med. *8:*55, 1980.

Wilmore, D.W., Long, J.M., and Mason, A.D., et al.: Catecholamines: mediator of the hypermetabolic response to thermal injury. Ann. Surg. *180:*653, 1974.

Wilmore, D.W.: Carbohydrate metabolism in trauma. Clin. Endocrinol. *5:*731, 1976.

CHAPTER 19

Pathology and Pathophysiology of the Systemic Toxicants Carbon Monoxide and Cyanide

YALE H. CAPLAN

Systemic poisons (toxicants) include a variety of chemical substances which may come into contact with the human body through both accidental and incidental means. These include carbon monoxide (CO) and cyanide as well as drugs, pesticides, solvents, and other materials available to man by means of ingestion or environmental exposure.

Toxicants may be classified into three groups:

1. toxicants affecting biochemical pathways (chemical asphyxiants);
2. toxicants affecting the central and peripheral nervous systems; and
3. toxicants acting as simple asphyxiants or otherwise affecting pulmonary function.

Many toxicants as well as other medical conditions produce anoxia. These have been classified as follows (Wiener, 1970):

1. Anoxic anoxia. This results from a reduction in the amount of O_2 available in the air, an obstruction of air passages, or CO poisoning.
2. Histotoxic anoxia. This results in the inability of tissue cells to utilize O_2 such as is the case with cyanide inhibiting intracellular oxidative enzymes.
3. Anemic anoxia. This results in a diminished O_2 carrying capacity of the blood such as occurs in blood loss or anemia.
4. Stagnant anoxia. This results from total or partial arrest of cerebral circulation as occurs in hanging or cardiac arrest.

This chapter will deal with the two principal chemical asphyxiants affecting biochemical pathways, namely CO and cyanide.

CARBON MONOXIDE

Carbon monoxide (CO) is perhaps the oldest toxicologic problem that man has encountered. Awareness of the effects of this substance date to the time that fire was first used. Fires started in caves that were used as shelters resulted in accidental poisonings. Greek writers in the 3rd century hypothesized that fumes from fire caused a thinness of air which in man obstructed normal breathing and resulted in insensible disturbances of motion and the senses. In 18th century Western Europe, many deaths due to CO were ascribed to the devil.

Carbon monoxide is an odorless, colorless compound which has a density less than that of air. It is produced in all situations where incomplete combustion of carbon-containing materials occurs. It is produced in gasoline engine exhaust, some illuminating gases, blast furnace and railroad locomotive stack gases, flue gases from water heaters and furnaces, and burning buildings and conflagrations. The concentrations of CO are highly variable depending on the nature of the source. Gasoline engine exhaust comprises the greatest single source, since 1 gallon of fuel can produce about 3 pounds of CO. Diesel engines, on the other hand, produce somewhat less CO. This exhaust poses no threat for the average driver, although personnel working in tunnels, garages, or other closed areas must exercise extreme care and caution. Faulty automobiles may result in CO build-up in the passenger compartments and ensuing intoxication or death. The toxicity of CO is greatly underrated by the general public. Since considerable quantities are produced by automobile exhaust, people fail to associate the gas with danger; however, in confined spaces or under appropriate circumstances, it can be rapidly fatal. A person exerting himself during a fire may die as the result of one or two breaths.

Toxicity

Carbon monoxide, which is otherwise chemically inert, rapidly combines with hemoglobin (Hb) in the red blood cell, thus incapacitating the vital respiratory pigment. It serves as a ligand to metals and reacts to form metal carbonyls. It is highly selective in this regard to both the metal and the oxidation and spin states. The ferro form of iron which is found in Hb meets the necessary requirements and is a suitable receptor. The red blood cell is inhibited in its function of carrying O_2 to the tissues from the lungs as well as carbon dioxide (CO_2) back from the tissues to the lungs. The reactions of CO and O_2 with Hb are similar in that CO occupies the same site as O_2 (Fenn and Rahn, 1964). Hb reacts with O_2 to form oxyhemoglobin (HbO_2) and with CO to form carboxyhemoglobin (HbCO). The reactions are reversible, as shown by the equations:

$$Hb + O_2 \rightleftharpoons HbO_2$$
$$Hb + CO \rightleftharpoons HbCO$$
$$CO + HbO_2 \rightleftharpoons O_2 + HbCO$$

The blood or Hb when exposed to an atmosphere containing both O_2 and CO becomes saturated in the proportion of 1 mol of O_2 or CO per atom of iron in the molecule. O_2 and CO are different, however, in that the partial pressure required for CO is 1/200–1/300 of that required for O_2; hence, when both gases are present, an equilibrium will be reached which has been described in the following equation (Haldane and Priestley, 1935):

$$\frac{HbCO}{HbO_2} = M \frac{PCO}{PO_2}$$

The number of moles of each gas is related to the respective partial pressures, and M is constant. The value for M has been measured by many workers and in human blood at physiologic pH and temperature usually lies in the range of 200–250. While species variation may be marked, very little variation occurs for individuals within each species. This remarkable affinity of CO for Hb, which is measured by the value for M, demonstrates that CO has an affinity for Hb which is 200–250 times that of O_2. Hence, relatively small amounts of CO in air can immobilize rather significant amounts of Hb.

The net result is a decrease in the amount of O_2 carried by the Hb. However, the presence of CO on the Hb molecule causes, in addition, a shift in the HbO_2 dissociation curve. Not only does the amount of O_2 bound by Hb decrease, but the O_2 which is carried is not released to be effectively utilized in cellular respiration. The O_2 molecules are said to "cling to the Hb with abnormal tenacity" (Haldane and Priestley, 1935). CO, therefore, causes the O_2 dissociation curve to be displaced to the left, in effect making the blood low in PO_2 as if the ambient air were low in O_2 (Fenn and Rahn, 1964).

The body of an average adult male contains enough Hb to hold about 1 liter of O_2 (about a 4-min supply). During bodily rest, about 30% of the O_2 in arterial blood is used; however, during exertion, this may increase to 70 or 80%, thus reducing substantially the large reserve factor and decreasing the margin of safety. A man at rest can, therefore, tolerate a temporary 30% reduction of the O_2 carrying capacity of his blood with little effect, perhaps limited only to a headache. Under exertion, however, the O_2 supply to the brain and other tissues rapidly becomes inadequate and fainting will usually result. Increasing the rate of pulmonary ventilation will shorten the time necessary for the CO in the air and blood to reach equilibrium. The concentration of the gas in the air breathed, the length of time it is breathed, and the volume of breathing during rest and work are all essential factors in determining the amount of CO absorbed. Absorption of CO from contaminated air is at first rapid. Upon continued exposure to moderate CO concentrations, the rate of absorption becomes somewhat slower. Even on prolonged exposure, CO displaces O_2 up to a point of equilibrium, depending upon the relative amounts of the two gases in the air. The distribution of the two gases always tends to an equilibrium determined by the products of the tensions and affinities of the two gases. The amount of CO that can be bound by Hb is usually greater in proportion to the amount in the air because of its increased affinity. No equilibrium is reached in rapidly fatal cases of intoxication. Short exposures at low concentrations are generally harmless.

Two individuals exposed to the same atmosphere may vary drastically in response. If a smaller and younger child is compared to a larger normal adult, the child with a more active metabolism and relatively larger volume of respiration can absorb more CO and more rapidly approach saturation. There is a rapid fall in cerebral circulation and O_2 utilization from childhood through adolescence, which is followed by a slower but progressive decrease throughout the remaining life span as follows (Wiener, 1970):

Age (years)	5	45	68
Cerebral blood flow (ml/100 g/min)	104	55	43
O_2 consumption (ml/100 g/min)	5.1	3.5	2.4

The fact that the binding force of CO to Hb is 200–250 times that of O_2 results in CO not being readily displaced from Hb. Therefore, prolonged exposures may result in the development of toxicity even from relatively low ambient air concentrations (Table 19.1). The induced anoxemia persists in a diminishing degree until all the gas has been eliminated from the blood. The effects resulting from varying percent saturation levels of HbCO are shown in Table 19.2. Since CO is prevalent in our environment, all people are exposed in varying degrees, and a normal saturation level is to be expected. Nonsmokers generally show less than 2% saturation, with moderate smokers showing up to 5% saturation, and heavy smokers up to 9% saturation. At these levels, signs and symptoms of intoxication are not generally produced. However, recent concern has been raised regarding chronic toxicity at low levels. When driving skills at HbCO saturation levels of 6, 11, and 17% were compared, statistically significant differences were noted which suggested some decrement in performance as the result of the CO exposure; however, the ability to drive motor vehicles was not seriously affected (McFarland, 1973).

Decreases in oxygen tension were related to lower birth weights found in infants born to women who smoked or were exposed to severe air pollution (Longo, 1976). At elevated levels, the toxic symptoms described in Table 19.2 become evident. In addition, the aftereffects of anoxemia such as headaches and disturbances in judgement persist for some time after an ample supply of O_2 has been restored. This represents an added burden when CO toxicity is compared to that of simple asphyxiants. In untreated cases, the slow elimination exposes the subject to a long period of asphyxia and delays recovery.

The biochemical exchange of O_2 for the metabolite CO_2 at the cellular level is also affected. The physiochemical dissociation of HbO_2 induces the catalytic enzymatic action required to facilitate the O_2 for CO_2 exchange. Since HbCO induces no such effect, there results an intracellular retention of CO_2 and a concomitant decrease in blood CO_2 content. CO_2 is important in the stimulation of respiratory centers since it affects the hydrogen ion concentrations in the blood. Arterial PO_2 is thereby unchanged, and specific stimulus to increased ventilation is lacking. CO asphyxia differs from suffo-

Table 19.1
Carbon Monoxide Toxicity[a]

Concentration in Air	Response
% (v/v)	
0.01	Allowable for an exposure of several hours
0.04–0.05	Can be inhaled for 1 hr without appreciable effect
0.06–0.07	Causing a just noticeable effect after 1 hr exposure
0.10–0.12	Causing unpleasant but not dangerous symptoms after 1 hr exposure
0.15–0.20	Dangerous for exposure of 1 hr
0.40 and above	Fatal in exposure of less than 1 hr

[a] Reprinted with permission from W. B. Deichmann and H. W. Gerarde. Carbon monoxide toxicity. *Symptomatology and Therapy of Toxicological Emergencies*, p. 449. Academic Press, New York, 1964.

Table 19.2
Carbon Monoxide Toxicity[a]

HbCO	Effect
% saturation	
10	Shortness of breath on vigorous muscular exertion
20	Shortness of breath on moderate exertion and slight headache
30	Decided headache, irritation, ready fatigue, and disturbance of judgement
40–50	Headache, confusion, collapse, and fainting on exertion
60–70	Unconsciousness, respiratory failure, and death if exposure is long continued
80	Rapidly fatal
Over 80	Immediately fatal

[a] Reprinted with permission from W. B. Deichmann and H. W. Gerarde: Carbon monoxide toxicity. *Symptomatology and Therapy of Toxicological Emergencies*, p. 449. Academic Press, New York, 1964.

cation since HbCO interferes with both the dissociation of HbO_2 and the elimination of CO_2 from the cells.

Carbon monoxide does not separate from the Hb spontaneously; rather it is displaced only by the mass action of O_2. The anoxemia resulting from exposure to elevated concentrations of CO is suffered mainly following removal from a contaminated atmosphere. It is important, therefore, to facilitate elimination and shorten the period of asphyxia. The speed with which treatment is received is directly proportional to the severity of symptoms and the time required for recovery. The essential condition in CO asphyxia is the interruption of the supply of O_2 to the tissues, particularly the brain. It is not the cessation of the movements of breathing, as may be the case with drowning or electric shock.

Although the toxicity of CO acting through a mechanism involving interaction with Hb seems sufficiently documented, there remain situations in which exposure to CO and the resulting toxicity do not produce the expected HbCO saturation results. It has been suggested that CO binding to myoglobin in heart and skeletal muscle is significant even in low exposure situations producing HbCO saturations of less than 5%; however, no conclusive proof has been presented to ascertain whether this binding is a significant cause of CO toxicity or sensitization of the myocardium to CO (Coburn, 1979). It has been suggested, without conclusive documentation, that CO toxicity is manifest through interaction with the iron-containing enzymes as the cytochromes.

Treatment

Treatment consists of removing the subject to fresh air. If breathing, administer O_2 or O_2 containing 5–10% CO_2. If not breathing, administer artificial respiration followed by the application of O_2 or an O_2/CO_2 mixture, continuing for 30 min after spontaneous respiration occurs. CO_2 acts as a respiratory and cardiac stimulant. It is reported to replace the CO_2 that the body has lost and to increase respiration and is said to be more effective than the administration of O_2 alone (Henderson and Haggard, 1943). There is, however, disagreement concerning the value of CO_2; in fact, no beneficial effect is actually observed. Patients suffering from severe CO poisoning show a critical metabolic acidosis, and superimposing a respiratory acidosis with CO_2 seems unsound (Arena, 1979). Pure O_2 therapy should be instituted as rapidly as possible. Use of a face mask and O_2 under pressure of up to 2.5 atmospheres is preferable. If revival is necessary, the application of high partial pressures of O_2 or the use of a hyperbaric chamber can be considerably beneficial. It takes 250 min of breathing ordinary air or 40 min of breathing pure O_2 to reduce the HbCO saturation level to one-half of its value (Arena, 1979).

Oxygen toxicity should be avoided. A too high partial pressure of O_2 can cause convulsions and add to the CO toxicity. A suggested treatment schedule in a severe case consists of the administration of 100% O_2 in a pressure chamber as follows (Arena, 1979): 1) 25 psi for 20 min; 2) 15 psi for 20 min; 3) 5 psi for 90 min; and 4) 6 hr at normal atmospheric pressure. During the 2-hr period, 75–80% of the CO should be eliminated.

Delayed aftereffects are possible, and after serious poisoning the prognosis is guarded and hospitalization advisable. Myocardial toxicity should be monitored, using serial EKGs and LDH, SGOT, and CPK determinations. This includes mild cases since myocardial toxicity does not correlate well with the HbCO saturation level.

The maximum allowable concentration permitted in industrial situations is 50 ppm. Although this figure is relatively low, it may still be too high for prolonged exposures. The following rule of thumb has been applied to assess safety. Multiply the hours of exposure by parts per 10,000. If the result is 3, no perceptible affect should be expected; if 6, symptoms are mild; if 9, symptoms become pronounced; if 15, death may ensue. This rule is particularly applicable when short periods of time are to be considered (Arena, 1979).

Laboratory Diagnosis

Diagnosis in cases of CO poisoning is largely a function of a review of history and circumstances surrounding the finding of the patient. If the CO saturation level exceeds 30%, a carmine coloration to the skin becomes evident. Milder cases can only be diagnosed by laboratory analysis of the blood. Acute symptoms resemble alcohol intoxication, whereas chronic exposures may be mistaken for epilepsy. Laboratory tests, therefore, become an important indicator to both facilitate diagnosis and monitor treatment.

A number of techniques are available for determining the HbCO saturation level of blood. For clinical situations, photometric methods are sufficiently precise and accurate as well as relatively simple and quick to perform. While many methods and variations have been reported, one reliable method (Tietz and Fiereck, 1973) employs a blood hemolysate prepared by diluting a blood sample with 0.4% ammonium hydroxide. Sodium dithionite is added to deoxygenate the HbO_2 without affecting the HbCO. The reduced sample is then measured in a spectrophotometer at 541 and 555 nm. The absorbance ratio of the 541/555 nm peaks is compared with standards containing known amounts of HbCO, and the percentage of HbCO in the sample is determined. This method is readily adaptable to any laboratory possessing a spectrophotometer but is highly dependent upon the calibration of the spectrophotometer. A more complicated technique which can produce instantaneous answers is the CO-Oximeter. Here, a spectrophotometer is coupled with a special minianalog computer. A blood sample is automatically diluted, and the absorption at three wavelengths (548, 568, 578 nm) is read simultaneously. The three absorbances are programmed in an electronic computational matrix which computes the HbCO and HbO_2 saturation levels as well as the percentage of hemoglobin. This commercially available instrument system is exceptionally rapid and requires only limited laboratory skills.

CYANIDE

Hydrogen cyanide (HCN) is one of the most lethal substances known to man. It was available to assassins from the earliest of times and has been used medicinally as well. It was employed as a war gas by the British and French during World War I and by the Germans in their mass extermination programs during World War II. It has found favor for the execution of criminals in the United States and other countries. As a drug, its use as a sedative was eventually deleted on the basis of its toxicity. It was used intravenously in the form of a 0.1% solution as a respiratory stimulant. Certain fruits, such as the pits or seeds from peaches, apricots, almonds, plums, cherries, chokeberries, apples, jet beads, and cassava beans, and some older pharmaceutical preparations, such as oil of bitter almond and cherry laurel water, contained cyanogenetic glycosides like amygdalin. It has been demonstrated that the cyanide content of 100 g of moist peach seed is 88 mg, cultivated apricot is 8.9 mg, and wild apricot is 217 mg (Arena, 1979). This glycoside is also the principal component of the questionable drug Laetrile, purported to be useful in the treatment of cancer. Laetrile has been reported to be responsible for the death of an 11-month old girl whose father was taking the drug—the child ingested 1 to 5 tablets (500 mg) of amygdalin (Laetrile) (Humbert et al., 1977).

Cyanide in the form of the free acid (HCN) is also known as prussic or hydrocyanic acid and is commonly available as potassium and sodium salts. HCN is a colorless volatile liquid which has a boiling point near room temperature at 25.6–26.1°C. It is a weak acid which is miscible with water and alcohol. The salts, on the other hand, are odorless; however, they readily deliquese and upon reaction with water form HCN, which possesses the characteristic almond odor. The salts are strong bases and cause direct caustic damage to the tissues to which they come into contact. Cyanide products are readily available since they are sold in hardware stores as common rodenticides. Cyanide derivatives such as acrylonitrile, cyanamide, and cyanogen chloride are used as fumigants and metal cleaners, in the refining of ores, and in the production of synthetic rubber. Cyanides are used in the home and in a number of industries such as in the process of electroplating, silver polishing, and photography. They are also produced by the burning of polymeric materials such as wool, silk, nylon, and polyurethane foam.

Toxicity

Hydrogen cyanide is highly toxic, and following the inhalation of sufficient quantities, symptoms usually appear within seconds. Through oral ingestion and skin contact, symptoms are delayed for minutes. Death occurs almost immediately with larger doses. The average lethal dose of HCN taken by mouth is thought to be from 60 to 90 mg (Gettler and Baine, 1938), which corresponds to about 1 tsp of 2% solution of HCN, or about 200 mg of KCN (Gettler and Baine, 1938; Gettler and St. George, 1934). The minimum fatal dose is approximately 50 mg, and the minimal acceptable concentration in air is 10 ppm (Arena, 1979).

Cyanide is a chemical asphyxiant, depriving tissues of their ability to utilize O_2 by inhibition of the electron transport system. Cyanide reacts reversibly with the ferric ion of cytochrome oxidase to form a cytochrome oxidase-cyanide complex, which is incapable of participating in the electron transport system of the cell. The result is a histotoxic anoxia, which causes cellular respiration to be inhibited. This mechanism was elucidated using a cytochrome c-cytochrome oxidase complex to oxidize hydroquinone. It was noted that when cyanide was added to this system, oxidation stopped; however, when more cytochrome oxidase was added, the oxidation was resumed (Stotz et al., 1938). The inhibiting effect of cyanide is due to the combination of cyanide with the iron of the prosthetic group of cytochrome oxidase. Therefore, cyanide action has been described as "internal asphyxia." The respiratory center of the medulla is affected and ceases to function. Its nerve cells can no longer obtain the O_2 required for their respiration. The venous blood becomes bright red, resembling arterial blood, since the tissues have not been able to use the O_2 delivered to them.

Hydrogen cyanide is of low molecular weight and poorly ionized. It is rapidly absorbed through the skin and all mucosal surfaces including the lungs and gastrointestinal tract. The bronchial mucosa and alveoli are particularly expedient in this regard. The effects of various concentrations of HCN in the atmosphere when inhaled by man are shown in Table 19.3. The lower the concentration inhaled the higher the total dose that is required to produce toxicity or death. This is because at high concentrations, there is a rapid overloading of endogenous detoxification mechanisms. However, at lower concentrations the rate of detoxification may be adequate, thus reducing the rate of accumulation in the body. The alkali salts (KCN, NaCN) are only toxic following oral ingestion.

Metabolism and Treatment

The principal route of detoxification by the body is the enzymatic conversion to the thiocyanate radical (CNS), which is relatively nontoxic. The two enzymes responsible for this process are rhodanese and β-mercap-

Table 19.3
Effects of Various Concentrations of Hydrogen Cyanide (HCN) in the Atmosphere[a]

Atmospheric concentration of HCN	Remarks
ppm	
10	Maximum permissible concentration
20	Slight symptoms after several hr
100	Very dangerous within 1 hr
200–400	Lethal within 30 min
2000	Immediately lethal

[a] Reprinted with permission from B. Ballantyne: *Forensic Toxicology*. John Wright and Sons, Ltd., Bristol, England, 1974.

topyruvate-cyanide transsulphurase (Sorbo, 1962). Rhodanese, or thiosulphate/cyanide sulphurtransferase (EC 2.8.1.2), is found mainly in the liver and kidney and catalyzes the reaction of cyanide to thiocyanate as follows:

$$CN^- + S_2O_3^{2-} \rightarrow CNS^- + SO_3^{2-}$$

β-Mercaptopyruvate-cyanide transulphurase, or 3-mercaptopyruvate:cyanide sulphurtransferase (EC2.8.1.2), is found in the blood, liver, and kidney and catalyzes the conversion of cyanide to thiocyanate as follows:

$$HSCH_2COCOO^- + CN^- \rightarrow CNS^- + CH_3COCOO^-$$

Some cyanide combines with Hb to form a stable non-O_2-bearing compound, cyanhemoglobin. This reaction occurs slowly, and only a small amount of cyanhemoglobin is formed. The toxicity is, therefore, not due to the formation of cyanhemoglobin (Arena, 1979), as is the case with the formation of HbCO in CO poisoning. Toxicity from cyanide is due strictly to inhibition of tissue cell respiration.

Acute cyanide intoxication is one of the most rapid modes of death. In general, a few breaths from a contaminated atmosphere or even a single breath may fall a man. Breathing may continue at greatly increased volume for a brief period, but death occurs almost immediately. In less acute situations, the symptoms of ordinary anoxia are seen more clearly. These include giddiness, headache, palpitation, dyspnea, and ultimately unconsciousness. Death usually occurs within 1 hr but may be delayed up to 3 hr. If a patient can be kept alive and treated, his chances for recovery are improved, although mortality from cyanide intoxication is near 95%.

Treatment must be rapid. If poisoning is the result of ingestion, gastric lavage using large amounts of water is mandatory. Potassium permanganate 1:5000 or hydrogen peroxide, 1% of the official preparation, may be used as chemical antidotes for this purpose; however, their value is limited. It is more important to facilitate detoxification through biochemical means. Amyl nitrite pearls are broken in a handkerchief or gauze and held over the patient's nose until sodium nitrite solution (10 ml, 3%) can be administered intravenously. This is followed by a solution of sodium thiosulfate (50 ml, 25%). Such treatment is dependent upon the nitrite's ability to oxidize the Hb (ferro) to methemoglobin (ferri) and the successful competition for cyanide ions by the methemoglobin. Hence, the cyanide will be prevented from interacting with the cytochrome oxidase (ferri). It has been demonstrated that methemoglobin competes with cytochrome oxidase for the cyanide ion (Album, et al., 1946). Cyanmethemoglobin, once formed, is metabolized slowly, predominantly in the liver and kidney (Westley, 1973). Then as an aid to the cyanmethemoglobin metabolism, thiosulfate is administered to provide a source of sulfur, facilitating conversion to the nontoxic thiocyanate, which is then excreted in urine. If symptoms recur, the treatment may be repeated. Epinephrine or ephedrine may be administered if blood pressure should drop sharply.

Cobalt ethylenediaminetetraacetate (Kelocyanor) and aminophenols have been used in Europe, replacing the nitrite-thiosulfate procedure, and appear to produce methemoglobin more rapidly with less risk of toxicity. Two ampuls of Kelocyanor solution (20 ml, 1.5%) are injected intravenously followed by glucose (20 ml, 50%). A cobalt chelate is formed, producing ultimately vitamin B_{12}. Methylene blue has also been used in the past but was less effective, since it produced methemoglobin much more slowly. O_2 is generally more available than other modes of treatment and should always be considered. Some experimental data have shown that high O_2 tension blocks the respiratory gasp reaction to intravenous cyanide in man, partially revises electrocardiographic anoxic changes in dogs, and protects goldfish from lethal doses (Arena, 1979). Since the methemoglobenia induced by the nitrite-thiosulfate treatment also reduces the ability of the blood to transport O_2 to the brain, O_2 therapy is recommended as an adjunct to the nitrite-thiosulfate therapy.

Nitroprusside sodium (Nipride) is used intravenously as a hypotensive agent. It is a potent, immediate acting compound whose action is probably due to the nitroso group. The effect of the drug is immediate and terminates when the infusion is stopped. The brief duration of action is due to its rapid metabolism to cyanide and thiocyanate. With excessive use, signs of thiocyanate toxicity appear; however, in gross overdose situations or in patients with hepatic insufficiency, cyanide intoxication is possible. More recently, the drug has been used chronically, and human fatalities have been reported. Dog studies have been described which recommend that drug administration should not exceed 0.5 mg/kg/hr, that thiosulfate be administered simultaneously to protect against toxicity, and that serum thiocyanate levels do not predict or reflect cyanide toxicity (Michenfelder and Tinker, 1977).

Pathology

Animals killed by intramuscular injections of HCN do not present specific anatomical or histological lesions at autopsy (Ballantyne et al., 1970). When death is rapid, the only changes observed may be slight cyanosis of the face, frothing at the lips, and mild congestion of the stomach. The only diagnostic clue might be the smell of burnt almonds in the body, but it is estimated that 20–40% of the population are unable to detect the odor of HCN (Gwilt, 1961). The color of HbO_2 may not be present when death is rapid (Pryce and Ross, 1963). These findings are consistent with HCN deaths in man where HCN was inhaled or injected.

Poisoning by the alkali metal (sodium and potassium) cyanides, on the other hand, provides greater diagnostic information regarding the cause of death. For example, the blood in some cases takes on a brick red color due to cyanmethemoglobin that was produced postmortem from HbO_2. The color of cyanmethemoglobin is a deeper red than HbCO. Internally, a bright red coloration of muscles and capillaries may be apparent. Although a small amount of cyanhemoglobin may exist, its presence is clearly not implicated in the cause of death (Arena, 1979). The stomach wall will exhibit burns and bleeding from contact with the highly alkaline salts.

Postmortem findings in a decomposed body are not reliable due to the disappearance of cyanide. The production of cyanide by putrefaction has been shown to be negligible (Gettler and Baine, 1938). Cyanide loss is due to its reaction with putrefaction aldehydes and ketones to form cyanohydrins, which are converted to α-hydroxy acids and finally to α-amino acids during putrefaction. If a body has been embalmed or tissue stored in formaldehyde preparations, the cyanide analysis would be unreliable (Svirbely and Roth, 1953, 1954). However, this is not the case with refrigerated or frozen samples, where cyanide has been shown to increase or decrease substantially (Svirbely and Roth, 1953; Caplan and Altman, 1976). No mechanism has been postulated to elucidate the cause of cyanide loss or production at reduced temperatures.

To demonstrate the instability of cyanide in biological fluids, 36 female albino rabbits were injected with a lethal dose of potassium cyanide. Half of the animals were stored (10–15°C) in situ in sealed plastic bags, and the other half were autopsied and the organs stored (10–15°C) in airtight containers (Ballantyne, 1974). Analysis of these samples showed a higher cyanide concentration in blood than in any other tissue, as was expected. Over a 3-week period, analyses for cyanide were performed at various time intervals. Samples that were isolated at time of death were more stable than those left in the body for storage, since the concentration of cyanide in the latter decreased at a faster rate. All concentrations of cyanide decreased with time.

Laboratory Diagnosis

The presence of cyanide can often be detected by the burnt almond odor imparted to the blood or other specimen. It can further be detected by the increases noted in serum or urine thiocyanate determinations. Since these do not always follow cyanide intoxication in a predictable fashion, it may become necessary to determine cyanide directly in the blood. Prior to chemical analysis, the cyanide must be separated from the blood. Under acidic conditions, as achieved by diluting blood three–five fold with solutions of tartaric or sulfuric acid (0.1 N), any cyanide ions are converted to the acid form (HCN), which is volatile, and can be separated by aeration or diffusion into a 0.1 N solution of KOH. Cyanide is unstable in blood, hence, the separation should be completed as soon as possible; however, after separation the KCN is appreciably more stable and can be analyzed after standing for several days.

A number of methods have been employed for the quantitative analysis. These include colorimetry, gas chromatography, and potentiometry using an ion selective electrode. An established colorimetric method is that in which chloramine T reacts with the HCN to form cyanogen chloride (Epstein, 1947). The cyanogen chloride is reacted with pyridine, which hydrolyzes to glutaconic aldehyde. This aldehyde is condensed with 1-phenyl-3-methyl-2-pyrazolin-5-one to form a blue dye, which is measured quantitatively at 630 nm. This method is specific; however, it lacks sensitivity and may require a larger specimen.

A gas chromatographic method with specificity of the colorimetric method and a sensitivity to 0.01 mg/liter has been reported (Valentour et al., 1974). HCN is reacted with chloramine T to form cyanogen chloride which is chromatographed by using a 5% Hallcomid M-18 column and detected with an electron capture detector. This method is suitable for both forensic and clinical applications, although it requires equipment not generally available in a clinical laboratory.

More recently, several potentiometric methods using an ion-specific electrode have been reported (McAnalley et al., 1979; Egekeze and Oehme, 1979). These methods are comparatively simple in that they require only an appropriate potentiometer such as an expanded scale pH meter and one of several commercially available electrodes. The diffused cyanide in a KOH solution is measured directly and compared to a series of standards. The method is sensitive to 0.01 mg/liter; however, it is not as specific as the other methods. Sulfides, for example, will interfere. Confirmation would be required for forensic cases; however, for clinical situations such as a rapid technique for monitoring nitroprusside therapy, these methods are well suited.

Cyanide may be present as a normal constituent of blood specimens; hence, an estimation of these concentrations is necessary to facilitate interpretation. Foods containing cyanocobalamin (vitamin B_{12}), conversion of thiocyanate formed as a by-product of cystine metabolism, and cigarette smoking produce low concentrations of cyanide in blood. Several studies indicated that these normal concentrations ranged up to 0.5 mg/liter. A study of 118 normal subjects including postmortem cases and healthy living subjects (smokers and nonsmokers) established a mean ranging from 0.05–0.07 mg/liter and an upper limit of 0.22 mg/liter (Caplan and Altman, 1976). Although fatal concentrations are usually above 10 mg/liter, this is the result of the excessive overdosage often encountered. Toxicity and lethality may occur from concentrations approximating 2 mg/liter.

CARBON MONOXIDE AND CYANIDE IN FIRE CASUALTY

Injury or fatality as the result of fires affects a significant and large portion of the population. In Maryland, approximately 100 people die in fires each year and hundreds more are injured. The causes of these casualties are not as simple as they may appear. What causes these deaths and the failure of people to escape from fires has been the subject of extensive research over the last 6 years (Birky et al., 1979). Many of the casualties result from "smoke inhalation," an insult to the respiratory system by the products of combustion. Combustible materials produce many toxic gases and vapors including CO, nitrogen oxide, HCN, formic acid, acetic acid, acrolein, sulphur dioxide, halogen acids, ammonia, aldehydes, benzene, phenol, and azo-bis-succino-nitrile (Rabash, 1966). "Smoke" in fires is generally considered to be comprised of irritants, such as hydrochloric acid, causing inflammation of the respiratory tract; asphyxiants such as CO and HCN affecting O_2 transport or utilization; and other materials which may affect the central nervous system.

Carbon monoxide is the major contributor in most fire fatalities; however, more recently, with the advent of increased use of plastic and synthetic materials by the home building and furnishing industries, concern has focused on HCN. Any nitrogen-containing material on combustion will produce cyanide. The toxic atmosphere in a fire will vary as a function of the materials burning, the temperature, the amount of O_2 available, as well as other factors. When coupled with individual biological variations and responses to a fire situation, the outcome is difficult to predict. The increased use of synthetic materials correlates with a three-fold increase in fire-related deaths recorded since 1955; however, there is little direct evidence linking these events. Several government-sponsored studies have reported the concentrations of CO and HCN produced by the combustion of 1 g of various materials in 1 m^3 of air space (Wagner, 1972; Ives et al., 1972). These are shown in Table 19.4. The polymeric materials contribute to the hazard of a fire by producing more smoke and toxic gases. In the case of polyurethane, the smoke generated is more dense than that produced by wood. Smoke density could be a critical factor for the panicked adult or child trying to escape a fire. Simply not being able to find an exit may result in death. If escape is also prevented or delayed by the presence of a toxic gas, the increased time of exposure to CO will increase the risk to life.

The Maryland study focused on CO and cyanide (Birky et al., 1979). CO was studied in 530 fatal cases. A HbCO saturation level of 50% or greater was found in 60% of these cases. The 50% saturation level was defined as that sufficient in and of itself to cause death. In those cases where the 50% saturation level was not reached, other factors were considered. In 20% of the cases, a combination of CO plus pre-existing cardiovascular disease was responsible for death, whereas burns were the cause in 11% of the cases. The 9% of cases which were listed as unexplained by CO or disease were the result of a combination of CO with other toxicants such as HCN, alcohol, or drugs.

Blood cyanide concentrations were determined in 272 fatalities. The toxicological significance of cyanide is difficult to assess since it is not well known from the literature or other animal experimental studies what environmental cyanide concentration will produce a corresponding blood concentration and physiological effect. A blood cyanide concentration of 0.25 mg/liter was established as normal for the purposes of determining exposure in these cases. Table 19.5 shows the distribution of blood cyanide concentrations in the 272 fire fatalities in Maryland. Normal concentrations would not be expected to elicit any biological effect, although concentrations exceeding 0.26 mg/liter are indicative of the presence of cyanide produced from burning building materials. Concentrations exceeding 1.0 mg/liter could be suspected of toxic implications. Evaluation of these results, by computing the mean cyanide concentrations on a yearly basis, showed no change in the pattern as a function of the introduction of more synthetic furnishings (1975–1978).

A correlation of blood cyanide concentrations in these cases with CO saturation levels shows that potentially dangerous cyanide concentrations were associated with high CO saturation levels. When cyanide was high, CO was high. No low CO levels were associated with high cyanide concentrations. Deaths could not be explained by the cyanide concentrations that were not otherwise explained. However, it is expected that cyanide and other toxicants could have played an intermediate role leading to early incapacitation which prevented escape. As a consequence the victim continued to be exposed to high levels of CO.

When the relationship between CO and cyanide is correlated by dividing all cases into 4 categories based on those which were normal or abnormal in cyanide and those which were above or below a 30% HbCO saturation level, the results are as follows:

1. 58% of cases show CO above 30% saturation and abnormal cyanide, reflecting exposure to both CO and cyanide;

Table 19.4
Concentration of Hydrogen Cyanide (HCN) and Carbon Monoxide (CO) Produced by Combustion of 1 g of Various Materials in m^3 Air Space[a]

Materials	Concentration	
	CO	HCN
	ppm	
Wool	5,000–50,000	13,000–26,000
Silk	30,000–44,000	22,000–68,000
Phenolic resins	41	2.7
Melamine resins with fillers	68	225
Foamed polyvinyl chloride	36	2.7
Polyurethane foam		6,000
Nylon		3,900
Douglas Fir	9,400	30

[a] Condensed from Ives et al., National Bureau of Standards Report No. 10807, 1972 and Wagner, Johns Hopkins University Applied Physics Laboratory Topical Report FPP TR11, 1972.

Table 19.5
Distribution of Blood Cyanide Concentrations in 272 Fire Fatalities Occurring in Maryland During the Period January 1, 1975–December 31, 1977

Cyanide concentration	Degree of toxicity	%
mg/liter		
0.00–0.25	None (normal)	31
0.26–1.00	Subtoxic	35
1.01–2.00	Possible toxic	24
2.01 and above	Probable toxic	10
		100

2. 13% of cases show CO above 30% and normal cyanide, reflecting the absence of cyanide-producing materials in the fire;
3. 21% of cases show CO below 30% and normal cyanide, which reflects fires in which the gases were not a factor, that is, death occurred prior to the fire or from natural causes.
4. 8% of cases show CO below 30% and abnormal cyanide. If cyanide were a principal factor, this number would be significant; however, the low number represents borderline cases which were explained by other factors.

The role of cyanide in fire fatalities is as an intermediary intoxicant, or it is merely a marker showing the presence of cyanide precursor materials in a fire. It was observed during the study of these fires that when multiple fatalities occurred, the cyanide concentrations found in the victims was proportional to the distance from which they were removed from the center of the fire, that is, the further away, the higher the concentration. Although this seems paradoxical, the phenomenon is consistent with what is known regarding fire chemistry. When nitrogen-containing materials burn, cyanide is produced in the fire rapidly and before CO. The cyanide produced is unstable to further heating at high temperatures; thus cyanide would break down as a function of the temperature of the fire environment. Therefore, the closer to the fire source, the lower the concentration that is expected for cyanide. On the other hand, the closer to the fire source, the concentrations and risk from CO become greater.

Some animal experimentation has been conducted which supports the concept that cyanide may act as an intermediary intoxicant. Experiments using rats showed that an atmosphere of 50 ppm HCN alone caused no fatalities and that 2000 ppm CO alone caused no fatalities, but 10–20 ppm HCN and 2000 ppm CO combined caused fatalities. It was postulated that HCN increased the respiration rate of the rats, resulting in an increased CO intake which could cause death in a relatively short period (Moss et al., 1951). The synergistic effect of CO and HCN in mice exposed to gas mixtures has also been reported (Pryor et al., 1969). In a real fire situation, the toxic potential is the sum, either additive or synergistic, of all the various factors that may cause death or incapacitation. Hence, the production of HCN could be significant in a fire containing such polymeric materials.

A study of the effects of CO and intravenous cyanide on cerebral circulation and metabolism in the dog has been reported (Pitt et al., 1979). Cerebral blood flow increased to 130 and 200% of control with elevations in HbCO to 30 and 51% or with elevations in blood cyanide concentrations to 1.0 and 1.5 mg/liter, respectively. Cerebral O_2 consumption remained unchanged until the higher level of CO or cyanide was reached. When CO and cyanide were administered simultaneously, cerebral blood flow increased in an additive manner, but significant decreases in cerebral O_2 consumption occurred at the combination of the lower concentrations. This suggests that CO and cyanide are physiologically additive in producing changes in cerebral blood flow but may act synergistically on cerebral metabolism.

References

Album, H., Tepperman, J., and Bodansky, O.: A spectrophotometric study of the competition of methemoglobin and cytochrome oxidase for cyanide in vitro. J. Biol. Chem. *163:* 641, 1946.

Arena, J.M.: *Poisoning—Toxicology, Symptoms, Treatments,* ed. 4, p. 827. Charles C Thomas, Springfield, IL, 1979.

Ballantyne, B.: The forensic diagnosis of acute cyanide poisoning. In: *Forensic Toxicology,* edited by B. Ballantyne, p. 99. John Wright and Sons, Ltd., Bristol, England, 1974.

Ballantyne, B., Bright, J., and Williams, P.: Levels of cyanide in whole blood and serum following lethal intramuscular injections to experimental animals. Med. Sci. Law *10:*225, 1970.

Birky, M.M., Halpin, B.M., Caplan, Y.H., Fisher, R.S., McAllister, J.M., and Dixon, A.M.: Fire fatality study. Fire and Materials *3:*211, 1979.

Caplan, Y.H., and Altman, R.: Microdetermination of cyanide in fire fatalities. Presented at the 25th Annual Meeting of the American Academy of Forensic Sciences, Washington, DC, 1976.

Coburn, R.F.: Mechanisms of carbon monoxide toxicity. Prev. Med. *8:*310, 1979.

Egekeze, J.O., and Oehme, F.W.: Direct potentiometric method for the determination of cyanide in biological materials. J. Analyt. Toxicol. *3:*119, 1979.

Epstein, J.: Estimation of microquantities of cyanide. Anal. Chem. *19:*272, 1947.

Fenn, W.O., and Rahn, H.: *Respiration,* vol. 1. American Physiological Society, Washington, DC, 1964.

Gettler, A.O., and Baine, J.O.: The toxicology of cyanide. Am. J. Med. Sci. *195:*182, 1938.

Gettler, A.O., and St. George, A.V.: Cyanide poisoning. Am. J. Clin. Pathol. *4:*420, 1934.

Gwilt, J.R.: Odour of (potassium) cyanide. Med. Leg. J. *29:*98, 1961.

Haldane, J.S., and Priestley, J.G.: *Respiration.* Yale University Press, New Haven, CT, 1935.

Henderson, Y., and Haggard, H.: *Noxious Gases and the Principles of Respiration Influencing Their Action,* (American Chemical Society Monograph Series) ed. 2, 294 pp. Reinhold, New York, 1943.

Humbert, J.R., Tress, J.H., and Braico, K.T.: Fatal cyanide poisoning: accidental ingestion of amygdalin. J.A.M.A. *238:* 482, 1977.

Ives, J.M., Hughes, E.E., and Taylor, J.K.: Toxic atmospheres associated with real fire situations. *National Bureau of Standards Report 10807.* U. S. Government Printing Office, Washington, DC, 1972.

Longo, L. D.: Carbon monoxide: Effects on oxygenation of the fetus in utero. Science *194:*523, 1976.

McAnalley, B.H., Lowrey, W.T., Oliver, R.D., and Garriott, J.C.: Determination of inorganic sulfide and cyanide in blood using specific ion electrodes: application to the investigation of hydrogen sulfide and cyanide poisoning. J. Analyt. Toxicol. *3:*111, 1979.

McFarland, R.A.: Low level exposure to carbon monoxide and driving performance. Arch. Environ. Health *27:*355, 1973.

Michenfelder, J.D., and Tinker, J.H.: Cyanide toxicity and thiosulfate protection during chronic administration of sodium nitroprusside in the dog. Anesthesiology *47:*441, 1977.

Moss, R.H., Jackson, C.F., and Saberlick, J.: Toxicity of carbon monoxide and hydrogen cyanide gas mixtures. Arch. Ind. Hyg. Occup. Med. *4:*53, 1951.

Pitt, B.R., Radford, E.P., Gurnter, G.H., and Traystman, R.J.: Interaction of carbon monoxide and cyanide on cerebral circulation and metabolism. Arch. Environ. Health *34:*354, 1979.

Pryce, D.M., and Ross, C.F.: *Ross's Postmortem Appearances,* ed. 6. Oxford University Press, London, 1963.

Pryor, A.J., Johnson, D.E., and Jackson, N.N.: Hazards of smoke and toxic gases produced in urban fires. Southwest Research Institute, OCD Work Unit 2537 B, San Antonio, Texas, 1969.

Rasbash, D.J.: Smoke and toxic gas. Fire, pp. 174–175, 1966.

Sorbo, B.: Enzymatic conversion of cyanide to thiocyanate. In *Proceedings of the First International Pharmacology Meeting,* vol. 6, p. 121. Stockholm, 1962.

Stotz, E., Atshcul, A., and Hogness, T.R.: The cytochrome *c*-cytochrome oxidase complex. J. Biol. Chem., *124:*745, 1938.

Svirbely, W.J., and Roth, J.F.: Carbonyl reactions. I. The kinetics of cyanohydrin formation in aqueous solution. J. Am. Chem. Soc. *75:*3106, 1953.

Svirbely, W.J., and Roth, J.F.: Analytical applications of the cyanohydrin reaction. Anal. Chem. *26:*1377, 1954.

Tietz, N.W., and Fiereck, E.A.: The spectrophotometric measurement of carboxyhemoglobin. Ann. Clin. Lab. Sci. *3:*36, 1973.

Valentour, J., Aggarwal, V., and Sunshine, I.: Sensitive gas chromatographic determination of cyanide. Anal. Chem. *46:*924, 1974.

Wagner, J.P.: Survey of the toxic species evolved in the pyrolysis and combustion of polymers. Topical Report FPP TR11. Applied Physics Laboratory, Johns Hopkins University, Silver Spring, MD, 1972.

Westley, J.: Rhodanese. In *Advances in Enzymology,* edited by A. Meister, vol. 39, p. 327. Wiley-Interscience, New York, 1973.

Wiener, M.F.: Carbon monoxide poisoning: basic concepts and current clinical-pathologic implications. In *Laboratory Diagnosis of Diseases Caused by Toxic Agents,* edited by F.W. Sunderman and F.W. Sunderman, Jr., ch. 26A. Warren H. Green, St. Louis, 1970.

PART 2

ORGAN DYSFUNCTIONS IN SHOCK

EDITORS' SUMMARY

Reduction in tissue perfusion and oxygenation secondary to a drop in systemic blood pressure are characteristic of the shock process. Once set into action, shock can trigger an irrevocable cycle of events which can cause organ, tissue, and cell failure and eventually death, even if the precipitating cause is eventually corrected.

While most organ systems are involved to a lesser or greater extent, space only allows discussion of those organs which are of most interest to the editors; one should not conclude that these are the only organs involved in shock. This section deals with organ dysfunction in shock and, as described, we have selected several organ systems for study because of their important role in the shock process. Shock is not a single etiological entity, but rather is a complex process which, if allowed to continue untreated or only partially treated, can result in dysfunction and/or failure of virtually any organ system. For a variety of circulatory and metabolic reasons, however, some organs are much more susceptible; skeletal muscle is one example of a tissue that is extremely resistant to ischemia and anoxia.

Whether or not failure occurs in one or more organ systems in shock depends on the length of time at risk and the severity of the shock process. To most observers, when organ failure occurs it is an indication that this process was either not identified initially or that the therapy was inadequate. Whatever the reason, when organ dysfunction or failure occurs, therapy becomes prolonged or unattainable for survival. The patient's demise is frequently attributed to some other cause or event.

Generally, organ dysfunction is difficult to assess because of the masking effect of the shock process itself. In the past 15 years, especially during the Viet Nam War, most physicians concluded that the major underlying focus of organ failure in patients during shock occurred in the lung, resulting in the vague and controversial term of "shock lung." It became evident later that the "shock lung syndrome" often resulted from fluid overload in treating military personnel. During this time, there was little discussion of the role played by the liver, a long overlooked organ in the shock process, and one wonders why this "biochemical energy and detoxification factory" was not an earlier subject for intensive shock research. Beecher (1949), however, noted the possible role of liver dysfunction in his studies of wounded men in World War II.

In the chapter on the liver, we review our clinical and experimental experience. Hepatic parenchymal cell alterations occur very early in both hemorrhagic and septic shock, though the effects on energy charge are initially the opposite, at least in experimental animals. The energy charge is decreased in hemorrhagic shock and is initially increased in septic shock. Later, however, both are depressed. We infer that this is the result of primary damage from ischemia and hypoxia in hemorrhagic shock and initial cell membrane damage with septic shock. Later, in septic shock, ischemia probably also occurs. Another difference between the two types of shock is the massive increase of autophagic vacuoles in septic shock. This probably correlates with the greatly increased protein degradation that occurs in septic shock and certainly explains the large cytoplasmic inclusions seen by light microscopy. Many of these latter changes are related to modulation of hormones—especially the marked increase in glucagon that occurs. Many of these changes in hepatocellular structure and function have not been emphasized in the past, probably because they are not visible without ultrastructural methods.

Clearly these are significant changes from the standpoint of the liver cell; their overall significance to the patient is less clear. It is evident, however, that such alterations may make major contributions to altered body economy, such as increased gluconeogenesis, increased protein degradation, altered blood coagulation, and altered serum protein levels.

The chapter by Mittermayer and Riede extends the consideration of injury to the gastrointestinal tract in shock. This area is largely neglected by clinicians because diagnosis is very difficult and usually not accomplished. On the other hand, these lesions are quite familiar to the pathologist who performs autopsies on patients dying from hemorrhagic and septic shock. Unfortunately, in the past, pathologists have usually regarded these as "terminal events," as if terminal events did not typically indicate that shock was indeed a terminal event in the patient.

This chapter emphasizes the role of microcirculatory disorders in the pathogenesis of a variety of mucosal lesions in the stomach, duodenum, and large intestine. Though they may often be very mild, they can also be extremely severe, culminating in death. The authors emphasize the role of proteolytic enzymes and ischemic epithelial necrosis in their pathogenesis.

Jones and Linhardt, in discussing the exocrine pancreas in shock, suggest that the "dying pancreas" has a role in perpetuating or exacerbating "shock." Certainly the changes in acinar cells are similar to those in the liver. They conclude that there is increased autophagy in the exocrine pancreas, as there is in other cells. If pancreatic perfusion could be isolated and maintained and survival was found, this could enhance the conclusion that pancreatic changes, including autophagy, constitute a major spoke in the "wheel of shock." The organ is of great interest and may play a greater role in the shock process than we think. More needs to be known concerning the modulation of insulin and glucagon secretions in the initial phase.

In addition to increased autophagy, the pancreatic acinar cells also show reversible and irreversible cell injury, roughly correlating with the severity and duration of shock. These changes could represent the cellular basis of the release of myocardial depressant factor, as discussed by Lefer (Ch. 12).

Barnes and McDowell review the pathophysiology of acute renal failure (ARF). This condition is still associated with a mortality of about 50%. Although it can result from ischemia, today it is more commonly associated with septic shock and/or chemical toxicity, e.g., aminoglycoside antibiotics. Although both oliguric and nonoliguric forms can occur, decreased glomerular filtration rate (GFR) is a common feature of both and to many a *sine qua non* for the diagnosis of ARF.

A single pathophysiologic mechanism for all types of ARF has not been established. Many toxins may act through tubuloglomerular feedback involving interactions between decreased sodium chloride reabsorption in the proximal tubule and the juxtaglomerular apparatus (JGA). The latter is triggered to secrete renin locally, resulting in decreased GFR through the action of angiotensin. This mechanism may help explain at least two types of protective interventions: those that improve sodium chloride resorption in the proximal tubule and those that deplete the JGA of renin prior to the initiating event. The distal acting "loop" diuretics might act in a similar fashion by reducing the "chloride signal" at the macula densa.

It is quite clear that conventional light microscopic techniques and renal function tests will not solve the problem. Recent studies from our laboratory clearly show that tubular necrosis and ARF can be readily dissociated. Necrosis of the tubule (usually the pars recta) can exist with or without ARF in the rat (for references, see Ch. 23). In the study of immediate autopsies from human traumatized patients, no correlation could be found between tubular necrosis and ARF (Sato et al., 1979). Proximal tubular dilation may correlate with ARF in patients studied at autopsy because of obstruction or because of inhibition of sodium transport in the pars convoluta. Application of current techniques including scanning and transmission electron microscopy, micropuncture, biochemical studies and studies of flow and pressure kinetics in the nephron will be needed to resolve this problem.

Recently, one line of evidence implicates the cytoskeleton in the pathophysiology of some or all types of ARF, especially as it is modulated by changes in cell ion content, especially ionized calcium. In acute ischemia, large blebs of apical proximal tubular cytoplasm protrude into the lumen, detach and may obstruct the lower nephron by forming casts. This cast formation could be affected by tubular flow, pH, and filtered proteins, e.g., hemoglobin. In addition, modification of the cytoskeleton seems to affect renin secretion in the JGA. Necrosis or even sublethal changes involving the permeability of cell junctions may influence the so called "back-leak," which is part of another hypothesis. The experimental evidence for back-leak, however, remains controversial. Our view, however, is straight forward in the sense that even total necrosis of the pars recta does not result in ARF. If back-leak is indeed a problem, one might imagine that total necrosis of such a significant segment of every nephron should uniformly result in ARF. Additionally, initiation of ARF, as evidenced by decreased GFR, precedes significantly the occurrence of any necrosis. Some investigators have attempted to implicate structural changes in the glomerular capillary wall in the pathogenesis of ARF. This has not, however, been supported by further critical studies.

The main theme that emerges from this excellent review is that tubular dysfunction is a central theme. Tubular dysfunction can begin within seconds or minutes of initiation. Interventions should, therefore, be designed to modify this seemingly important feature. The role of renal prostaglandins as a modifying factor needs much more study.

Gehr and associates critically review the early diagnosis and treatment ARF. As they discuss, the definition of ARF is based in part on the exclusion of a number of other causes of diminished renal function that can accompany syndromes involving shock, ischemia, and anoxia. These authors stress that the diagnosis and therapy must be correlated with and appropriate to the phases of ARF. These phases are: 1) initiation, 2) maintenance, and 3) recovery.

In the initiation phase, prevention must be considered—the details depending on the type of patient. Diuretics may be useful; their beneficial effects may be explainable on at least two hypotheses. "Loop" diuretics remain controversial in established ARF and precautions must be exercised to be sure that the patient is not suffering from volume depletion. If this is not done, such diuretics may well aggravate ARF. The efficacy of mannitol in modifying ARF is unquestioned, but its mechanism is controversial. Its efficacy appears best when given early—especially before the initiating insult.

In the maintenance phase, therapy is much more difficult and includes management of fluid and electrolyte problems, maintenance of nutrition, and various forms of dialysis. Each of these is critical with a potential for harm as well as help. Control of potassium is one critical requirement. Particular efforts must also be made to control serum ionized calcium, dangerous elevation of which may occur, especially in the recovery phase (see

Ch. 1). The control of nutrition in this phase is also critical as well as difficult. This is especially so because many patients are in severe negative nitrogen balance. In view of excretory deficiencies with the type of hormonal imbalance explained by Bessman and Renner in Chapter 3, new therapies must be developed if we are to be truly effective in this problem.

Therapy in the recovery phase requires constant attention to fluid and electrolyte problems since salt and water losses may be excessive.

All in all, treatment of patients with ARF has great significance; if successful, most patients die not from ARF per se but from concurrent problems such as infection and bleeding difficulties. In the future, we should look for better primary therapies directed against the primary tubular dysfunction. These might include ATP-Mg, as discussed by Chaudry and Baue in Chapter 15.

In their chapter, Riede et al. present an excellent and concise summary of the pathology and pathophysiology of the shock lung. The authors stress the primary role of altered cell junctions in the endothelium, which appear to initiate the transfer of fluid into the interstitium. The initiators of this endothelial damage may be multiple, including anoxia, cell membrane damage resulting from complement activation and endotoxin and vascular mediators discussed by Lefer (Ch. 12). It is probable that the cytoskeleton of the endothelial cell plays an important role in this process and that this, in turn, is modulated by modification of ionized calcium in the cytosol, as discussed in Chapter 1. Increased ionized calcium in the cytosol can also decrease adhesion of cell junctions and this increases the permeability of the endothelium. It is probable that simultaneous, thin filament contraction also occurs, which contributes to the widening of such junctions. Irreversibility may correlate with type II epithelial proliferation and proliferation of fibroblasts in the interstitium.

Riede et al. stress that the edema is first seen in peribronchial and perivascular connective tissue and that it is associated with lymphangiectasis. Eventually, this results in discharge of fluid into the alveolar interstitium, decreasing alveolar compliance and interfering with oxygenation. This edema in turn results from loosening of contacts between endothelial cells. This occurs even more rapidly in septic shock. In septic shock, the events soon lead to neutrophil adherence, which further contributes to the damage. The pulmonary endothelial cells react quickly to injury. These reactions transcend those of impaired O_2 diffusion and include fibrinolysis, lipolysis, and effects on angiotensin. These three reactions are likely to be destroyed in shock. Hypotension, fat embolism, and microthrombus formation may, therefore, relate to such alterations. Later changes include type I epithelial necrosis, type II epithelial cell proliferation, and interstitial fibrosis.

The authors, however, assert that respiratory insufficiency is related primarily to disturbances of perfusion. The utilization of aggressive respiratory therapy, including early intubation and use of positive end expiratory pressure (PEEP), may ameliorate many of these microcirculatory factors. We do not presently know of methods to control the fibrosis which occurs during the chronic phase, although Riede et al. discuss its possible reversibility.

Sibbald and Driedger continue this discussion emphasizing adult respiratory distress (ARD) syndrome in sepsis. As high as 23% of cases with gram-negative bacteremia may have this condition. Their review of basic mechanisms complements and extends that of Riede et al. In view of the subatmospheric pressure in the interstitium and permeability characteristics, the hydrostatic and osmotic processes favor the egress of fluid from the vessel to the interstitium. The major defense against this is the pulmonary lymphatic system. In septic shock, a pathological increase in vascular permeability occurs, beginning at the level of the bronchial venules. The effect of this on water movement, however, must be normalized for the amount of shock. This increased conductance of the pulmonary alveolo-capillary barrier membranes is the principal difference of this type of edema from that occurring in cardiac failure. Even here, however, the protein reflection coefficient is not zero.

The subcellular basis of the increased permeability not only includes slight gaps and structural changes in endothelium but also areas of complete destruction, especially involving type I cells, in the alveolar epithelium. Endothelial lesions were more pronounced in the subacute and chronic phases. The amount of damage is reduced in the presence of leukopenia or by treatment with glucocorticoids. Evidence also indicates that the leukocyte aggregation may be followed by basophil and/or mast cell release of histamine.

Demling and Flynn review more about the mechanisms involved in ARD syndrome. They again emphasize that the syndrome does not normally occur in uncomplicated hemorrhagic shock in man or most experimental animals other than dogs. It does, however, characteristically occur with burns and sepsis, and a number of factors may be implicated in the increased vascular permeability.

Lysosomal enzymes derived from leukocytes may be related to the capillary barrier damage. These enzymes increase in the pulmonary lymph and roughly parallel the increased permeability. Ratliff (1980) recently reviewed this effect in another publication. Recent progress has been made in the cellular mechanisms of lysosomal enzyme release from leukocytes (Weissman, 1980). This is closely associated with generation of a number of oxidation and peroxidation products, including the superoxide anion. The entire sequence involves influx of calcium and changes in the cytoskeleton and is modulated by cyclic nucleotides. Both prostaglandins and glucocorticoids also modify the process. For example, prostaglandin (PGE)-treated lung tissue has resulted in amelioration of hemodynamic changes, and it is known that PGE_1 minimizes leukocyte enzyme secretion. Glucocorticoids may exert an inhibitory effect through modification of the calcium-induced phospholipase activation. Consistent with this, as reviewed by the authors, aspirin and indomethacin treatment exacerbated the permeability changes. Obviously, much more work is needed to delineate the effects of pharmacological interventions on ARD. At the present time, it would appear that steroids are more effective than nonsteroidal antiinflammatory agents, as the steroids may protect against the initial interaction.

References

Beecher, H.K.: *Resuscitation and Anesthesia for Wounded Men; The Management of Traumatic Shock.* Charles C Thomas, Springfield, IL, 1949.

Blaisdell, F.W.: Pathophysiology of the respiratory distress syndrome. Arch. Surg. *108:*44, 1974.

Burns, B., and Stiff, J.L.: Membrane diffusion and gas exchange in pulmonary fibrosis caused bleomycin. *Proceedings of the 28th International Congress of Physiological Sciences.* Budapest, 1980.

DeFouw, D.O., and Berendsen, P.B.: A morphometric analysis of isolated perfused dog lungs after acute oncotic edema. Microvasc. Res. *17:*90–103, 1979.

Kirby, R.R., Down, J.B., Ciuetta, J.M., Modell, J.H., Dannemiller, F.J., Klein, E.F., and Hodges, M.: High level positive end expiratory pressure (PEEP) in acute respiratory insufficiency. Chest *67:*157–163, 1975.

McCabe, W.R.: Serum compliment levels in bacteremia due to gram negative organisms. N. Engl. J. Med. *288:*21, 1973.

Ratliff, N.B.: In *Pathobiology of Cell Membranes,* B.F. Trump and A.U. Arstila, vol. II, pp. 382–417. Academic Press, New York, 1980.

Sato, T., Kamiyama, Y., Jones, R.T., Cowley, R.A., and Trump, B.F.: Ultrastructural study on kidney cell injury following various types of shock in 26 immediate autopsy patients. Adv. Shock. Res. *1:*55–69, 1979.

Schumer, W., et al.: Mechanisms of protection in septic shock. Surgery *72:*119, 1972.

Wagner, P.D., Laravuso, R.B., Goldzimmer, E., Naumann, P.F., and West, J.B.: Distributions of ventilation—Perfusion ratios in dogs with normal and abnormal lungs. J. Appl. Physiol. *38:*1099–1109, 1975.

Weismann, G.: Prostaglandins in acute inflammation. *Current Concepts.* Upjohn, Kalamazoo, 1980.

CHAPTER 20

Pathology and Pathophysiology of the Liver

R ADAMS COWLEY
JOHN R. HANKINS
RAYMOND T. JONES
BENJAMIN F. TRUMP

Excluding the brain, the kidneys, lungs, liver, and heart are the four major organ systems generally affected by shock. If only functional reversible damage is suffered and the affected organ system is properly supported, complete recovery is possible. However, if perfusion deficits are profound and prolonged before they are corrected, severe organ failure may subsequently result. Shoemaker (1976) has emphasized this point beautifully in his treatise on the pathobiology of death as it relates to structural and functional interactions in various shock syndromes. Although several reports have shown that preventive measures and maximum support have reduced the incidence of acute renal failure and lung shock, the problem of liver failure is difficult to resolve when shock (either hemorrhagic or septic) is severe and/or prolonged. When liver failure is accompanied by sepsis, recovery can be greatly delayed and death usually results.

Among the known sequelae of deterioration of liver function during shock are decreased efficiency of protein and carbohydrate metabolism accompanied by the breakdown of the body's primary detoxification mechanism (see Ch. 3). Severe impairment of the coagulation process has been shown by Attar et al. (1966). Ollodart et al. (1963, 1965, 1967) and Blair et al. (1969) have described breakdown of bacterial defense mechanisms in patients suffering from shock.

Clinical manifestations of liver injury do not occur early in the onset of shock, although damage can be documented at the cellular level. It is not until late in the recovery period that physiopathological changes become clinically apparent; by this time, severe complications may occur, and death of the patient is often wrongly attributed to causes other than hepatic dysfunction. Our analysis of this problem has been described by Champion et al. (1976), especially as it relates to septic shock.

If one uses only light microscopic (LM) techniques, early hepatic architectural changes are not detected in those dying in shock. This also applies to surgical biopsy of the liver during or after shock, as it takes several days for the centrilobular necrosis to appear. However, current use of the electron microscope (EM) in the immediate autopsy procedure (Trump et al., 1973a and b, 1975; Cowley, 1975) shows that subtle changes in liver architecture can be seen as early at 15 min to 2 hr after trauma and/or hemorrhage. These EM findings have also been demonstrated in the surgical biopsy.

In recent years, the hemodynamic and metabolic mechanisms of shock have been partially defined, first in studies with experimental animals and now increasingly with human subjects.

HEPATIC PERFUSION AND FUNCTION DURING SHOCK

Portal Circulation

Relying on the portal bed and hepatic arteries making up the splanchnic bed for its dual blood supply, the liver is at great potential risk in the event of general circulatory failure. Guyton, in describing the liver in shock, concludes that nearly 30% of the body's total blood flow reaches the liver via the splanchnic system, three-quarters of which originates in the portal system with the remainder coming from the hepatic arteries. Thus, it is obvious that hepatic function can be drastically impaired by any mechanism that adversely affects the flow of blood through the liver.

In times of excess blood volume, the liver appears to serve as a reservoir for the storage of large quantities of venous blood. However, extra blood can be released from the liver to the general circulation by vasoconstrictive stimulation activated by the sympathetic nervous system. This mechanism is capable of expelling up to 400 ml of blood into the general circulation in less than 4 min.

Unlike other capillary systems, the hepatic endothelium has unique properties of permeability. This is manifested in its ability to permit the diffusion of most blood proteins into the extravascular spaces. Sinusoidal pressure is only about 6–8 mm Hg, permitting most of the proteins that diffuse out of the sinusoids to readily return, with the remainder passing into the lymphatic system. Because of this ready vascular permeability, nutrient materials may be exchanged rapidly between the blood and liver cells.

Of vital importance to the circulation of blood in the liver is the sinusoidal reticuloendothelial system and Kupffer cells, which quickly remove bacteria and other particulates from the intestinal capillary blood as it flows through this organ. The volume of bacteria entering into the systemic circulation via the hepatic veins is generally held to no more than 1% (Guyton, 1976). The role of the Ito cells in altered liver function is not presently known.

In the event of circulatory collapse, there is a drop in pressure and flow of both the hepatic artery and the portal vein, and a probable vasoconstrictor response within the liver may be triggered by these changes. Ternberg and Butcher (1965) explain hepatic artery-portal vein flow relationships as a simple mechanical effect. By using square wave electromagnetic flow meter techniques, they found that hepatic arterial flow increased the portal venous flow; when the hepatic artery flow decreased, the portal venous flow also decreased. Thus, it is important to evaluate the effects on both systemic and portal circulation when studying hepatic changes in shock.

In many patients, we have used perumbilical catheters for manometric studies of the portal venous system. The effect of external influences, such as contraction of thoracic and abdominal muscles, on portal venous pressure has been documented by these studies. The studies have shown a consonance between the portal venous pressure and the central venous pressure (Hankins et al., 1972). An increased portal venous pressure-central venous pressure gradient was found in three of five patients studied during the course of shock.

Effects of Hypoperfusion

The insertion of perumbilical catheters along with central venous and arterial catheters made it possible to perform serial determinations, in both nonshocked and shocked patients, of blood gases, pH, lactate, ammonia, and other metabolites simultaneously in blood from all three circulatory systems (Hankins et al., 1973, 1974) (Fig. 20.1).

Liver Pathology

Among the findings in portal vein blood during and after shock are the occurrence of hypoxia, hypercarbia, and acidosis, an elevation of blood lactic acid and ammonia, a rise in the arterial-portal oxygen saturation difference, and elevated portal venous pressure. These findings strengthen the hypothesis of an obstruction of portal flow within the liver in some shock victims. The stasis which ensues may account for the ischemic hypoxia and cellular changes observed.

Alterations in the human liver resulting from a perfusion deficit have been examined. With the enlargement of the hepatic sinusoids, particularly those in the region

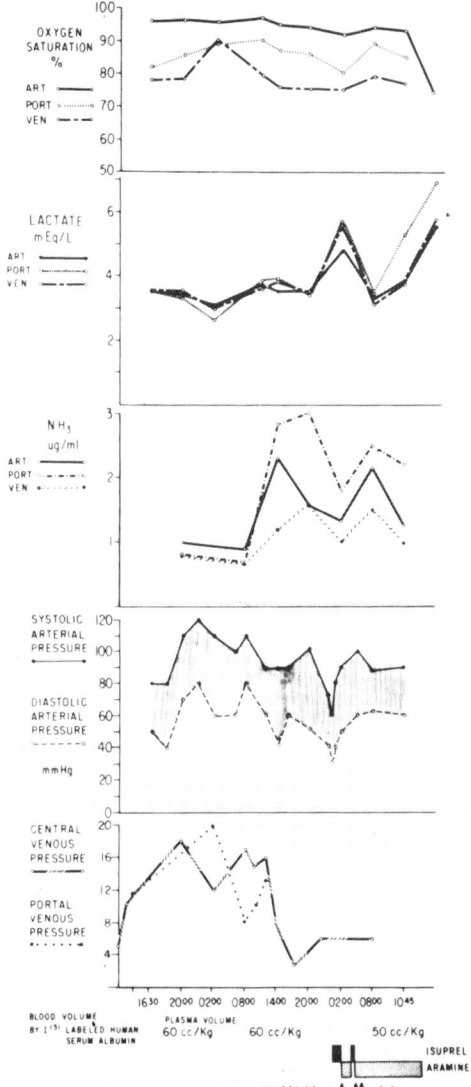

Figure 20.1. Physiological parameters in shock. A 50-year-old man with hypovolemic and bacteremic shock (bacteroides) resulting from complications of a thoracoabdominal gunshot wound sustained on Day 1. The umbilical catheter was inserted during a laparotomy performed to control delayed bleeding from the diaphragm on Day 13. The patient died in refractory shock on Day 15.

of the central veins, the appearance of red cell aggregates is noted. As stasis increases in the sinusoids, the flow of portal blood is further obstructed and the likelihood of hepatic ischemia becomes greater. Carlson and Lefer (1976) found, while working with isolated perfused cat livers, that the impairment of liver cell integrity (i.e., of Kupffer and parenchymal cells) occurred after 60–90 min of stimulated shock conditions, indicating that the liver is stable for 60 min when it is exposed to hypoperfusion. It is generally accepted that the human liver is not very tolerant to warm ischemia for longer than 15 min. However, clinical observations made by Huguet et al. (1978) parallel recent experimental work in that the human liver in three cases could tolerate normothermic ischemia for 50 min or longer. The results of this work could greatly affect the surgical management of severe hepatic trauma.

The perfused liver is sensitive to local stimuli that predominates circulatory shock, particularly hypoxia. These stimuli promote the release of lysosomal and cytoplasmic enzymes, as well as depressed phagocytosis by the reticuloendothelial system—phenomena that exacerbate the shock state. On the other hand, White et al. (1973) concluded that hypoxia alone is not responsible for generating the swollen mitochondrial matrices common to endotoxemia and hemorrhage.

Further changes include generalized intracellular edema; compression of the hepatic plates; increased dilatation of the central veins, portal tracts, and lymphatics; and congestion of the sinusoids with erythrocytes. Eventually, necrosis occurs in the cells around the central veins, and the parenchymal cells disappear. On pathological examination, the liver lobule assumes an architectural appearance similar to that of carbon tetrachloride poisoning (Brody et al., 1961). Such centrilobular necrosis presents a classical representation of the liver in shock and does not appear if the animal is treated with sympatholytic drugs.

It is likely that during stasis, the already hypoxic blood, passing slowly from the periphery of the liver lobule to the central vein, leaves less oxygen available for extraction by those cells nearer to the central vein. Thus, greater central lobular damage occurs, as demonstrated by increased peripheral spread of cellular necrosis.

Oxygen Availability

Baseline studies of patients by Hankins et al. (1973, 1974) substantiated other researchers' findings of a high oxygen content in portal venous blood. The oxygen saturation of portal venous blood can be increased to 95–96% by the administration of oxygen. In nonshocked patients not receiving oxygen, the mean values for portal venous oxygen saturation and for arterial-portal venous oxygen content differences resemble those reported by Symthe et al. (1951) and Stori et al. (1966).

To further illustrate the vital importance of oxygen availability in shock, we have demonstrated experimentally in several animal models that the survival rate improves when using hyperbaric oxygen (OHP) techniques during the therapy phase (100% oxygen at three atmospheres) (Cowley et al., 1965 a and b; Attar et al., 1962, 1964). For example, when drum-shocked rats were divided and placed in an environment of 100% oxygen at three atmospheres and then compared to those treated at one atmosphere breathing air, the survival rate of the latter group was 40%, as compared to 80% for patients treated with 100% oxygen at three atmospheres (Moulton et al., 1962).

In the group of shock patients, the most notable observation was the presence of some degree of portal venous oxygen desaturation in all patients examined. In comparing the shock patients with the nonshock group, we observed that among the former the mean portal venous oxygen saturation was significantly lower, and the mean arterial-portal venous oxygen saturation difference was significantly greater than that in the nonshock patients. The shock patients also showed a higher PCO_2 and a lower pH in the portal venous blood than did patients who had never been in shock.

Metabolic Changes

In three of four shock patients who died, the total blood lactate showed a greater rise in portal venous blood than was seen in arterial or central venous blood. The fourth patient did not exhibit an increased portal venous pressure-central venous pressure gradient. These findings supply evidence for impairment of splanchnic circulation or, more specifically, for anaerobic metabolism within the gastrointestinal tract. White (1968) noted high portal venous blood lactate levels in patients suffering from portal hypertension. He thought this indicated stasis in the splanchnic circulation caused by portal venous obstruction.

This correlates with the finding of an increased portal venous pressure-central venous pressure gradient in three of our five shock patients, which suggests impedance to portal venous blood flow through the liver.

Also, a rise in portal venous blood ammonia levels was observed in the shock patients. In all three fatal shock cases that had ammonia levels determined, the rise in portal venous blood ammonia was later accompanied by lesser increments in arterial and central venous blood ammonia. This phenomenon suggests impairment of hepatic urea-synthesizing mechanisms, which allows the escape of ammonia through the liver (Cowley et al., 1960).

These findings, along with those indicating an increase in portal venous pressure in certain shock patients, strengthen our hypothesis that in some cases of shock there occurs an increased impedance to portal venous blood flow through the liver. This results in stasis in the portal-splanchnic circulation. Because the liver is thus deprived of part of the oxygen supplied to it by the portal vein, this portal circulatory stasis is at least a contributory factor toward hypoxic hepatocellular injury.

LIVER PATHOPHYSIOLOGY OF THE PATIENT IN SHOCK

Some microscopic evidence (at the EM or LM level) of hepatocellular damage will be observed in all shock victims. The duration and severity of the shock episode will determine the extent of the injury. In shock patients who suffer from preexisting hepatic disease, the insult to the liver during circulatory collapse will accordingly be more extensive.

Over 9000 severely injured patients have been admitted to our clinical shock trauma center (Cowley, 1975, 1976 a and b; Cowley et al., 1979, 1980) since it opened in 1961. The majority of these patients (80%) have suffered from some type of shock. Standard methods were used in treating all patients. Autopsies (standard or immediate) were performed on most of those who died (Cowley et al., 1969).

Patients admitted to the shock trauma center are evaluated according to significant physiological (hemodynamics, hematology, and coagulation) and biochemical parameters (electrolytes and nonelectrolytes, blood gases, metabolites, and enzymes). Readings are taken on admission, during the patient's hospitalization, and at the time of discharge or death. Distinct differences between shock patients who survive and those who die may be revealed by analysis of such data, especially as they relate to pathological lesions found in the liver.

To further the understanding of the pathophysiology of the liver, it is instructive to use the following parameters to elaborate on the differences noted between shock patients who live and those who die.

Hemodynamics

Most of the variables studied in this group were under the direct control of the physician. Normal readings were often maintained for blood pressure, pulse, temperature, and central pressure in shock patients because these were controlled by the clinician during therapy. However, the cardiac output and total peripheral resistance were greatly significant and served as a means for determining perfusion abnormalities. Cardiac function, as it relates to the sufficiency of the central circulatory system, is collected by cardiac output. Such measurements cannot accurately determine segmental flow to specific organs, but a suspicion of diminished flow to certain organs may be indicated. To illustrate how hemodynamic indicators may yield valuable data on shock patients, it has been noted that, of those who died, the cardiac output was lower both on admission to the center and throughout their stay. Lower values of cardiac output were considered an indicator that perfusion to certain organs was also depressed, thus causing tissue hypoxia and the ensuing biochemical and morphological changes observed at the time of the biopsy or autopsy. It is possible that newer noninvasive radiographic techniques may contribute to the understanding of the phenomenon. Following hemorrhage or other causes of shock, the body attempts to maintain blood pressure by increasing catecholamine production. The sympathetic stimulation increases vascular tone and results in increased total peripheral resistance. Following prolonged hypoxia, however, the accumulation of lactic acid decreases pH, which counteracts constriction of the venules but not the arterioles. This finally results in venous stasis and congestion. This defense mechanism may be responsible for producing centrizonal hypoxia and resultant central necrosis in the liver.

Hematology

Among the values examined during hematological studies, the counts for red and white blood cells and for platelets and hematocrit did not differ significantly between shock patients who lived and those who died. These values were thought to be secondary to transfusion therapy. Significant differences were, however, seen in hemoglobin studies. We have not yet determined whether this phenomenon is due to hemolysis or sludging, a condition that is present in a number of our critically ill patients (Knisely et al., 1970; Knisely, 1975).

Coagulation

Great interest has been generated by coagulation studies because such data have shown marked differences between shock patients who live and those who die (Attar et al., 1966 a–c, 1969, 1970; Attar, 1967). Both prothrombin production and prothrombin time are related to the clotting time. Observation of the fibrinogen level indicates either a drop in production or a rise in utilization of the substance. All clotting factors, as well as the fibrinolytic inhibitors, are controlled by the liver. From our study of shock patients, we have observed a decrease in clotting factors and an acceleration in fibrinolytic activity. A rise in consumption or a drop in production may explain the clotting factor decrease. The rise in fibrinogen consumption has been explained by an intravascular clotting mechanism, but we have not been able to verify this on autopsy.

The coagulation and fibrinolytic changes observed in shock patients are approximately the same as those seen in subjects who suffer from liver disease. In our studies, the difference in clotting time and fibrinogen levels have been significant at the 1% level; however, we have noted that neither of these parameters are markedly different on initial admission samples.

Blood Gases

Interpretation of these values is difficult because every effort is made by respiratory therapy to clinically regulate oxygen tension within the range of 90–150 mm Hg (McAslan, 1976). Enriched concentrations of oxygen are administered to most patients, particularly in conjunction with intermittent positive pressure respiration techniques. The presence of high concentrations of oxygen in blood that was observed even at the time of the patient's death may be a result of physiological shunting (McLaughlin, 1967, 1971) and/or the failure of the injured cell to utilize oxygen, as well as the clinical attempt in keeping the patient oxygenated.

In animal studies, it has been shown by *polarographic techniques* that when oxygen electrodes are inserted in the liver and muscle, both undergo a drop in oxygen tension during shock. When the animal is exposed to hyperbaric oxygen, recovery occurs (Fig. 20.2).

The finding of low *standard bicarbonate* is of real significance in that every effort is made to buffer the blood to within the normal pH range with sodium bicarbonate. It is noted, however, that both bicarbonate and pH values are always lower in terminal patients despite the fact that they receive more bicarbonate than do surviving patients. It is interesting and possibly significant in this context that extracellular acidosis (pH 5.9–6.5) appears to be protective against cellular anoxia.

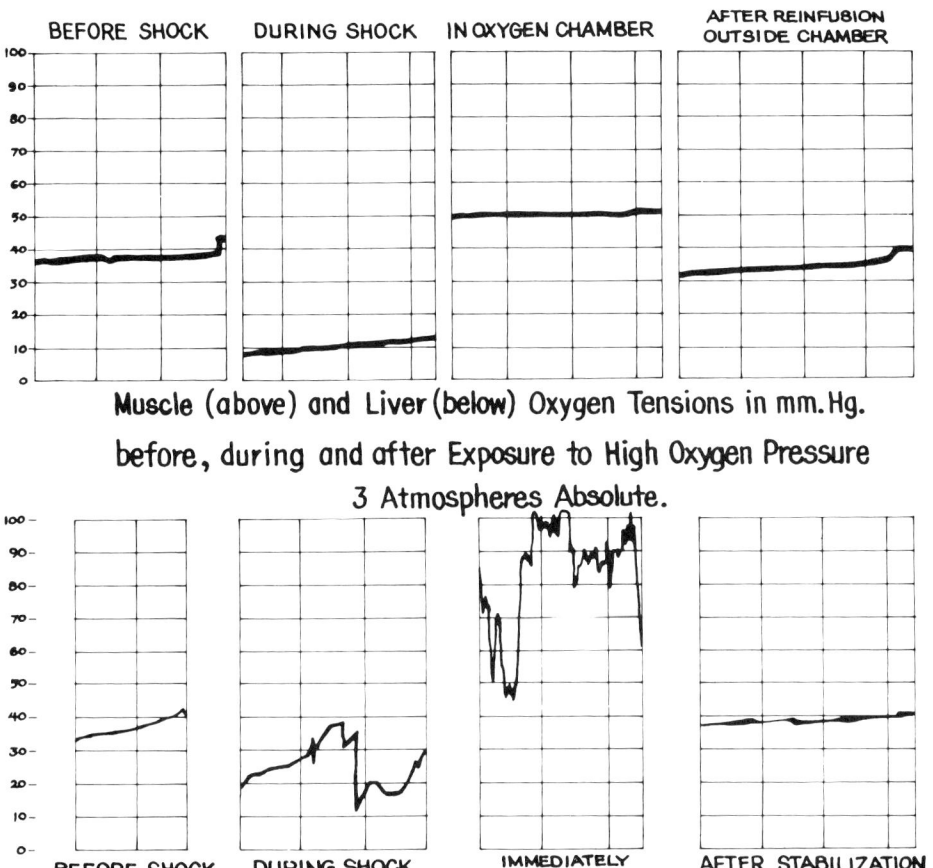

Figure 20.2. This figure demonstrates relatively what happens to muscle and liver organ tensions measured with needle electrodes before, during, and after exposure to high oxygen pressure. Note that there is recovery of tissue oxygen tension without any further therapy.

Electrolytes and Nonelectrolytes

Such indicators add little because of clinical manipulation. However, a rise in potassium was observed in most patients, which might be explained by the decreased function of cell membrane ATPase triggered by an intracellular energy deficit. Measurements of serum glucose and osmolality were observed to differ markedly between shock patients who lived and those who died, with rises in these factors closely paralleling the intensity of shock. It was observed that the total serum protein and solids fell in all patients. This might well relate to decreased albumin and fibrinogen synthesis in the liver.

In a comparison of the two groups of patients, the availability of blood glucose for transformation of energy was highest in those who died, with an elevation in blood glucose evident even at the time of admission (Cowley et al., 1969). From such observations, we suspect that the high concentration of catecholamines released during stress plays a role in the gluconeogenesis process (LaBrosse and Cowley, 1973).

Utilization of oxygen and glucose apparently decrease gradually, as indicated by a rise in blood glucose levels and increased anaerobic metabolism with elevated levels of lactate.

Fluctuations of serum bilirubin levels paralleled the occurrence of septicemia or perihepatic bilirubin loads following blood transfusion. This aspect of septicemia correlated closely with extreme hepatic dysfunction when defined by the bilirubin peak, as described by Champion et al. (1976 a and b) (Fig. 20.3).

Nunes et al. (1970) found bilirubin peaked either early or late in most of their patients. Late elevations were thought to be related to subsequent operations, renal failure, or bacteremia. Nunes and coworkers have also described other factors that contribute to postoperative jaundice, including anesthesia, massive transfusion, hemolysis, congestive heart failure, extravasated blood, liver disease, and hepatic anoxia. Centrilobular necrosis, described by these authors, was not unlike ours.

Volume Replacement

Because of our concern regarding tissue edema and thus oxygen transport, in all shock resuscitation efforts, we emphasize utilization of colloids in preference to crystalloids. Lambotte and Wojcik (1978) have measured cellular edema in anoxia and have studied its prevention by using hyperosmolar solutions. They conclude that in addition to preserving membrane functions, inhibition of cellular swelling also can protect intracellular structures. The use of hyperosmolar solutions can maintain a

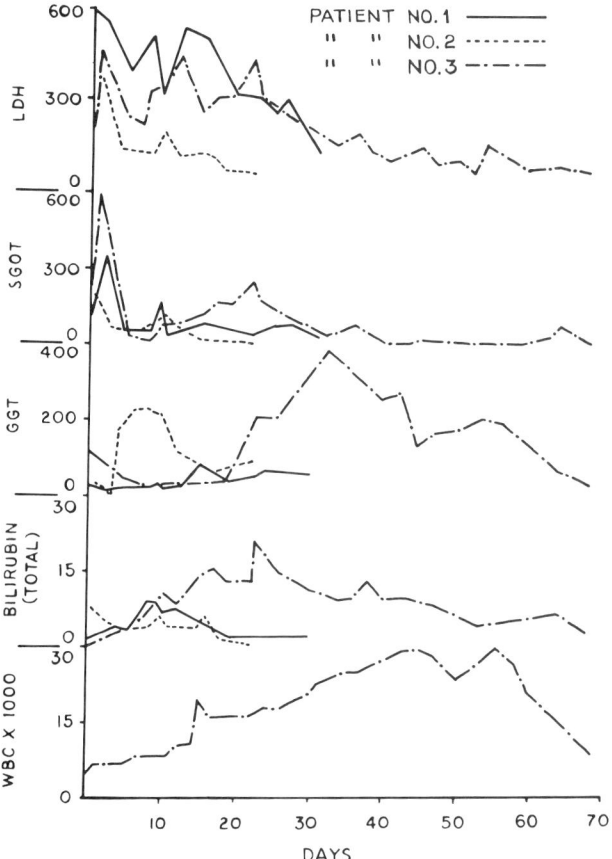

Figure 20.3. Examples of bilirubin peaks in three severely traumatized patients in shock.

normal cellular volume. Therefore, attempts to preserve a normal cell volume is justified. Using refractometry and osmometry techniques, Boyd and Mansberger (1968) and Mansberger et al. (1969) described serum water and osmolal changes in shock patients. The results of these studies point out that the movement of water is governed by the colloidal oncotic pressure in addition to sodium and osmolal shifts. During recovery, all patients must have restoration of water solute, protein, and osmolal hemostasis. If this does not occur, water logging of the tissue results, compounding the problem of tissue oxygenation.

Metabolites

Of all the parameters studied, the most marked differences between patients who lived and those who died were found to be their level of metabolites. Patients who died always manifested significantly higher levels of metabolite measures.

Ammonia

In shock, all patients showed elevated arterial-ammonia levels as compared with those found in normal subjects, indicating the liver in shock loses its capacity to convert ammonia into urea (Cowley et al., 1960; Hankins et al., 1959). These levels might also indicate that the quantity of ammonia coming from the gut overwhelms the mechanism of urea production. We thus conclude that there is a strong correlation between liver damage and blood ammonia concentration.

The major origin of ammonia can be traced to bacterial putrefaction of nitrogenous compounds in the gut along with tissue catabolism; it is generally eliminated from the portal system via a single passage through the liver, where it undergoes conversion mainly to urea. The average level of arterial ammonia in a normal subject is under $2\ \gamma/ml$. In our examination of this variable in shock patients who survived and those who died, we found that arterial levels of both groups were higher than normal ($1.3 \pm 1.5\ \gamma/ml$), evidencing an escape of ammonia through the liver. Oxidative energy is required for synthesis of urea. Thus, it appears that the urea synthesizing mechanism is damaged during shock, possibly as a result of anoxia of the liver due to stasis.

Blood Urea Nitrogen (BUN)

Elevation of levels of BUN and creatinine may reflect increased protein catabolism. Such an acceleration in protein breakdown is a typical reaction to shock and can be further compounded by widespread tissue injury. Since various amino acids and other protein products of catabolism are produced, (LaBrosse et al., 1967) elevated BUN levels are not necessarily a positive indicator of renal failure (for example, in the instance of elevated BUN with levels approaching 60 mg/100 ml). However, it has been our experience that patients in shock evidence a severe drop in urea clearance.

Lactate

In studies on acidosis, we have observed that metabolic acidosis occurring in conjunction with both clinical and experimental shock is thought to be related to the accumulation of lactic acid. The development of acidosis during times of accelerated anaerobic metabolism is likewise associated with the poor perfusion of tissues with oxygen-carrying blood. Therefore, the development of lactacidemia is characteristic of all types of shock (Blair et al., 1965; Vitek and Cowley, 1971, 1978; Tranquada et al., 1966). Although high lactate concentrations may be induced by chemical stimuli under clinical conditions (e.g., an increase in blood pH following bicarbonate injection, high glucose concentration, etc.), the major factor, and usually the determining factor, causing high lactate concentrations is the insufficiency of oxygen with its concomitant tissue hypoxia.

There is ample documentation of lactate mortality relationships during shock, a finding concordant with those of Broder and Weil (1964), Duff (1966), and Blair et al. (1965). A dependable index of the intensity of defective perfusion may be gained by regular determinations of lactate, with depth and duration constituting one of the most important predictors of survival. Maintenance of elevated lactic levels over a long time, as well as increased levels despite therapy, are unfavorable signs even if the blood pressure rises about 90 mm Hg. Conversely, if the blood pressure stabilizes above the normal range, there is usually a drop in blood lactate concentrations. In our experience, variances in lactate level among different forms of clinical shock are of prognostic value. The primary cause of these differences is that metabolic and physiological alterations existing in the underlying disease cause circulatory failure and continue even with the recovery from shock. They continue to contribute in varying degrees toward the overall impact of hypoxia on the cell. Our research has shown that the rate of survival declines with increasing lactate. The upper limit of normality was estimated as 1.5 mEq/liter lactate level, and we found that about 40% of the patients fell in the highest lactate range of 1.5–4.5 mEq/liter, with a similar percentage falling in the range of 4.5–9.0 mEq/liter. Among patients with lactates exceeding 10 mEq/liter, none survived (Vitek and Cowley, 1971, 1978).

Our calculations of the likelihood of survival for patients suffering from four of the most common types of shock where the lactate level was set for 50% survival are computed as follows:

1. hemorrhage, consisting of traumatic shock in combinations, 7.3 mEq/liter;
2. pure septic shock, 5.5;
3. septic shock with combinations, 3.5; and
4. cardiogenic shock with combinations, 2.4.

For all groups pooled, the measure is 4.9 mEq/liter. Such findings are of benefit to use because they underscore the value of blood lactate as an indicator of the severity of shock. If lactate changes are monitored carefully and if the etiopathogenic background of hypotension is respected, the prognosis for recovery of shock patients may be greatly enhanced.

Enzymes

In 300 consecutive shock patients, serum enzyme levels of asparate aminotransferase (AST) [formerly glutamate oxaloacetate transaminase (GOT)], alanine aminotransferase (ALT) [formerly glutamate pyruvate transaminase (GPT)], lactate dehydrogenase (LDH), and malate dehydrogenase (MDH) revealed that the mean serum levels of each of these enzymes were higher in the dying patients as compared with survivors. All differences were significant at the 1% level (Cowley et al., 1969).

These enhanced levels of enzymes are a result of their leaking from destroyed or damaged cells into the extracellular fluids. This may result from injury, hypoxia,

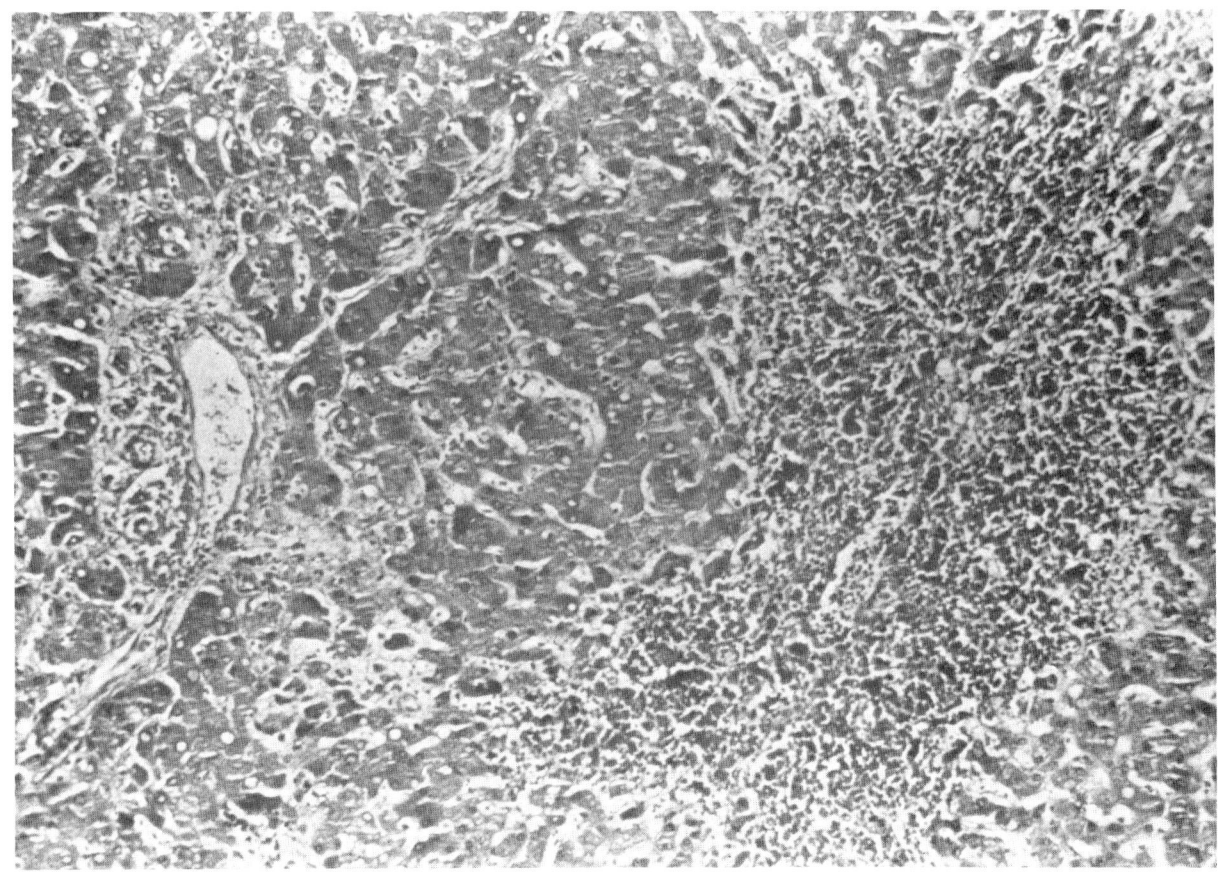

Figure 20.4. The centrizonal cells have largely disintegrated and have been replaced by a sea of red blood cells. Hidden among the red blood cells are the Kupffer cells of the sinusoids. Many of the nuclei of the hepatic cells in the periportal areas seem vacuolated and are apparently filled by glycogen. Only very minimal inflammatory reaction is seen in the liver adjacent to the centrizonal change. Hematoxylin and eosin ×110.

sepsis, cardiac failure, endogenous toxins, chemicals, disrupted lysosomes, etc., that produce increased permeability of the cellular membrane, which leads to further release of intracellular enzymes.

Following the above study, we decided to improve detection specificity and sensitivity to further define liver impairment by examining another set of enzymes, isocitrate dehydrogenase (ICDH) and sorbitol dehydrogenase (SDH), both richly present in liver parenchyma. Creatine phosphokinase (CPK) was used to improve the differential diagnosis, since this enzyme is not found in liver tissue.

In both groups of patients studied on admission, CPK demonstrated a 10-fold elevation when its activity was compared with normal reference values. The enzyme primarily reflects muscle damage and, to a lesser degree, myocardial and cerebral damage. In contrast to other enzymes listed above, liver specific enzymes ICDH and SDH show a higher mean admission value in patients who died. For ICDH the difference was substantial ($p = 0.02$). A comparison of the levels in the final sample of those who lived and those who died revealed that there was still higher activity of ICDH in nonsurvivors ($p = 0.02$), whereas the difference in SDH was less pronounced.

Our findings indicate that liver-specific serum enzymes are substantially enhanced on admission or shortly afterwards. Such an increase is not always the result of mechanical or hypoxic hepatic injury, but in many cases it may reflect only liver irritation by blunt impact without clinically detectable liver damage. Presence of high blood alcohol levels or trauma stress may also potentiate the effect on a hepatic enzyme system. Apparently, the latter temporarily increases membrane permeability by an unknown mechanism that may involve the action of hormones. It is a regular phenomenon to find a mild-to-moderate elevation of hepatic enzymes in patients with a pure head injury and no history of shock.

In the final samples taken, the activity of hepatic enzymes declines in both survivors and nonsurvivors. In both, the mechanism for the decrease is different. In surviving patients, a decline is expected in accordance with the improved clinical condition, since the effect of the initial stress of trauma on cellular permeability has already subsided. Through the natural healing process, the initial mechanical or hypoxic damage might have resolved or disappeared after reaching its maximum intensity. A decline in the activity of hepatic serum enzymes in patients who expired is paradoxical. It does not correspond to clinical reality in which hepatic cellular damage that was sustained in the original trauma does not resolve but frequently continues and intensifies as

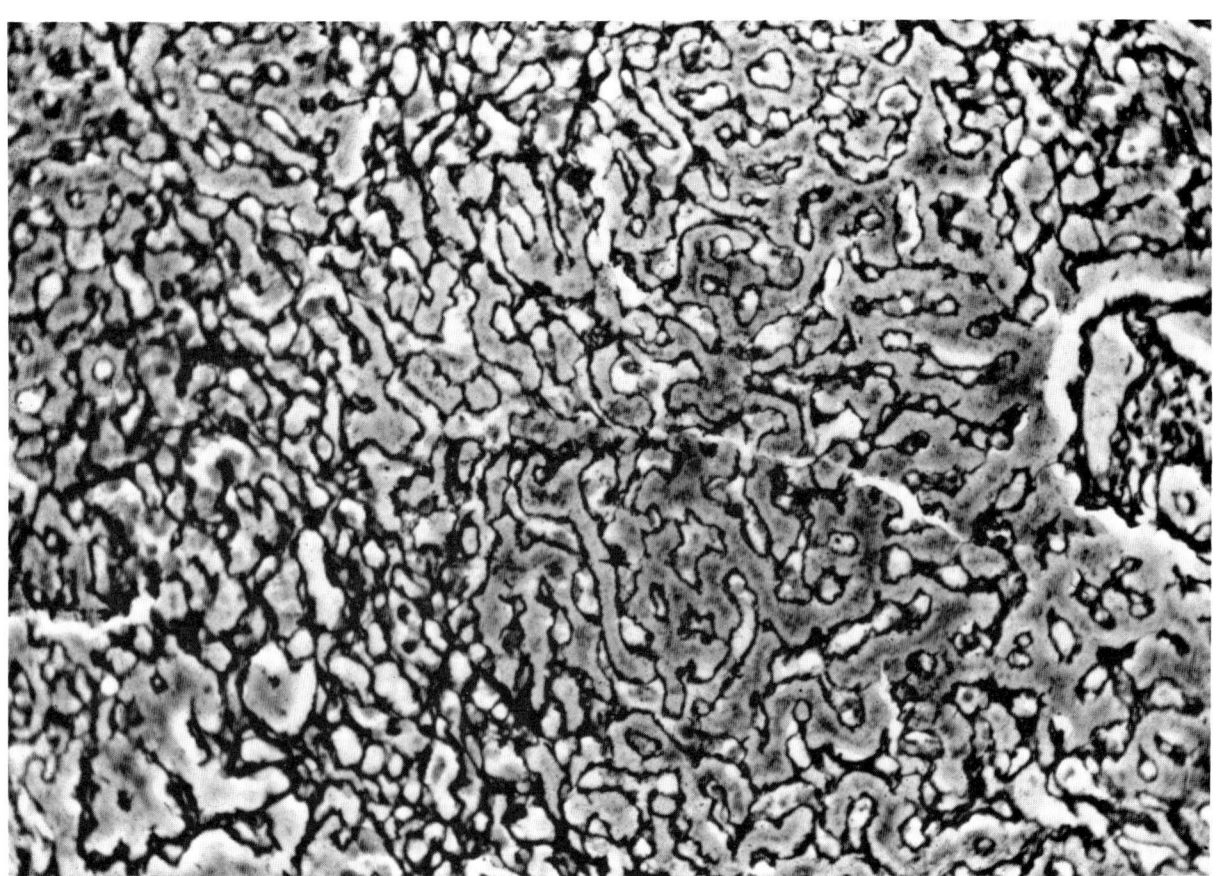

Figure 20.5. The prominent condensation of reticulum in the central lobar zone corresponding to the area of necrosis. Modified Hortega reticulum ×110. This is thought to be the template for regeneration (see text).

the patient's general condition deteriorates. Findings reveal that the intensity and extent of the affected areas continue to progress with centrilobular necrosis and degeneration increasing markedly. A large upsurge of serum hepatic enzymes being released from affected cells would be expected. Our results, however, demonstrate that this does not happen since, contrary to our expectation, the enzyme levels decline. We suggest that the failure of hepatic serum enzymes to respond to such a profound disorder is the result of a marked metabolic derangement that makes hepatocytes unable to synthesize and replenish exhausted or reduced intracellular

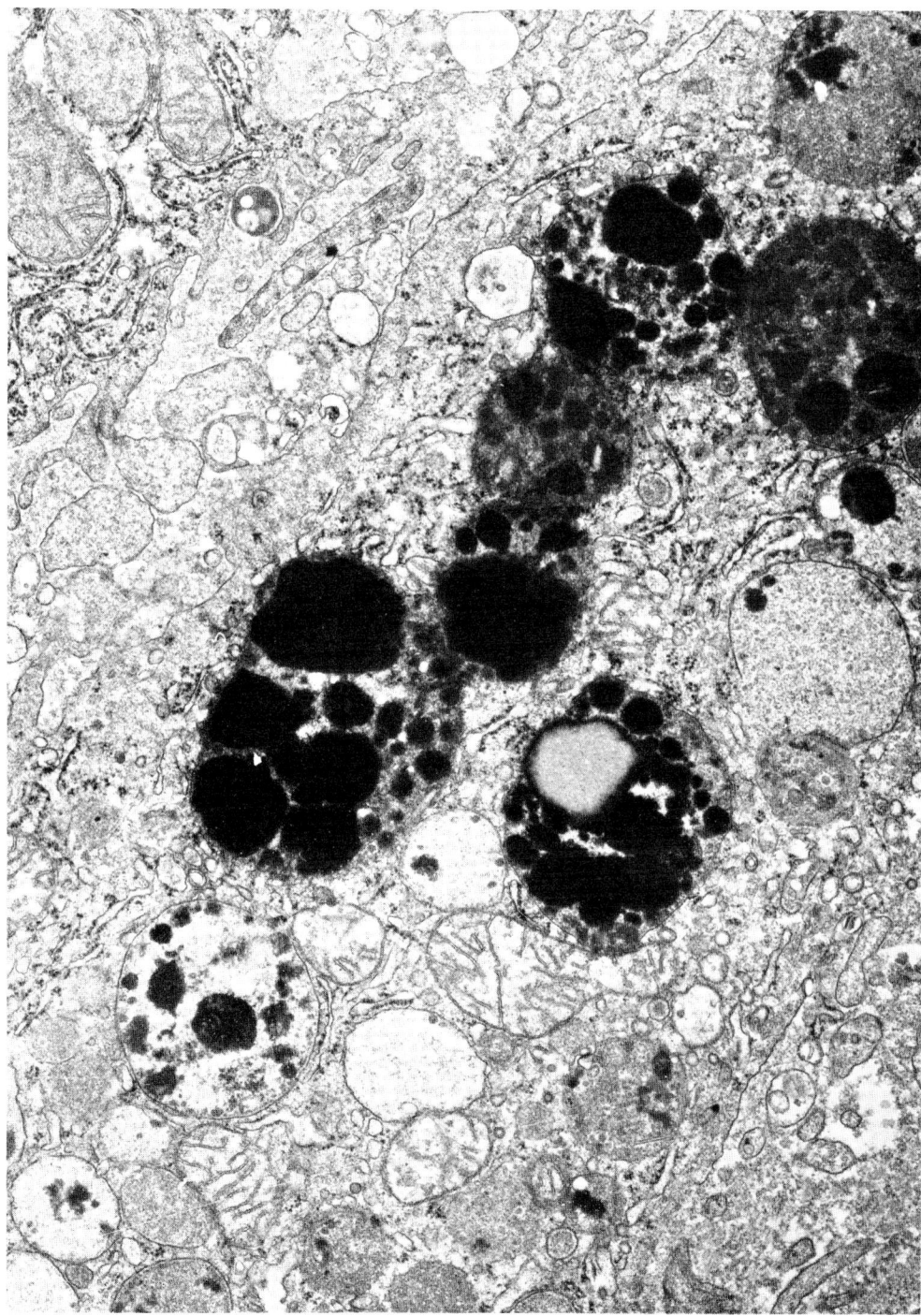

Figure 20.6. Electron micrograph of liver obtained at autopsy from a 62-year-old male who suffered irreversible brain injury following self-inflicted gunshot wounds to the head. This patient had several shock episodes. Note the numerous residual bodies.

stores. It is likely that inhibited proteosynthesis is the common denominator not only here but also for the other metabolic phenomena found, including coagulopathies (poor prothrombin synthesis), impaired plasma protein synthesis, low levels of energy rich substrates, etc.

In summary, we believe that interpretation of serum enzyme values must be done selectively on an individual basis in conjunction with the results of other biochemical laboratory and clinical parameters and with a respect for the time that has elapsed since injury.

Thus, we have been studying various parameters in our trauma patients to improve clinical care. We have found that seemingly unrelated measurements in the trauma patient can be applied to understanding liver pathophysiology as it relates to liver dysfunction in shock.

MORPHOLOGY OF THE LIVER IN SHOCK

Clinical Studies

LIGHT MICROSCOPY

In studies of patients conducted between 2 and 24 hr following the onset of shock, LM of the liver was employed, revealing a consistent increase in intracellular lipid. In some patients, a minimal number of acute inflammatory cells were found. Focal necrosis was observed only in those patients who subsequently exhibited a severe hepatic dysfunction (Fig. 20.4).

Dilatation and congestion of the sinusoids and hepatic veins were the most striking histological changes observed in these shock patients. Dilatation of the sinusoids was most marked in the area of the central zone and was coupled with a narrowing of the liver cords. The distension spread to involve the midzone in more severe cases, with linking of one central zone to the next in the plane of section 6–8 ml thick. In some instances, the sinusoidal dilatations nearly reached the portal zone, but in the majority of cases, the periportal areas were normal. This lesion is also described by Birgens et al. (1978) in their study of five patients with cardiogenic shock. Since the reticular framework of the necrotic parts of the liver lobule persists, these authors think that this structure serves as a template for regeneration. Korb et al. (1969) saw signs of regeneration within 48 hr.

The most severe cases evidenced pyknosis of the nuclei of the centrizonal and, at times, of the midzonal cells. Dense eosinophilia was observed in the cell cytoplasm. It was presumed that the centrizonal parenchymal cells were subsequently lost and replaced by a number of red blood cells. In instances of centrizonal or midzonal necrosis, the Kupffer's cell nuclei were usually less involved.

The affected zones also showed a significant increase in reticulum (Birgens, 1978), corresponding to the congestive and necrotic changes. Some thickening of the fibers was observed in the most severe cases, as evidenced by their ability to stain more collagen (Fig. 20.5). In some patients, fatty changes were detected, but we could not correlate these with the degree of shock sustained or with any of the other manifestations or changes described above.

Little indication was observed of intravascular fibrin

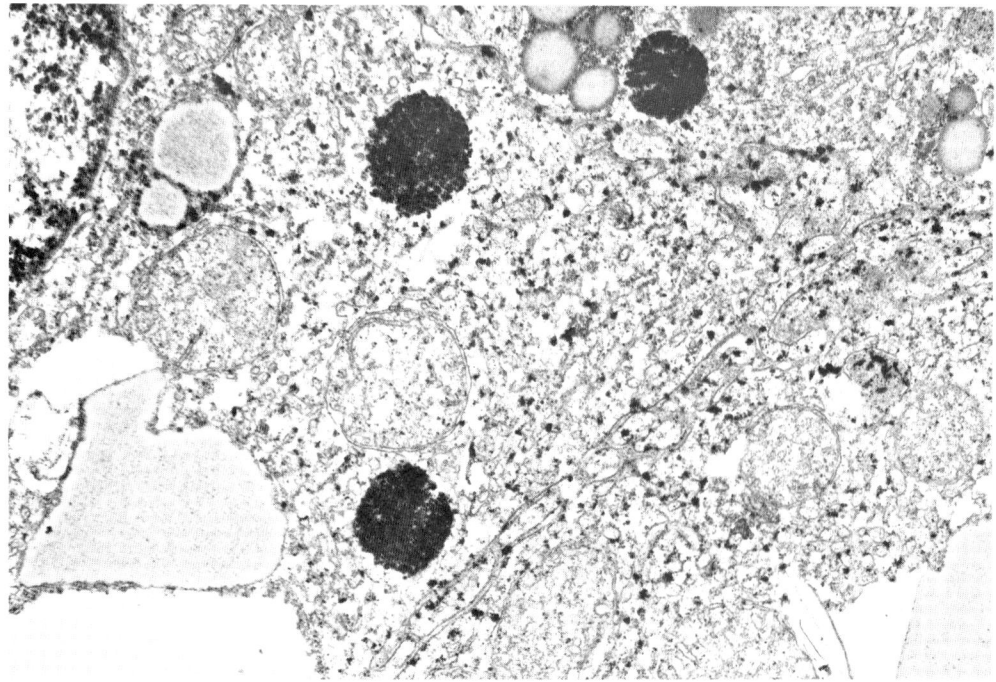

Figure 20.7. The reaction product for acid phosphatase can be seen in this liver sample obtained at autopsy from a 72-year-old male who suffered multiple injuries in a motor vehicle accident.

in the liver, lungs, or kidneys. Nor did we find the multiple foci, cardiac necrosis, or hemorrhagic enteropathy of the gut that have been noted in patients suffering from cardiac disease. Some patients maifested small focal areas of acute necrosis in the brain.

In prolonged cases, especially in those patients who develop septic shock, the parenchymal changes are often dramatic. At the LM level, they include an increased number of mitotic figures, fibroblastic repair, bile duct proliferation, and hypertrophy of hepatocytes with the presence of large intracytoplasmic eosinophilic acid-fast inclusions. The latter are especially prominent in the centrilobular regions. These inclusions are best interpreted as "residual bodies"—the presumed result of multiple autophagic events that lead to the sequestration of organelle debris within the lysosomal system (Fig.

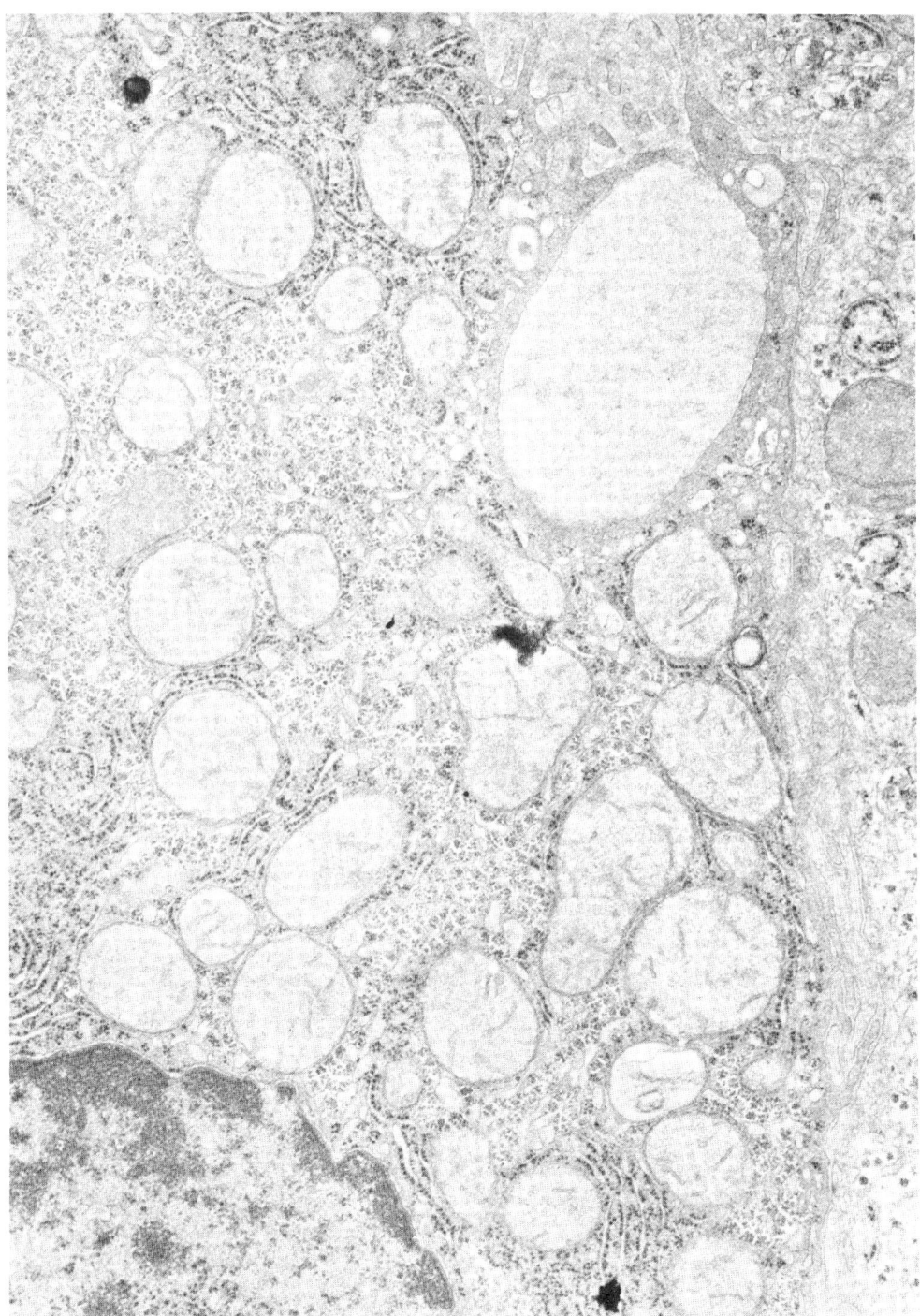

Figure 20.8. A hypoxic vacuole (*HV*) can also be seen in the liver of the patient described in Fig. 20.6.

20.6). These have acid phosphatase activity and may replace much of the cytoplasm (Fig. 20.7).

Electron Microscopy

We have studied numerous specimens of human liver that were obtained at biopsy or immediate autopsy at various intervals after hemorrhagic or septic shock (Trump et al., 1973a and b, 1975; Champion et al., 1976 a and b; Cowley et al., 1979). As discussed in this chapter, changes in humans have been compared with those seen in experimental animals. Biopsies taken soon after the primary injury, usually within the first 2 hr, show predominantly reversible, but significant changes in hepatic parenchymal cells. These changes, clearly definable at the ultrastructural level, typically occur in the absence of any LM changes with the possible exception of centrilobular congestion. The principal changes observed are those reversible stages of cell injury (see Ch. 1 for a description of these stages). Briefly, these stages consist of a clumping of nuclear chromatin (probably a result of decreased pH), dilatation of the endoplasmic reticulum, condensation or swelling of mitochondria, and distortion of plasmalemmal contours, including the formation of hypoxic vacuoles at the cell periphery (Fig. 20.8). These hypoxic vacuoles show a cytoplasmic border of contractile microfilaments, probably reflecting alteration of the cytoskeleton. Irreversible changes are seldom seen at this time interval; on the other hand, in the cases of patients in whom resuscitation is delayed for three or more hours, we have observed total irreversible changes in almost every hepatic parenchymal cell (Fig. 20.9). This was always associated with irreversible shock. It must be emphasized that at the gross and LM levels, these and normal livers were indistinguishable except for slight centrilobular congestion. As mentioned above, however, the latter may be significant insofar as it indicates altered hepatic blood flow. Thus, pathologists in the past were not able to observe severe cellular changes in the liver because they did not have the aid of EM.

Another early change in the acute stage is the formation of autophagic vacuoles (Fig. 20.10). In experimental animals, these readily form in response to elevated levels of plasma glucagon (Deter and deDuve, 1967). In shock patients, glucagon increases may well be the causative agent; on the other hand, cyclic AMP levels may also be stimulated by cellular ischemia, and both may relate to cellular failure to regulate ionized calcium. The formation of these autophagic vacuoles may well be the initial cellular reflection of increased protein catabolism and negative nitrogen balance.

The mechanisms responsible for the increased number of mitotic figures in the liver are not presently known. Increases in liver cell mitosis occur after necrosis or hepatectomy; however, in shock, the number of dividing cells seems out of proportion to these causes. Again, glucagon levels occur in the serum during the acute phase after hemorrhagic shock and therefore could play a role in both increased mitosis as well as the increased number of autophagic vacuoles.

In our experience, the extent of fibrosis and bile duct

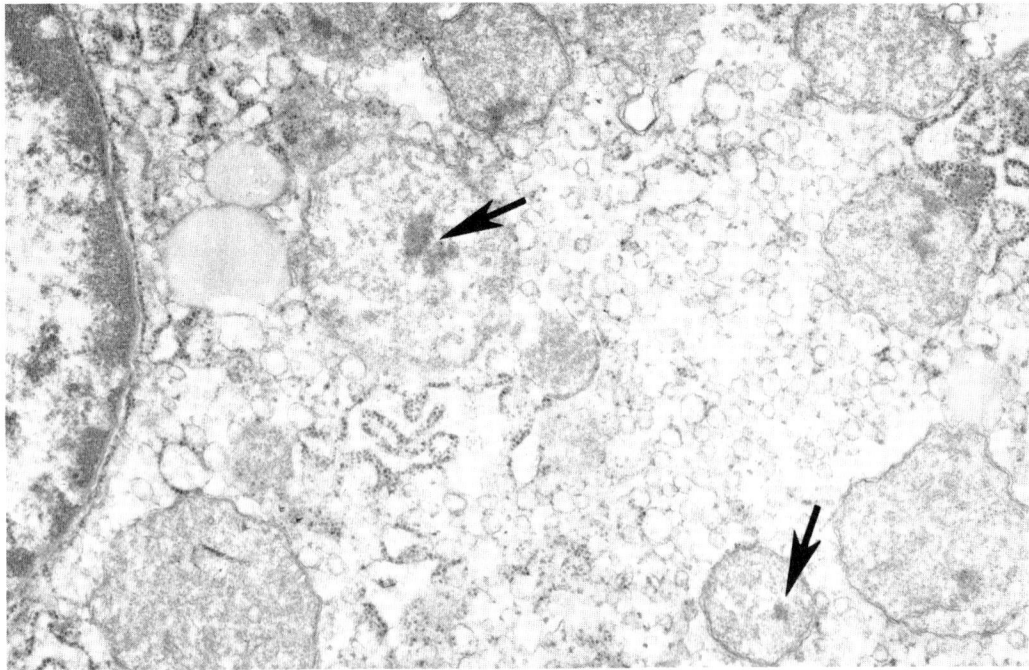

Figure 20.9. Liver biopsy from a 27-year-old male following a gunshot wound through the liver, esophagus, and aorta. This patient subsequently died. Flocculent densities (*arrows*), hallmarks of irreversibly injured cells, can be seen in these cells.

proliferation seems presently to be out of proportion to the amount of documented hepatic cell necrosis. Since 50% of our patients admitted for acute trauma have elevated blood alcohol levels (Benner et al., 1979), it may be valuable to explore the relationship of chronic alcohol ingestion to this phenomenon.

EXPERIMENTAL SHOCK MODELS

As discussed previously, it is our philosophy that improvements in clinical therapy can be made most rapidly by developing animal models of the human problem. Therefore, we have been carefully comparing

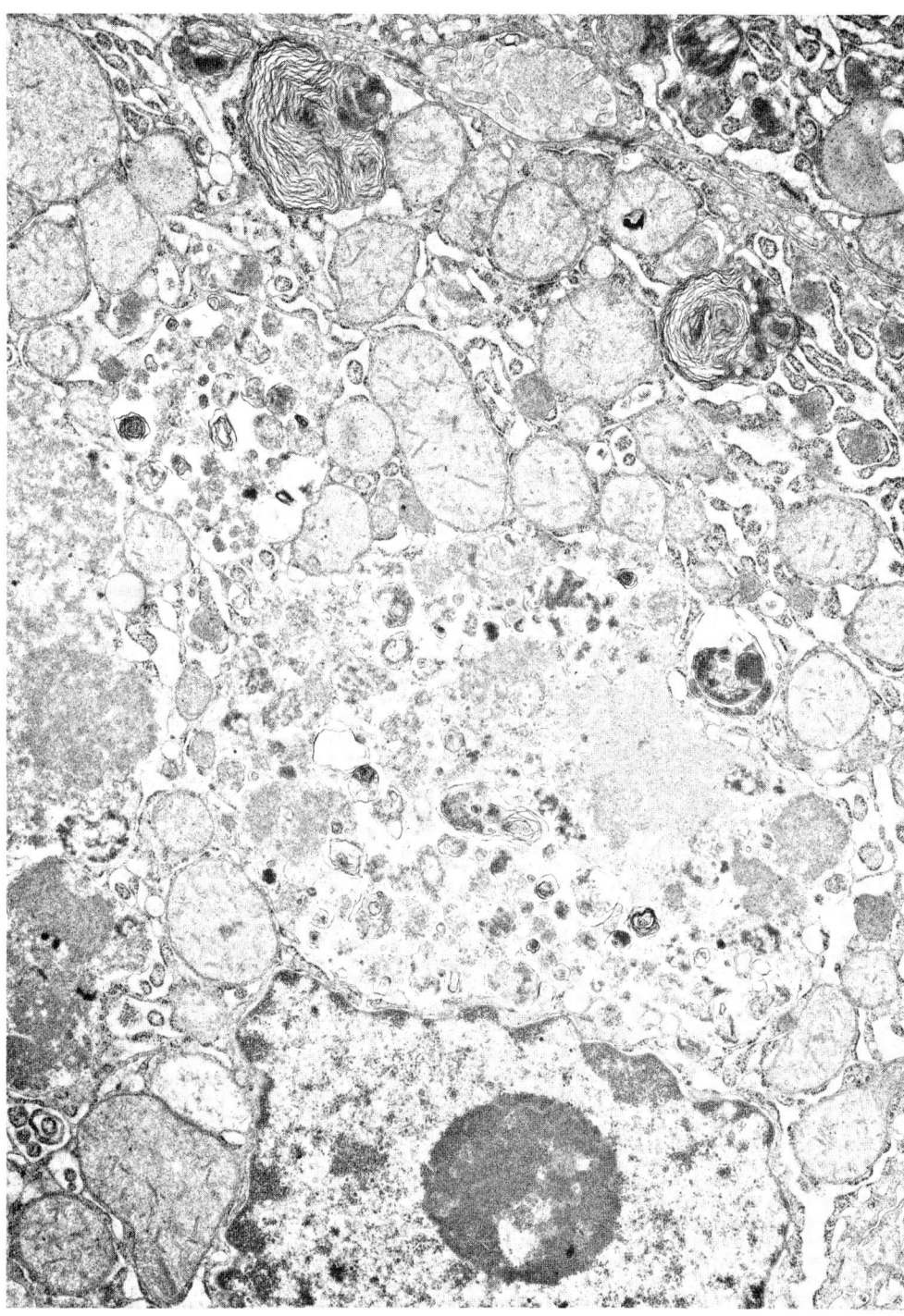

Figure 20.10. Numerous autophagic vacuoles can be seen in this liver biopsy specimen from a 24-year-old male who suffered blunt abdominal trauma as a result of a motor vehicle accident.

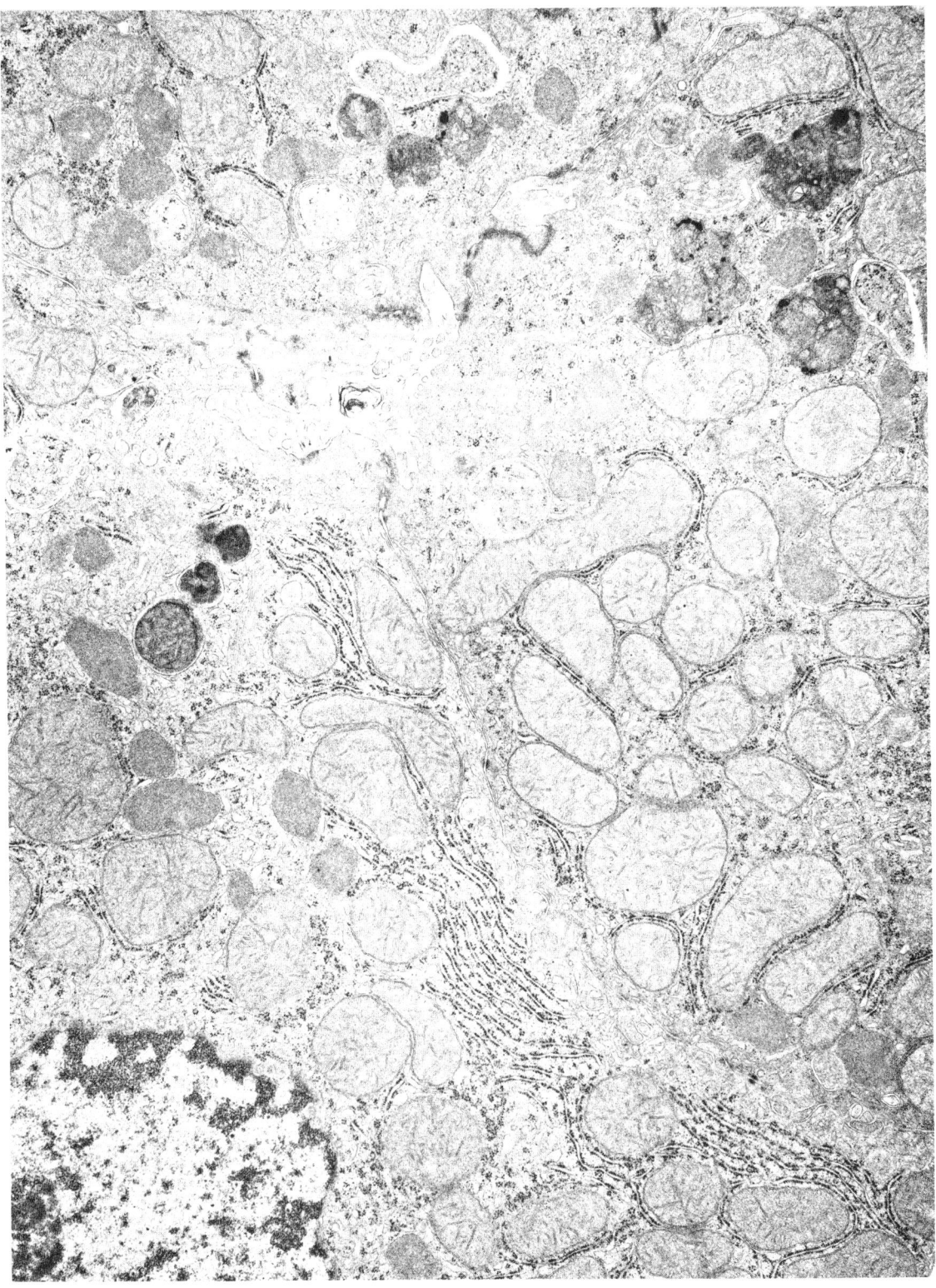

Figure 20.11. Rat liver from an experimental septic shock experiment. Numerous autophagic vacuoles can be seen.

experimental models with our studies of human shock, ischemia, and anoxia.

Hemorrhagic Shock

In our studies, we have employed a fixed volume hemorrhagic model similar to that described by Flenker and Greupner (1974). Rats were used in all of our studies. Reproducible values were obtained for the amount of blood loss which correlates with mortality (Sato et al., 1981). In these studies, there was a significant correlation between the amount of blood loss, the mean arterial blood pressure, and the hepatic energy charge (Atkinson, 1968). Significantly, further anaerobic incubation of the livers of animals shocked to the 84% lethality level showed no further reduction, indicating maximal ischemic reduction of hepatic energy charge (Ukikusa et al., 1981). This 84% lethality level is probably similar to many patients at the beginning of resuscitation. These findings, also indicated previously by Ozawa et al. (1976), suggest that the cellular homeostasis in the liver after hemorrhagic shock bears a reproducible relationship to the actual survival of the animal. Unfortunately, at the present time we have no way, except by EM or adenine nucleotide measurements, to assess this in a clinical patient in a shock trauma unit.

The parallel relationship between hepatic energy charge and mortality observed in this model is highly consistent with our observations and conclusions on human patients. At the ultrastructural level, the changes in the experimental liver are similar to those seen in humans immediately before resuscitation. That is, there was widespread mitochondrial swelling, dilatation of the endoplasmic reticulum, increased autophagy, and nuclear chromatin clumping.

Septic Shock

In our studies of septic shock, we have elected to utilize a live *Escherichia coli* model; we believe that this better represents the situation in humans (Tanaka et al., 1980). This type of shock is a major life-threatening syndrome. In this model, adult male Sprague-Dawley rats were injected with a bolus of live *E. coli* adjusted to concentrations that would produce standard mortality rates. It was obvious from our studies that a good dose-response curve could be obtained that was dependent on the number of organisms injected (normalizing for body surface area).

There was a marked drop in the hepatic energy charge in fatally dosed animals, even though in the mild or sublethal dose the hepatic oxidoreduction state actually increased. On the other hand, in the fatal stage, a marked decrease did occur in this hepatic oxido reduction state.

Our results suggest that the decrease in energy charge in septic shock is not due to a reduction of hepatic blood flow but that it might be due to more direct effects of endotoxin or the live bacteria on the parenchymal cells. Similar effects were suggested by the work of Mela et al. (1971).

Ultrastructural examination of the hepatic parenchymal cells from these animals revealed a striking increase in the number of autophagic vacuoles (Fig. 20.11), which was extremely reminiscent of the situation in human patients, as described earlier.

Although our studies seem to have established a correlation between parenchymal cell injury (especially in the liver) and the mortality of septic shock, the precise mechanism(s) of cellular damage remains unknown. Studies by Mela et al. (1971) on in vitro systems suggest a possible direct action of endotoxin. We have performed similar studies in vitro with isolated rodent hepatic parenchymal cells; *E. coli* endotoxin rapidly inhibits respiration in isolated liver cells.

Morphological changes detected by EM within a few hours of shock were generally found to correlate with the measure of uncomplicated hepatic dysfunction (using serum bilirubin as an index of the severity of shock), observed 5–10 days later. The onset of septicemia markedly increased the severity of the jaundice or triggered a deterioration of hepatic function.

Acknowledgment. This work was supported in part by National Institutes of Health Grant No. AM-15440-08A.

References

Atkinson, D.E.: Enzymes as control elements in metabolic regulation. In *The Enzymes*, edited by P. D. Boyer, vol. 1, p. 461. Academic Press, New York, 1970.

Attar, S.: Coagulation in human shock. Md. State Med. J. *16:* 69, 1967.

Attar, S., Esmond, W., and Cowley, R.A.: Hyperbaric oxygenation in vascular collapse. J. Thorac. Cardiovasc. Surg. *44:* 759, 1962.

Attar, S., Esmond, W., and Cowley, R.A.: Hyperbaric oxygenation in massive pulmonary embolism. Surg. Forum *15:*200, 1964.

Attar, S., Kirby, W.H., Masaitis, C., et al.: Coagulation changes in clinical shock: I. Effect of hemorrhagic shock on clotting time in humans. Ann. Surg. *164:*34, 1966a.

Attar, S., McLaughlin, J.S., Mansberger, A.R., et al.: Prognostic significance of coagulation studies in clinical shock. Surg. Forum *17:*8, 1966b.

Attar, S., Mansberger, A.R., Irani, B., et al.: Coagulation changes in clinical shock. II. Effect of septic shock on clotting times and fibrinogen in humans. Ann. Surg. *164:*41, 1966c.

Attar, S., Boyd, D.R., Layne, E., et al.: Alterations in coagulation and fibrinolytic mechanisms in acute trauma. J. Trauma *9:*939, 1969.

Attar, S., Hanashiro, P., Mansberger, A., et al.: Intravascular coagulation—Reality or myth? Surgery *68:*27, 1970.

Benner, C., Brown, T.C., and Cowley, R.A.: Drinking and driving in Maryland: A special report, 1979. Md. State Med. J. *28:*57, 1979.

Birgens, H., Henriksen, J., Matzen, P., et al.: The shock liver: Clinical and biochemical findings in patients with centrilobular liver necrosis following cardiogenic shock. Acta Med. Scand. *204:*417, 1978.

Blair, E., Cowley, R.A., and Tait, M.K.: Refractory septic shock in man: Role of lactate and pyruvate metabolism and acid-base balance in prognosis. Am. Surg. *31:*537, 1965.

Blair, E., Cowley, R.A., Wise, A., et al.: Clinical physiology of late (refractory) gram-negative bacteremic shock. Am. J. Surg. *117:*573, 1969.

Boyd, D.R., and Mansberger, A.R.: Serum water and osmolal changes in hemorrhagic shock: An experimental and clinical study. Am. Surg. *34:*744, 1968.

Broder, G., and Weil, M.H.: Excess lactate: An index of reversibility of shock in human patients. Science *143:*1457, 1964.

Brody, T.M., Calvert, D.N., and Schneider, A.F.: Alteration of carbon tetrachloride-induced pathologic changes in the rat by spinal resection, adrenalectomy and adrenergic blocking agents. J. Pharmacol. Exp. Ther. *131:*341, 1961.

Carlson, R.P., and Lefer, A.M.: Hepatic cell integrity in hypodynamic states. Am. J. Physiol. *231:*1408, 1976.

Champion, H.R., Jones, R.T., Trump, B.F., et al.: A clinicopathologic study of hepatic dysfunction following shock. Surg. Gynecol. Obstet. *142:*657, 1976a.

Champion, H.R., Jones, R.T., Trump, B.F., et al.: Post-traumatic hepatic dysfunction as a major etiology in post-traumatic jaundice. J. Trauma *16:*650, 1976b.

Cowley, R.A.: A total emergency medical services system for the state of Maryland. Md. State Med. J. *24:*37, 1975.

Cowley, R.A.: Maryland's Med-Evac program. In *Collected Papers in Emergency Medical Services and Traumatology*, edited by R.A. Cowley, p. 78. 20th Century Press, Baltimore, 1976a.

Cowley, R.A.: The resuscitation and stabilization of major multiple trauma patients in a trauma center environment. Clin. Med. *83:*14, 1976b.

Cowley, R.A.: Maryland's Med-Evac helicopter program. Conference Proceedings No. 255, Operational Helicopter Aviation Medicine, 1979.

Cowley, R.A., and Bond, S.: The Mid-Atlantic Emergency Medical Services Council, Inc. Emergency *9:*71, 1980.

Cowley, R.A., Mansberger, A.R., Rudo, F., et al.: A comparison of the levels of blood ammonia and other metabolites in the portal and systemic circulation during shock. Surg. Forum *10:*405, 1960.

Cowley, R.A., Attar, S., Esmond, W., et al.: Prevention and treatment of shock by hyperbaric oxygenation. Ann. N.Y. Acad. Sci. *117:*673, 1965a.

Cowley, R.A., Blair, E., Ollodart, R.M., et al.: Hyperbaric oxygen (OHP) therapy in shock. In *Shock and Hypotension*, p. 678. Grune & Stratton, New York, 1965b.

Cowley, R.A., Attar, S., LaBrosse, E., et al.: Some significant biochemical parameters found in 300 shock patients. J. Trauma *9:*926, 1969.

Cowley, R.A., Mergner, W.J., Fisher, R.S., et al.: The subcellular pathology of shock in trauma patients: Studies using the immediate autopsy. Am. Surg. *45:*255, 1979.

Deter, R.L., and deDuve, C.: Influence of glucagon, an inducer of cellular autopathy, on some physical properties of rat liver lysosomes. J. Cell Biol. *33:*437, 1967.

Duff, J.H., Scott, H.M., Peretz, D.K., et al.: The diagnosis and the treatment of shock in man based on hemodynamic and metabolic measurements. J. Trauma *6:*145, 1966.

Flenker, H., and Greupner, E.: Reversibler and irreversibler haemorragisher schock bei der ratte. Methode und ergebnisse eines standarisierten modells. Beitr. Pathol. *153:*339, 1974.

Guyton, A.C.: *Textbook of Medical Physiology*, ed. 5, p. 375. W. B. Saunders, Philadelphia, 1976.

Hankins, J.R., Bessman, S., Mansberger, A., et al.: The origin and utilization of ammonia in shock: A comparison of the levels of blood ammonia in the portal and systemic circulation during shock induced by the Fine Technique. Bull. Soc. Int. Chir. *1:*1, 1959.

Hankins, J.R., Cowley, R.A., Zipser, M.E., et al.: Use of the umbilical vein for manometric and radiographic studies of the splanchnic and portal beds in shock and trauma. Ann. Surg. *176:*111, 1972.

Hankins, J.R., Ayella, R.J., Gill, W., et al.: Umbilical vein portohepatography in hepatic trauma. Surg. Gynecol. Obstet. *137:*200, 1973.

Hankins, J., Gill, W., Zipser, M.E., et al.: Use of the umbilical vein to study the splanchnic and portal beds in shock and trauma: II. Metabolic studies. Ann. Surg. *180:*110, 1974.

Huguet, C., Nordlinger, B., Bloch, P., et al.: Tolerance of the human liver to prolonged normothermic ischemia; a biological study of 20 patients submitted to extensive hepatectomy. Arch. Surg. *113:*1448, 1978.

Knisely, M.H.: Intravascular erythrocyte aggregation (blood sludge). In *Handbook of Physiology, Circulation, Vol. III*, edited by W. F. Hamilton and P. Dow, ch. 63. American Physiological Society, Washington, DC, 1965.

Knisely, M.H., Cowley, R.A., Hawthorne, I., et al.: Separation of shock types. Experimental and clinical separation of hypovolemic and septic shock. Angiology *21:*728, 1970.

Korb, G., Müller, R., Gedigk, P., et al.: Über die entstehung und abheilung von lebernekrosen nach einem schock. Virchows Arch. [Pathol. Anat.] *348:*374, 1969.

LaBrosse, E.H., Beech, J.A., McLaughlin, J.S., et al.: Plasma amino acids in normal humans and patients with shock. Surg. Gynecol. Obstet. *125:*516, 1967.

LaBrosse, E.H., and Cowley, R.A.: Tissue levels of catecholamines in patients with different types of trauma. J. Trauma *13:*61, 1973.

Lambotte, L., and Wojcik, S.: Measurement of cellular edema in anoxia and its prevention by hyperosmolar solutions. Surgery *83:*94, 1978.

McAslan, T.C.: Automated respiratory gas monitoring of critically injured patients. Crit. Care Med. *4:*255, 1976.

McLaughlin, J.S.: The treatment of shock in a research facility. Md. State Med. J. *16:*73, 1967.

McLaughlin, J.S.: Physiologic consideration of hypoxemia in shock and trauma. Ann. Surg. *173:*667, 1971.

McLaughlin, J.S., LeeLacer, R., Attar, S., et al.: Pulmonary dysfunction in shock. South. Med. J. *62:*674, 1969.

Mansberger, A.R., Boyd, D.R., Cowley, R.A., et al.: Refractometry and osmometry in clinical surgery. Ann. Surg. *169:*672, 1969.

Mela, L., Bacalzo, L.V., and Miller, L.D.: Defective oxidative metabolism of rat liver mitochondria in hemorrhagic and endotoxin shock. Am. J. Physiol. *220:*571, 1971.

Moulton, G.A., Esmond, W., and Michaelis, M.: Effect of hyperbaric oxygenation on noble collip drum shock in the rat. Bull. Univ. Md. Sch. Med. *47:*42, 1962.

Nunes, G., Blaisdell, F.W., and Margaretten, W.: Mechanism of hepatic dysfunction following shock and trauma. Arch. Surg. *100:*546, 1970.

Ollodart, R.M.: Immunobacterial defense in humans in shock. Surg. Forum *14:*21, 1963.

Ollodart, R.M., and Mansberger, A.R.: Effect of hemorrhage and reinfusion on bacterial clearance in the dog. Surg. Forum *16:*76, 1965.

Ollodart, R.M., Hawthorne, I., and Attar, S.: Studies in experimental endotoxemia in man. Am. J. Surg. *113:*599, 1967.

Ozawa, K., Ida, T., Kamano, T., et al.: Different response of hepatic energy charge and adenine nucleotide concentrations to hemorrhagic shock. Res. Exp. Med. *169:*145, 1976.

Sato, T., Kamiyama, Y., Kamano, T., et al.: Pathophysiology of hemorrhagic shock. I. A model for studying the effects of acute blood loss in the rat. Pathol. Res. Pract., in press, 1981.

Shoemaker, W.C.: Pathobiology of death: Structural and functional interactions in shock syndromes. Pathobiol. Annu. *6:* 365, 1976.

Smythe, C.McC., Fitzpatrick, H.F., and Blakemore, A.H.: Studies of portal venous oxygen content in unanesthetized man (abstract). J. Clin. Invest. *30:*674, 1951.

Stori, E., Lusvarghi, E., Lenzi, M., et al.: La catheterisme portal: Porto-manometrie et porto-hepatographie trans-ombilicale: Ramarques physiopathologiques et cliniques. Presse Med. *74:*207, 1966.

Tanaka, J., Sato, T., Jones, R.T., et al.: Bacteremic shock: Aspects of high-energy metabolism in rat liver following living *E. coli* bacteremia. Circ. Shock *7:*207, 1980.

Ternberg, J.L., and Butcher, H.R.: Blood-flow relation between hepatic artery and portal vein. Science *150:*1030, 1965.

Tranquada, R.E., Grant, W.J., and Peterson, C.R.: Lactic acidosis. Arch. Intern. Med. *117:*1972, 1966.

Trump, B.F., Valigorsky, J., Dees, J.H., et al.: Cellular changes in human disease: A new method of pathological analysis. Hum. Pathol. *4:*89, 1973a.

Trump, B.F., Valigorsky, J., Dees, J.H., et al.: The modernization of the autopsy: Application of ultrastructural and biochemical methods to human disease. Med. Col. VA Q. *9:* 323, 1973b.

Trump, B.F., Valigorsky, J.M., Jones, R.T., et al.: The application of electron microscopy and cellular biochemistry to the autopsy; observations on cellular changes in human shock. Hum. Pathol. *6:*499, 1975.

Ukikusa, M., Kamiyama, Y., Sato, T., et al.: Pathophysiology of hemorrhagic shock. II. Anoxic metabolism of the rat liver following acute blood loss. Circ. Shock, in press, 1981.

Vitek, V., and Cowley, RA.: Blood lactate in the prognosis of various forms of shock. Ann. Surg. *173:*308, 1971.

Vitek, V., and Cowley, RA.: Lactic acid in blood as indicator of prognosis in hypotensive shock. Clin. Res. *16:*519, 1978.

White, J.J.: Direct portal hepatography and metabolic studies via the re-opened umbilical vein: Effect of vasoactive drugs on portal pressure, blood gases and lactates. Am. Surg. *34:* 852, 1968.

White, R.R., Mela, L., Bacalzo, V., et al.: Hepatic ultrastructure in endotoxemia, hemorrhage, and hypoxia: Emphasis on mitochondrial changes. Surgery *73:*525, 1973.

CHAPTER 21

Human Pathology of the Gastrointestinal Tract in Shock, Ischemia, and Hypoxemia

CHRISTIAN MITTERMAYER

URS N. RIEDE

Disorders of the gastrointestinal organs (pancreatitis, gastric or duodenal ulcers, esophageal ruptures) are one of the serious causes of septic or hemorrhagic shock in man.

Generalized circulatory shock can have different repercussions to the integrity of the intestinal tract. The lesions can be classified as uncharacteristic signs or as shock specific disorders. Among these, certain forms of the Mallory-Weiss syndrome associated with microthrombosis (embolism) or diffuse capillary bleeding of the stomach associated with hyperactivation of fibrinolysis in the gastric vessels may be mentioned. Shock-induced gastric and duodenal erosions are among the least effective clinically diagnosed causes of gastrointestinal hemorrhages, as investigations of the autopsy material show.

GENERAL CONSIDERATIONS

Disorders of the gastrointestinal tract (e.g., pancreatitis, duodenal or gastric ulcers, esophageal ruptures) are liable to cause septic or hemorrhagic shock. On the other hand, ischemia and shock of different etiologies can have various repercussions to the integrity of gastrointestinal organs. The stomach, intestines, pancreas, liver, and even the spleen can be involved. Those lesions are a neglected area of medical research for two reasons: in man, life-terminating disorders in shock or ischemia originate regularly from the lung ("shock lung"), the kidney ("shock kidney"), or the brain. Furthermore, the organs of the gastrointestinal tract undergo very fast postmortal autolysis, thus hampering the exactness of pathohistological diagnosis. Therefore, the knowledge of lesions induced by shock, hypoxemia, and ischemia in the gastrointestinal tract are based mainly on experimental data in animals. Only recently has biopsy diagnosis acquired increasing importance. Species specific reaction must be taken into consideration. In carnivorous animals, severe erosions of the mucosa of the small intestine dominate the clinical picture. In rodents, primates, and man the derangement of kidney and lung functions is the decisive factor for survival. This review deals with diseases in man. Only in very important and characteristic examples will animal experiments be quoted.

In order to understand these continuous changes, which manifest themselves as special appearances of shock hypoxia or ischemia, the original clinical picture of the shock syndrome and general pathological findings should be referred to.

Insufficiency of microcirculation must be considered to be the main cause for the onset of shock, and as a result, the effective balance between the contents of the blood vessels, the vessel wall, and the blood flow is disturbed (Lasch, 1978). Pathological and anatomical observations by light microscopy concentrate particularly on changes which are seen in the contents of the blood vessels and the vessel wall. Findings obtained from the blood-flow during a shock-induced state (Neuhof et al., 1978) reveal valuable supplementary aspects, in particular those following intravital microscopic investigations of the terminal blood flow. Four important phenomena may be observed in connection with these investigations (Fig. 21.1). Each of these general phenomena may produce special diseases in man. The adhesion of parietal thrombi may decrease the blood flow, thus inducing ischemia (A). Due to obstructing microthrombosis, which occurs within the tissues and organs, focal necroses accompanied by subsequent hemorrhages, e.g,

within the gastric mucosa, may be produced within areas where the anastomotic circulation is poor (B). Fibrinolysis near the endothelia will ensue when the intima has been damaged and/or when thrombi have been eliminated. Excessive fibrinolysis may be an additional cause for diffuse gastric mucosal bleedings (C). During the shock-induced event, ruptures of small vessels are liable to suddenly destroy entire organs or their parts, for example, hemorrhagic necroses of the intestine or the pancreas (D).

An analysis made of the general fundamental phenomena of shock shows that various forms of injury to the endothelium play an essential role (Freudenberg, 1978).

Observation of the microcirculation in the intravital microscope in the animal experiment demonstrates the features of platelet aggregation, parietal thrombosis (Fig. 21.2) and hemorrhage (Fig. 21.3) in the mesentery of the rabbit.

Besides the pure microcirculatory aspect of ischemia, hypoxemia, and shock, the role of endotoxin should be taken into consideration. Shock-induced tissue damage in the intestine may lead to invasion of gram-negative intestinal bacteria and/or their toxic constituents (endotoxins) into the blood circulation. Circulating endotoxin was demonstrated during various forms of shock by using the limulus test (Fine et al., 1971). Dependent on the intensity of endotoxemia, a great number of pathophysiological mechanisms may be induced like activation of blood coagulation and of complement system as well as liberation of endogenous mediators (histamine, serotonine, plasmakinines, catecholamines, prostaglandines, and others). The activation of humoral systems and mediators leads to an intensification of still existing shock or to a renewed occurrence of shock due to endotoxemia (endotoxin shock). Therefore, the importance of elimination and detoxification of endotoxin is obvious. The mechanisms leading to the elimination and detoxification of endotoxin are not completely understood. However, it was shown in animal experiments that the phagocytic activity of the reticuloendothelial system (RES) plays an important role in this process, with the liver representing the main organ (Policard, 1962) and

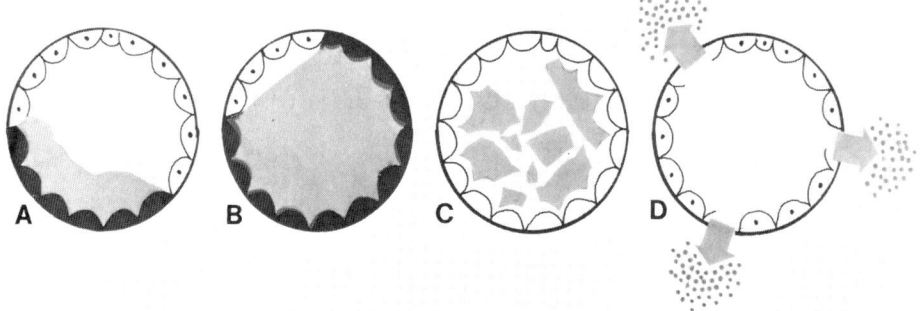

Figure 21.1. Endothelial lesions as characteristic feature of the shock-induced event. A, parietal thrombosis; example: gastrointestinal petechial hemorrhage. B, obstructive thrombosis; example: Mallory-Weiss syndrome. C, increased fibrinolysis; example: diffuse petechial gastric hemorrhage. D, toxic hemorrhagic rupture of a vessel; example: hemorrhagic necroses of the pancreas.

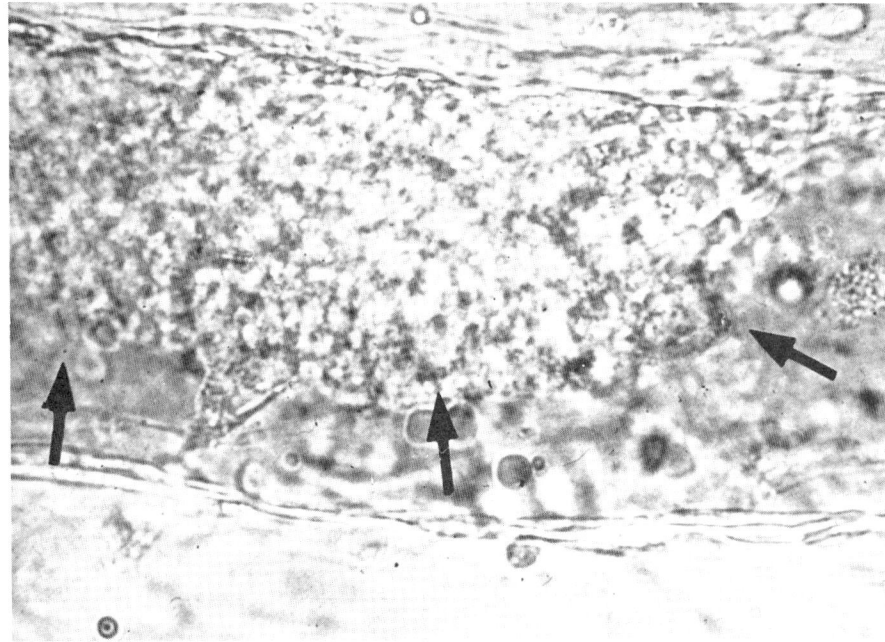

Figure 21.2. Intravital microscopy. Hemorrhagic shock in the rabbit. Small mesenteric vein with intravascular clotting consisting mainly of thrombocytes. A few strings of fibrin are visible on the right portion of the figure. The plasma exhibits a pinkish color because of hemolysis. ×690.

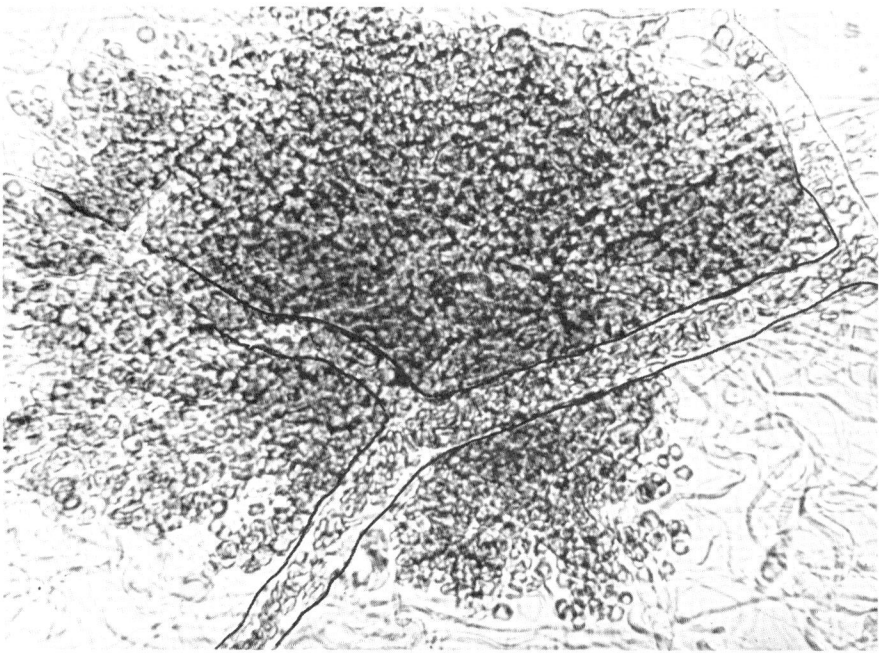

Figure. 21.3. Intravital microscopy. Endotoxic shock in the rabbit. Venole crossing the figure diagonally. Several capillaries flow into the venole. Rupture and perivascular accumulation of erythrocytes. ×140.

the Kupffer cells representing the main cell population (Freundenberg et al., 1980) in this activity. Circulating endotoxin in near lethal doses influences the phagocytic function of RES dramatically. During the first 12 hr after parenteral endotoxin application in experimental animals, a decreased phagocytic activity of the RES can be observed (Gospos et al., 1977). This coincides with morphological signs of cell injury of the Kupffer cells in the liver (De Palma, 1967), which are believed to be the main representatives of the RES system. Damage of these cells may therefore be the reason for the observed decrease in the velocity of RES clearance in the first 12 hr after endotoxin-induced shock.

INTESTINES

Because of the high α-receptor activity in the splanchnic area, shock can induce a pronounced vasoconstriction (Zweifach and Fronek, 1975; Reynolds and Swan, 1972; Messmer, 1968; Marston, 1977). The blood circulation in the stratum mucosum is almost selectively decreased, while stratum submucosum and muscularis propria are spared of the decrease in blood supply.

Thus, the transitory vasoconstriction induces ischemia in the mucosa of the stomach and the gut likewise. Preferential localizations for this damage are the mucosa of the stomach, the jejunum, and the ileum in decreasing order. Very seldom is the colonic mucosa involved. Older patients are more often struck by these phenomena, especially if the superior mesenteric artery is partly or totally obliterated by arteriosclerosis. Very often the damage is segmentally localized, as seen in the autopsy corresponding to the anatomical organization of the vascular supply. The initial necrotizing process may end in pseudomembranous enteritis (Fig. 21.4).

The colon is frequently damaged in the ascending part and in the left flexure, where the watershed of the superior and inferior mesenteric arteries is situated. Flenker and Liehr (1978) found 24 such cases in 1037 autopsies. Findings of animal experiments cannot be transferred to man without some reservation. Endotoxin leads to splanchnic vasoconstriction in dogs while in primates, vasodilatation ensues (Brobmann et al., 1970).

Disturbances of the intestines may have two important repercussions. First, the damage of the mucosa leads to a loss of water, electrolytes, and proteins through the intestinal lumen. Second, the mucosal damage may be the cause of irreversibility of shock. There is no unanimosity of how the mucosal erosions arise. Microthrombosis and micronecrosis may be the decisive factor in certain cases. Enzymatic tryptic activity may conceivably destroy the mucosal layer (Bounous, 1967; Marston, 1977), although mucosal damage also occurs in pancreatectomized animals.

Derangement of the barrier function of the gut may prepare for the invasion of gram-negative bacteria or their endotoxins. Necrotizing lesions of the intestines (Marston, 1962) end lethally in 70% of the cases. Shock-induced lesions of the gut are probably responsible for the final cause of shock in many instances (Fine et al., 1971; Lillehei, 1957; Marston, 1977). Recent progress in the assay of endotoxin with the aid of the limulus test (Liehr et al., 1976) and immunohistochemistry (Freudenberg et al., 1980) confirm the important role of the intestines in bringing about irreversibility of shock. The pattern of damage during ischemia occurs in phases: in the earliest phase cristolysis in mitochondria can be observed; 15 min after onset of shock, apical edema of the cell takes place. After 60 min, edema extends to the basis of the cells and leads to the shedding of superficial cell layers. Epithelia of the crypts, especially their undifferentiated stem cells, are less sensitive towards ischemia and hypoxia than is their differentiated counterpart at the surface. The possibility of mucosal renewal exists since regeneration of cells occurs through proliferation of crypt epithelia to replace the epithelia of villi.

STOMACH AND DUODENUM

These organs are frequently exposed to shock-induced lesions in man. Early lesions are not life-threatening, but the shock lesions in the stomach and duodenum pose difficult diagnostic and therapeutic problems. The cen-

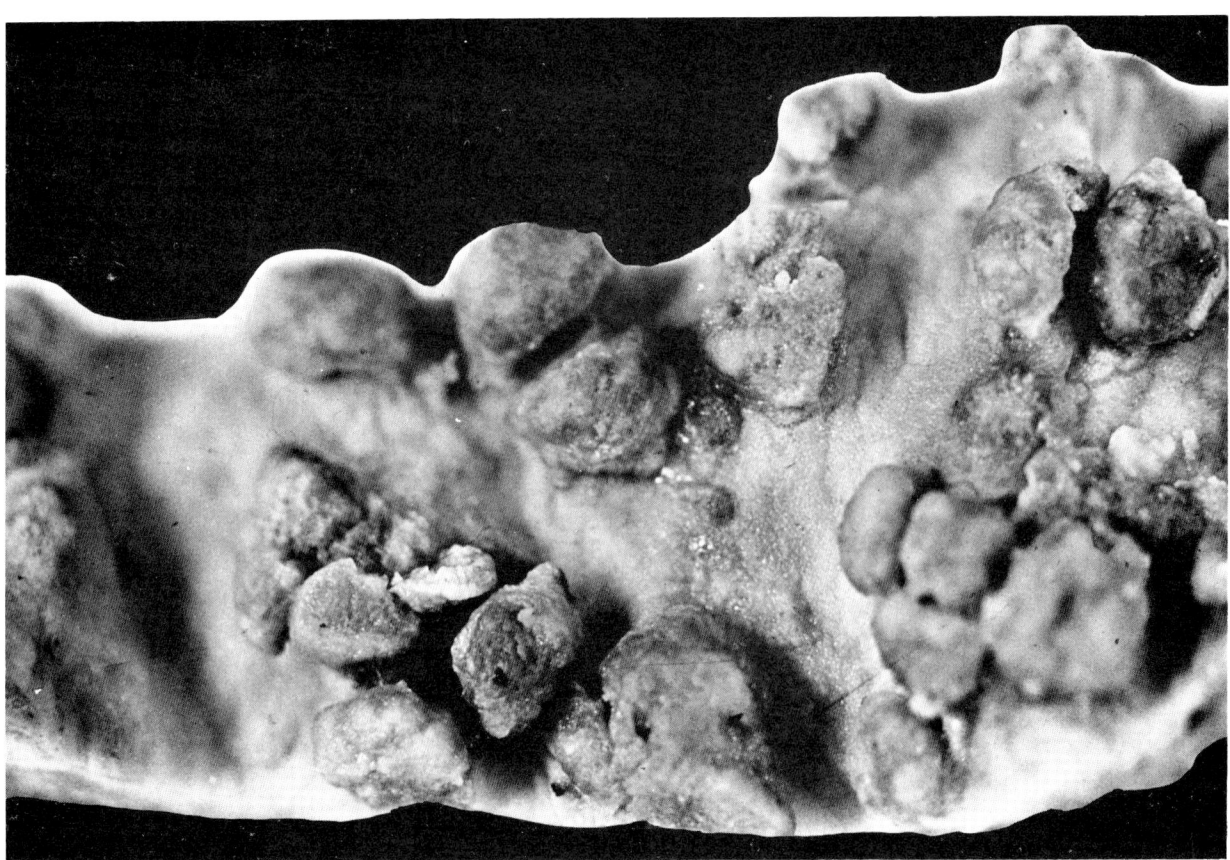

Figure 21.4. Pseudomembranous colitis after septic shock of 2-weeks duration. 62-year-old man.

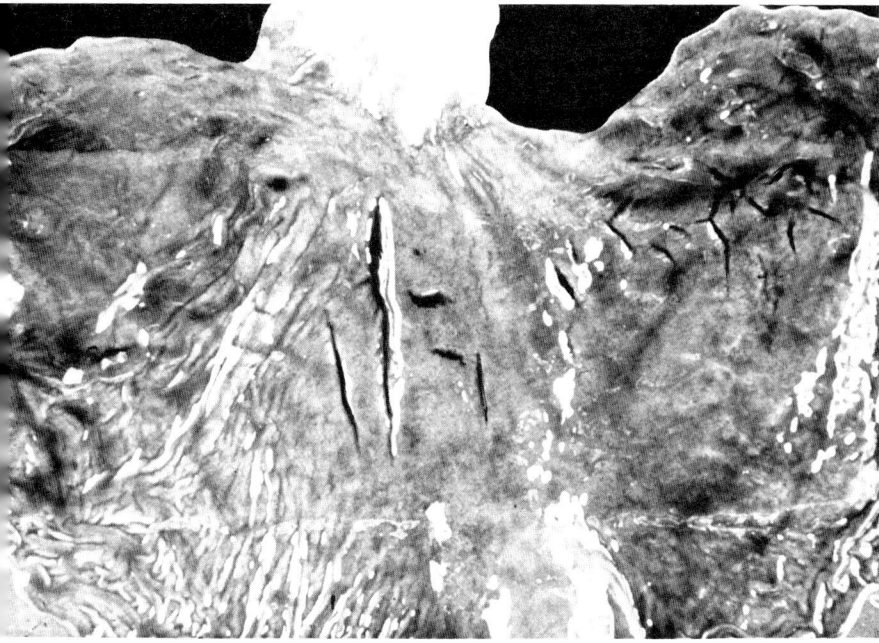

Figure 21.5. Mallory-Weiss Syndrome. Several longitudinal fissures in the cardia region radiating from gastro-eosophageal junction. Thirty-seven-year-old alcoholic in septic shock. The gastric and enteric vessels were obliterated with microthrombosis.

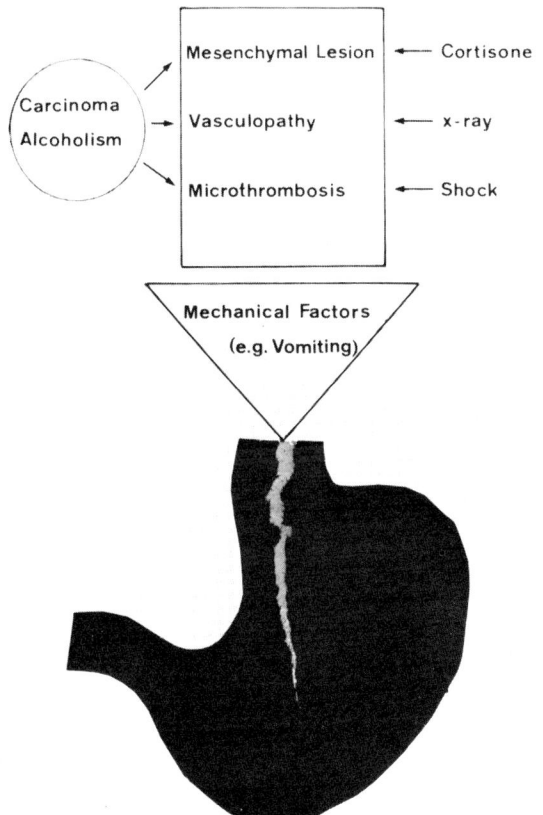

Figure 21.6. Pathogenetic factors observed in the Mallory-Weiss Syndrome. Some of the well known pathogenetic manifestations, caused either by the abuse of alcohol, the presence of a carcinoma of the esophagus or of the stomach, or by cortisone or x-ray treatment, may be aggravated by a shock-induced

tral feature here appears to be vasoconstriction in the initial phases. Endotoxin is able to evoke a segmental decrease of blood supply in areas of the corpus ventriculi. Hemorrhagic shock leads to the generalized decrease of blood supply in all regions of the stomach (Richardson et al., 1973). The blood supply and shock conditions are disproportionally reduced in the stomach, if one takes the cardiac output into consideration. Not surprisingly, in severe burns, multiple gastric erosions are found mainly in the corpus ventriculi. Shock-induced mucosal hemorrhages in the stomach and duodenum have been well known since the last century (Curling, 1842; Billroth, 1867). The sequential steps in pathogenesis have been amply described (Flenker and Liehr, 1978). The earliest morphological signs of ischemic or shock-induced damage can be seen in gastric mucosal cells as apical edema. This edema extends to the basis and appears as subepithelial edema. After 30 min, parts of the mucosal cells are extruded, mitochondria begin to swell, cristolysis occurs, and platelets aggregate in capillaries. Two hours after onset of shock or ischemia, superficial necrosis of epithelia ensues. As a consequence, interstitial edema of the lamina propropria and endothelial damage in the small mucosal vessels, diffuse microthrombosis can be observed. Extensive erosions of mucosa appear after 6 hr. Necrosis now reaches a depth of about one-half the mucosa. One day after onset of the damage, the basal third of the mucosa is destroyed. On the 2nd day, progressive shallow ulcers can be registered. Among gastrointestinal hemorrhages in man one can discern between fatal and nonfatal cases. In both classes, shock-incident and microthromboses. When the mucosa has been damaged by microthrombosis and micronecrosis, ruptures may occur that are brought about by an increased intragastric pressure.

induced hemorrhages play a role (Mittermayer et al., 1978). Most of shock-induced hemorrhages are not clinically diagnosed. Two shock-derived conditions may deserve attention.

Microthrombosis and Manifestation of the Mallory-Weiss Syndrome

During the initiating shock-triggering incident, microthrombosis occurs within the tissues and organs. Because of this, focal necroses within areas depending on blood supply may be produced by obstruction of end arterial blood vessels. Numerous intravital investigations carried out under the light microscope show that microthrombosis occurs in vivo and must not be considered as a postmortal phenomenon (Hagedorn et al., 1975; Mittermayer et al., 1972). Thrombocyte thrombi are prevailing in an intact rapid blood flow and in the presence of an exceeding coagulation instability (Fig 21.3), whereas fibrin thrombi occur in a slowly running blood flow. Gastric bleedings during shock can be seen rather frequently, although they are rarely diagnosed since the nonfatal cases are usually not noticed by the

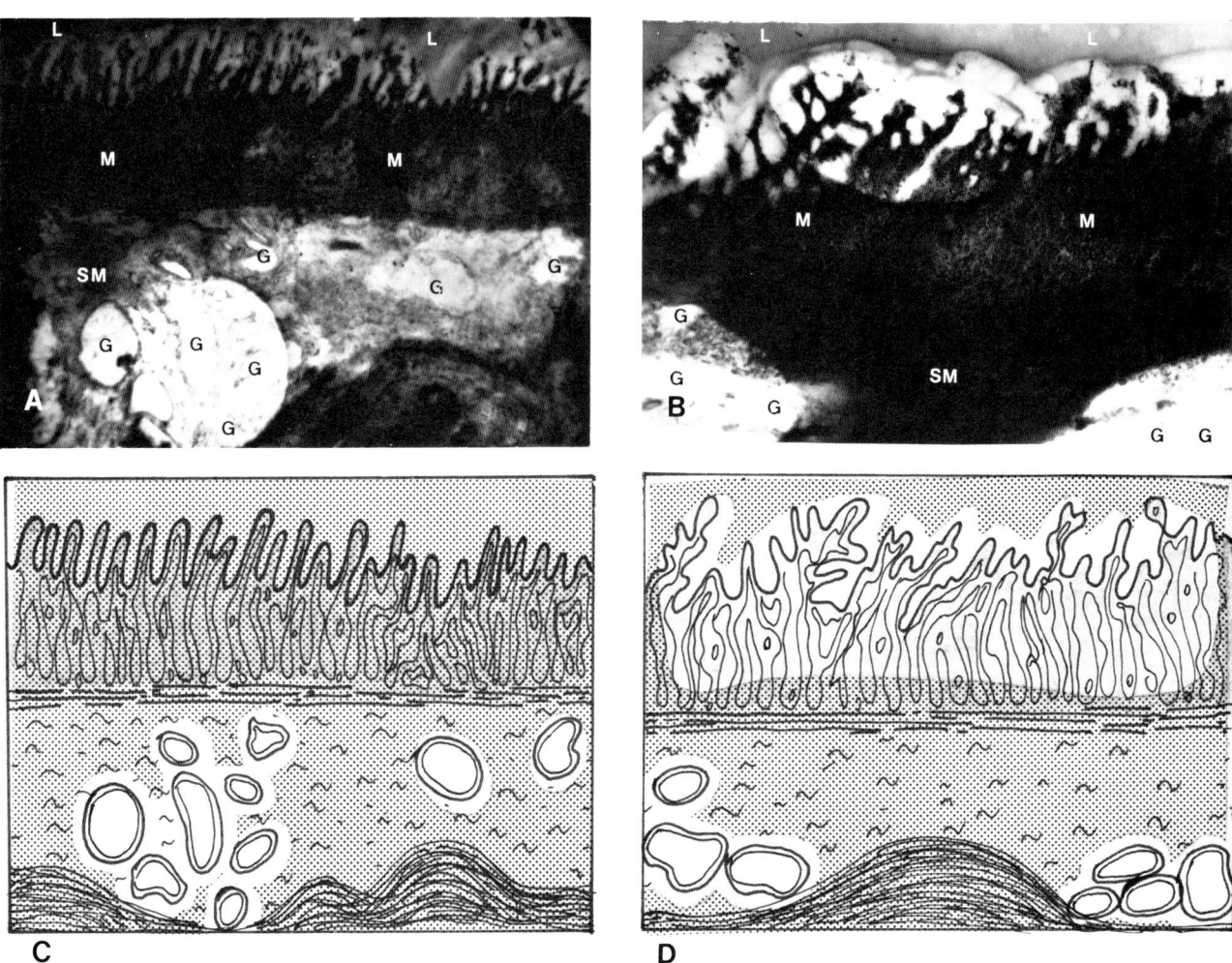

Figure 21.7. Fibrinautography of the gastric wall A, healthy stomach. The determination of tissue-bound plasminogen-activator is performed by plasmin rich fibrin film (Blümel, 1972; Schlag et al., 1973; Denk et al., 1976). A thin, faintly red-stained film of fibrin is layered over frozen sections of a normal (A) and bleeding stomach (B). According to the distribution and concentration of the plasminogen-activator in the tissue, plasminogen is converted to plasmine. The fibrin film is lysed. The zones of lysis are indicated as bright halos. In the normal gastric wall, the fibrinolytic activity is localized exclusively over blood vessels of the submucosa. In contrast, the mucosa shows almost no activity. ×36. B, diffuse capillary gastric hemorrhage ("weeping stomach"). The fibrinautography shows large bright halos over the mucosa, indicating increased fibrinolytic activity in the mucosal layer. ×36. C, schematic demonstration of fibrinautography of normal gastric wall. Fibrinolytic activity is characterized by bright halos. C, schematic demonstration of fibrinautography with diffuse capillary bleeding. Abbreviations: M, gastric mucosa; L, gastric lumen; SM, submucosal layer, G, blood vessel.

clinician. Among 1000 autopsies that were observed in a large university hospital within the period of 1 year, two cases were attributed to the Mallory-Weiss syndrome. The characteristic mucosal ruptures of this syndrome (Fig. 21.5) differ in size and length. During the past years, we investigated 18 cases and found that the Mallory-Weiss syndrome is frequently associated with the state of shock or with disseminated intravascular coagulation. In two-thirds of the cases which were observed, findings obtained from histological examinations revealed extensive microthrombosis (Mittermayer et al., 1971) within the mucosal vessels. One could assume microthrombosis to be a secondary effect following laceration. In the above mentioned cases, however, a diffuse occurrence of microthrombosis was found to be present not only in the stomach but also in the entire intestinal tract. The characteristic mucosal ruptures of the Mallory-Weiss syndrome were also obtained in shock-induced animal experimental models (Linder et al., 1971; Linder, 1972). Microthrombosis and subsequent focal necroses are, however, unlikely to cause the Mallory-Weiss syndrome by themselves. Prior publications list a large number of well known pathogenetic factors (Nielsen et al., 1970) (Fig. 21.6) to which we would like to add obstructive microthrombosis. It is suggested that this clinical picture is produced by additional aggravating factors which result from microthrombosis, e.g., raise of intragastric pressure.

Increased Fibrinolysis and Diffuse Gastric Hemorrhages

Another type of bleeding may occur in the stomach, i.e., diffuse petechial hemorrhage. Five cases which we investigated showed this type of bleeding in fatal shock (Mittermayer et al., 1978). Our investigation method was based on fibrin-histoautography (Todd, 1972; Denk, 1976; Blümel, 1972), which allows the activity of fibrinolysis to localize within the tissue. Fibrin, which had been stained faintly (Fig. 21.7), was deposited on top of gastric tissue sections. Clear zones indicated the activity of fibrinolysis and showed the area where fibrin was digested. Except for the mucosal vessels, normal gastric mucosa develops no activity. Considerably increased fibrinolysis, which spread throughout the gastric surface, can be seen in the mucosa of diffusely bleeding stomachs. Inasmuch as no microthrombosis could be detected in the cases investigated, it must be assumed that fibrinolytic activity either increases in the absence of pre-existing thrombotic deposits or that deposits which might have been present were completely digested before and could no longer be seen.

It should be pointed out again that during shock-induced incidents, hemorrhages are likely to occur within the gastric mucosa which may have been brought about by different pathogenetic pathways (Eder and Castrup, 1969; Eichfuss et al., 1976; Fahrtmann and Eichen, 1977; Feifel and Heberer, 1977; Katz and Siegel, 1968; Martinoli and Ganther, 1970; Oehlert et al., 1978) that cannot be enumerated in detail here.

Toxic Ruptures of Blood Vessels and Manifestation of Diffuse Gastric Bleeding

It has been demonstrated by experiments that excessive endotoxinemia (Fig. 21.3) may produce direct and sudden ruptures of small blood vessels in the absence of any pre-existing visible endothelial damage or thrombosis. The course of events appears to be progressing so rapidly that our methods merely allow time to indicate the final stage during which disruption occurs. In this stage, the walls of the small blood vessels, particularly those of the small veins, are torn suddenly and unexpectedly.

Human pathology suggests that gastric diffuse bleeding, hemorrhagic necroses of the pancreas, and the Waterhouse-Friderichsen syndrome (Mittermayer et al., 1979) are manifestations of general septic hemorrhages.

Acknowledgment. Supported by the Sonderforschungshererich 46 of The Deutsche Forschungsgemeinschaft.

References

Billroth, T.: Über Duodenalgeschwüre bei Septicämie. Wien. Med. Wochenochr. *17*:705, 1867.

Blümel, G.: Experimentelle und klinische Untersuchungen zum posttraumatischen Geschehen. *Neue Aspekte der Trasylol-Therapie*, Edited by W. Brendel und G.L. Haberland, pp. 95-106. F.K. Schattauer Verlag, Stuttgart, 1972.

Bounous, G.: Role of the intestinal contents in the pathophysiology of acute intestinal ischemia. Am. J. Surg. *114*:368, 1967.

Brobmann, G., Ulano, H.B., Hinshaw, L.B., and Jacobson, E.D.: Mesenteric vascular responses to endotoxin in the monkey and dog. Am. J. Physiol. *219*:1464, 1970.

Curling, T.B.: On acute ulceration of the duodenum in cases of burn. Med.-chirurg. Trans. *25*:260, 1842.

Denk, S., Kujat, R., Schlag, G., Wriedt-Lübbe, I., Blümel, G.: Das Verhalten gewebeständiger Plasminogenaktivatoren nach Poly-trauma. Med. Welt *27*:876, 1986.

De Palma, R.G., Coil, J., Davis, J.H., and Holden, W.D.: Cellular and ultrastructural changes in endotoxemia: A light and electron microscopic study. Surgery *62*:505, 1967.

Eder, M., and Castrup, H.J.: Die gastrointestinale Blutung aus der Sicht des Pathologen. Chirurg *40*:97, 1969.

Eichfuss, H.P., Fahrtmann, E., Horatz, K., and Schreiber, H.W.: Die grosse Blutung aus Magen und Zwölffingerdarm. Dtsch. med. Wochenschr. *101*:753, 1976.

Fahrtmann, E.H., and Eichen, R.: Chirurgische Behandlung der intestinalen Blutungen. Chirurg *48*:219, 1977.

Feifel, G., and Heberer, G.: Die Prolematik der akuten oberen gastrointestinalen Blutung. Chirurg *48*:204, 1977.

Fine, J., Caridis, D.T., Cuevas, P., Ishijama, M., and Reinhold, R.: Therapeutic implications of new developments in the study of refractory nonseptic shock. Shock in low- and high-flow states. Excerpta Med. Int. Congr. Ser. 247, 1971.

Flenker, H., and Liehr, H.: Schockmanifestationen in Magen, Darm, Pankreas und Leber, Klinik und Pathologie. Verh. Dtsch. Ges. Pathol. *62*:127, 1978.

Freundenberg, M., Freudenberg, N., and Galanos, C.: Immunhistochemischer Nachweis von Endotoxin in den Ausscheidungs-organen der Ratte. Verh. Dtsch. Ges. Pathol. *64*:437, 1980.

Freudenberg, N.: Endothel und Schock. Pathol. Res. Pract. *162:*105, 1978.

Gospos, Ch., Freudenberg, N., Bank, A., and Freudenberg, M.A.: Effect of endotoxin-induced shock on the reticuloendothelial system. Phagocytic activity and DNA-synthesis of reticuloendothelial cells following endotoxin treatment. Beitr. Pathol. *161:*100, 1977.

Hagedorn, M., B. Pfrieme, Ch. Mittermayer, and Sandritter, W.: Intravitale und pathologisch-anatomische Beobachtungen beim Verbrennungsschock des Kaninchens. Beitr. Pathol. *155:*398–409, 1975.

Katz, D., and Siegel, H.: Erosive Gastritis and Acute Gastrointestinal Mucosal Lesions. Progr. Gastroenterol. *1:*67, 1968.

Lasch, H.G.: Klinik und Pathophysiologie des Schocks. Verh. Dtsch. Ges. Pathol. *62:*2, 1978.

Liehr, H., Grün, M., Brunswig, D., and Sautter, T.: Endotoxinämie bei Leberzirrhose. Z. Gastroenterol. *14:*14, 1976.

Lillehei, R.C.: The intestinal factor in irreversible hemorrhagic shock. Surgery *42:*1043, 1957.

Linder, M.M., and McKay, D.G.: An experimental study of thrombotic ulceration of the gastrointestinal mucosa. Surg. Gynecol. Obstet. *133:*21, 1971.

Linder, M.: Über die mögliche pathogenetische Rolle der intravasalen Gerinnung beim Mallory-Weiss-Syndrom. Chirurg *43:*503, 1972.

Marston, A.: The bowel in shock, the role of mesenteric arterial disease as a cause of death in the elderly. Lancet *1:*365, 1962.

Marston, A.: *Intestinal Ischaemia.* Edward Arnold Publishers, London, 1977.

Martinoli, E., and Ganter, J.: Die hämorrhagischen Erosionen von Magen und Duodenum im Vergleich mit den akuten und chronischen Ulzera in einem Sektionsgut von 11.352 Erwachsenen. Schweiz. Med. Wochenschr. *100:*37, 1970.

Messmer, K.: Die Bedeutung des Interstinums beim Schock. Anaesthesist *12:*386, 1968.

Mittermayer, C., Halbfa, J., Mack, T., and Staubesand, J.: Pathologische und anatomische Aspekte der gastrointestinalen Blutung. *Diagnose—Therapie—Verhütung—Chirurgische Naht. Symposium Kassel,* Hrsg.: H. Bartelheimer, K. Horatz, H.W. Schreiber, and P. Eckert. p. 33. Bibliomed, Kassel, 1978.

Mittermayer, C., Riede, U.N., and Sandritter, W.: Rare manifestations of shock in man. Pathol. Res. Pract. *165:*287, 1979.

Mittermayer, C., Rolffs, J., Pfrieme, B., Schönbach, G., Huth, K., and Sandritter, W.: Intravitale und pathologisch-anatomische Beobachtungen beim generalisierten Sanarelli-Shwartzman-Phänomen des Kaninchens. Beitr. Pathol. Anat. *145:*149, 1972.

Mittermayer, C., Thiele, H., Spillner, G., and Ostendorf, P.: Über die Pathogenese des Mallory-Weiss-Syndroms. Beitr. Pathol. Anat. *144:*44, 1971.

Neuhof, H., Mittermayer, C., and Freudenberg, N.: Makro- und Mikrozirkulation im Schock. Verh. Dtsch. Ges. Pathol. *62:*80, 1978.

Nielsen, P.E., and Zacharias, F.: The Mallory-Weiss-Syndrome. Acta Pathol. Microbiol. Scand. (Suppl.) *212:*166, 1970.

Oehlert, W., Dischler, W., Henke, M., and Straub, M.: Die akute Erosion der Magenschleimhaut in Biopsiematerial, ihre Ätiologie und Pathogenese. Med. Welt. *29:*1149, 1978.

Policard, A.: Le système réticuloendothélial. Sa position actuelle. C.R.Soc. Biol. *156:*984, 1962.

Reynolds, D., and Swan, K.G.: Intestinal microvascular architecture in endotoxin shock. Gastroenterology *63:*601, 1972.

Richardson, R.S., Norton, L.W., Sales, J.E.L., and Eiseman, B.: Gastric blood flow in endotoxin-induced stress ulcer. Arch. Surg. *106:*191, 1973.

Schlag, G., Blümel, G., and Regele, H.: The use of percutaneous needle biopsy of the lung in experimental animals and in severely injured patients. *New Aspects of Trasylol Therapy,* edited by G.L. Haberland and D.H. Lewis. p. 247. F.K. Schattauer Verlag, Stuttgart, 1973.

Todd, A.S.: Endothelium and Fibrinolysis Atherosclerosis *15:* 137, 1972.

Zweifach, B.W., and Fronek, A.: The interplay of central and peripheral factors in irreversible hemorrhagic shock. Prog. Cardiovasc. Dis. *18:*147, 1975.

CHAPTER 22

Pathology and Pathophysiology of the Exocrine Pancreas in Shock

RAYMOND T. JONES
GEORGE E. LINHARDT, Jr.

The pancreatic acinar cell has been postulated to play an important role in the pathophysiology of shock, based on data from biochemical and morphological studies (see Ch. 12; Seifert, 1970; Lefer and Glenn, 1972a and b; Manabe et al., 1978). However, little is known about the subcellular changes which occur during and following shock, especially in the human pancreas. Several hypotheses have been proposed in attempts to explain the cellular changes in shock (Shanbour, 1972; Baue et al., 1974; Trump et al., 1974). These hypotheses were based on the assumption that shock and ischemia result in similar cell responses (Trump et al., 1980). These hypotheses are quite similar and can be summarized as follows. In shock, decreased tissue and cell perfusion occurs which may lead to a decrease in cellular ATP. Changes in cellular cyclic AMP levels, which could relate to an increased autophagy, may result from alterations in circulating insulin, glucagon, catecholamines, and corticosteroids. The ion pumps at the plasma membrane could be inactivated due to lack of ATP, thereby causing derangement of physiological concentration gradients with sodium and calcium entering the cell and potassium and magnesium leaving the cell. Ion shifts also result in loss of cellular and organellar volume control. Damage to lysosomal membranes could occur and might induce widespread cellular damage due to the release of proteolytic enzymes. Ultimately the cell is destroyed, and potentially toxic factors might be released. These toxic factors may then contribute to the shock state or damage the membranes of other cells.

While the above scheme remains to be established, it does provide a tentative context in which to interpret many cellular changes which occur in profound shock states. The type and severity of shock and the animal species considered are likely to influence the relative importance of the events summarized in this scheme.

Trump and his coworkers (Ginn et al., 1968; Trump et al., 1971, 1974, 1980; Arstila et al., 1974) have studied the subcellular pathophysiology of both acute lethal cell injury and sublethal chronic cell injury in a variety of model systems.

Acute lethal injuries are defined as injuries that result in cell death within a relatively short period of time (minutes or hours) (Trump et al., 1974). Following an acute lethal injury, the cell has been postulated to pass through a series of morphological stages (see Ch. 1 for a full description of these stages). Various types of injuries, such as those resulting from anoxia, ischemia, and chemical toxins, can cause acute lethal cell injury (Trump and Mergner, 1974).

Chronic sublethal cell injury has been defined by Artila et al. (1974) "as the cell's reaction(s) to one or more small chemical or physical stimuli which do not kill instantaneously and to which the cell is able to maintain its homeostasis approximately at the normal level for long periods ... (days, months, or years)." A very common type of cell response to sublethal injury is autophagy (Arstila et al., 1974). Autophagy is the phenomenon of the lysosomal system digesting the cell's own organelles in bodies termed autophagic vacuoles (de Duve and Wattiaux, 1966; Ericsson, 1969). Many compounds including glucagon (Ashford and Porter, 1962), various antimetabolites, and toxins (Holtzman et al., 1967) induce the formation of autophagic vacuoles. Increased autophagy also is seen in neoplastic cells, bacterial or viral infected cells (Dales, 1969), and hypoxic cells (Abraham et al., 1967).

Many animal models have been studied in order to elucidate the sequence of pathological, physiological, and biochemical events in human circulatory shock. These include dogs, rats, cats, pigs, rabbits, and subhuman primates (Fine, 1962; Bertelli and Back, 1970; Bacalzo et al., 1971; Hinshaw and Cox, 1972; Manabe et al., 1978; Sato et al., 1981). Inadequate perfusion of certain tissue beds in different parts of the body is a phenomenon common to all forms of circulatory shock in all species of mammals. However, it is still uncertain which particular cells must sustain injury and to what extent before hypotensive states become progressive and irreversible and finally result in myocardial damage, which may be the ultimate cause of somatic death (Visscher, 1972). It has been proposed that toxic humoral factors, produced within an animal during shock, play a role in initiating this myocardial damage (Gomez and Hamilton, 1964; Lefer and Glenn, 1972b). Toxic factors may also play a role in the pathogenesis of shock by acting on other components of the cardiopulmonary system (Lefer, 1973). Lefer has reviewed the available data on these humoral factors (Ch. 12) and their role in the pathophysiology of shock and believes that the pancreas is the source of one of the most active agents.

Since blood flow to the pancreas can be drastically reduced during shock (Lau et al., 1972; Spath et al., 1974) and as the pancreas is a source of several proteases (i.e., cathepsins), lethal or sublethal injuries to the pancreas could play an important role in the systemic consequences of shock. Similarly, the intrinsic vascular resistance of this organ is extremely labile when subjected to hypoxic or hypercapnic episodes. Such fluctuation substantially inhibit perfusion selectively when compared to surrounding organs (Broadie et al., 1979). A comparison of liver adenine nucleotide and mitochondrial metabolisms in hemorrhagic shock of normal and pancreatectomized rats showed that the pancreas plays an important role in maintaining hepatic energy metabolism in hemorrhagic shock (Sato, 1978). Seifert (1970) has called the pancreas "the shock organ," that is, the organ which is the primary cause of shock. Furthermore, the effect of fibrotic and normal pancreata during shock has shown that the pancreas may have governance over splanchnic and celiac blood flow (Manabe et al., 1978). Two ultrastructural studies of the pancreas upon which Seifert based his concept of the pancreas as a shock organ were those of Moser et al. (1967) and Donath et al. (1970). The ultrastructural changes observed by Donath and his coworkers in rat pancreatic acinar cells from animals made hypovolemic by cardiac punctures ranged from mitochondrial alterations to dissolution of zymogen granules noted after 24 hr. From their results, they concluded that vascular hypoxic factors led to an initial mitochondrial lesion associated with myelin figures in the matrix. However, identical appearing myelin figures in acinar cells were interpreted by Nevalainen (1970) to be fixation artifacts due to slow penetration of glutaraldehyde. Moreover, such myelin figures are well known artifacts following glutaraldehyde fixation of many cells and tissues.

Although Moser et al. (1967) used 28 dogs to study total pancreatic ischemia, they only showed two electron micrographs (one control and one experimental). The ultrastructural alterations found at 2 hr were swollen mitochondria, a dilated endoplasmic reticulum (ER), and what they have termed "swollen, pale secretion granules." Herlihy and Lefer (1975) found minimal responses in ultrastructural changes of lysosomes in response to splanchic artery occlusive shock if previous pancreatic duct ligation was undertaken. Untreated pancreatic lysosomes were identified to have larger lysosomes with clear vacuoles present. All fractionization studies showed increased fragility of zymogen granules in the unligated and shocked group.

In an attempt to further elucidate the subcellular changes occurring during shock in the pancreatic acinar cells and to further the general fundamental understanding of subcellular reaction to injury, the human pancreas has been studied at autopsy (Jones et al., 1975), as well as the pancreas from experimental animals. Since the morphological changes presented must be compared to control or "normal" cells, the structure and function of the acinar cells of the exocrine pancreas will be reviewed.

STRUCTURE AND FUNCTION OF THE PANCREAS

Although the pancreas is both an exocrine and an endocrine gland, it is the acinar cells of the exocrine portion of the pancreas which have been proposed to play a major role in shock (Seifert, 1970; Lefer and Glenn, 1972a and b). The structure and function of acinar cells will be discussed in general terms below, since Webster and his coworkers (1977) have recently written an excellent review of their metabolism and function.

Light Microscopy

The secretory cells of the mammalian exocrine pan-

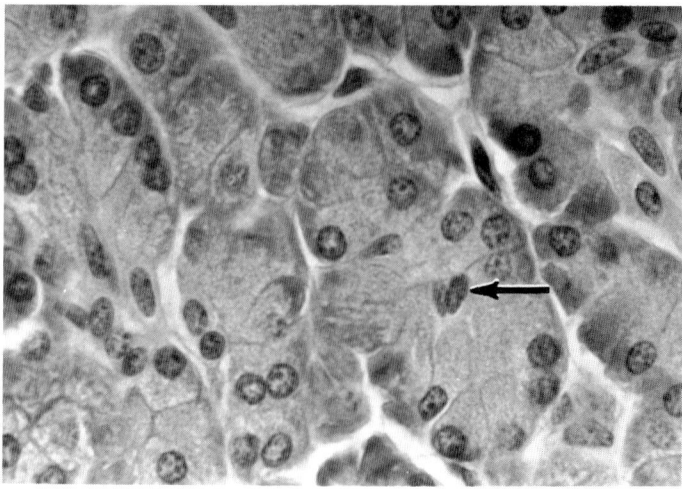

Figure 22.1. Human exocrine pancreas showing a typical acinus surrounding a centroacinar cell (*arrow*). Note the pyramidal shape of the acinar cells and the basal nucleus. The glanular material at the apex of the cells is zymogen.

creas are grouped into ellipsoid aggregates of several cells, termed acini. These acini are separated from each other by connective tissue. Two kinds of cells are found in acini: 1) the true exocrine cells or acinar cells, and 2) the centroacinar cells which form the beginning of the pancreatic ductal system. Both of these can be identified by light microscopy (Fig. 22.1).

Acinar cells are pyramidal-shaped with a basal nucleus. Their apical portions are filled with acidophilic granules, which are increased in quantity during the fasting state. The proteolytic enzymes which hydrolyze proteins in the digestive tract are synthesized as precursors called zymogens, which are concentrated in these granules. In addition to zymogens, the granules contain active digestive enzymes (i.e., amylase and lipase). The basal portion of the acinar cell is basophilic due to a high

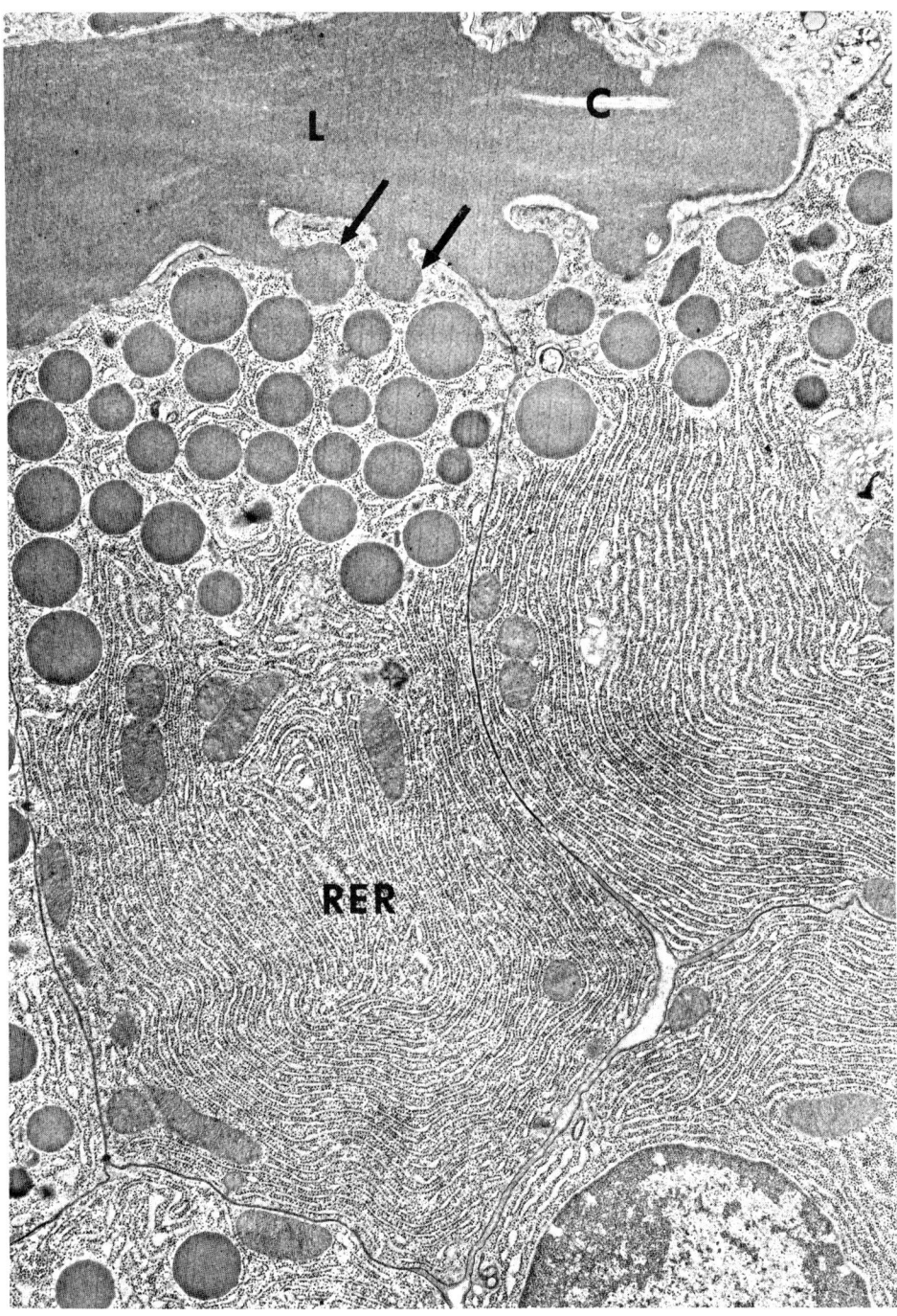

Figure 22.2. Rat pancreatic acinar cells. Zymogen granules fused with the apical plasma membrane (*arrows*). Note the similar appearance of the matrix in the lumen (L) to that within zymogen granules. Abundant RER is apparent in the basal portion of the cells.

concentration of ribonucleic acid in the form of ribosomes.

Electron Microscopy

At both the light and electron microscopic levels, there is a marked similarity between acinar cells of the rat, guinea pig, and man. The main ultrastructural features of these cells are concentrations of zymogen granules at the apex, rough endoplasmic reticulum (RER) at the base, and the nucleus, which is slightly eccentrically located toward the base of the cell (Fig. 22.2).

Secretory Process

Our knowledge of the secretory process of pancreatic acinar cells is due to the work of Jamieson and Palade (Jamieson and Palade, 1971a and b; 1977) who used the

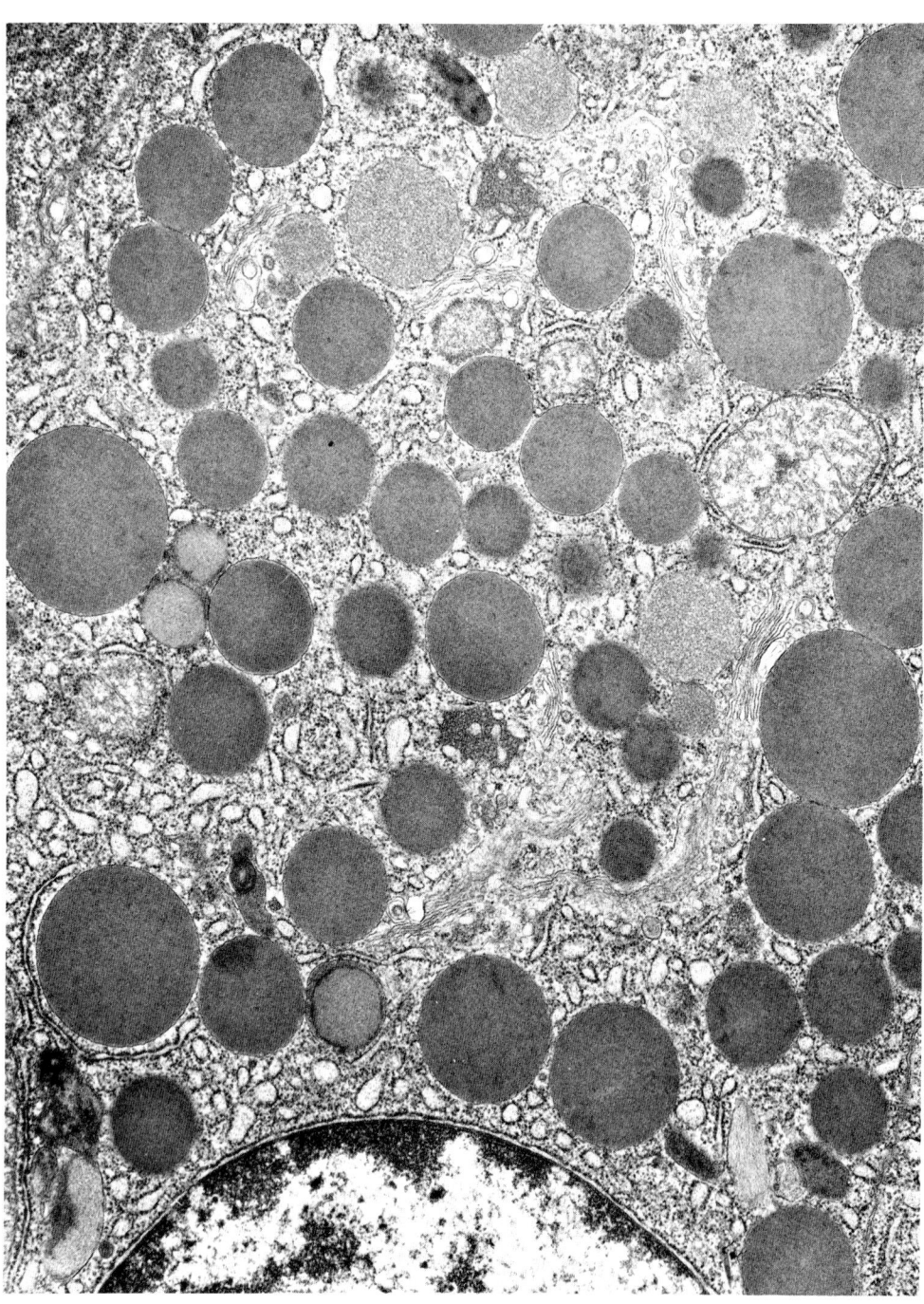

Figure 22.3. This patient was a 43-year-old male admitted to the Maryland Institute for Emergency Medical Services Systems (MIEMSS) following a gunshot wound to the head. This patient was declared brain dead 48 hr after admission and underwent immediate autopsy. Initial stages of reversible cell injury are seen with clumping of the chromatin and swollen mitochondria.

technique of electron microscopic autoradiography with guinea pig acinar cells. Briefly, their technique utilized tissue slices incubated in a medium containing a labeled amino acid such as leucine (Jamieson and Palade, 1971a). This label becomes incorporated into the secretory protein during synthesis. The cells are then washed to remove any unincorporated label, and the cells are reincubated in a label-free medium. This chase medium prevents further incorporation of the label into the protein. The result is a labeled protein pulse which can be traced as it moves from one organelle to another by removing, fixing, and autoradiographing tissue samples at various intervals. Guinea pigs were used because their pancreas was larger and more sharply delineated than that of the rat (Palade and Siekevitz, 1956).

The normal discharge of pancreatic secretory products is cyclic in the sense that there is a period when zymogen granules are discharged from the cells in response to

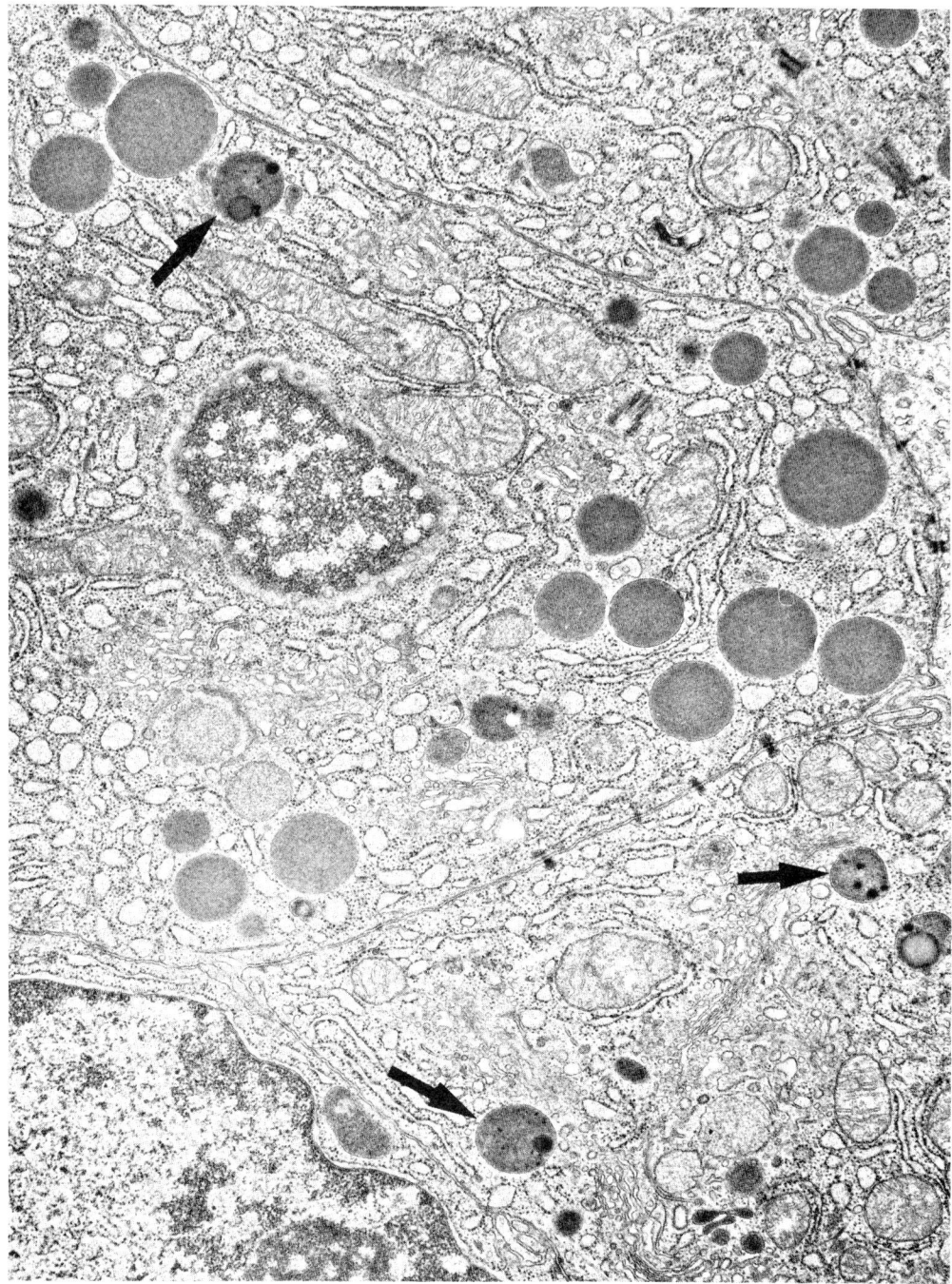

Figure 22.4. This patient, a 25-year-old male, sustained a close range gunshot wound to the head. The patient was declared brain dead within the first 24 hr after admission and was a donor for renal transplantation. At no time was the patient hypotensive. Numerous autophagic vacuoles (*arrows*) are present.

secretagogues. Scheele and coworkers (1978), making measurements of leakage and redistribution of endogenous label during fractionation, have provided the necessary information for the accurate interpretation of Jamieson and Palade's studies and have shown that secretory proteins are indeed transported successfully from the RER to the Golgi complex and then to the zymogen granules. The secretory pathway in the pan-

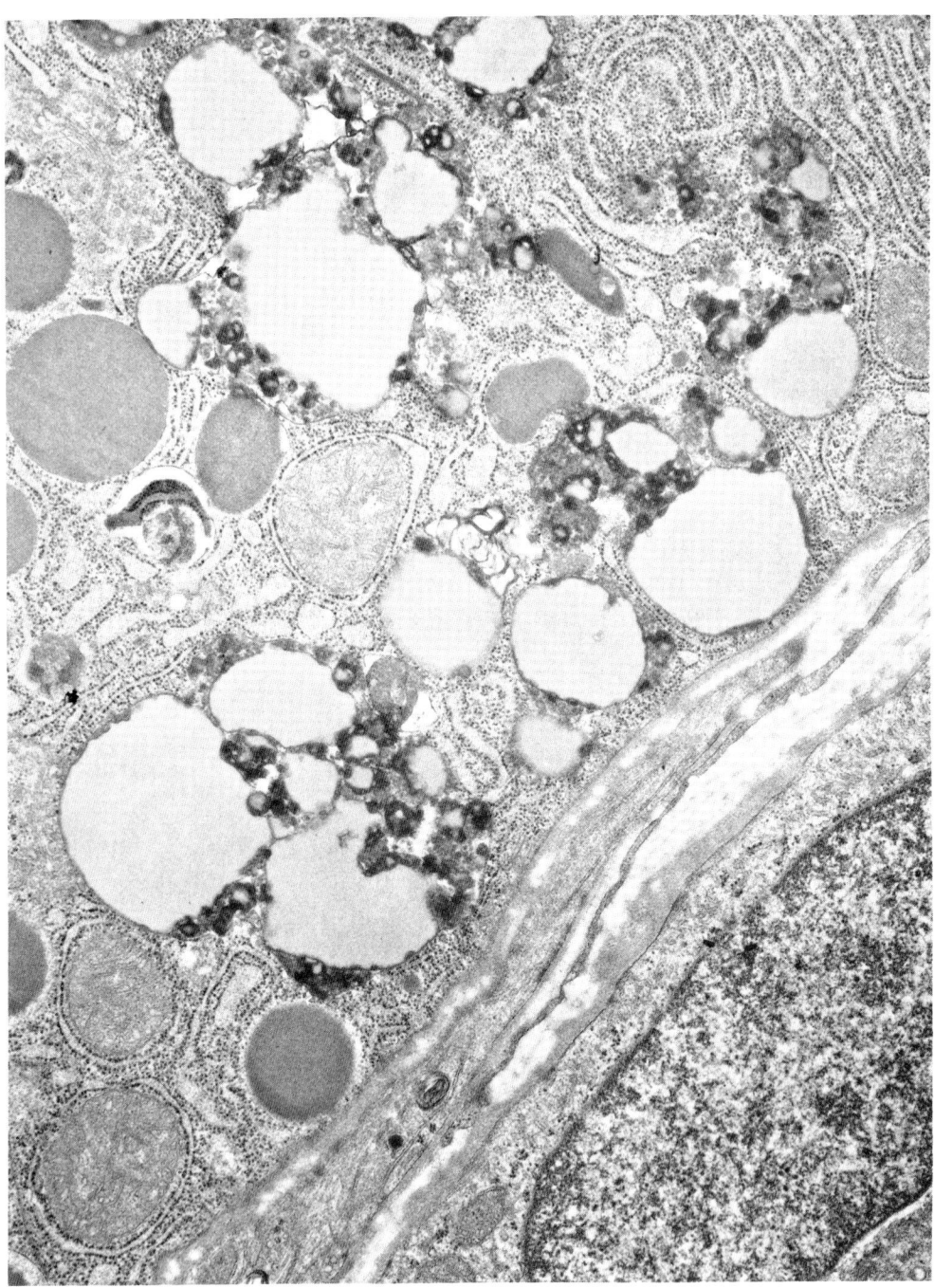

Figure 22.5. This patient was a 25-year-old male struck on the roadside by a passing motor vehicle. The patient was brought by helicopter to Maryland Institute for Emergency Medical Services Systems (MIEMSS) and was found to have a severe closed head injury and a ruptured spleen. Additional injuries included multiple fractures of the upper and lower extremities. On admission, the patient was in profound shock and required multiple transfusions of uncrossed matched blood. The patient continued to deteriorate neurologically and was declared brain dead 24 hr postadmission. In this electron micrograph, multiple residual bodies are present.

creatic acinar cell has been divided into six steps by Jamieson and Palade (Jamieson and Palade, 1977; Palade, 1975) and are listed by Scheele (1980) as follows:

1. Secretory proteins are synthesized on membrane-bound ribosomes.

2. The proteins are vectorially transported across the microsomal membrane during synthesis, resulting in their segregation within the RER cisternal space.

3. The proteins are transported from the RER to the Golgi complex by an energy-dependent process.

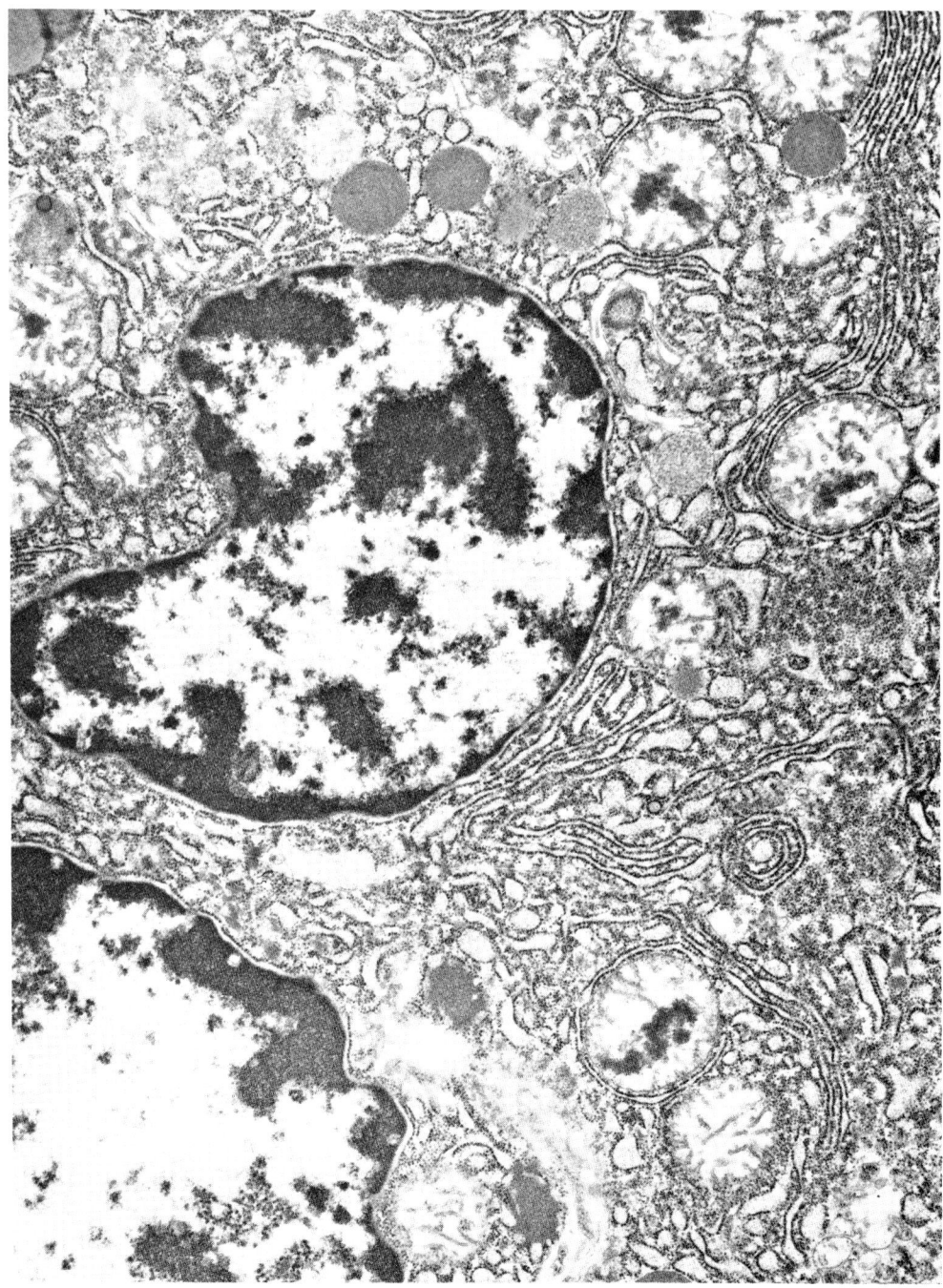

Figure 22.6. This electron micrograph demonstrates severe subcellular injury with flocculent densities, the hallmark of cellular death. Following a motor vehicle accident this patient sustained a severe open head injury requiring cranectomy for decompression. Despite maximal operative methods and therapeutic coma, the cerebral intraventricular pressure could not be controlled. Refractory hypotension ensued and the patient suffered a cardiac arrest 8 hr later.

4. The secretory proteins are then packaged within condensing vacuoles.

5. The secretory proteins are then packaged within condensing vacuoles.

6. The final step is the discharge of the granules from the apical portion of the acinar cell by the energy-dependent and hormone-responsive process of exocytosis.

The human exocrine pancreas has been shown to be very susceptible to injury in shock (Jones et al., 1975; Warshaw and O'Hara, 1978). The cellular alterations observed in all cases studied could be correlated with the severity, duration, and cause of shock (Jones et al., 1975). In cases with isolated head injury or relatively mild shock, only reversible alterations were seen (Fig. 22.3). Shock of short duration of neurogenic etiology selectively generated autophagic vacuoles (Fig. 22.4), while those

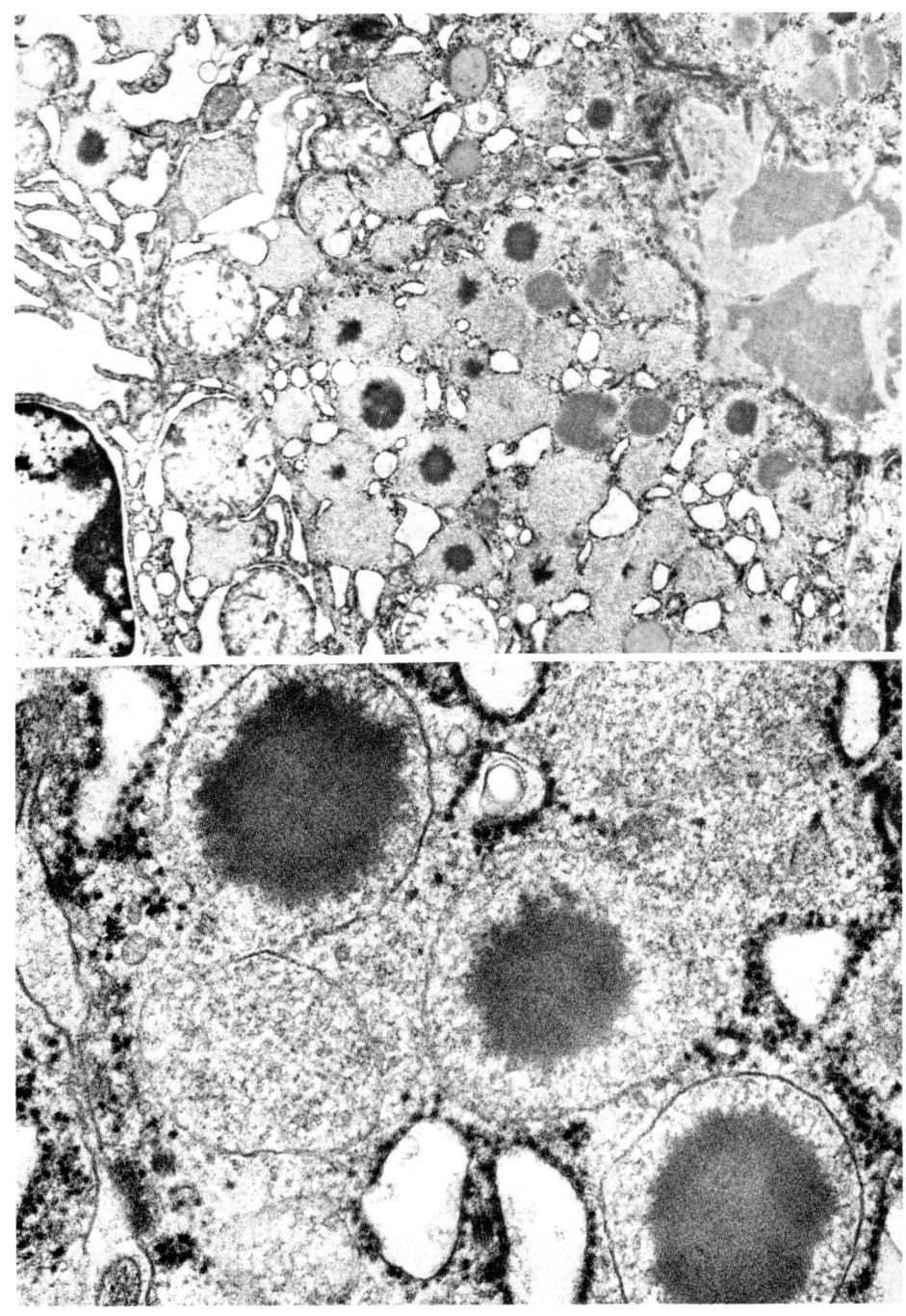

Figure 22.7. Electron micrograph from a patient who suffered a ruptured aortic aneurysm. There is an apparent breakdown and fusion of the zymogen granules (*top* micrograph). *Bottom* micrograph is a higher power view demonstrating a breakdown of the limiting membranes.

patients suffering repeated shock insults over long periods of time displayed residual bodies in their exocrine pancreas (Fig. 22.5). The subcellular alterations seen in those patients with severe shock were those considered to reflect irreversible stages of cell injury (Fig. 22.6). The pancreatic acinar cells were observed to follow the cascade of necrosis, beginning with zymogen granule activation and digestion of the granule limiting membrane. Sequentially, the granules aggregated, although this was primarily elicited in those patients with severe hemorrhagic shock (Fig. 22.7). A similar breakdown of zymogen granules has been shown in electron micrographs of totally ischemic pancreas in dogs by Moser et al. (1967).

EXPERIMENTAL ANIMAL STUDIES

in Vitro

Most of the cellular alterations observed in the human exocrine pancreas in shock were similar to those seen in total ischemic injury to the rat and guinea pig pancreas

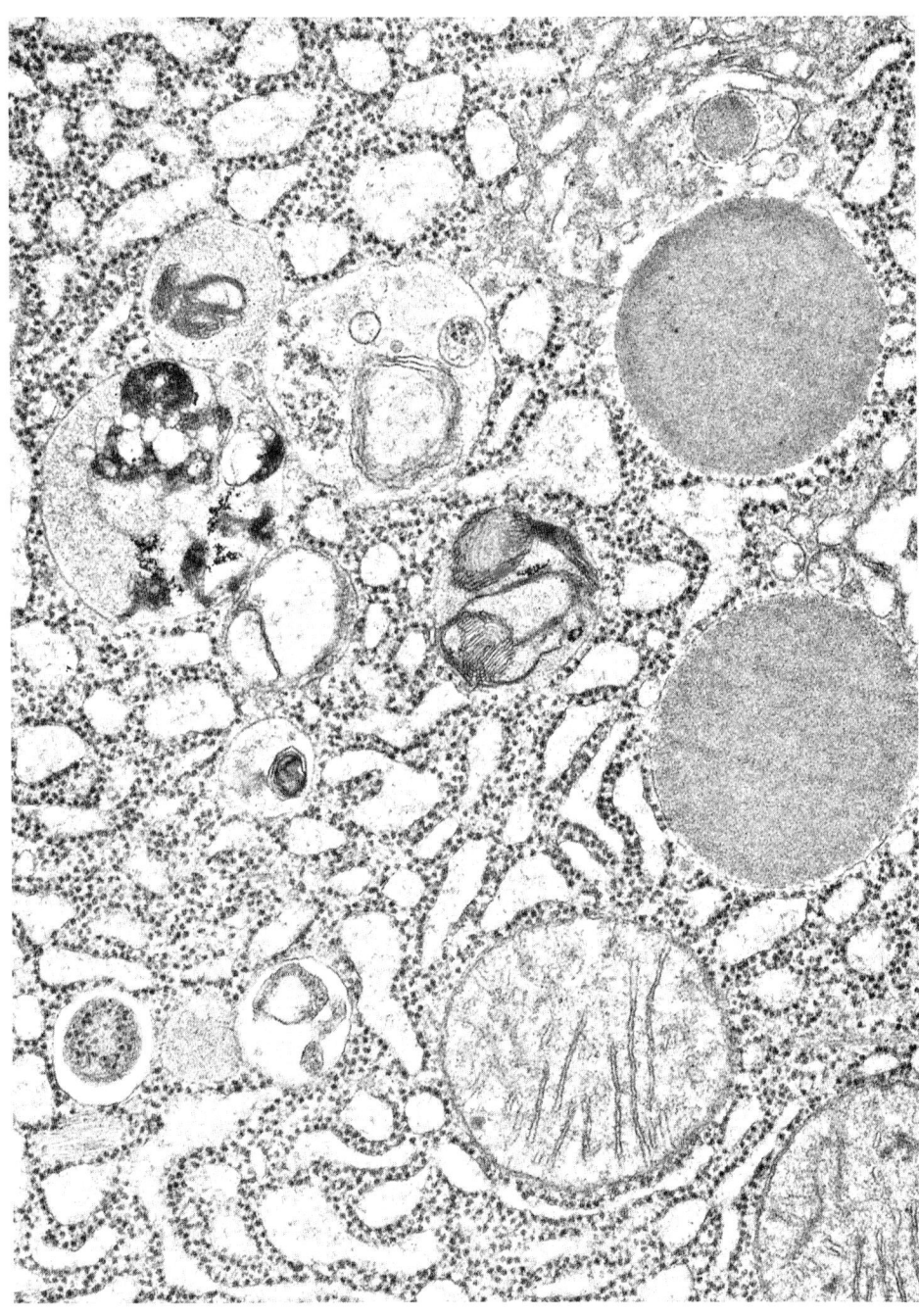

Figure 22.8. Guinea pig pancreatic slice following 1 hr incubation in vitro. Several autophagic vacuoles containing recognizable cellular debris are present. Note the swollen mitochondria and intact zymogen granules.

(Jones and Trump, 1975). Pancreatic slices were incubated at 37° in vitro and then studied in the electron microscope. This experimental system has the advantage over an in vivo system in that the cellular effects of ischemia can be studied under controlled conditions free of complicating factors such as collateral blood flow, inflammation, and regeneration.

Good morphological correlation is found between the ultrastructural changes seen in this system and those seen in the human exocrine pancreas in hemorrhagic shock (Jones et al., 1975) as well as in the pancreas from experimental hemorrhagic shock models (Jones et al., 1979). The well known progression through the stages of cell injury (see Ch. 1) were seen in these in vitro studies. These changes range from dilated endoplasmic reticulum and swollen mitochondria (reversible changes) to mitochondrial flocculent densities and other indicators of cell death. As previously mentioned, the pancreas has been

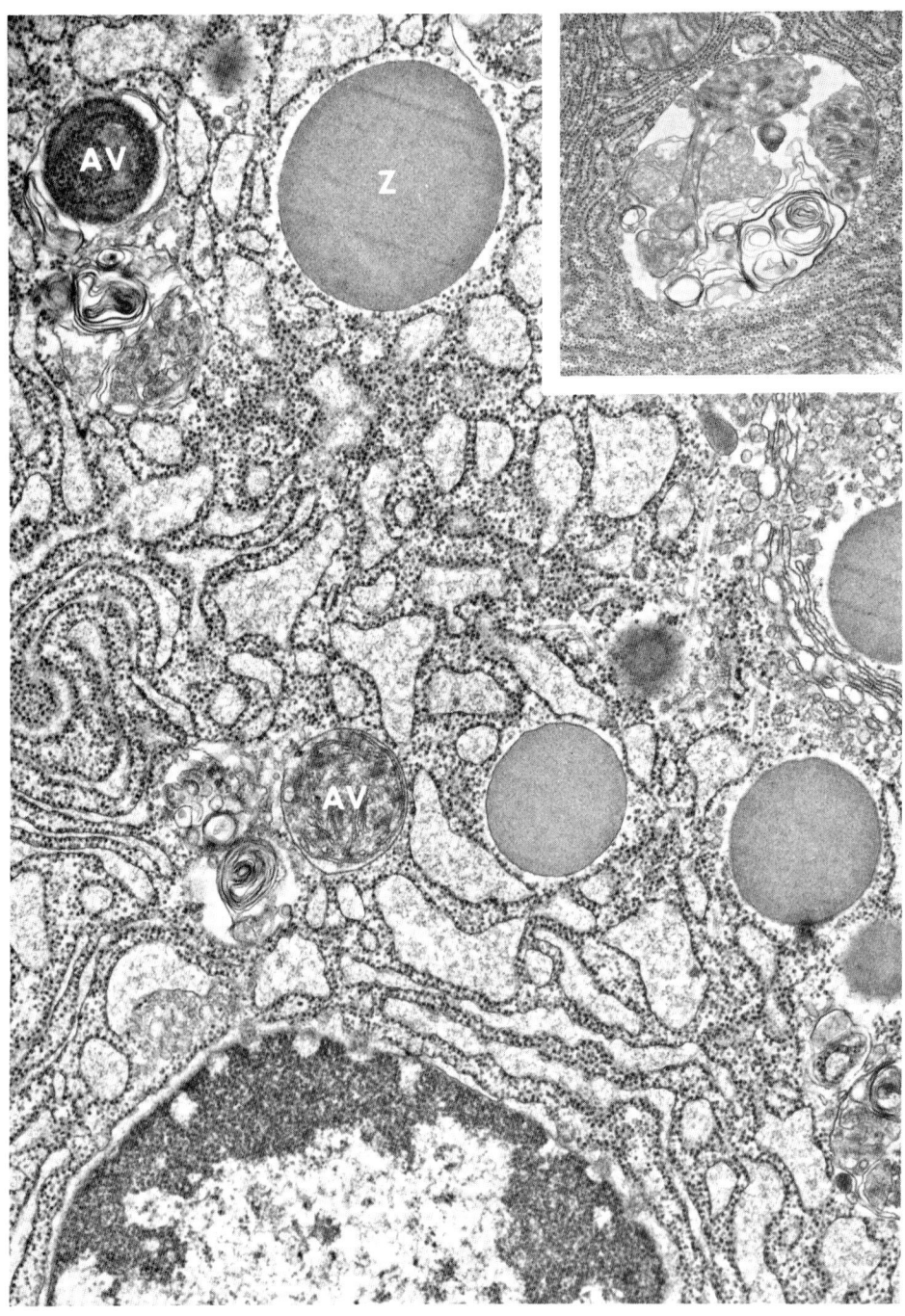

Figure 22.9. Electron micrograph of a rat pancreatic acinar cell 4 hr after induction of hypovolemia. Here the endoplasmic reticulum is markedly dilated. (*AV*) autophagic vacuole, (*Z*) zymogen granule. Also note the mitochondria with flocculent densities in an autophagic vacuole (*inset*).

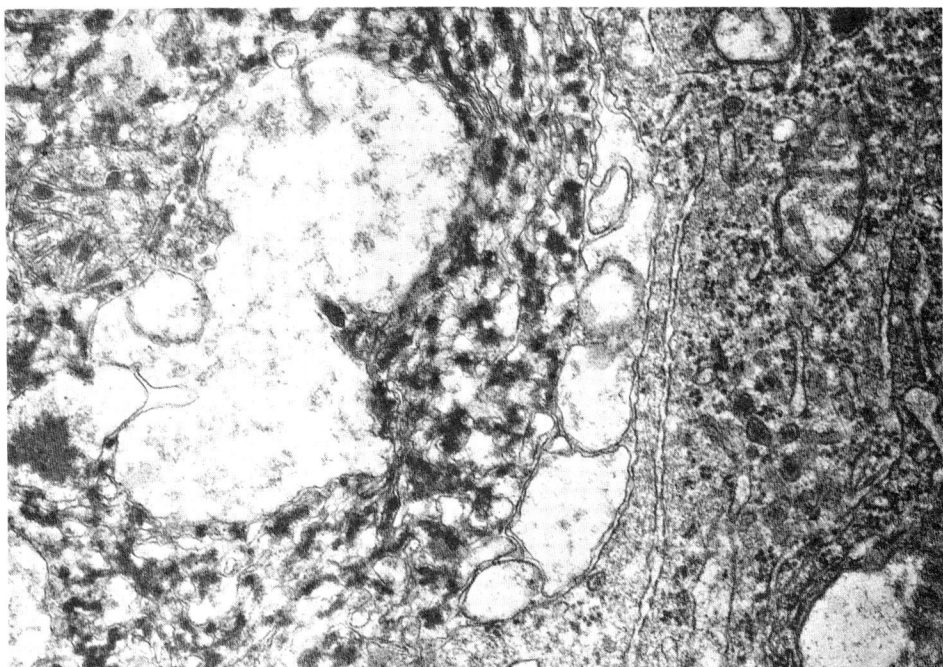

Figure 22.10. Electron micrograph from an animal 4 hr after being subjected to hypovolemic shock. This rat had a high plasma lipase level. Some focal areas of necrosis, as shown here, were present.

postulated to be an important shock organ, and these studies provide evidence to its strength in resisting the progression to cellular death. After 1 hr of complete ischemia, numerous autophagic vacuoles were seen in the pancreatic slices (Fig. 22.8). However, Nevalainen and Anttinen (1977) did not see this increase in autophagic vacuoles when they incubated rat pancreatic slices at room temperature (18–20°C). The reason for this lack of autophagy is perhaps due to the lower temperature during the complete ischemic incubation, inasmuch as autophagy requires ATP (Arstila et al., 1974).

Increased numbers of residual bodies were not seen in any of the incubated slices. This is in contrast to the large numbers of residual bodies seen in the cases of human shock (Jones et al., 1975). Since residual bodies are thought to be the end stage of autophagic vacuoles, they are therefore indicative of prior injury, playing a protective function in regenerating cells. It is not surprising that they were not observed under these conditions of study. Nor was there any indication of an early release of enzymes into the cell, as has been postulated by Lefer and Glenn (1972) in their hypothesis for the formation of myocardial depressant factor. However, the findings based on the complete ischemia studies using pancreatic slices do not contradict the work of Lefer, since if the breakdown of pancreatic exocrine cells is accelerated, hydrolylic enzymes released from the necrotic cells would further damage other cells, thereby continuing the degeneration of the pancreas.

in Vivo

Numerous animal models have been used to study the effect of both hemorrhagic and septic shock on the

Table 22.1
Initial and Final Plasma Lipase Levels in Hypovolemic Rats

Animal No.	Initial Lipase[a]	Final Lipase	Time Between Initial and Final Sampling
	I.U.	I.U.	Hr
1	42	42	4
2	52	73	4
3	42	115	4
4	2	11	17
5	52	73	16
6	94	104	16

[a] Lipase was determined by the method of Shihabi and Bishop (1971). *I.U.*, International Units.

pancreas, as mentioned at the beginning of this chapter. The majority of the experimental studies of hemorrhagic shock have been done using the dog as a model. However, the high cost of these animals and the lack of homogenous colonies have caused investigators to look at other animal models. The rat is being used more and more as a model to study hemorrhagic and septic shock (Donath et al., 1970; Balcalzo et al., 1971; Flenker and Greupner, 1974; Sato et al., 1981; Tanaka et al., 1980).

Experimental hemorrhagic shock is produced by either of two basic techniques. One is the reservoir technique of Wiggers (1950). In this model, blood is shed into a reservoir to monitor a predetermined blood pressure for a set period. At the end of the shocked period, the blood is reinfused. The second technique is to withdraw a percentage of the total blood volume by either single or multiple hemorrhages (Donath et al., 1970; Balcalzo et al., 1971; Flenker and Greupner, 1974; Sato et al., 1981).

Following removal of approximately one-half of the total blood volume of the rat or maintenance of the blood pressure at 40 torr for 60 min, the pancreas shows evidence of chronic sublethal injury (Jones et al., 1979). Similar to what was seen in both the human studies as well as in the in vitro studies described above, there was a formation of numerous autophagic vacuoles within 1 hr of shock with a maximal number reached at 4 hr (Fig. 22.9). Okuda and coworkers (1974) also report an increase in autophagic vacuoles in dog pancreas following cardiogenic shock. However, they do not provide electron microscopic evidence.

The number of autophagic vacuoles decreased in the rat pancreas 24 hr following hemorrhagic shock. Other prelethal ultrastructural alterations such as dilated ER and swollen mitochondria were also present in the exo-

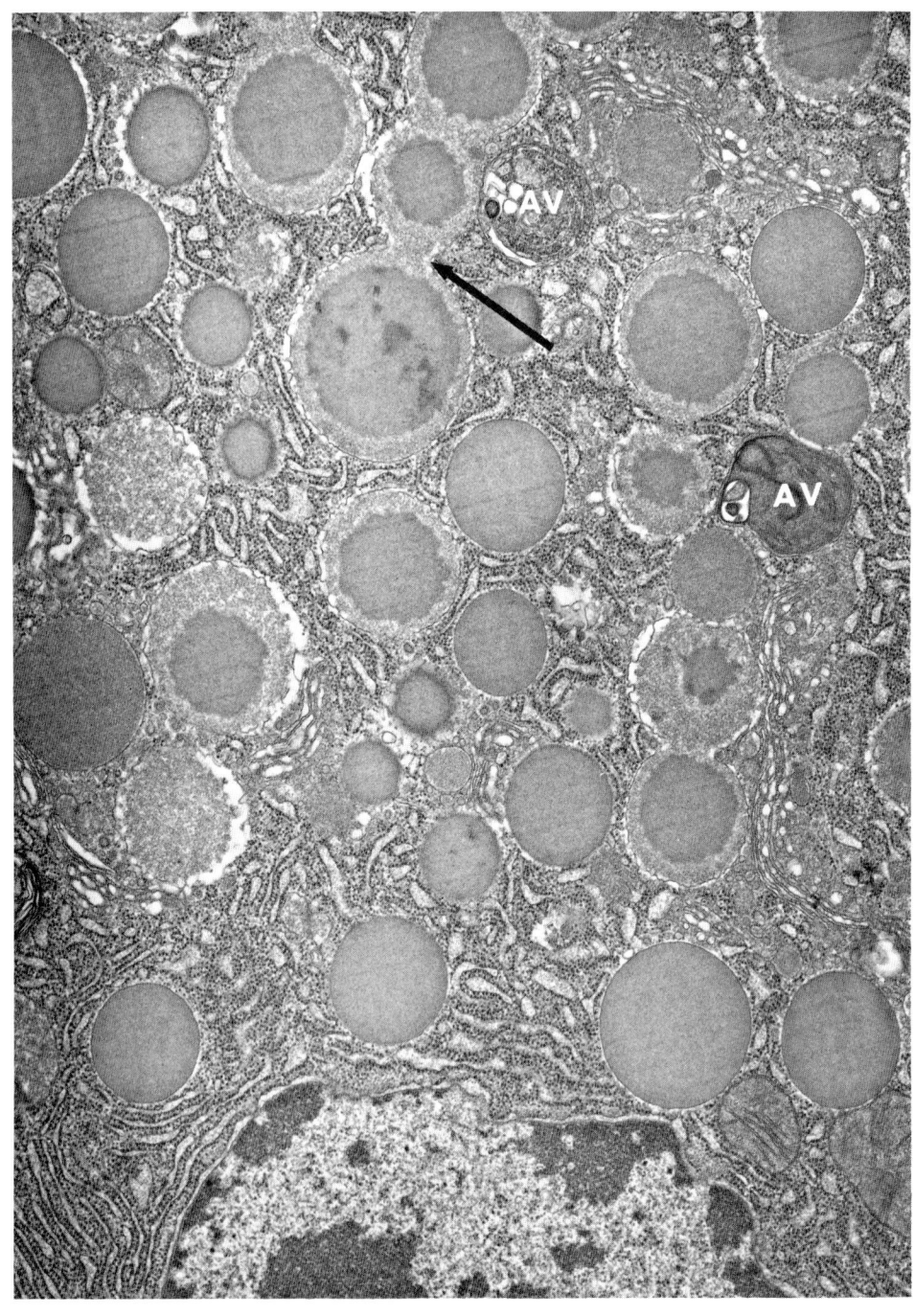

Figure 22.11. After 4 hr of sustained hypotensin, the zymogen granules in this rat pancreas appear to be breaking down and fusing with one another. One such area is indicated by an *arrow*. *AV*, autophagic vacuoles.

crine pancreatic cells of these animals. In some samples, there were small focal areas of necrosis. These were especially evident in animals with high plasma lipase levels. Figure 22.10 is such an example and is from animal number 3 (Table 22.1). From these studies and those of others, it appears that the rat is able to compensate for hypovolemic episodes of short duration or to the loss of 50% blood volume. The ultrastructural changes in the rat pancreas are similar to those found in the human pancreas in cases of mild to moderate shock (Jones et al., 1975). However, when rats are maintained in a shocked state for 4 hr, residual bodies and fusion of zymogen granules occurs (Fig. 22.11). These are the same changes seen in human pancreas in cases of marked shock.

There is a paucity of studies in the literature on the effects of septic shock on the exocrine pancreas. Wagenstein et al. (1971) show an increase in plasma cathep-

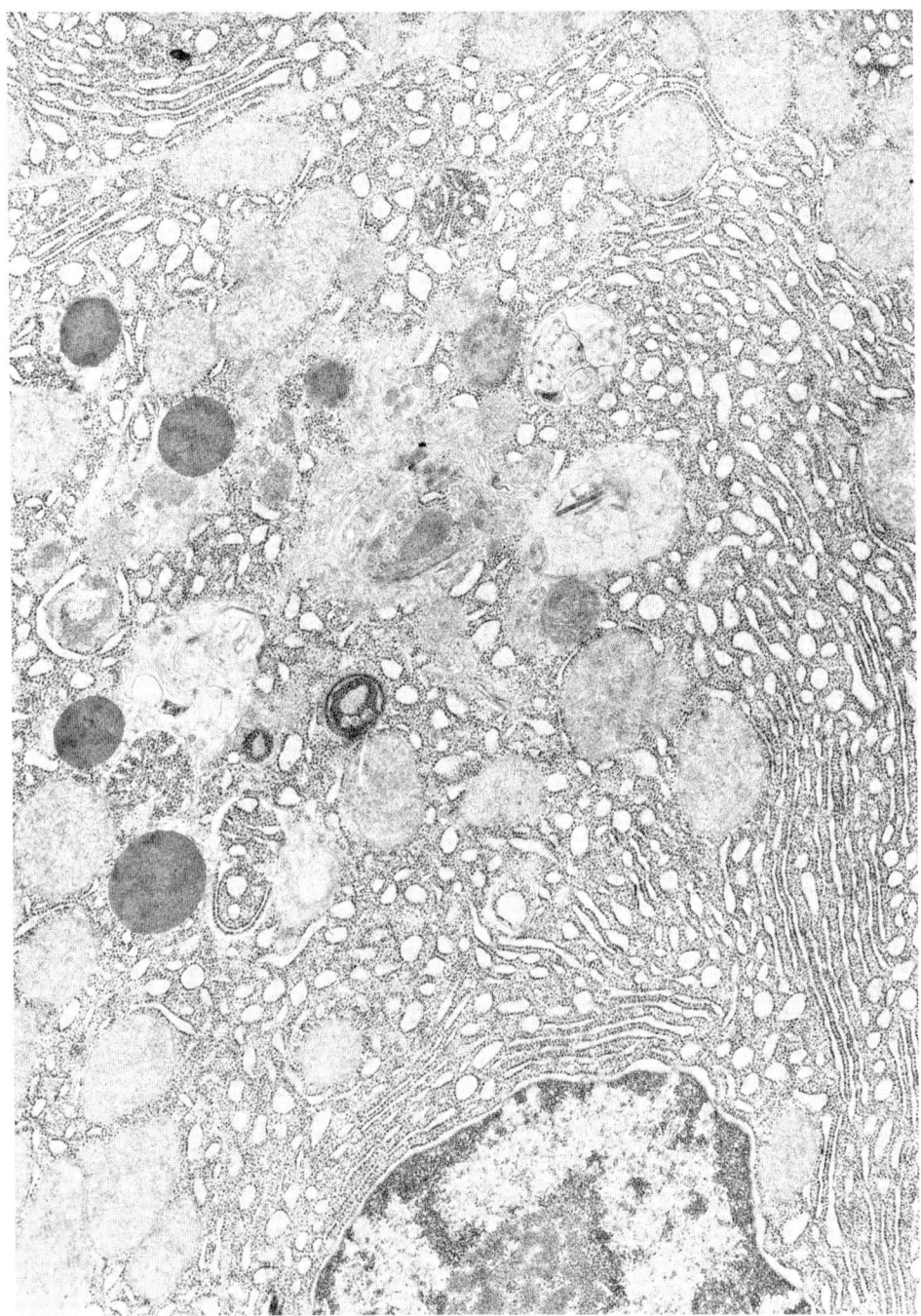

Figure 22.12. Rat exocrine pancreas 3 hr following an injection of $1.5 \times 10^5/100$ g body wt live *E. coli* organisms demonstrates numerous autophagic vacuoles in this electron micrograph.

sin-like activity and mitochondrial depressant factor in cats following endotoxin shock. The injection of 1.5 × 10^5/100 g body wt live *Escherichia coli* organisms (Tanaka et al., 1980) into the rat caused a wave of autophagy in the pancreas within 3 hr of injection (Fig. 22.12). These autophagic vacuoles became larger and more like residual bodies just prior to the death of the animals (Fig. 22.13). There was no fusion of zymogen granules nor any evidence of pancreatic acinar cell death in these preliminary studies. However, this intense formation of autophagic vacuoles in the pancreas makes this an area for further study, since the most severely damage pancreatic tissue studied by electron microscopy is that from those patients dying with fulminating septic shock (Trump et al., 1974; Cowley et al., 1979).

SUMMARY AND CONCLUSIONS

Although shock is a multiorgan problem, numerous studies have shown the pancreas to play an important

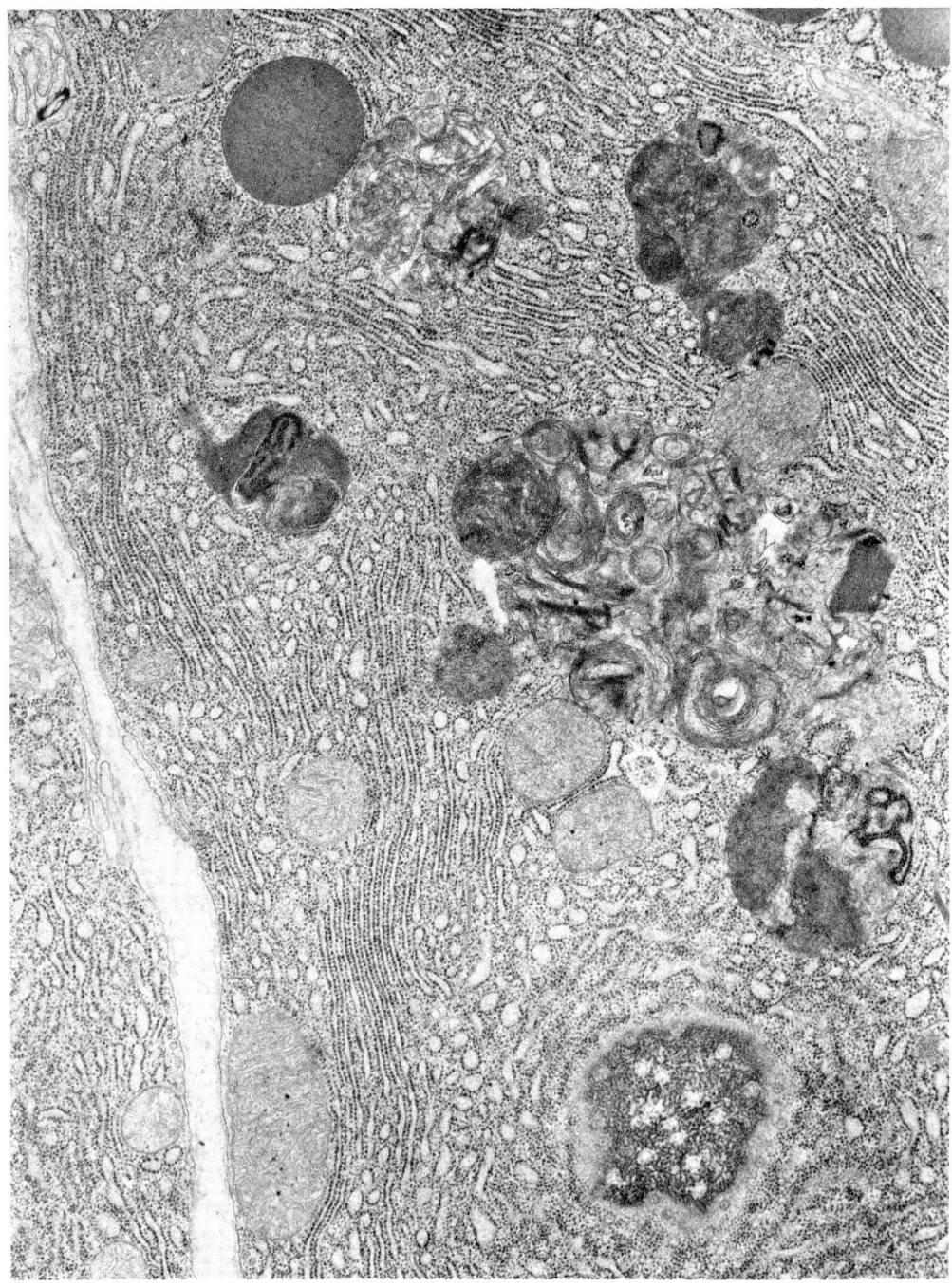

Figure 22.13. Twelve hours after injection of the same number of *E. coli* organisms as in Fig. 22.12, larger residual bodies are present.

role in the pathophysiology of shock. In hemorrhagic and hypovolemic shock there is a reduction of blood flow in the splanchnic region and the pancreas becomes ischemic. Catabolism of the acinar cells occurs as indicated by the formation of autophagic vacuoles. If the injury is removed and the shock episode treated, the autophagic vacuoles go on to become residual bodies, otherwise the cell continues destroying itself which in turn releases enzymes and other toxic factors such as myocardial depressant factor.

Acknowledgments. Supported in part by the Pangborn Fund and the Dean's Summer Fellowship Fund of the University of Maryland School of Medicine and the National Institute of Health Grant AM15440. This is publication no. 990 from the shock laboratory.

References

Abraham, R., Goldberg, L., and Grasso, P.: Hepatic response to lysosomal effects of hypoxia, neutral red and chloroquine. Nature (Lond.) *215:*194–196, 1967.

Arstila, A.U., Hirsimaki, P., and Trump, B.F.: Studies on the subcellular pathophysiology of sublethal chronic injury. Beitr. Pathol. *152:*211–242, 1974.

Ashford, T.P., and Porter, K.R.: Cytoplasmic components in hepatic cell lysosomes. J. Cell Biol. *12:*198–202, 1962.

Bacalzo, L.V., Cary, A.L., Miller, L.D., and Parkins, W.M.: Methods and critical uptake volume form hemorrhagic shock in rats. Surgery *70:*555–560, 1971.

Baue, A.E., Chaudry, I.K., Wurth, M.A., and Sayeed, M.M.: Cellular alterations with shock and ischemia. Angiology *25:* 31–42, 1974.

Bertelli, A., and Back, N. (Eds.): *Shock: Biochemical, Pharmacological, and Clinical Aspects.* Plenum Press, New York, 1970.

Broadie, T.D., Devedas, M., Rysavy, J., Leonard, A.S., and Delaney, J.P.: The effect of hypoxia and hypercapnia on canine pancreatic blood flow. J. Surg. Res. *27:*114–118, 1979.

Cowley, R.A., Mergner, W.J., Fisher, R.S., Jones, R.T., and Trump, B.F.: The subcellular pathology of shock in trauma patients; studies using the immediate autopsy. Am. Surg. *4:* 255–269, 1979.

Dales, S.: Role of lysosomes in cell-virus interactions. In *Lysosomes in Biology and Pathology,* edited by J.T. Dingle and H.B. Fell, vol. 2, p. 69. North-Holland, Amsterdam, 1969.

de Duve, C., and Wattiaux, R.: Functions of lysosomes. Ann. Rev. Physiol. *28:*435–467, 1966.

Donath, K., Mitschke, H., and Seifert, G.: Ultrastrukturelle veranderungen am rattenpaukreas beim hamorrhagischen schock. Beitr. Pathol. *141:*33–51, 1970.

Ericsson, J.L.E.: Mechanism of cellular autophagy. In *Lysosomes in Biology and Pathology,* edited by J.T. Dingle and H.B. Fell, vol. 2, p. 345. North-Holland, Amsterdam, 1969.

Fine, J.: Comparison of various forms of experimental shock. In: *Shock: Pathogenesis and Therapy,* edited by K.D. Bock, p. 32. Springer-Verlag, Berlin, 1962.

Flenker, H., and Greupner, E.: Reversibler und irreversible haemorrhagisher shock bei der Ratte. Methode und ergebnisse eines standardisierten Modells. Beitr. Pathol. *153:*339–352, 1974.

Ginn, F.L., Shelburne, J.D., and Trump, B.F.: Disorders of cell volume regulation. I. Effects of inhibition of plasma membrane adenosine triphosphatase with ouabain. Am. J. Pathol. *53:*1041–1071, 1968.

Gomez, O.H., and Hamilton, W.F.: Functional cardiac deterioration during development of hemorrhagic circulatory deficiency. Circ. Res. *14:*327–336, 1964.

Herlihy, B.L., and Lefer, D.M.: Alterations in pancreatic acinar cell organelles during circulatory shock. Circ. Shock *2:*143–153, 1975.

Hinshaw, L.B., and Cox, B.G. (Eds.): *The Fundamental Mechanisms of Shock.* Plenum Press, New York, 1972.

Holtzman, E., Novikoff, A.B., and Villaverde, H.: Lysosomes and gerl in normal and chromatolytic neurons of the rat ganglion nodosum. J. Cell Biol. *33:*419–435, 1967.

Jamieson, J.D., and Palade, G.E.: Condensing vacuole conversion and zymogen granule discharge in pancreatic exocrine cells: metabolic studies. J. Cell Biol. *48:*503–522, 1971a.

Jamieson, J.D., and Palade, G.E.: Synthesis, intracellular transport, and discharge of secretory proteins in the pancreatic exocrine cell. II. Transport to condensing vacuoles and zymogen granules. J. Cell Biol. *34:*597–615, 1977.

Jones, R.T., and Trump, B.F.: Cellular and subcellular effects of ischemia on the pancreatic acinar cell. *In vitro* studies of rat tissue. Virchows Archiv. B Cell Pathol. *19:*325–336, 1975.

Jones, R.T., Garcia, J.H., Mergner, W.J., Pendergrass, R.E., Valigorsky, J.M., and Trump, B.F.: Effects of shock on the pancreatic acinar cell. Cellular and subcellular effects in humans. Arch. Pathol. Lab. Med. *99:*634–644, 1975.

Jones, R.T., Kreisberg, J.I., Linhardt, G.E., and Trump, B.F.: Studies of the ischemic pancreas in shock. Adv. Shock Res. *1:*197–207, 1979.

Lau, T.S., Tauberfligel, W., Levene, R., Farago, G., Chan, H., Koven, I., and Drucker, W.R.: Pancreatic blood flow and insulin output in severe hemorrhage. J. Trauma *12:*880–884, 1972.

Lefer, A.M., and Glenn, T.M.: Interaction of lysosomal hydrolases and a myocardial depressant factor in the pathogenesis of circulatory shock. In *Shock in Low- and High-flow States,* edited by B.K. Forscher, R.C. Lellehei and S.S. Stubbs, p. 88. Excerpta Medica, Amsterdam, 1972a.

Lefer, A.M., and Glenn, T.M.: Role of the pancreas in the pathogenesis of circulatory shock. In *The Fundamental Mechanisms of Shock,* edited by L.B. Hinshaw and B.G. Cox, p. 311. Plenum Press, New York, 1972b.

Lefer, A.M., and Glenn, T.M.: Letter to the editor. J. Trauma *13:*746–747, 1973.

Manabe, T., Suzuki, T., and Honjo, I.: Role of the pancreas in organ blood flow during shock. Surg. Gynecol. Obstet. *146:* 577–582, 1978.

Moser, R., Neil, H.U., and Largiader, F.: Die ischamietoleranz des Pankreas. Z. Gesamte Exp. Med. *143:*266–274, 1967.

Nevalainen, T.J.: Effects of pilocarpine stimulation on rat pancreatic acinar cells. Acta Pathol. Microbiol. Scand. (Suppl.) 210, 1970.

Nevalainen, T.J., and Anttinen, S.: Ultrastructural and functional changes in pancreatic acinar cells during autolysis. Virchows Arch. [Cell Pathol.] *24:*197–207, 1977.

Okada, K., Kosugi, I., Kitagaki, T., Yamaguchi, Y., Yoshikawa, Y., Kawakami, S., and Senoh, Y.: Pathophysiology of shock. Jpn. Circ. J. *41:*346–361, 1977.

Okuda, M., Yamada, T., and Hosono, K.: Activity of a myocardial depressant factor and associated lysosomal abnormalities in experimental cardiogenic shock. Circ. Shock *1:* 17–29, 1974.

Palade, G.: Intracellular aspects of the process of protein synthesis. Science *189:*347–358, 1975.

Palade, G.E., and Siekevitz, P.: Pancreatic microsomes: an integrated morphological and biochemical study. J. Biophys. Biochem. Cytol. *2:*671–707, 1956.

Sato, M., Yamamoto, M., Ozawa, K., and Honjo, T.: Role of

the pancreas in stability of mitochondrial function in hemorrhagic shock. J. Surg. Res. 25:226–231, 1978.
Sato, T., Kamiyama, Y., Kamano, T., Rutkowski, J., Jones, R.T., Cowley, R.A., and Trump, B.F.: Pathophysiology of hemorrhagic shock. I. A model for studying the effects of acute blood loss in the rat. Pathol. Res. Pract., in press, 1981.
Scheele, G.A.: Biosynthesis, segregation, and secretion of exportable proteins by the exocrine pancreas. Am. J. Physiol. 238:467–477, 1980.
Scheele, G.A., Palade, G.E., and Tarakoff, A.M.: Cell fractionation studies on the guinea pig pancreas: redistribution of exocrine proteins during tissue homogenization. J. Cell Biol. 78:110–130, 1978.
Seifert, V.G.: Das Pankreas als Schockorgan. Leber-und Pankreas-schaden durch Schock und Narkose, edited by K. Horatz, p. 17. Geog Thieme, Stuttgart, 1970.
Shanbour, L.L.: Biochemical-biophysical basis of shock. In The Fundamental Mechanisms of Shock, p. 437. Plenum Press, New York, 1972.
Shihabi, Z.K., and Bishop, C.: Simplified turbidimetric assay for lipase activity. Clin. Chem. 17:1150–1153, 1971.
Spath, J.A., Gorczynski, V.J., and Lefer, A.M.: Pancreatic perfusion in the pathophysiology of hemorrhagic shock. Am. J. Physiol. 226:443–451, 1974.
Tanaka, J., Sato, T., Jones, R.T., Trump, B.F., and Cowley, R.A.: Aspects, high-energy metabolism in rat liver following E. coli bacteremia. Circ. Shock 7:207, 1980.
Trump, B.F., and Mergner, W.J.: Cell injury. The Inflammatory Process, edited by B.W. Zweifach, L. Grant, and J.T. McClusky, vol. 1, ed. 2, pp. 115–257. Academic Press, New York, 1974.
Trump, B.F., Croker, B.P., and Mergner, W.J.: The role of energy metabolism, ion, and water shifts in the pathogenesis of cell injury. In Cell Membranes: Biological and Pathogical Aspects, edited by G.W. Richter and D.G. Scarpelli, p. 84. Williams & Wilkins, Baltimore, 1971.
Trump, B.F., Laiho, K.U., Mergner, W.J., and Arstila, A.U.: Studies on the pathophysiology of acute lethal cell injury. Beitr. Pathol. 151:243–271, 1974.
Trump, B.F., Jesudason, M.L., and Jones, R.T.: Ultrastructure of diseased cells. Diagnostic Electron Microscopy, edited by B.F. Trump and R.T. Jones, vol. 1. pp. 1–88. John Wiley & Sons, New York, 1978.
Trump, B.F., McDowell, E.M., and Arstila, A.U.: Cellular reaction to injury and cell death. Principles of Pathobiology, edited by R.B. Hill and M.D. LaVia, pp. 20–111. Oxford University Press, New York, 1980.
Visscher, M.B.: Introduction: an overview of the shock problem. The Fundamental Mechanisms of Shock, edited by L.B. Hinshaw and B.G. Cox, p. 3. Plenum Press, New York, 1972.
Wagensteen, S.L., Geissinger, W.T., Lovett, W.L., Glenn, and Lefer, A.M.: Relationship between splanchnic blood flow and a myocardial depressant factor in endotoxin shock. Surgery 69:410–418, 1971.
Warshaw, A.L., and O'Hara, P.J.: Susceptibility of the pancreas to ischemic injury in shock. Ann. Surg. 188:197–201, 1978.
Webster, P.D., Black, O., Mainz, D.L., and Singh, M.: Pancreatic acinar cell metabolism and function. Gastroenterology 73:1434–1449, 1977.
Wiggers, C.J.: Physiology of shock. Commonwealth Fund, p. 1–137. New York, 1950.

CHAPTER 23

Pathology and Pathophysiology of Acute Renal Failure—A Review

JEFFREY L. BARNES
ELIZABETH M. McDOWELL

Acute renal failure (ARF) can be defined as an abrupt deterioration in renal function, characterized by rapid rises in blood urea nitrogen and creatinine and associated with fluid overload, hyperkalemia, and acidosis (Rees, 1976). The syndrome is frequently associated with oliguria, characterized by diminutions in urine volume to less than 400 ml daily (Levinsky and Alexander, 1976), although a nonoliguric variant is now being recognized with increasing frequency (Vertel and Knochel, 1967; Meyers et al., 1974; Singh et al., 1974; Anderson et al., 1977). Despite the disparity of urine outputs in oliguric and nonoliguric ARF, both are characterized by positive solute balances believed to result from reduction in the glomerular filtration rate (GFR). In patients there are two main types of ARF; the first resulting from ischemia following shock, cardiac arrest, or renal artery occlusion, and the second resulting from a variety of nephrotoxins. The most important nephrotoxins today are the aminoglycoside antibiotics and various cancer chemotherapeutic agents such as cis-platinum. In addition, septic shock continues to be an important cause of ARF which may have both ischemic and toxic components. The ischemic and toxic types of ARF may be similar or different in their pathogenesis. In spite of considerable work done over the years, the pathophysiology of this syndrome remains incompletely understood.

The mortality rate from ARF remains high, despite the advancement of dialysis technology, ranging from 20 to 50% in the general clinical setting (Swann and Merrill, 1953; Hamburger, 1968) to 53 to 63% following post traumatic episodes (Teschan et al., 1955; Whelton and Donadio, 1969; Lordon and Burton, 1972; Stone and Knepshield, 1974). Several theories concerning the pathogenesis of ARF have been postulated through the use of a variety of experimental models, but as yet, no single theory has established unifying acceptance. Existing data suggest that multiple mechanisms are involved, depending on the etiology of ARF and the phase of ARF being studied. It is obvious that any future development in the treatment of ARF relies on further advancements into the pathophysiologic mechanisms of this syndrome.

The recognition of ARF as a clinical entity began during World War II (Bywaters and Dible, 1942). In spite of the effort of many eminent pathologists in attempting to define the histopathologic basis of this syndrome, pathological findings remain controversial. Part of this is because many of the earlier studies were based on routine autopsies, in which postmortem alterations probably obscured many of the important changes. Furthermore, most studies have utilized classic light microscopic techniques which are able to detect lesions only in a relatively late stage. In addition, the time of tissue obtainment was random and not based on the course of the disease, which can be divided into initiation, maintenance, and recovery phases. The key findings that are important in the pathogenesis of ARF occur during the initiation phase, while patients are typically biopsied during the maintenance or recovery phases or studied at autopsy.

Review of the literature reveals that the findings in human patients with this condition are as follows. The glomeruli are for the most part normal (Olsen and Skjoldborg, 1967), although some have argued that defects in the capillary wall, including changes in the organization of the foot processes, occur and that fibrin deposits are significant (Clarkson et al., 1970). Both of these latter events seem to occur in too focal a fashion and too infrequently to be of real significance. Proximal tubules show a variety of changes which are often difficult to separate from the artifactual background. A recent study by Bohle et al. (1976) suggests that dilatation of proximal tubules is a common feature, a finding often utilized on an anecdotal basis by older anatomical pathologists. Bohle attributes this dilatation, not to tubular obstruction since casts were relatively few, but to defective Na^+ and water resorption in the nephron. In the typical case of ARF where a toxic factor is not implicated, extensive necrosis in the pars convoluta usually does not occur. This is not to say that changes do not occur in this part of the nephron at the subcellular level but only that typical coagulation necrosis with its ensuing inflammatory response is seldom seen. Casts, often of a characteristic ropey or coarsely granular type, are seen especially in the distal nephron. The distal nephron is also dilated according to Bohle's measurements and pigmented material in the lumen is seen in cases with obvious transfusion reactions as well as in some cases without. Tubulovenous anastomoses and tubulorrhexis are relatively rare. Goormaghtigh (1945), looking at the region of the afferent arteriole in kidneys of crush injury casualties, noted changes in this region which he attributed to interactions between the tubule, especially in the region of the macula densa, and the arterioles. These observations, made a number of years ago, anticipated current findings concerning tubuloglomerular feedback which, according to many, is an important feature of the syndrome, leading other investigators to term this condition "vasomotor nephropathy" (Oken, 1971). Interactions between the tubular fluid content in the macula densa and the afferent arteriole are theorized by many to be extremely important in the initiation phase of this disease (Flamenbaum, 1973; Thurau et al., 1976). The presence of interstitial edema can be marked in some cases, and this is probably dependent on duration. Inflammatory reactions in the interstitium are seen later in the course of ARF and are often accompanied by tubular regeneration.

EXPERIMENTAL THEORIES ON THE PATHOGENESIS OF ARF

ARF can be divided into three phases. The first, the initiation phase, is defined as the interval of time between the initiating event and the clinical appearance of ARF. The second, the maintenance phase, is defined as the interval during which renal function is deteriorating, until it is reduced to a stable level. The third is the recovery phase, defined as the interval of time during which renal function returns to normal. Therefore, when evaluating any experimental model of ARF, consideration must be made of the pathophysiological mechanisms which account for all phases of the syndrome. These are likely to be multiple and complex.

Thus, it is not surprising that no one simple animal model adequately recapitulates the human syndrome. The mechanism(s) responsible for the pathophysiology of ARF continues to be a controversial issue, which may result from individual investigators seeking a simple mechanism to account for all parameters of the syndrome at all phases during the course of ARF. Multiple mechanisms are probably responsible, taking different priorities at different times during the clinical course.

There are several mechanisms that may play a role in the pathophysiology of ARF and could be responsible for a reduction of GFR.

Effective glomerular filtration is normal; however, passive backleak of a normally formed filtrate leads to oliguria and under estimation of GFR—or—effective glomerular filtration is actually diminished as a result of:
1. an increased intratubular hydrostatic pressure caused by obstruction or tubular compression;
2. altered glomerular permeability due to toxic and/or ischemic events;
3. diminished glomerular capillary hydrostatic pressure caused by: a) capillary endothelial and/or epithelial cell swelling; b) efferent arteriolar dilatation; or c) afferent arteriolar vasoconstriction.

As stated previously, it has not been ascertained whether one or all of the above mechanisms is/are primarily involved in the development of ARF or at what phase these factors may interfere with normal renal function.

The potential roles of passive backleak and obstruction will be discussed in some detail. Passive backleak and obstruction of tubules are interrelated to the extent and severity of renal tubular necrosis. However, the precise relationship between tubular epithelial necrosis and ARF remains obscure. In the toxic animal models of ARF, as well as in toxic ARF in human patients, necrosis typically occurs only in a particular region of the nephron. For example, following $HgCl_2$, it may occur only in the pars recta of the proximal tubule. In humans, following volume depletion, necrosis is scattered and often difficult to find, a feature that was pointed out elegantly some years ago by Oliver (1953). It is complicated even further by the fact that in some experimental models of ARF, necrosis can occur in the pars recta without marked alterations in renal function (see below).

The role of necrosis, therefore, is confounding at present and demands further study. Necrosis has been postulated to contribute by obstructing the tubules, elevating hydrostatic pressure in excess of glomerular transcapillary pressure, permitting a passive backflow or leak through the tubular epithelium, and releasing toxic materials such as peptides, which exert deleterious effects on the microcirculation. It appears, however, from numerous human studies that have been conducted as well as from recent experiments on rat models, that the extent of necrosis bears an uncertain relationship to ARF, at least in the pars recta, but that it may complicate the picture. It is certainly not essential and, indeed, may not occur as part of the basic mechanism. This would indicate that much more attention should be directed toward a definition of the earlier proximal tubular changes, many of them reversible, which in turn would have the advantage that therapeutic approaches could be devised to potentiate their reversibility or to minimize their occurrence.

Normal Effective Glomerular Filtration—Passive Backleak

Azotemia and oliguria have been theorized to be the result of unselective passage or backleak across damaged tubular epithelia. The hypothesis is that GFR is normal but oliguria and azotemia result from tubular fluid returning to the systemic circulation across damaged epithelia, resulting from ischemia or the action of nephrotoxins. Thus, exogenous or endogenous molecules routinely used to assess filtration function leak out of the tubules giving erroneously low clearance values and a false impression of reduced GFR. Some evidence exists both for and against this mechanism playing a major role in the pathophysiology of ARF.

One of the earliest observations of a tubular leak was made by Richards (1929). With the aid of micropuncture, Richards was able to demonstrate leakage of the dye, phenosulfonphthaline, out of renal tubules of frogs poisoned in vivo with $HgCl_2$. Similarly, Bank et al. (1967) provided evidence for backleak in proximal tubules of rats by the use of intravenously injected lissamine green 24 hr following $HgCl_2$. Steinhausen et al. (1969) were also able to show a disappearance of lissamine green between split oil droplets along the length of the proximal tubule 24 hr after administration of $HgCl_2$ to rats; Huguenin et al. (1978) demonstrated a rapid reabsorption of saline, 20% mannitol and 20% albumin, through necrotic proximal convoluted tubules of the rat 48 hr after administration of $HgCl_2$. Others, however, have not been able to demonstrate leakage of lissamine green through proximal tubules of rats given nephrotoxins (Ruiz-Guinazu et al., 1967; Flanigan and Oken, 1965; Oken et al., 1966).

Morphological evidence in support of backleak has been afforded by Wada et al. (1974) through the use of a qualitative Hanssen technique, which converts sodium ferrocyanide into a visible precipitate (Prussian blue). Sodium ferrocyanide is filtered by the glomerulus and is neither reabsorbed nor secreted by normal proximal tubular epithelia. Thus, in controls, Prussian blue was confined to tubular lumens and stained with high intensity. However, 24–30 hr after the administration of $HgCl_2$ to rabbits, the dye was less intense and was observed to be diffuse within the tubular cells. Donohoe et al. (1978) microinjected horseradish peroxidase into proximal tubules and cytochemically demonstrated this tracer throughout the cytoplasm of necrotic proximal tubule cells and in the interstitium at 1–3 hr following clamping of the renal artery for a duration of 25 and 60 min. Similar localizations were observed after intravenous injection of horseradish peroxidase, thus indicating that abnormal permeability after microinjection was not artifactually induced.

Quantitative physiological evidence for backleak has been afforded by the finding of reduced creatinine/inulin clearance ratios in dogs poisoned with uranium (Hayman et al., 1939), an observation one would expect if passage of the two markedly different molecules, with regard to size, molecular weight and diffusion coefficients, pass through damaged epithelia incongruently. Similar results were reported after the administration of uranium acetate to rabbits (Nomiyama and Foulkes, 1968). However, Flamenbaum et al. (1971), using micropuncture, and

DiBona et al. (1971) were not able to confirm these results in rats treated with $HgCl_2$. Both groups described clearance of [^{14}C]inulin to be reduced to the same degree as [^{3}H] or [^{14}C]mannitol clearance 24 hr following administration of $HgCl_2$ in rats.

Further support for the role of backleak in rats given $HgCl_2$ was provided by Steinhausen et al. (1969). Increases in tubular permeability to inulin were alluded to by finding [^{14}C]inulin in the urine of the contralateral kidney following microinjection of this glomerular marker in proximal tubules of the ipsilateral kidney. Tanner et al. (1973) demonstrated 98% recovery of [^{14}C]inulin from the urine of the microinjected control kidneys but only 0.6% from uninjected contralateral kidneys. At 0.5–3 hr following 1 hr of occlusion of the renal artery, [^{14}C]inulin recovery averaged 36.4% from urine of microinjected kidneys and 27.3% recovery from contralateral kidneys. Similar data were reported by Eisenbach and Steinhausen (1973) and Donohoe et al. (1978) after 1 hr of renal ischemia.

Data generated from microinjection techniques, however, have been under considerable skepticism due to the possibility of artifactual "leakiness" from the tip of the micropipet or through the effects of abnormally high microperfusion pressures on fragile tubular epithelia following nephrotoxic or ischemic episodes (Oken, 1965a and b). Furthermore, Olbricht et al. (1977) studied the recovery of microperfused [^{14}C]ferrocyanide and [^{14}C]- and [^{3}H]inulin along various lengths of the nephron following methemoglobin and ischemic- and nephrotoxic-induced ARF. Late proximal recovery of [^{14}C]ferrocyanide was reduced by a maximum of 6% when compared to controls, while distal recoveries of [^{14}C] and [^{3}H]inulin were depressed by a maximum of 11%. They concluded that tubular leakage was not a significant feature in the early phase of ARF and attributed reductions in whole kidney inulin or polyfructosan clearance as true reflections of reduced GFR. The marginal decrease in the recovery of labeled markers was suggested to be unrelated to ARF since elevated intratubular pressures, as observed during the early stages of nephrotoxic and ischemic-induced ARF (Mason et al., 1977), have been shown to augment the passage of usually impermeable molecules across tubular epithelia in normal kidneys (Lorentz et al., 1972).

Although backleakage may contribute during the maintenance phase of ARF, numerous studies have minimized the role of backleakage during initiation of the syndrome. For example, a number of physiological parameters generally associated with ARF become evident long before anatomical evidence of proximal tubular necrosis. Flanigan and Oken (1965) observed reduced GFR to values 45% of controls in rats 6 hr after administration of $HgCl_2$, before gross disruption of tubular epithelia which was noted at 24 hr. Also, Barenberg et al. (1968) described a diminution in GFR and increases in fractional excretion of sodium (FE_{Na^+}) at 30 min after administration of $HgCl_2$. No apparent differences in kidney morphology were noticed between experimentals and controls. Data from a number of other studies described similar functional impairment prior to advanced lesions of the proximal tubules (Flamenbaum et al., 1972b, 1974; Kleinman et al., 1975; McDowell et al., 1976).

In contrast, there are also a number of studies reported in experimental animals where a poor correlation exists between extensive pars recta necrosis and the development of ARF (DiBona et al., 1971; Ryan et al., 1973; Kreisberg et al., 1976; Dobyan et al., 1977a and b; Solez et al., 1977a and b; Barnes et al., 1980a and b), strongly suggesting that backleak has little if any role in the pathophysiology of ARF. Such a dissociation between necrosis and ARF is also compatible with the morphology of the varied forms of ARF in humans, where tubular necrosis may not be widespread and is not even a consistent feature (Lucké, 1946; Brun and Munck, 1957; Finckh et al., 1962; Bohle et al., 1976; Olsen, 1976).

Further evidence that the role of backleakage is minimal has been furnished by experiments utilizing chronic NaCl loading. ARF induced by a variety of nephrotoxins is markedly ameliorated by chronic NaCl loading, a maneuver that does not prevent tubular necrosis (DiBona et al., 1971; Ryan et al., 1973; Richards and DiBona, 1974; Lameire et al., 1976; Barnes et al., 1980b). If necrosis were the equivalent of leak, one would expect comparable impairment of renal function in NaCl drinking rats as in H_2O drinking rats, following administration of these nephrotoxins.

Diminished Effective Glomerular Filtration

INCREASED INTRATUBULAR HYDROSTATIC PRESSURE CAUSED BY OBSTRUCTION

A role for intratubular obstruction has been postulated as either a primary or contributing factor in ARF even though many human cases do not show evidence of necrosis. This, however, could result from altered morphology of tubular epithelium, with blebs and protrusions into the lumen. Several workers have found significant increases in intratubular pressure in ischemic models (Arendshorst et al., 1976; Tanner and Steinhausen, 1976), in contrast to the heavy metal models, including $HgCl_2$ (Flanigan and Oken, 1965). Looking at electron micrographs of tubules with altered cell shape and lumens filled with debris and blebs, it is difficult to imagine how they could *not* cause obstruction. It is of interest that following reflow these elements of the tubular epithelium apparently rapidly revert to normal and continuity is rapidly re-established, even at the subcellular level. This leads to the impression, shared by many, that tubular obstruction may well be a result rather than the cause of the same factors that initiate the entire syndrome. The subject, however, cannot be closed at present, and it needs more study in particular with regard to the relationship between the extent of these tubular changes and their correlation with functional parameters such as azotemia, changes in GFR, and survival.

As early as 1911, Yorke and Nauss injected hemoglobin solutions into rabbits and observed pigment precipitates in renal tubules implicating intratubular obstruction. Subsequently, diminished GFR in ARF has been proposed to be a result of tubular obstruction due to the accumulation of intratubular debris and/or interstitial edema (Baker and Dodds, 1925; Peters, 1945; Meroney and Rubini, 1959; Mason et al., 1963). If tubular obstruction were instrumental in diminishing GFR to the extent of producing oliguria, one would expect intratubular hydrostatic pressures high enough to compromise effective glomerular filtration pressure measured to be 45 mm Hg in Munich rats (Brenner et al., 1971; Deen et al., 1974) and 62.5 mm Hg in Sprague-Dawley rats (Kallskög et al., 1975). Indeed, intratubular hydrostatic pressures of proximal tubules approach these values when stop-flow conditions are instituted by blocking normal kidney tubules by microinfusion of castor oil (Allison 1972) or ureteral obstruction (Jaenike, 1969). Control values for proximal convoluted tubular pressures range from 13 to 16 mm Hg.

Numerous micropuncture measurements of intraluminal hydrostatic pressure have been conducted on several experimental models of ARF. However, the data reflect conflicting results. Ruiz-Guinazu et al. (1967) measured an increase of intratubular pressure, 8 mm Hg higher than controls, in dilated tubules 1 hr after injection of methemoglobin into the rat. However, intratubular pressure returned to normal or subnormal values at later time intervals. Similarly, Jaenike (1969) described increases above control values in 81% of the tubules measured 24 hr following methemoglobin-induced ARF. Also, Tanner et al. (1973) observed proximal tubular pressures of 46 mm Hg, 2–3 hr after 1 hr occlusion of the left renal artery by clamping. Obstruction and backleak were suggested to be primarily responsible for reduced inulin clearance, based on the observation of increased proximal tubular pressure, dilated proximal tubules, and impeded movement of lissamine green down microinfused nephrons. Subsequent studies repeated these observations and also described moderate increases in intratubular pressure (5 mm Hg over controls) at 24 hr following the release of the clamp (Tanner and Sophasan, 1976). Again, decreased GFR was attributed to obstruction, which was supported by proximal tubular dilation and numerous eosinophilic casts in 92% of distal tubules examined in rats shortly after release of the clamp.

However, Mason et al. (1977) were not able to consistently correlate ARF with increased intratubular pressures in either ischemic or nephrotoxic models of ARF. They concluded that obstruction was not a consistent feature of experimental ARF and that the obstruction hypothesis may only be applicable in a few instances. Oken et al. (1966) reported reductions in proximal tubular hydrostatic pressures by approximately 40% at 15 min to 4 hr and at 18–26 hr following intramuscular injection of glycerol in rats. Reductions in pressure were associated with low tubular flow and tubules were collapsed, despite the presence of intratubular casts. Similar reductions in intratubular hydrostatic pressure were reported in the glycerol model (Wilson et al., 1967, 1969) and after intravenous injection of methemoglobin (Ruiz-Guinazu et al., 1967; Cirksena, 1971). Numerous studies that used heavy metals rather than pigment-induced ARF also failed to demonstrate increases of intratubular hydrostatic pressure (Flanigan and Oken, 1965; Bank et al., 1967; Barenberg et al., 1968; Flamenbaum et al., 1971, 1974; Stein et al., 1975). Oken et al. (1966) also noted that the introduction of fluid through a micropipet, at pressures less than that of glomerular filtration, was able to dislodge accumulated casts and debris. The authors concluded that obstruction exists as a secondary event following a diminished GFR. Arendshorst et al. (1976) also described intratubular hydrostatic pressures below control values in collapsed tubules at 22–24 hr following 1 hr renal ischemia. The rats were oliguric, and numerous casts were observed in necrotic tubules concomitant with reduced renal blood flow (RBF) and increased renal vascular resistance, thus supporting obstruction to be secondary to hemodynamic mechanisms. However, when RBF and vascular resistance were returned to normal or slightly higher than normal values by acute volume expansion, reduced GFR and oliguria persisted and intratubular pressures increased moderately. Arendshorst et al. (1976) concluded that tubular obstruction is the primary cause of ARF but occurred simultaneously with backleak and hemodynamic mechanisms.

The role of interstitial edema causing tubular compression has been essentially ruled out, because dogs with experimentally induced ARF lacked increased interstitial pressure (de Wardener, 1955). Also, therapeutic renal decapsulation, a maneuver designed to relieve interstitial pressure due to edema does not necessarily negate renal failure (Abeshouse, 1945). Conversely, some investigators have recommended renal decapsulation in the prophylactic treatment of ARF (Stone and Fulenwider, 1977). However, Bohle et al. (1976) observed a poor correlation between interstitial edema and tubular compression. In fact, tubular lumens were observed to be dilated in human cases of ARF and were observed to be widest in kidneys with the most expanded interstitial space. Dilatation of the tubular lumens was suggested to be due to a defect in electrolyte reabsorption since they observed no relation between the number of tubular casts and the severity of ARF.

If obstruction were operational in ARF, anuria (in extreme cases), or at least oliguria, would be expected, especially during times when tubular necrosis is widespread and cast formation is most likely to occur. However, a number of studies have found a poor correlation between urine volumes and severe functional impairment. For example, Finckh (1960) described polyuria in rats 24 hr after administration of glycerol and in temporary ischemia at 24 hr, when necrosis was clearly established. Likewise, nonoliguric ARF has been described concomitant with functional impairment during at least the first few hours following 30 to 60 min renal ischemia (Tanner et al., 1973; Tanner and Sophasan, 1976; Mason, 1976) or after administration of glycerol (Finckh, 1960; DiBona and Swain, 1971; Flamenbaum et al., 1973b) and heavy metals (Barenberg et al., 1968;

Flamenbaum et al., 1971, 1972b, 1974; Stein et al., 1975; McDowell et al., 1976; Mason et al., 1977).

Also, the observation that severe renal impairment may occur well before advanced lesions are noted (discussed in the passive backleak section) does not support the obstruction theory.

Evidence exists both in support and against obstruction in the development of ARF. Obviously, more work is needed to define what role obstruction has in the pathophysiology of ARF in experimental animals. However, it seems clear that mechanical factors associated with necrosis, that is backleak and obstruction, play only a secondary role in the pathogenesis of ARF in humans, since necrosis and casts are not always observed in histological preparations (Oliver et al., 1951; Finckh et al., 1962; Bohle et al., 1976).

Collectively, the above observations minimize the roles of backleak and obstruction in the pathophysiology of ARF, pointing towards a significant role played by hemodynamic factors.

ALTERED GLOMERULAR PERMEABILITY

Cox et al. (1974) have postulated a decrease in glomerular permeability as a primary event for decreased glomerular filtration in ARF. By infusing norepinephrine (0.75 µg/kg/min.) for 2 hr into the renal artery of dogs, they were able to demonstrate diminished cortical RBF measured with microspheres. Anuria developed and persisted after termination of the infusion and upon re-establishment of cortical RBF to normal values by infusion of Ringer's solution. Conger and Robinette (1976) have reported similar findings with an infusion of norepinephrine followed by acetylcholine or prostaglandin E_1. Also, Baehler et al. (1977) reported reduced RBF, GFR, and urine flow in dogs at 48 hr following $HgCl_2$. However, after infusion of saline (10% body weight), RBF increased above normal, but GFR and urine flow remained markedly depressed. The above investigators attributed the persistence of low urine volumes, despite normal RBF, to an alteration in the K_f, which is a measure of capillary permeability expressed as the product of glomerular capillary surface area and hydraulic conductivity across glomerular capillary membranes. Indeed, direct measurements have assessed a reduction in K_f following uranyl nitrate- (Blantz, 1975) and gentamicin- (Baylis et al., 1977) induced ARF.

Studies by transmission and scanning electron microscopy revealed abnormalities in the epithelial structure of glomeruli following infusion of norepinephrine (Cox et al., 1974) and renal ischemia by renal artery occlusion (Barnes et al., 1979), supporting this hypothesis. Stein et al. (1975) have also reported abnormalities in glomerular epithelia in dogs treated with uranyl nitrate, suggesting glomerular permeability changes as a responsible factor for diminished GFR in ARF. Baehler et al. (1977) showed a slight swelling of podocytes in glomeruli 48 hr following $HgCl_2$, concomitant with depressed renal function. However, NaCl-loading, a maneuver that ameliorates ARF, failed to relieve this lesion. Thus, cessation of filtration following administration of $HgCl_2$ was concluded to be unrelated to the slight structural alterations observed in glomerular podocytes.

With regard to ARF in humans, Dalgaard and Pederson (1961), Olsen and Skjoldborg (1967), Olsen (1976), and Bohle et al. (1976), failed to show ultrastructural changes in glomeruli in renal biopsy tissue from patients with various forms of ARF. If diminished glomerular permeability was a primary factor in the pathogenesis of ARF, one would expect cortical RBF to remain at normal levels, which is not consistent with the observations in experimental and human cases of ARF, where RBF is markedly depressed (discussed below). The current concensus is that change in glomerular perfusion, related to afferent arteriolar constriction and/or efferent dilatation, are probably more important in causing the decreased GFR.

DIMINISHED GLOMERULAR CAPILLARY HYDROSTATIC PRESSURE

Numerous studies using a variety of methods have described marked reductions in effective glomerular filtration to be associated with decreases in total RBF in ARF both in man (Shaldon et al., 1963; Reubi et al., 1966, 1973; Hollenberg et al., 1968, 1970, 1973) and in that induced in animals by ischemia (Selkurt, 1946; Eisenbach et al., 1974; Daugherty et al., 1974; Arendshorst et al., 1976), glycerol (Ayer et al., 1971; Chedru et al., 1972; Kurtz et al., 1976), and heavy metals (Flamenbaum et al., 1972b, 1974, 1976b; Baehler et al., 1977; Hsu et al., 1977). The possibility that alterations in renal hemodynamics play an important role in ARF has long been recognized. Changes in total RBF during the initiation and maintenance phases, with a return to normal during the recovery phase, have been noted with older as well as with more current techniques. The most significant recent conceptual change has been that even the diminished total RBF cannot perhaps account for the severe decreases in GFR that are found. Hollenberg et al. (1968), using washout techniques, indicated that this discrepancy may be explained by altered RBF distributions, the consensus being a shift away from the outer cortical nephrons. Cortical ischemia with diminished perfusion has been observed in a number of experimental models. Despite these observations, others have failed to describe similar reductions in total RBF in a variety of experimental models (reviewed by S. Churchill et al., 1977).

Three major vascular events that might lead to a decreased glomerular hydrostatic pressure have been proposed, and these are discussed in some detail below.

Capillary Endothelial and/or Epithelial Cell Swelling

According to this theory, cellular swelling may lead to diminutions in glomerular capillary patency, thus impeding plasma flow through these vessels (Leaf, 1970). If such a mechanism were operating, RBF and effective GFR would be reduced.

Indeed, obstructed glomerular capillaries due to cellular swelling have been described by light (Summers and Jamison, 1971) and electron microscopy (Flores et al., 1972; Frega et al., 1976; Johnston and Latta, 1977), following total renal ischemia of 15 min to 1 hr duration. After 1 hr ischemia, cloudy swelling in glomeruli was noted by light microscopy. By electron microscopy, swollen glomerular endothelial and mesangial cells were observed compressing erythrocytes in capillary lumens, thus giving the impression of obstruction. Summers and Jamison (1971) observed decreased and incomplete filling of the lumens of glomeruli by carbon particles after infusion in the rat following induction of ischemia. However, if the erythrocytes were flushed out of the kidney by saline prior to the induction of ischemia, the carbon particles were distributed uniformly throughout the capillary lumens, as in controls. Reperfusion of erythrocytes into the kidney resulted in failure of the carbon particles to completely fill the glomerular tufts. The authors then concluded that the primary event in total renal ischemia was swelling of the capillary epithelial or endothelial cells and that trapping of erythrocytes completed the obstruction. These studies were recently repeated using electron microscopy and similar results were reported (Johnston and Latta, 1977). Frega et al. (1976) described a diffuse patchy ischemia as judged by silicone-rubber injections following 1 hr ischemia. However, the administration of hypertonic mannitol after release of the clamp improved flow, as demonstrated by reversal of the ischemia pattern of silicone casts. Also, cell swelling within the capillaries was alleviated, as observed by electron microscopy. Mannitol does not penetrate cell membranes, thus the authors concluded that protection against cell swelling was afforded by prevention of osmotic fluid flow into endothelial and epithelial cells of the glomerulus. Similar observations were made by Sherwood, et al. (1974) in $HgCl_2$-induced ARF. In these studies, $HgCl_2$ caused an immediate and lasting fall in RBF, accompanied by severe cortical ischemia. However, upon infusion of hyperosmolar mannitol prior to administration of $HgCl_2$, renal vascular shutdown was prevented (Sherwood et al., 1974). Russell (1975) reported similar observations with mannitol but was unable to protect against $HgCl_2$-induced increased vascular resistance by various vasodilators, including adrenergic blocking agents (phentolamine and propranolol), bradykinin, and low concentrations of mannitol. Thus, a primary role for endothelial cell swelling was suggested, excluding other vasomodulating mechanisms.

As mentioned above, the extrapolation of these results to humans should be done with caution because glomeruli are generally normal in appearance in biopsy and autopsy tissue of human ARF cases.

Efferent Arteriolar Dilatation

Little evidence exists for efferent arteriolar dilatation as a primary event in the pathogenesis of ARF. Ruiz-Guinazu et al. (1967) measured efferent arteriolar pressures in normal control rats as well as in rats with methemoglobin-induced ARF and found a decrease in intraarteriolar hydrostatic pressure. However, if efferent arteriolar dilatation alone were responsible for decreased GFR, one would expect a normal cortical RBF, which would be inconsistent with a decreased superficial cortical RBF documented to occur in various forms of experimental ARF and in humans with ARF (see above). Conversely, Venkatachalam et al. (1976) described vasoconstriction of the efferent arteriole and afferent arteriole in rats 24 hr following glycerol-induced ARF.

Afferent Arteriolar Vasoconstriction

Data concerning RBF have lead a number of investigators to conclude that vasoconstriction of the afferent arteriole leads to diminished glomerular filtration pressure, concomitant with decreased formation of filtrate. Several investigations, using a variety of techniques, have shown that cortical RBF is decreased while medullary flow remains the same or increases. Histologically, a pallor of the cortical region is a common observation in kidneys of patients with ARF (Finckh et al., 1962; Heptinstall, 1974), an observation which may well correlate with the studies of Hollenberg et al. (1968, 1970), demonstrating inadequate filling of the terminal cortical vasculature in renal arteriographs of human ARF cases. Hollenberg et al. (1968, 1970) also demonstrated decreased cortical perfusion in humans by the Xenon washout technique. Similarly, reductions in superficial cortical RBF have been documented in experimental animals in ARF induced by heavy metals (Thiel et al., 1973; Flamenbaum et al., 1974, 1976b; Lameire et al., 1976), glycerol (Ayer et al., 1971; Chedru et al., 1972) and ischemia (Kashgarian et al., 1976). Vasoconstriction of the afferent arteriole has been implicated in diminished superficial cortical RBF since glomeruli are more abundant in the superficial cortex. Furthermore, a structural-functional correlation has been implicated involving the renin-angiotensin system. Juxtaglomerular (JG) cells present in the media of the afferent arteriole are known to contain renin, a proteolytic enzyme involved in the production of angiotensin II, a potent vasoconstrictor. Glomeruli in the superficial cortex have been associated with a more abundant renin content when compared with those of the juxtamedullary region (Cook, 1962; Granger et al., 1972; deRouffignac et al., 1974; Flamenbaum and Hamburger, 1974), an observation which correlates well with superficial cortical ischemia associated with ARF, as discussed above. Moreover, Venkatachalam et al. (1976) demonstrated afferent arteriolar vasoconstriction by morphometric evaluation following glycerol-induced ARF.

Alternatively, other vasoconstrictor substances may have a role in ARF. For instance, catecholamines have been shown to be released after administration of $HgCl_2$ (Solomon and Hollenberg, 1975). Oken (1976) suggested that some undefined vasoconstrictor substance may be released by injured tubular epithelial cells into the interstitial spaces surrounding glomeruli.

An alternative hypothesis to augmentation of afferent arteriolar vasoconstriction is a diminution of vasoactive modulating substances such as prostaglandins (Fine, 1970; Oken, 1975c). According to this hypothesis, ARF may be the result of damage to the medulla where prostaglandin synthesis takes place. Inasmuch as prostaglandins are vasodilators, their absence may alter the balancing effect they could have on arteriolar vasoconstriction, thus enhancing cortical ischemia. Indeed, Torres et al. (1975) blocked prostaglandin synthesis by indomethacin and enhanced glycerol-induced ARF in rabbits. However, Oken (1976) was not able to repeat these results in rats. Renal medullary autotransplants, which may release prostaglandins, have been shown to protect rabbits against ischemic ARF (Held, 1976). However, direct administration of prostaglandins failed to protect experimental animals against ARF induced by glycerol or uranyl nitrate (Cioffi et al., 1975; Mauk et al., 1977) and ischemia (Eliahou et al., 1977). Conversely, others have observed a beneficial effect of prostaglandin infusion in the glycerol model of ARF (Werb et al., 1978).

RENIN-ANGIOTENSIN AXIS AS A MEDIATOR OF ARF

Hypothesis

The first suggestion that vasoconstriction might be involved in the pathogenesis of ARF was made by Goormaghtigh (1945) when increased granularity and hypertrophy of JG cells were noted in four human cases of anuric crush syndrome. Goormaghtigh postulated that a "liberation of a vasopressor substance occurs in the anuric crush syndrome, causing arteriolar spasm at the vascular pole of the glomerular tufts." He indicated that the pressor substance also acts on neighboring smooth muscle cells near arterioles with an overflow in the general circulation. He concluded that the renal tubules must not be considered independently, since a connection at the level of the macula densa suggests a possible functional relationship between the two parts of the nephron.

The concept of tubuloglomerular feedback originally hypothesized in Goormaghtigh's studies has since been well documented (Thurau et al., 1967, 1972; Schnermann et al., 1970; Davis et al., 1972; Schnermann et al., 1973, 1979; Burke et al., 1974; Hierholzer et al., 1974; Wright and Schnermann, 1974; Schnermann, 1975).

Schnermann et al. (1966) proposed that vasoconstriction of the afferent arteriole, leading to ARF, is the result of tubular dysfunction that results from ischemia or a nephrotoxic injury. According to this hypothesis, ARF results from augmentation of a normal tubuloglomerular feedback mechanism, proposed by Thurau (1966) where an increase in intratubular NaCl is sensed at the level of the macula densa and signals a local release of renin from JG cells located within the media of the afferent arteriole, leading to angiotensin II production. Angiotensin II mediates vasoconstriction of the afferent arteriole leading to a reduction in GFR and filtered Na^+, thus completing a feedback mechanism which is capable of maintaining NaCl balance. Recently, Schnermann et al. (1979) have provided data suggesting involvement of prostaglandins in tubuloglomerular feedback since inhibitors of prostaglandin synthesis diminished feedback responses. However, the precise role of prostaglandins or angiotensin in tubuloglomerular feedback has not been elucidated.

It has been postulated that proximal convoluted tubular injury, resulting from a nephrotoxic or ischemic event, leads to impairment of fluid and electrolyte reabsorption. Since 60-70% of the filtered NaCl load is normally reabsorbed by the proximal tubule, such a dysfunction could increase $[Na^+]$ or $[Cl^-]$ at the level of the macula densa and lead to prolonged vasoconstriction and renal cortical ischemia, which would exaggerate proximal tubular dysfunction and initiate a vicious cycle (Flamenbaum, 1973). Indeed, a number of investigators have described elevated plasma renin or angiotensin activity in patients with ARF (Massani et al., 1966; Kokot and Kuska, 1969; Ochoa, et al., 1970; Brown et al., 1970). Similar elevations of plasma renin have been described in the glycerol model (Hayes et al., 1968; DiBona and Swain, 1971) and in the methemoglobin model (Ruiz-Guinazu et al., 1967) of experimental ARF.

Thus, evidence has been obtained in both human patients and in experimental models favoring this general mechanism, although the details remain obscure. The general failure to correlate circulating renin levels or angiotensin levels with ARF has led to correlations based on intrarenal levels and especially of renin measured within an individual juxtaglomerular apparatus (JGA). This is now possible through sensitive radioimmunoassay techniques and microdissection of injected kidneys (Flamenbaum and Hamburger, 1974). Such findings indicate very rapid elevations in JGA renin after either ischemia or administration of a toxin. Correlative morphological studies (Sato et al., 1977) demonstrated that these increases in JGA renin are paralleled by changes in the JG index and in the ultrastructural appearance of the afferent arteriole within 30 min after a subcutaneous injection of $HgCl_2$.

Prerequisites for the Initiation of a Tubuloglomerular Feedback Mechanism in ARF

Recently, Mason (1976) enumerated three prerequisites necessary for the tubuloglomerular feedback mechanism to work in initiation of ARF: 1) a defect in proximal tubular reabsorption; 2) increased $[Na^+]$ or $[Cl^-]$ at the macula densa; and 3) an intact JGA to make tubuloglomerular feedback operational.

DEFECT IN PROXIMAL TUBULAR REABSORPTION

Numerous studies have described reduced transport functions across a variety of epithelial surfaces by uranyl compounds and $HgCl_2$ (Newey et al., 1966; Frizzell and Schultz, 1970; Armstrong and Dugue, 1975; Stirling, 1975; Schwartz and Flamenbaum, 1976) and in tissue slices following ischemia (Berndt, 1976). Reduced fluid or electrolyte reabsorption has been observed in vivo following ARF that was induced by a variety of nephrotoxins including glycerol (Oken et al., 1966), dichromate (Henry et al., 1968), $HgCl_2$ (Bank et al., 1967; Barenberg et al., 1968; Flamenbaum et al., 1971), uranyl nitrate (Flamenbaum et al., 1974; Kleinman et al., 1977) and ischemia (Tanner et al., 1973; Mason, 1976).

Evidence for a very early proximal tubular lesion in $HgCl_2$-induced ARF was demonstrated by McDowell et al. (1976) and Zalme et al. (1976). At early time intervals (30 min onwards) changes were described both histochemically and ultrastructurally in all segments of the proximal tubule. Marked dispersion of polysomes as well as condensation of mitochondrial matrices in proximal tubules occurred 30 min after administration of $HgCl_2$ (McDowell et al., 1976). Zalme et al. (1976) noted the inhibition of membrane marker enzymes, alkaline phosphatase, and 5'-nucleotidase as early as 15 min following the same dose of $HgCl_2$. These studies supported a structural-functional correlation between early proximal tubular injury and the development of functional impairment.

Recently, the direct effects of heavy metals on membrane function have been studied in vitro, using isolated urinary bladders of freshwater turtles (Schwartz and Flamenbaum, 1976). Bladders were prepared in such a way as to expose mucosal and serosal surfaces to separate compartments of lucite chambers. Upon addition of 10^{-5} M $HgCl_2$ to the mucosal side, a decrease in active Na^+ transport was noted without measurable changes in passive flow of small ions. Diminished transport remained even after rinsing the bladder with fresh Ringer's solution. However, upon addition of dithiothreitol (DTT), a dithiol sugar that chelates heavy metals as well as maintains sulphydryl groups in their reduced state (Cleland, 1964), transport returned towards normal. Likewise, amphotericin B, a compound that increases membrane permeability, also returned transport towards normal when added to the mucosal side. Since the addition of $HgCl_2$ to the serosal side had no effect on transport, an apical site of Na^+ entry was hypothesized as being initially affected by $HgCl_2$. It may be possible to extrapolate this information to the in vivo situation. Rothstein (1959) and Webb (1966) have stated that $HgCl_2$ is preferentially bound to sulphydryl groups of intact tissues. Since membrane components of the brush border of proximal tubules are richly endowed with sulphydryl groups, the initial decrease in membrane enzyme activity noted by Zalme et al. (1976) may represent a similar phenomenon.

In vivo studies have recently been conducted to examine the effects of DTT on the course of heavy metal-induced ARF (Kleinman et al., 1977). Rats were administered either uranyl nitrate or $HgCl_2$ at 10 or 4 mg/kg, respectively, and compared physiologically with rats given the same dosage of heavy metal followed by DTT 30 min later. When heavy metal was administered alone, azotemia, diminished C_{Cr}, and increased FE_{Na^+} resulted. Animals given DTT 30 min after admininstration of the heavy metal showed a nearly complete amelioration of renal dysfunction. Involvement of the renin-angiotensin system was implicated by a marked increase in plasma and JGA renin activity 6 hr after administration of heavy metal. However, activity of both parameters was prevented with DTT, suggesting that DTT alters the effect of heavy metals on epithelial transport functions, preventing an increased $[Na^+]$ at the level of the macula densa and subsequent involvement of the renin-angiotensin system.

Structural-functional correlations in the kidneys of rats that are largely protected against $HgCl_2$-induced ARF by administration of DDT were recently studied (Barnes et al., 1980a). Rats were given $HgCl_2$ alone, DTT alone, or $HgCl_2$ followed by DTT 30 min later. The kidneys were studied by light and electron microscopy and enzyme histochemistry throughout the initiation phase of ARF. Rats receiving $HgCl_2$ alone developed a nonoliguric form of ARF, apparent at 12 hr and progressive through 48 hr. All segments of the proximal tubules of these rats showed morphological and enzymatic changes as early as 1 and 3 hr. By 6, 12, 24, and 48 hr, morphological changes in the first portion of the pars convoluta (P_1) tended to be reversible, whereas injury which occurred in the more terminal portions of pars convoluta (P_2) was sublethal in some rats but progressed to necrosis in others. Activities of all enzymes studied were reduced throughout P_1 and P_2 at 6, 12, 24, and 48 hr. By 24 and 48 hr, all pars recta (P_3) tubules were necrotic and enzyme activities were minimal. Rats given $HgCl_2$ and DTT were largely protected against ARF and this paralleled near total protection of the pars convoluta (P_1 and P_2) against morphological and enzymatic changes. Nevertheless, extensive necrosis developed in P_3 of rats given $HgCl_2$ plus DTT. The results of this study supported the hypothesis that structural-functional correlations do exist between injury to P_1 and P_2 and the development of $HgCl_2$-induced ARF, which is unrelated to necrosis of P_3. According to this hypothesis, $HgCl_2$-induced alterations in proximal tubular handling of Na^+ and Cl^- lead to augmentation of a tubuloglomerular feedback mechanism involving the renin-angiotensin system. This results in vasoconstriction of the afferent arteriole and subsequent filtration failure. DTT ameliorates ARF by altering the effect of $HgCl_2$ on Na^+ and Cl^- transport functions of P_1 and P_2 and the subsequent initiation of such a feedback mechanism.

INCREASED NaCl CONCENTRATION AT THE MACULA DENSA

Further support for a tubuloglomerular feedback mechanism rests with the observation of an elevation of $[Na^+]$ at the level of the macula densa, as measured by early distal tubular punctures. Increases in early distal tubular $[Na^+]$ have been reported in heavy metal-induced ARF (Flamenbaum et al., 1976a; Mason, 1976) and in ischemia-induced ARF (Schnermann et al., 1966). Indeed, increases in $[Na^+]$ have been associated with elevated JGA renin activity following heavy metal-induced ARF (Flamenbaum et al., 1976a; Kleinman et al., 1977), a finding which correlates well with the elevated JGA renin activity after microperfusion with high NaCl to the macula densa of untreated rats (Thurau and Mason, 1974). Using microtechniques, they observed that injection of solutions containing Na^+ and Cl^- into the distal tubular regions of the macula densa was associated with a diminution of GFR in the same nephron. This would imply that failure of the proximal tubule to reabsorb NaCl would be followed by a compensatory reduction of glomerular filtration.

According to Thurau and Boylan (1976), this has great survival value, since in the face of inadequate reabsorption of ions in the nephron, failure to reduce GFR could lead to excessive urine production. Failure of this mechanism to operate might even be responsible for the excessive production of up to 50 liters of urine by some patients with ARF. In the presence of diminished tubular function with diminished salt reabsorption, the system operates according to this concept, as if it is better to retain substances such as urea than to produce excessive urine volumes (Thurau and Boylan, 1976). This would mean that an important initiating event would be alterations, caused by toxins or ischemia, in the proximal convoluted tubule which might well be reversible. This would alter Na^+, Cl^-, and water reabsorption, leading to an increased load in the macula densa with feedback on the afferent arterioles with constriction and diminished GFR, initiating a vicious cycle.

FUNCTIONALLY INTACT JGA

Initiation of the renin-angiotensin system by tubuloglomerular feedback relies on the local presence of renin substrate and on all the necessary enzyme systems for angiotensin production. Indeed, renin, angiotensin I converting enzyme and/or angiotensin II have been located in renal lymph, suggesting a renal locus for all components of angiotensin II production (Lever and Peart, 1962; Higgins et al., 1964; Skinner et al., 1963; Bailie et al., 1971; Horky et al., 1971). Moreover, Finkielman et al. (1972) demonstrated the production of angiotensin I and II from isolated glomeruli in vitro, thus suggesting the presence of renin substrate at this locus. Granger et al. (1972) also demonstrated the presence of converting enzyme activity and renin activity in individually dissected JGAs. Such an intrarenal locus has been further supported by the finding of a subcellular location of converting enzyme (Oshima et al., 1974) and renin substrate in granules from rat kidney cortex (Morris and Johnston, 1976).

As mentioned above, increases in $[Na^+]$ have been associated with elevated JGA renin activity, following heavy metal-induced ARF (Flamenbaum et al., 1976a). Moreover, feedback responses were shown by Mason (1976) to remain intact following the administration of uranyl nitrate, $HgCl_2$ or total renal ischemia of 45 and 75 min duration. These observations may well correlate with the fine structure of the JGA which has been shown to remain intact and apparently stimulated following administration of $HgCl_2$ (Rojo-Ortega et al., 1974; Sato et al., 1977). Typically the JG cells develop an increase in granularity, hypertrophied Golgi apparatus, and dilatation of the endoplasmic reticulum, suggesting a stimulation of a secretory process that most likely involves renin release, since these granules have been related to pressor activity (Pitcock et al., 1959).

Amelioration of ARF by Interruption of the Renin-Angiotensin System

In attempts to implicate the renin-angiotensin system in the pathophysiology of ARF, a variety of maneuvers involving interruption of this system have been performed. For example, chronic NaCl-loading prior to administration of a variety of nephrotoxins has been shown to ameliorate ARF (Henry et al., 1968; McDonald et al., 1969; DiBona and Swain, 1971; Ryan et al., 1973). Conversely, a low sodium diet enhances ARF. Since chronic NaCl-loading depletes renin content in renal cortical tissue (Gross et al., 1964; Cockett et al., 1967; deRouffignac et al., 1974) as well as in individual glomeruli or JGAs (Gavras et al., 1970; Granger et al., 1972; Flamenbaum and Hamburger, 1974; Kaufman et al., 1976) and a low sodium diet increases renal and JGA renin content, a role for the renin-angiotensin system in ARF is strongly implicated. Moreover, partial renin suppression by KCl-loading results in only partial amelioration of $HgCl_2$-induced ARF (Flamenbaum et al., 1973a). Nearly all secondary factors associated with high NaCl diets have been excluded as the mechanism of protection against experimentally induced ARF, thus suggesting a primary role for the renin-angiotensin system. For example, increased plasma volume (which accompanies NaCl loading) can be ruled out because sodium bicarbonate increases plasma volume but does not protect against $HgCl_2$-induced ARF (Beaumont et al., 1977). Conversely, KCl-loading does not expand plasma volume but ameliorates $HgCl_2$-induced ARF (Flamenbaum et al., 1973a). Other factors such as serum and urine osmolarity, or urine volume have also been ruled out as protective agents against ARF (Thiel et al., 1967; McDonald et al., 1969; Wilson et al., 1969). However, a correlation between amelioration of ARF and diuresis or solute excretion independent of renal renin content has been observed (Thiel et al., 1976; Bidani et al., 1978; Mason et al., 1979).

Structural-functional correlations in NaCl-loaded rats treated with $HgCl_2$, in which ARF was ameliorated, were recently made (Barnes et al., 1980b). Rats were maintained on a 1% sodium chloride solution instead of water for 3 weeks prior to the administration of $HgCl_2$. Kidneys were studied by light and electron microscopy and enzyme histochemistry at intervals between 1 and 48 hr. Despite amelioration of ARF, saline-loaded rats given $HgCl_2$ were not protected against proximal convoluted tubular injury and developed lesions similar to rats given $HgCl_2$ alone. These results supported the hypothesis that $HgCl_2$-induced ARF was initiated by activation of the renin-angiotensin system. It was argued that since saline-loading results in the depletion of intrarenal renin, saline-loaded $HgCl_2$-treated rats were protected against the development of ARF despite injury to proximal convoluted segments, because in this case tubular dysfunction and increases in electrolyte concentration could not trigger the renin-angiotensin system.

Powell-Jackson et al. (1972) and Rauh et al. (1975) prevented glycerol-induced ARF by passive immunization with angiotensin II antibodies. However, Powell-Jackson et al. (1973) and Oken et al. (1975) were not able to reproduce these findings. Moreover, passive immunization against renin does not prevent experimental ARF induced by glycerol or $HgCl_2$ (Flamenbaum et al., 1972a). Also, synthetic competitive inhibitors of angiotensin II fail to prevent glycerol- (Powell-Jackson et al., 1973) and ischemia (Eliahou et al., 1977)-induced ARF. Maneuvers known to suppress plasma renin activity but not renal renin do not prevent experimentally induced ARF. For example, NaCl-loading for 30 hr prior to initiation of glycerol-induced ARF has been found not to be preventative, despite a suppression in plasma renin (Flamenbaum et al., 1973b). Also, sodium bicarbonate reduced plasma renin but not renal renin and does not prevent $HgCl_2$-induced ARF (Beaumont et al., 1977). Moreover, phentolamine, which induces a blockade of α-receptors and suppresses renin secretion, reduced plasma renin activity but not renal renin activity and does not ameliorate $HgCl_2$-induced ARF (Birbari and Haidar, 1976). It has been suggested by Flamenbaum et al. (1972a) that the vasoactive mechanism involved in the renin-angiotensin system works at a local intrarenal site and is independent of circulating renin levels. Failure of immunization or competitive inhibition against the renin-angiotensin system to protect against ARF may reflect the inability of antibodies or inhibitors to penetrate cell membranes at the level of the JGA. Indeed, recent studies by Forssmann and Taugner (1977) have observed that the endothelial junctions of cells within the afferent arteriole of tree shrews exhibit a highly developed zonular arrangement of tight junctions (indicating a tight blood-tissue barrier) in comparison to other systemic arterioles, as described by Simionescu et al. (1976).

However, the sympathetic nervous system has also been implicated in renin release and the development of ARF. For example, propranolol, an α-blocker, has been suggested to suppress renin release in dogs (Yun et al., 1977). Recently, Eliahou et al. (1977) and Solez et al. (1977a and b) have described an alleviation of post-ischemic-induced ARF by propranolol in rats and rabbits, respectively. Solez et al. (1977b) were able to eliminate propranolol's beneficial effect by chemical renal denervation using phenol. The authors concluded that the probable action of propranolol is interference with neurogenically stimulated renin release. This is of considerable interest because Holst (1972) has reported that psychosocial stress may lead to chronic renal failure in the tree shrew. Indeed, Forssmann and Taugner (1977) reported an extremely extensive innervation of the JGA in this same species.

It is important to point out that the precise role of the renin-angiotensin system in ARF remains to be elucidated. Several investigators have recently studied the development of ARF in the two kidney Goldblatt rat. In this model, the left kidney was made partially ischemic for several weeks by partially clamping the renal artery. This maneuver results in an increased intrarenal renin content in the stenotic kidney but reduced intrarenal renin content in the untouched contralateral kidney with respect to controls. Administration of glycerol (P.C. Churchill et al., 1977), $HgCl_2$ (Churchill et al., 1978) or occlusion of the renal artery (Ploth et al., 1978; Mason et al., 1979) induced ARF of equal severity in the stenotic kidney when compared to the contralateral kidney or in controls receiving the same treatment. If intrarenal renin content were a major factor in the development of ARF, one would expect a more severe functional impairment in the stenotic (high renin) kidney than in the contralateral (low renin) kidney or in controls. It is obvious that roles of the renin-angiotensin system, prostaglandins, or other vasomodulating substances in the pathophysiology of ARF will require further investigation.

SUMMARY

It seems clear that of the numerous models that have been devised for the study of ARF, none matches exactly the picture seen in the human. Even this last statement needs to be tentatively made, since exact data concerning findings with newer subcellular techniques in the human are not entirely clear. Of the models, the two which seem most worthy of further study are the toxic model and the ischemic model. Other models of ARF, such as glycerol-induced, could be more complex because of the uncertain nature of the initiating event. The toxic and ischemic models at least have a reasonably clear starting point. Differences between the rat, dog, and the human, especially with respect to blood flow distribution need to be taken into account. For example, the uniform necrosis of the pars recta which occurs in the rat may not have any consistent relationship to ARF.

Another central theme that emerges from the review of the current literature and symposia on the subject (Kidney International Supplement No. 6, 1976) is the importance of tubular dysfunction, which is generally the most controversial part of most models. Tubular dysfunction can begin within seconds or minutes following ischemic injury and probably following toxic damage as well. It is very important to keep in mind that this tubular dysfunction need not lead to tubular necrosis and, indeed, infrequently does so extensively in the human condition. The early occurrence of tubular alterations may well incite other mechanisms such as glomerular tubular feedback, obstruction, and backleak. It would appear that efforts at modifying the tubular lesion may be the most effective way to reduce morbidity and mortality in this disease. Such efforts might be directed toward preventing the development of the early initiating lesions and toward promoting recovery of these, if they have already occurred. Further understanding of the interaction of reversible ischemic or toxic lesions with those resulting from bacterial sepsis, especially endotoxin, need much more study. Accurate definition of tubular changes is needed at the morphological level and correlation of these changes with metabolic changes is essential. There is a need for the development of therapeutic interventions at the initiation, maintenance, and recovery phases in order to more effectively modify the course of ARF in man. Presently, greater understanding of the syndrome in man is certainly needed in order to validate experimental models or parts thereof which are most relevant to clinical medicine.

References

Abeshouse, B.S.: Renal decapsulation: A review of the literature and a report of ten cases. J. Urol. 53:27–84, 1945.

Allison, M.E.M., Lipham, E.M., and Gottschalk, C.W.: Hydrostatic pressure in the rat kidney. Am. J. Physiol. 223:975–983, 1972.

Anderson, R.J., Linas, S.L., Berns, A.S., Henrich, W.L., Miller, T.R., Gabow, P.A., and Schrier, R.W.: Nonoliguric acute renal failure. N. Engl. J. Med. 296:1134–1138, 1977.

Arendshorst, W.J., Finn, W.F., and Gottschalk, C.W.: A micropuncture study of acute renal failure following temporary renal ischemia in the rat. Kidney Int. 10:S100–S105, 1976.

Armstrong, W.M., and Dugue, J.: Effect of UO^{2++} on sugar-induced potential (P.D.) and short circuit current (I_{sc}) across isolated bullfrog small intestine. Fed. Proc. 34:469, 1975.

Ayer, G., Grandchamp, A., Wyler, T., and Truniger, B.: Intrarenal hemodynamics in glycerol-induced myohemoglobinuric acute renal failure in the rat. Circ. Res. 29:128–135, 1971.

Baehler, R.W., Kotchen, T.A., Burke, J.A., Galla, J.H., and Bhathena, D.: Considerations on the pathophysiology of mercuric chloride-induced acute renal failure. J. Lab. Clin. Med. 90:330–340, 1977.

Bailie, M.D., Rector, F.C., and Seldin, D.W.: Angiotensin II in arterial and renal venous plasma and renal lymph in the dog. J. Clin. Invest. 50:119–126, 1971.

Baker, S.L., and Dodds, E.C.: Obstruction of the renal tubules during excretion of hemoglobin. Br. J. Exp. Pathol. 6:247–260, 1925.

Bank, N., Mutz, B.F., and Aynedjian, H.S.: The role of "leakage" of tubular fluid in anuria due to mercury poisoning. J. Clin. Invest. 46:695–704, 1967.

Barenberg, R.L., Solomon, S., Papper, S., and Anderson, R.: Clearance and micropuncture study of renal function in mercuric chloride treated rats. J. Lab. Clin. Med. 72:473–484, 1968.

Barnes, J.L., Osgood, R.W., Reinick, H.J., and Stein, J.H.: Glomerular alterations in the ischemic model of acute renal failure. Kidney Int. 16:771, 1979.

Barnes, J.L., McDowell, E.M., McNeil, J.S., Flamenbaum, W., and Trump, B.F.: Studies on the pathophysiology of acute renal failure. IV. Protective effect of dithiothreitol following administration of mercuric chloride. Virchows Arch. [Cell Pathol.] 32:201–232, 1980a.

Barnes, J.L., McDowell, E.M., McNeil, J.S., Flamenbaum, W., and Trump, B.F.: Studies on the pathophysiology of acute renal failure. V. Effect of chronic saline loading on the progression of proximal tubular injury and functional impairment following administration of mercuric chloride. Virchows Arch. [Cell Pathol.] 32:233–260, 1980b.

Baylis, C., Rennke, H.R., and Brenner, B.M.: Mechanisms of the defect in glomerular ultrafiltration associated with gentamicin administration. Kidney Int. 12:344–353, 1977.

Beaumont, J.E., Kotchen, T.A., Galla, J.H., and Luke, R.G.: Failure of loading with sodium bicarbonate to protect against acute renal failure induced by mercuric chloride in the rat. Clin. Sci. 53:149–154, 1977.

Berndt, W.O.: Effects of acute anoxia on renal transport processes. J. Toxicol. Environ. Health 2:1–11, 1976.

Bidani, A.K., Fleischmann, L.E., Churchill, P., and Becker-McKenna, B.: Naturesis-induced protection in acute myohemoglobinuric renal failure without renal cortical renin content depletion in the rat. Nephron 22:529–537, 1978.

Birbari, A., and Haidar, G.A.: Renin-angiotensin system and acute renal failure. Johns Hopkins Med. J. 139:73–77, 1976.

Blantz, R.C.: The mechanism of acute renal failure after uranyl nitrate. J. Clin. Invest. 55:621–635, 1975.

Bohle, A., Jahnecke, J., Meyer, D., and Schubert, G.E.: Morphology of acute renal failure: Comparative data from biopsy and autopsy. Kidney Int. 10:S9–S16, 1976.

Brenner, B.M., Troy, J.L., and Daugharty, T.M.: The dynamics of glomerular ultrafiltration in the rat. J. Clin. Invest., 50:1776–1780, 1971.

Brown, J.J., Gleadle, R.I., Lawson, D.H., Lever, A.F., Linton, A.L., Macadam, R.F., Prentice, E., and Robertson, J.I.S., and Tree, M.: Renin and acute renal failure: Studies in man. Br. Med. J. 1:253–258, 1970.

Brun, C., and Munck, O.: Lesions of the kidney in acute renal failure following shock. Lancet 1:603–607, 1957.

Burke, T.J., Navar, L.G., Clapp, J.R., and Robinson, R.R.: Response of single nephron glomerular filtration rate to distal nephron microperfusion. Kidney Int. 6:230–240, 1974.

Bywaters, E.G., and Dible, J.H.: Renal lesion in traumatic anuria. J. Pathol. Bacteriol. 54:111–120, 1942.

Chedru, M.-F., Baethke, R., and Oken, D.E.: Renal cortical blood flow and glomerular filtration in myohemoglobinuric acute renal failure. Kidney Int. 1:232–239, 1972.

Churchill, P.C., Bidani, A., Fleischman, L., and Becker-McKenna, B.: Glycerol-induced acute renal failure in the two-kidney Goldblatt rat. Am. J. Physiol. 233:F247–F252, 1977.

Churchill, P.C., Bidani, A., Fleischmann, L., and Becker-McKenna, B.: $HgCl_2$-induced acute renal failure in the Goldblatt rat. J. Lab. Clin. Med. 91:660–665, 1978.

Churchill, S., Zarlengo, M.D., Carvalho, J.S., Gottlieb, M.N., and Oken, D.E.: Normal renocortical blood flow in experimental acute renal failure. Kidney Int. 11:246–255, 1977.

Cioffi, R.F., O'Connell, J.M.B., and Shalhoub, R.J.: Effect of prostaglandin A_1 on acute renal failure in the rat. Nephron 15:29–34, 1975.

Cirksena, W.J.: Pathogenetic studies in a model of pigment nephropathy in the rat. In *Pathogenesis and Clinical Findings with Acute Renal Failure*, edited by U. Gessler, K. Schroder, and H. Weidinger, pp. 105–117. Thieme, Stuttgart, 1971.

Clarkson, A.R., MacDonald, M.K., Fuster, V., Cash, J.D., and Robson, J.S.: Glomerular coagulation in acute ischemic renal failure. Q. J. Med. 39:585–599, 1970.

Cleland, W.W.: Dithiothreitol, a new protective reagent for SH groups. Biochemistry 3:480–482, 1964.

Cockett, A.T.K., Moore, R.S., Kazmin, M., and Roberts, A.P.: Extraction and bioassay of renin from kidneys of sodium-depleted and sodium-loaded rats. J. Urol. 97:168–171, 1967.

Conger, J.D., and Robinette, J.B.: Pathogenetic events in ischemic acute renal failure (ARF). Kidney Int. 10:555, 1976.

Cook, W.F.: Renin and the juxtaglomerular apparatus. Mem. Soc. Endocrinol. 13:247–254, 1962.

Cox, J.W., Baehler, R.W., Sharma, H., O'Dorisio, T., Osgood, R.W., Stein, J.H., and Ferris, T.F.: Studies on the mechanism of oliguria in a model of unilateral acute renal failure. J. Clin. Invest. 53:1546–1558, 1974.

Dalgaard, O.Z., and Pedersen, K.J.: Ultrastructure of the kidney in shock. *Proceedings of 1st International Congress of Nephrology*, p. 165. Karger, Basel, 1961.

Daugherty, T.M., Ueki, I.F., Mercer, P.F., and Brenner, B.M.: Dynamics of glomerular ultrafiltration in the rat. V. Response to ischemic injury. J. Clin. Invest. 53:105–116, 1974.

Davis, J.M., Schnermann, J., and Horster, M.: Micropuncture

method for the determination of nephron filtration rate. Pflüegers Arch. *333:*271–280, 1972.

Deen, W.M., Robertson, C.R., and Brenner, B.M.: Glomerular ultrafiltration. Fed. Proc. *33:*14–20, 1974.

deRouffignac, C., Bonvalet, J.P., and Menard, L.: Renin content in superficial and deep glomeruli of normal and salt-loaded rats. Am. J. Physiol. *426:*150–154, 1974.

de Wardener, H.E.: Intrarenal pressure in experimental tubular necrosis. Lancet *1:*580–584, 1955.

DiBona, G.F., and Swain, L.L.: The renin-angiotensin system in acute renal failure in the rat. Lab. Invest. *25:*528–532, 1971.

DiBona, G.F., McDonald, F.D., Flamenbaum, W., Dammin, G.J., and Oken, D.E.: Maintenance of renal function in salt loaded rats despite severe tubular necrosis induced by $HgCl_2$. Nephron *8:*205–220, 1971.

Dobyan, D.C., Nagle, R.B., and Bulger, R.E.: Acute tubular necrosis in the rat kidney following sustained hypotension. Physiologic and morphologic observations. Lab. Invest. *37:*411–422, 1977a.

Dobyan, D.C., Nagle, R.B., and Bulger, R.E.: Hypovolemic models of acute tubular necrosis in the rat kidney. Virchows Arch. [Cell Pathol.] *25:*271–280, 1977b.

Donohoe, J.F., Venkatachalam, M.A., Bernard, D.B., and Levinsky, N.G.: Tubular leakage and obstruction after renal ischemia: Structural-functional correlations. Kidney Int. *13:*208–222, 1978.

Eisenbach, G.M., Klitzlinger, B., and Steinhausen, M.: Renal blood flow after temporary ischemia of rat kidneys. Pflüegers Arch. *347:*223–234, 1974.

Eisenbach, G.M., and Steinhausen, M.: Micropuncture studies after temporary ischemia of rat kidneys. Pflüegers Arch. *343:*11–25, 1973.

Eliahou, H.E., Iaina, A., Solomon, S., and Gavendo, S.: Alleviation of anoxic experimental acute renal failure in rats by β-adrenergic blockade. Nephron *19:*158–166, 1977.

Finckh, E.S.: The failure of experimental renal tubulonecrosis to produced oliguria in the rat. Aust. Ann. Med. *9:*283–288, 1960.

Finckh, E.S., Jeremy, D., and Whyte, H.M.: Structural renal damage and its relation to clinical features in acute oliguric renal failure. Q. J. Med. *31:*429–446, 1962.

Fine, L.G.: Acquired prostaglandin E_2 (medullin) deficiency as the cause of oliguria in acute tubular necrosis: A hypothesis. Ir. J. Med. Sci. *6:*346–350, 1970.

Finkielman, S., Goldstein, D.J., Fischer-Fenaro, C., and Nahnol, V.F.: In vitro production of angiotensin and renin release by isolated glomeruli. Medicine (Buenos Aires) *32:*37–39, 1972.

Flamenbaum, W.: Pathophysiology of acute renal failure. Arch. Intern. Med. *131:*911–928, 1973.

Flamenbaum, W., and Hamburger, R.J.: Superficial and deep juxtaglomerular apparatus renin activity of the rat. Effect of surgical preparation and NaCl intake. J. Clin. Invest. *54:*1373–1381, 1974.

Flamenbaum, W., McDonald, F.D., DiBona, G.F., and Oken, D.E.: Micropuncture study of renal tubular factors in low dose mercury poisoning. Nephron *8:*221–234, 1971.

Flamenbaum, W., Kotchen, T.A., and Oken, D.E.: Effect of renin immunization on mercuric chloride and glycerol-induced renal failure. Kidney Int. *1:*406–412, 1972a.

Flamenbaum, W., McNeil, J.S., Kotchen, T.A., and Saladino, A.J.: Experimental acute renal failure induced by uranyl nitrate in the dog. Circ. Res. *31:*682–698, 1972b.

Flamenbaum, W., Kotchen, T.A., Nagle, R., and McNeil, J.S.: Effect of potassium on the renin-angiotensin system and $HgCl_2$-induced acute renal failure. Am. J. Physiol. *224:*305–311, 1973a.

Flamenbaum, W., McNeil, J.S., Kotchen, T.A., Lowenthal, D., and Nagle, R.B.: Glycerol-induced acute renal failure after acute plasma renin activity suppression. J. Lab. Clin. Med. *82:*587–596, 1973b.

Flamenbaum, W., Huddleston, M.L., McNeil, J.S., and Hamburger, R.J.: Uranyl nitrate-induced acute renal failure in the rat: Micropuncture and renal hemodynamic studies. Kidney Int. *6:*408–418, 1974.

Flamenbaum, W., Hamburger, R., and Kaufman, J.: Distal tubule [Na^+] and juxtaglomerular apparatus renin activity in uranyl nitrate induced acute renal failure in the rat. An evaluation of the role of tubulo-glomerular feedback. Pflüegers Arch. *364:*209–215, 1976a.

Flamenbaum, W., Hamburger, R.J., Huddleston, M.L., Kaufman, J., McNeil, J.S., Schwartz, J.H., and Nagle, R.: The initiation phase of experimental acute renal failure: An evaluation of uranyl nitrate-induced acute renal failure in the rat. Kidney Int. *10:*S115–S122, 1976b.

Flanigan, W.J., and Oken, D.E.: Renal micropuncture study of the development of anuria in the rat with mercury-induced acute renal failure. J. Clin. Invest. *44:*449–457, 1965.

Flores, J., DiBona, D.R., Beck, C.H., and Leaf, A.: The role of cell swelling in ischemic renal damage and a protective effect of hypertonic solute. J. Clin. Invest. *51:*118–126, 1972.

Forssmann, W.G., and Taugner, R.: Studies on the juxtaglomerular apparatus. V. The juxtaglomerular apparatus in *Tupaia* with special reference to intercellular contacts. Cell Tissue Res. *177:*291–305, 1977.

Frega, N.S., DiBona, D.R., Guertler, B., and Leaf, A.: Ischemic renal injury. Kidney Int. *10:*S17–S25, 1976.

Frizzell, R.A., and Schultz, S.G.: Effects of monovalent cations on the sodium-alanine interactions in rabbit ileum. Implications of anionic groups in Na^+ binding. J. Gen. Physiol. *56:*462–490, 1970.

Gavras, H., Brown, J.J., Lever, A.F., and Robertson, J.I.S.: Changes of renin in individual glomeruli in response to variations of sodium intake in the rabbit. Clin. Sci. *38:*409–414, 1970.

Goormaghtigh, N.: Vascular and circulatory changes in renal cortex in the anuric crush-syndrome. Proc. Soc. Exp. Biol. Med. *59:*303–305, 1945.

Granger, P., Dahlheim, H., and Thurau, K.: Enzyme activities of the single juxtaglomerular apparatus in the rat kidney. Kidney Int. *1:*78–88, 1972.

Gross, F., Schaechtelin, G., Brunner, H., and Peters, G.: The role of the renin-angiotensin system in blood pressure regulation and kidney function. Can. Med. Assoc. J. *90:*258–262, 1964.

Hamburger, J.: Acute tubular and interstitial nephritis ("Acute tubular necrosis"). In *Nephrology*, pp. 501–575. W.B. Saunders, Philadelphia, 1968.

Hayes, J.M., O'Connell, J.M.B., Siegel, L., Pryce, F.A., and Schreiner, G.E.: Renal renin and renin release in acute renal failure in the rat. Fed. Proc. *27:*629, 1968.

Hayman, J.M., Shumway, N.P., Dumke, P., and Miller, M.: Experimental hyposthenuria.: J. Clin. Invest. *18:*195–212, 1939.

Held, E.: Protective effects of renomedullary autotransplants upon the course of postischemic acute renal failure in rabbits. Kidney Int. *10:*S201–S207, 1976.

Henry, L.N., Lane, C.E., and Kashgarian, M.: Micropuncture studies of the pathophysiology of acute renal failure in the rat. Lab. Invest. *19:*309–314, 1968.

Heptinstall, R.H.: *Pathology of the Kidney*, pp. 781–820. Little, Brown, Boston, 1974.

Hierholzer, K., Muller-Suur, R., Gutsche, H.-U., Butz, M., and Lichtenstein, I.: Filtration in surface glomeruli as regulated by flow rate through the loop of Henle. Pflüegers Arch. *352:* 315–337, 1974.

Higgins, J.T., Davis, J.O., and Urquhart, J.: Demonstration by pressor and steriodogenic assays of increased renin in lymph of dogs with secondary hyperaldosteronism. Circ. Res. *14:* 218–227, 1964.

Hollenberg, N.K., Epstein, M., Rosen, S.M., Basch, R.I., Oken, D.E., and Merrill, J.P.: Acute oliguric renal failure in man: Evidence for preferential renal cortical ischemia. Medicine (Baltimore) *47:*455–474, 1968.

Hollenberg, N.K., Adams, D.F., Oken, D.E., Abrams, H.L., and Merrill, J.P.: Acute renal failure due to nephrotoxins. Renal hemodynamic and angiographic studies in man. N. Engl. J. Med. *282:*1329–1334, 1970.

Hollenberg, N.K., Sandor, T., Controy, M., Adams, D.F., Solomon, H.S., Abrams, H.L., and Merrill, J.P.: Xenon transit through the oliguric human kidney: Analysis by maximum likelihood. Kidney Int. *3:*177–185, 1973.

Holst, D. Von.: Renal failure as the cause of death in *Tupaia belangeri* exposed to persistent social stress. J. Comprehensive Physiol. *78:*236–273, 1972.

Horky, K., Rojo-Ortega, J.M., Rodriguez, J., Boucher, R., and Genest, J.: Renin, renin substrate, and angiotensin I converting enzyme in the lymph of rats. Am. J. Physiol. *220:* 307–311, 1971.

Hsu, C.H., Kurtz, T.W., Rozenweig, J., and Weller, J. M.: Renal hemodynamics in $HgCl_2$-induced acute renal failure. Nephron *18:*326–332, 1977.

Huguenin, M., Thiel, G., and Brunner, F.P.: $HgCl_2$-induced acute renal failure studied by split drop micropuncture technique in the rat. Nephron *20:*147–156, 1978.

Jaenike, J.R.: Micropuncture study of methemoglobin-induced acute renal failure in the rat. J. Lab. Clin. Med. *73:*459–468, 1969.

Johnston, W.H., and Latta, H.: Glomerular mesangial and endothelial cell swelling following temporary renal ischemia and its role in the no-reflow phenomenon. Am. J. Pathol. *89:*153–166, 1977.

Källskog, Ö., Lindbom, L.O., Ulfendahl, H.R., and Wolgast, M.: Kinetics of the glomerular ultrafiltration in the rat kidney. An experimental study. Acta Physiol. Scand. *95:* 293–300, 1975.

Kashgarian, M., Siegel, N.J., Ries, A.L., DiMeola, H.J., and Hayslett, J.P. Hemodynamic aspects in development and recovery phases of experimental postischemic acute renal failure. Kidney Int. *10:*S160–S168, 1976.

Kaufman, J.S., Hamburger, R.J., and Flamenbaum, W. Tubuloglomerular feedback: Effect of dietary NaCl intake. Am. J. Physiol. *231:*1744–1749, 1976.

Kleinman, J.G., McNeil, J.S., and Flamenbaum, W.: Uranyl nitrate acute renal failure in the dog: Early changes in renal function and hemodynamics. Clin. Sci. *48:*9–16, 1975.

Kleinman, J.G., McNeil, J.S., Schwartz, J.H., Hamburger, R.J., and Flamenbaum, W.: Effect of dithiothreitol on mercuric chloride and uranyl nitrate-induced acute renal failure in the rat. Kidney Int. *12:*115–121, 1977.

Kokot, F., and Kuska, J.: Plasma renin activity in acute renal insufficiency. Nephron *6:*115–127, 1969.

Kreisberg, J.I., Bulger, R.E., Trump, B.F., and Nagle, R.B.: Effects of transient hypotension on the structure and function of rat kidney. Virchows Arch. [Cell Pathol.] *22:*121–133, 1976.

Kurtz, T.W., Maletz, R.M., and Hsu, C.H.: Renal cortical blood flow in glycerol-induced acute renal failure in the rat. Circ. Res. *38:*30–35, 1976.

Lameire, N., Ringoir, S., and Leusen, I.: Effect of variation in dietary NaCl intake on total and fractional renal blood flow in the normal and mercury-intoxicated rat. Circ. Res. *39:* 506–511, 1976.

Leaf, A.: Regulation of intracellular fluid volume and disease. Am. J. Med. *49:*291–295, 1970.

Lever, A.F., and Peart, W.S.: Renin and angiotensin-like activity in renal lymph. J. Physiol. (Lond.) *160:*548–563, 1962.

Levinsky, N.G., and Alexander, E.A.: Acute renal failure. In *The Kidney*, edited by B.M. Brenner and F.C. Rector, pp. 806–837. W.B. Saunders, Philadelphia, 1976.

Lordon, R.E., and Burton, J.R.: Post tramatic renal failure in military personnel in Southeast Asia. Am. J. Med. *53:*137–147, 1972.

Lorentz, W.B., Lassiter, W.E., and Gottschalk, C.W.: Renal tubular permeability during increased intrarenal pressure. J. Clin. Invest. *51:*484–492, 1972.

Lucké, B.: Lower nephron nephrosis (The renal lesions of the crush syndrome of burns, transfusion and other conditions affecting the lower segments of the nephron). Mil. Surg. *99:* 371–396, 1946.

Mason, A.D., Teschan, P.E., and Muirhead, E.E.: Studies in acute renal failure. III. Renal histologic alterations in acute renal failure in the rat. J. Surg. Res. *3:*450–456, 1963.

Mason, J.: Tubulo-glomerular feedback in the early stages of experimental acute renal failure. Kidney Int. *10:*S106–S114, 1976.

Mason, J., Olbricht, C., Takabatake, T., and Thurau, K.: The early phase of experimental acute renal failure. I. Intratubular pressure and obstruction. Pflüegers Arch. *370:*155–163, 1977.

Mason, J., Kain, H., Shiigai, T., Welsch, J., Schlecker, H., and Steff, M.: The early phase of experimental acute renal failure. V. The influence of suppressing the renin-angiotensin system. Pflüegers Arch. *380:*233–243, 1979.

Massani, Z.M., Finkielman, S., Worcel, M., Agrest, A., and Paladini, A.C.: Angiotensin blood levels in hypertensive and non-hypertensive diseases. Clin. Sci. *30:*473–483, 1966.

Mauk, R.H., Patak, R.V., Fadem, S.Z., Lifschitz, M.D., and Stein, J.H.: Effect of prostaglandin E administration in a nephrotoxic and a vasoconstriction model of acute renal failure. Kidney Int. *12:*122–130, 1977.

McDonald, F.D., Thiel, G., Wilson, D.R., DiBona, G.F., and Oken, D.E.: The prevention of acute renal failure in the rat by long-term saline loading. A possible role of the renin-angiotensin axis. Proc. Soc. Exp. Biol. Med. *131:*610–614, 1969.

McDowell, E.M., Nagle, R.B., Zalme, R.C., McNeil, J.S., Flamenbaum, W., and Trump, B.F.: Studies on the pathophysiology of acute renal failure. I. Correlation of ultrastructure and function in the proximal tubule of the rat following administration of mercuric chloride. Virchows Arch. [Cell Pathol.] *22:*173–196, 1976.

Meroney, W.H., and Rubini, M.E.: Kidney function during acute tubular necrosis: Clinical studies and a theory. Metabolism *8:*1–15, 1959.

Meyers, C., Roxe, D.M., and Hano, J.: The clinical course of nonoliguric acute tubular necrosis. Kidney Int. *6:*76A, 1974.

Morris, B.J., and Johnston, C.I.: Renin substrate in granules from rat kidney cortex. Biochem. J. *154:*625–637, 1976.

Newey, H., Sanford, P.A., and Smyth, D.H.: The effect of uranyl nitrate on intestinal transfer of hexoses. J. Physiol. (Lond.) *186:*493–502, 1966.

Nomiyama, K., and Foulkes, E.C.: Some effects of uranyl acetate on proximal tubular function in rabbit kidney. Toxicol. Appl. Pharmacol. *13:*89–98, 1968.

Ochoa, E., Finkielman, S., and Agrest, A.: Angiotensin blood levels during the evolution of acute renal failure. Clin. Sci. *38:*225–231, 1970.

Oken, D.E.: Nosologic considerations in the nomenclature of acute renal failure. Nephron *8:*505–510, 1971.

Oken, D.E.: On the passive backflow theory of acute renal failure. Am. J. Med. *58:*77–82, 1975a.

Oken, D.E.: Acute renal failure (vasomotor nephropathy): micropuncture studies of the pathogenetic mechanisms. Annu. Rev. Med. *26:*307–319, 1975b.

Oken, D.E.: Role of prostaglandins in the pathogenesis of acute renal failure. Lancet *1:*1319–1322, 1975c.

Oken, D.E.: Local mechanisms in the pathogenesis of acute renal failure. Kidney Int. *10:*S94–S99, 1976.

Oken, D.E., Arce, M.L., and Wilson, D.R.: Glycerol-induced hemoglobinuric acute renal failure in the rat. I. Micropuncture study of the development of oliguria. J. Clin. Invest. *45:*724–735, 1966.

Oken, D.E., Cotes, S.C., Flamenbaum, W., Powell-Jackson, J.D., and Lever, A.F.: Active and passive immunization to angiotensin in experimental acute renal failure. Kidney Int. *7:*12–18, 1975.

Olbricht, C., Mason, J., Takabatake, T., Hohlbrugger, G., and Thurau, K.: The early phase of experimental acute renal failure. II. Tubular leakage and the reliability of glomerular markers. Pflüegers Arch. *372:*251–258, 1977.

Oliver, J.: Correlations of structure and function and mechanisms of recovery in acute tubular necrosis. Am. J. Med. *15:*535–557, 1953.

Oliver, J., MacDowell, M., and Tracy, A.: The pathogenesis of acute renal failure associated with traumatic and toxic injury. Renal ischemia, nephrotoxic damage and the ischemuric episode. J. Clin. Invest. *30:*1307–1351, 1951.

Olsen, S.: Renal histopathology in various forms of acute anuria in man. Kidney Int. *10:*S2–S8, 1976.

Olsen, T.S., and Skjoldborg, H.: The fine structure of the renal glomerulus in acute anuria. Acta. Pathol. Microbiol. Scand. *70:*205–214, 1967.

Oshima, G., Gecse, A., and Erdös, E.G. Angiotensin I-converting enzyme of the kidney cortex. Biochim. Biophys. Acta *350:*26–37, 1974.

Peters, J.T.: Oliguria and anuria due to increased intrarenal pressure. Ann. Intern. Med. *23:*221–236, 1945.

Pitcock, J.A., Hartroft, P.M., and Newmark, L.N.: Increased renal pressor activity (renin) in sodium deficient rats and correlation with juxtaglomerular cell granulation. Proc. Soc. Exp. Biol. Med. *100:*868–869, 1959.

Ploth, D.W., Thomas, C.E., Roy, R.N., and Rudulph, J.G.: Ischemic acute renal failure in DOCA-salt loaded and Goldblatt hypertensive rats. J. Lab. Clin. Med. *92:*1009–1018, 1978.

Powell-Jackson, J.D., Brown, J.J., Lever, A.F., MacGregor, J., MacAdam, R.F., Titterington, D.M., Robertson, J.I.S., and Waite, M.A.: Protection against acute renal failure in rats by passive immunization against angiotensin II. Lancet *1:*774–776, 1972.

Powell-Jackson, J.D., MacGregor, J., Brown, J.J., Lever, A.F., and Robertson, I.S.: The effect of angiotensin II antisera and synthetic inhibitors of the renin-angiotensin system on glycerol-induced acute renal failure in the rat. In *Proceedings, Acute Renal Failure Conference,* edited by E.A. Friedman and H.E. Eliahou, pp. 281–289. DHEW Publication No. [NIH] 74-6081, Washington, DC, 1973.

Rauh, W., Oster, P., Dietz, R., and Gross, F.: The renin-angiotensin system in acute renal failure of rats. Clin. Sci. *48:*467–473, 1975.

Rees, A.J.: Acute renal failure. In: *Scientific Foundations of Urology,* edited by D.I. Williams and G.D. Chisholm, pp. 47–54. Year Book Medical Publishers, Chicago, 1976.

Reubi, F.C., Gossweiler, N., and Gurtler, R.: Renal circulation in man studied by means of a dye-dilution method. Circulation *33:*426–442, 1966.

Reubi, F.C., Vorburger, C., and Tuckman, J.: Renal distribution volumes of indocyanine green, [^{51}Cr] EDTA, and ^{24}Na in man during acute renal failure after shock. Implications for the pathogenesis of anuria. J. Clin. Invest. *52:*223–235, 1973.

Richards, A.N.: Direct observations of change in function of the renal tubule caused by certain poisons. Trans. Assoc. Am. Physicians *44:*64–74, 1929.

Richards, C.J., and DiBona, G.F.: Acute renal failure: Structural-functional correlation. Proc. Soc. Exp. Biol. Med. *146:*880–884, 1974.

Rojo-Ortega, J.M., Hatt, P.-Y., and Genest, J.: The juxtaglomerular apparatus in mercury intoxication in rats. Light and electron microscopic studies. Lab. Invest. *30:*696–703, 1974.

Rothstein, A.: Cell membrane as site of action of heavy metals. Fed. Proc. *18:*1026–1035, 1959.

Ruiz-Guinazu, A., Coelho, J.B., and Paz, R.A.: Methemoglobin-induced acute renal failure in the rat. Nephron *4:*257–275, 1967.

Russell, S.B.: The mechanism of action of mercuric chloride on the isolated perfused rat kidney. Eur. J. Clin. Invest. *5:*319–325, 1975.

Ryan, R., McNeil, J.S., Flamenbaum, W., and Nagle, R.: Uranyl nitrate induced acute renal failure in the rat: Effect of varying doses and saline loading. Proc. Soc. Exp. Biol. Med. *143:*289–296, 1973.

Sato, T., McDowell, E.M., McNeil, J.S., Flamenbaum, W., and Trump, B.F.: Studies on the pathophysiology of acute renal failure. III. A study of the juxtaglomerular apparatus of the rat nephron following administration of mercuric chloride. Virchows Arch. [Cell Pathol.] *24:*279–293, 1977.

Schnermann, J.: Regulation of single nephron filtration rate by feedback. Clin. Nephrol. *3:*75–81, 1975.

Schnermann, J., Nagel, W., and Thurau, K.: Die frühdistale natrium-konzentration in rattennieren nach renaler ischämie und hämorrhagischer hypotension. Pflüegers Arch. *287:*296–310, 1966.

Schnermann, J., Wright, F.S., Davis, J.M., Stackelberg, W. von, and Grill, G.: Regulation of superficial nephron filtration rate by tubuloglomerular feedback. Pflüegers Arch. *318:*147–175, 1970.

Schnermann, J., Persson, A.E.G., and Agerup, B.: Tubuloglomerular feedback. Nonlinear relation between glomerular hydrostatic pressure and loop of Henle perfusion rate. J. Clin. Invest. *52:*862–869, 1973.

Schnermann, J., Schubert, G., Hermle, M., Herbst, R., Stowe, N.T., Yarimizu, S., and Weber, P.C.: The effect of inhibition of prostaglandin synthesis on tubuloglomerular feedback in the rat kidney. Pflüegers Arch. *379:*269–279, 1979.

Schwartz, J.H., and Flamenbaum, W.: Heavy metal-induced alterations in ion transport by turtle urinary bladder. Am. J. Physiol. *230:*1582–1589, 1976.

Selkurt, E.E.: Comparison of renal clearances with direct renal blood flow under control conditions and following renal ischemia. Am. J. Physiol. *145:*376–386, 1946.

Shaldon, S., Silva, H., Lawson, T.R., and Walker, J.G.: Measurement of renal red cell and plasma transit times in acute renal failure. Proc. Soc. Exp. Biol. Med. *112:*359–362, 1963.

Sherwood, T., Lavender, J.P., and Russell, S.B.: Mercury-induced renal vascular shutdown: observations in experimental acute renal failure. Eur. J. Clin. Invest. *4:*1–8, 1974.

Simionescu, M., Simionescu, N., and Palade, G.E.: Segmental differentiations of cell junctions in the vascular endothelium. Arteries and veins. J. Cell Biol. *68:*705–723, 1976.

Singh, R., Leb, D., and Brooks, D.: Nonoliguric acute tubular necrosis. Kidney Int. *6:*98A, 1974.

Skinner, S.L., McCubbin, J.W., and Page, I.H.: Angiotensin in blood and lymph following reduction in renal arterial perfusion pressure in dogs. Circ. Res. *13:*336–345, 1963.

Solez, K., Freshwater, M.F., and Su, C.-T.: The effect of propranolol on postischemic acute renal failure in the rat. Transplantation *24:*148–151, 1977a.

Solez, K., D'Agostini, R.J., Stawowy, L., Freedman, M.T., Scott, W.W., Siegelman, S.S., and Heptinstall, R.H.: Beneficial effect of propranolol in a histologically appropriate model of postischemic acute renal failure. Am. J. Pathol. *88:*163–192, 1977b.

Solomon, H.S., and Hollenberg, N.K.: Catecholamine release: Mechanism of mercury-induced vascular smooth muscle contraction. Am. J. Physiol. *229:*8–12, 1975.

Stein, J.H., Gottschall, J., Osgood, R.W., and Ferris, T.F.: Pathophysiology of a nephrotoxic model of acute renal failure. Kidney Int. *8:*27–41, 1975.

Steinhausen, M., Eisenbach, G.M., and Helmstadter, V.: Concentration of Lissamine green in proximal tubules of antidiuretic and mercury poisoned rats and the permeability of these tubules. Pflüegers Arch. *311:*1–15, 1969.

Stirling, C.E.: Mercurial perturbation of brush border membrane permeability in rabbit ileum. J. Membr. Biol. *23:*33–56, 1975.

Stone, H.H., and Fulenwider, J.T.: Renal decapsulation in the prevention of postischemic oliguria. Ann. Surg. *186:*343–355, 1977.

Stone, W.J., and Knepshield, J.H.: Post-traumatic acute renal insufficiency in Vietnam. Clin. Nephrol. *2:*186–190, 1974.

Summers, W.K., and Jamison, R.L.: The no reflow phenomenon in renal ischemia. Lab. Invest. *25:*635–643, 1971.

Swann, R.C., and Merrill, J.P.: The clinical course of acute renal failure. Medicine (Baltimore) *32:*215–292, 1953.

Tanner, G.A., and Sophasan, S.: Kidney pressures after temporary renal artery occlusion in the rat. Am. J. Physiol. *230:*1173–1181, 1976.

Tanner, G.A., and Steinhausen, M.: Tubular obstruction in ischemia-induced acute renal failure in the rat. Kidney Int. *10:*S65–S73, 1976.

Tanner, G.A., Sloan, K.L., and Sophasan, S.: Effects of renal artery occlusion on kidney function in the rat. Kidney Int. *4:*377–389, 1973.

Teschan, P.E., Post, R.S., and Smith, L.H.: Post-traumatic renal insufficiency in military casualties. I. Clinical characteristics. Am. J. Med. *18:*172–186, 1955.

Thiel, G., Huguenin, M., Brunner, F., Peters, L., Peters, G., Eckert, H., Torhorst, J., and Rohr, H.P.: Étude du mechanisme de l'insuffisance renale aique à $HgCl_2$ chez le rat. J. Urol. Nephrol. *79:*967–977, 1973.

Thiel, G., Wilson, D.R., Arce, M.L., and Oken, D.E.: Glycerol induced hemoglobinuric acute renal failure in the rat. II. The experimental model, predisposing factors, and pathophysiologic features. Nephron *4:*276–297, 1967.

Thiel, G., Brunner, P., Wunderlich, M., Hugenin, B., and Peters, G.: Protection of rat kidneys against $HgCl_2$-induced acute renal failure by induction of high urine flow without renin suppression. Kidney Int. *10:*S191–S200, 1976.

Thurau, K.: Influence of sodium concentration at macula densa cells on tubular sodium load. Ann. N.Y. Acad. Sci. *139:*388–399, 1966.

Thurau, K., and Boylan, J.W.: Acute renal success. The unexpected logic of oliguria in acute renal failure. Am. J. Med. *61:*308–315, 1976.

Thurau, K., and Mason, J.: The intrarenal function of the juxtaglomerular apparatus. In *MTP International Review of Science, Kidney and Urinary Tract Physiology*, edited by A.C. Guyton and K. Thurau, vol. 6, pp. 357–409. University Park Press, Baltimore, 1974.

Thurau, K., Schnermann, J., Nagel, W., Horster, M., and Wahl, M.: Composition of tubular fluid in the macula densa segment as a factor regulating the function of the juxtaglomerular apparatus. Circ. Res. (Suppl. 2) *20/21:*79–90, 1967.

Thurau, K., Dahlheim, H., Gruner, A., Mason, J., and Granger, P.: Activation of renin in the single juxtaglomerular apparatus by sodium chloride in the tubular fluid at the macula densa. Circ. Res. (Suppl. 1) *30:*182–186, 1972.

Thurau, K., Vogt, C., and Dahlheim, H.: Renin activity in the juxtaglomerular apparatus of the rat kidney during postischemic acute renal failure. Kidney Int. *10:*S177–S182, 1976.

Torres, V.E., Strong, C.G., Romero, J.C., and Wilson, D.M.: Indomethacin enhancement of glycerol-induced acute renal failure in rabbits. Kidney Int. *7:*170–178, 1975.

Venkatachalam, M.A., Rennke, H.G., and Sandstrom, D.J.: The vascular basis for acute renal failure in the rat. Preglomerular and postglomerular vasoconstriction. Circ. Res. *38:*267–279, 1976.

Vertel, R.M., and Knochel, J.P.: Nonoliguric acute renal failure. J.A.M.A. *200:*598–602, 1967.

Wada, T., Aizawa, K., Kan, K., Kitamoto, K., Kuroda, S., Ogawa, M., and Kato, E.: Morphologic evidence to support the role of tubular leakage as a cause of anuria induced by mercury poisoning. Am. J. Pathol. *77:*175–184, 1974.

Webb, J.L.: *Enzyme and Metabolic Inhibitors*, vol. 2. Academic Press, New York, 1966.

Werb, R., Clark, W.F., Lindsay, R.M., Jones, E.O.P., Turnbull, D.I., and Linton, A.L.: Protective effect of prostaglandin [PGE_2] in glycerol-induced acute renal failure in rats. Clin. Sci. *55:*505–507, 1978.

Whelton, A., and Donadio, J.V.: Post-traumatic acute renal failure in Vietnam. A comparison with the Korean War experience. Johns Hopkins Med. J. *124:*95–105, 1969.

Wilson, D.R., Thiel, G., Arce, M.L., and Oken, D.E.: Glycerol-induced hemoglobinuric acute renal failure in the rat. III. Micropuncture study of the effects of mannitol and isotonic saline on individual nephron function. Nephron *4:*337–355, 1967.

Wilson, D.R., Thiel, G., Arce, M.L., Oken, D.E.: The role of the concentration mechanism in the development of acute renal failure: Micropuncture studies using diabetes insipidus rats. Nephron *6:*128–139, 1969.

Wright, F.S., and Schnermann, J.: Interference with feedback control of glomerular filtration rate by furosemide, triflocin and cyanide. J. Clin. Invest. *53:*1695–1708, 1974.

Yorke, W., and Nauss, R.W.: The mechanism of the production of suppression of urine in blackwater fever. Ann. Trop. Med. Parasitol. *5:*287–312, 1911.

Yun, J.C.H., Kelly, G., and Bartter, F.C.: Effect of propanolol on renin release in the dog. Can. J. Physiol. Pharmacol. *55:*747–754, 1977.

Zalme, R.C., McDowell, E.M., Nagle, R.B., McNeil, J.S., Flamenbaum, W., and Trump, B.F.: Studies on the pathophysiology of acute renal failure. II. A histochemical study of the proximal tubule of the rat following administration of mercuric chloride. Virchows Arch. [Cell Pathol.] *22:*197–216, 1976.

CHAPTER 24

Treatment of Acute Renal Failure

MARC GEHR
MICHAEL GROSS
GUNTHER SCHMITT
WALTER FLAMENBAUM

Acute renal failure (ARF) is a complex disease of diverse etiology (Flamenbaum, 1977). It has, at various times, also been termed lower nephron nephrosis, acute tubular necrosis (ATN), and vasomotor nephropathy. For the present review, term ARF will be used, a general description for a disease process during which there is a sudden diminution or loss of renal function, rather than other terms having histopathologic or pathophysiologic attributes. The generality of the term ARF presupposes the necessity of making the diagnosis by exclusion of other processes resulting in an abrupt change in renal function. The diagnosis of ARF requires exclusion of prerenal, obstructive, renovascular, and renal parenchymal alteration, which could also decrease renal function (Levinsky and Alexander, 1976; Finn, 1979). This requires use of appropriate diagnostic techniques, as well as the patient's clinical history and physical examination, to establish a diagnosis of ARF.

Having arrived at the diagnosis of ARF, the clinician may proceed to select the appropriate therapy. The clinical course of ARF, however, precludes a set pattern of treatment because of the different therapeutic approaches required during various phases of ARF. ARF may be subdivided into the initiation, maintenance, and recovery phases. Each of these subdivisions of the clinical course of ARF has important clinical and experimental implications. Since therapy relative to the temporal course or phase of ARF will be discussed, it will be useful to briefly describe and define each phase:

1. Initiation phase. The interval between the etiologic event (e.g., hypotension, nephrotoxin) and the first clinical manifestations (azotemia, with or without oliguria) of ARF, this phase covers the period from "incipient" ARF, during which appropriate therapy may reverse underlying pathophysiology and prevent the development of ARF, to early ARF, during which therapy may only shorten the course or change the severity of ARF rather than abort its development.

2. Maintenance phase. ARF is established, with or without oliguria (Anderson et al., 1977), and treatment is directed at fluid, electrolyte, and acid-base imbalances and nutrition. It covers the interval of progressive azotemia until the onset of the recovery phase.

3. Recovery phase. Gradual and progressive return of the renal function, which is initially marked by an increasing urine volume if the patient has been oliguric and characterized by a slower return of tubular function, concludes when renal function reaches its new plateau and may occur for as long as 12–18 months. With these intervals in mind, one may consider therapy in relation to a specific conceptual point in the clinical course of ARF.

THERAPY OF THE INITIATION PHASE

Prevention

We would be remiss if we failed to indicate that preventive measures are worthwhile in certain clinical situations known to precede ARF. These range from achieving rehydration or volume replacement in patients with prerenal azotemia to prevent its eventual progression to ARF to avoiding known nephrotoxins. One may also anticipate potential problems under specific circumstances such as uric acid nephropathy in patients receiving chemotherapy for lymphomatous processes or the possible enhancement on the nephrotoxicity of antibiotics by the concomitant use of diuretic agents. Thus, a combination of hydration, alkalinization of the urine, and possibly allopurinol can prevent uric acid nephropathy. Furthermore, cognizance of the nephrotoxic potential of therapeutic agents and an understanding of their appropriate use, including required monitoring or safeguards, can prevent or minimize ARF in many patients. Of particular interest in this regard are the instances of ARF occurring after the administration of radiologic contrast agents in general as well as in particular circumstances (e.g., patients with diabetes mellitus or multiple myeloma).

At the present time, there are no specific maneuvers that serve as prophylaxis against the development of

ARF. Maintenance of adequate hydration and volume status is generally accepted. There are, however, no *specific* drugs which may be administered to prevent the development of ARF even in well recognized high risk situations. At best, the astute physician may have only a limited opportunity, based on a high index of suspicion in a particular clinical situation, to try and prevent the development of ARF in patients with incipient ARF or to modify the course of ARF in patients during the initiation phase of ARF.

Diuretic Treatment of ARF

The efficacy of diuretics in the management and treatment of ARF in its initiation phase remains a controversial issue (Early and Gottschalk, 1979). Before specifically discussing the use of diuretic therapy in ARF, a brief review of the theories concerning its pathophysiology is in order. This review is necessary to relate the proposed use of diuretics in ARF to the mechanisms that it may be affecting.

Several pathophysiologic mechanisms have been proposed to account for the observed changes in renal function in ARF. These include the following: tubule obstruction (Arendshorst et al., 1975; Jaenike, 1969; Tanner et al., 1973; Tanner and Sophason, 1976); passive backflow of a normally formed filtrate (Bank et al., 1967; Blantz, 1975; Arendshorst et al., 1975); and a primary failure of glomerular filtration (Cox et al., 1974; Daugharty et al., 1974; Flanigan and Oken, 1965; Oken et al., 1966). It has been suggested that any primary failure of the formation of glomerular filtrate may be associated with increased preglomerular vascular resistance. Similarly, factors effecting renal blood flow have also been implicated in the pathogenesis of acute renal failure. These renal hemodynamic alterations may be due to changes in sympathetic nervous system tone (Flamenbaum, 1973), alterations in renin-angiotensin system activity (Goormaghtigh, 1945; J. J. Brown et al., 1970, 1973), synthesis and release of renal prostaglandins (Finn and Arendshorst, 1976; McGiff et al., 1970; Phillips and Silvers, 1969; Kotchen and Miller, 1974), and activation of the coagulation system (Koffler and Paronetto, 1966; Larsson et al., 1971; Wardle, 1973; Kincaid-Smith, 1972).

Diuretics may be a useful therapy of ARF if intratubular obstruction plays a role in its pathogenesis. According to this theory, the increase in intratubular pressure secondary to intratubular obstruction, with accumulation of intracellular debris and protein, would increase to a level so that effective filtration pressure is diminished, resulting in a decline in the glomerular filtration rate. Diuretics would inhibit salt and water reabsorption proximal to such an intratubular obstruction. This would lead to an increased amount of tubular fluid which would "flush" the tubule, remove the intratubular obstruction, and result in an increase in urine flow (Epstein et al., 1975). Furthermore, Hollenberg et al. (1968) have demonstrated that ARF is characterized hemodynamically by preferential renal cortical ischemia. Furosemide has been demonstrated to have a vasodilator property which may offset this cortical ischemia (Birtch et al., 1967; Ludens et al., 1968).

It has also been suggested that ARF may, during its initiation phase, be due to activation of tubuloglomerular feedback (Flamenbaum, 1973). This mechanism proposes that alterations in proximal handling of filtrate results in enhanced delivery of filtrate to the macula densa or some change in the tubular fluid composition at the macula densa, causing the local release of renin and generation of angiotensin. This increase in renin-angiotensin system activity would diminish glomerular plasma flow and glomerular filtration rate. In contrast to normal physiology, the tubuloglomerular feedback mechanism has an interruption in its loop which does not allow it to be turned off due to a decreased glomerular filtration rate and enhanced proximal reabsorption of salt and water. Central to this concept is the requirement for chloride transfer across macula densa cells to activate the tubuloglomerular feedback mechanism. Diuretics, in particular "loop" diuretics, have been shown to interfere with activation of the tubuloglomerular feedback and the subsequent increase in renin-angiotensin system activity (Linton et al., 1973; T. C. Brown et al., 1966; Fraser et al., 1965). Thus, diuretics may effect the course of ARF by removing intratubular obstruction, directly vasodilating the renal vasculature, or inhibiting the activation of the renin-angiotensin system via the tubuloglomerular feedback mechanism. The pathophysiology of ARF may be characterized as being multifactorial, with various mechanisms having a relatively greater degree of importance depending upon when in the course of acute renal failure they are examined. In this regard, the time of administration of diuretics relative to the etiologic event for ARF becomes an important question. Linton et al. (1973) have demonstrated that furosemide when administered more than 5 hr prior to a nephrotoxic insult (mercuric chloride, cephaloridine) protected experimental animals from both the biochemical and histological features of ARF. The concomitant administration of furosemide and a nephrotoxic agent, however, resulted in an enhancement of the observed nephrotoxicity (Linton et al., 1973). In contrast, in clinical situations diuretics are administered only as specific therapy for ARF after the etiologic event. Clinical evidence suggests that diuretics, either mannitol or loop diuretics, must be administered early in the initiation phase of ARF, especially to those patients with incipient ARF, if attempts are being made to prevent its development (Kjellstrand, 1972; Luke et al., 1970).

LOOP DIURETICS

The efficacy of the administration of loop diuretics early in the course of ARF has been demonstrated (Kjellstrand, 1972). Kjellstrand observed that ethacrynic acid administered to patients having ARF of less than 22 hr in duration and a serum creatinine concentration of less than 4.5 ml/dl resulted in a decrease in the rapidity of rise of blood urea nitrogen concentration and in an arrest or slowing of the progression of the renal insufficiency. While a mortality rate of approximately 50% was seen in both responders and nonresponders to diuretic therapy having ARF, all nonresponders died as a consequence of uremia, whereas responders died a nonuremic death. Additional support for the utility of furosemide in clinical ARF is available (Cantarovich et al., 1973). Patients with well established ARF that required dialysis received high doses of furosemide (2000 mg/day), which resulted in increased urine volume (conversion to nonoliguric ARF), decreased number of anuric days, decreased number of days during recovery phase, and a decline in the time required to reach normal renal function (serum creatinine concentration of 1.5 mg/day).

In addition to the apparent importance of the time of administration of loop diuretics, the appropriate dosage of these diuretics has also been the subject of question. Large doses of furosemide have been initially used by some investigators (2000 mg/day) who continue to give this dose, regardless of the change in urine volume, until the patient no longer requires dialysis. As noted above, this routine of furosemide administration demonstrated a beneficial effect of loop diuretic therapy in ARF. Lower doses of furosemide have been used (Kleinknecht et al., 1976), up to 1200 mg/day, with adjustments in the dose of loop diuretic dependent upon urine flow. This study, however, demonstrated no effect on short-term furosemide administration on established ARF (i.e., during the maintenance phase). It is thus difficult to conclude from the available data specifically when in the course of ARF loop diuretics should be administered, the appropriate dosage of diuretics to be used, and the overall effect in ARF. It is apparent that it is unrealistic to use loop diuretics prior to the occurrence of the etiologic event, whether it be nephrotoxic or ischemic in nature, because of the problems associated with the use of potent diuretics. These problems include dehydration, hypokalemia, activation of the renin-angiotensin system due to volume depletion, and a decline in glomerular filtration rate (Linton et al., 1973). This is underscored by the fact that many of these factors may be expected to increase the subsequent renal damage from nephrotoxins or systemic hypotension.

As a general guideline, it would appear most efficacious, at the present time, to use loop diuretics as early in the course of ARF as is possible, with moderate to large dosages. That this use of loop diuretics may not be associated with a positive clinical response is apparent from a review of the literature. There are several studies which indicate that loop diuretics either do not materially affect the course of ARF or may potentially enhance the associated nephrotoxicity of other pharmaceutical agents. A randomized study (Kleinknecht et al., 1976) did not show any benefit of furosemide in established ARF. Administration of furosemide directly into the renal artery (Epstein et al., 1975) at a dose of 300 mg in 30 min did not result in any detectable alterations in mean renal blood flow or its intrarenal distribution. In a large study, no salutary effect of furosemide on the course of ARF could be demonstrated (Minuth et al., 1976), except for a decrease in the number of hemodialyses required for the control of volume overload. The recent literature (Grevin and Klein, 1976; Lopez-Nova et al., 1977; Papadimitriou, 1978; Borirakchamyavat et al., 1978) similarly supports an absence of the therapeutic effect of furosemide in ARF.

Some of the apparent failure to demonstrate a beneficial effect of loop diuretics in ARF may relate to inappropriate use, as well as to some of their potential toxic effects. Before commencing the use of loop diuretics in the treatment of ARF, the clinician must be certain that the patient is not suffering from true volume depletion (prerenal failure). This can usually be ascertained with a careful history, physical examination, and routine laboratory parameters. Recently, some attention has been paid to the use of urinary diagnostic indices to help differentiate between the oliguria of ARF and that associated with prerenal azotemia. The "renal failure index" has been used (Miller et al., 1978), as well as the fractional excretion of sodium, to help differentiate between these two forms of oliguria. In our hands, it has been extremely useful to obtain determinations of urine sodium concentration and urine and plasma creatinine concentrations and to calculate the renal failure index prior to institution of therapy. More importantly, these urinary parameters should be obtained prior to beginning loop diuretic therapy because these agents are known to affect the fractional excretion of sodium as well as the concentration of urine (Harrington, 1975) and may yield results indicative of ARF due to the induced alterations in the handling of fluid and electrolytes. It should also be stated that the administration of any diuretics, including the loop diuretics, in the face of volume depletion may aggravate rather than ameliorate the associated renal insufficiency (Miller et al., 1978).

The loop diuretics in general and furosemide in particular are not without their own toxicities, which may be directly related to the diuretic per se or to the use of diuretics with other agents otherwise not having an associated nephrotoxicity. In a recent study of 533 inpatients receiving furosemide, there were documented adverse reactions in 40% (Naranjo et al., 1978). The bulk of these adverse reactions were electrolyte disturbances, although a 0.5% occurrence of ototoxicity was observed. Both ethacrynic acid and furosemide, the currently available loop diuretics, have been associated with ototoxicity, with and without renal failure (Linton et al., 1973; Schwartz et al., 1970; Merriwether et al., 1971). Furthermore, the concurrent use of aminoglycoside antibiotics along with loop diuretics has been shown to potentiate the ototoxicity of these diuretics (Mathog and Klein, 1969). Loop diuretics may in addition increase the nephrotoxicity of antibiotics (Lawson et al., 1972). Evidence has been obtained (R. D. Brown, 1975) indicating that ethacrynic acid is more ototoxic than furosemide. Ohtani et al. (1978) have concluded that the synergistic ototoxicity of furosemide and aminoglycosides is related to the inhibitory effect of loop diuretics on the excretion of aminoglycoside antibiotics by the kidneys. The ototoxicity, which manifests itself as a hearing loss, with both diuretics usually occurs within 10-20 min after intravenous administration. It is usually reversible, but permanent hearing losses have been reported. The ototoxicity of furosemide has been clearly related to the rate of intravenous administration, and it has been recommended (Cooperman and Rubin, 1973) that an intravenous administration rate of no greater than 4 mg/min be used.

This review of the literature suggests that the patients at greatest risk for developing ototoxicity from loop diuretics are those with uremia as well as those receiving aminoglycoside antibiotics. The incidence of aminoglycoside nephrotoxicity is clearly increasing (Anderson et al., 1977), although it may be related to the specific antibiotic utilized. Acute allergic interstitial nephritis after the administration of furosemide has been observed (Lyons et al., 1974). Last, loop diuretics, with their potent effect on volume, may through reduction in intravascular volume stimulate the renin-angiotensin system activity and aggravate the underlying renal insufficiency (J. J. Brown et al., 1970; Linton et al., 1973; McDonald et al., 1969; Powell-Jackson et al., 1972).

The previous literature suggests that it is difficult to come to a current conclusion concerning the efficacy of loop diuretics in the treatment of ARF. As in many clinical situations, the physician must carefully weigh the risks and benefits of the drug being administered to that particular patient. Recent data (Anderson et al., 1977) suggests that in a well conducted, prospective study the benefits clearly outweigh the potential risks of diuretic therapy. The hospital course, the morbidity, and the mortality of oliguric versus nonoliguric ARF were compared. Included among their patients who demonstrated nonoliguric ARF were 18 individuals who were converted from oliguric to nonoliguric renal disease by the administration of furosemide. This represents approximately ⅓ of all patients presenting with nonoliguric ARF. The nonoliguric group of patients required a shorter interval of hospitalization and had fewer instances and shorter courses of hemodialysis and a decreased morbidity and mortality (26 versus 50%). This data is quite compelling, and it is our belief that all patients with oliguric ARF, especially early in the course of their disease, should be given a trial of furosemide therapy at a dose of 2-10 mg/kg by slow intravenous administration. Furthermore, these doses should be continued on a regular basis once the urine volume has increased in order to maintain a urine volume of greater than 1 liter/day if required.

MANNITOL

The use of mannitol in clinical states of oliguria and diminished renal function has been credited with protecting the kidney from structural damage, preventing the establishment of ARF, or altering its course. This apparent efficacy of mannitol must be interpreted in view of the clinical situation in which it has been used. Thus, claims of maintaining high urine volume subsequent to the exposure of the kidney to nephrotoxic agents or products must be separated from those instances in which mannitol has been observed to promote improvement in renal function, as denoted by clearances, or to prevent histopathological alterations. Whereas the effects of mannitol on alterations in renal function which have been observed are extremely varied, only a few have been studied in detail.

Mannitol is a form of mannose, a reduced 6-carbon sugar. It has the beneficial properties of being confined to the extracellular space, being freely filtered by the glomerulus, and not being absorbed or secreted by the tubules. These are the characteristics which make it an excellent osmotic diuretic. When compared to similar substances which may be used to maintain glomerular filtration rate and urine flow, mannitol has been demonstrated to be equal or superior. The effect of various osmotically active solutions on an experimental model of renal failure in dogs has been examined (Barry et al., 1963). The solutions used were 4% urea, 20% mannitol, and 5% dextrose and water, which were administered prior to an ischemic event. The animals that received 20% mannitol or 5% dextrose and water had a lower mortality and developed a lesser degree of axotemia. Mannitol's superiority over urea suggests that properties other than osmotic activity play a significant role in this protective effect. One obvious difference is that mannitol is distributed in the extracellular space, while urea is freely diffusable into cells. Mannitol, therefore, can reduce cellular swelling and interstitial edema (Flores, 1972).

Therapeutic claims attributed to mannitol may be divided into three areas: dilution and removal of toxic substances from the renal circulation and tubules; prophylaxis against the development of renal failure during surgical procedures; and prevention or alteration in the course of ARF. One of the most consistent aspects of mannitol infusions is the resultant diuresis. General agreement is available, therefore, concerning the use of mannitol to promote the excretion of direct nephrotoxic substances which include myoglobin, released through rhabdomyolysis; acid hematin, released during hemolytic states; uric acid; and contrast agents (Silverberg and Johnson, 1966; Barry and Crosby, 1963; Bourne and Cerny, 1964).

A large degree of positive experience has been obtained with mannitol in the prevention of renal impairment when it is administered prior to situations carrying a high risk for the development of renal failure. The urine flow in two groups of patients undergoing resection of abdominal aneurysms (Barry et al., 1961) has been studied. One group of patients received a 20% mannitol solution, while the second group was given 5% dextrose and water prior to undergoing surgery. Estimates of urine flow were obtained prior to anesthesia, prior to the cross clamping of the aorta, during cross clamping of the aorta, as well as 1 and 3 hr after the cross clamp was removed. The mannitol group of patients had a two- to three-fold greater urine output in all periods after the preanesthetic interval. However, this improvement in urine flow does not necessarily imply an improvement in renal function. Additional studies were performed during which glomerular filtration rate and renal plasma flow were determined in surgical patients having a known depression in these parameters. (Levitin et al., 1963; Barry, 1960). Mannitol, when administered prior to the surgical event, resulted in an increased glomerular filtration rate and renal plasma flow. In addition, a recent micropuncture study (Blantz, 1974) demonstrated consistent improvement in both renal blood flow and glomerular filtration rate, as well as urine flow, after mannitol infusion.

A number of parameters in 18 patients undergoing cardiopulmonary bypass (Levitin et al., 1963) were also studied. These patients received 10% mannitol as a constant infusion in order to maintain a urine output greater than 30 ml/hr. The infusion was continued throughout the postoperative period in those patients who developed hemoglobinuria and was only discontinued after the urine cleared of hemoglobin. The parameters examined during this study were: creatinine and urea clearance; fractional excretion of sodium; total sodium excretion; urine output; renal blood flow; and serum electrolytes. These parameters were examined prior to the administration of mannitol infusions, prior to the administration of anesthesia, during cardiopulmonary bypass, and subsequent to the discontinuation of cardiopulmonary bypass. When mannitol was administered, glomerular filtration rate and renal blood flow increased during anesthesia, a stimulus known to reduce renal function. The patients had a decrease in glomerular filtration rate and fractional excretion of sodium during cardiopulmonary bypass, except for a few whose urine flow and fractional excretion of sodium increased despite a fall in glomerular filtration rate. These latter patients appeared to have suffered tubular damage during the procedure. None of the patients, however, went on to develop classical ARF. It may be concluded from this study that mannitol given prior to an ischemic event can improve renal hemodynamics when a known stimulus to depress these parameters (anesthesia) is administered, but it does not appear to be totally protective against the development of renal failure during cardiopulmonary bypass. There is additional experimental evidence, however, suggesting that after an episode of renal ischemia with arterial reperfusion ("the reflow phenomenon") mannitol may reduce the amount of resulting histological and functional damage (Franklin et al., 1974). Although mannitol reduces the amount of histological damage in general, it did not prevent necrosis in the subcortical area, and its beneficial effects only occurred if it was administered prior to the ischemic event.

In contrast, a subsequent study (Beall et al., 1965) suggested that mannitol was not beneficial in an ischemic model of renal failure. In these experiments, which involved 24 dogs during 3 days of observation after renal arterial occlusion, a similar degree of reduction in glomerular filtration rate, renal blood flow, and urine output was observed when mannitol was used as compared to dogs that received only 5% dextrose. These observations would support the occasional clinical observation that mannitol may not have a beneficial effect.

The overall efficacy of mannitol administered prior to events with known high risk for the development of acute renal failure may be related more to its ability to maintain urine volume and clear potentially toxic substances. There is evidence, however, to suggest that renal hemodynamics may improve during infusion of mannitol. The long-lasting effects of mannitol on renal function remain controversial.

The use of mannitol has been advocated to "reverse" ARF. However, as noted earlier, one must be careful concerning specifics of the time of administration of any therapeutic agent during the course of ARF in discussing its potential activity to reverse this disease process. It has been proposed (Barry and Malloy, 1962) that there are two phases in development of ARF: the first phase constitutes an alteration in renal function without histological damage, which is considered reversible; the second phase is characterized by the appearance of histological damage. These authors indicated that changes in renal function persist through an undefined period of time, which is dependent upon many unknown factors including host response. Mannitol, they believe, reverses ARF when administered during the first phase of ARF. This would coincide with the incipient interval of the initiation phase of ARF discussed above. Inasmuch as this period is variable and unpredictable, mannitol should be given as early as possible in the course of ARF, and its administration should be continued to maintain urine volumes above normal. Barry and Malloy believed that the reversal of ARF was an improvement in urine output, which facilitated the medical management of patients with ARF, as regards the administration of fluid, acid-base and, electrolyte status. This latter reversal would be more consistent with conversion of oliguric to nonoliguric ARF, since the patients continued to have decreased clearances of a variety of substances. It has been demonstrated (Eliahou, 1964) that the administration of mannitol improved the renal concentrating ability of patients with ARF. However, the effect of mannitol on clearances was not examined, leaving the question open as to whether mannitol reversed functional renal failure or converted oliguric to nonoliguric ARF.

A number of mechanisms have been proposed to account for the increased urine volume, improved renal hemodynamics, and other alterations in renal function observed when mannitol was administered to patients with ARF (Blantz, 1974; Barry and Malloy, 1962; Flores et al., 1972). The properties noted above, which allow mannitol to act as an excellent osmotic diuretic capable of removing toxic substances from the kidney, may also by the same osmotic action, reduce interstitial edema within the renal parenchyma. This interstitial edema could compress renal tubules, resulting in an offsetting of glomerular filtration rate. Mannitol may also improve glomerular filtration rate by decreasing arteriolar resistance (Goldberg and Lilienfield, 1965; Morris et al., 1972; Coelho and Bradley, 1964). Furthermore, vascular resistance within the renal vasculature is regulated in part by the activity of the renin-angiotensin system, and the macula densa may play a role in controlling the synthesis and release of renin. By altering the flux of sodium chloride, or other constituents of tubular fluid, mannitol may alter the signal at the macula densa due to its osmotic effects on tubular fluid handling and, thus, diminish renin release and synthesis. An alternative mechanism has been suggested (Blantz, 1974). Formation of ultrafiltrate by the glomerulus is regulated by a variety of factors, including modification of Starling's law. In these experiments, the effect of mannitol on oncotic and hydrostatic pressures, as well as on glomerular permeability, were evaluated. Results indicated that mannitol did not consistently increase renal plasma flow, suggesting that a direct effect of mannitol on arterial resistance may not occur. The most consistent observation, however, was a decrease in systemic oncotic pressure, which accounted for more than a 60% increase in effective filtration pressure. This increase in effective filtration pressure would lead to improvement in glomerular filtration rate. At the very least, these results suggest that the mechanisms by which mannitol asserts its effects on renal function in the face of developing ARF are multifactorial.

The method of administration of mannitol depends on the goals set by the clinician. Infusions of mannitol solution may be particularly useful in aiding in the removal of toxic substances or in the prophlaxis against ARF in high risk surgical procedures (e.g., cardiopulmonary bypass, aneurysm resection, and surgery of the biliary system). One method would be to dissolve 25–50 g of mannitol in 500 ml of intravenous fluid and infuse it at a rate resulting in a urine flow at or slightly above 1 ml/min (Dawson, 1965; Silverberg and Johnson, 1966). This type of administration would be appropriate prior to the administration of an anesthetic agent in patients about to undergo surgical procedures or shortly after it has become apparent that a toxin is involved in the patients' course. In contrast, mannitol is usually administered as a bolus when attempting to prevent the development of ARF or change oliguric to nonoliguric ARF. In these instances, usually shortly after recognizing oliguria exists, a bolus of 12.5 g of mannitol in 50 ml (a 25% solution) is given by intravenous "push" over a 3- to 5-min interval. If the urine flow has not increased to greater than 40 ml/hr at the end of 3 hr, a second dose of up to 25 g should be given by intravenous administration over 6–10 min. If urine flow is established at a rate greater than 40 ml/hr, the clinician may continue this enhanced urine volume by constant mannitol infusion designed to maintain urine flow at or above 50–100 ml/hr. In any event, it is inadvisable to administer more than 100 g of mannitol within a 24-hr period unless there is maintenance of urine volume.

Mannitol is a relatively safe drug with few complications. Hyponatremia may occur subsequent to the administration of mannitol in a patient with a persistent low urine output by osmotically "drawing" fluid into the intravascular space. In contrast, a good therapeutic response to mannitol, as noted by marked increase in urine volume, may be accompanied by hypernatremia, as well as hypokalemia, due to its osmotic diuretic effect. Mannitol may also precipitate congestive heart failure in patients with compromised cardiac function. It has also been observed that the administration of mannitol in patients with hepatic cirrhosis may result in deterioration of their mental status (Silverberg and Johnson, 1966). When mannitol alone is ineffective it may be used in conjunction with a loop diuretic, such as ethacrynic acid or furosemide, which may promote an additional diuresis (Auger et al., 1968). However, the concomitant administration of loop diuretic may result in the potential toxicities, noted above, of these diuretic agents. In general, mannitol is a safe drug which is easy to administer. It is particularly useful in states of toxin-induced renal failure and for the protection of renal function in high risk situations. Most clinical evidence would suggest that mannitol's main benefit is to convert oliguric ARF to a high output state rather than prevent the development of ARF. The exception to this is its administration in high risk surgical patients. The achievement of an improved urine volume, however, facilitates the management of the patient with ARF. If it has been decided to treat incipient or early ARF with mannitol, the patient should receive these agents as early as possible in their clinical course.

MAINTENANCE PHASE

The onset of the maintenance phase of ARF is variable. Many clinicians will conclude that the patient has entered the maintenance phase of ARF after an unsuccessful attempt with diuretics to prevent or change the course of the initiation phase of ARF. Alternatively, the maintenance phase may be characterized as a period of continuing decline in renal function, with or without oliguria. Regardless of how one defines its onset, the maintenance phase is characterized by continued reduction in renal function until it reaches a new plateau. The proper management of patients in the maintenance phase of ARF requires attention to several fundamental aspects of their clinical care. These include traditional conservative management of patients with ARF, concentrating on problems of fluid electrolyte balances as well as nutritional status, and extend to the various methods available for dialysis of patients during this phase of ARF.

Fluid and Electrolyte Management

FLUID BALANCE

There are two major determinants of fluid balance in patients with ARF. These determinants are concerned with fluid losses and the endogenous production of water. In the patient with oliguric ARF, fluid losses are limited to those occurring in diffusion and evaporation of water through the skin, as well as the losses associated with the water content of expired air. While urinary losses of fluid must be considered, they are relatively small in the patient with oliguric ARF.

As reviewed by Gambos (1973) "insensible water loss"

amounts to approximately 0.5–0.6 ml/kg body wt/hr in the basal state. Atmospheric pressure as well as humidity will affect insensible loss, with atmospheric temperatures in excess of 30°C increasing the loss of water at a rate of 10–13% for each degree centigrade. Similarly, a rise in humidity from 0–50% will decrease insensible loss by approximately 50% (Merrill, 1965). The relationship between atmospheric temperature and water loss is not a simple one, since fever, which may be a direct consequence of environmental temperature, raises the basal metabolic rate. This increase in basal metabolic rate simultaneously increases insensible loss to a greater degree as well as increases endogenous production of water. With rare exceptions, variations in respiratory rate or pattern do not effect insensible water loss. The major exception to this would be Kussmaul respirations, which are observed in patients with severe metabolic acidosis and result in a marked increase in insensible water loss At the other extreme, shallow respirations tend to result in reduction in insensible water loss.

In the absence of marked changes in environmental temperature or in respiratory pattern, the figure of 0.5–0.6 ml/kg body wt/hr may be used as a good approximation of insensible water loss. To this must also be added volume loss resulting from urine excreted, water losses due to vomiting or gastric drainage, and/or diarrhea. It must be underscored that when the patient is febrile and sweating ensues, insensible water loss may increase by 1–2 liters/24 hr, reaching a level of 15–30 ml/kg body wt/24 hr.

To calculate water balance in a patient with oliguric ARF, one must take into account not only insensible losses, which contribute to negative fluid balance, but also endogenous water production. This endogenous water production results from the metabolic pathways utilized when fats, proteins, and carbohydrates are oxidized. The approximations of endogenous water production may be obtained by using the information available on the rates of protein and fat utilization during periods of fasting in normal individuals subjected to an exhaustion of their carbohydrates stores. Available calories from external sources, such as glucose, will decrease protein oxidation and the accompanying endogenous water formation. Based on the data of Lawson et al. (1962), one may assume that a 70-kg patient will burn 1 g of protein and 2 g of fat per kilogram of body weight, without carbohydrate supplementation. Furthermore, 100 g of carbohydrate supplementation results in a reduction in protein metabolism of 50%, and it has been calculated that some 564 ml of water will be produced from endogenous metabolism without carbohydrate supplementation, and 425 ml of water results from the addition of carbohydrate supplement. It must be underscored that these figures are theoretical and are derived from normal subjects under basal conditions. Direct application, therefore, to patients with ARF is not fully justified. Based on balance studies, it appears as though acutely ill or traumatized patients, similar to those with ARF, produce a far greater amount of endogenous water than can be estimated from the above experiments. These studies indicate that during the oliguric phase of ARF, water replacement should be limited to approximately 400 ml/day for an average 70-kg patient plus additional fluid for overt losses as noted above.

It is not unusual for a patient with ARF to be in an extremely catabolic state, due to either infection or recent surgery. In these patients, it may be more practical to estimate fluid replacement therapy based on daily measurements of body weight. For this purpose, it is required that an accurate daily measurement of body weight be performed with the same scale at the same time of day. A useful general rule to prevent overhydration is to set as an objective a daily weight loss of 0.2–0.3 kg. Weight loss due to starvation does not approach the value of 1–2 kg/day, and therefore should weight loss of this magnitude be observed it is highly suggestive of a fluid volume deficit. On the other hand, constant weight in these individuals may portend the development of fluid overload, such as pulmonary edema, requiring additional fluid restriction and/or therapy for removal of fluid (see below). A sound principle for fluid balance in the patient with ARF is to err on the side of a volume deficit rather than create a situation of overhydration. Fluid deficits can easily be replaced, whereas fluid removal in a patient with oliguria may require a more complex intervention such as dialysis. One source of fluid gain which is occasionally overlooked is that of the volume associated with the administration of medication. This must be included in any estimate of daily fluid balance to avoid iatrogenic overhydration.

SODIUM BALANCE

During the maintenance phase of ARF, the injudicious intake of sodium leads to the predictable consequences of volume expansion, hypertension, and congestive heart failure. Prior to the recognition of this difficulty, congestive heart failure was the leading cause of death during oliguric ARF (Swann and Merrill, 1953). In contrast, as will be noted below, failure to liberalize sodium intake during the recovery phase of ARF may result in volume depletion and hypotension.

The most practical and readily available guide to sodium requirements in the patient with ARF revolves around a daily clinical assessment of the patient, including measurement of body weight. In addition, it may be useful in many patients to measure sodium excretion in the urine. Early in the maintenance phase, especially in the oliguric patient, urinary sodium excretion is low. Later in the course, and in patients with nonoliguric ARF, urine sodium excretion may reach a level requiring consideration of this parameter in efforts to avoid sodium excess or deficit. Measurements of urine sodium excretion may, therefore, be required to achieve this clinical goal. The "typical" urinary sodium concentration of the patient with oliguric ARF is approximately 70 mEq/liter, as compared to 50 mEq/liter in patients with nonoliguric ARF (Anderson et al., 1977). If a patient is oliguric and has a 24-hr urine volume of 300 ml, then the total predicted sodium excretion would be approximately 20 mEq/day. To achieve dietary replacement, therefore, a 500-mg sodium diet is suggested (Gambos, 1973) since 1 g of sodium is the equivalent of 43 mEq of sodium. Hyponatremia is not uncommon during the course of ARF and is almost always due to failure to take into account endogenous water production and exogenous fluid administration. Hypernatremia may also occur and is usually due to excess sodium intake in the form of sodium bicarbonate, which is used to correct the acidosis occurring during the maintenance phase of ARF. Last, it must also be recognized that many of the medications given to patients with ARF contain sodium (i.e., sodium penicillin), which may lead to sodium excess.

POTASSIUM BALANCE

Hyperkalemia is the leading biochemical cause of death in patients with ARF (Levinsky, 1966). During the maintenance phase of ARF, with few exceptions, the intake of potassium should be avoided. Potassium intake should be limited to that contained in dietary protein, which is approximately 1 mEq of potassium per gram of protein. Due to the inability of the kidney to excrete potassium, there is a tendency for potassium released from cell destruction, adsorption of degraded blood cells, or as a result of endogenous metabolism to reach toxic and occasional fatal concentrations. Acidosis and uremia favor the accumulation of potassium in the extracellular fluid at the expense of the intracellular fluid. Thus, in severe acidosis, normal serum potassium concentration may represent a state equivalent to potassium depletion. Loss of potassium during ARF may occur by the gastrointestinal tract in association with vomiting, nasogastric suction, or diarrhea.

The final common pathway for the deleterious effects of hyperkalemia is in the disturbance of neural conduction, and the immediate causes of death are alterations in the conducting system of the heart. The ratio of intracellular to extracellular potassium concentrations is a critically important factor in determining neuromuscular function. Since under the usual circumstances, only 2% of total body potassium content is extracellular, it becomes apparent that relatively small changes in the extracellular fluid potassium concentrations will markedly alter this ratio and have profound effects on neuromuscular excitability. Hyperkalemia should be considered as a clinical syndrome rather than simply in terms of serum potassium concentration. This is amply demonstrated by considering the effect of potassium concentration on an EKG, in which EKG abnormalities do not correlate well with the absolute level of serum potassium. Furthermore, EKG changes in potassium intoxication may be aggravated by concomitant hyponatremia as well as hypocalcemia. In contrast, one may find a normal EKG tracing in the face of hyperkalemia when it occurs in a patient with hypercalcemia. The sequence of EKG changes observed with potassium intoxication has been reviewed by Levine (1953) and by Marriot (1972).

The earliest EKG changes associated with potassium intoxication consist of slightly asymmetric and peaked T waves. Later in the course of potassium intoxication, the P-R interval is prolonged, RST segments become depressed, and QRS intervals lengthen. The latest changes to occur consist of the disappearance of the P waves and further widening of the QRS complex, resulting in a sine wave appearance in the electrocardiogram until ventricular fibrillation occurs. Several modes of therapy for hyperkalemia are available (Thomson, 1973), which may be broken down into the following categories: prophylactic, acute emergent, and chronic.

The prophylactic treatment of hyperkalemia includes elimination of potassium intake, treatment of concurrent infections, drainage of blood and/or fluid accumulations, debridement of necrotic tissue, and provision of adequate nonprotein calories.

Prior to specific considerations of the emergency treatment of hyperkalemia, a brief review of the electrophysiology of the action potential and how electrolyte abnormalities are reflected in the EKG is in order. In association with hyperkalemia the transmembrane potential gradient is reduced, and, as such, the resting membrane potential of any neural conducting tissue is less negative than normal, or partially depolarized. With moderate increases in serum potassium concentration (6–7 mEq/liter), the principle effect observed is on the repolarization of neuroconduction and is observed on the EKG as peaked T waves. As a result of partial depolarization, the membrane becomes less able to effect the rapid inward flux of sodium and the action potential is slowed, leading to a prolonged QRS complex. A serum potassium concentration greater than 6.5 mEq/liter is associated with a prolonged QRS, and a serum potassium concentration greater than 8 mEq/liter demands emergency treatment even in the absence of an abnormal QRS complex.

The emergency treatment of choice is calcium gluconate (Levinsky, 1966), usually in the dose of 10–30 ml of a 10% solution infused intravenously over a 1–5 min interval under constant EKG monitoring. Although calcium does not alter plasma potassium concentration, it often reverses rapidly the electrocardiographic manifestations of potassium toxicity. The mechanism by which calcium acts is to raise the threshold potential of any excitable neuromuscular tissue, thereby opposing the effect of hyperkalemia which had resulted in a partial depolarization of the membrane bringing it closer to threshold. Hypocalcemia has exactly the opposite effect and, therefore, enhances the cardiac toxicity of hyperkalemia. Other methods for actually reducing serum potassium concentration within a relatively short period of time (1 hr) may be obtained through the use of glucose and insulin infusions, as well as the infusion of sodium bicarbonate. Both of these methods are based on the enhanced transfer of potassium from the extracellular to the intracellular fluid compartments. Insulin and glucose infusions have been demonstrated to promote the transfer of both potassium and phosphate into the cell (Fenn, 1939). Sodium bicarbonate, by raising the pH of the extracellular fluid, promotes the shift of potassium from extra- to intracellular fluid compartments. It has been specifically recommended that 25–50 g of glucose, as a 50% solution, be administered with 5–10 units of regular insulin (1 unit of insulin per 5 g of glucose) intravenously. A "hyperkalemia cocktail" can be made by adding 1 ampule of sodium bicarbonate solution (44 mEq of sodium bicarbonate) to the glucose insulin solution. The effects of glucose and sodium bicarbonate can be observed within ½ hr after their administration and may last as long as 4-6 hr. It must be noted that these measures act fairly promptly but do not actually lower total body potassium concentration.

A longer lasting reduction in serum potassium concentration, as well as a decrease in total body potassium, can be achieved by removal of potassium through the gastrointestinal tract. Using a cation exchange resin, such as sodium polystirene sulfonate (Kayexylate) potassium may be exchanged for sodium. The usual oral dose of this agent is 20-30 g mixed in 30 ml of 70% sorbitol, the latter being used to prevent fecal impaction. In patients who cannot take medication by mouth, because of uremic nausea, this exchange resin may be given as a retention enema utilizing 50 g of Kayexylate suspended in 50 ml of 70% sorbitol and 100 ml of tap water. The enema should be retained for approximately ½ hr. Kayexylate therapy is not without problems as it can cause massive diarrhea with associated fluid and electrolyte losses, and because of the exchange of sodium for potassium, it can lead to volume overload. A most efficient way to reduce total body potassium is dialysis, which may be necessary for the control of hyperkalemia when it is associated with severe acidosis and/or fluid overload, which prohibits the use of sodium bicarbonate.

CALCIUM AND PHOSPHATE

Increases as well as decreases in serum calcium concentration have been associated with patients in the maintenance phase of ARF. The hypocalcemia noted in patients with ARF (Schreimer, 1967; Kovithavongs et al., 1972) can be accounted for by various theoretical factors. These include hyperphosphatemia (Scatopolsky et al., 1971), hypomagnesmia (Estep et al., 1969), hypoalbuminemia or alterations in calcium binding by serum proteins (Nordin and Smith 1965; Kleeman et al., 1971), failure of parathyroid gland function, and skeletal resistance to parathyroid hormone (Massry et al., 1976). Massry et al. (1974) demonstrated that hypocalcemia during ARF occurs with elevated levels of parathyroid hormone, suggesting skeletal resistance to the hormone. This study also indicated that a decrease in the production of 1,25-dihydroxycholecalciferol during ARF may render the skeleton less responsive to parathyroid hormone. It has also been observed that the conversion of the parent vitamin D compound to its active metabolite (1,25-dihydroxy vitamin D_3), occurs in the kidney (Gray et al., 1971). These investigators (Massry et al., 1976) demonstrated that the lack of production of 1,25-dihydroxy vitamin D_3 is at least partially responsible for the skeletal resistance to the calcium mobilization action of parathyroid hormone during the maintenance phase of ARF. Recently, it has been observed that low levels of the liver metabolite of vitamin D (25-hydroxy vitamin D) can be demonstrated in patients with ARF. These investigators propose that the deficiency observed in 25-hydroxy vitamin D makes less substrate available for the synthesis of the active vitamin D metabolite, with a subsequent decrease in calcium absorption from the gastrointestinal tract, leading to hypocalcemia, secondary hyperparathyroidism, or skeletal resistance to parathyroid hormone. It is noteworthy that all of these may contribute to the hypocalcemia of ARF.

Hypercalcemia has also been observed during the course of ARF (de Torrente et al., 1976; Grossman et al., 1974; Leonard and Nelms, 1970; Leonard and Eichner, 1970; Tavill et al., 1964; Turkington et al., 1968). Some authors (Leonard and Eichner, 1970; and Leonard and Nelms, 1970) have suggested that increased levels of parathyroid hormone observed in ARF (Massry et al., 1974) are maintained throughout its course and account for the hypercalcemia observed. All cases of reported hypercalcemia occurring during ARF have been preceded by hypocalcemia, which is the probable stimulus for parathyroid hormone synthesis and release. Two groups of investigators (Turkington et al., 1968; and de Torrente et al.,1976) have documented suppressed parathyroid hormone levels in the face of hypercalcemia. From a clinical point of view, many cases of hypercalcemia in ARF have been preceded by rhabdomyolysis. The occurrence of hypocalcemia and hypercalcemia during the course of rhabdomyolysis has been studied recently (Akman et al., 1976). Calcium deposition, which was observed in injured muscle tissue during the oliguric phase of ARF, was attributed to metastatic calcification due to a high calcium-phosphate product brought about by the initial hyperphosphatemia of renal insufficiency. The resolution of these calcific deposits was also demonstrated during the recovery (diuretic) phase of ARF, when the serum phosphate began to decline towards more normal levels. It is during the recovery (diuretic) phase of ARF that hypercalcemia usually occurs.

Nutrition

The nutritional balance of patients is severely threatened by ARF. Part of the lack of improvement in mortality statistics for patients with ARF may be related to disturbances in nutrition. Currently available therapeutic modalities have allowed severely ill, traumatized, or elderly patients with multiple organ dysfunctions to develop ARF. One of the limiting factors in improving the mortality statistics in these groups of patients may be the severe catabolism associated with these clinical states. In patients with ARF, the problem of supplying nutrients is compounded by the necessity to prevent the ravages of concurrent catabolism without aggravating the build-up of toxic nitrogenous wastes. In addition, fluid and electrolyte imbalances place a further limitation on the replacement of deficient nutrients. Although dialysis may alleviate some of these limitations, it also contributes to septic and pulmonary complications of ARF, as well as aggravates an already precarious nutritional balance. Early attempts at dietary therapy in patients with ARF recognized the need to restrict substances that added to toxic nitrogenous wastes, fluid overload, and electrolyte imbalances. However, these diets failed to supply adequate nutritional support, and it was only with the increased understanding of the minimal requirements for nutrition that new directions and supplementation evolved.

Adequate nutrition was long recognized as a major clinical consideration in the treatment of uremic patients. The inappropriate management of nutritional status exacerbated the build-up of nitrogenous wastes in patients with renal insufficiency. The effects of uremia on the gastrointestinal tract and CNS further complicated the clinician's ability to provide an adequate diet to these patients. Early attempts utilized carbohydrates and fats exclusively in recognition of the need to supply calories without adding to the nitrogen load to patients with renai insufficiency. Furthermore, provision of glucose, 200 g, and fats led to a protein-sparing effect. These diets proved to be nauseating and the fat had to be removed, which led to an inadequate caloric intake. In addition, evidence was presented that uremic patients exhibited a certain degree of carbohydrate intolerance (Horton et al., 1968). Horton and associates developed a glucose tolerance test curve similar to that observed in diabetics after an oral glucose load which caused a blunted insulin response as well as a persistently elevated plasma insulin level in the presence of normal glucose concentration. These observations led to the reinstitution of protein as part of the nutritional therapy of patients with ARF.

The addition of high "biological value" proteins (i.e., eggs, meat, and milk products) was accomplished without adverse effects (Blagg et al., 1962; Maddock et al., 1968). Nitrogen balance could be improved further with the use of anabolic steroids (McCracken and Parsons, 1958), although this was not a consistent observation (Berlyne et al., 1967a). Using proteins that are high in biological value improved nitrogen balance, and daily increments in blood urea nitrogen concentration were reduced by 10–50% (Lawson et al., 1962). The most comprehensive study of these benefits in patients with ARF matched a group of patients on a low protein diet with a control group on carbohydrates only (Berlyne et al., 1967a). The low protein diet supplied 16 g of the minimal essential amino acids while controlling fluid intake, calories, and electrolytes. The carbohydrate diet supplied approximately 1000 calories. The patients receiving low protein diet exhibited an improved overall state of well being with less nausea and fewer episodes of vomiting per patient days. This effect was most evident after 12 days of therapy. Biochemically, the low protein group of patients had a significant decrease in urea rise per day (11.8 versus 34 mg/100 ml) as compared to the control group. Utilizing total balance studies, the mean daily protein catabolism could be calculated. The patients on the low protein diet had a significant decrease in daily protein catabolism (14.29 g/day) as compared to the control group (31.3 g/day). However, the frequency of dialysis was unchanged and creatinine continued to rise at an equal rate in the two groups. This study focused on the requirements for at least 1200–1800 calories/day, while supplying 20–35 g protein/day in patients with ARF characterized by prolonged periods of anuria. As a result of this study, it also became obvious that not all of the protein required to maintain nutritional status at an optimal level needed to be supplied exogenously as long as a certain minimal amount of essential amino acids were available.

The quantity of the eight essential amino acids required to achieve a positive nitrogen balance was established as 8.65 g of protein or 1.42 g of nitrogen. In addition, 2.28–2.55 g of nitrogen are needed to make the nonessential amino acids (Rose and Wixom, 1955), which may be supplied by other sources of nitrogen such as urea or glycine. Therefore, only small quantities of nitrogen were required as long as the eight essential amino acids were supplied in their minimal daily amounts. Furthermore, the production of protein proceeded only if all of the essential amino acids were supplied in the proper proportion, either exogenously or endogenously.

In this regard, a special case has been made for histidine in patients with uremia (Abel, 1976). This extra requirement for histidine in patients with ARF remains controversial. Histidine is not an essential amino acid in normal adults. Serum histidine levels are decreased in patients with chronic renal failure. It has been demonstrated that the addition of extra histidine to the diet results in an increased incorporation of this amino acid into the hemoglobin, leading to the speculation that histidine may play a role in the anemia of renal disease. Other studies have not demonstrated a decreased plasma level of histidine, but they have demonstrated an increased level of 1 or 3 methalhistadine in patients with uremia (Condon and Asatoor, 1971), suggesting that the abnormality may be in the metabolism of histidine rather than in the quantitative absorption of this amino acid. Since histidine is not decreased in patients with ARF, there is probably no need to supply an extra amount of this amino acid in this particular clinical state (Abel et al., 1974a).

Ideally, the nitrogen accumulating as waste products in patients with ARF could be utilized to provide the nitrogen necessary for a positive nitrogen balance beyond that achieved by the administration of essential amino acids. Substantial evidence has been obtained that urea is not an inert compound and may participate metabolically in the synthesis of protein (Richards et al., 1967; Rose and Dekker, 1956). Animals fed only essential amino acids fail to gain weight unless urea is added to their diet. In addition, the administration of radio-labeled urea results in the appearance of radio-labeled carbon dioxide in their expired graft, suggesting that urea does undergo metabolism and participates in growth and anabolism. Further support to this conclusion was provided in studies comparing rats fed essential amino acids alone with a separate group of rats receiving a casein hydrolysate (Rose and Dekker, 1956). Both groups of rats were given radio-labeled urea, but only those animals fed essential amino acids were able to incorporate urea nitrogen into nonessential amino acids to any degree. Thus, urea nitrogen is utilized best when urea is the sole source of nitrogen for the production of nonessential amino acids. This process can be blocked by the addition of only small amounts of nonessential amino acids. When healthy humans were given labeled urea and the nitrogen compounds were studied in their urine, the urea recovered was 20% less than that predicted. Ten percent of the label appeared on other nitrogenous compounds, while the urea in the plasma was newly synthesized with radio-labeled carbon (Walser and Bodenlos, 1959). These findings confirm the fact that urea is metabolized and utilized in the human. Additional evidence in support of this conclusion was observed by comparing the fate of labeled urea in patients on a no-protein restriction diet as compared with patients on a 21 g/day protein diet (Richards et al., 1967). The patients on a protein restricted diet have the greatest amount of albumin labeled, suggesting that these patients utilized more nitrogen from urea since they had less nitrogen available for competition from their diet. In comparing nonuremic to uremic patients, nonuremic patients incorporate more label into their albumin, presumably because the labeled urea would not have to compete with a large amount of nonlabeled urea that is available in uremic patients. It seems clear, therefore, from both animal and human data that urea is metabolically active and contributes to the nitrogen pool required for protein synthesis. The evidence from these studies suggests that the most important condition for the utilization of urea nitrogen is a limited supply of other sources of nitrogen.

Metabolism of urea is of interest in this regard. The urea is hydrolyzed by bacterial urease in the gut, and this hydrolysis is abolished when animals are treated with an antibiotic cocktail (Walser, 1959). The requirement for bacterial ureases is further demonstrated by an analysis of the utilization of labeled urea in germ-free mice (Levenson et al., 1959). Germ-free mice expire 1% as much labeled carbon dioxide as normal mice, an amount which can be accounted for solely by the spontaneous hydrolysis in the gut. Supporting data were obtained in humans after injecting labeled urea and collecting urine to quantitate its recovery (Walser, 1959). The recovery of injected label was incomplete in the intact human, suggesting metabolic conversion of urea, but was complete in those patients who had received neomycin. Approximately 25% of the administered urea is hydrolyzed by the intestinal bacteria of normal man.

With the establishment of the essential nutritional requirement of normal man, interest increased in giving only the essential nutrients to patients who do not excrete nitrogenous wastes. The observation that urea could participate in the metabolic pathways that are required to protect protein production suggested that these patients could go into a positive nitrogen balance without increasing nitrogenous waste. In an early attempt, 1.24 g of essential amino acids were administered to patients, with extra calories provided by carbohydrates available from hard candies (Schloerb, 1966). Berlyne (Berlyne et al., 1967a) provided an in depth study of the clinical and biochemical benefits of such an oral regimen in patients with ARF. With the advent of parenteral nutrition techniques, the composition of nutritional supplements could be adjusted more precisely, and the amounts given could be regulated in a careful fashion. The problems of anorexia, lethargy, and vomiting could be avoided, which gave new impetus to the development of formulas designed specifically for patients with nitrogen-accumulating diseases (Ryan et al., 1974; Abel et al., 1972a). The original parenteral solutions were composed of casein hydrolysates, which added a significant load to the accumulation of nitrogenous wastes. Purer forms of essential amino acids proved far superior in providing nutritional support without increasing azotemia (Abel et al., 1971). Investigations of these solutions revealed that the patients developed a feeling of well being and had less nausea and vomiting, an improved appetite, and decreased stomatitis. In addition, lethargy diminished and the patients gained weight, and wound healing was consistently improved. (Abel et al., 1974a and b; Dudrick et al., 1970; Schloerb, 1966; Wilmore and Dudrick, 1969). It was also observed that the salt and water balance was usually easier to maintain in these patients, although there was an occasional increase in edema secondary to the loss of the osmotic diuretic effect of endogenous urea. The most consistent chemical improvement observed in these patients was a decrease in serum urea nitrogen concentration, which occurred even in patients with a postoperative catabolic state. While some of the earlier studies suggested an improvement in nitrogen balance, the latter studies indicated a reduction in blood urea nitrogen concentration of as much as 50%, with a consistent improvement in nitrogen balance so that an occasional patient demonstrated a positive nitrogen balance. Furthermore, the observed increase in nitrogen requirements for uremics could be reduced with the addition of essential amino acids to their diets (Schloerb, 1966).

Indirect support that amino acids were incorporated into new tissue was provided by the analysis of changes in serum chemical composition. Patients receiving the specifically designed parenteral and oral nutritional supplements demonstrated a positive potassium balance with a fall in serum potassium concentration (Abel et al., 1971, 1972a; Dudrick et al., 1970; Wilmore and Dudrick, 1969). Since potassium is essential to tissue production, this observation provided indirect evidence that amino acids were being incorporated into new protein (Cannon et al., 1952). A more detailed study revealed a consistent fall of potassium concentration within 8 hr of initiating therapy, and that none of the patients required dialysis or cation exchange resins to control hyperkalemia and even an occasional supplementation of potassium was necessary. Intracellular shifts of magnesium and phosphorus with consistent lowering of the serum levels of these ions provided further indirect evidence for protein synthesis (Abel et al., 1971, 1972a; Dudrick et al., 1970; Wilmore and Dudrick, 1969). Both phosphorus and magnesium serum concentrations decreased within 48 hr of the initiation of nutritional therapy. The patients demonstrated a consistent weight gain and improved wound healing. None of these patients had evidence of improved renal function with increased urinary excretion of these substances. When amino acids were measured in patients receiving this parenteral nutrition, the serum level remained unchanged from preinfused levels. It should be noted that these patients were not dialyzed, nor was there an increase in the urinary excretion of amino acids. The weight gain, intracellular shifts of ions known to be necessary for protein synthesis, and the unchanged serum amino acid levels constitute indirect evidence that the administered amino acids were utilized for protein synthesis. None of these beneficial metabolic effects occurred with the use of protein hydrolysates (Baek et al., 1975).

Evidence has also been obtained that treatment with essential amino acids of patients with ARF changes requirements for dialysis and alters the mortality statistics in these patients (Dudrick et al., 1970; (Wilmore and Dudrick, 1969). In a controlled study of matched patients with or without essential amino acids, the interval and frequency of hemodialysis was unchanged in patients with ARF, but the survival rate of these patients was increased from 30% in the control group to 50% for those receiving amino acids supplementations (Abel et al., 1972a). The need for hemodialysis was greater in the absence of amino acid therapy. Similar observations have been made in other studies (Abel et al., 1973; Dudrick et al., 1970). Using a selected population of patients with ARF, the survival figures for patients receiving amino acids was 75–80%, while in the control group not receiving essential amino acids the survival rate was 40–44% (Abel et al., 1972b, 1973, 1974b). Survival after ARF or therapy with essential amino acids seemed to be related to the duration of therapy with nutritional supplementation, and the best survival statistics correlated with a 8–14 day course of therapy. Therapy for less than 8 days or for more than 2 weeks was associated with a decrease rate of survival. However, those patients dying early may have had more severe multiple organ failure, and those dying at a later interval may have had irreversible disease. There is also evidence that the morbidity of patients with ARF receiving amino acids may also be decreased. The administration of amino acids was associated with a decreased incidence of sepsis and hypotension. Those patients who developed these complications had an improved survival as compared to control matched patients developing the same complication (Baek et al., 1975). In a separate but similar study, patients who received amino acids survived the complications of pneumonia, sepsis and gastrointestinal hemmorhage to a better degree than did the matched control group (Abel et al., 1973).

A more controversial claim concerns an improved rate of recovery of patients with ARF undergoing treatment with nutritional supplements. In early studies, there was a progressive rise in serum creatinine concentration while the urea nitrogen concentration in serum fell, suggesting that nitrogen balance was enhanced but that improvement in filtration rate was not occurring. More recently, the administration of essential amino acids to patients with ARF resulted in a slower rate of rise in creatinine per day than in untreated patients (Abel et al., 1973), suggesting an improvement not only in general tissue repair but perhaps also in renal tubular repair. However, the study design excluded patients on hemodialysis, resulting in a small number of individuals in each of the various study groups. The difference in the rate of rise in creatinine could be accounted for by a decreased endogenous creatinine production due to a positive nitrogen balance. A more detailed account of clearance data would be necessary prior to reaching the conclusion that essential amino acids result in an improved rate of recovery from ARF.

The improvements observed with amino acid administration, an enhanced knowledge of the metabolism of urea per se, and improved biochemical synthetic abilities led investigators to go a step further towards reducing nitrogen administration to patients with ARF. If humans were supplied with the basic building blocks for protein synthesis (specific essential amino acids but without nitrogen, α-keto analogues), could they reaminate these analogue amino acids? Three steps appear to be involved in reamination: 1) urea must be hydrolyzed by gastrointestinal bacterial urease to ammonium; 2) the ammonium must be utilized to reaminate the glutarate to glutamate; and 3) the nitrogen must be transaminated from the glutamate to the α-keto acid of the essential amino acid being produced. The rate-limiting factor in these processes would be the availability of the α-keto acid, as well as the unavailability of nitrogen compounds in a form other than urea. Lysine and threonine cannot be reaminated by this process and are true essential amino acids (Abel, 1976). Subsequent to the elucidation of the involved biochemical processes, animal or human experiments were performed. Animals given α-keto analogues had a weight gain and a positive nitrogen balance (Abel, 1976), and isolated tissue perfused with keto analogues demonstrated a linear decline of keto acids with a concomitant increase in amino acid content (Walser et al., 1973b). These investigators also studied patients separated into two groups: one group received keto acid analogues, while a separate group received essential amino acids over an 18-day period (Walser et al., 1973a). All patients were in negative nitrogen balance during the control interval, while nitrogen balance was variable during the administration of keto acids. The urea appearance rate was less in patients on keto analogues than that in patients receiving essential amino acids, and the rate of urea appearance abruptly rose with cessation of keto analogue therapy or substitution of essential amino acids. The process of reamination is approximately 49% efficient and utilizes 1.6 g of ammonia per day at its maximum. There seems to be no accumulations of keto acids or other deleterious effects, and the technique clearly promotes anabolism as evidenced by the improvement of negative nitrogen balance. However, the keto acid analogues may not promote anabolism to a significantly greater degree than did essential amino acids, although decreasing urea concentration may promote better utilization of nitrogen and further improve nitrogen balance. While α-keto analogues can lower urea concentration beyond that observed with essential amino acids, there may be no associated clinical improvement, and the quest for a lower serum urea nitrogen concentration may not justify the increased effort and cost required to supply keto analogues. Consequently, most efforts have been directed towards utilization of the less expensive and more readily available essential amino acid mixtures.

As noted above, dialysis in patients with ARF adds an additional stress to the already over burdened nutritional status due to the effects of uremia. Both peritoneal and hemodialysis deplete the patient of amino acids, which are cleared during the process of dialysis and lost into the dialysate, although plasma levels of amino acids remain normal. The maintenance of normal plasma amino acid levels presupposes an enhanced metabolism of protein and release of amino acid into the circulation, since during 12 hr of hemodialysis amino acid clearance may be up to eight times greater than the total plasma amino acid content (Rubini and Gordon, 1968). In quantitative terms, this represents the loss of 4.79 g of amino acids, or 50% of the minimal daily requirements of amino acids. It should be noted that these observations were obtained by using older more porous dialysis membranes. Newer currently available artificial kidneys may result in smaller losses of amino acids into the dialysate. Peritoneal dialysis is even more deleterious to protein balance, and hypoproteinemia is a well recognized complication. For example, it has been reported that as much as 11.02 g of amino acids may be removed in 27 liters of peritoneal dialysate exchange, with an average loss of 4.96 g per peritoneal dialysis treatment (Berlyne et al., 1967b). In general, the amount of amino acids lost during peritoneal dialysis is directly related to the duration of the procedure and the frequency with which peritoneal dialysis is performed. In addition to amino acid removal, protein may also be lost during peritoneal dialysis, up to 20–60 g per peritoneal dialysis treatment. Included in the proteins lost into the peritoneal dialysate are immunoglobulins, especially IgG, which may contribute to the increase incidence of infections during this procedure. While amino acid losses may be prevented by adding amino acids to the peritoneal dialysate fluid, whole protein losses must be replaced by providing additional protein in the diet. As a general estimate, it would require approximately five whole eggs to replace the amino acids and whole protein losses which occur during a 27-liter peritoneal dialysis.

In general, the nutritional requirements of acutely ill patients with ARF are extremely specialized. These patients have increased requirements for substances necessary for tissue repair after trauma and the negative nitrogen balance characteristic of their clinical status. Because of their renal insufficiency, these patients have a severe limitation in their ability to handle nitrogenous waste, fluid overload, and electrolyte imbalances which may accompany the usual replacement modalities for meeting their nutritional requirements. Meeting these specific clinical needs requires a further understanding of the metabolic contribution of urea nitrogen to their overall metabolic state. The final extension of this concept leads to the use of α-keto analogues in the treatment of patients with ARF. By supplying the necessary carbon structures required for nutritional replacement, full advantage of recycling of urea nitrogen for metabolism can be realized without adding to the total burden of nitrogenous wastes in patients with ARF. While this concept is scientifically sound, there are practical and economical limitations to achieving this goal which are not harmonious with the clinical needs set as the objective for the nutritional replacement of patients with ARF. Furthermore, the goal set in association with improvement of nutrition for a lowering of blood urea levels does not appear to have any great clinical benefit. It would seem more appropriate, therefore, to provide a diet which meets the nutritional needs of the patient with ARF, while at least stabilizing the rise in urea nitrogen concentration observed in these patients. This may be accomplished with demonstrated clinical benefits by using available essential amino acid mixtures. In addition, for those patients who are "gastrointestinal cripples," secondary to surgery of uremic complications, parenteral solutions would also provide adequate nutritional support for the correction of their underlying metabolic abnormalities.

Dialysis

Dialysis has been shown to have a significant role in the management of ARF (Teschan et al., 1960). In a study comparing "conservative," or nondialytic therapy with a regimen including early and frequent dialysis, Kleinknecht et al. (1976) demonstrated that the patients undergoing dialysis had a lower overall mortality. The incidence as well as the mortality due to gastrointestinal bleeding was reduced in those patients with ARF treated with dialysis. Likewise, dialysis appeared to reduce the mortality of ARF patients developing sepsis. Peritoneal dialysis was shown to be less effective in reducing mortality in these patients than hemodialysis. This may be due to its relatively lower overall efficiency, especially in patients who are hypercatabolic (Nolph et al., 1969). The reasons for the improvement in the clinical course of ARF are probably multiple. On the one hand, uremic patients who have undergone dialysis are better able to tolerate an optimum protein and caloric intake. They therefore derive obvious salutory effects on wound healing and the sense of well being of an improved nutritional status. For this reason, when patients are unable to ingest an adequate diet, dialysis therapy should be supplemented with intravenous amino acids (Blackburn et al., 1978). In addition, dialysis therapy is associated with an improvement in platelet function.

The choice of peritoneal dialysis as opposed to hemodialysis for the treatment of ARF depends upon: 1) availability of either modality; 2) the condition of the peritoneal cavity; 3) whether the patient is hypercatabolic; 4) whether the patient has on-going or potential blood loss; 5) whether the patient is stable from a cardiovascular standpoint; and 6) the presence or absence of gastric and/or bowel distention.

When hemodialysis is available, it is the modality of choice in patients who do not have an intact peritoneal cavity even though peritoneal dialysis may in some instances still be feasible. Likewise, hemodialysis, rather than peritoneal dialysis, is advisable when the patient is hypercatabolic or when bowel or gastric distention are present and it cannot be easily decompressed. On the other hand, as peritoneal dialysis does not require the systemic infusion of heparin, it is safer in those patients who are actively bleeding. In addition, since peritoneal dialysis is carried out in a space external to plasma volume, it places much less stress on cardiovascular homeostasis. Therefore, it should be preferentially employed in those patients who are having problems with maintaining their blood pressure or who have sustained cardiac damage. Even though the efficiency of peritoneal dialysis will be adversely affected by hypotension because of decreased mesenteric perfusion, it is still safer than hemodialysis under these circumstances.

The indications for dialysis in ARF are similar to those for renal failure in general. The presence of uremic symptoms and signs, especially pericarditis, a plasma creatinine of 10 mg/dl or higher, fluid over-load, electrolyte and/or acid/base imbalance not correctable by more conservative measures, suggests the need for dialysis. It should be emphasized that one should not wait for the development of overt uremia to initiate dialysis. It should be instituted when the patient clearly has severe renal failure (i.e., plasma creatinine of 10 mg/dl or greater) and shows no signs of imminent improvement in renal function. Dialysis should be maintained until there is clear evidence of spontaneous decline in plasma creatinine and improvement in renal function.

RECOVERY PHASE

Treatment in the recovery phase of patients with ARF parallels that described above for the maintenance phase. Continued attention to fluid and electrolyte management, nutrition, and the provision of dialysis are hallmarks of therapy during this phase. It must be emphasized that during this phase, recovery of renal function lags behind the return of urine volume, creating an apparent contradiction. Thus, uremic symptoms requiring dialysis may persist or develop despite a dramatic increase in urine volume, which is similar to the situation existing in patients with nonoliguric ARF. Primary considerations must be given to fluid and electrolyte balance during this phase since salt and water losses can be significant and, if not adequately replaced, may result in clinical deterioration due to hemodynamic alterations. The significance of this phase cannot be underestimated since up to 25% of the morbidity observed in ARF occurs during this phase.

SYNTHESIS AND FUTURE EVENTS

Treatment of ARF when placed in perspective assumes great clinical importance. It is a process from which the patient has a great potential for recovery with adequate management and attention to their medical problems. Indeed, its major clinical significance is related to the inherent reversibility of the ongoing disease process. The concept has been accepted, from a clinical standpoint, but the vast majority of patients dying after having developed ARF do so not from renal failure but from the associated complications of infection and bleeding difficulties. While these complications are directly related to the occurrence of renal insufficiency, the general availability of dialysis techniques usually precludes death from renal failure itself.

Future considerations for the therapy of patients with ARF will be directed towards the nutritional status of these patients, as well as to searching for agents which may modify or reverse the underlying pathophysiology. Currently, diuretics, as noted above, are the mainstay of agents used to modify the course of ARF. A large number of experiments have been performed using models of ARF in animals to evaluate the potential efficacy of other agents. For the most part, these are vasoactive substances which interfere with what is assumed to be the primary pathophysiologic event, an alteration in renal hemodynamics. These agents include: angiotensin inhibitors, prostaglandins, dopamine, acetylcholine, bradechinine, α- and β-adrenergic blocking agents, as well as drugs designed to alter intraglomerular coagulation (i.e., heparin, an antiplatelet agent). The newest of these therapeutic endeavors involves the use of adenosine triphosphate and magnesium chloride (Osias et al., 1977). The experimental model utilized was ischemic ARF, and the administration of adenosine triphosphate and magnesium chloride resulted in a more rapid recovery in cortical renal blood flow and renal function. While additional studies are awaited confirming the experimental utility of these agents, they represent a significant advance in the approach to the basic underlying pathophysiology through the recognition of a basic defect in cellular metabolism. The common denominator, after all, of both ischemic and nephrotoxic ARF would seem to be interference with cellular function involving the renal tubules. The use of these agents would appear to be designed to directly return cell metabolism to normal.

References

Abel, R.M.: Parenteral nutrition in the treatment of renal failure. In *Total Parenteral Nutrition*, edited by Josef E. Fisher, ed. 1, pp. 143–170. Little, Brown, Boston, 1976.

Abel, R.M., Abbott, W.M., and Fischer, J.E.: Acute renal failure: Treatment without dialysis by total parenteral nutrition. Arch. Surg. *103:*513, 1971.

Abel, R.M., Abbott, W.M., and Fischer, J.E.: Intravenous essential L-amino and hypertonic dextrose in patients with acute renal failure. Am. J. Surg. *123:*632, 1972a.

Abel, R.M., Beck, C.H. Jr., Abbott, W.M., Ryan, J.A., Barnett, G.O., Fischer, J.E.: Treatment of acute renal failure with intravenous administration of essential amino acids and glucose. Surg. Forum *23:*77, 1972b.

Abel, R.M., Beck, C.H., Jr., Abbott, W.M., Ryan, J.A., Jr., Barnett, G.O., and Fischer, J.E.: Improved survival from acute renal failure after treatment with intravenous essential L-amino acids and glucose. N. Engl. J. Med. *288:*695, 1973.

Abel, R.M., Shih, V.E., Abbott, W.M., Beck, C.H., Jr., and Fischer, J.E.: Amino acid metabolism and acute renal failure. Ann. Surg., *180:*350, 1974a.

Abel, R.M., Abbott, W.M., Beck, C.H., Ryan, J.A., and Fisher, J.E.: Essential L-amino acids for hyperalimentation in patients with disordered nitrogen metabolism. Am. J. Surg. *128:*317, 1974b.

Akman, M., Goldstein, D.A., Telfer, M., Wilkinson E., and Massry, S.G.: Resolution of muscle calcification in rhabdomyolysis and A.R.F. Ann. Intern. Med. *89:*928, 1976.

Anderson, R.J., Linas, S. L., Berns, A. S., Henrich, W. L., Miller, T. R., Gabow, P. A., and Schrier, R. W.: Nonoliguric acute renal failure. N. Engl. J. Med. *296:* 1134, 1977.

Arendshorst, W.J., Finn, W.F., and Gottschalk, C.W.: Pathogenesis of acute renal failure following temporary renal ischemia in the rat. Circ. Res. *37:*558, 1975.

Auger, G., Dayton, A., Harrison, C.E., Tucker, M., and Anderson, F.: Use of ethacrynic acid in mannitol resistant oliguric renal failure. J.A.M.A. *206:*891, 1968.

Baek, Se-Min., Makabali, G.G., Bryan-Brown, C.W., Kusek, J., and Shoemaker, W.C.: The influence of parenteral nutrition on the course of acute renal failure. Surg. Gynecol. Obstet. *141:*405, 1975.

Bank, N., Mutz, B.F., and Aynedjian, H. S.: Role of "leakage" of tubular fluid in anuria due to mercury poisoning. J. Clin. Invest. *46:*695, 1967.

Barry, K.G., and Crosby, W.H.: The prevention and treatment of renal failure following transfusion reactions. Transfusion (Phila.) *3:*34, 1963.

Barry, G., and Malloy, P.: Oliguric renal failure: Evaluation and therapy by the intravenous infusion of mannitol. J.A.M.A. *179:*134, 1962.

Barry, G., Cohen, K.P., Ehelan, J., Beisel, W.R., Vargas, C.A., and LaBlanc, P.C.: The prevention of acute functional renal failure during resection of an aneurism of the abdominal aorta. N. Engl. J. Med. *264:*967, 1961.

Barry, G., Schwartz, D., and Doberneck, D.: A comparison of the prophylactic value of 20% mannitol, 4% urea and 5% dextrose on the effect of renal ischemia. J. Urol. *89:*300, 1963.

Beall, A.C., Hall, C., Morris, C., and DeBakey, E.: Mannitol-induced osmotic diuresis during renal artery occlusion. Ann. Surg. *161:*46, 1965.

Berlyne, G.M., Bazzard, F.J., Booth, E.M., Jandbi, K., and Shaw, A.B.: The dietary treatment of acute renal failure. Q.J. Med. *35:*59, 1967a.

Berlyne, G.M., Lee, H.A., Giordano, C. de Pascale, C., and Esposito, R.: Amino acid loss in peritoneal dialysis. Lancet *1:*1339, 1967b.

Birtch, A.G., Zakheim, R.M., Jones, L.G., and Barger, A.C.: Redistribution of renal blood flow produced by furosemide and ethacrynic acid. Circ. Res. *21:*869, 1967.

Blackburn, G.L., Etter, G., and MacKenzie, T.: Criteria for choosing amino acid therapy in acute renal failure. Am. J. Clin. Nutr. *31:*1841, 1978.

Blagg, C.R., Parsons, F.M., and Young, G.A.: Effect of dietary glucose and protein in acute renal failure. Lancet *2:*612, 1962.

Blantz, R.C.: Effect of mannitol on glomerular ultrafiltration in the hydropenic rat. J. Clin. Invest. *54:*1135, 1974.

Blantz, R.C.: The mechanism of acute renal failure after uranyl nitrate. J. Clin. Invest. *55:*621, 1975.

Borirakchamyavat, V., Longsthongsri, M., and Sitprija, V.: Furosemide and acute renal failure. Postgrad. Med. J. *53:*30, 1978.

Bourne, C.W., and Cerny, J.C.: The role of mannitol in acute trauma. Univ. Mich. Med. Cent. J. *80:*109, 1964.

Brown, J.J., Gleadle, R.I., Lawson, D.H., Lever, A.F., Linton, A.L., Macadam, R.F., Prentice, E., Robertson, J.S., and Tree, M.: Renin and acute renal failure. Br. Med. J. *1:*253, 1970.

Brown, J.J., Garvas, H., Drenes, D., Levin, A., MacGregar, J., Powell-Jackson, J.D., and Robertson, I.S.: Renin and acute renal failure. In *Proceedings of the Conference on Acute Renal Failure*, edited by E. Friedman and H. Eliahou. DHEW Publication No. (NIH) 74-608, Washington, DC, 1973.

Brown, R.D.: Comparison of the cochlear toxicity of sodium ethacrynate, furosemide and the cysteine adduct of sodium ethacrynate in cats. Toxicol. Appl. Pharmacol. *31:*270, 1975.

Brown, T.C., Davis, O.J., Johnston, O.J.: Acute response in plasma renin and aldosterone secretion to diuretics. Am. J. Physiol. *211:*437, 1966.

Cannon, P.R., Frazier, L.E., and Hughes, R.H.: Influence of potassium on tissue protein synthesis. Metabolism *1:*49, 1952.

Cantarovich, F., Galli, C., Benedetti, L., Chena, C., Castro, L., Correa, C., Petez-Loredo, J., Fernandez, J.C., Loctelli, A., and Tizado, J.: High-dose fursemide in established acute renal failure. Br. Med. J. *4:*449, 1973.

Coelho, J.B., and Bradley, S.E.: Function of the nephron population during hemorrhagic hypotension in the dog, with special reference to the effect of osmotic diuresis. J. Clin. Invest. *43:*386, 1964.

Condon, J.R., and Asatoor, A.M.: Amino acid metabolism in uremic patients. Clin. Chim. Acts. *32:*333, 1971.

Cooperman, L.B., and Rubin, I.L.: Toxicity of ethacynic acid and furosemide. Am. Heart J. *85:*831, 1973.

Cox, J.W., Baehler, R.W., Sharma, H., O'Dorisio, T., Osgood, R.W., Stein, J.H., and Ferris, T.F.: Studies on the mechanism of oliguria in a model of unilateral acute renal failure. J. Clin. Invest. *53:*1546, 1974.

Daugharty, T.M., Ueki, J.F., Mercer, P.F., and Brenner, B.M.: Dynamics of glomerular ultrafiltration in the rat. V. Response to ischemic injury. J. Clin. Invest. *53:*105, 1974.

Dawson, J.: Post operative renal function in obstructive jaundice: Effect of mannitol diuresis. Br. Med. J. *1:*82, 1965.

de Torrente, A., Berl, T., Cohn, P.D., Kawametes, E., Hertz, P., and Schrier, R.W.: Hypocalcemia of ARF: Clinical significance and pathogenesis. Am. J. Med. *61:*119, 1976.

Dudrick, S.J., Steiger, E., and Long, J.M.: Renal failure in surgical patients treatment with intravenous essential amino acids and hypertonic glucose. Surgery *68:*180, 1970.

Earley, L.E., and Guttschalk, C.W. (Eds.): *Strauss and Welt's Disease of the Kidney*, vol. 1, ch. 5, p. 191. Little, Brown, Boston, 1979.

Eliahou, H.E.: Mannitol therapy in oliguria of acute onset. Br. Med. J. *1:*807, 1964.

Epstein, M., Schneider, M., and Befeler, B.: Effect of intrarenal furosemide on renal function and intra renal hemodynamics in acute renal failure. Am. J. Med. *58:*510, 1975.

Estep, H., Shaw, W., Waltington, C., Hobe, C., Hellano, W., and Tucker, H.: Hypocalcemia due to reversible hypomagnesemia and parathyroid hormone unresponsiveness. J. Clin. Endocrinol. Metab. *29:*842, 1969.

Fenn, W.O.: Deposition of potassium and phosphate with glycogen in rat livers. J. Biol. Chem. *128:*297, 1939.

Finn, W.F.: Acute renal failure. In *Diseases of the Kidney*, edited by L. E. E. Farley and C. W. Gottschalk, ed. 3, pp. 167–210. Little, Brown, Boston, 1979.

Finn, W.F., and Arendshorst, W.J.: Effect of prostaglandin synthetase inhibitors on renal blood flow in the rat. Am. J. Physiol. *231:*1541, 1976.

Flamenbaum, W.: Acute renal failure. Arch. Intern. Med. *131:* 911, 1973.

Flamenbaum, W.: Pathophysiology of acute renal failure. In *Pathophysiology of the Kidney*, edited by N. Kurtzman and M. Martinez-Maldonado, pp. 795–841. Charles C Thomas, Springfield, IL, 1977.

Flanigan, W.J., and Oken, D.E.: Renal micropuncture study of the development of anuria in the rat with mercury-induced acute renal failure. J. Clin. Invest. *44:*449, 1965.

Flores, J., DiBona, D.B., Beck, C.H., and Leaf, A.: The role of cell swelling in ischemic renal damage and the protective effect of hypertonic saline. J. Clin. Invest. *51:*118, 1972.

Franklin, A., Ganote, C. E., and Jennings, B.: Blood reflow after renal ischemia. Arch. Pathol. Lab. Med. *198:*100, 1974.

Fraser, R., James, V.H.T., Brown, J.J., and Isaac, T.: The effect of furosemide on plasma aldosterone, corticosterone, cortisol and renin in man. Lancet *2:*989, 1965.

Gambos, E.A.: Acute renal failure. Principles of management. N.Y. State J. Med. *73:*2055, 1973.

Goldberg, A.H., and Lilienfield, L.S.: Effects of hypertonic mannitol on renal vascular resistance. Proc. Soc. Exp. Biol. Med. *119:*635, 1965.

Goormagtigh, N.: Vascular and circulatory changes in renal cortex in the anuric crush-syndrome. Proc. Soc. Exp. Biol. Med. *59:*303, 1945.

Gray, R., Boyle, I., Deluca, H.F., and Litamin, D.: Metabolism the role of the kidney. Tissue Sci. *172:*1232, 1971.

Grevin, I., and Klein, H.: Renal effects of furosemide in glycerol induced acute renal failure of the rat. Pflueger Arch. *365:*81, 1976.

Grossman, R.A., Hamilton, R.W., Morse, R.M., Penn, A.S., and Goldberg, M.: Nontraumatic rhabdomyolysis and A.R.F. N. Engl. J. Med. *291:*807, 1974.

Harrington, J.: Drug therapy reviews: Diuretics. Am. J. Hosp. Pharm. *32:*316, 1975.

Hollenberg, N.K., Epstein, M., Rosen, S.M., Basch, R.I., Oken, D.E., and Merrill, J.P.: Acute oliguric renal failure in man and evidence for preferential renal cortical ischemia. Medicine *47:*455, 1968.

Horton, E.S., Johnson, C., and Lebovit, H.E.: Carbohydrate metabolism in uremia. Ann. Intern. Med. *68:*63, 1968.

Jaenike, J.R.: Micropuncture study of methemoglobin-induced acute renal failure in the rat. J. Lab. Clin. Med. *73:*459, 1969.

Kincaid-Smith, P.: Coagulation and renal disease. Kidney Int. *2:*183, 1972.

Kjellstrand, C.M.: Ethacynic acid in acute tubular necrosis: Indication and effect on natural course. Nephron *9:*337, 1972.

Kleeman, C.R., Massry, S.G., and Coburn, J.W.: The clinical physiology of calcium homeostatis, parathyroid hormone and calcitonin. Calif. Med. *114:*14, 1971.

Kleinknecht, D., Ganeval, D., Gonzalez-Duque, L.A., and Fermanian, J.: Furosemide in acute oliguric renal failure: A controlled trial. Nephron *17:*61, 1976.

Koffler, D., and Paronetto, F.: Fibrinogen deposition in acute renal failure. Am. J. Pathol. *47:*383, 1966.

Kotchen, T.A., and Miller, M.C.: Effect of prostaglandins in renin reactivity. Am. J. Physiol. *226:*384, 1974.

Kovithavongs, T., Becker, F.O., and Img, T.S.: Parathyroid hyperfunction in A.R.F. Nephron *9:*349, 1972.

Larsson, S.W., Hedner, U., and Nilsson, I.M.: On fibrinolytic split products in serum and urine in uremia. Scand. J. Urol. Nephrol. *5:*234, 1971.

Lawson, D.H., MacAllan, R.F., Singh, H., Garvas, H., Hartz, S., Turnbull, D., and Linton, A.L.: Effect of furosemide on antibiotic induced renal damage in rats. J. Infect. Dis. *126:* 593, 1972.

Lawson, L.J., Blaney, J.D., Dawson-Edwards, P., Tonge, S.M.: Dietary management of acute oliguric renal failure. Br. Med. J. *3:*293, 1962.

Leonard, A., and Nelms, R.: Hypercalcemia in the diuretic phase of A.R.F. Ann. Intern. Med. *73:*173, 1970.

Leonard, C.D., and Eichner, E.R.: A.R.F. and transient hypercalcemia in idiopathic rhabdomyolyses. J.A.M.A. *211:*1539, 1970.

Levenson, S.M., Crowley, L.U., Horowitz, R.E., and Malm, O.J.: The metabolism of carbon-labeled urea in the germ free rat. J. Biol. Chem. *234:*2061, 1959.

Levine, H.D.: Electrolyte imbalance and the EKG. Mod. Concepts Cardiovasc. Dis. *23:*246, 1953.

Levinsky, N.G.: Management of emergencies: VI hyperkalemia. N. Engl. J. Med. *274:*1076, 1966.

Levinsky, N.S., and Alexander, E.A.: Acute renal failure. In *The Kidney*, edited by B. Brenner and F. Rector, pp. 806–837. W.B. Saunders, Philadelphia, 1976.

Levitin, H., Etheredge, E.E., Nakamure, K., and Glen, W.W.L.: Effect of mannitol on renal function during open-heart surgery. Ann. Surg. *161:*53, 1963.

Lilien, O.M., Jonas, S.G., and Mueller, C.B.: The mechanism of mannitol diuresis. Surg. Gynecol. Obstet. *117:*221, 1963.

Linton, A.L., Bailey, R.R., Natale, R., Turnbull, D.I., and Graswell, P.W.T.: Protective effect of furosemide in acute tubular necrosis and acute renal failure. In: *Proceedings of the Conference on Acute Renal Failure*, edited by E. Friedman and H. Eliahou, DHEW Publication No. (NIH) 74-608, Washington, DC, 1973.

Lopez-Nova, J.M., Rodico-Diaz, L., and Hernando-Avendano, L.: Negative effect of furosemide pre-treatment in glycerol induced acute renal failure. Biomedicine *26:*117, 1977.

Ludens, J.H., Hook, J.B., Brody, M.J., and Williamson, H.E.: Enhancement of renal blood flow by furosemide. J. Pharmacol. Exp. Ther. *163:*456, 1968.

Luke, R.G., Briggs, J.D., Allison, M.E., and Kennedy, A.C.: Factors determining response to mannitol in acute renal failure. Am. J. Med. Sci. *259:*168, 1970.

Lyons, H., Pinn, V.W., Cortell, S., Cotton, J.J., and Harrington, J.T.: Allergic interstitial nephritis causing reversible renal failure in 4 patients with idiopathic nephrotic syndrome. N. Engl. J. Med. *288:*124, 1974.

Maddock, R.K., Jr., Blommer, H.A., de St. Jeor, S.W.: Low protein diets in the management of renal failure, Ann. Intern. Med. *69:*1003, 1968.

Marriot, H.J.L.: *Practical Electrocardiography*, ed. 5. Williams & Wilkins, Baltimore, 1972.

Massry, S.G., Arieff, A.I., Coburn, J.W., Patmieri, G., and Kleeman, C.R. Divalent ion metabolism in patients with A.R.F.: Studies on the mechanism of hypocalcemia. Kidney Int. *5:*347, 1974.

Massry, S.G., Stein, R., Garty, J., Arieff, A.I., Coburn, J.W., Norman, A.W., and Fried, R.M.: Skeletal resistance to the calcemic action of parathyroid hormone in uremia: Role of 1,25(OH)$_2$D$_3$. Kidney Int. *9:*467, 1976.

Mathog, R.H., and Klein, W.: Ototoxicity of ethacrynic acid and amino-glycoside antibiotic in uremia. N. Engl. J. Med. *280:*1223, 1969.

McCracken, B.H., and Parsons, F.M.: Use of anabolic hormones to improve nitrogen balance. Lancet *2:*885, 1958.

McDonald, F.D., Thiel, G., Wilson, D.R., Di Bona, G.F., and Oken, D.E.: The prevention of acute renal failure in the rat by long-term saline loading: A possible role of the renin-angiotensin axis. Proc. Soc. Exp. Biol. Med. *131:*610, 1969.

McGiff, J.C., Crowshaw, K., Terragno, R.A., and Lonigro, A.J.: Release of prostaglandin-like substances into renal venous blood in response to angiotensin. Circ. Res. (Suppl. 1) *27:*121, 1970.

Merrill, V.P.: *The Treatment of Renal Failure*, Grune & Stratton, New York, 1965.

Merriwether, W.D., Nange, R.J., and Serpick, A.A.: Deafness following standard intravenous doses of ethacrynic acid. J.A.M.A. *216:*795, 1971.

Miller, T.R., Anderson, R.J., Linas, S.C., Henrich, W.L., Burns, A.S., Gabow, D.A., and Schrier, R.W.: Urinary diagnostic indices in acute renal failure: A prospective study. Ann. Intern. Med. *89:*47, 1978.

Minuth, A.N., Terrell, V.B., and Suki, W.N.: Acute renal failure: A study of the course and prognosis of 104 patients and of the role of furosemide. Am. J. Med. Sci. *271:*317, 1976.

Morris, C.R., Alexander, E.A., Bruns, F.J., and Levinsky, N.G.: Restoration and maintenance of glomerular filtration by mannitol during hypoperfusion of the kidney. J. Clin. Invest. *51:*1555, 1972.

Naranjo, C.A., Busto, U., and Cassis, L.: Furosemide induced adverse reactions during hospitalization. Am. J. Hosp. Pharmacol. *35:*514, 1978.

Nolph, K.D., Whitcomb, N.E., Shrier, R.W.: Mechanisms for inefficient parenteral dialysis in acute renal failure. Ann. Intern. Med. *71:*316, 1969.

Nordin, B., and Smith, D.A.: *Diagnostic Procedures in Disorders of Calcium Metabolism*, ed. 1, pp. 8–18. Little, Brown, Boston, 1965.

Ohtani, I., Ohtsuki, K., Omata, J., Ouchi, J., and Saito, T.: Potentiation and its mechanism of cochlear damage resulting from furosemide and amino glycoside antibiotic. ORL *40:*53, 1978.

Oken, D.E., Arce, M.L., and Wilson, D.R.: Glycerol-induced hemoglobinuric acute renal failure in the rat. I. Micropuncture study of the development of oliguria. J. Clin. Invest. *45:*72, 1966.

Osias, M.B., Srgel, N.J., Chandrey, I., Lyton, B., and Bare, A.: Postischemic renal failure. Accelerated recovery with adenosine triphosphate-magnesium chloride infusion. Arch. Surg. *112:*729, 1977.

Papadimitriou, M., Milionis, A., Eakellariou, G., and Metayas, P.: Effect of furosemide on acute ischemic renal failure in the dog. Nephron *70:*157, 1978.

Phillips, S.M., and Silvers, N.P.: Glucose-6-phosphate-dehydrogenase deficiency, infectious hepatitis, acute hemolysis and renal failure. Ann. Intern. Med. *70:*99, 1969.

Powell-Jackson, J.D., Brown, J.J., Lever, A.F., MacGregor, J., Macadam, R.F., Titterington, D.M., Robertson, J.I.S., and Waik, M.A.: Protection against acute renal failure in rats by passive immunization against angiotensin II. Lancet *1:*774, 1972.

Richards, P., Metcalge-Gibson, A., Ward, E., Wrong, O., and Houghton, B.J.: Utilization of ammonia nitrogen for protein synthesis in man, and the effects of protein restriction and uremia. Lancet *2:*845, 1967.

Rose, W.C., and Dekker, E.E.: Urea as a source of nitrogen for the biosynthesis of amino acids. J. Biol. Chem. *223:*107, 1956.

Rose, W.C., and Wixom, R.L.: The amino acid requirements of man XVI. The role of the nitrogen intake. J. Biol. Chem. *217:*997, 1955.

Rubini, M.E., and Gordon, S.: Individual plasma-free amino acids in uremics: Effect of hemodialysis. Nephron *5:*339, 1968.

Ryan, J.A., Jr., Abel, R.M., and Abbott, W.M.: Catheter complications of total parenteral nutrition. A prospective study of two hundred consecutive patients. N. Engl. J. Med. *290:*757, 1974.

Schloerb, P.R.: Essential L-amino acid administration in uremia. Am. J. Med. Sci. *252:*650, 1966.

Schreimer, G.E.: Acute renal failure in renal disease, edited by B. Dak, ed. 2. F. A. Davis, Philadelphia, 1967.

Schwartz, G.H., David D.S., Riggio, R.R., Sterzel, K.H., and Rubin, A.L.: Ototoxicity induced by furosemide. N. Engl. J. Med. *282:*1413, 1970.

Silverberg, S., and Johnson, J.: The use of mannitol in oliguric renal failure. Med. Clin. North Am. *50:*1159, 1966.

Slatopolsky, E., Caglars, S., Pennell, J.P., Taggart, D.B., Canterbury, J.M., Reiss, E., and Bruker, N.S.: On the pathogenesis of hyperparathyroidism in chronic renal insufficiency in the dog. J. Clin. Invest. *50:*492, 1971.

Swann, R.C., and Merrill, J.P.: The clinical course of acute renal failure. Medicine (Baltimore) *32:*215, 1953.

Tanner, G.A., and Sophason, S.: Kidney pressures after temporary renal artery occlusion in the rat. Am. J. Physiol. *230:*1173, 1976.

Tanner, G.A., Sloan, K.L., and Sophason, S.: Effect of renal artery occlusion on kidney function in the rat. Kidney Int. *4:*377, 1973.

Tavill, A.S., Evanson, J.M., Baker, S.B. de C., and Hewitt, V.: Idiopathic paroxysmal myoglobinuria with A.R.F. and hypercalcemia. N. Engl. J. Med. *271:*283, 1964.

Teschan, P.E., Baxter, C.R., O'Brien, J.S., Freyhoff, J.N., and Hall, W.H.: Prophylactic hemodialysis in the treatment of acute renal failure. Ann. Intern. Med. *53:*992, 1960.

Thomson, G.E.: Acute renal failure. Med. Clin. North Am. *57:*1579, 1973.

Turkington, R.W., Delcher, H.K., Meelon, F.A., and Gitelman, H.J.: Hypercalcemia following ARF. J. Clin. Endocrinol. Metab. *28:*1224, 1968.

Walser, M., and Bodenlos, L.: Urea metabolism in man. J. Clin. Invest. *38:*1617, 1959.

Walser, M., Coulter, A., W., Dighe, S., Crontz, F.R.: The effect of keto-analogues of essential amino acids in severe chronic uremia. J. Clin. Invest. *52:*678, 1973a.

Walser, M., Lund, P., Ruderman, V.B.: Synthesis of essential amino acids from their alpha-keto analogues by perfused rat liver and muscle. J. Clin. Invest. *52:*2865, 1973b.

Wardle, E.N.: Fibrinogen catabolism studies in patients with renal disease. Q. J. Med. *42:*205, 1973.

Wilmore, D.W., and Dudrick, S.J.: Treatment of acute renal failure with intravenous essential L-amino acids. Arch. Surg. *99:*669, 1969.

CHAPTER 25

Pathobiology of the Alveolar Wall in Human Shock Lung

URS N. RIEDE
CHRISTIAN MITTERMAYER
R. HORN
WALTER SANDRITTER

The discussion of the pathogenesis of shock lung, causes many misunderstandings, resulting from the fact that the late stages of this condition are considered under the same aspects as the early stage (Fischer, 1972; Herzog, 1976).

The early phase of shock lung is characterized by the consecutive development of the following changes seen in the alveolar wall: a) interstitial edema; b) necrosis of the endothelium; c) microthrombi; and d) necrosis of the epithelium.

WHEN IS THE SHOCK-INDUCED PULMONARY EDEMA PRODUCED AND WHERE IS THE PLACE OF ORIGIN?

In order to be able to answer this question we investigated the lungs of patients who had survived the shock-producing event for only a short period of time (cf., Joachim et al., 1978). Histomorphometric investigations of these lungs revealed that the interstitial edema is first seen within the peribronchial and perivascular connective tissue associated with lymphangiectasis and only at a later stage within the alveolar septa. This may be explained by the fact that during normal conditions of rest the extra-alveolar interstitium shows a more pronounced negative pressure as compared to that found in the alveolar interstitium. As a result, the interstitial fluid is discharged into the extra-alveolar interstitium and is stored in the lymphatic vessels (Lauweryns and Baert, 1977).

The removal of the fluid is, however, also due in part to the expansion of the lungs and is therefore less pronounced in the hilar segments of the lung (Ferner, 1977). In addition, the subpleural pulmonary tissue lying above the pleural lymphatic plexus is drained directly into the venous system (Lauweryns and Baert, 1977). For this reason, at first, no edema develops in the peripheral sections of the lung (Figs. 25.1 and 25.2).

If the interchange between the fluid produced by the alveolar capillaries and the fluid removed by the lymphatic vessels is disturbed, pulmonary edema will develop within the extra-alveolar interstitium, i.e., within the peribronchovascular connective tissue, because the original negative pressure has increased at this site. The continuously developing interstitial edema finally causes a reflux of the fluid into the alveolar interstitium, thereby decreasing the alveolar compliance (Hurley, 1978).

HOW IS THE INTERSTITIAL PULMONARY EDEMA PRODUCED?

Normally, the alveolar interstitial space consists of a virtual fissure. A few minutes following the onset of shock, the interstitium is enlarged; no cytoplasmic damage to the alveolar epithelial and endothelial cells can, however, be noticed. Only the binding between the interendothelial cell contacts is loosened. From this we may conclude that the alveolar endothelial cells play a decisive role, allowing interstitial pulmonary edema to spread (Riede et al., 1978) from the capillaries into the alveolar interstitium due to the permeability of the vessels (Riede et al., 1978; Hurley, 1978).

This observation is supported by morphological findings showing the alveolar epithelial cells to be tightly linked with desmosomes, whereas the endothelial cells of the capillaries are only loosely connected (Schneeberger, 1977; Mittermayer et al., 1978). In addition to this functional endothelial disturbance a disturbance of the epithelium can be observed due to a defective development of the surfactant (v. Wichert, 1978). As a direct result, the surface of the pulmonary alveoli shows an increased tension, a negative pressure is seen in the alveolar interstitium, and the drainage of fluids from the pulmonary capillaries into the alveolar interstitium has increased (v. Wichert, 1978). Consequently, in the initial phase of the shock-producing event, a functional distur-

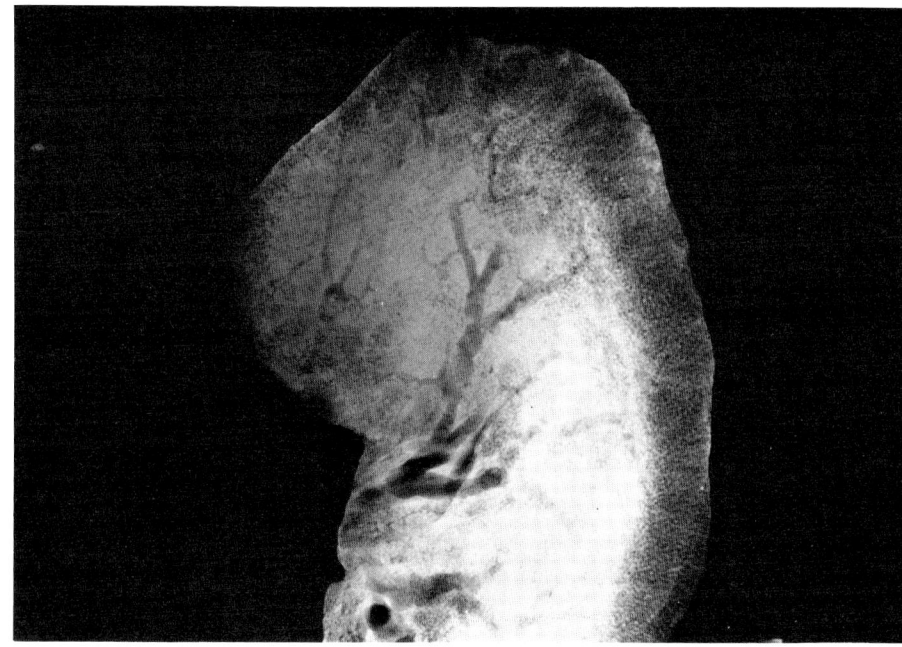

Figure 25.1. Radiograph of the lung after fixation in formalin vapor of a patient in the initial phase of hemorrhagic shock (for technique see Mittermayer et al., 1978).

bance in the barrier of the blood-gas exchange is produced, which occurs even before an underlying pathomorphological condition of this disturbance has developed (Joachim et al., 1976). This abnormal and increased permeability of the capillaries explains the extremely sensitive reaction of shock lung to an accumulation of fluids (Derks and Peters, 1973). The damage to the endothelium resulting from this disturbance will, however, only be recognized at a later stage (Riede et al., 1978). It starts with a swelling and vacuolization of the cytoplasm (Riede et al., 1978). In septic shock, this process is initiated within 2–3 min following the onset of endotoxemia (Myrvoll and Svalander, 1977) and is terminated when the damaged endothelial cells become detached from their bases (Gerrity et al., 1976). Simultaneous with the launching of the serogenous inflammatory mediators, owing to endotoxin, the complement system becomes activated. As a result, a C5 fragment is produced, C5-des-Arg, which attracts chemotactic neutrophil granulocytes within the terminal vascular bed (Henson, 1979).

In septic-hemorrhagic shock, the granulocytes sticking to the terminal vascular bed also cause leukopenia (Pingleton et al., 1972; Mittermayer et al., 1978).

WHAT ROLE DOES GRANULOCYTE STICKING PLAY?

The significance of the granulocytes being trapped within the terminal vascular bed in septic and hemorrhagic shock is not yet fully understood (Neuhof et al., 1977; Riede et al., 1978). There is, however, no doubt that the lysosomes (the granules themselves) of the granulocytes contain proteolytic enzymes which can, on the one hand, cause depolymerization, resulting in a swelling of the alveolar ground substance (Ackermann and Bebee, 1974), and on the other hand, activate the kinin and clotting mechanisms (Pingleton et al., 1972; Haberland, 1968, 1970).

WHAT ROLE DOES THE DAMAGED ENDOTHELIUM PLAY?

Recent investigations have shown that the role of the capillary endothelial cells is not restricted to that of a physical blood gas barrier, since these cells are capable of showing a great number of metabolic reactions (Ryan and Ryan, 1977).

Fibrinolysis

While the pulmonary endothelial cells, possess the ability to transform plasminogen into plasmin they also enclose tissue thrombocinases.

Lipolysis

The pulmonary endothelial cells contain a specific esterase which may be incorporated by the chylomicrons, because the lipids are initially drained from the intestines through the thoracic duct into the lung by the venous system.

Influence on the Blood Pressure

In addition, the pulmonary endothelial cells contain an enzyme capable of transforming angiotensin (kinase II) which can decompose bradykinin and transform angiotensin I to angiotensin II. Subsequently, angiotensin II is discharged into the general circulation. Therefore, the lung possesses the ability to regulate both the volume density and the tone of the vessels within the entire circulation (Ryan and Ryan, 1977).

In shock-induced endothelial necrosis, these three functions of the pulmonary endothelial cells are likely to be destroyed. Hypotension, fat embolism, and the presence of microthrombi must therefore be considered to be

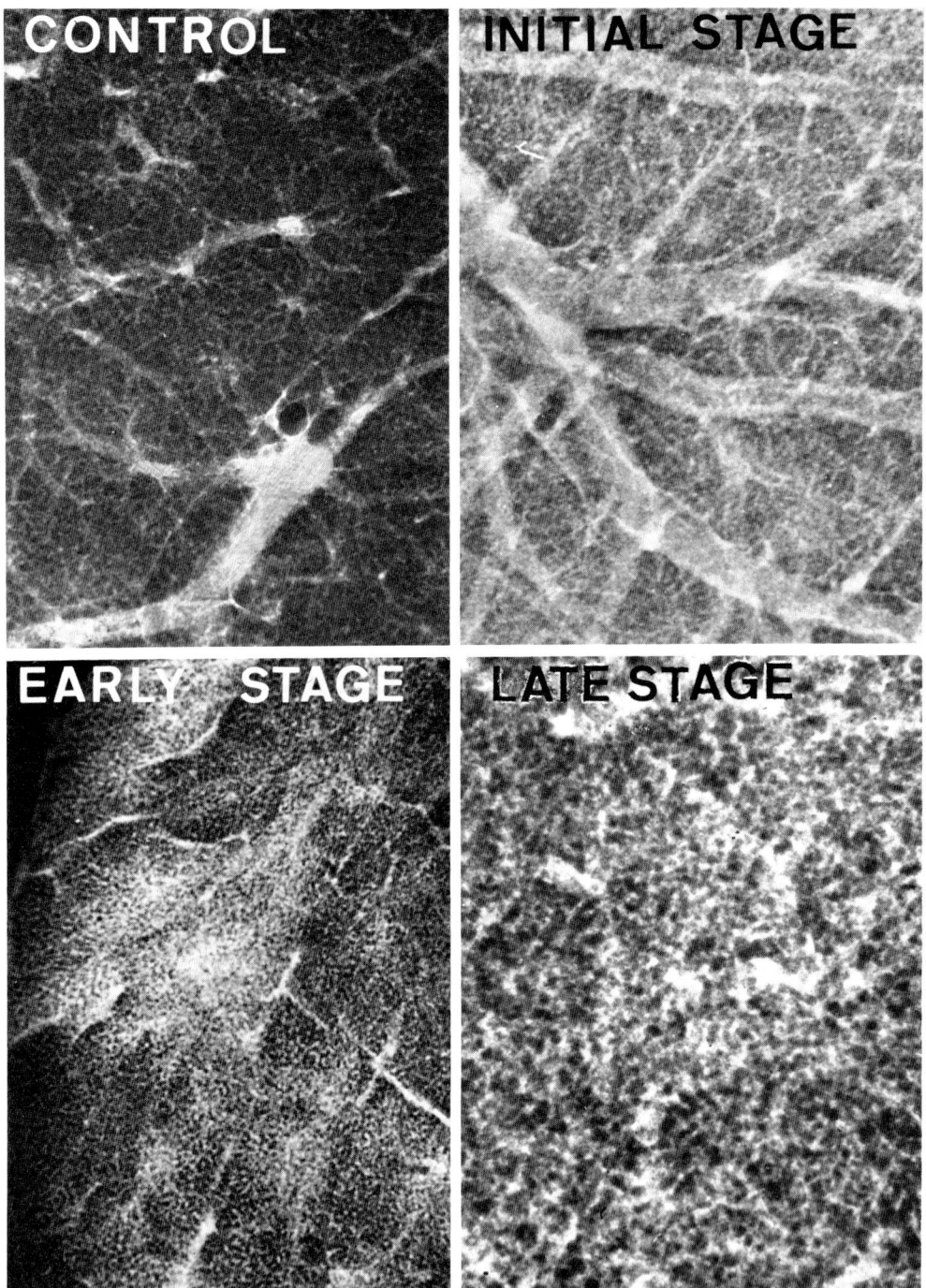

Figure 25.2. Radiograph of the lung in controls and during the initial phase of shock with "rail-track"-widening of the bronchi and blood vessels due to peribroncho-vascular edema. The lung edema extends during the early phase of shock into the alveolar interstitium. An interstitial lung fibrosis characterizes the late phase of shock.

at least partly caused by the damage to the endothelium in the terminal vascular bed. However, correlation between endothelial necrosis (Figs. 25.3 and 25.4) and the presence of microthromboemboli cannot be found in every individual case (Horwitz et al., 1972; Vogel et al., 1973; Coalson et al., 1975; Mittermayer et al., 1977).

MICROTHROMBI AS MORPHOLOGICAL EQUIVALENTS OF SHOCK

The reversible aggregates of the thrombocytes occurring in the terminal vascular bed associated with thrombocytopenia seen in the peripheral circulation are the

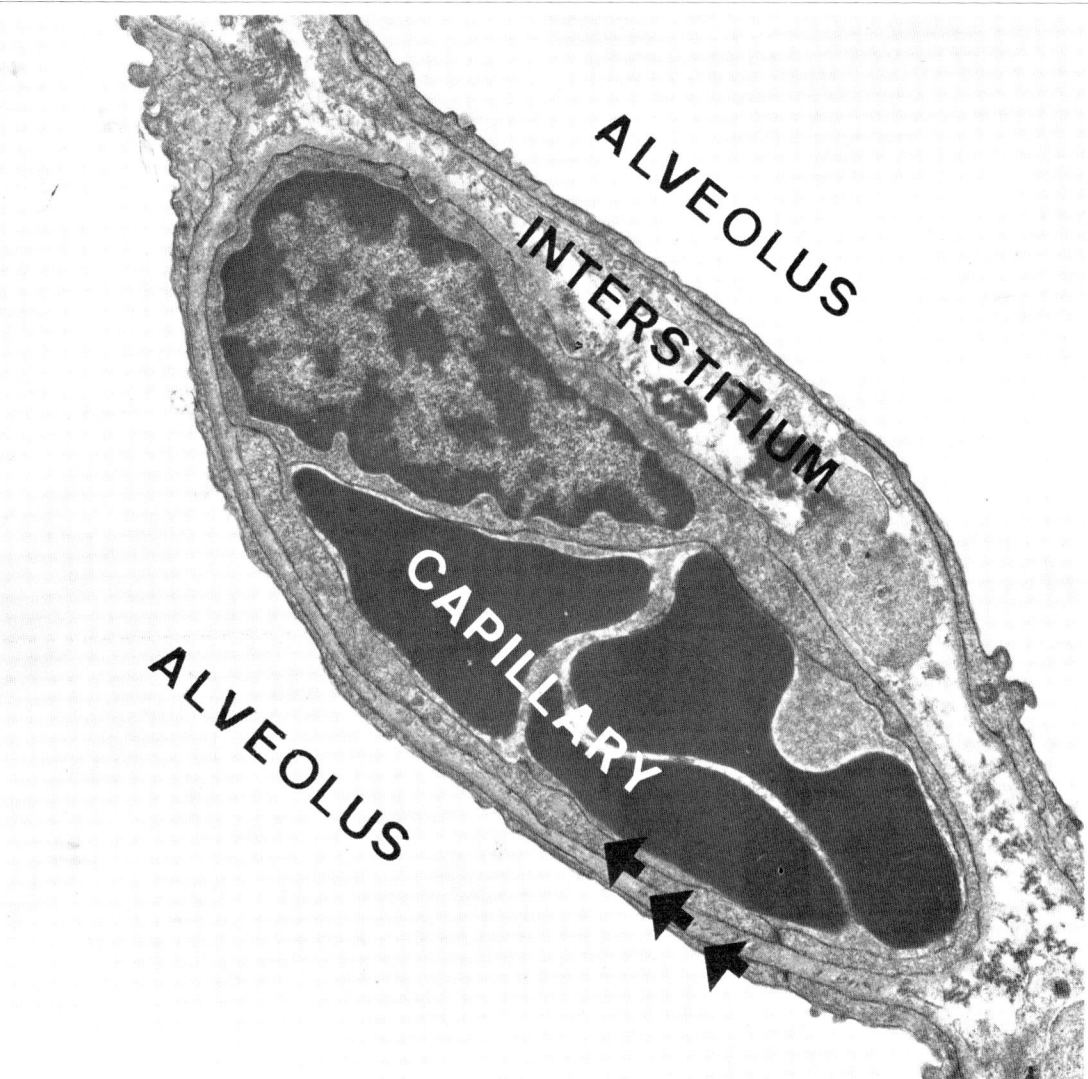

Figure 25.3. Ultrastructure of a normal human alveolar wall (biopsy specimen). Note the thin, three-layered blood-exchange barrier (*arrows*), which consists of a thin layer of endothelium, a narrow interstitial space, and a thin epithelial layer of membranous alveocytes. ×8.500.

first underlying morphological conditions of the generalized microcirculatory disturbance that is characteristic of shock. At first, some of these aggregates of the thrombocytes reenter the general circulation. Only at a later stage do the irreversible aggregates of the thrombocytes develop in the peripheral circulation. They release the vasoactive peptides, ADP, serotonin, histamine, catechol amines, prostaglandines, and other substances during the viscous metamorphosis. After having been drained into the terminal vascular bed, the thrombocytes cause a temporary vasoconstriction associated with an increased pressure within the region of the pulmonary artery and an acute overload of the right heart (Neuhof et al., 1977). A generalized plasmatic hypercoagulability is the first sign of activated blood clotting observed within the peripheral circulation. It is characterized by fibrin monomers that have been discharged from the peripheral circulation into the terminal vascular bed. At a later stage, soluble fibrinoligomers are present, and because of them fibrin is precipitated by means of microthrombi. Both the soluble fibrin monomers and the fibrinoligomers that show a transverse cross linking are stopped in the cells of the reticuloendothelial system (RES) (Bleyl, 1978). This process is composed of two phases. The fibrin monomers are first absorbed at the surface of the cells of the RES in order to enable intracellular digestion following phagocytosis. During intracellular digestion, the ability of the cells of the RES to continue absorption is lost; there is a blockage of the RES. The circulating fibrin complexes seen within the terminal vascular bed are removed, on the one hand, because of the proteolytic property of the granulocytes and, on the other, because of the fibrinolytic capacity of the pulmonary endothelial cells (Fig. 25.5) If, however, the intravascular activation of the clotting mechanisms within the periphery of the circulation proceeds very rapidly, both the granulocytes

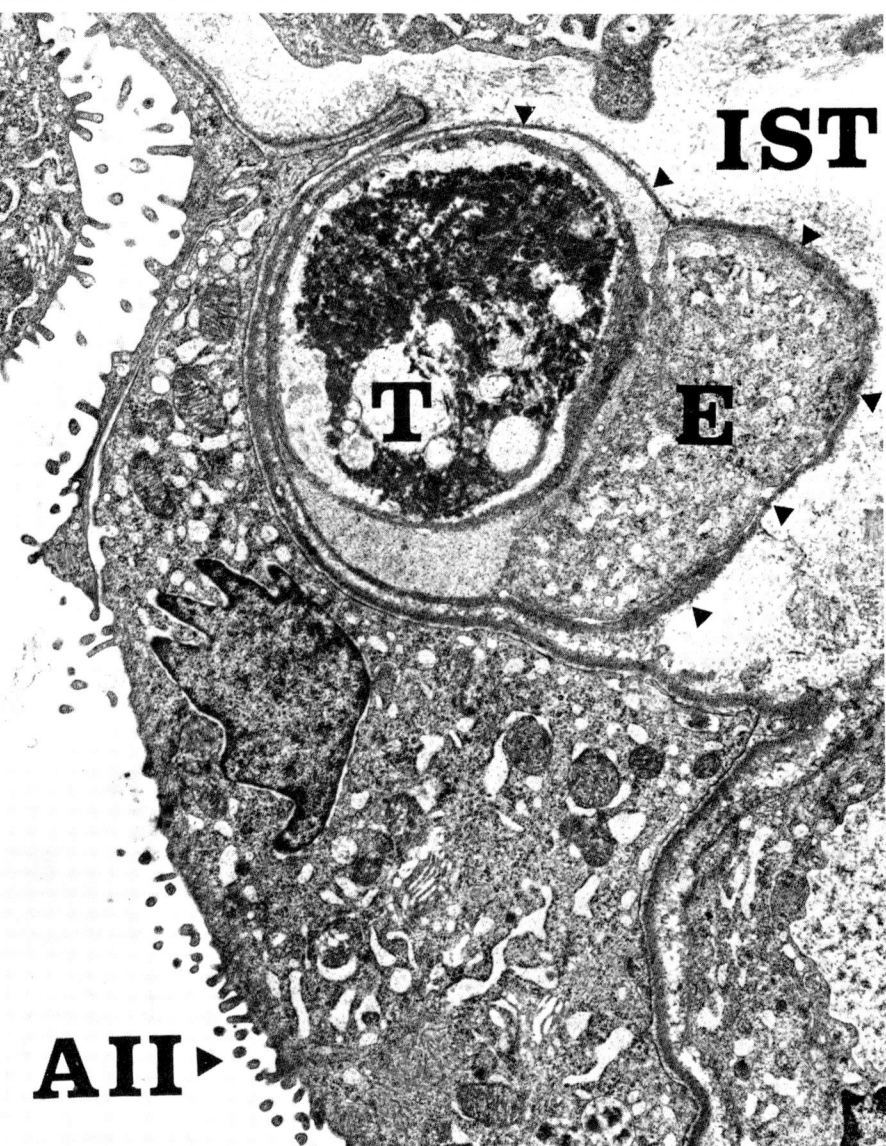

Figure 25.4. Case of early shock; "Ultra-microscopical thrombus" (*T*) in a damaged capillary of which only cell debris (*E*) and an empty basement membrane (*arrow*) remains. The interstitium is dispersed (*Ist*). Alveocytes type II (*A II*). ×9.500.

and the RES are no longer in a position to remove the fibrin complexes that are circulating within the vessels; as a result, there is an occurrence of highly polymerous microthrombi in the terminal vascular bed (Fig. 25.6). These intravascular formations of thrombi are the morphological correlative of consumption coagulopathy, and their appearance may vary depending on the particular type of shock (Mittermayer et al., 1977)

WHAT ARE THE CONSEQUENCES OF EPITHELIAL NECROSIS?

Shock-induced injury to the cells does, however, involve not only the cells of the pulmonary endothelium but also those of the alveolar capillary epithelium. It is first seen to affect the sensitive membranous alveocytes type I, thus destroying the epithelial layer specialized for the gas exchange in the pulmonary alveoles. The contacts of the cells lying between the alveolar epithelium burst (Fig. 25.7). This is followed by a necrosis of the more resistant granular alveocytes type II. As a result, both the capacity of the alveolar wall to regenerate and the development of the antiatelectatic factor (surfactant) are reduced. Consequently, fibrin monomers and oligomers leaving the pulmonary capillaries first enter the alveolar interstitium. When necrosis has reached a more advanced stage in the alveolar epithelial layer and in the adjoining basal membrane, fibrin monomers and oligomers will also project into the alveolar lumen. There the fibrin links the cellular debris to the pulmonary hyaline membranes. Furthermore, the alveolar walls are getting sticky, thereby increasing the inclination of the lung parenchyma to produce atelectases (Fig. 25.8).

WHAT ARE THE CHARACTERISTIC FEATURES OF THE LATE STAGE?

A chance exists in about 50% of the patients who have

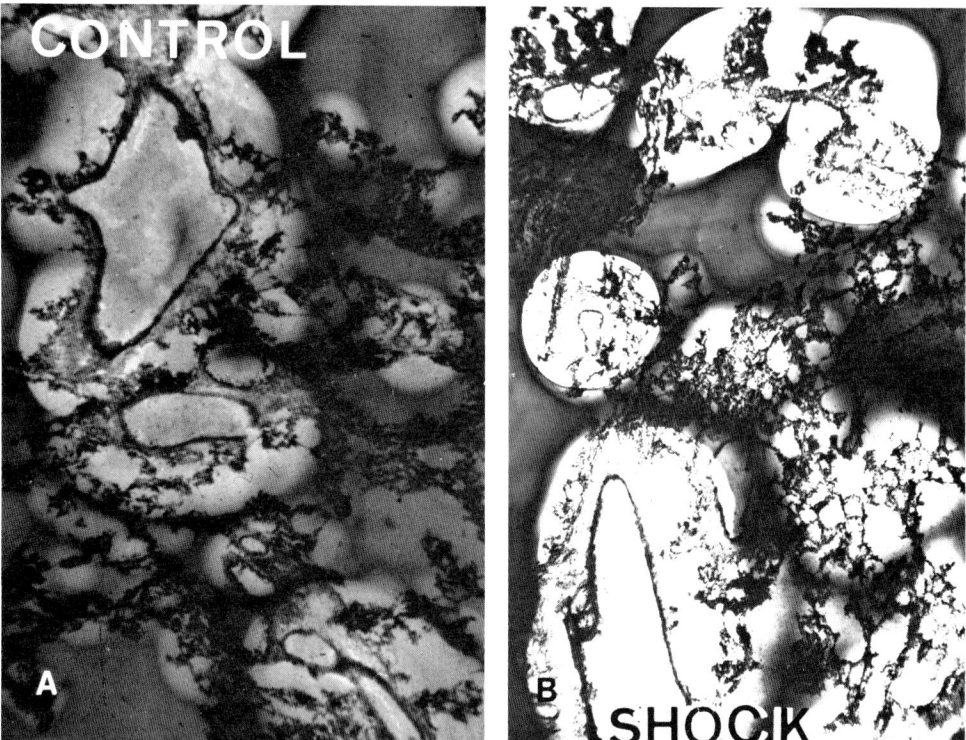

Figure 25.5. *A*, fibrin-histoautogram of a normal lung: the fibrin covering the lung parenchyma is carried away by the fibrinolytic capacity of the blood vessels. ×40. *B*, fibrin-histoautogram in shock lung: in early shock, the fibrinolytic activity of the lung parenchyma is increased, so that the degree of fibrinolysis in situ is intensified. ×40.

survived the shock-induced injury to the lung parenchyma up to this stage that the radiological and histological changes seen in the lung may be healed and that a satisfactory functioning of the lung will be regained (Ostendorf et al., 1975; Yernault et al., 1975). In the cases of severe shock, the pathological process will, however, take a progressive course. A reticularly striped pattern within the pulmonary fields is seen in the radiographs (Fig. 25.2) (Ostendorf et al., 1975). This is in accordance with the clinical picture of respiratory insufficiency resistant to therapy. The reticular pattern seen in the chest film may be explained histologically both by a proliferation of fibroblasts and by an increased fibroplasia within the peribronchovascular connective tissue of the alveolar interstitium (Riede et al., 1977). Based on ultrastructural and morphometric findings, the onset of the interstitial fibrosis of the lung is initiated by a considerable widening of the endothelial and epithelial gas exchange barrier (Reide et al., 1977). This indicates the beginning of cell regeneration in the epithelium and endothelium of the alveolar wall at the end of the 1st week. Both processes result in an overshooting cell repair in the alveolar wall which will have serious consequences in those patients who survive the shock-producing event for longer than 1 week (Bachofen and Weibel, 1974; Riede et al., 1977, 1978). Due to this incidence, the structural and functional integrity of the alveolar wall is destroyed. A thickening is seen in the alveolar wall which is rarefied because of a destruction of the capillaries in the vessels. The small number of remaining lung capillaries are pushed away from the gas-exchanging surface of the alveolus and are surrounded by a fibrosed connective tissue (Riede et al., 1978). A regeneration takes place, and the gaps in the alveolar wall that are being produced by the necrosis of the membranous alveocytes become overgrown with bulky alveocytes type II which are useless for the exchange of gases (Fig. 25.9). This incidence and the presence of the hyaline membranes that can be observed frequently are the reason for a decreasing partial pressure of oxygen in the arteries in shock patients with a simultaneously increasing thickening of the barrier of the alveolar interstitium. Due to the exponential and not linear nature of this process, this critical threshold of respiratory insufficiency is not reached gradually by the patients but is unexpected and sudden (Fig. 25.10).

CAN RESPIRATORY INSUFFICIENCY IN SHOCK BE CONSIDERED A PROBLEM OF DIFFUSION?

The morphometric findings obtained reveal that in the early stage of shock lung the arithmetic mean thickness of the barrier of the alveolar capillary membrane is hardly enlarged, although it shows a considerable increase in the late stage (Riede et al., 1978). From this we can conclude that because of the narrowed gas exchange

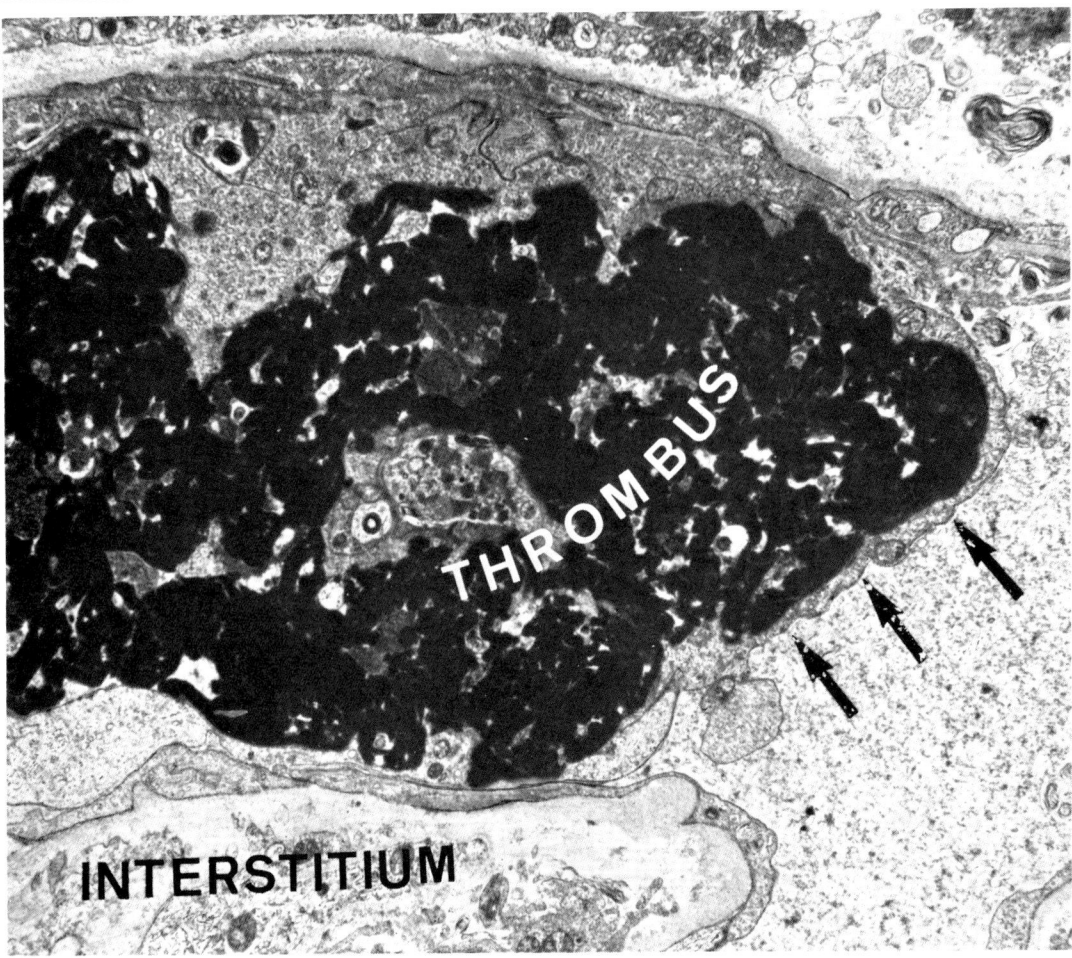

Figure 25.6. Hyaline thrombus in a pulmonary alveolar capillary. The thrombus in the lumen has already been covered with a layer of endothelium (*arrow*); the microvascular clotting is therefore already a few days old. ×7.500.

barrier, diffusion remains virtually unaltered regarding the structures in the early stage of shock. In the late stage of shock, however, when, due to fibrosis, the alveolar septa are enlarged as much as 10-fold in comparison with the normal value, a disturbed diffusion must be expected to be the cause of respiratory insufficiency. When comparing the capacity of diffusion obtained from ultrastructural measurements in shock lungs with that found in lungs affected by fibrosis (Fig. 25.11), the latter show a significantly increased thickening of the alveolar wall that is associated with an improved oxygen saturation of the blood as compared to that seen in shock lungs. It can therefore be concluded that shock-induced fibrosis of the lung develops on the basis of a mechanism other than fibroses of different etiology and that shock-induced respiratory insufficiency results only partly from a disturbed diffusion. It can rather be assumed that respiratory insufficiency is produced by a disturbance of the perfusion.

This assumption is based on the following arguments: 1) in shock microcirculation is partly obstructed by microthrombi, 2) there is a continuously decreasing reduction of the capillary content in the alveolar septa with increasing duration of shock; and 3) particularly in the late phase of shock, postmortem angiograms of the lungs show a rarefication of the vascular tree (Fig. 25.12).

IS SHOCK-INDUCED FIBROSIS OF THE LUNG REVERSIBLE?

Today we are in a position to affirm definitely that shock-induced interstitial fibrosis of the lung is capable of regression. This is suggested by findings obtained from animal experiments (Gross et al., 1962) and is to be expected from the results seen in patients that could be observed over a long period of time (Lamarre et al., 1973; Yernault et al., 1975). This process of reversibility in human shock lung could be demonstrated in one case by a study combining radiological and pathohistological findings (Mittermayer et al., 1979). In this case, the traumatic shock-producing event was followed by an interstitial fibrosis of the lung. The final condition showed occasional scarred fields that could not be distin-

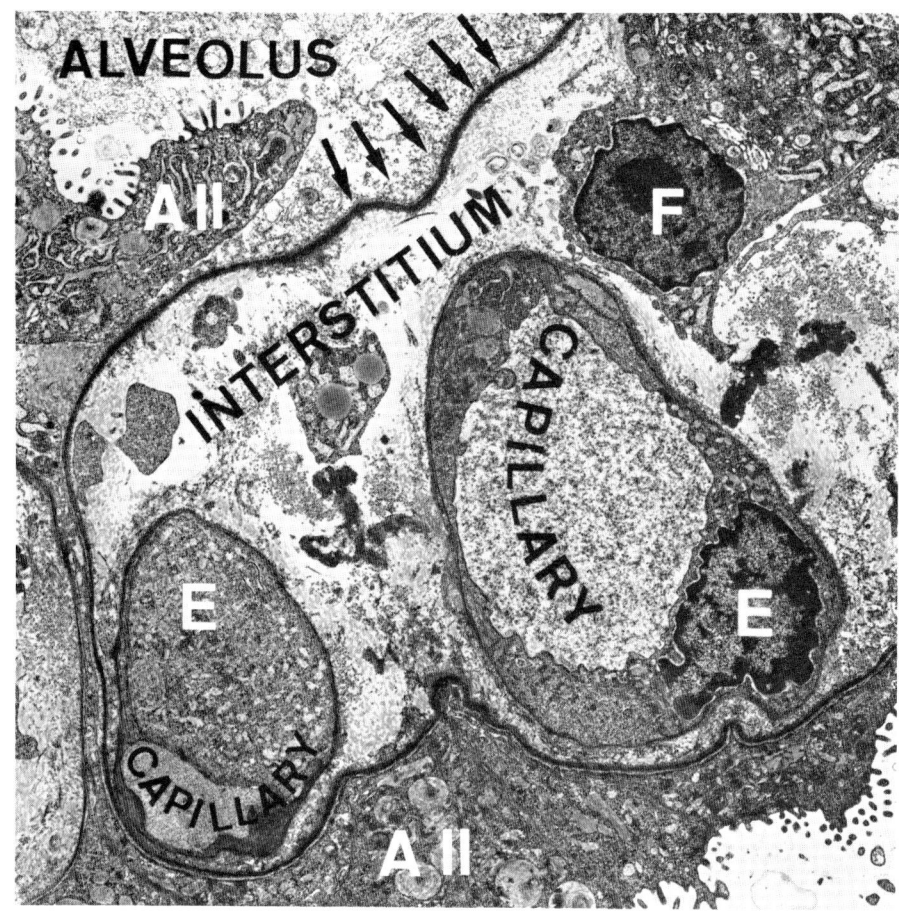

Figure 25.7. Ultrastructure of a alveolar wall in the case of traumatic shock 4 days after onset of shock. The injured capillaries float in the alveolar interstitial space in a pool of edema fluid. *E*, endothelium; *F*, fibroblasts. The injured alveocytes are removed from their as yet intact basal membrane (*arrows*). ×6.500.

guished from tuberculous scars. In the meantime, four other cases of shock-induced fibrosis of the lung (Fig. 25.13), having reached the stage of regression, have been analyzed. In all cases a persisting diffuse interstitial fibrosis of the alveolar septa could be seen. Correspondingly, a reticular pattern of the pulmonary fields may be recognized in the chest film after a number of years. The alveolar septa are morphometrically enlarged in correspondence with a focal interstitial increase of collagenous, elastic fibrous material. The normal collagenous fibrous tissue of the lung is composed of collagen types I and III. The latter is mainly synthesized by the smooth muscle cells (cf. to literature by Huang, 1977). In shock-induced pulmonary fibrosis, the immature collagen fibers most likely consist of collagen type III, since in these lungs a proliferation of myofibroblasts can be observed in addition to an increase of fibers.

WHAT ARE THE DECISIVE FACTORS FOR THE REVERSIBILITY OF SHOCK LUNG?

This question has still to be elucidated for there is only a small number of cases known in which shock lung has reached the stage of reversibility. The following comments can, however, be made:

1. All cases reported so far of patients who had survived a shock-induced respiratory insufficiency showed the following characteristics: all patients had suffered from traumatic shock; they were between 18 and 35 years of age (mostly nonsmokers); and their history did not include a preceding affection of the lung (Lakshminarayan and Hudson, 1978; Yernault et al., 1975; Rotman et al., 1977; Klein et al., 1976; Mittermayer et al., 1978). These characteristics are in accordance with the four cases which we observed.

2. Findings obtained from animal experiments revealed that a damage to the lung parenchyma will only heal completely as long as the basal membrane remains intact (Vracko, 1972). We were able to confirm these findings by producing endotoxin shock in the domesticated hog (Riede and Schäfer, unpublished data). In the four cases which we observed, the alveolar basal membrane had also remained intact during the acute stage of shock; this must be considered as a true gleam of hope for the affected patient (cf. Schnells et al, 1979).

HOW CAN LUNG FIBROSIS IN SHOCK BE GROUPED WITHIN THE SYSTEM OF LUNG FIBROSES?

Shock-induced pulmonary fibrosis of the interstitial-proliferative type is mainly found in the perialveolar parts of the lung but does involve, to a lesser extent, the bronchioles and perilobular septa of the connective tis-

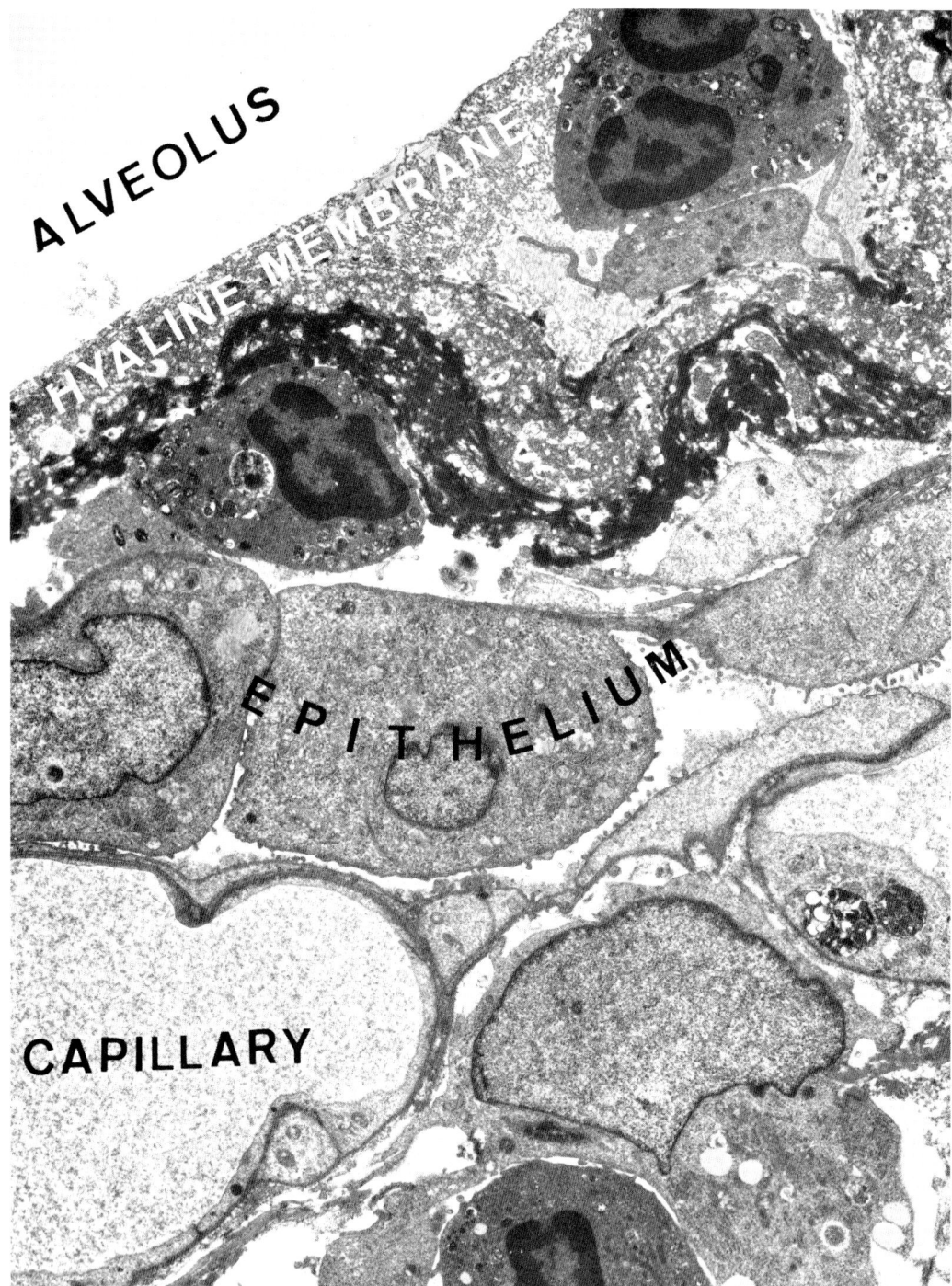

Figure 25.8. Ultrastructure of a hyaline membrane in a shock lung from a case of septic shock. ×7.500.

sue. This process of fibrosis is preceded by exudative alveolitis. In contrast to the types of interstitial pulmonary fibroses described so far (Otto, 1975), shock-induced fibrosis takes a rapid and progressive course (Bohlig, 1975; v. Wichert, 1979). The advancing disease is composed of several phases. It will be found only in a certain part of the lung, and therefore a variety of different simultaneously occurring stages of this clinical picture may be seen in the same lung. Shock-induced pulmonary fibrosis is classified on the basis of a histological grading into grades I–V. It is noteworthy that the condition progresses rapidly within 14–21 days by passing through all grades I–IV (IV = destruction of the lung structure) without ever reaching grade V (V = atelectatic-indurative fibrosis, emphysematous pulmonary sclerosis) (Spencer, 1977). Because of its formal pathogenesis,

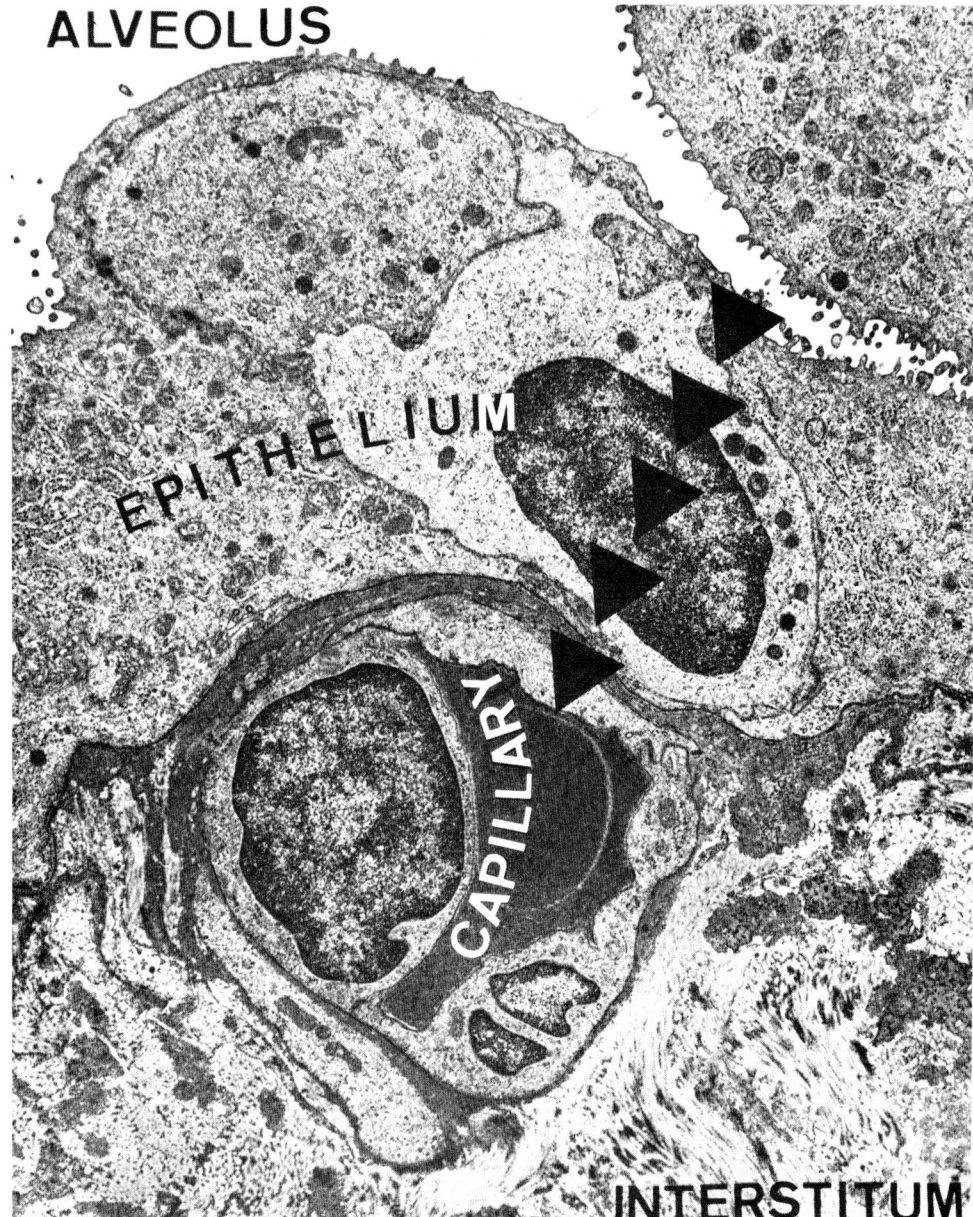

Figure 25.9. Ultrastructure of human alveolar wall in the late stage of shock. The alveolar wall is diffusely thickened. Capillaries lie in a fibrosed and thickened interstitial space and have been forced away from the alveolar surface by the cuboidal epithelium. Because of this, gaseous exchange is impaired and compliance is reduced to a level which threatens the life of the patient. ×6.500.

shock-induced pulmonary fibrosis must therefore be included in the category of "alveolitic pulmonary fibrosis."

IS A RESTITUTIO AD INTEGRUM SEEN IN SHOCK-INDUCED PULMONARY FIBROSIS?

The cases investigated also showed that shock-induced pulmonary fibrosis cannot be completely healed as far as the structure and the function of the lung are concerned. This observation is in agreement with the investigations performed by other authors. According to their observations, about 40% of all patients who survived a shock-induced respiratory insufficiency showed an impaired capacity of diffusion. In about 30% of the patients, the partial pressure of oxygen in the arteries was reduced in the case of physical exercise (Yernault et al., 1975; Lakshminarayan et al., 1976). Furthermore, 25% of the patients showed an obstruction of the gaseous exchange (Lakshmina-Rayan and Hudson, 1978). This is in agreement with the four cases we observed, so that a possible correlation may be assumed in regard to the proliferation of those myofibroblasts within the alveolar interstitium

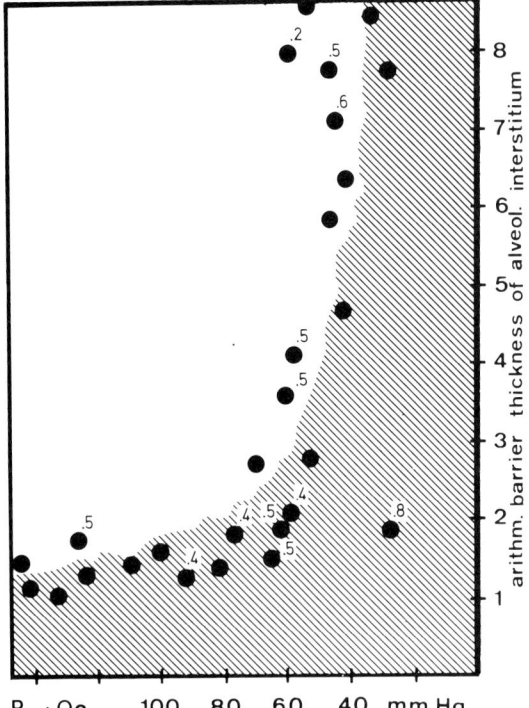

Figure 25.10. Correlation between thickness of the interstitial barrier of the alveolar wall (cf. Figs. 25.3 and 25.9) and the PaO_2 in patients who survived the original shock-producing event for different periods of time. The PaO_2 is reduced with increased duration of shock. Note the exponential nature of the reduction in blood gas levels alongside the reduction of respiratory function.

having contractile properties (Kapanci et al., 1974). This assumption is also supported by the fact that an administration of bronchospasmolysants gives a relief to the breathing mechanism in this condition of shock-induced obstruction (Lakshminarayan and Hudson, 1978).

DOES A RELATIONSHIP EXIST BETWEEN PULMONARY EDEMA AND PULMONARY FIBROSIS DURING SHOCK?

If one considers the fact that in the early stage of shock both the alveolar and the extra-alveolar interstitium are enlarged due to an edema and, in the late stage of shock due to a proliferation of fibroblasts, the question arises as to whether these two events are produced by a common cause that may explain the observation. This assumption is supported by animal experiments. Findings obtained from these experiments revealed that in shock the thoracic lymph contains a growth-stimulating factor which has a proliferating effect on the lung fibroblasts in vitro (Mittermayer et al., 1977; Mittermayer and Riede, 1978). The observation is particularly noteworthy because this proliferation-stimulating characteristic of the thoracic lymph must be attributed to a low molecular fraction possibly being produced by proteolysis of larger molecules (Mittermayer et al., 1978; Riede et al., 1979). Such an assumption coincides with the observation of an increased activity of lysosomal enzymes in shock lymph (Clermont and Williams, 1972).

Besides the proliferated fibroblasts seen in the fibrosed alveolar walls, so called matrix vesicles are also present. Although the lysosomal nature of some of these matrix vesicles has been confirmed morphologically and functionally (cf. Riede and Staubesand, 1977), their role is not yet fully understood. They are invariably lying outside the cytoplasmic regulation because of their extra-

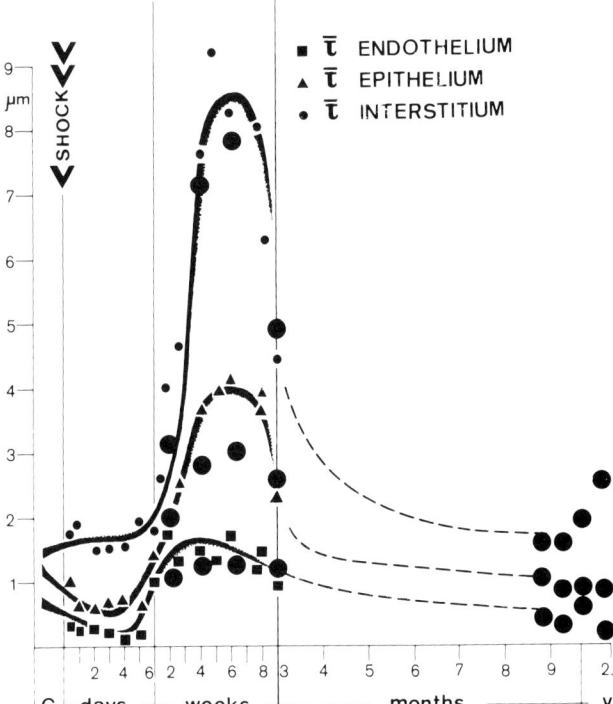

Figure 25.11. Morphometric analysis of human lung parenchyma in shock patients. Morphometric values from patients who died as a result of the shock are indicated in small black symbols. Values from patients who survived are shown in large dots. The thickness of the capillary endothelial barrier shows a reduction due to necrosis during the 1st day, followed by an increase after the 1st week due to regeneration. The thickness of the alveolar epithelial barrier (*triangles*) was also reduced during the 1st day and then increased owing to reepithelialization with cuboidal cells. The thickness of the alveolar interstitial barrier (*triangles*) showed a small but recognizable increase. In the late stage of shock, however, it increased to seven-fold its normal value due to fibrosis. In four cases, biopsies taken at least 1 year later showed gradual return of morphometric values to the gas-exchange barrier (arithmetic mean thickness) to normal.

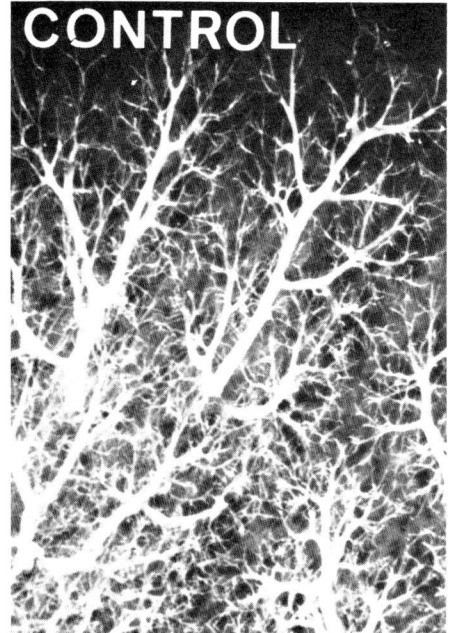
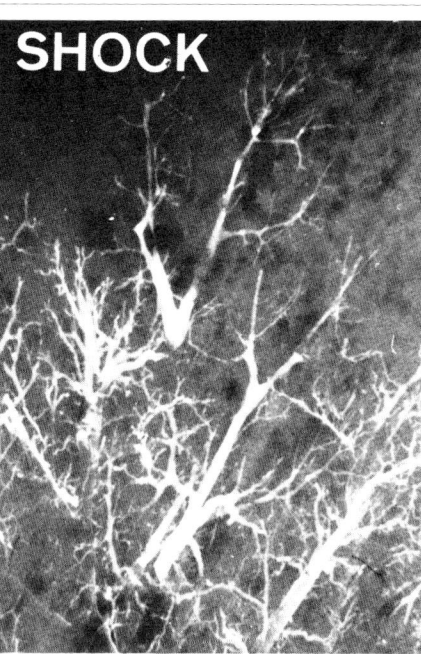

Figure 25.12. Microangiogram (fixation with formol vapor) of control and shock lung. Control shows well developed vascular tree. The shock lung shows a rarefaction of the vascular tree.

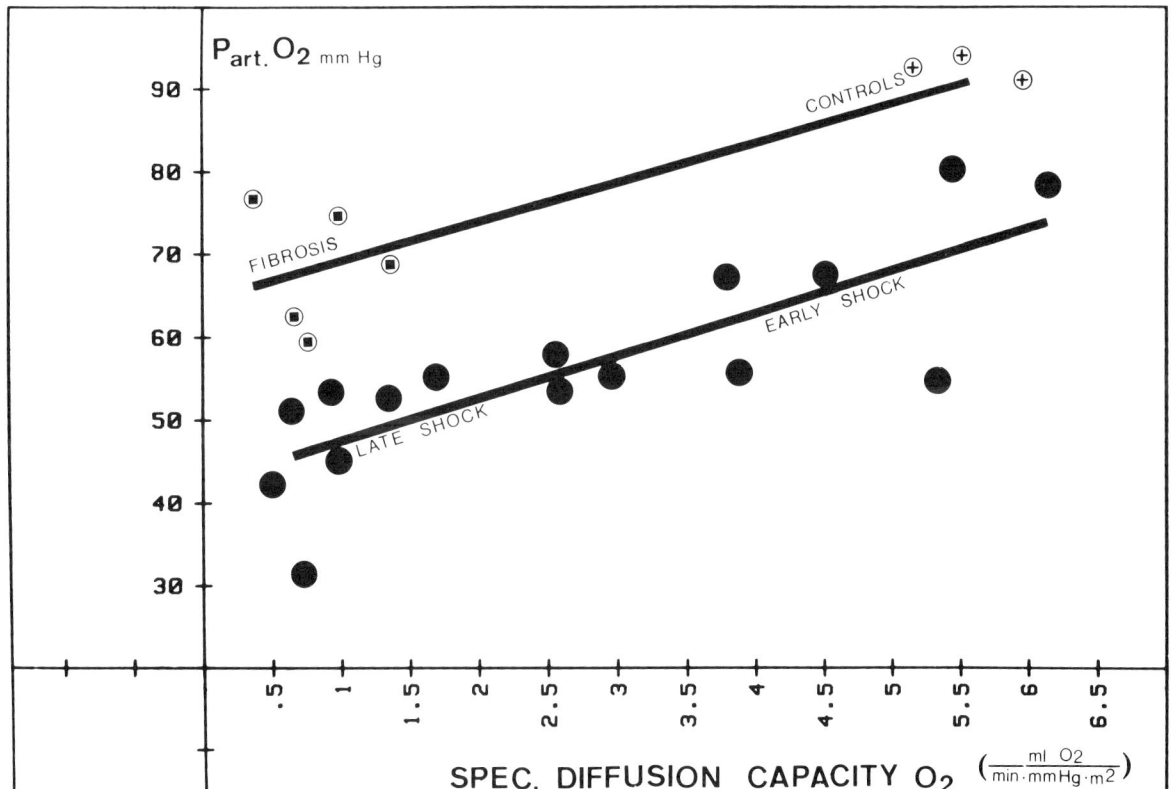

Figure 25.13. Correlation between specific diffusion capacity of the alveolar wall (computer plot) (method, Weibel, 1973) and the PaO_2 in shock patients, in controls, and in patients with idiopathic lung fibrosis. The diffusion capacity is reduced with increased duration of shock. The fibrotic alveoli as well as the alveoli in the late stage of shock reveal similar values of the diffusion capacity but decreased values of PaO_2. Therefore, in shock a disturbance of lung perfusion rather than diffusion must be assumed.

cellular position between the collagen fibers. Due to their catabolic capacity, they would be able to maintain the self-perpetuating process of shock-induced lung fibrosis by way of a permanent damage to the connective tissue. Patients having reached this late stage of shock are inclined to spontaneously develop a progressive lung fibrosis.

SUMMARY

Interstitial edema in the alveolar septa is the first morphologically recognizable change to be observed in cases of shock. It is brought about by the altered function of the membranes of the damaged epithelium and endothelium in the alveolar wall. At the same time, there is an impairment of gas exchange, which is rendered more difficult by the exudative process in the interstitium. Pari passu with these events, there is injury to the cells of both the alveolar epithelium and the alveolar capillary endothelium. Both of these processes are still reversible. The point of irreversibility appears to be reached, at the end of the 1st week; after which the injurious effects on the cell are established, since the thin alveolar wall necessary for the exchange of gases becomes overgrown with bulky alveocytes (type II), and the fibroblasts in the alveolar interstitium crowd the capillaries away from the surface of the alveolus. In most of the advanced cases of shock, this process of thickening of the alveolar wall exceeds the critical value, and respiratory exchange is so impaired that satisfactory functioning of the lungs is no longer possible.

Acknowledgments. This paper was selected for the F.K. Frey prize, 1980, from the German Society of Anesthesiology and Intensive Medicine and was translated into English from the original German by Lilo Riedel, Institute of Pathology, University of Freiburg, Freiburg, West Germany.

References

Ackermann, N.R., and Bebee, J.R.: Release of lysosomal enzymes by alveolar mononuclear cells. Nature 247:475–477, 1974.

Bachofen, M. and Weibel, E.R.: Basic pattern of tissue repair in human lungs following unspecific injury. Chest 65:14–19, 1974.

Bergmann, H.: Die Pathophysiologie der Beatmungslunge (Einführungsreferat). In *Kongreßbericht DGAW Jährestagung Erlangen,* 2.–5.10.1974, edited by E. Rügheimer, pp. 419–442. Perimed, Erlangen, 1975.

Bleyl, U., Rieger, R., and Rossner, J.A.: Identification of soluble fibrinogen monomer complexes by nonenzymatic polymerization in the tissue. Virchows. Arch. [Pathol. Anat.] 378:67–83, 1978.

Bohlig, H.: Die Lungenfibrose im Röntgenbild. In *Tuberkulose-Bücherei. Monographien zur Monatsschrift "Praxis der Pneumologie" vereinigt mit "Der Tuberkuloseaarzt"* edited by R. Griesbach und R.W. Müller and Interstitielle Lungenerkankungen-Lungenfibrosen, edited by J. Hamm, pp. 74, 75. Georg Thieme Verlag, Stuttgart, 1975.

Clermont, G.H., and Williams, J.S.: Lymph lysosomal enzyme acid phosphatase in hemorrhagic shock. Ann. Surg., 176:90–96, 1972.

Coalson, J.J., Hinshaw, L.B., Guenter, C.A., Berrel, E.L., and Greenfield, L.J.: Pathophysiologic responses of the subhuman primate in experimental septic shock. Lab. Invest. 32:561–569, 1975.

Derks, C.M., and Peters, R.M.: The role of shock and fat embolus in leakage from pulmonary capillaries. Surg. Gynecol. Obstet. 137:945–948, 1973.

Ferner, H.: Die lunge. In *Lehrbuch der Anatomie des Menschen,* vol. II, edited by Eingeweide und Kreislauf, p. 226. Urban & Schwarzenberg, München, 1977.

Fischer, H.: Schock und schockbekämpfung. Münch. Med. Wochenschr. 114:2091–2096, 1972.

Gerrity, R.G., Richardson, M., Caplan, B.A., Cade, J.F., Hirsh, J., and Schwartz, C.J.: Endotoxin-induced vascular endothelial injury and repair. II. Focal injury, en face morphology, (3_H) thymidine uptake and circulating endothelial cells in the dog. Exp. Mol. Pathol. 24:59–69, 1976.

Gross, P., McNerney, J.M., Westrick, M.L., and Babyak, M.A.: Resolution of chronic interstitial pneumonitis; Experimental observation. Arch. Pathol. 74:81–87, 1962.

Haberland, G.L.: Einleitende Bemerkungen zu den Grundlagen der Trasylolherapie. In *Neue Aspekte der Trasylol-Therapie II,* edited by R. Marx, H. Imdahl, and G.L. Haberland, pp. 1–9. Schattauer Verlag, Stuttgart, 1968.

Haberland, G.L.: Die Wirkung von Trasylol im Schockgeschehen In *Neue Aspekte der Trasylol-Therapie IV,* edited by G.L. Haberland, P. Huber, and P. Matis, pp. 109–116. Schattauer Verlag, Stuttgart, 1970.

Henson, P.M., McCarthy, K., Larsen, G.L., Webster, R.O., Giclas, P.C., Dreisin, R.B., King, T.E., and Shaw, J.O.: Complement fragments alveolar macrophages and alveolitis, Am. J. Pathol. 97:93–110, 1979.

Herzog, H.: Akute respiratorische Insuffizienz. Intensivmedizin. (Suppl. I) 13:69, 1976.

Horwitz, D.L., Moquin, R.B., and Herman, C.M.: Coagulation changes of septic shock in the subhuman primate and their relationship to hemodynamic changes. Ann. Surg. 1975:417–428, 1972.

Huang, T.W.: Chemical and histochemical studies of human alveolar collagen fibers. Am. J. Pathol., 86:81–98, 1977.

Hurley, J.V.: Current views on the mechanisms of pulmonary edema. J. Pathol. 125:59–79, 1978.

Joachim, H., Vogel, W., and Mittermayer, C.: Untersuchungen zum Phänomen der Schocklunge. Z. Rechtsmed. 78:13–23, 1976.

Joachim, H., Riede, U.N., and Mittermayer, C.: The weight of human lungs as a diagnostic criterion. Pathol. Res. Pract. 162:24–40, 1978.

Kapanci, Y., Assimacopoulos, A., Irle, C., Zwahlen, A., and Gabbiani, G.: "Contractile interstitial cells" in pulmonary alveolar septa: A possible regulator of ventilation/perfusion ratio. J. Cell. Biol. 60:375–392, 1974.

Klein, J.J., vanHaeringen, J.R., Sluiter, H.J., et al.: Pulmonary function after recovery from the adult respiratory distress syndrome. Chest 69:350–355, 1976.

Lakshminarayan, S., and Hudson, L.D.: Pulmonary function following the adult respiratory distress syndrome. Chest 74:489–490, 1978.

Lakshminarayan, S., Stanford, R.E., and Petty, T.L.: Prognosis after recovery from adult respiratory distress syndrome. Am. Rev. Respir. Dis. 113:7–16, 1976.

Lamarre, A., Linsao, L., Reilly, B.J., Swyer, P.R., and Levison, H.: Residual pulmonary abnormalities in survivors of idiopathic respiratory distress syndrome. Am. Rev. Respir. Dis. 108:56–61, 1973.

Lauweryns, J.M., and Baert, J.H.: Alveolar clearance and the role of the pulmonary lymphatics. Am. Rev. Respir. Dis. *115*:625-683, 1977.

Mittermayer, C., and Sandritter W.: Besondere Manifestationen des Schocks beim Menschen. *Blutgerinnüng, Kreislauf, Stoffwechsel. Giessener Gerinnungsgespräche,* edited by H.G. Lasch and H. Neuhof, pp. 279-291. Schattauer Verlag, Stuttgart, 1971.

Mittermayer, C., Ostendorf, P., and Riede, U.N.: Pathologisch-anatomische Untersuchungen bei der respiratorischen Insuffizienz durch Schock. I. Lichtmikroskopische und Biochemische Analyse. Intensivmedizin *14*:252-262, 1977.

Mittermayer, C., Riede, U.N., Bleyl, U., Herzog, H., v. Wichert, P., Riesner, K.: Schocklunge Verh. Dtsch. Ges. Pathol. *62:* 11-65, 1978.

Mittermayer, C., Riede, U.N., and McEwan, J.R.: II. Morphologie der Spätphase. *Pathologisch-anatomische Untersuchungen der Schocklunge: Spätschäden und Irreversibilität.* INA-Reihe (Intensivmedizin, Notfallmedizin, Anästhesiologie), vol. 16, pp. 163-170. Georg Thieme Verlag, Stuttgart, 1979.

Myrvold, H.E., and Svalander, C. Pulmonary microembolism in early experimental septic shock. J. Surg. Res. *23*:65-74, 1977.

Neuhof, H., Platt, D., Braehler, A. and Müller, P.: Die Wirkung von Prednisolon auf Letalität, Aktivität lysosomaler Enzyme und Haemodynamik bei Endotoxinaemie. Intensivmedizin *14*:378-386, 1977.

Ostendorf, P., Birzle, H., Vogel, W. Mittermayer, C.: Pulmonary radiographic abnormalities in shock. Radiology *115:* 257-263, 1975.

Otto, H.: Zur Morphologie des Endbildes und der behandlungsbedürftigen Frühphasen interstitieller Lungenfibrosen. In *Tuberkulose-Bücherei. Monographien zur Monatsschrift "Praxis der Pneumologie" vereingtt mit "Det Tuberkuloseaarzt,"* edited by R. Griesbach und R.W. Müller and Interstitielle Lungenerkrankungen-Lungenfibrosen, edited by J. Hamm, pp. 1-9. Georg Thieme Verlag, Stuttgart, 1975.

Pingleton, W.W., Coalson, J.J., Hinshaw, L.B., and Guenter, C.A.: Effect of steroid pretreatment on development of shock lung. Lab. Invest., *27*:445-456, 1972.

Riede, U.N., and Staubesand, J.: A unifying concept for the role of matrix vesicles and lysosomes in the formal pathogenesis of disease of connective tissue and blood vessels. Beitr. Pathol. *160*:3-37, 1977.

Riede, U.N., Mittermayer, C., Hassenstein, J., and Bensing, K.: Pathologisch-anatomische Untersuchungen bei der respiratorischen Insuffizienz durch Schock. II. Ultrastrukturell-morphometrische befunde. Intensivmedizin *14*:263-273, 1977.

Riede, U.N., Joachim, H., Costabel, U., Hassenstein, J., Sandritter, W., Augustin, P., and Mittermayer, C.: The pulmonary air-blood barrier of human shock lung (A clinical, ultrastructural and morphometric study). Pathol. Res. Pract. *162*:41-72, 1978.

Riede, U.N., Mittermayer, C., Friedburg, H., Wybitul, K. and Sandritter, W.: Morphologic development of human shock lung. Pathol. Res. Pract. *165*:269-286, 1979.

Rotman, H.H., Lavelle, T.F., Jr., Dimcheff, D.G., et al.: Long-term physiologic consequences of the adult respiratory distress syndrome. Chest *72*:190-192, 1977.

Ryan, S.F., and Ryan, U.S.: Pulmonary endothelial cells. Fed. Proc. *36*:2683-2690, 1977.

Schneeberger, E.E.: Ultrastructure of intercellular junctions in the freeze fractured alveolar-capillary membrane of mouse lung. Chest *71*:299-300, 1977.

Schnells, G., Voigt, H.W., Redl, H., Schlag, G., and Glatzl, A.: Elektronenmikroskopische Untersuchungen an menschlichen Lungenbiopsien zum Verlauf der posttraumatischen respirattorischen insuffizienz. INA-Reihe (Intensivmedizin, Notfallmedizin, Anaesthesiologie), vol. 16, pp. 171-180. Georg Thieme Verlag, Stuttgart, 1979.

Spencer, H.: *Pathology of the Lung.* ed. 3, pp. 235-240. Pergamon Press, New York, 1977.

Vogel, W., Walter, F., Mittermayer, C., Böttcher, D., Zimmerman, W.E., and Birzle, H.: Pulmonale mikrothrombosierung bei hyperkoagulabilität. In *International Symposium in Freiburg, 1971,* edited by K. Wiemers, and K.L. Scholler, pp. 289-298. Georg Thieme Verlag, Stuttgart, 1973.

Vracko, R.: Significance of basal lamina for regeneration of injured lung. Virchows Arch. [Pathol. Anat.] *355*:264-274, 1972.

Weibel, E.R.: Morphological basis of alveolar-capillary gas exchange. Physiol. Rev. *53*:419-495, 1973.

v. Wichert, P.: Alveolarwandphysiologie und Surfactant. Verh. Dtsch. Ges. Pathol. *62*:29-34, 1978.

v. Wichert, P.: Die Schocklunge. Med. Klin. *74*:1-8, 1978.

Yernault, J.C., Englert, M., Sergysels, R., DeCoster, A.: Pulmonary mechanics and diffusion after shock lung. Thorax *30*:252-257, 1975.

CHAPTER 26

Pulmonary Alveolarcapillary Permeability in Human Septic Respiratory Distress Syndrome

WILLIAM J. SIBBALD
A. A. DRIEDGER

The adult respiratory distress syndrome (ARDS) has been recognized as a clinical entity for at least three decades. ARDS characterized by pulmonary insufficiency secondary to pulmonary edema, excluding that which occurs due to acute myocardial disease, complicates acute medical and surgical illness. In 1946, Brewer et al., on the basis of experience in World War II, for the first time recorded that the lung was unique in its ability to respond to severe trauma to the chest, and to other parts of the body, by an increase in its water content, without apparent myocardial failure. Subsequently, a number of clinical reports have documented the high incidence of ARDS complicating systemic human sepsis (Fulton et al., 1975; Sibbald et al., 1978; Vito et al., 1974). In 1974, Vito and associates (Vito et al.) reported that of the surgical patients with acute respiratory insufficiency, 40% were subsequently shown to have systemic sepsis, mostly infradiaphragmatic. ARDS complicating systemic human sepsis may be a more frequent complication of gram-negative or gram-positive bacteremia than was previously appreciated. Kaplan et al. noted (1979) that 20 of 86 (23%) consecutive cases of gram-negative rod bacteremia were complicated by ARDS. Further, the mortality of patients developing ARDS complicating gram-negative rod bacteremia appears significantly greater than the reported mortality of ARDS from all other causes. In Vito's series of ARDS complicating sepsis, the mortality rate was 68% and was directly related to the ability to effectively manage the underlying sepsis (Vito et al., 1974).

Pulmonary edema secondary to sepsis is not an infrequent complication of a serious illness that requires hospitalization, which initially does not have a primary pulmonary impact. There is usually a latent period of several hours to a few days, described after hospitalization, during which time respiratory involvement is minimal or absent. After this latent period, if the underlying sepsis is not found and treated, acute respiratory failure may develop and progress to ultimately cause the patient's death (Murray, 1977). Not all people who develop septicemia will develop ARDS; however, the difference between those who do and those who do not is not known.

ARDS is clinically characterized by arterial hypoxemia secondary to an increase in intrapulmonary shunting; a reduction in compliance of the pulmonary parenchyma; a decrease in the functional residual capacity; a pattern of diffuse alveolar infiltrates on the chest roentgenograph, and the absence of any clinical or historical evidence to suggest heart failure (Sibbald et al., 1979a). Although many of these clinical sequelae are interrelated, all are the result of a diffuse, acute injury to the alveolo-capillary unit, which results in a loss of it's normal barrier function to the flux of fluid from vessels to the pulmonary interstitium and alveoli. Therefore, the basic lesion in ARDS complicating human sepsis is an increased permeability of the pulmonary alveolarcapillary membrane(s) so that intravascular fluid and solutes may freely traverse this barrier membrane, resulting in interstitial and alveolar edema or an increase in lung water (Gump et al., 1971). As a result of the increased lung water, the functional residual capacity will fall, as will the compliance. Hence, the lungs become "stiff" and manifest a requirement for high inspiratory pressures to generate adequate expansion. The fall in pulmonary compliance is due to an increase in elasticity, which is associated with pulmonary parenchymal congestion as well as decreased surfactant metabolism and increased surfactant destruction (Petty and Ashbaugh, 1971).

It is a frequent clinical observation that there is a spectrum of ARDS complicating human sepsis, which in all probability is related to the severity of the underlying septic process and the rapidity with which the septic process is recognized and clinically managed. However, despite the increased awareness of this complication of human sepsis, the morbidity and mortality of respiratory failure complicating human sepsis remains significant (Kaplan et al., 1979; Vito et al., 1974).

This chapter will review human and animal data which have accumulated to identify that the cause of pulmonary edema complicating human sepsis is a primary defect in the permeability of the barrier to transvascular flux of water and solutes at the level of the alveolarcapillary membrane(s). In addition, the potential agents responsible for this increased permeability and the pathological aberrations of the barrier membrane in sepsis that in part explain the cause of the pulmonary edema will be reviewed.

FLUID AND SOLUTE EXCHANGE IN THE LUNG

To develop the concept of an increase in permeability of the pulmonary microvasculature as the primary cause of the pulmonary edema accompanying human sepsis, a thorough understanding of the movement of solutes and water within the human lung in both normal and abnormal situations is required.

The flux of water and other solutes from the intravascular compartment to the interstitium and/or alveoli of the human lung is determined by an interplay of hydrostatic and osmotic pressures within the vessel and interstitium, as well as the conductance of the limiting barrier membranes. The principle of this relationship was initially described by Starling (1896) as:

$$\text{fluid flux} = \text{pressure} \times \text{conductance.} \quad (1)$$

However, with the appreciation that the pulmonary barrier membranes were not totally impermeant to proteins (Drenker and Field, 1931), the equation has been expanded and is more completely stated as:

$$Qf = K(Pmv - Ppmv) - \sigma(\pi mv - \pi pmv)* \quad (2)$$

where
- Qf = net transvascular fluid flow;
- K = fluid filtration coefficient or endothelial conductance;
- Pmv = hydrostatic pressure within the pulmonary vessels where fluid exchange takes place;
- $Ppmv$ = hydrostatic pressure within the interstitium;
- πmv = plasma protein osmotic pressure;
- πpmv = osmotic pressure in the interstitium; and
- σ = protein reflection coefficient, which determines the "effective" transvascular protein osmotic pressure difference (Staverman, 1951).

Another equation, derived by Kedem and Katchalsky (1958), describes protein flux across a homogeneous membrane. This parallel equation for protein flux describes net protein flux as equal to diffusive flux plus convective flux. Solute movement across the barrier endothelial membrane in the pulmonary microvasculature can occur by passive diffusion in response to concentration gradients on either side of the membrane or in response to water movement. Bulk flow of solute occurring by this latter method is related to the concentration of the particular molecule, its reflection coefficient, and the flow rate across the membrane. In symbols:

$$\dot{Q}s = \omega(\pi mv - \pi pmv) + (1 - \sigma)CsQf \quad (3)$$

where
- $\dot{Q}s$ = net protein flux;
- ω = true permeability coefficient for protein diffusion; and
- Cs = average concentration of protein across the microvascular membrane.

The majority of protein flux in the pulmonary microvasculature is diffusive.

Vischer et al. (1956) has described pulmonary edema as simply an increase in lung water. Filtration of water or solutes from the pulmonary microvasculature to the interstitium depends upon the balance of the Starling forces acting across the alveolocapillary barrier membrane. Even in health, Staub's group (1974) has shown that a net outward summation of forces exists from the intravascular compartment to the interstitium, thus normally favoring movement of fluid into the interstitium (Erdmann et al., 1975).

The Pmv is affected by gravity and increases vertically from the apex to the base of the lungs or from the anterior to posterior aspects of the lung when the patient is in the supine position. It is probable that because of resistance offered at the postcapillary venular level, the Pmv is not exactly equal to the left atrial pressure in zone III of the lung. Since the pulmonary capillary wedge pressure (PCWP) reflects the left atrial pressure (LAP) in a broad range of clinical situations in man (Lappas et al., 1973), it is often used as an indirect estimate of either the Pmv or the LAP for clinically deriving equation 4. However, in certain patients this may not be reasonable since gross discrepancies between the PCWP and the left ventricular end-diastolic pressure have been recorded, particularly in hyperdynamic human sepsis (Lefcoe et al., 1979). In animal and human studies (Brigham et al., 1974, 1979b), the Pmv has been calculated according to:

$$Pmv = Pla + 0.4(Ppa - Pla) \quad (4)$$

This equation has been derived from estimations of postcapillary venous resistance in isolated lung preparations in the animal model. It is not yet known whether this relationship may be applied to the human situation, where a similar appreciation of the magnitude of the pulmonary venous resistance in zone III remains largely unknown (Taylor and Drake, 1977). In zone II of the lung, the Pmv is influenced by the fact that through part of the cardiac cycle, alveolar pressure exceeds venous pressure. However, equations have also been described for this situation, where the Pmv may be estimated in experimental conditions (Staub, 1974). Again, there is little evidence to support the applicability of this equation in the human situation. Hence, the Pmv is difficult to measure accurately in human states and varies from

---

* In an attempt to maintain uniformity within the literature of the graphical description of the Starling equation, we have chosen to use the symbols for the description of the hydrostatic and osmotic pressures within the pulmonary microvasculature and interstitium, as described by Staub (1978).

the apex to base of the lungs, being relatively smaller in the apex as compared to the base. This variation in pressure no doubt determines the clinical finding of early roentgenographic changes of pulmonary edema in cardiac disease occurring in the lung bases. However, for lack of a better method, it is probably reasonable to "estimate" *Pmv* by the PCWP in human studies (Fein et al., 1979; Weil et al., 1978).

The πmv probably has a uniform distribution within the lung and is one of the major forces opposing the influence of the *Pmv* on increasing fluid movement from the intravascular to extravascular space. The osmotic pressure may be derived from the equation of Landis and Pappenheimer (1963), where:

$$\pi c = 2.1C + 0.16C^2 + 0.009C^3 \quad (5)$$
and C = total plasma proteins (g/dl),

or measured by a Hansen-Prather type osmometer (Hansen, 1961). In health, πmv averages 25–27 mm Hg (Weil et al., 1974), and it is unknown whether there is any major gradient between the pulmonary artery and the left atrium within the human lung.

The *Ppmv* has not been measured in the human lung. However, in animal experiments, despite considerable controversy, a review of the evidence sugggests that the interstitial pressure is subatmospheric with a gradient between the upper and lower lung regions, with a mean value of -7 to -8 mm Hg (Staub, 1974).

The πpmv again is unknown in the human situation. However, in animals, evidence suggests that the protein concentration in the interstitium is equivalent to the protein concentration of lung lymph fluid (Erdman et al., 1975). Based on this assumption, measurements of pulmonary lymph protein concentration and subsequent measures of interstitial protein concentration by micropipetting (Vreim et al., 1976a) have indicated that the πpmv is about two-thirds that of the πmv and averages 16–19 torr (Staub, 1978a).

The protein reflection coefficient (σ) which determines the effective transvascular protein osmotic pressure difference is about 0.8 in health. Were the barrier membrane between vessel and interstitium in the lung to be totally impermeable to protein, the value for this factor would be unity. However, were the barrier membrane to be totally permeable to protein, no effective osmotic pressure gradient would exist across the barrier membrane, and σ would be one.

Based on these considerations, and in an idealized situation, a schematic diagram of net flow of water from the intravascular compartment to the interstitium can be described (Fig. 26.1). In this figure, it can be seen that in the presence of no change in permeability of the barrier membrane (conductance), the hydrostatic and osmotic pressures favor the egress of fluid from the vessel to the interstitium. The major defense in the maintenance of a 'relatively' dry interstitium is the pulmonary lymphatic system (Staub, 1974), which actively returns water and protein from the interstitium to the systemic circulation by the major thoracic lymph channels.

In summary, the Starling equation adequately describes the transvascular flux of water from the intravascular compartment to the interstitium in the human lung. Any increase in lung water or pulmonary edema is adequately explained by a change in any one or a combination of the factors described by the Starling equation.

HYDROSTATIC (CARDIAC) EDEMA

In pulmonary edema on the basis of heart failure, an increase in the microvascular hydrostatic pressure (*Pmv*) is all that is needed to define the pathophysiological sequence for fluid accumulation in the lungs. In an isolated lung experiment, Garr et al. (1967) demonstrated that an increase in the LAP (*Pmv*) resulted in no increase in lung fluid until the pressure was 28 mm Hg, described as the "critical pressure" for fluid accumulation. By decreasing plasma protein concentration to 50% of normal, and hence the πmv, the critical pressure for fluid transudation was reduced to 35% of normal, indicating the importance of the πmv in the Starling equation. Because the upward slopes (pulmonary edema) in his experiments were parallel at both normal and reduced πmv, Garr et al. (1967) concluded that the rate of fluid transudation was not a function of capillary pressure per se but rather a function of *Pmv* minus πmv within the vessel. Levine and associates (Levine et al., 1967) also documented this interrelationship between the *Pmv* and πmv. By maintaining a constant *Pmv* minus πmv gradient over a range of high and low *Pmvs*, they showed that the rate of lung water accumulation was indeed dependent on the intravascular gradient of the *Pmv* and πmv (Fig.

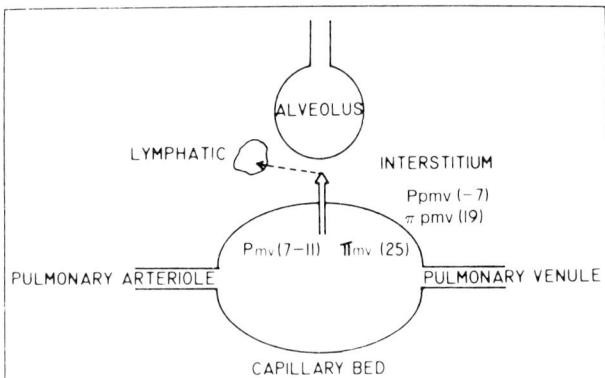

Figure 26.1. Normal pressure relations in the lung favor the movement of an ultrafiltrate of plasma from the microvasculature to the perimicrovascular space since $Qf = K(Pmv - Pi) - K\sigma(\pi mv - \pi i) = K(11 - (-7)) - K\sigma(25 - 19) = 12$. Although these pressure values are not absolute in the whole lung, they are generally representative of zone III. (Reprinted with permission from W. J. Sibbald, R. R. Anderson, and R. L. Holliday: Canadian Medical Association Journal 120:445, 1979.)

26.2). However, their data also showed that the initial phase of lung water accumulation was slower at small differences than at large differences of *Pmv* minus πmv. This nonlinearity of the formation of pulmonary edema is now readily explained by the changes that occur in the *Ppmv*, πpmv, and lymph flow, in response to an increased flux of water and solutes across the barrier membrane.

These latter three variables are part of the adaptive mechanism to reduce the egress of fluid, once begun from the vessels, and hence are meant to "defend" the interstitium against an excessive accumulation of lung water. In the first place, the pulmonary lymphatics may increase their absorptive capacity of water and solutes moving into the interstitium many times over. Increased lymphatic flow is a characteristic of pulmonary edema on a hydrostatic basis (Staub, 1974). It was this function of the lymphatics that allowed Staub et al. (1975), to establish an animal model for study of the transvascular movement of water and solutes in health and disease. In an elegant experiment, Staub cannulated the main right pulmonary lymphatic duct of the sheep, after previously negating all contributions to this lymph from abdominal sources. By increasing the LAP, Staub's group showed that pulmonary lymph flow increased and when compared to the baseline state, its protein content had decreased (Erdmann et al., 1975). In addition to showing the dependence of pulmonary edema on the *Pmv* in his model, Staub demonstrated other defense mechanisms which become operative in states of increased egress of water from the vascular compartment to the interstitium (Fig. 26.3). Accompanying an increase in lymph flow, a dilution of the πpmv occurs, which further operates to retard the egress of fluid from the vascular compartment (Erdmann et al., 1975). Together with this, a change in the *Ppmv* occurs so that, rather than being negative, as in the normal state, it is likely to become slightly positive (Parker et al., 1978; Staub, 1974). Recently, an appreciation of the compliance of the pulmonary interstitium has indicated that early on an increase in the transvascular flux of fluid results in a large change in pressure. But, as transvascular fluid flux continues, the pressure change is only minimal. This allows the interstitium to eventually accommodate large quantities of fluid which have crossed the alveolarcapillary barrier membrane with only slight changes in pressure. Hence, in response to a change in intravascular pressures which favor the egress of fluid from the intravascular to the interstitial compartments, the *Ppmv* becomes more positive; the πpmv falls, and the lymph flow increases. It is only when the capacity of this interstitial space and the pulmonary lymphatics is exceeded that alveolar flooding or edema occurs (Staub, 1974). This does not mean that the entire pulmonary interstitium must be filled before alveolar

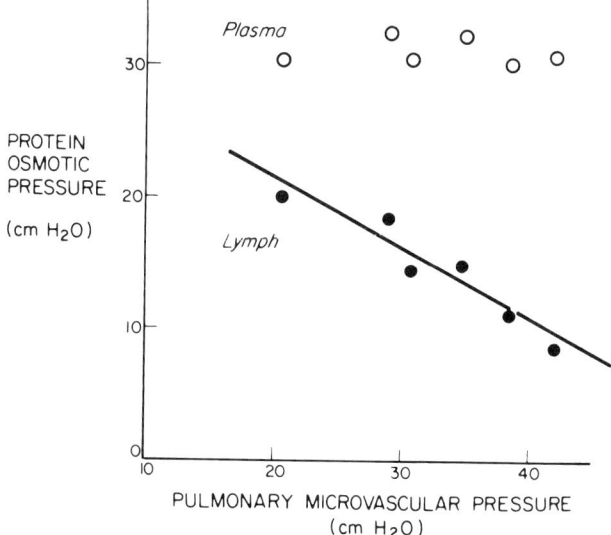

Figure 26.3. As the *Pmv* is increased the πpmv falls; a reflection of the "washout" phenomenon seen in early pulmonary edema, which acts as a protective mechanism against further extravascular movement of fluid. This defense reaction may be attenuated in permeability edema since increased transvascular flux of water is accompanied by increased flux of protein. (Reprinted with permission from A. J. Erdmann, T. R. Vaughn, Jr., K. L. Brigham et al.: Circulation Research 37:271, 1975.)

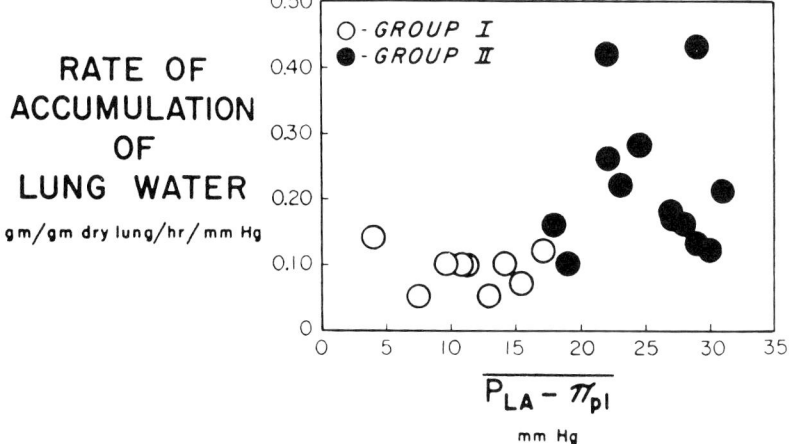

Figure 26.2. In animal experiments, performed by Levine, the rate of accumulation of water in the lungs is seen to increase in an exponential fashion when the mean "transcapillary pressure difference" ($P_{LA} - \pi_{PI}$) exceeds 20 mm Hg. (Reprinted with permission from O. R. Levine, R. B. Mellins, R. M. Senior et al.: Journal of Clinical Investigation 46:934, 1967.)

flooding occurs in some regions because of the regional disparities in pressure that occur. Once alveolar flooding does occur, the collapsed air fluid interface in the alveolus provides for an increased extravascular driving pressure, thus further augmenting fluid flux from the vascular compartment (Albert, 1979).

The study of pulmonary edema formation in the human has been much more difficult to characterize than in the animal, because of the inability to maintain constancy of experimental conditions during study and more importantly because of the lack of an acceptable technique in humans. Brigham et al. (1979b) have recently described the application of multiple isotopic tracer disappearance curves for the calculation of extravascular lung water in patients without permeability edema. In this model, using patients with cardiac disease, Brigham et al. (1979b) showed that the formation of extravascular lung water is indeed dependent on the Pmv minus πmv gradient (Fig. 26.4).

We recently described a technique which appears to adequately relate the intravascular Starling forces to the egress of a small molecular weight solute from blood into pulmonary edema fluid in patients with cardiac edema (Sibbald et al., 1979b and c). A small molecular weight water soluble nonvolatile solute, such as a radiolabeled chelate (Cr-51, In-III or TC-99m, DTPA), will rapidly equilibrate across vascular membranes into extracellular water after intravenous injection. Such a tracer, when infused into blood, is recoverable from bronchoalveolar secretions of patients with pulmonary edema, and a clearance rate may be calculated. Preliminary results (Sibbald et al., 1979c) indicate that the clearance rate is dependent upon the Pmv minus πmv gradient (Fig. 26.5) in a curvilinear fashion. These findings apparently satisfy certain inherent criteria which have been established in animal experiments. Namely, since there is always a flux of fluid from vessel to interstitium and alveolus in health, which is simply augmented in disease states, any technique which measures the formation of pulmonary edema by measuring either a change in lung water or the movement of a small molecular weight solute from blood to bronchoalveolar secretions should not intercept the line describing the Pmv minus πmv gradient. In our studies, we have assumed that the Pmv is equal to the measured PCWP and that the πmv is equal to the osmotic pressure calculated from the equation 5. Although the latter assumption may not be difficult to accept, the first may be. As mentioned previously, resistance at the postcapillary venular level may influence Pmv and hence the PCWP may not be representative of the absolute Pmv (Gabel and Drake, 1979). However, the postcapillary resistance often decreases as venous pressure becomes elevated (Taylor & Drake, 1977) so that a different ratio of pre- to postcapillary resistance might exist at higher venous pressures and hence negate clinical application of the equation described by Brigham for calculating Pmv. Although our data may not relate to the exact Pmv minus πmv gradient, because of potential errors in assuming that the Pmv equals the PCWP, we do feel that any errors introduced in this assumption would likely be the same in the population as a whole and would only shift the curvilinear relationship between clearance of the tracer and the pressure gradients horizontally.

Other clinical studies (Da Luz et al., 1975; Weil et al., 1978) have attempted to relate chest roentgenographic appearances of pulmonary edema to the colloid osmotic pressure (COP) minus PCWP gradient. Although these data indicate that maximum pulmonary edema occurs at the same range of intravascular pressure as shown by Brigham et al. (1979b) and Sibbald et al. (1979c), it is emphasized that the chest roentgenograph is a poor means of assessing lung water formation or content (Kanto et al., 1978) in other than clinical situations, where a gross approximation of the mechanism for pulmonary edema is required.

Anderson et al. (1979) and others (Levine et al., 1967) have shown that protein (I-125-albumin) flux from blood into pulmonary edema fluid occurs in hydrostatic edema.

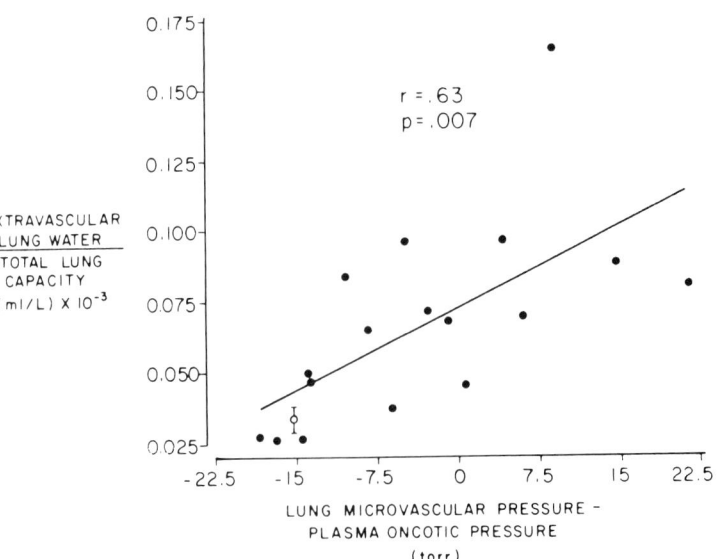

Figure 26.4. When expressed as a function of the intravascular Starling forces ($Pmv - \pi mv$), extravascular lung water increases as this gradient becomes more positive. (Reprinted with permission from K. L. Brigham, J. D. Snell, T. R. Harris et al.: Circulation Research 44: 523, 1979.)

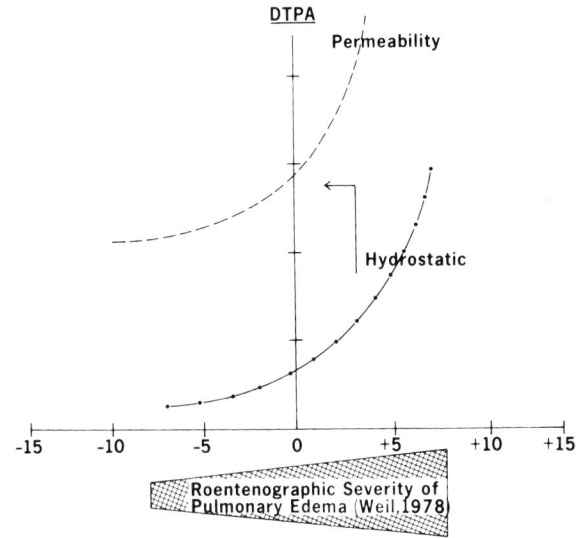

Figure 26.5. A comparison of the clearance of In-111-DTPA from blood to pulmonary edema fluid shows clear descrimination between patients with hydrostatic (—·—) versus permeability (septic) (– – –) edema and their dependence on the Pmv − πmv gradient. When compared to the Pmv − πmv gradient, the relationship between chest roentgenographic severity of pulmonary edema and the Pmv − πmv gradient is shown, as described by Weil et al. (1978).

However, the major characteristic of this type of edema is that its genesis is dependent on the *Pmv* minus *πmv* gradient, with changes in the *Ppmv* and *πpmv* due to the initial increased movement of water from the intravascular to the interstitial space, initially acting in a protective mechanism to retard this increased flux of water across the barrier membranes. Also, the bulk flow of water from the intravascular to extravascular compartments is not primarily due to a permeative mechanism.

PERMEABILITY (NONCARDIAC) EDEMA IN SEPSIS

A number of clinical (Anderson et al., 1979; Fein et al., 1979) and animal (Brigham et al., 1974, 1979a) studies have now established the pulmonary edema occurring in association with systemic human sepsis is due to a primary increase in permeative (conductive) transport across the pulmonary microvascular membrane. However, it would appear that even in the presence of an increased permeability of the pulmonary barrier membrane, the Starling pressures *Pmv* and *πmv* still play a significant role in modulating the transvascular flux of water and protein (Sibbald, 1979c).

Animal Studies

In animal models, the majority of work which has delineated the effect of septic states on the pulmonary microvascular barrier membrane(s) has utilized the chronic lymphatic cannulated sheep model described by Staub. Brigham et al. (1974) infused *Pseudomonas aeruginosa* bacteria into unanesthetized sheep and then compared lung lymph flow and lymph protein concentration to values obtained where the LAP (*Pmv*) had been artificially increased by the inflation of a balloon in the left atrium. *Pmv* was estimated by equation 4. The infusion of *Pseudomonas* resulted in a sustained early increase in mean pulmonary artery pressure which later fell towards baseline. Importantly, lung lymph flow increased dramatically in the animals infused with *Pseudomonas*, in whom a low *Pmv* had been maintained. In contradistinction, lung lymph flow also increased in the hydrostatic model where the *Pmv* was acutely increased, but not to the same degree as noted in the *Pseudomonas* model. Also, the lung lymph protein was markedly increased in the *Pseudomonas* model as compared to the hydrostatic model, where it was reduced. When the *Pmv* was allowed to increase in this permeability model, a dramatic increase in edema formation was noted. In this study, a mathematical analysis of the changes in membrane structure that would be required to predict the observed changes in lung lymph protein flow was also performed. It was noted that the mathematical model best described an increase in intermediate pore radius and an increase in small pore area, suggesting that large changes in fluid and protein filtration could result from small changes in the structure of exchanging vessels. Further studies by Brigham et al. (1976b) showed that the barrier membranes in permeability edema, although damaged, still retain their ability to sieve proteins. He measured the filtration of a number of plasma proteins of different molecular weights into the lung lymph during permeability edema and noted that during the period of increased lung vascular permeability, lung lymph clearance of proteins ranging from 36 to 96 Å was increased, but their clearance still decreased with increasing molecular radius. Such data was again not consistent with the view that either marked endothelial membrane destruction or large intercellular gaps are necessarily the main physical change causing increased microvascular filtration when permeability is increased. Brigham (1976b), therefore, concluded that large increases in lung transvascular fluid and protein movement could result from increased vascular permeability even when changes in microvascular porosity were not large enough to preclude sieving of proteins less than 100 Å molecular radius. In other studies, Brigham et al. (1979a) demonstrated that an infusion of live *Escherichia coli* endotoxin also increases microvascular permeability within the lung, although the permeability increase is relatively larger in the *Pseudomonas* model. (Fig. 26.6)

Sturm et al. (1979) examined the effect of septic shock in the same sheep model and, unlike Brigham et al. (1979a), were unable to demonstrate an increase in the permeability of the exchanging vessels. Their experiment, however, was remarkably different from that of Brigham's. They created a shock model and only studied

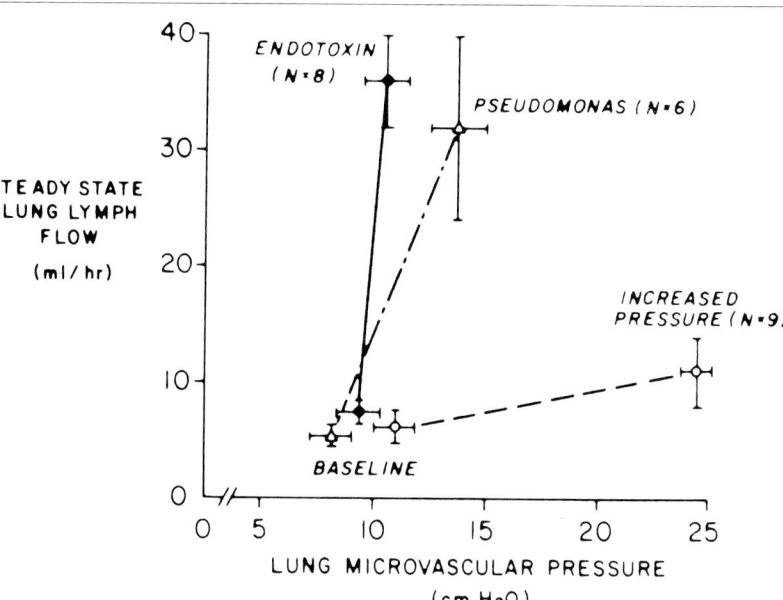

Figure 26.6. The increase in lung lymph flow associated with permeability edema for any given change in Pmv is greater with *E. coli* endotoxin than with *Pseudomonas* infusion, indicating the more damaging effect of endotoxin on the barrier exchanging membrane than live *Pseudomonas*. (Reprinted with permission from K. L. Brigham, R. E. Bowers, and J. Haynes: Circulation Research 45:292, 1979.)

the animal model for 4 hr after infusion of *E. coli*. Shock by itself will increase lung water but probably only through an effect on the Pmv (Demling et al., 1979), by increasing pulmonary venular resistance. Only when resuscitated from shock, with improved perfusion, will the permeability defect of the sheep model become profoundly evident (Brigham et al., 1979a). Therefore, septic shock may cause an increase in lung water for completely different reasons than does systemic sepsis without hypotension (↑ pressure versus ↑ permeability). Hence, studies on the cause of an increase in lung water in sepsis must be carefully designed to obviate the effect of hypotension on the Pmv at the exchanging vessel level.

In other animal work, Pietra infused *E. coli* into dogs and then injected colloid carbon intravenously to detect the sites of the pathological increase in vascular permeability (Pietra et al., 1974). During the 1st hr following infusion, bronchial venules allowed carbon and blood elements to traverse their walls, whereas no leakage of these large particles or any ultrastructural changes could be detected within the alveolar walls. These findings suggest that the site of increased permeability edema or the site of the loss of barrier membrane function may be at the bronchial venular level and not necessarily at the capillary level. A number of other animal models, utilizing different techniques, have also confirmed that a primary change of permeability in the pulmonary exchanging vessels is the likely cause of increased lung water in septic-like states. Fischer et al. (1977) studied the movement of specific molecular species from pulmonary capillary blood to saline-filled alveoli in an in vivo dog lung model. Their results confirmed an increase in alveolocapillary membrane permeability following endotoxin infusion to substances up to a molecular weight of 10,400. Unlike the studies in the sheep model, no increase in permeability to dextran (MW 20,000) or albumin (MW 69,000) was found. The reasons for these differences in effect of endotoxin on the permeability of the exchanging vessels may be related to differences in species or in the hemodynamic response to endotoxin.

Using a double indicator dilution technique to assess changes in lung waer (I-131-Human Serum Albumin and tritiated water), Snell and Ramsay (1969) showed that a sublethal dose of endotoxemia increased perivascular lung water.

Brigham et al. (1977b; Harris et al., 1978) have also utilized indicator dilution experiments in awake, instrumented sheep to determine calculated permeability times surface area products. They compared them to the increase in permeability that was determined in the cannulated lymphatic sheep model with its change in lymph protein flow. Their data showed good qualitative agreement between the indicator and lymph estimates of lung vascular permeability.

From these animal experiments, it may be concluded that permeability edema is indeed due to a decrease in the resistance of the walls of the exchanging vessels within the pulmonary microvasculature to the passage of fluid and solutes; the endotoxin shock model may not reflect the true events occurring in the pulmonary microvasculature in systemic human sepsis without shock where large increases in the postcapillary resistance which would increase the Pmv are not uniformally observed; and, more importantly, animal studies should be carefully controlled with particular reference to the presence or absence of shock. Brigham (1977a) has thus summarized the prerequisites for documenting an increase in permeability of the exchanging vessels as compared to an increase in Pmv (hydrostatic edema) as: 1) the transvascular movement of fluid and solute across the barrier membranes is markedly increased with changes not completely explained by any concomitant change in driving pressures; and 2) for a given increase in Pmv, the transvascular movement of fluid and solute is greater in permeability than hydrostatic edema (Fig. 26.7).

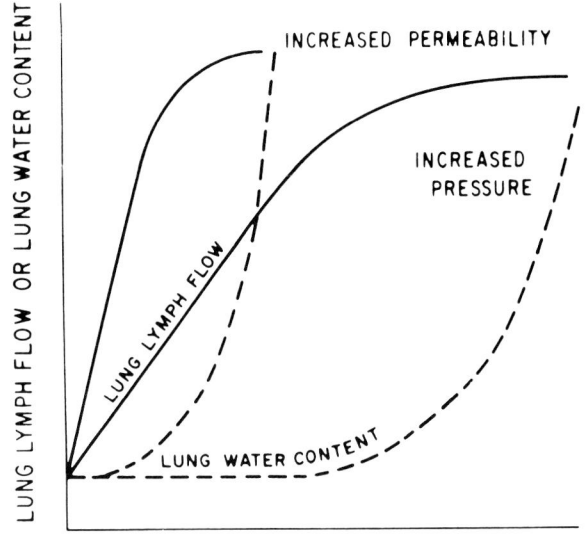

Figure 26.7. Increased permeability edema is characterized by a greater increase in transvascular movement of water, here indicated as lung water content for any given change in Pmv, than in pulmonary edema secondary only to hydrostatic factors. (Reprinted with permission from K. H. Brigham: *Lung Biology in Health and Disease, Vol. 9, Lung Solute Exchange.* Marcel Dekker, New York, 1977.)

Human Studies

Despite these elegant studies in animal models to show an increase in permeability of the pulmonary exchanging vessels during septic-like states, it must be emphasized that a great deal of controversy surrounds the assumption that the use of endotoxin or live bacteria infusion in an animal bears any resemblance to the human state of pulmonary edema associated with systemic sepsis. However, a considerable body of evidence does indeed support the notion that human septic pulmonary edema is accompanied by a true increase in permeability of the exchanging vessels within the pulmonary microvasculature.

Finley et al. (1975), in a comparative study of patients with pulmonary edema secondary to systemic sepsis or cardiac disease, found that when judging pulmonary edema by roentgenographic criteria, the two groups (when manifesting similar degrees of pulmonary edema by chest x-ray), were dissimilar in that the measured PCWP minus COP gradient was significantly higher in the septic group than in the cardiac group. For the most part, this was due to the presence of an elevated PCWP in the cardiac group. They were left to conclude that changes in the Pmv or πmv could not completely explain pulmonary edema in sepsis (Finley et al., 1975) as it might logically do in cardiac disease (Sibbald et al., 1979a).

Robin et al. (1972) analyzed the chemical composition of pulmonary edema fluid to plasma in a case of sepsis and found a number of solutes including various plasma proteins were in clear chemical equilibrium between plasma and the edema fluid (Table 26.1). They were left to conclude that the accumulation of these substances in the edema fluid of their patient was consistent with increased conductance of the pulmonary microvessels. Riordan and Walters (1968) also felt that pulmonary edema in five patients studied at necropsy was due to preceding nonpulmonary bacterial infections, with a presumed increase in microvascular permeability. Gelb and Klein (1976) studied 11 patients, 2 of whom were septic with ARDS, and confirmed a high protein content in the alveolar fluid, approaching values similar to concurrent plasma protein concentrations. Only in one patient was the alveolar protein greater than the plasma protein. In all patients, the PCWP was less than 15 mm Hg. Since an excellent correlation has been found between pulmonary lymph protein, interstitial protein, and protein in secretions, obtained by deep suctioning of the endobronchial tree in animal models of permeability (Vreim and Staub, 1976) and cardiac edema (Vreim et al., 1976b), Fein and associates (1979) have also sampled pulmonary edema fluid in cases of ARDS and cardiac edema and assumed that the osmotic pressure calculation from protein concentration in the pulmonary edema fluid was an approximate indicator of the πpmv. In three patients with sepsis, they found the ratio of edema fluid concentration to plasma protein concentration to be 0.58, 0.62, and 2.68. However, in hydrostatic pulmonary edema, this ratio averaged 0.51. When they took into account the intravascular Starling forces ($Pmv-\pi mv$), the septic patients were all greater than -4.8 mm Hg (average -8.6), while in the cardiac patients the Pmv minus πmv gradient was greater than $+2.5$ mm Hg (average $+9.9$). Adding the assumption that osmotic

Table 26.1
Composition of Pulmonary Edema Fluid to Plasma in a Patient with Sepsis[a]

	Plasma	PEF
Na+, mEq/liter	137	141
K+, mEq/liter	4.0	4.2
Cl−, mEq/liter	93	97
Glucose, mg/100 ml	123	114
Total protein, gm/100 ml	3.1	2.9
Albumin, gm/100 ml	2.1	2.0
α Globulin, gm/100 ml	0.2	0.2
α Globulin, gm/100 ml	0.2	0.2
β = globulin, gm/100 ml	0.2	0.3
γ = globulin, gm/100 ml	0.4	0.2
Dextran 70, mg/100 ml	611	545
Fibrinogen, mg/100 ml	48	54
Dextran (MW 500,000), mg/100 ml	1,309	680

[a] Increased permeability of the barrier membrane still shows some sieving properties, in that progressively less solute was obtained from pulmonary edema fluid (*PEF*) as the molecular weight of the solutes increased. (Reprinted with permission from E. D. Robin, L. C. Corey, A. Gremik et al.: *Archives of Internal Medicine 130:*66, 1972. Copyright, American Medical Association.)

pressure calculated from the protein content of the edema fluid approximated the πpmv in the septics, the average net face favoring fluid flux was less than +12 mm Hg and in the cardiacs was greater than +10 mm Hg. Hence, in many clinical studies, analysis of pulmonary edema fluid and consideration of the Starling forces within the limits of measurement in intact man favor the conclusion that pulmonary edema in association with sepsis differs from that due to cardiac disease primarily by an increase in conductance of the pulmonary alveolarcapillary barrier membranes in sepsis.

Other human studies have employed isotope tracer flux within the lung to assess the degree of permeability of the exchanging vessels. In part, this is because patients with pulmonary edema secondary to sepsis, when ventilated with PEEP often do not have sufficient sputum for easy biochemical analysis of protein, as described by Robin et al. (1972), Fein et al. (1979), and Gabel and Drake (1979). Gorin et al. (1978) have described a noninvasive method of determining the increase in permeability of the barrier membrane, which is potentially applicable in clinical states of sepsis. Using two isotopes, one which would remain intravascularly at all times and one which would remain intravascularly only during conditions of no increase in permeability, they measured the accumulation of this latter tracer with a portable scintillation detection probe that was fitted with a collimator and compared their results to protein flux in the chronically instrumented sheep model (Staub et al., 1975). They showed good correlation between the two methods, suggesting that the use of isotopic flux quantification was indeed applicable to the diagnosis of a permeability change of the barrier membrane in the human situation. Brigham and associates (Brigham, 1979; Brigham et al., 1979b) have used four isotopes to measure simultaneously the lung extravascular water volume and the permeability surface product of urea in patients with cardiac and septic edema. From these studies, they have demonstrated that permeability of the exchanging vessels is increased in sepsis when compared to patients with heart failure (Fig. 26.8) (Brigham, 1979).

As described previously, we have employed a method of assessing the clearance of an injected tracer in the human situation, from blood to bronchoalveolar secretions, to determine the integrity of the pulmonary microvascular barrier membranes. Following the injection of a tracer molecule, pulmonary edema fluid is collected on an hourly basis by deep suctioning through an endotracheal tube. Using a generalized clearance equation:

$$\frac{\text{sputum tracer concentration (counts/ml)} \times \text{sputum volume (ml/hr)}}{\text{plasma tracer concentration (counts/ml)}}$$

a value is obtained for the clearance of the tracer from blood into bronchoalveolar secretions [representing pulmonary edema fluid (Fein et al., 1979; Vreim and Staub, 1976)] on an hourly basis. Utilizing I-125-HSA, we found a greater clearance in human septic ARDS than in cardiac edema (Fig. 26.9) (Anderson et al., 1979).

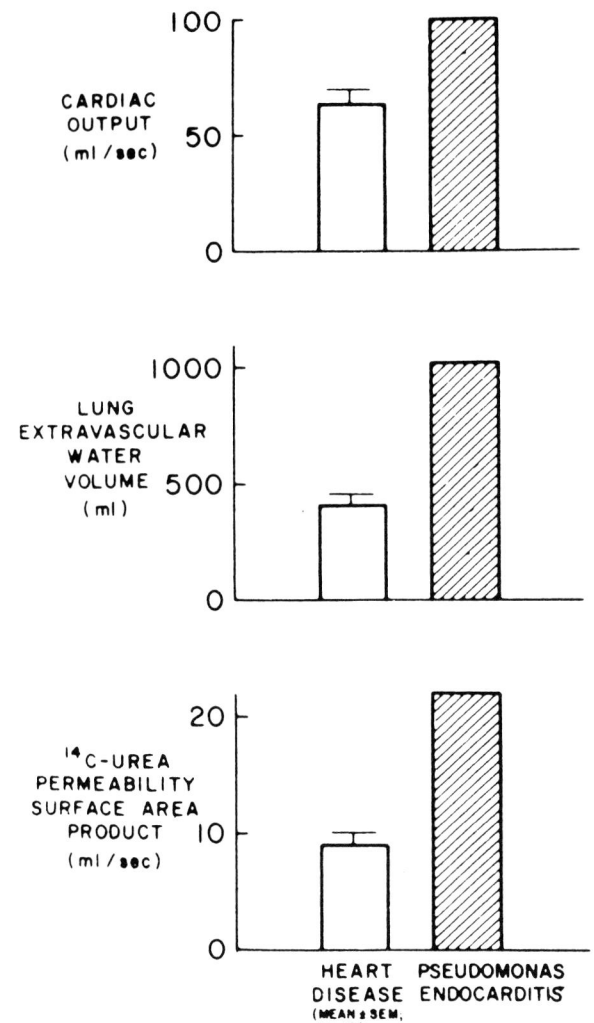

Figure 26.8. Pulmonary indicator dilution data in a patient with *Pseudomonas* endocarditis compared with average data from patients with heart failure. Heart failure shows the applicability of C14 urea permeability surface area product in the clinical diagnosis of septic ARDS. (Reprinted with permission from K. L. Brigham: American Journal of Surgery 138: 361, 1979.)

Subsequently, utilizing two tracers, I-125-HSA and In-111-DTPA, we calculated the clearance of these large (69,000) and small (502) molecular weight tracers, respectively, from blood to bronchoalveolar secretions in a number of patients with pulmonary edema secondary to systemic sepsis or congestive heart failure. We compared the clearance values to the PCWP minus COP gradient, as a measure of the Pmv minus πmv gradient, again assuming that the measured PCWP was a close reflection of the Pmv. In these studies, as we have shown in human cardiac edema, there was an exponential relationship between the PCWP minus COP gradient and the clearance of the small molecular weight tracer (In-

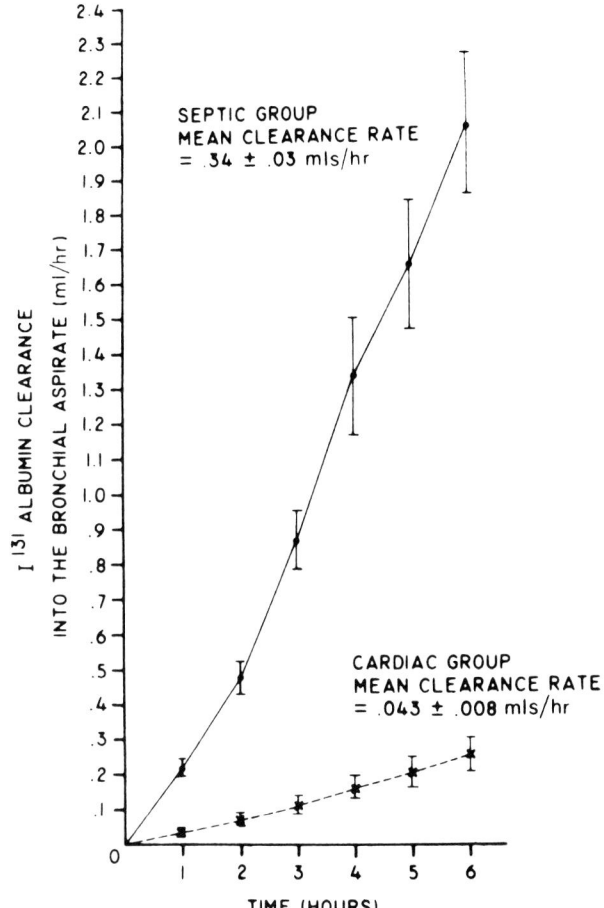

Figure 26.9. Cumulative clearance of ^{131}I-labeled human serum albumin (^{131}I-HSA) into the bronchial aspirate for 10 patients with pulmonary edema associated with sepsis (septic group) and for 10 patients with pulmonary edema associated with cardiac disease (cardiac group). These data reflect the increased permeability of the alveolarcapillary membrane in septic as compared to cardiac pulmonary edema.

111-DTPA) (Fig. 26.5) (Sibbald et al., 1979c). When examining the effect of the hydrostatic pressure alone on the clearance of DTPA, the slope of this relationship was significantly greater than the slope of a similar relationship obtained in cardiac edema (Sibbald et al., 1979c). Further, in addition to having shown previously that large molecular weight solutes appear in greater concentration in pulmonary edema fluid in sepsis than in pulmonary edema fluid in hydrostatic edema, we found that the clearance of I-125-HSA was similarly dependent on the PCWP minus COP gradient (Sibbald et al., 1979b). Our studies would then fulfill the criteria elucidated by Brigham (1979) for the definition of an increase in permeability of the pulmonary microvascular barrier membrane as the primary cause of pulmonary edema, in that 1) when compared to patients with cardiac edema, patients with septic edema are characterized by the finding of solutes of greater molecular weight in pulmonary edema fluid; and 2) the movement of these solutes from the intravascular compartment to the pulmonary edema fluid is greater for any given change in the hydrostatic pressure than in cardiac edema. These studies also document that, despite an increase in permeability of the pulmonary microvascular barrier membrane in human sepsis, the intravascular hydrostatic minus osmotic pressure gradient still remains clinically operative in affecting the transvascular flux of water and albumin.

In human septic edema, there is no reason to believe that there is any major alteration in the initial defense reaction to the transvascular flux of water and solutes. In other words, all experimental data reported supports the concept that the primary response to an increased movement of fluid from the intravascular to the interstitial compartment within the lung is a change in Pmv to more positive values which, as in cardiac edema, would then oppose any further increase in interstitial volume. Similarly, pulmonary lymphatics are capable of increasing flow, providing their very necessary function of trying to maintain a "dry" pulmonary interstitium in septic as well as in cardiac edema. Halmagyi (1977) has suggested that in human sepsis, the pulmonary lymphatics may not function as well as in hydrostatic edema, an interesting yet clinically unproved speculation. In sepsis, the permeability of the exchanging membranes is increased to both water and solutes and the concentration of albumin in the pulmonary interstitial space is increased. This would be expected to result in smaller difference between the πmv and πpmv in septic edema and thus reduce the effect of increased flux of water to decrease the πpmv, as seen in hydrostatic edema. Hence, the effect of any change in the πpmv to aid in reducing the egress of fluid from the intravascular to extravascular compartment would be blunted in septic edema. However, most studies in septic edema to date have shown that interstitial protein concentration is less than intravascular protein (Fein et al., 1979; Gelb and Klein, 1976) ($\pi mv > \pi pmv$), indicating that a functional gradient of the osmotic pressure must exist across the exchanging membranes and that the protein reflection coefficient is not zero, although certainly less than the normal situation.

Therefore, it is hypothetically argued that in septic edema the defense within the lung to reduce the transvascular flux of water and solute, once edema formation begins, is less effective than in hydrostatic edema but is still operative. Data presented from our work showing the maintenance of the exponential relationship between the intravascular hydrostatic minus osmotic pressure gradients and the clearance of small and large molecular weight tracers would support this theoretical concept (Sibbald et al., 1979c).

In summary, animal and human studies are supportive of the concept that a primary increase in permeability of the pulmonary microvascular membranes is the primary cause of pulmonary edema in sepsis. This is in contradistinction to hydrostatic or cardiac edema where an increase in the intravascular hydrostatic pressure is all that is required to explain the genesis of increased lung water in this condition (Staub, 1978b). However, the data would suggest that even in states of increased permeability edema, with its known increase in large molecular weight solute flux across the barrier membranes, the protein reflection coefficient (σ) is not zero and that there is still an effect of osmotic pressure being manifested across the barrier membrane. It could be argued however, that there is a spectrum of injury to the barrier membrane in septic edema and that with severe or agonal sepsis, a total loss of integrity may be seen, allowing the free transfer of fluid and solutes of all molecular weights across the barrier membranes. Clinically, this is seen infrequently, when the pulmonary edema fluid is voluminous and the protein concentration is equal to or greater than simultaneous plasma protein concentration. However, in our experience this occurs only in the premorbid state of septic edema. It is emphasized that under most clinical conditions, the protein reflection coefficient, although reduced, cannot be zero, and that the hydrostatic minus colloid osmotic pressure gradient within the pulmonary microvasculature still influences the transvascular flux of water and solutes, even though the primary cause of the edema is an increase in the conductivity of the pulmonary microvasculature. The clinical implications of this are obvious. With a reduced, yet still effective transvascular osmotic pressure gradient, and in the presence of the maintenance of an effect of the Starling forces, some beneficial effect of the maintenance of a large intravascular hydrostatic minus colloid osmotic pressure gradient must accrue in septic pulmonary edema. The argument that albumin infusions in septic ARDS increase the transmicrovascular flux of fluid and solutes by virtue of a "reversed" osmotic pressure gradient (Weaver et al., 1979) would seem untenable with the presence of a clinically demonstrated protein reflection coefficient (σ), which, although less than normal, is not zero. If albumin infusions, or any fluid whether it be colloid or crystalloid, were to increase the transmicrovascular flux of fluid and solutes, it would do so only insofar as the fluid increases the Pmv or decreases the πmv.

PATHOLOGICAL CORRELATIONS IN SEPTIC PULMONARY EDEMA

Normal Lung

In normal human lung, the alveolar epithelium is the main restrictive barrier to the passage of water soluble molecules from within the capillary lumen to the alveolus (Taylor and Gaark, 1970). The capillary network is surrounded first by a connective tissue sheet and then by the alveolar spaces. On one side of the capillary, the interstitium is reasonably thick (mean 2 μm), and hence the air-blood barrier separating the alveolus capillary is rather wide. However, there is a "thin" section on the opposite side of the capillary where very little interstitium separates the capillary and the alveolus so that only the fused endothelial and epithelial basement membranes separates the epithelial type 1 cells of the alveolus and the endothelial cell. The majority of gas exchange occurs across this very thin alveolarcapillary barrier.

Intravascular endothelial cells are joined together by tight junctions with a structural arrangement, suggesting that the endothelial cell junctional complex becomes progressively less well developed from the arterial to the venous side of the pulmonary circulation (Schneeberger and Karnovsky, 1976). The endothelial cells of the lung are nonfenestrated and are permeable to lipid soluble molecules, yet impermeable to lipid insoluble molecules. In contradistinction to fenestrated endothelium, in the lungs, extracellular pathways provide most of the hydraulic conductivity. The interendothelial junctions appear to be small water-filled pathways between these cells, from one side to the other, the size of these channels is small enough to progressively restrict passage of larger molecules. These small pores will not explain the passage of albumin, which has previously been shown to traverse this barrier membrane even in health (Drinker and Field, 1931). Hence, when examining the potential pathways for the movement of water and solute from the capillary to the interstitium either in health or disease states, it is probable that larger pores do exist, although their exact anatomical location is not known with certainty. Renkin (1978) has summarized that in health there are four potential mechanisms for the movement of water and solutes, including: 1) a transendothelial cell pathway; 2) by micropinocytotic vesicles; 3) through interendothelial (intercellular) cell junctions; and 4) by chains of fused micropinocytotic vesicles.

Barrier Membrane in Pulmonary Edema

Largely because of the lack of a reproducible animal model for septic pulmonary edema and the difficulties in interpreting postmortem sections of lung, it has been only recently that microscopic and theoretical data have been applied to explain the sites of increased permeability within the fluid and solute exchanging barrier membranes of the pulmonary microvasculature in pulmonary edema associated with sepsis. As noted earlier, increased permeability could occur either at the arteriolar, capillary, or venular level. Pietra et al. (1971) produced permeability edema by the intravenous infusion of histamine into dogs and used colloidal carbon as an electron dense tracer to show that bronchial venules became leaky at the same time that capillaries within the microcirculation remained unaffected. Based on these findings and after reproducing similar data with the infusion of endotoxin in dogs Pietra et al. (1974), suggested that it was at the venular level where maximal permeability likely occurs. Staub (1978b), however, disputes this and suggests that it is within the capillary bed that the major permeability defect occurs. Work by Blake and Staub (1976) has suggested that intercellular junctions between endothelial cells vary in radius from approximately 20 Å to 1000 Å, a small and large pore concept, with intermediate sized pores between these limits. They then proceeded to mathematically calculate the change in these pores that would be necessary to explain the permeability changes noted in the sheep model of chronic *Pseudomonas* infusion. The data were compared to normal, where the intermediate sized pore was felt to be the major site for protein transport. Fluid and solute transfer were reasonably equivalent between small and intermediate pores, with the large pores contributing only very little. When creating a model of increased hydrostatic pressure, a significant increase in fluid transport and the osmotic pressure gradient across the exchanging membrane tended to decrease the relative amount transported through the intermediate pores. With increased permeability using the *Pseudomonas* model, the mathematical applications suggested that both small and intermediate sized pores increased in number, and only modest loosening of the intercellular junctions was required to explain the data. Hence, relatively large changes in fluid and solute movement across the exchanging membranes can occur with relatively minor changes in the functional or pathological sense—changes that may not be seen even by quantitative electron microscopy. This would suggest that the pulmonary edema of systemic sepsis may not necessarily be due to the result of extensive or irreversible damage to the exchanging membranes.

This conclusion is supported by electron microscopy in a permeability edema model. Horig et al. (1971), by electron microscopy, were unable to find any obvious structural changes in the pulmonary microvascular endothelium including the intercellular junctions.

The experimental data are supported by the recent elegant studies of Bachofen and Weibel (1977). Using an ingenious fixative technique shortly after a patient's death, they were able to obtain specimens from patients with pulmonary edema secondary to sepsis at various stages of their illness. In what they term acute phases, death having occurred within 24 hr of admission, they noted pulmonary edema with alveolar fluid containing white and red blood cells and protein. Areas of complete destruction of the epithelial surface over the thinnest areas of the gas exchanging membrane were noted and type II pneumocytes were better preserved than type I pneumocytes. Generally, structural changes in the endothelium were much less than in the epithelium, although there was an occasional gap in the endothelial layer. In subacute and chronic phases of the disease process, patients who had died more than 48 hr after the initiation of pulmonary edema secondary to systemic sepsis, alveolar edema was less widespread, and proliferation of type II cells was noted. The capillaries were sometimes collapsed by surrounding edema, and endothelial lesions were more prominent than they were in the acute phase. Their data then supported the mathematical modeling of Blake and Staub (1976), where interendothelial junctional changes would have to be of only a small degree to explain the increased transvascular flux of fluid and solute. It is emphasized that no open junction could be found in the acute phase of septic ARDS in Bachofen's study and that data for the first time provided a graphical illustration of how fluid and solute could move from interstitium to the intraalveolar spaces. In Staub's previous studies on the pathological sequence of fluid accumulation in hydrostatic edema, he was concerned that there were few changes in the alveolar membrane to account for the gross alveolar flooding seen in this type of edema (Staub, 1974). He proceeded to postulate that the early collection of fluid in the peribronchiolar areas of the interstitium then overflowed into the distal alveolar spaces in hydrostatic edema. This explanation is not necessary in pulmonary edema secondary to sepsis with the morphological studies of Bachofen and Weibel. Egan et al. (1977) have also suggested, even in acute hemodynamic edema in dogs, that the air space epithelial sheet ruptures at a few relatively discrete sites and bulk flow of interstitial fluid into the air space occurs, a thesis at divergence with Staub (1978b).

The pathological changes required to explain the increased transvascular flux of fluid and solutes in edema secondary to sepsis may not necessarily be the same as those required to explain permeability under other conditions. Conditions such as acid aspiration, which will likewise cause permeability edema, will create gross alveolar and endothelial cell destruction easily visible by light and electron microscopy.

Therefore, in septic pulmonary edema, theoretical studies tend to support early electron microscopic studies, suggesting that increased flux of large molecules probably occurs through the interendothelial junctions and that only small changes in pore sizes and number are required to explain the large increase in fluid and solute flux. Under abnormal conditions, such as in septic pulmonary edema, other modes of transport may account for increased water movement, such as pinocytosis or increased transport transendothelially.

ETIOLOGY OF THE PERMEABILITY DEFECT: EVIDENCE AND SPECULATIONS

The Adult Respiratory Distress Syndrome (ARDS) is simply a description of an apparent common reaction of the lung to many different clinical conditions (Petty, 1975). Increased permeability, or noncardiac edema (ARDS), has been noted in a number of clinical situations, the most common being systemic human sepsis, aspiration of liquid gastric contents, fat embolism, head injury with intracranial hypertension, overdose with aspirin, and inhalation of toxic fumes (Table 26.2). Its occurrence in such a diverse list of diseases has left Brigham (1977b) to speculate that there are three potential mechanisms for the development of increased pulmonary microvasculature permeability: humoral, cellular, and neural, acting singly or in combination.

Postmortem examination of ARDS secondary to sepsis shows aggregates of leukocytes occluding the pulmonary microvasculature. Coalson et al. (1975) have suggested that in ARDS secondary to sepsis, complement activation, and in particular C5a generation, enhance such white cell aggregation (Craddock et al., 1977). It has also

Table 26.2
Some of the More Common Causes of Pulmonary Edema, Classified by the Change in the Microvascular Hydrostatic Pressure (Pmv) or the Permeability of the Exchanging Membranes

    Cardiac
        Left ventricular failure
            Pressure overload (hypertensive heart disease)
            Volume overload (valvular heart disease)
            Myocardial disease (cardiomyopathy, myocarditis, etc.)
        Other
            Constrictive pericarditis
    Noncardiac (Permeability)
        Sepsis (gram-positive and gram-negative)
        Aspiration
        Trauma
            Fat embolism
            Pulmonary contusion
        Pancreatitis
        Drug overdose
        Viral pneumonia
        Intracranial hypertension ("neurogenic")
        Cardiopulmonary bypass
        Inhalation of toxins
        Disseminated intravascular coagulation
        Shock

been noted that the permeability defect following the *Pseudomonas* infusion model of Brigham et al. (1974) is not fully expressed in the presence of leukopenia (Heflin and Brigham, 1978). Subsequently, Brigham was able to reproduce the permeability defect characteristic of septic ARDS in an animal model, with the intravenous infusion of histamine (Brigham et al., 1976a), an action which could be blocked by treatment of up to 4 hr following infusion with an antihistamine of the H-1 but not the H-2 variety (Brigham and Owen, 1975a). Similarly, utilizing a different technique and a different animal species, Propst et al. (1978) found that histamine would increase pulmonary alveolocapillary permeability. Further, the infusion of endotoxin for a period exceeding 4 hr has caused pulmonary edema on the basis of a defect in permeability of the alveolocapillary membrane(s) (Fischer et al., 1977). More importantly, it results in the outpouring of pulmonary edema fluid, which is rich in histamine (Propst et al., 1978). Endotoxin is known to result in complement activation and subsequent aggregation of leukocytes, which physically occlude capillaries in the pulmonary microvasculature (Fischer et al., 1977).

Experimental models show that the permeability defect in ARDS can be blunted markedly by prior depletion of leukocytes (Heflin and Brigham, 1978) as well as with the use of corticosteroids in pharmacological doses (Anderson et al., 1977; Bowers and Brigham, 1978). We have also found previously, using our technique of documenting the permeability defect in human sepsis with pulmonary edema, that high dose corticosteroid therapy reduces the recovery of labeled I-125 human serum albumin from bronchoalveolar secretions a finding interpreted as substantiating animal work in which corticosteroids reduce the pulmonary alveolarcapillary permeability defect in septic ARDS (Anderson et al., 1977).

Therefore, animal data suggest that pulmonary edema accompanying sepsis could be related to the generation of histamine. It is not known whether the histamine is derived from mast cells within the pulmonary parenchyma or blood-borne basophils. It might be logically hypothesized that in human sepsis, a disease characterized by complement activation (Feraron et al., 1975), leukocyte aggregates develop which subsequently microembolize to the small vessels of the lung (Murray, 1977). Then, histamine released from mast cells or blood-borne basophils (acting at a local level) could be the factor responsible for the increased permeability noted in experimental and human ARDS secondary to sepsis. It is not without precedence to suggest that histamine may be responsible for the increase in permeability in ARDS secondary to sepsis (Brigham et al., 1976a; Murray, 1977). It might be logically explained that since C5a attracts basophils, their accumulation will result in histamine release (Lett-Brown et al., 1976). Therapeutic changes noted in ARDS with corticosteroids might be explained by a depression in basophil count, which occurs with corticosteroids, the net expression being a decrease in histamine levels (Parwaresche, 1975). Corticosteroids may also increase intracellular cyclic AMP levels, a situation in both human lung and basophils which parallels a reduction in histamine release (Bevans, 1977).

This argument for the mediation of the increase in pulmonary endothelial permeability in human sepsis by histamine does not by any means negate other possible etiological factors. In sepsis, many other potential vasoactive mediators are present in the systemic circulation, including bradykinin, serotonin, and various components of the prostaglandin system (Clowes et al., 1970). Serotonin increases transvascular flux only by increasing microvascular pressures in the animal model, and hence is not felt to be a prime cause of permeability increase in the human septic lung lesion (Brigham and Owen, 1975b). Similarly, there is little data from animal models to suggest any major contribution of bradykinin in septic-like states. Workers from Brigham's unit have investigated some of the prostaglandins and have found no major contribution from prostaglandin F-2α in enhancing pulmonary permeability (Brigham, 1977b). The exact vasoactive mediator of the increased barrier membrane permeability in human sepsis is as yet unknown. However, it is probably related to complement-induced leukocyte aggregation.

It is well appreciated that patients with pulmonary hypertension who have systemic sepsis are at risk for increased morbidity (Sibbald et al., 1978). It is in this area where Staub has provided some interesting data by showing that with increased pulmonary artery pressures there occurs increased sheer forces which may physically cause an increase in permeability within the pulmonary microvasculature (Ohkuda et al., 1978). This is supported by other studies in which increased permeability edema was noted to be associated with high central venous pressures and hence an implied increase in pulmonary artery pressures (Miller et al., 1978). In our data, we have not been able to explain increased permeability on this physical theory. If increased hydrostatic pulmonary artery pressures were a cause for the increased permeability of human sepsis, they might enhance permeability through a "stretched pore phenomenon," as described by Shirley (Shirley et al., 1957), who felt that increased hydrostatic pressures would stretch interendothelial junctions.

The cause of the increased permeability of the exchanging vessels within the lung in pulmonary edema associated with sepsis must at this time remain only speculative. Elsewhere, Demling (Ch. 28) discusses the metabolic function of the lung in sepsis and the release of mediators in animal models that are meant to reproduce a situation compatible with human septic ARDS. The identification of the agent(s) responsible for the increased permeability of the pulmonary exchanging vessels in septic ARDS must be found to permit a more rational approach to treatment of the lung lesion.

SUMMARY

Pulmonary edema accompanying systemic human sepsis is characterized by an increase in lung water that is secondary to an increase in the conductance or permeability of the exchanging vessels within the lung. Permeability to solutes of varying molecular weight is increased, and, indeed, the more severe or chronic the septic process, the potentially more severe the permeability defect in allowing the transvascular flux of solutes of greater molecular weight. Regardless of the increased permeability, there are no data that have shown concomitantly a total absence of effect of the intravascular Starling forces. Indeed, initial data have been presented to show that the Starling forces remain clinically operative even in states of increased permeability within the pulmonary exchange vessels (Sibbald et al., 1979b). The increased permeability can be explained mathematically by an increase in the number of small pores and by an increase in the size of the intermediate pores (Blake and Staub, 1976). Mathematical modeling of increased transvascular flux of fluid and solutes in permeability septic edema has been confirmed recently by electron microscopy in the human. The alveolar membrane has been shown to be so severely injured that it can no longer provide the barrier to movement of water and solutes from the capillary to the intraalveolar space, as it does in health (Bachofen and Weibel, 1977). The cause of the increased permeability in septic pulmonary edema remains speculative but may involve activation of the complement system with subsequent generation of vasoactive mediators, such as histamine. At this point in our knowledge, the most effective primary therapy for the lung lesion accompanying systemic human sepsis must remain as the control of the underlying septic focus, either by antibiotic therapy, surgical drainage, or both.

Acknowledgments. Part of the work reported in this paper was supported by a grant from the Physicians Services Incorporated (Ontario) and a Development Grant from the Upjohn Company of Canada.

References

Albert, R.K.: Increased surface tension favours pulmonary edema in anesthetized dogs lungs. J. Clin. Invest. *63*:1015, 1979.

Anderson, R.R., Sibbald, W.J., Holliday, R.L., et al.: Increased pulmonary capillary permeability in human sepsis. Eur. J. Int. Care Med. *3*(3):110, 1977.

Anderson, R.R., Sibbald, W.J., Holliday, R.L., et al.: Documentation of pulmonary capillary permeability in human adult respiratory distress syndrome (ARDS) secondary to sepsis. Am. Rev. Respir. Dis. *119*:869, 1979.

Bachofen, M., and Weibel, E.R.: Alterations of the gas exchange apparatus in adult respiratory insufficiency associated with septicemia. Am. Rev. Resp. Dis. *116*:589, 1977.

Beaven, M.A.: Histamine. N. Engl. J. Med. *294*:30 and 320, 1977.

Blake, I., and Staub, N.C.: Pulmonary vascular transport in sheep: A mathematical model. Microvasc. Res. *12*:197, 1976.

Bowers, R., and Brigham, K.L.: Methylprednisolene prevents endotoxin induced high lung vascular permeability in the awake sheep. Clin. Res. *26*:444A, 1978.

Brewer, L.S., Samson, P.C., Burbank, B. et al.: The wet lung in war casualities. Ann. Surg. *123*:343, 1946.

Brigham, K.L.: Lung edema due to increased vascular permeability. In *Lung Biology in Health and Disease, Vol. 9, Lung Solute Exchange*, edited by N. C. Staub. Marcel Dekker, New York, 1977a.

Brigham, K.L. Factors affecting lung vascular permeability. Am. Rev. Respir. Dis. *115*:165, 1977b.

Brigham, K.L.: Pulmonary edema: Cardiac and non-cardiac. Am. J. Surg. *138*:361, 1979.

Brigham, K.L., and Owen, P.J.: Increased sheep lung vascular permeability caused by histamine. Circ. Res. *37*:647, 1975a.

Brigham, K.L., and Owen, P.J.: Mechanism of the serotonin effect on lung transvascular fluid and protein movement in awake sheep. Circ. Res. *36*:761, 1975b.

Brigham, K.L., Woolverton, W., Blake, L., et al.: Increased sheep lung vascular permeability caused by pseudomonas bacteremia. J. Clin. Invest. *54*:792, 1974.

Brigham, K.L., Bowers, R.E., and Owen, P.J.: Effect of antihistamines on lung vascular response to histamine in unanaesthetized sheep. J. Clin. Invest. *158*:391, 1976a.

Brigham, K.L., Harris, T., and Owen, P.: ^{14}C-Urea and ^{14}C-sucrose as permeability indicators in histamine pulmonary edema. J. Appl. Physiol. *43*:99, 1977a.

Brigham, K.L., Harris, T., Rowlett, T., et al.: Comparisons of ^{14}C-urea and ^{3}H-mannitol as lung vascular permeability indicators in awake sheep: Evidence against red cell urea trapping. Microvasc. Res. *13*:97, 1977b.

Brigham, K.L., Bowers, R.E., and Haynes, J.: Increased sheep lung vascular permeability caused by *Escherischia coli* endotoxin. Circ. Res. *45*:292, 1979a.

Brigham, K.L., Snell, J.D., Harris, T.R., et al.: Indicator dilution lung water and vascular permeability in humans: Effects of pulmonary vascular pressure. Circ. Res. *44*:523, 1979b.

Clowes, G.H., Farrington, G.H., Zuschneid, W., et al.: Circulating factors in the etiology of pulmonary insufficiency and right heart failure accompanying severe sepsis. Ann. Surg. *171*:663, 1970.

Coalson, J.J., Hinshaw, L.B., et al.: Pathophysiological response of the subhuman primate in experimental septic shock. Lab. Invest. *32*:561, 1975.

Craddock, P.R., Hammerschmidt, L., White, J.C., et al.: Complement (C5a) induced granulocyte aggregation in vitro. J. Clin. Invest. *60*:260, 1977.

Da Luz, P.L., Shubin, H., and Weil, M.H.: Pulmonary edema

related to changes in colloid osmotic and pulmonary artery wedge pressure in patients after acute myocardial infarction. Circulation *51:*350, 1975.

Demling, R.H., Niehaus, G., and Will, J.A.: Pulmonary microvascular response to hemorrhagic shock, resuscitation and recovery. J. Appl. Physiol. *46:*498, 1979.

Drinker, C.E., and Field, M.E.: The protein content of mammalian lymph and the relation of lymph to tissue fluid. Am. J. Physiol. *97:*32, 1931.

Egan, E.A., Nelson, R.M., and Gessner, I.H.: Solute permeability of alveolar epithelium in acute hemodynamic edema in dogs. Am. J. Physiol. *233:*80, 1977.

Erdmann, A.J., Vaughn, T.R., Jr., Brigham, K.L., et al.: Effect of increased vascular pressure on lung fluid balance in unanesthetized sheep. Circ. Res. *37:*271, 1975.

Fein, A., Grossman, R.F., Jones, J.G., et al.: The value of edema fluid protein measurements in patients with pulmonary edema. Am. J. Med. *67:*32, 1979.

Feraron, D.T., Ruddy, S., Schur, P.H., and McCabe, W.C.: Activation of the properdin pathology of complement in patients with gram negative bacteremia. N. Engl. J. Med. *292:*937, 1975.

Finley, R.L., Holliday, R.H., Lefcoe, M., et al.: Pulmonary edema in patients with sepsis. Surg. Gynecol. Obstet. *140:*851, 1975.

Fischer, P., Millen, J.E., and Glauser, F.L.: Endotoxin induced increased alveolar capillary membrane permeability. Cir. Shock. *4:*387, 1977.

Fulton, R.L., and Jones, C.E.: The cause of post traumatic pulmonary insufficiency in man. Surg. Gynecol. Obstet. *140:*179, 1975.

Gabel, J.C., and Drake, R.E.: Pulmonary capillary pressure and permeability. Crit. Care Med. *7:*92, 1979.

Garr, K.A., Jr., Taylor, A.E., Owens, L.J., et al.: Pulmonary capillary pressure and filtration coefficient in the isolated, perfused lung. Am. J. Physiol. *213:*910, 1967.

Gelb, A., and Klein, E.: Hemodynamic and alveolar protein studies in noncardiogenic pulmonary edema. Am. Rev. Resp. Dis. *114:*831, 1976.

Gorin, A.B., Weidner, W.J., Demling, R.H., et al.: Noninvasive measurement of pulmonary transvascular protein flux in sheep. J. Appl. Physiol. *45:*225, 1978.

Gump, F.E., Mashima, T., Ferencyz, A., et al.: Pre- and postmortem studies of lung fluids and electrolytes. J. Trauma *11:*474, 1971.

Halmagyi, D.R.: Role of lymphatics in the genesis of "shock lung": A hypothesis. In: *Lung Biology in Health and Disease*, vol. 9, Lung Solute Exchange, edited by N. C. Staub. pp. 423. Marcel Dekker, New York, 1977.

Hansen, A.T.: A self-recording electronic osmometer for quick, direct measurement of collois osmotic pressure in small samples. Acta. Physiol. Scand. *53:*197, 1961.

Harris, T.R., Brigham, K.L., and Rowlett, R.D.: Pressure, serotonin and histamine effects on lung multiple-indicator curves in sheep. J. Appl. Physiol. *44:*245, 1978.

Heflin, A.C., and Brigham, K.L.: Granulocyte depletion prevents increased lung vascular permeability after endotoxemia in sheep. Clin. Res. *26:*399A, 1978.

Horig, T., Nicolaysen, A., and Nicolaysen, G.: Ultrastructural studies of the alveolar capillary barrier in isolated plasma-perfused rabbit lungs. Effects of EDTA and of increased capillary pressure. Acta. Physiol. Scand. *82:*417, 1971.

Kanto, W.P., Jr., Kuhns, L.P., Borer, R.C., Jr., et al.: Failure of serial chest radiographs. Am. J. Obst. Gynecol. *131:*757, 1978.

Kaplan, R.L., Sahn, S.A., and Petty, T.L.: Incidence and outcome of the respiratory distress syndrome in gram negative sepsis. Arch. Intern. Med. *139:*867, 1979.

Kedem, O., and Katchalsky, A.: Thermodynamic analysis of the permeability of biological membranes to non-electrolytes. Biochim. Biophys. Acta *27:*229, 1958.

Landis, E.M., and Pappenheimer, J.R.: Exchange of substances through capillary walls. In *Handbook of Physiology, Vol. II*, pp. 961. American Physiological Society, Washington, D.C., 1963.

Lappas, D.G., Leu, W.A., and Gabel, J.C.: Indirect measurement of left atrial pressure in surgical patients: a comparison of pulmonary capillary wedge and pulmonary artery end-diastolic pressure measured via a flow-directed pulmonary artery catheter (Swan Ganz) to left atrial pressure. Anaesthesia *38:*394, 1973.

Lefcoe, M., Sibbald, W.J., and Holliday, R.L.: Wedged balloon catheter angiography in the critical care unit. Crit. Care Med. *7:*449, 1979.

Lett-Brown, M.A., Boetcher, D.A., and Leonard, E.J.: Chemotactic response of normal human basophils to C5a and to lymphocyte derived chemotactic factor. J. Immunol. *117:*246, 1976.

Levine, O.R., Mellins, R.B., Senior, R.M., et al.: Application of Starlings law of capillary exchange to the lungs. J. Clin. Invest. *46:*934, 1967.

Miller, W.C., Simi, W.W., and Rice, D.L.: Contribution of systemic venous hypertension to the development of pulmonary edema in dogs. Circ. Res. *43:*598, 1978.

Murray, J.F.: Conference Report. Mechanisms of acute respiratory failure. Am. Rev. Respir. Dis. *115:*1071, 1977.

Ohkuda, K., Nakahara, K., Weidner, W.J., et al.: Lung fluid exchange after uneven pulmonary artery obstruction in sheep. Circ. Res. *43:*152, 1978.

Parker, J.C., Guyton, A.C., and Taylor, A.E.: Pulmonary interstitial and capillary pressure estimated from intra-alveolar fluid pressures. J. Appl. Physiol. *44:*267, 1978.

Parwaresch, M.R.: *The Human Blood Basophil*. Springer, Berlin, 1976.

Petty, T.: The adult respiratory distress syndrome (confessions of a "lumper") (E). Am. Rev. Respir. Dis. *111:*713, 1975.

Petty, T.L., and Ashbaugh, D.G.: The adult respiratory distress syndrome. Clinical feature, factors influencing prognosis and principles of management. Chest *60:*233, 1971.

Pietra, G.G., Szidon, J.P., Leventhal, M.M., et al.: Histamine and interstitial pulmonary edema in the dog. Circ. Res. *29:*323, 1971.

Pietra, G.G., Szidon, J.P., Carpenter, H.A., et al.: Bronchial venular leakage during endotoxin shock. Am. J. Pathol. *77:*387, 1974.

Propst, K., Millen, J. E., and Glauser, F.L.: The effects of endogenous and exogenous histamine on pulmonary alveolar membrane permeability. Am. Rev. Respir. Dis. *117:*1063, 1978.

Renkin, E.M.: Transport pathways through capillary endothelium. Microvasc. Res. *15:*123, 1978.

Riordan, J.F., and Walters, G.: Pulmonary oedema in bacterial shock. Lancet *1:*719, 1968.

Robin, E.D., Carey, L.C., Grenvik, A., et al.: Capillary leak syndrome with pulmonary edema. Arch. Intern. Med. *130:*66, 1972.

Schneeberger, E.E., and Karnovsky, M.J.: Structure of intercellular junctions in freeze-fractured alveolar-capillary membranes of mouse lung. Circ. Res. *38:*404, 1976.

Shirley, H.H., Wolfram, C.G., Wasserman, K., et al.: Capillary permeability to macromolecules: Stretched pore phenomenon. Am. J. Physiol. *190:*189, 1957.

Sibbald, W.J., Paterson, N.A.M., Holliday, R.L., et al.: Pulmonary hypertension in sepsis. Chest 73:583–591, 1978.
Sibbald, W.J., Anderson, R.R., and Holliday, R.L.: Pathogenesis of pulmonary edema associated with the adult respiratory distress syndrome. Can. Med. Assoc. J. 120:445, 1979a.
Sibbald, W.J., Moffat, J., Calvin, J., et al.: Alveolo-capillary permeability to large and small molecules in human septic pulmonary edema (abstract). Crit. Care Med. 7:126, 1979b.
Sibbald, W.J., Myers, M.L., Moffat, J., et al.: Demonstrations of the clinical significance of intravascular starling forces in human cardiac and non-cardiac edema (abstract). Chest 76:367, 1979c.
Snell, J., and Ramsay, L.: Pulmonary edema as a result of endotoxemia. Am. J. Physiol. 217:170, 1969.
Starling, E.H.: On the absorption of fluids from connective tissue spaces. J. Physiol. (Lond.) 19:312, 1896.
Staub, N.C.: Pulmonary edema. Physiol. Rev. 54:678, 1974.
Staub, N.C.: The forces regulating fluid filtration in the lung. Microvasc. Res. 15:45, 1978a.
Staub, N.C.: Pulmonary edema due to increased permeability to fluid and protein. Circ. Res. 43:143, 1978b.
Staub, N.C., Bland, R.D., Brigham, K.L., et al.: Preparation of chronic lung lymph fistules in sheep. J. Surg. Res. 19:315, 1975.
Staverman, A.J.: The theory of measurement of osmotic pressure. Rec. Trav. Chem. 70:344, 1951.
Sturm, J.A., Carpenter, M.A., Lewis, F.R., et al.: Water and protein movement in the sheep lung after septic shock: Effect of colloid versus crystalloid resuscitation. J. Surg. Res. 26:233, 1979.
Taylor, A.E., and Drake, R.E.: Fluid and protein movement across the pulmonary microcirculation. In: *Lung Biology in Health and Disease, Vol. 9, Lung Solute Exchange*, edited by N.C. Staub. Marcel Dekker, New York, 1977.
Taylor, A.E., and Gaark, A.: Estimation of equilivant pore raddi of pulmonary capillary and alveolar membranes. Am. J. Physiol. 218:1133, 1970.
Visscher, M., Haddy, F., and Stephens, G.: The physiology and pharmacology of lung edema. Pharmacol. Rev. 8:389, 1956.
Vito, L., Dennis, R.C., Weisel, R.D., et al.: Sepsis presenting as acute respiratory insufficiency. Surg. Gynecol. Obstet. 138:896, 1974.
Vreim, C.E., and Staub, N.C.: Protein composition of lung fluids in acute alloxan edema in dogs. Am. J. Physiol. 230:376, 1976.
Vreim, C.E., Snashall, P.D., Demling, R.H., et al.: Lung lymph and free interstitial fluid protein composition in sheep with edema. Am. J. Physiol. 230:1650, 1976a.
Vreim, C.E., Snashall, P.D., and Staub, N.C.: Protein composition of lung fluids in anesthetized dogs with acute cardiogenic edema. Am. J. Physiol. 231:1466, 1976b.
Weaver, D.W., Ledgerwood, A., and Lucas, C.: Pulmonary effects of albumin resuscitation for severe hypovolemic shock. Arch. Surg. 113:387, 1979.
Weil, M.H., Morrisette, M., and Michaels, S.: Routine plasma colloid osmotic pressure measurements. Crit. Care Med. 2:229, 1974.
Weil, M.H., Hennins, P.J., Morrissette, M., et al.: Relationship between colloid osmotic pressure and pulmonary artery wedge pressure in patients with acute cardiorespiratory failure. Am. J. Med. 64:643, 1978.

CHAPTER 27

Treatment of the Adult Respiratory Distress Syndrome

STEPHEN M. AYRES

Two distinct streams of inquiry have converged on the problem of acute respiratory failure: one seeks to understand the processes leading to diffuse alveolar injury, and the other believes that mechanical attempts to alter lung inflation can improve survivorship. The dual approach is surprisingly similar to the parallel lines of research that led to a remarkable decline from 80 to 20% in the mortality from respiratory distress of the newborn. Comroe (1977) has told in trenchant prose how continuous positive airway pressure applied to a sick infant by an imaginative resident physician accomplished what a decade of fundamental investigation could not—the maintenance of lung inflation at the bedside. The story may be prophetic and significant; history need not always be relived.

Forty years before Gregory et al. (1970) applied positive airway pressure to an infant with respiratory distress, the father of modern oxygen therapy, Alvan et al. (1938), used a crude motor blower to deliver oxygen by continuous positive pressure to eight patients with either hydrostatic or permeability induced pulmonary edema. He noted that six survived and suggested that "the function of positive pressure in these cases as in the experimental production of pulmonary edema was to exert a direct opposing physical force on the external capillary wall tending to counteract the tendency to ooze serum and to decrease the inlet of blood into the right heart diminishing pulmonary congestion." The problem of capillary leakage impairing oxygenation was then forgotten as Pearl Harbor and the Second World War dramatically shifted priorities.

The idea that failure to breathe is not synonymous with death began to gain credence with the war-inspired development of demand valves and positive pressure resuscitation equipment between 1941–1945 and with the use of positive and negative pressure ventilators to maintain ventilation during the poliomyelitis epidemics of 1948 through 1952. McCann et al. (1952) developed the concept of the failing lung in a prescient little essay published in 1952, pointing out that extrapulmonary events could cause the lung to fail and that either hypocapnia or hypercapnia could occur, depending upon the distribution of pulmonary lesions. Noehren (1955) described the use of mechanical ventilation in patients with hypoxemia and hypercapnia secondary to severe emphysema. Miller et al. (1960) used a tank respirator to successfully treat a 37-year-old man with overwhelming staphylococcal pneumonia and suggested that respirator breathing might be helpful with severe inflammatory or chemical pneumonitis and for individuals with life-threatening respiratory insufficiency from other causes.

The almost simultaneous development of pump oxygenators, volume-cycled ventilators, and electrodes for rapidly measuring oxygen and carbon dioxide tensions in small samples of arterial blood ushered in a new era of ventilatory support of seriously ill medical and surgical patients. The "pump lung" syndrome following open heart surgery provided a human model for diffuse lung injury, and Dammann et al. (1963) demonstrated that elective postoperative mechanical ventilation could reduce the frequency of pulmonary complications.

Our own experience in a combined medical and surgical intensive care unit at the Saint Vincent's Hospital in New York City led us to distinguish between *hypoxemia without hypercapnia* and *hypoxemia with hypercapnia* (Ayres and Giannelli, 1967). The former syndrome was observed to develop in patients with a variety of acute situations including shock, trauma, and sepsis. Marked venoarterial shunting and overall alveolar hyperventilation were observed. Hypercapnic hypoxemia developed in individuals with chronic pulmonary disease; hypoxemia was caused by both venoarterial shunting and by regional hypoventilation with persistence of perfusion, hypercapnia by overall hypoventilation and the presence of multiple regions with low ventilation/perfusion characteristics.

Ashbaugh et al. (1969) christened hypoxemia without hypercapnia the adult respiratory distress syndrome. This creative group emphasized the importance of expiratory alveolar collapse with reduction of functional residual capacity and demonstrated the ability of expiratory airway pressure to maintain alveolar integrity. Investigators from the same group provided important experimental evidence that positive pressure ventilation could prevent as well as treat the respiratory distress syndrome (Uzawa and Ashbaugh, 1969). Acute hemorrhagic pulmonary edema produced by the injection of oleic acid into the right ventricle in the dog was uniformly fatal. More than 80% of the animals survived when mechanical ventilation was initiated immediately after injection of oleic acid.

ADULT RESPIRATORY DISTRESS SYNDROME

Lumping all patients with acute respiratory failure that developed in previously normal lungs into a new nosologic pigeonhole, the adult respiratory distress syndrome, was a satisfying tour-de-force that focused attention on a group of stereotyped abnormalities. Whether the initial problem was trauma, sepsis, shock, hypoxemia, head injury, aspiration pneumonitis, or viral pneumonitis, the final result appeared to be diffuse lung injury with decreased pulmonary compliance and massive venoarterial shunting. More recent studies have shown some differences among patients with different etiologic events. Patients with sepsis or pneumonitis, for example, appear resistant to positive end-expiratory pressure and have a substantially higher mortality.

Bachofen and Weibel (1977), in an ultrastructural and morphometric study made possible by the early postmortem transthoracic injection of stained glyceraldehyde solution, have shown that the earliest stages are characterized by a massive capillary leak. Granular leukocytes, red blood cells, macrophages, cell debris, and proteinacous material fill the alveolar spaces, whereas the alveolar septa bulge with edema fluid and migrated cells. The type I membranous pneumocytes that line the alveoli are destroyed so that the basement membrane is denuded; in contrast, the type II granular pneumocytes seem impervious and increase in number, often protruding into the alveolar space. Capillaries are distended and frequently plugged with leukocytes. Later, the interalveolar septa become thickened or replaced by massive structures which are unrecognizable as the previously delicate alveolar septa. Plasma cells, clusters of histiocytes, fibrosis, and edema all serve to distort lung architecture. In many sections, massive proliferation of type II pneumocytes are a striking finding.

These ultrastructural data together with a group of lung biopsy and physiologic observations made by Lamy et al. (1976) permit reasonable correlation of morphologic and functional events. In the early stages, marked impairment of gas exchange is caused primarily by the filling of alveoli with edema fluid and formed elements of the blood. A large venoarterial shunt, arterial hypoxemia, decreased pulmonary compliance, and modest elevation of pulmonary vascular resistance are observed. Positive end-expiratory pressure is effective in increasing lung volume and decreasing the venoarterial shunt. In later stages, the lungs become progressively less compliant as chronic inflammatory changes and fibrosis occur. The lungs require increasingly higher inflation pressures; pulmonary vascular resistance and alveolar dead space increase, and positive end-expiratory pressure becomes less effective in decreasing the venoarterial shunt. The morphometric data of Bachofen and Weibel (1977) suggest that in the later stages of diffuse lung injury, decrease in surface area and septal thickening may make diffusion the limiting factor for gas exchange.

Biopsies from patients with pneumonitis represent an important subset. Four of the patients studied by Lamy et al. (1976) had diffuse pneumonitis with alveoli filled with necrotic or hemorrhagic material; in these patients the venoarterial shunt appeared fixed and unresponsive to elevation of end-expiratory pressure. In contrast to these patients are those with viral pneumonitis who seem to respond to end-expiratory pressure. Presumably, these patients have changes predominantly located in the interstitium so that enhancement of alveolar expansion is possible.

Two sequential biopsies and an autopsy specimen from a patient with burn trauma and shock demonstrate the sequence described above and emphasize the impact of trauma on the entire organism. The first biopsy taken at 9 days reveals hyaline membranes, indicating capillary leakage, interstitial proliferation and open alveoli; arterial oxygen tension at that stage was improved by positive end-expiratory pressure. On day 18, cellular and fibrotic changes limited the ability of that technique to augment alveolar expansion. The autopsy specimen on day 56 revealed areas of attempted alveolar reconstruction alternating with large areas of fibrosis.

The common pathway linking all of these situations seems to be the presence of increased capillary permeability, hence the descriptive term, "the leaky capillary syndrome." A number of lines of evidence suggest that sepsis, hypoxemia, hypotension and other factors can initiate an immunologic sequence that produces diffuse lung injury. As early as 1927, for example, Landis (1943) found that the pulmonary capillary permeability for proteins was increased following a 3-min period of oxygen deprivation. More recent studies with endotoxin administration or following hemodialysis have suggested activation of a complex series of defense responses that may be more devastating than the initial insult.

The mammalian defense system, evolved over millions of years of vertebrate development, is particularly well equipped to deal with blood loss and infection; the coagulation proteins and platelets attempt to repair rents in the vascular system while the complement and kinin systems have an opposite action; they increase vascular permeability so that specially constructed attack units can reach infected tissue. Their explosive detonation probably underlies the development of the adult respiratory distress syndrome.

While much remains to be learned, the initial step appears to be the activation of a humoral factor (Hageman factor, or factor 12) by certain antigens and antibodies or by vascular injury. The two may be linked since fragments of vascular wall could be recognized as "foreign" by the immune surveillance system. Regardless of the initial step, at least four discrete pathways began to operate: activation of complement, generation of kinins, blood coagulation, and fibrinolysis. These systems mobilize formed elements of the blood, directing leukocytes to areas of infection and platelets to areas of hemorrhage.

A variety of substances destroy lung tissue and increase capillary permeability. The complement cascade unfolds much as a military organization sends out special squads for specific tasks. Two components, C3a and C5a have a specific effect on vascular permeability, allowing formed elements to be mobilized to tissue areas. Activated Hageman factor mobilizes the kinin system as well as the complement cascade, however, enhancing the formation of kallikrein. Kallikrein then converts kininogen to bradykinin producing vasodilatation, enhancing circulation to distressed regions. C3a, C5a, and other complement fragments direct polymorpholeukocytes to the same extravascular regions and cause those cells to release a group of lysosomal proteases which attack infectious agents as well as normal tissue. At the same time, the turbulence within the vascular system and the leaks created by the antiinflammatory efforts further activate the coagulation system and its counterpoise, the fibrinolytic network. Disseminated intravascular coagulation, when it occurs, is another example of activation of an inappropriate defense system.

MAINTENANCE OF ALVEOLAR INTEGRITY IN THE NORMAL AND DISEASED LUNG

The distending pressure of the whole lung and the myriad lung units is the difference between pressure at the mouth and pressure in the pleural space—the transpulmonic pressure. A diagram of lung volume and transpulmonic pressure is sigmoid. With a completely gas-free or atelectatic lung, volume does not enter until a critical opening pressure of 6–10 cm H_2O is reached. At that point, gas flows in and the relationship between pressure change and volume changes is relatively linear until close to maximum inflation. The critical opening pressure appears to be the force necessary to overcome surface forces and allow inflation to proceed. Obviously, if the lung emptied completely with each expiration, extremely high pressure would always be necessary for the subsequent inspiration.

The transpulmonic pressure does not fall to zero at the end of each expiration but is about 5 cm H_2O. This distending pressure is sufficient to overcome the tendency of the lung to collapse and is the force creating the functional residual capacity. Opposing this negative distending force is the elastic force stored within the alveolar wall.

The ability of a distending force of about 5 cm H_2O to maintain expansion during expiration when a force of more than twice that is necessary to produce inflation in a completely collapsed lung is a function of the surface-lining material secreted by the type II pneumocytes. When ordinary bubbles grow smaller, the pressure exerted within the cavity of the bubble by the membrane increases, since pressure equals four times surface tension/diameter (LaPlace Law). As the diameter decreases, pressure increases if surface tension is unchanged and the bubble soon collapses. Surfactant, a complex lipoprotein, has the fortunate property of changing its surface tension with a change in its dimensions. As the layer thickens during expiration, the change in molecular orientation leads to a decrease in surface tension which reduces the pressure within the alveolar units and thus the tendency to collapse.

It is convenient to view alveolar collapse during expiration as a contest between the elastic properties of the lung, which favor collapse, and the transpulmonic or distending pressure, which favors continued expansion. Opening the thorax of an experimental animal leads to a sudden reduction in transpulmonic pressure with consequent sudden reduction of functional residual capacity. Adding positive expiratory pressure permits maintenance of functional residual capacity by preventing collapse. Factors which increase the elastic recoil of the lung or destroy the surface-tension reduction properties of the alveolar wall favor collapse.

Mead and Collier (1959) first observed that certain alveoli progressively collapsed if an anesthetized animal or human was allowed to breathe at a constant tidal volume for several hours. This collapse was evidenced by a decrease in compliance and an increase in venoarterial shunting. It was also discovered that normal individuals interrupt this cycle of progressive collapse by sighing every 5–15 min. These brief, deep inspirations increased transpulmonic pressure, exceeding critical opening pressures and opening the previously atelectatic units. General anesthesia, sedation, the pain associated with recent surgery, general debility, and the shock state decrease the frequency of sighing. Many of these same situations also decrease the antiatelectasis properties of surfactant. The combination of an increased tendency towards collapse and a diminution of the frequency of deep breaths with associated increases in transpulmonic pressure lead to progressive atelectasis.

Early approaches to maintenance of lung expansion in patients with the acute respiratory distress syndrome were based on reliably high volume inspirations delivered by a volume-cycled ventilator and with automatic deep inspirations or sighs (Bendixen et al., 1965). The first Emerson volume ventilators embodied these principles. Persistence of hypoxemia in spite of the "inspiratory" approach lead to a re-evaluation of maintaining transpulmonic pressure during expiration by positive end-expiratory pressure.

EFFECTS OF POSITIVE END-EXPIRATORY PRESSURE ON LUNG EXPANSION

Respirator theorists of the early 1960s followed the doctrine enunciated by Cournand et al. (1948) and shunned elevation of airway pressure during expiration. Important studies performed 15 years earlier had shown that when positive pressure occupied more than 50% of the entire breathing cycle, mean intrathoracic pressure was raised to a degree capable of impeding venous return to the right ventricle. Faced with an unacceptable mortality in patients with acute respiratory failure, several groups of investigators cautiously applied expiratory pressure in a sporadic manner. Ashbaugh et al. (1969) systematically applied the technique to 14 patients with severe respiratory failure and observed improved oxygenation and a substantial decrease in overall mortality. Cardiac output did not fall, apparently because most of the positive airway pressure was spent in distending the rigid lung and not transmitted to the pleural space. The authors enunciated their own principle and wrote that "absolute control of ventilation in these patients is mandatory."

Positive and expiratory pressure works because it maintains an increased transpulmonic pressure at all times, leading to an increased lung volume. Consider two alveolar units, one with normal surface properties and compliance, the other with reduced compliance and absent surfactant. When fully expanded, both are capable of oxygenating pulmonary capillary blood. As the individual expires, intrathoracic pressure becomes less negative approaching −5 cm H_2O. At that point, the transpulmonic pressure difference is 5 cm H_2O since airway pressure is zero. This distending pressure allows the normal unit to remain one-quarter inflated. Depending upon the pressure generated inwards by the diseased lung unit, it may completely collapse or may reduce itself to a lower than normal functional residual capacity. With end-expiratory pressure maintained at a greater than atmospheric level, transpulmonic pressure is increased and expiratory collapse is obviated.

After the initial enthusiasm over the advantages of positive pressure ventilation had somewhat leveled, a number of investigators theorized that air distributed by a single pressure wave at the mouth could not reach all units as evenly as a similar breath produced by negative pressure applied uniformly over the pleural surface. One consequence of this was that compliance during intermittent positive pressure breathing appeared to be flow dependent (Ayres et al., 1963). With lower flow rates, compliance increased and the inspired air appeared to be better distributed. Dammann and McAsland (1979) studied a group of patients with extrapulmonary trauma and relatively normal lungs during mechanical ventilation. Positive end-expiratory pressure reduced the alveolar-arterial oxygen difference and venoarterial shunt. Alveolar and arterial washout of argon revealed that positive end-expiratory pressure improved distribution of the inspired air and increased the functional residual capacity.

That the maintenance of lung expansion is not a magical function of positive end-expiratory pressure itself but a consequence of increasing transpulmonic or alveolar distending pressure throughout the breathing cycle is shown by the approach developed by Vidyasagar and Chernick (1971). Continuous negative pressure applied to the thorax of newborn infants maintained an increased gradient between atmospheric mouth pressure and the negative extrathoracic pressure. Chernick was later to name this continuous distending pressure. Important for the development of new techniques is the observation that the maintenance of an increased transpulmonic pressure difference maintains alveolar inflation and appears to reverse progressive lung injury in the respiratory distress syndrome.

HEMODYNAMIC EFFECTS OF POSITIVE END-EXPIRATORY PRESSURE

Rhythmic changes in intrapleural pressure consequent to changes in position of the respiratory muscles affect cardiac function by changing systemic venous flow, pulmonary vascular resistance, and the dimensions of the cardiac chambers. Figure 27.1 shows schematically the interrelationships among airway and lungs, cardiac structures, and the intrapleural space. During spontaneous respiration, intrapleural pressure becomes progressively more negative, overcoming the retractive or collapsing tendency of the lung and producing airflow and alveolar expansion. The increasing negative pressure increases the gradient between the systemic venous reservoir and the right atrium, enhancing venous return.

These upstream-downstream gradients that promote air and blood flow must be distinguished from the transmural pressure differences acting across vessel and chamber walls. The negative intrapleural pressure is transmitted to the right atrium, for example, so that it is lower than it would be if intrapleural pressure were at atmospheric levels. A problem ensues since the usual hemodynamic measurements relate vascular pressure to atmospheric pressure rather than to intrapleural pressure. This convention leads to right atrial pressure falling during inspiration, although the atrial pressure relative to intrapleural pressure is essentially unchanged. The major reason for considering these transmural pressure gradients is their effect on chamber or vessel size. A negative intrapleural pressure can be viewed as increasing atrial, ventricular, and vascular dimensions while positive intrathoracic pressure decreases them.

During positive pressure ventilation, the driving pressure for alveolar expansion is the positive pressure delivered to the airway; part of this pressure is transmitted to the intrapleural space, but intrapleural pressure is less than airway pressure so that alveolar expansion occurs. Lung volume is determined by this transpulmonic pressure and is independent of whether intrapleural pressure is less than (spontaneous ventilation) or more than (positive pressure ventilation) airway pressure. While the mode of producing the transpulmonic pressure gradient

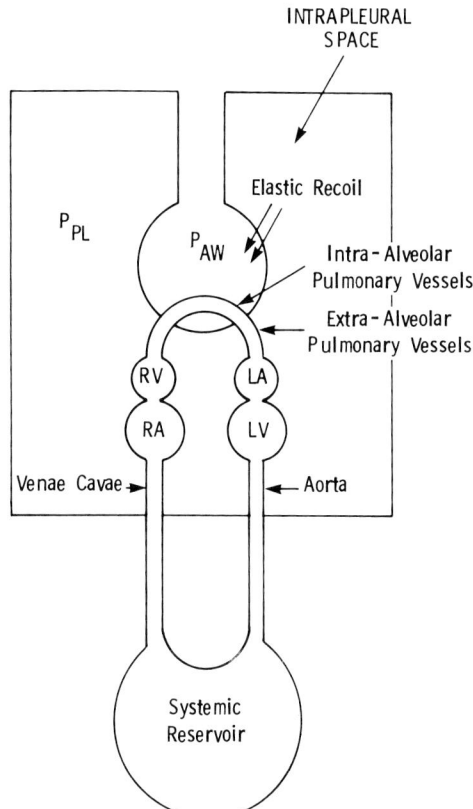

Figure 27.1. Pressure relationships among airways (P_{AW}), pleural space (P_{PL}), and circulatory system. Pressure in alveolar units is considered identical with that in airways when gas is not flowing. Lung inflation is determined by gradient between pressure at mouth and that in the alveolar spaces. Cardiac filling is determined by the gradient between pleural pressure and pressure in the extrathoracic veins.

is of no consequence for lung inflation, it has a profound effect on cardiac function.

Positive airway and alveolar pressures are transmitted to the intrapleural space; the fraction transmitted depends upon the retractile force of the alveolar wall or the pulmonary compliance. When the lung is highly distensible, much of the airway pressure is transmitted to the intrapleural space; when compliance is reduced, substantially less is transmitted. This phenomenon accounts for the ability to use high levels of positive pressure in patients with the adult respiratory distress syndrome. Marked reductions in pulmonary compliance obviate the rises in intrapleural pressure that would occur in individuals with normal compliance.

The effects of raising intrathoracic pressure on cardiac output can be visualized from the venous return curves described by Guyton (1963). Venous return is normal when systemic venous pressure is 4 mm Hg or more than right atrial pressure. Venous return falls as this difference disappears and when right atrial pressure is about 8 mm Hg higher than peripheral pressure (in the dog), venous return ceases. The sensitivity of venous return to venous volume is shown by the effects of bleeding or infusion. When moderate hypovolemia is produced, venous return ceases when right atrial pressure is 4–6 mm Hg above peripheral pressure; with hypervolemia, adequate venous return may be maintained even when right atrial pressure is 4–8 mm Hg greater than peripheral pressure. Similar results may be produced by venodilator or venoconstrictor agents; administration of an α-blocking agent during positive pressure ventilation produces a profound decrease in cardiac output, which may be reversed by the administration of a pressor amine.

CLINICAL USE OF POSITIVE PRESSURE VENTILATION

Accumulated experience over the past two decades has demonstrated that early intubation together with positive pressure ventilation maintain alveolar integrity and provide the best chance for patient survival. The earlier emphasis on large tidal volumes with frequent even larger tidal volumes or sighs gave way to the realization that increasing functional residual capacity was more useful to increasing tidal volume (Bendixen et al., 1965). As most centers turned to positive end-expiratory pressure to improve oxygenation and reduced inspired oxygen concentrations in the adult respiratory distress syndrome, other investigators continued to worry about the effects on cardiac output and blood pressure. Lutch and Murray (1972) focused that view by showing that positive end-expiratory pressure increased arterial oxygen tension but decreased cardiac output, venous oxygen tension, and overall oxygen delivery (oxygen content times cardiac output). Attempting to determine the level of positive end-expiratory pressure that would improve oxygenation without affecting cardiac output, Suter et al. (1975) hit on the idea of using total compliance for an end-point in the titration of end-expiratory pressure. They noted that when compliance increased to its maximum, cardiac output, oxygen transport, and venous oxygen tension were higher than they were initially. Increasing end-expiratory pressure from that point led to a decrease in compliance and a decrement in blood flow.

Early success with positive pressure ventilation has been obtained with heavy sedation and total control of ventilation. Several observations led many to question this approach: 1) controlled ventilation led to rapid deconditioning of systemic and ventilatory muscles; 2) the inspired air was not distributed as well with positive pressure ventilation as with spontaneous ventilation leading to increased atelectasis; 3) increased systemic venous pressure led to increased transvascular fluid filtration requiring the addition of replacement fluids such as albumin to maintain vascular volume.

Since mechanical ventilation was used to augment alveolar ventilation, *when it was reduced*, and positive expiratory pressure was indicated to increase functional residual capacity and improve oxygenation, Kirby et al. (1975) introduced positive end-expiratory pressure with intermittent mandatory ventilation (IMV). With IMV, patients breathe spontaneously and a variable number of respiratory breaths are added each minute to maintain alveolar ventilation. Figures 27.2 and 27.3 show the spectacular results obtained with this approach. Arterial oxygen tension was much higher than with controlled ventilation, presumably because the patients' own breaths did a better job of distributing the inspired air; cardiac output did not fall because mean intrathoracic pressure was close to atmospheric most of the time.

In patients who appear to be ventilating adequately and who do not have excessive secretions, the same

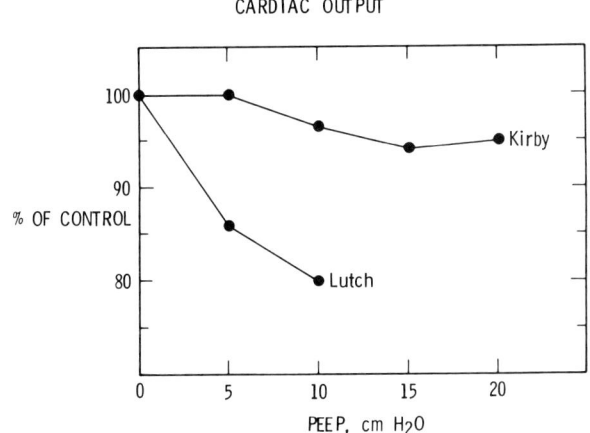

Figure 27.2. Effect of progressive increments in positive end-expiratory pressure on arterial oxygen tension (the PaO_2/FIO_2 ratio). Note that the use of IMV with PEEP leads to strikingly greater oxygenation in patients with the adult respiratory distress syndrome.

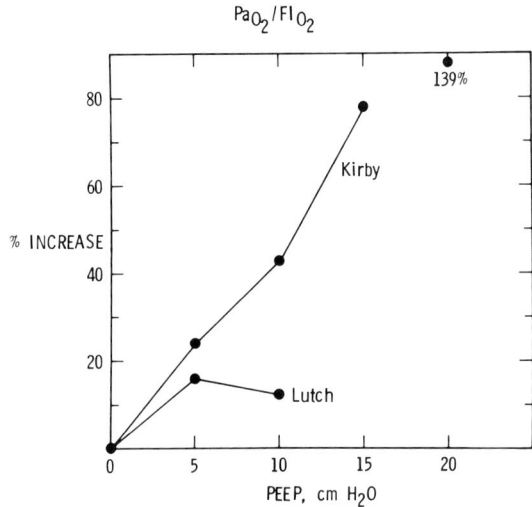

Figure 27.3. Effect of progressive increments in positive end-expiratory pressure on cardiac output. IMV with PEEP blunts the substantial decrease in cardiac output observed with PEEP and controlled ventilation.

technique used to great advantage in the newborn may be indicated. Taylor et al. (1976) used a simple mask technique and showed striking improvement in oxygenation in two patients with severe viral pneumonitis. Similar results have been reported by other investigators (Shah et al., 1977).

TREATMENT OF THE ADULT RESPIRATORY DISTRESS SYNDROME

Correction of the Original Problem

While many aspects of treatment are the same regardless of the cause, specific problems must be corrected. Gram-negative or gram-positive sepsis must be rapidly treated with appropriate antibiotics. Specific fluid losses in patients with trauma must be eliminated. Viral pneumonitis should be treated with appropriate antiviral agents as they become available; amantadine seems effective in influenzal pneumonitis at this time (NIH, 1979). Severe left ventricular failure should be treated with mechanical assistance techniques such as intra-aortic balloon counterpulsation (Mueller et al., 1971).

Specific Pharmacologic Agents

A common pathway for the development of increased vascular permeability appears to be the activation of the complement pathways with release of a variety of potent mediator substances. Eventually it should be possible to administer specific pharmacologic agents aimed at cooling down the complement cascade. Until their availability, many believe that patients should receive one or two large doses of corticosteroid.

The use of corticosteroid in high doses for the treatment of the vascular injury characteristic of septic shock gained further credence when Schumer (1976) showed in a prospective study that mortality could be strikingly reduced. He administered either 30 mg/kg of methyl prednisolone or 3 mg/kg of dexamethasone and repeated it once, if necessary, after 4 hr. Nine of the 77 patients treated with steroid died (10.4%), while 33 of 53 treated with a saline placebo died. While this data can correctly only be applied to patients with septic shock, it is suggestive evidence that corticosteroids may be useful in the microcirculatory injury found in the adult respiratory distress syndrome.

Positive Pressure Ventilation

At the present writing, most adult patients should probably be intubated as early as possible. If alveolar hypoventilation evidenced by a rising carbon dioxide tension and respiratory acidosis is not present, patients should be ventilated by intermittent mandatory ventilation with positive end-expiratory pressure, added in increments of 5 mm Hg until the arterial oxygen tension divided by the fraction of inspired oxygen is greater than 300. Positive end-expiratory pressure should be continued until there is clear evidence that pulmonary mechanics and gas exchange are substantially improved.

Vascular Volume

Ideally, the patient should be neither hypervolemic nor hypovolemic. There is considerable empiric evidence that furosemide reduces lung water, in part by its diuretic effect and in part by a direct vascular effect that appears to decompress lung vessels. It should be tried, provided that central venous pressure is within normal limits. If central venous pressure is reduced, adequate fluids must be administered.

There is still no general agreement regarding the role of crystalloid or colloid solutions. There is no evidence that colloid can lead to a worsening of pulmonary gas exchange, but there is suggestive evidence that it may improve the alveolar-arterial oxygen difference in certain situations. Generally, it is wise to begin with normal saline; if venous pressure does not rise with this solution, albumin or other colloid solutions should be used. Keeping systemic venous pressure down with intermittent mandatory ventilation rather than with ventilatory control appears to obviate the need for colloid solutions.

Maintenance of Blood Pressure

Vasopressor agents are contraindicated since they increase pulmonary and systemic vascular pressures and lead to increased fluid losses into the interstitial space. If raising venous pressure does not increase blood pressure or if left atrial pressures as estimated from pulmonary wedge measurements are elevated, direct inotropic support is indicated. Dobutamine, a recently synthesized catecholamine with inotropic and vasodilator properties, is probably more useful than a digitalis drug. Cardiac glycosides act by a direct effect on the sarcolemma sodium-potassium ATPase so that serious cardiac arrhythmias limit the therapeutic range. The presence of acidosis and hypoxia make the myocardium even more sensitive to the arrhythmogenicactivity of digitalis glycosides. In one study (Mikulic et al., 1977), dobutamine, in an average dose of 10 μg/kg/min, led to a 28% decrease in wedge pressure and a 96% increase in stroke output.

RESULTS OF TREATMENT

Both patient selection and method of treatment seem to influence outcome. Bone (1978), for example, reviewed the literature and reported the mortality to vary from 32 to 80%; mortality was 67% in the 12 patients treated by his group. The importance of pathologic changes to the response to positive end-expiratory pressure and ultimate mortality was demonstrated by Lamy et al. (1976). Mortality was 52% in those patients who responded to end-expiratory pressure and who had pathologic changes such as alveolar edema and atelectasis; mortality was 75% in the nonresponders who also tended to have either fibrosis or alveolar replacement. Cotev et al. (1976) described 57 patients treated with positive end-expiratory pressure delivered by conventional methods. All but two of 28 nonseptic patients increased arterial oxygenation with positive end-expiratory pressure; the overall mortality was 18%. Only 20 of 29 septic patients responded with increased oxygenation, and the increase was one-third that of the nonseptic patients; the overall mortality was 62%.

The results of investigators using the intermittent mandatory ventilation method of Kirby et al. (1975) are in striking contrast to the rather gloomy data reported above. Douglas and Downs (1977) treated 54 patients with the adult respiratory distress syndrome admitted to the Wilford Hall United States Air Force Medical Center; initial measurements of arterial oxygenation and gas exchange were similar to those reported by Cotev et al. (1976). Eighty percent were alive 3 months after leaving the hospital; pulmonary function testing on 10 was relatively normal, suggesting that near complete recovery is the rule. Since the mean age was 38, the useful years salvaged, assuming a life expectancy of 75, was 1591 person-years.

Of importance was the observation that the 11 patients who died were able to maintain an arterial oxygen tension of greater than 60 mm Hg while breathing 60% oxygen. Nine patients died from septicemia and low cardiac output and two died from other causes; hypoxemia was not considered contributory in any of the deaths. Autopsies were performed on six patients who died and revealed minimal alveolar capillary interstitial narrowing and edema. Proliferation of alveolar type II cells was present in all documenting repair and recovery from the initial injury. These data must be interpreted as strongly supporting the early use of positive end-expiratory pressure and intermittent mandatory ventilation will reverse the pathologic changes characteristic of the acute respiratory distress syndrome. Patients still die, but they die from conditions such as sepsis that produced lung injury in the first place.

References

Ashbaugh, D.G., Petty, T.L., Bigelow, D.B., and Harris, T.M.: Continuous positive-pressure breathing (CPPB) in adult respiratory distress syndrome. J. Thorac. Cardiovasc. Surg. 57: 31, 1969.

Ayres, S.M., and Giannelli, S., Jr.: *Care of the Critically Ill*, Appleton-Century-Crofts, New York, 1967.

Ayres, S.M., Kozam, R.L., and Lukas, D.S.: The effects of intermittent positive pressure breathing on intrathoracic pressure, pulmonary mechanics, and the work of breathing. Am. Rev. Respir. Dis. 87:370, 1963.

Bachofen, M., and Weibel, E.R.: Alterations of the gas exchange apparatus in adult respiratory insufficiency associated with septicemia. Am. Rev. Respir. Dis. 116:589, 1977.

Barach, A.L., Martin, J., and Eckman, M.: Positive pressure respiration and its application to the treatment of acute pulmonary edema. Ann. Int. Med. 12:754, 1938.

Bendixen, H.H., Egbert, L.D., Hedley-Whyte, J., Laver, M.B., and Pontoppidan, H.: *Respiratory Care*. C. V. Mosby, St. Louis, 1965.

Bone, R.G.: Treatment of adult respiratory distress syndrome with diuretics, dialysis, and positive end-expiratory pressure. Crit. Care Med. 6:136, 1978.

Comroe, J.H., Jr.: *Retro Spectro Scope—Insights into Medical Discovery*. Von Gehr, Menlo Park, CA, 1977.

Cotev, S., Perel, A., Katzenelson, R., and Eimerl, D.: The effect of PEEP on oxygenating capacity in acute respiratory failure with sepsis. Crit. Care Med. 4:186, 1976.

Cournand, A., Motley, H.L., and Werko, L., et al.: Physiological studies of the effects of intermittent positive pressure breathing on cardiac output in man. Am. J. Physiol. 152:162, 1948.

Dammann, J.F., and McAslan, T.C.: PEEP: its use in young patients with apparently normal lungs. Crit. Care Med. 7:14, 1979.

Dammann, J.F., Thung, N., Christlieb, I.I., Littlefield, J.B., and Muller, W.H., Jr.: The management of the severely ill patient after open-heart surgery. J. Thorac. Cardiovasc. Surg. 45:80, 1963.

Douglas, M.E., and Downs, J.B.: Pulmonary function following severe acute respiratory failure and high levels of positive end-expiratory pressure. Chest 71:18, 1977.

Gregory, G.A., Kitterman, J.A., Phibbs, R.H., Tooley, W.H., and Hamilton, W.K.: Continuous positive airway pressure with spontaneous respiration: a new method of increasing arterial oxygenation in the respiratory distress syndrome. Pediatr. Res. 4:469, 1970.

Guyton, A.C.: In *Handbook of Physiology, Section 2, Circulation*, p. 1099. American Physiological Society, Washington, DC, 1963.

Kirby, R.R., Downs, J.B., Civetta, J.M., Modell, J.H., Dannemiller, F.J., Klein, E.F., and Hodges, M.: High level positive end expiratory pressure (PEEP) in acute respiratory insufficiency. Chest 67:156, 1975.

Lamy, M., Fallat, R.J., Koeniger, E., Harm-Peter, D., Ratliff, J.L., Eberhart, R.C., Tucker, H.J., and Hill, J.D.: Pathologic features and mechanisms of hypoxemia in adult respiratory distress syndrome. Am. Rev. Respir. Dis. 114:267, 1976.

Landis, E.M.: Micro-injection studies of capillary permeability. Am. J. Physiol. 387:1927, 1943.

Lutch, J.S., and Murray, J.F.: Continuous positive-pressure ventilation: effects on systemic oxygen transport and tissue oxygenation. Ann. Int. Med. 76:193, 1972.

McCann, W.S., Lovejoy, F.W., Jr., and Yu, P.N.G.: Failing lung. N.Y. State J. Med. 52:1983, 1952.

Mead, J., and Collier, C.: Relationship of volume history of lungs to respiratory mechanics in anesthetized dogs. J. Appl. Physiol. 14:669, 1959.

Mikulic, E., Cohn, J.N., and Franciosa, J.A.: Comparative hemodynamic effects of inotropic and vasodilator drugs in severe heart failure. Circulation 56:528, 1977.

Miller, F.L., Zerbi-Ortiz, A., and Elkins, J.T.: Use of the tank respirator in overwhelming bacterial pneumonia. N. Engl. J. Med. 262:1264, 1960.

Mueller, H.S., Ayres, S.M., Conklin, E.F., et al.: The effects of intra-aortic counterpulsation on cardiac performance and metabolism in shock associated with acute myocardial infarction. J. Clin. Invest. 50:1885, 1971.

NIH Consensus Development Conference Summary: Amantadine: does it have a role in the prevention and treatment of influenza? Sponsored by the National Institute of Allergy and Infectious Diseases, assisted by the Office for Medical Applications of Research, NIH, October, 1979.

Noehren, T.: Relief of carbon dioxide narcosis by simple intermittent positive pressure breathing therapy. Dis. Chest 28:515, 1955.

Schumer, W.: Steroids in the treatment of clinical septic shock. Ann. Surg. 184:333, 1976.

Shah, D.M., Newell, J.C., Dutton, R.E., and Powers, S.R.: Continuous positive airway pressure versus positive end-expiratory pressure in respiratory distress syndrome. J. Thorac. Cardiovasc. Surg. 74:557, 1977.

Suter, P.M., Fairley, B., and Isenberg, M.D.: Optimum end-expiratory airway pressure in patients with acute pulmonary failure. N. Engl. J. Med. 292:284, 1975.

Taylor, G.J., Brenner, W., and Summer, W.R.: Severe viral pneumonia in young adults. Therapy with continuous positive airway pressure. Chest 69:722, 1976.

Uzawa, T., and Ashbaugh, D.G.: Continuous positive-pressure breathing in acute hemorrhagic pulmonary edema. J. Appl. Physiol. 26:427, 1969.

Vidyasagar, D., and Chernick, V.: Continuous positive transpulmonic pressure in hyaline membrane disease: Simple device. Pediatrics 48:296, 1971.

CHAPTER 28

Humoral Factors and Lung Injury During Shock, Trauma, and Sepsis

ROBERT H. DEMLING
JOHN T. FLYNN

Pulmonary cellular injury following severe trauma complicated by hemorrhagic shock or sepsis is well described. The pathologic response consists of alterations in the permeability of the capillary endothelium and alveolar epithelium leading to increasing interstitial and alveolar fluid and sometimes progressing to intra-alveolar hemorrhage and atelectasis. Although the physiologic response of the lung to this injury is well described, the actual mechanism of injury is only beginning to be understood.

In this chapter we will discuss pulmonary injury caused by hemorrhagic shock, trauma, and sepsis. A number of vasoactive substances are found in the lung during these insults. Some are believed to act as mediators of cellular injury, whereas others seem to be released in response to the injury and correlate temporally with a number of physiologic alterations. Each of these substances will be discussed in relation to pulmonary injury and the pertinent literature summarized. We will preface these remarks with a brief characterization of the basic disease state and physiologic alterations of each of the clinical syndromes.

HEMORRHAGIC SHOCK

Hemorrhagic shock alone does not seem to produce any significant, clinically evident lung injury in humans or in most animal models with the exception of the dog. Lung damage in humans after hemorrhage is usually associated with a superimposed insult of either soft tissue trauma, burns, or sepsis. Experimentally, there remains some controversy over the pulmonary response to pure hemorrhagic shock. In the sheep with chronic lung lymph fistula, a permeability change was not found during either fatal or nonfatal shock (Demling et al., 1979) and lactic dehydrogenase activities in lymph draining the lung were not elevated, indicating no major cell injury (Figs. 28.1 and 28.2). Other investigators (Todd et al., 1978) have reported finding an increase in permeability in the dog lung following hemorrhage which was associated with increased lymph flow but minimal histologic evidence of injury. Under these conditions, lung lymph flow reflects the transvascular fluid filtration rate (Staub, 1971). Pulmonary cell damage following hemorrhage can be produced by rapidly returning the shed blood which acutely increases capillary pressure, probably due to increased venous resistance, and leads to interstitial hemorrhage and edema. Controlled resuscitation also produces a modest but transient increase in lung lymph flow with increased red cell content, an indication of increased transvascular fluid filtration due to high pressure but with no evidence of increased protein permeability (Fig. 28.1). It may well be that a very subtle lung injury is produced during hemorrhagic shock that leads to severe cellular damage when a second type of injury is superimposed.

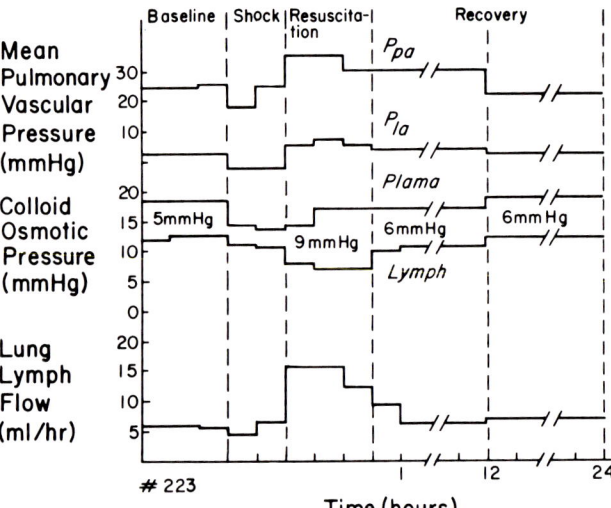

Figure 28.1. The pulmonary microvascular response of an unanesthetized sheep to severe hemorrhagic shock, resuscitation, and a 24-hr period of recovery is shown. Lymph flow and vascular pressures decreased during early shock then returned to baseline. Lymph flow increased during resuscitation, as did vascular pressures; however, the lymph/plasma protein ratio decreased, indicating that the sieving effect for protein was intact and no protein permeability change was evident. The increase in lymph flow was most likely due to an increase in capillary hydrostatic pressure. This would occur if the venous resistance were increased, increasing capillary pressure despite a baseline left atrial pressure. All microvascular parameters quickly returned to baseline after resuscitation. (Reprinted with permission from R. H. Demling, M. Manohar, J. A. Will, and F. O. Belzer: Surgery 86:323–328, 1979.)

TRAUMA—BURNS

Severe soft tissue trauma and multiple fractures, usually with superimposed shock, can lead to the clinical syndrome of post-traumatic respiratory failure (Blaisdell and Schlobohm, 1973). The lung damage is usually delayed 24 hr or more after injury, with progressing interstitial and intra-alveolar edema and hemorrhage being the pathologic findings. Cellular injury has been reported to have been produced by emboli of platelets, fibrin, or fat and by vasoactive substances released from the damaged tissue. Thermal injuries produce two types of lung injury. Severe body burns lead to an indirect lung injury similar to that seen with trauma (Demling et al., 1978). Smoke inhalation is a direct injury to the bronchial mucosa and epithelial lining. Both cellular injuries are delayed in onset from 24 hr to 7 days after the initial insult, strongly suggesting an embolic or humoral agent as being causative. Sepsis is almost always present, compounding the injury (Pruitt et al., 1970).

SEPSIS—ENDOTOXEMIA

Sepsis alone or associated with trauma or shock is the most common cause of the adult respiratory distress syndrome (Fulton and Jones, 1975). The lung injury is characterized by pulmonary hypertension (Sibbald et al., 1978) and increased pulmonary vascular permeability to large molecules. The pathologic picture is similar to that described after trauma and burns. The cause of the injury is considered by many to be due to endotoxins released from the cellular membranes of gram-negative bacteria. Sepsis-induced lung injury has been studied experimentally using either live bacteria or, more frequently, purified endotoxin. Although still controversial, the endotoxin-induced lung injury is considered by many to be the same as that seen clinically in sepsis (Christy, 1971). Animal lung lymph models have added considerably to our knowledge of pulmonary microvascular permeability changes (Staub, 1978). Lymph flow is considered equal to the capillary transvascular fluid filtration rate, and the lymph contents of proteins, enzymes, humoral substances, and other materials are representative of their concentrations in interstitial fluid. In the unanesthetized sheep model, both live *Pseudomonas* bacteria and *Escherichia coli* endotoxin have been used to produce a very similar lung injury (Brigham et al., 1974; 1979). A two phase response is characteristically seen. The acute phase consists of a severe pulmonary artery hypertension beginning about 30 min after injection and lasting for about 2 hr. Lymph flow increases significantly during this period, while the lymph protein content decreases slightly, indicating the injury to be a combination of increased capillary hydrostatic pressure and a moderate increase in pulmonary microvascular permeability. Lymph red blood cell content increases during this phase and is indicative of the increase in capillary hydrostatic pressure. The second, or delayed phase, occurs 3–6 hr after endotoxin or bacteria administration; it is characterized by a further increase in the flow rate of protein-rich lymph and only minimal to modest pulmonary artery hypertension (Fig. 28.3). This is the increased permeability phase which lasts for 24–36 hr, depending upon the degree of insult. Ultrastructural abnormalities are minimal (Staub, 1978). Except for the increased interstitial fluid, the endothelial membrane appears normal. The observed lung injury in the presence of normal histology may be explained by the fact that very minimal changes in pore size along the membrane, i.e., increases of 50–100 Å, are all that are necessary to produce a marked increase in water and protein flow (Staub, 1978).

MEDIATORS AND MODULATORS OF PULMONARY INJURY

A number of humoral agents and vasoactive substances appear in the lung or lung fluids in response to the injuries just described. The presence of several of these agents seems to correlate with cellular injury, and a number of these compounds have been suggested as

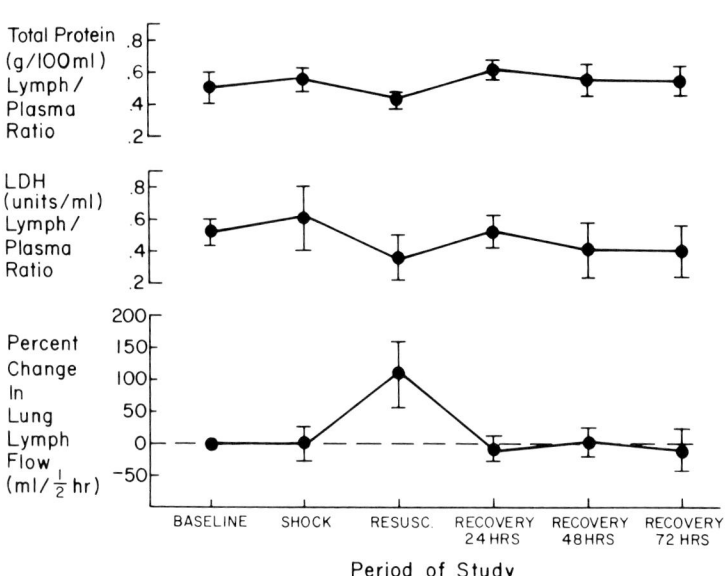

Figure 28.2. The pulmonary microvascular response of an unanesthetized sheep to severe hemorrhagic shock, resuscitation, and recovery is shown. Lung lymph flow increased during the resuscitation period but the lymph/plasma protein ratio decreased, indicating no significant increase in protein permeability. The lactic dehydrogenase activity of lung lymph was not increased. Lactic dehydrogenase is an intracellular enzyme released into interstitial fluid and lymph after severe cell ischemia. The fact that levels were not increased indicates no major lung cell injury. (Reprinted with permission from G. Niehaus and R. H. Demling: Lymphology 12:158–164, 1979.)

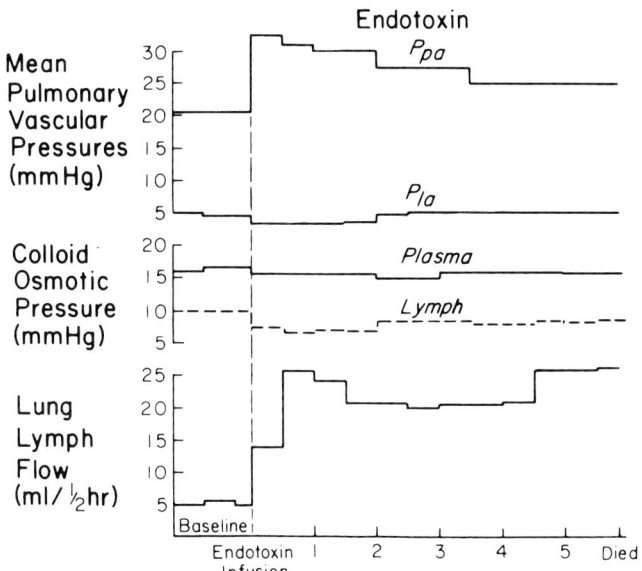

Figure 28.3. The pulmonary microvascular response of an unanesthetized sheep to E. coli endotoxin is shown. Pulmonary artery pressure increased acutely, as did lung lymph flow; lymph/plasma colloid osmotic pressure gradient increased slightly, indicating some sieving of protein to be intact. Five hours after endotoxin, as pulmonary artery pressure was decreasing, lung lymph flow again increased, while the lymph/plasma ratio returned to baseline, indicating a protein permeability change. (R. H. Demling, unpublished data.)

possible mediators of the lung damage. We will discuss the possible mechanisms of release of these agents and the evidence for their role in pulmonary injury.

Lysosomal Enzymes

Lysosomal enzymes are released from various cells into the interstitial fluid during shock and sepsis where the lymphatics carry these substances into the systemic circulation (Lefer, 1976). These enzymes are also released from leukocytes, macrophages, and platelets in response to injury (Goldstein et al., 1973). Increased activities of circulating lysosomal enzymes not only indicate cell injury, but have been reported to produce further cellular injury via their autolytic properties (Mela et al., 1973). Mitochondrial dysfunction has also been reported in the presence of free lysosomal enzymes. The splanchnic bed is considered to be a major source of plasma lysosomal enzymes following injury, with high concentrations being found in thoracic duct lymph. Lung injury has also been attributed to these enzymes, which are felt to be released into the lung by the leukocytes found sequestered in the pulmonary microcirculation during shock and sepsis. Leukocytes can be seen adhering to the endothelial cells and frequently obstructing capillaries both in animals and humans. Mast cells and circulating platelets found in the lung are also possible sources of lysosomal enzymes. Actual release of these enzymes into the lung has not been demonstrated in humans but has been measured in animals. The degree of lysosomal enzyme elevation seems to correlate with the magnitude of lung injury (Figs. 28.4 and 28.5).

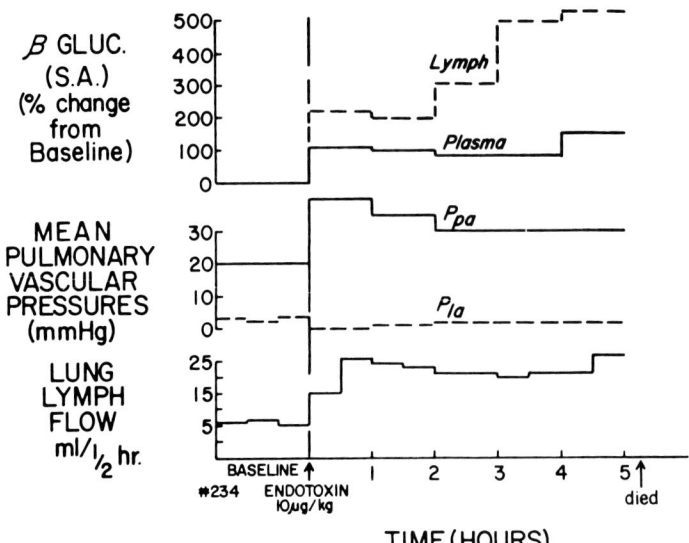

Figure 28.4. The pulmonary microvascular response to *E. coli* endotoxin (10 μg/kg) is compared with the lymph and plasma specific activity of the lysomal enzyme β-glucuronidase in an unanesthetized sheep. The two phase microvascular response is seen with the early pulmonary hypertension followed by a later permeability phase. Lymph enzyme specific activity (units activity/g of albumin) increased by 500% during the permeability phase. Lymph flow was increased four-fold, resulting in an actual increase in lymph transport (units/time) of 20 times baseline. Plasma values increased by 100% over baseline. The animal died at about 7 hr from endotoxin-induced systemic shock. (R. H. Demling, unpublished data.)

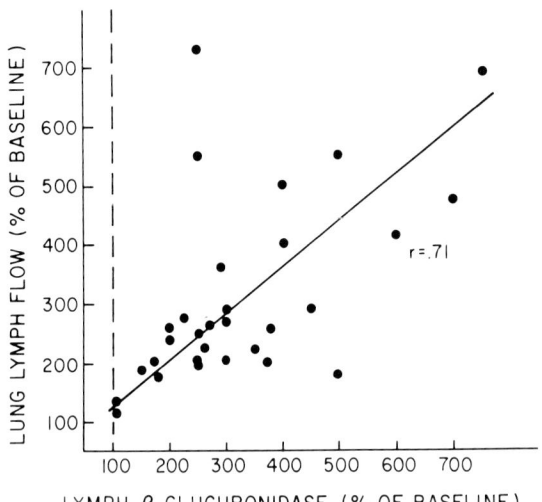

Figure 28.5. The percentage change in lung lymph flow is compared with that of lymph β-glucuronidase activity during the permeability phase after varying doses of *E. coli* endotoxin (2–10 μg/kg). Lymph lysosomal enzyme activity was three to five-fold greater than that seen in plasma, and the degree of activity correlated well with pulmonary microvascular injury ($r = .71$). Enzyme specific activity is defined as units of enzyme activity/g of albumin in lung lymph. This normalized the data and allowed comparison between animals. (R. H. Demling, unpublished data.)

HEMORRHAGIC SHOCK

As previously described, hemorrhagic shock alone does not seem to produce a major lung permeability injury. There is evidence of increased pulmonary venous resistance during hemorrhagic shock which is maintained during resuscitation and which may lead to an increase in capillary hydrostatic pressure. Animal studies monitoring the lung lymph and plasma concentrations of lysosomal enzymes during hemorrhagic shock have demonstrated that, while plasma activities increased during injury, lymph activities remained normal (Fig. 28.6). These findings correlate well with the lack of increased lymph protein transport following hemorrhage, an indicator of pulmonary vascular permeability and cellular injury (Fig. 28.1). Although leukocyte sequestration has been reported in the lung during hemorrhagic shock, degranulation probably does not occur.

TRAUMA—BURNS

Increased activities of systemic plasma lysosomal enzymes have also been observed after trauma. We are not aware of any direct measurement of lysosomal enzyme release into the lung or lung lymph after trauma, and these experiments need to be performed. Following burn injury in the sheep, lysosomal enzyme activity increases in lung lymph, as does the lymph flow rate and pulmonary vascular resistance (Fig. 28.7). The degree of change, however, is very small compared to that seen after endotoxin. White blood cells can be found sequestered in the lung after trauma and burns, but severe lung dysfunction often occurs only after superimposed sepsis (Fulton and Jones, 1975).

SEPSIS—ENDOTOXIN

Release of lysosomal enzymes from both tissue and circulating cells is well described after sepsis and endotoxemia with high concentrations of lysosomal enzymes reported in systemic plasma and thoracic duct lymph (Berman et al., 1969). Leukocyte sequestration in the lung is very prominent during endotoxemia. Platelet-fibrin emboli have also been reported. It has been postulated that the release of lysosomal enzymes into the lung from white cells produces the recognized permeability change (Kux et al., 1972). It has also been suggested that the initial pulmonary hypertension seen after endotoxin may be due to capillary obstruction by white cells or platelets. The authors have measured lysosomal enzyme activity in lung lymph and plasma of unanesthetized sheep after *E. coli* endotoxin administration (Demling et al., 1980). A 4- to 5-fold increase in lymph lysosomal enzyme activity and a 15- to 20-fold increase in the actual lymph transport of these enzymes after endotoxin was found, while plasma activities increased only 1- to 2-fold (Fig. 28.4). In the presence of a high dose of endotoxin (10 μg/kg), we were able with methylprednisolone (Solu-medrol) to block both the increase in plasma lysosomal enzymes and the observable systemic injury, but we were unable to completely block the increase in lung lymph enzyme activity or the lung injury (Fig. 28.8). The pulmonary injury was most likely produced by agents released from circulating cells or released by the lung itself. The white blood cell was a likely source, as a marked neutropenia was seen after endotoxin. The pulmonary injury was prevented by

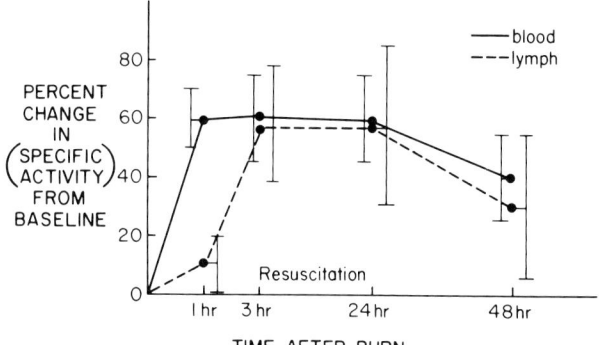

Figure 28.7. Mean changes ± standard error in plasma and lung lymph β-glucuronidase activity are shown after a 40% body surface burn in six sheep. Sheep were resuscitated, beginning 3 hr after the injury, with lactated Ringer's solution (3 cc/kg/% burn over 24 hr). Lung lymph flow increased by 200% during the 3- to 24-hr period of resuscitation. Pulmonary vascular resistance increased by 100%. Both lymph and plasma enzyme activity increased to comparable degrees after injury, with a gradual return toward baseline by 48 hr. The degree of change was not comparable to that seen after endotoxin in Fig. 28.4, and the pulmonary injury was less severe. (Reprinted with permission from R. H. Demling, N. Duy, M. Manohar, and J. Starling: *Journal of Trauma* 20: 791–794, 1980.)

methylprednisolone pretreatment when lower doses of endotoxin were used. Lymph lysosomal enzyme activity seemed to correlate reasonably well with the degree of permeability change as reflected by the increased lymph flow and protein transport rates (Fig. 28.5). Although lysosomal enzyme activity was concurrent with lung injury, a cause and effect relationship has not yet been determined, and the definitive study of removing or of infusing lysosomal enzymes and monitoring lung injury in this model has not been done. However, removing the white cells prior to endotoxin does seem to protect the lung. Further studies in this most interesting area are clearly needed.

Histamine

Histamine is a vasoactive agent present in large quantities in body tissues and particularly in white cells, platelets, and lung mast cells. Histamine has been reported to produce both increased vascular tone and increased vascular permeability in the lung (Brigham and Owen, 1975a). Histamine also constricts pulmonary venules. Brigham and Owen (1975a) demonstrated that an infusion of histamine (4 μg/kg/min) produced a modest pulmonary microvascular permeability change with an increase in lung lymph flow and lymph protein transport (Fig. 28.9). The lung response to histamine could be effectively blocked by diphenhydramine, an H_1 receptor blocker, but not by the H_2 receptor blocker,

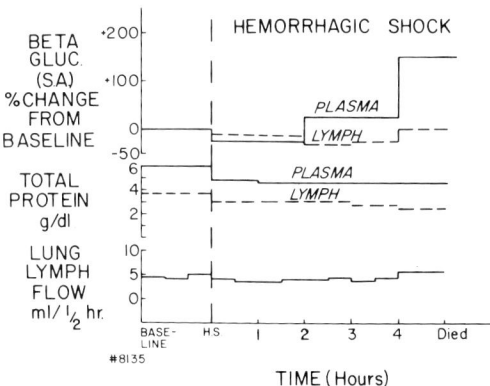

Figure 28.6. The response of an individual animal to fatal hemorrhagic shock is shown. Lung lymph flow decreased transiently initially then returned to baseline. Aortic pressure was maintained at a mean of 50 mm Hg. Both plasma and lung lymph protein content decreased, with the greatest decrease occurring in the 1st hr postshock. Plasma β-glucuronidase activity gradually increased, while the lymph value remained at baseline. (R. H. Demling, unpublished data.)

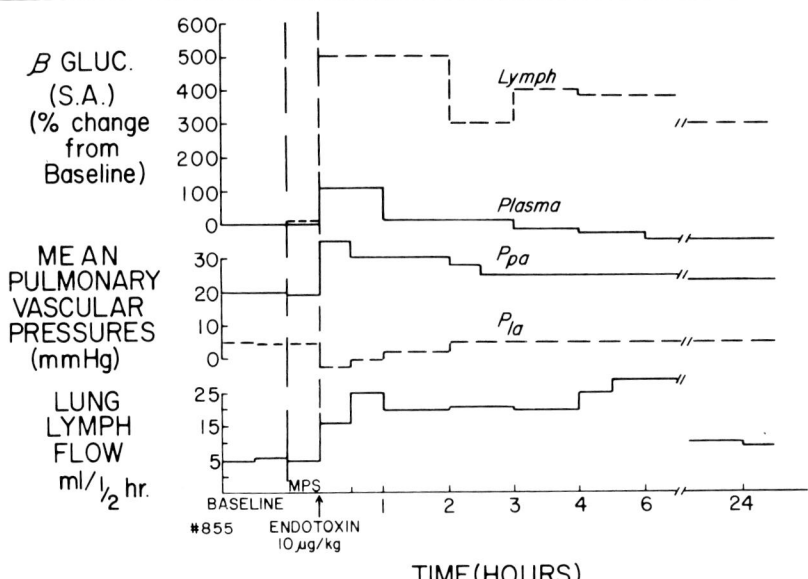

Figure 28.8. The pulmonary microvascular response to *E. coli* endotoxin (10 μg/kg) pretreated with methylprednisolone (Solu-medrol), 30 mg/kg, is compared with the lymph and plasma specific activity of the lysosomal enzyme β-glucuronidase in a sheep. The two phase microvascular response is seen, with the early pulmonary hypertension followed by a later permeability phase. Lymph enzyme activity increased 500% over baseline. Lymph flow increased by 4-fold, thereby increasing lymph enzyme transport 20-fold over baseline. After an initial increase, plasma enzyme activity returned to baseline. The animal demonstrated no systemic injury and survived. The lung injury was significant but reversible and appeared to be separate from the systemic response. The enzymes were most likely released from sequestered white cells or platelets. (R. H. Demling, unpublished data.)

metiamide. Therefore, the histamine effects on lung vascular permeability are H_1 receptor functions. The exact site of action of histamine remains controversial. Pietra et al. (1971) considered the bronchial venous system to be the major source of histamine-mediated fluid and protein leakage. The systemic effects of histamine seem to be much more pronounced, with hypotension and increased systemic vascular permeability. Histamine interacts with human lung tissue to increase cyclic GMP and AMP through H_1 and H_2 stimulation, respectively. Histamine has also been found to induce prostaglandin $F_{2\alpha}$ ($PGF_{2\alpha}$) synthesis in the lung (Platshon and Kaliner, 1978). $PGF_{2\alpha}$ is known to constrict pulmonary vessels. Interestingly, histamine has also been reported to be protective to cells during shock and sepsis (Fox and Lasker, 1962). The exact role of histamine in pulmonary injury remains undetermined.

HEMORRHAGIC SHOCK

Histamine has been found to be variably increased in plasma during hemorrhagic shock, but few specific measurements of histamine concentrations in lung tissue or lymph are available. Since no major pulmonary cellular injury is evident during hemorrhagic shock, the role of histamine is probably minimal except for possibly being involved in the increased pulmonary venous resistance seen during shock and resuscitation (Demling et al., 1979) (Fig. 28.1).

TRAUMA—BURNS

A more consistent increase in plasma histamine is present after trauma and particularly after burns. Markley et al. (1965) reported plasma concentrations of histamine to be increased by more than 50% after both tourniquet trauma and thermal injury in mice. These values were returning toward normal by 2 hr. Although both trauma and burns result in an early increase in pulmonary vascular resistance (Fig. 28.10), the vascular permeability changes and onset of clinical symptoms usually do not occur for hours to days after the initial insult. The early vascular resistance changes may well be due to histamine, although antihistamines have not always been successful in reversing the resistance changes. Luterman et al. (1977) reported that the severe lung injury produced in rabbits after fragment D infusion, a fibrin split product, was significantly attenuated by antihistamines of the H_1 type, but they suggested that this was involved with the effect of histamine on platelet aggregation. The effect of released histamine on lung injury may be more related to the effect of histamine on other systems—such as the prostaglandins, cyclic AMP and GMP, and platelets—rather than to its direct cellular effect. These types of interactions would explain the variability of response to antihistamines given after the traumatic insult. Measurements of histamine in lung lymph and lung tissue after injury need to be pursued and correlated with changes in these other systems.

SEPSIS—ENDOTOXIN

Systemic histamine release after endotoxin is well described (Hinshaw et al., 1961). Fisher et al. (1977) reported that lung histamine significantly increases in all lung liquid samples postendotoxin, even without significant increases in blood histamine concentrations. Indirect evidence that histamine may play a role in the lung injury during sepsis has been obtained by Padove et al. (1979), who noted an attenuation of the lung lymph flow response to endotoxin with H_1 antihistamines. Davis et al. (1963) considered the platelet to be the source of histamine release after endotoxin. This is a possibility since platelets appear to aggregate in the lung after endotoxin, and a local release of histamine may be in part responsible for the subsequent vasospasm and permeability change. Mast cells contain large amounts of histamine and may also be involved.

Serotonin

Serotonin is a vasoactive agent found in particularly high concentrations in circulating platelets. Like the previous substances, serotonin has been reported to play a role in lung injury. Brigham and Owen (1975b) reported that serotonin infused into sheep produced an increase in protein-poor lymph flow, indicative of increased vascular hydrostatic pressure but not increased vascular permeability (Fig. 28.11). Glazier and Murray (1971) reported that serotonin infusion in dogs produced an increase in pulmonary vascular resistance and pulmonary hypertension. This is consistent with the finding of increased pulmonary vascular resistance in patients with serotonin-producing tumors in the carcinoid syn-

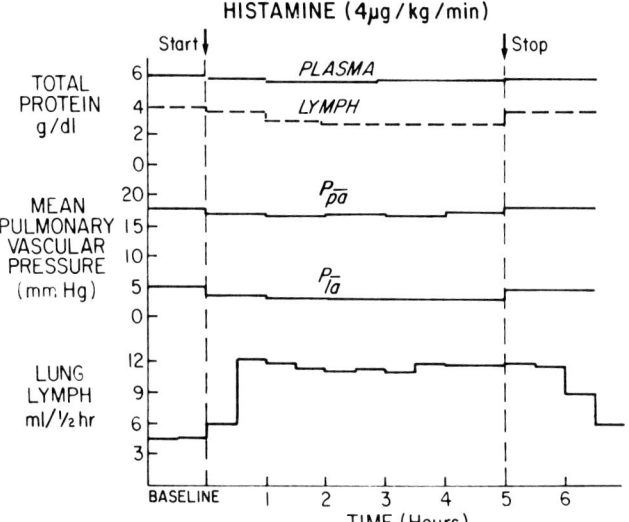

Figure 28.9. The pulmonary microvascular response to histamine infusion is shown. Lung lymph flow increased while vascular pressures and lymph/plasma protein ratio remained constant, indicating a modest increase in pulmonary vascular permeability.

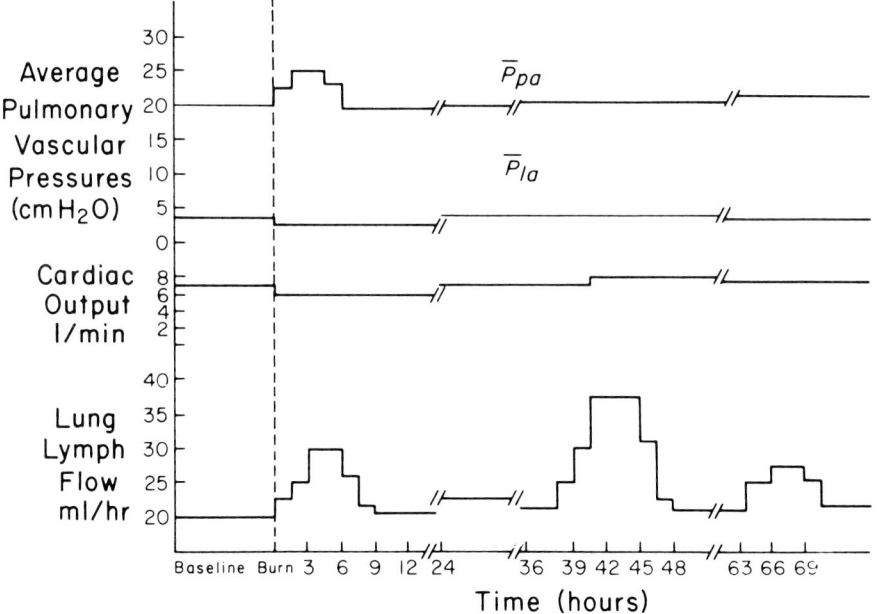

Figure 28.10. Time course of one experiment, before and after a 40% body burn in a sheep with lung lymph fistula, is shown. Immediately after burn there was a large increase in pulmonary vascular resistance as pulmonary artery pressure increased and left atrial pressure and cardiac output decreased. Lymph flow increased as lymph protein content decreased in this study, indicating no major permeability change but rather an increase in capillary hydrostatic pressure. At 36 and 63 hr, lymph flow again increased with lymph protein content decreasing, but total vascular resistance was close to baseline. Values then returned to baseline. (Reprinted with permission from R. H. Demling, J. A. Will, and F. O. Belzer: Surgery 83:746-751, 1978.)

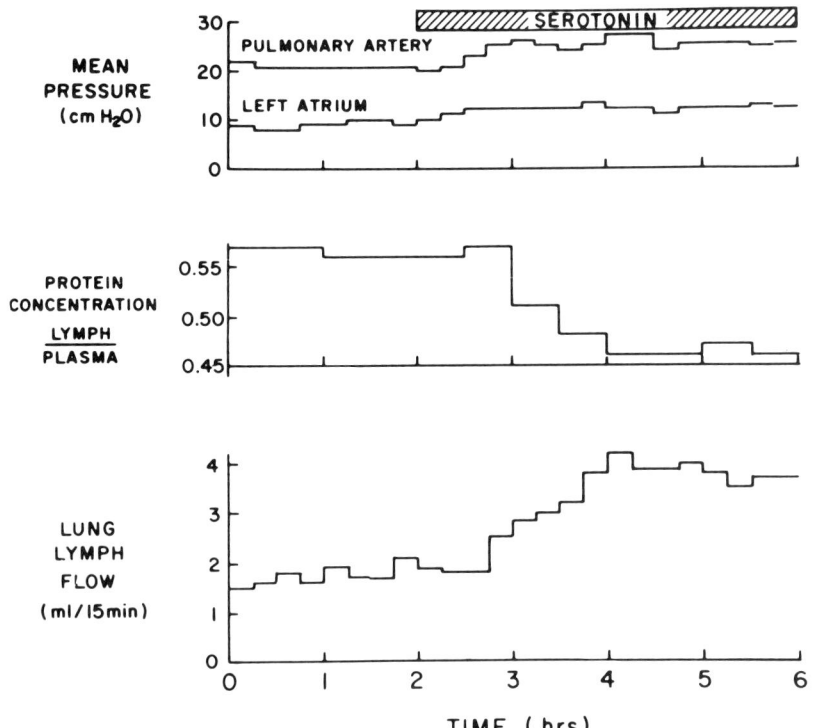

Figure 28.11. The pulmonary microvascular response to serotonin infusion is shown. Lung lymph flow and pulmonary artery pressure increase during infusion while the lymph/plasma protein ratio decreases, indicating that the increase in lymph flow is due to an increase in vascular hydrostatic pressure rather than a change in permeability. (Reprinted with permission from K. L. Bringham and P. J. Owen: Circulation Research 36:761–770, 1975a.)

drome. Pulmonary hypertension and increased pulmonary vascular resistance are characteristic of the lung injury seen after sepsis and trauma. Serotonin liberated from platelet sequestration may play a role in this aspect of lung injury.

Bradykinin

Kinins are a group of polypeptides with potent vasoactive properties, including systemic vasodilatation and changes in vascular permeability. Bradykinin is the prototype of the kinin system and is produced by the action of the enzyme kallikrein on kininogen. Bradykinin is generated after a number of insults but most prominently after endotoxemia. This may be precipitated by the granulocytes responding to endotoxin (Nies et al., 1968). The primary effect of the increased bradykinin seems to be a decrease in peripheral vascular resistance and hypotension. The release of kinins after endotoxin has also been documented in humans and is believed to be partly responsible for the bacteremia shock state (Robinson et al., 1975). Although bradykinin has severe systemic effects, it does not seem to alter the pulmonary circulation. Grega et al. (1971) and Wang et al. (1972) have infused bradykinin into the lung and have found no alterations in vascular pressures or permeability. The lung is of major importance, however, in that the pulmonary endothelial cell is responsible for the metabolic breakdown of bradykinin, with 80% of blood bradykinin being metabolized in one pass through the lung (Gillis and Roth, 1976). Any impairment in lung metabolic function due to endothelial injury could exaggerate the systemic circulatory abnormalities produced by the excess bradykinin.

Prostanoids

There is little doubt that products of the arachidonic acid cascade are involved in the series of events that accompanies cellular injury. Systemic, circulating concentrations of various prostanoids have been shown to be increased during hemorrhagic shock (Flynn et al., 1975; Jakschik et al., 1974), endotoxic shock (Anderson et al., 1975), anaphylactic shock (Anhut et al., 1978; Korbut et al., 1978), and burn shock (Anggard et al., 1970; Barac et al., 1975). The relationship between the prostanoid system and the lungs during these periods of injury is of importance for the following reasons. First, the lungs possess the enzymatic capability to synthetize all of the presently known prostanoids under a number of experimental conditions. Second, the lungs are responsible in large part for removing and catabolizing many prostaglandins in circulating blood. Third, prostanoids are very potent materials in regard to pulmonary hemodynamics, barrier properties, and respiratory function. Any change in the pattern or magnitude of prostanoid production following lung injury may be expected to have physiologic significance. However, the precise role which prostanoids may play in the pathophysiology of pulmonary injury is equivocal. Since a very large number of prostanoids exists within the lung, three theoretical possibilities exist. It is conceivable that certain prostanoids may act as causative factors and mediate the pulmonary damage that follows the original insult. The second possible role for pulmonary prostanoids is that they may represent a novel homeostatic mechanism. This concept was initially formalized by Markelonis and Garbus (1975) and recently restated in regard to the lung by Gryglewski et al. (1978). This hypothesis suggests that prostanoid production occurs as a concurrent process with cellular injury and that the prostanoids thus formed act to modulate or moderate the pathophysiologic events. The third theoretical possibility regarding a role for endogenous prostanoids during pulmonary injury is that their synthesis and release simply correspond temporally with injury, and the prostanoids have no significant role other than possibly acting as sensitive indicators of pulmonary injury. In reality, the diverse and often opposing biologic activities of individual prostaglandin-like materials suggest that all three of these theoretical roles may be being played simultaneously during lung injury, each by a different type of prostanoid.

HEMORRHAGIC SHOCK

There are a number of reports in the literature that demonstrate prostaglandin involvement in hemorrhagic shock. However, a few reports have dealt directly with pulmonary prostanoid involvement. Jakschik et al. (1974) reported that the carotid arterial blood concentration of E-type prostaglandins as measured by bioassay increased in dogs subjected to hemorrhage. Since E series prostaglandins (PGE) are normally almost completely removed from the circulation in one pass through the lung, these results suggested either an increased production of PGE by the lung or a decreased rate of pulmonary prostanoid extraction during hemorrhagic shock. Similar increases in arterial blood prostanoid concentrations were reported by Flynn et al. (1975), who observed significant increases in prostaglandins A_1, E_1, and $F_{2\alpha}$ concentrations in a canine hemorrhagic shock model. Confirmative evidence for enhanced pulmonary prostaglandin synthesis during hemorrhage was supplied by Blasingham and Selkurt (1976), who quantitated the net extraction of endogenous PGE by the lung. Prior to hemorrhage, the lungs had a positive venous-arterial (V-A) difference, whereas in the decompensatory phase of the experiment the (V-A) was significantly negative. These data strongly suggest de novo pulmonary prostaglandin synthesis following hemorrhage. The interpretation of these data as suggesting an increase in pulmonary prostanoid synthesis and release as opposed to a decrease in their rates of extraction from plasma and subsequent catabolism is strengthened by the following studies. Selkurt (1979) has demonstrated that the lungs of dogs in severe hemorrhagic shock were still able to extract and metabolize exogenously administered PGE, even when the concentrations administered far exceeded endogenous values. In addition, Flynn and Lefer (1977) have demonstrated that lung tissue taken from animals in hemorrhagic shock metabolized radiolabeled PGE and PGF at rates equivalent to those measured in lung tissue from control animals.

Although it appears that there is a net production of prostanoids by the lung during hemorrhagic shock, there are few data available to characterize their role in the lung following hemorrhage. Kazui et al. (1976) have reported that the administration of PGE_1 (20 μg/kg over 20 min) to dogs in hemorrhagic shock resulted in some amelioration of hemodynamic changes in the lung. PGE_1 significantly reduced pulmonary artery pressure, pulmonary vascular resistance, and the pressure gradient across the alveolar bed as compared to values in hemorrhaged animals receiving vehicle. In addition, PGE_1-treated lung tissue showed less histologic evidence of interstitial edema. To summarize, inadequate data are available to characterize the role of prostaglandin-like materials in the lung during hemorrhagic shock. It is known that there is enhanced prostanoid production following hemorrhage and that the ability of the lung to extract prostaglandins from the circulation and subsequently catabolize them is not significantly altered during this form of shock. It view of the lack of prominent lung injury in humans and most other species during hemorrhagic shock, the importance of the lung prostanoid relationship would seem to reside in the ability of the lung either to add or remove prostanoids from the systemic circulation. In addition, studies should be undertaken to investigate the mechanism of the enhanced prostanoid production during shock. These types of studies may determine whether pulmonary prostaglandins function to protect the lung against the effects of humoral factors that circulate in high concentrations in systemic blood during hemorrhagic shock. It is well established that such agents as histamine, angiotensin, and kinins directly stimulate prostanoid production.

BURNS—TRAUMA

Increased systemic plasma prostanoid concentrations have been reported during burn injury and trauma, but the origin of these materials is unknown. Recently, the authors have studied the effect of burn shock on the lung production of prostanoids by measuring the concentrations of PGE_2, $PGF_{2\alpha}$, and PGI_2 (as 6-keto $PGF_{1\alpha}$) in pulmonary lymph and venous blood (Fig. 28.12). These studies show that lung lymph concentrations of all three prostanoids increase following the burn injury, particularly during the period of increased pulmonary vascular resistance. Although it seems that the lung produces several prostanoids following burn injury and shock, their physiologic role in the lung under these circumstances remains to be elucidated.

Another form of lung trauma is microembolism with subsequent pulmonary hypoxia and interstitial edema. Weidner (1979) has reported that pretreatment of sheep with indomethacin, a prostaglandin synthetase inhibitor, significantly attenuates the pulmonary hypertension that normally results from embolization and thus reduces hydrostatic edema formation. These findings were quite similar to those reported by Tucker et al. (1976) following embolization in the dog. The data suggest that a vasoconstrictive prostaglandin may partially mediate the pulmonary hypertension following microembolization. The nature of the stimulus that provokes de novo prostanoid production during embolism is not clear. Scott et al. (1979) and Gee, Spath, and Flynn (unpublished observation) have demonstrated that neither rate of transcapillary fluid flux following a fluid load stimulates pulmonary prostanoid biosynthesis. Thus, the stimulus for embolism-provoked prostanoid biosynthesis in the lung

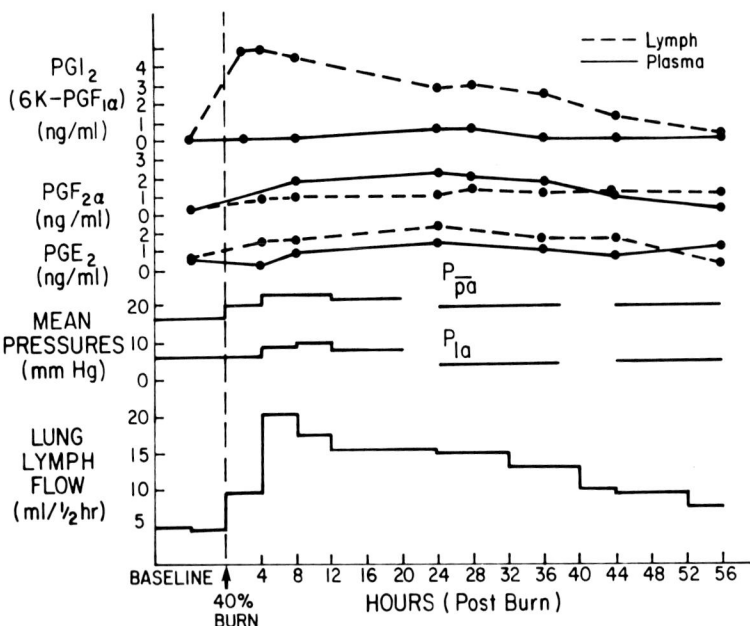

Figure 28.12. Lymph and plasma prostanoid concentrations are compared to lung lymph and vascular pressures after a major body burn. Lymph PGI_2, $PGF_{2\alpha}$, and PGE_2 levels were increased during the peak increase in lung lymph flow and pulmonary hypertension. Values remained elevated for approximately 48 hr, returning to baseline with lymph flow. Plasma levels of $PGF_{2\alpha}$ were consistently higher than in lymph, as opposed to PGI_2 and PGE_2, which were higher in lymph. A cause and effect relationship between prostanoid output and physiologic change remains to be determined. (R.H. Demling, M.H. Gee, and J.T. Flynn, unpublished data.)

may be mechanical, mediated by hypoxia, or involve circulating blood cells such as platelets. The role that pulmonary hypoxia subsequent to embolism may play in stimulating prostanoid production is equivocal. Wiberg et al. (1978) reported that hypoxia was not an adequate stimulus for prostaglandin production in isolated cat and rat lung preparations. In contrast, Vaage et al. (1975) reported two findings. First, prostaglandin synthetase inhibitors did not affect the pulmonary pressor response to hypoxia, which argues that prostanoid synthesis was not involved in hypoxia-mediated pulmonary vasoconstriction. Second, these investigators observed that nonsteroidal anti-inflammatory drugs induced a moderate potentiation of the vasoconstrictor effect of hypoxia. These results suggest that the lungs may be producing a pulmonary vasodilator type of prostaglandin in response to hypoxia. These speculations are in agreement with work by Said and Yoshida (1974), who noted prostaglandin-like biologic activity in the effluent perfusate from hypoxic lungs. Thus, it seems that there may be preferential production of specific prostanoids during different forms of lung injury. Additional studies are necessary to characterize the pattern of arachidonic acid metabolism during these various lung pathologies so that an understanding of their significance can be gained.

SEPSIS—ENDOTOXEMIA

Brigham et al. (1979) described the pulmonary response to endotoxin as having two relative phases. The initial phase is characterized by pulmonary vasoconstriction and a moderate increase in microvascular protein permeability, whereas the long term effect of endotoxin is primarily a permeability defect. Although a transient increase in pulmonary vascular resistance does not necessarily constitute lung injury, it can lead to hydrostatic edema with subsequent lung damage. Therefore, we will discuss pulmonary prostanoids as they relate to both phase I and II pulmonary responses to endotoxin.

Regarding pulmonary production of prostanoids during endotoxemia, Anderson et al. (1975) measured pulmonary arterial and venous concentrations of PGE and PGF following endotoxin-induced hypertension in calves. They reported significant increases in pulmonary venous PGF but not PGE concentrations, which correlated temporally with increases in pulmonary vascular resistance. These investigators presented no data on the second permeability phase response. Recently, Frölich et al. (1979) presented preliminary data showing a sevenfold increase in the thromboxane B_2 (TXB_2) concentration in sheep lung lymph during the initial hypertensive phase response to endotoxin. Pulmonary venous plasma concentrations of TXB_2 did not change during this period. Some very good data documenting prostanoid production by the lung following endotoxin were published by Hirose et al. (1978). Measurements of PGE and PGF concentrations in lung lymph reveal significant increases in PGF during the initial phase, which slowly returned toward baseline values during the later permeability phase. PGE did not seem to change significantly during the experiment. Although these data suggest lung prostanoid synthesis, this is not certain because plasma prostaglandin concentrations were not well documented and a question exists in the dog as to the precise origin of right duct lymph. Thus, increases in right duct lymph prostaglandin concentrations could simply reflect increased systemic plasma prostanoid concentrations or reflect a cardiac contribution. The authors have recently completed a study of unanesthetized sheep that characterizes the lung prostanoid response during endotoxin-mediated pulmonary injury. As shown in Fig. 28.13, the lung lymph concentrations of PGI_2, a pulmonary vasodilator, and $PGF_{2\alpha}$ and TXB_2, both pulmonary vasoconstrictors, increased significantly during the initial hemodynamic permeability phase. During the later permeability phase of injury, the concentrations of all three prostanoids decreased and were not significantly different from the baseline period values. There were also early increases in plasma concentrations of the prostaglandins. Neither lymph nor plasma concentrations of PGE were found to change significantly during any phase of the endotoxin injury. These data, gathered in unanesthetized sheep where the purity of lung lymph is well established, definitely demonstrate that enhanced pulmonary prostanoid production occurs following endotoxin administration. The magnitude of this enhanced production varies with the specific prostanoid measured, and the large increases in pulmonary thromboxanes and prostacyclin warrant further attention.

In view of the importance of the lung in clearing and catabolizing certain circulating prostanoids, a study was carried out to determine whether endotoxin-mediated pulmonary injury has any effect on the ability of the lung to perform this task (Flynn and Lefer, 1977). It was found that lung tissue removed from animals in the second phase of endotoxic shock possessed the ability to metabolize both tritium-labeled PGE_2 and $PGF_{2\alpha}$ at rates equivalent to control lung tissue. It can be concluded that the ability of the lung to catabolize prostanoids during endotoxemia is not impaired.

The precise role that endogenous prostaglandin-like materials might play in the lung during sepsis or endotoxemia is unclear. Many studies have been carried out using various prostaglandin synthetase inhibitors, such as indomethacin, aspirin, and meclofenamate. Unfortunately, many technical and interpretative difficulties make it extremely tenuous to come to any conclusion regarding what these agents might be doing in the lung. Most of the available studies relate to the possible involvement of such pulmonary vasoconstrictor prostanoids as PGH_2, PGG_2, TXA_2, and $PGF_{2\alpha}$ in the initial, hypertensive response to endotoxin (Reeves et al., 1972; Massion and Kux, 1973). Parratt and Sturgess (1977) have clearly demonstrated that various prostaglandin synthetase inhibitor and polyphloretin phosphate, an agent that interferes with the biologic activity of preformed prostanoids, can completely abolish the initial pulmonary hypertension following endotoxin. Although it is agreed that prostanoids may very well play a role in the hypertensive period of experimentally induced endotoxin shock, there is a question whether this is an important component of clinically observed septicemia. Of major importance is whether pulmonary prostanoids have any involvement in the microvascular permeability changes that are seen both clinically and experimentally during the shock state. In this regard, there is a relative paucity of data. Ogletree and Brigham (1979) reported that, in a limited study, indomethacin caused an exacerbation of the lung vascular permeability change following endotoxin. These authors did not measure lung lymph prostanoid concentrations, so it is not known whether the indomethacin effect was mediated by a removal of endogenous prostanoids or by some other

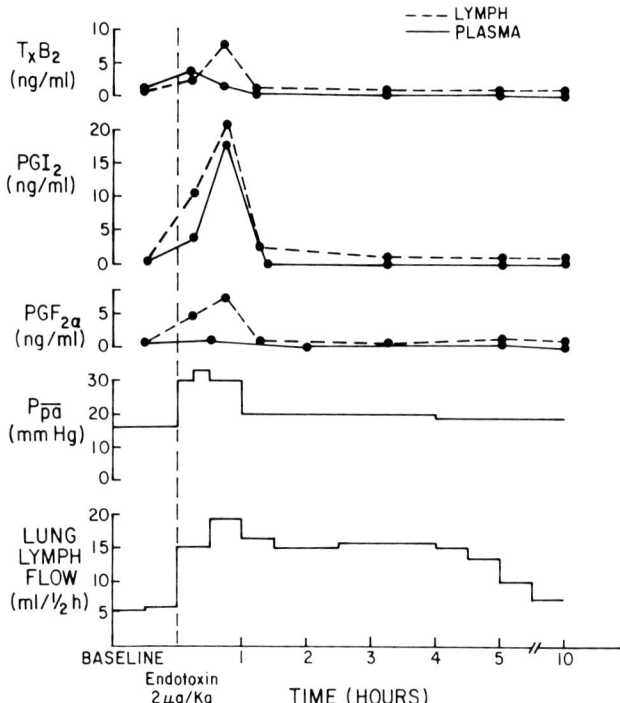

Figure 28.13. The pulmonary microvascular response to *E. coli* endotoxin is shown, comparing changes in prostanoid concentration with changes in vascular pressures and lung lymph flow. $PGF_{2\alpha}$, PGI_2 (6 keto-$PGF_{1\alpha}$), and thromboxane (TXB_2) contents in lung lymph rose sharply during the early hypertension phase of lung injury. Values began to return toward baseline, while lung lymph flow remained elevated during the later increased vascular permeability phase. Changes in plasma prostanoid contents followed a similar course. (R.H. Demling, M.H. Gee, and J.T. Flynn, unpublished data.)

mechanism. Hirose et al. (1978) have provided the most conclusive evidence for a role of endogenous prostanoid production in the microvascular permeability changes following endotoxin. These authors reported, as previously noted, that endotoxin (40 µg/kg) administered to dogs resulted in increased microvascular permeability and also an increase in endogenous pulmonary prostanoid production as reflected in lung lymph. Pretreatment with indomethacin or aspirin inhibited lung PGE and PGF production and exacerbated the permeability change in much the same way as reported by Ogletree and Brigham (1979) in the sheep. In addition, the infusion of arachidonic acid, the precursor for the bisenoic series of prostanoids, significantly increased pulmonary prostanoid synthesis and ameliorated the endotoxin-induced permeability change. As a further refinement, Hirose et al. (1978) administered prostacyclin to the animals both before and after the permeability change became evident. They found that PGI_2 pretreatment could inhibit the permeability change following endotoxin. More interestingly, if PGI_2 was administered after the permeability change was evident, the lung injury

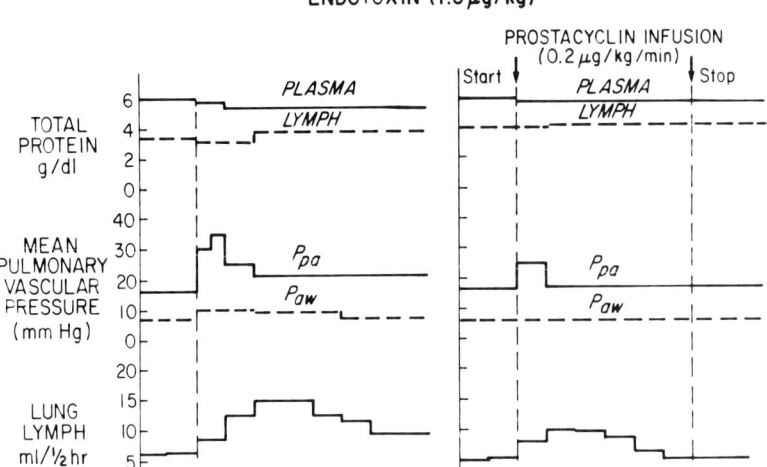

Figure 28.14. The pulmonary microvascular response to two doses of *E. coli* endotoxin given 1 week apart with the addition of prostacyclin infusion in one study, with the infusion beginning at the time of endotoxin injection. The pulmonary hypertension and the lung flow response were decreased with prostacyclin. The lymph/plasma protein ratio increased on both occasions. The mechanism of protection needs to be delineated. (R.H. Demling, M.H. Gee, and J.T. Flynn, unpublished data.)

could be decreased. The authors have also investigated the effect of prostacyclin infusion on endotoxin-induced lung injury in unanesthetized sheep (Fig. 28.14). Prostacyclin was seen to significantly ameliorate both the increase in pulmonary vascular resistance and the permeability effects of endotoxin and also to improve the overall survival rate (Demling, Gee, and Flynn, unpublished data). The studies just described suggest that certain endogenously produced prostaglandin-like materials may be acting to minimize the pulmonary injury following endotoxemia. Although these data are quite interesting in both a physiologic and clinical sense, much work needs to be done to establish a role for prostanoids in the pulmonary response to endotoxemia or septicemia.

References

Anderson, F.L., Tsagaris, T.J., Jubiz, W., and Kuida, H.: Prostaglandin F and E levels during endotoxin induced pulmonary hypertension in calves. Am. J. Physiol. *228:*1479, 1975.

Anggard, E., Arturson, G., and Jonsson, C.E.: Efflux of prostaglandins in lymph from scalded tissue. Acta Physiol. Scand. *80:*46, 1970.

Anhut, H., Peskar, B.A., and Bernauer, W.: Release of 15-keto-13, 14 dihydrothromboxane B_2 and prostaglandin D_2 during anaphylaxis as measured by radioimmunoassay. Arch. Pharmacol. *305:*247, 1978.

Barac, G., Van Caneghem, P., and Deby, C.: Prostaglandins in burn-induced acute olig-anuria and oedema. Arch. Int. Physiol. Biochem. *83:*612, 1975.

Berman, I.R., Moseley, R.C., Lamborn, P.B., and Sleeman, K.: Thoracic duct lymph in shock: Gas exchange, acid-base balance and lysosomal enzymes in hemorrhagic and endotoxin shock. Ann. Surg. *169:*202, 1969.

Blaisdell, F.W., and Schlobohm, R.M.: The respiratory distress syndrome: A review. Surgery *74:*251, 1973.

Blasingham, C., and Selkurt, E.E.: Changes in metabolism of prostaglandin E by the dog lung during hemorrhagic shock. Fed. Proc. *25:*608, 1976.

Brigham, K.C., Bowers, R.E., and Haynes, J.: Increased sheep lung vascular permeability caused by *Escherichia coli* endotoxin. Circ. Res. *45:*292–297, 1979.

Brigham, K.L., and Owen, P.J.: Increased sheep lung vascular permeability caused by histamine. Circ. Res. *37:*647, 1975a.

Brigham, K.L., and Owen, P.J.: Mechanism of the serotonin effect on lung transvascular fluid and protein movement in awake sheep. Circ. Res. *36:*761, 1975b.

Brigham, K.L., Woolverton, W.C., Blake, L.H., and Staub, N.C.: Increased sheep lung vascular permeability caused by *Pseudomonas* bacteremia. J. Clin. Invest. *54:*792, 1974.

Christy, J.H.: Pathophysiology of gram-negative shock. Am. Heart. J. *81:*694, 1971.

Davis, R.B., Bailey, W.L., and Hanson, N.P.: Modification of serotonin and histamine release after *E. coli* endotoxin administration. Am. J. Physiol. *205:*560, 1963.

Demling, R.H., Will, J.A., and Belzer, F.O.: Effect of major thermal injury on the pulmonary microcirculation. Surgery *83:*746, 1978.

Demling, R.H., Niehaus, G., and Will, J.A.: Pulmonary microvascular response to hemorrhagic shock, resuscitation and recovery. J. Appl. Physiol. *46:*498, 1979.

Demling, R.H., Proctor, R., Grossman, J., Duy, N., and Starling, J.: Comparison of the systemic and pulmonary vascular response to endotoxin with plasma and lung lymph lysosomal enzyme release. Circ. Shock *7:*317, 1980.

Fisher, P., Miller, J.E., and Glauser, F.L.: Endotoxin induced increased alveolar capillary membrane permeability. Circ. Shock *4:*387, 1977.

Flynn, J.T., and Lefer, A.M.: Prostaglandin metabolism during circulatory shock. Biochim. Biophys. Acta *497:*775, 1977.

Flynn, J.T., Appert, H.E., and Howard, J.M.: Arterial prostaglandin A_1, E_1, and $F_{2\alpha}$ concentrations during hemorrhagic shock in the dog. Circ. Shock *2:*155, 1975.

Fox, C.L., and Lasker, S.E.: Protection by histamine and metabolites in anaphylaxis, scalds and endotoxin shock. Am. J. Physiol. *202:*111, 1962.

Frölich, J.C., Ogletree, M., and Brigham, K.L.: Pulmonary hypertension correlated to pulmonary thromboxane synthesis. In *Abstracts of the 4th International Prostaglandin Conference*, edited by P.W. Ramwell, B. Samuelsson, and R. Paoletti, p. 38. Washington, DC, 1979.

Fulton, R.L., and Jones, C.E.: The cause of post traumatic pulmonary insufficiency in man. Surg. Gynecol. Obstet. *140:*179, 1975.

Gillis, N.C., and Roth, J.A.: Pulmonary disposition of circulating vasoactive hormones. Biochem. Pharmacol. 25:2547, 1976.

Glazier, J.C., and Murray, J.F.: Sites of pulmonary vasomotor reactivity in the dog during alveolar hypoxia and serotonin and histamine infusion. J. Clin. Invest. 50:2550, 1971.

Goldstein, I.M., Brai, M., Oster, A.G., and Weissman, G.: Lysosomal enzymes release from human leukocytes: Mediation of the alternate pathway of complement activation. J. Immunol. 111:33, 1973.

Grega, G., Daugherty, R., Scott, J., Radawski, D., and Haddy, F.: Effect of pressure, flow and vasoactive agents on vascular resistance and capillary filtration in canine, fetal, newborn. Microvasc. Res. 3:297, 1971.

Gryglewski, R.J., Korbut, R., Ocetkiewicz, A., Splawinski, J., Wojtaszek, B., and Swies, J.: Lungs as a generator of prostacyclin—hypothesis of physiological significance. Arch. Pharmacol. 304:45, 1978.

Hinshaw, L.B., Vick, J.A., Carlson, C.H., and Fan, Y.L.: Role of histamine in endotoxin shock. Proc. Soc. Exp. Biol. Med. 104:379, 1961.

Hirose, T., Ikeda, T., Aoki, E., and Hara, N.: The protective effect on PGI_2 on increased lung vascular permeability caused by endotoxin in dogs. Nippon Kyobu Shikkan Gakkai Zasshi 16:410, 1978.

Jakschik, B.A., Marshall, G.R., Kourik, J.L., and Needleman, P.: Profile of circulating vasoactive substances in hemorrhagic shock and their pharmacologic manipulation. J. Clin. Invest. 54:842, 1974.

Kazui, T., Webb, W.R., and Wax, S.D.: Effect of prostaglandin E_1 on the lung in hemorrhagic shock. Surg. Forum 27:187, 1976.

Korbut, R., Ocetkiewicz, A., and Gryglewski, R.J.: The influence of hydrocortisone and indomethacin on the release of prostaglandin-like substances during circulatory shock in cats which was induced by an intravenous administration of rabbit blood. Pharmacol. Res. Commun. 10:371, 1978.

Kux, M., Coalson, J.J., Masscon, W.H., and Guenter, C.A.: Pulmonary effects of E. coli endotoxin: Role of leukocytes and platelets. Ann Surg. 179:26, 1972.

Lefer, A.M.: The role of lysosomes in circulatory shock. Life Sci. 19:1803, 1976.

Luterman, A., Manwaring, D., and Curreri, P.W.: The role of fibrinogen degradation products in the pathogenesis of the respiratory distress syndrome. Surgery 82:703, 1977.

Markelonis, G., and Garbus, J.: Alterations of intracellular oxidative metabolism as stimuli evoking prostaglandin biosynthesis. Prostaglandins 10:1087, 1975.

Markley, K., Harakova, A., Smallman, E., and Beavan, M.: The role of histamine in burn, tourniquet and endotoxin shock in mice. Eur. J. Pharmacol. 33:255, 1965.

Massion, W.H., and Kux, M.: Protective effects of various inhibitor agents against pulmonary damage following shock. In New Aspects of Trasylol Therapy, The Shock Lung, edited by G.L. Haberland, W. Elberfeld, and D.H. Lewis, pp. 191–198. Shattauer Verlag, Stuttgart, 1973.

Mela, L., Miller, L.D., Bacalzo, L.V., Olofsson, K., and White, R.R.: Role of intracellular variations of lysosomal activity and oxygen tension in mitochondrial impairment in endotoxemia and hemorrhagic shock in the rat. Ann. Surg. 178:727, 1973.

Nies, A.S., Forsyth, R., Williams, H., and Melmon, K.: Contribution of kinins to endotoxin shock in unanesthetized rhesus monkeys. Circ. Res. 22:155, 1968.

Ogletree, M.L., and Brigham, K.L.: Indomethacin augments endotoxin induced lung vascular permeability in sheep. Am. Rev. Resp. Dis. 119:383, 1979.

Padove, S.J., Bryant, D.M., Brigham, K.L., and McKeen, C.R.: Diphenhydramine reduces endotoxin induced increased lung vascular permeability in unanesthetized sheep. Am. Rev. Resp. Dis. 119:384, 1979.

Parratt, J.R., and Sturgess, R.M.: The possible roles of histamine, 5-hydroxytryptamine and prostaglandin $F_{2\alpha}$ as mediators of the acute pulmonary effects of endotoxin. Br. J. Pharmacol. 60:209, 1977.

Pietra, G.G., Szidon, J.P., Leventhal, M.M., and Fishman, A.P.: Histamine and interstitial pulmonary edema in the dog. Circ. Res. 29:323, 1971.

Platshon, L.F., and Kaliner, M.: The effects of the immunologic release of histamine upon human lung cyclic nucleotide levels and prostaglandin generation. J. Clin. Invest. 62:1113, 1978.

Pruitt, B.A., Flemma, R.J., and DiVincenti, F.C.: Pulmonary complications in burn patients. J. Thorac. Cardiovasc. Surg. 59:7, 1970.

Reeves, J.T., Daoud, F.S., and Estridge, M.: Pulmonary hypertension caused by minute amounts of endotoxin in calves. J. Appl. Physiol. 33:739, 1972.

Robinson, J., Klodnycky, M., Loeb, H., Racic, M., and Gunnar, R.: Endotoxin, prekallikrein, complement and systemic vascular resistance: Sequential measurement in man. Am. J. Med. 59:61, 1975.

Said, S.I., and Yoshida, T.: Release of prostaglandins and other humoral mediators during hypoxic breathing and pulmonary oedema. Chest (Suppl.) 12, 1974.

Scott, E., Vaarge, J., and Wiberg, T.: Lack of release of prostaglandins from isolated perfused lungs during pulmonary hypertension and oedema. Br. J. Pharmacol. 65:197, 1979.

Selkurt, E.E.: Role of the kidney and lung in the handling of prostaglandin E in hemorrhagic shock. Adv. Shock. Res. 1:159, 1979.

Sibbald, W.J., Paterson, N.A.M., Holliday, R.L., Anderson, R.A., Lobb, T.R., and Duff, J.H.: Pulmonary hypertension in sepsis. Chest 73:583, 1978.

Staub, N.C.: Steady state pulmonary transvascular water filtration in unanesthetized sheep. Circ. Res. 28:135, 1971.

Staub, N.C.: Pulmonary edema due to increased microvascular permeability to fluid and protein. Circ. Res. 43:143, 1978.

Todd, T.R.J., Baile, E., and Hogg, J.C.: Pulmonary capillary permeability during hemorrhagic shock. J. Appl. Physiol. 45:298, 1978.

Tucker, A., Weir, E.K., Reeves, J.T., and Grover, R.F.: Pulmonary microembolism: Attenuated pulmonary vasoconstriction with prostaglandin inhibitors and antihistamines. Prostaglandins 11:31, 1976.

Vaage, J., Bjertnaes, L., and Hauge, A.: The pulmonary vasoconstrictor response to hypoxia: Effects of inhibitors of prostaglandin biosynthesis. Acta Physiol. Scand. 95:95, 1975.

Wang, C., Khaneja, S., Green, L., Jackson, S., and Emmanuel, G. Effects of bradykinin, bradykinin potentiating factor and serotonin on the pulmonary circulation. Circulation 65:234, 1972.

Weidner, W.J.: Effect of indomethacin on pulmonary hemodynamics and extravascular lung water in sheep after pulmonary microembolism. Prostaglandins Med. 3:71, 1979.

Wiberg, T., Vaage, J., Bjertnaes, L., Hauge, A., and Gautuik, K.M.: Prostaglandin content in blood and lung tissue during alveolar hypoxia. Acta Physiol. Scand. 102:181, 1978.

PART 3

CURRENT THERAPY OF SHOCK

EDITORS' SUMMARY

In this chapter, Safar reviews the history of modern resuscitation for shock, ischemia, and anoxia and gives an excellent and detailed historical account. The chapter is also extremely useful for his exposition of current resuscitation methods, including his classification of the stages of shock. The following subjects are covered: airway control, ventilation-oxygenation, CPR, control of hemorrhage, fluid resuscitation, drugs in shock, and CNS resuscitation.

He emphasizes that the CNS is one of the most susceptible organs to shock of all types and repeatedly emphasizes the problem that a trickle of blood flow may cause more serious effects than no flow at all (see also Ch. 6).

The comments on airway control, ventilation and oxygenation are especially useful, as is the review of cardiopulmonary resuscitation and open chest CPR. The author points out that although open chest CPR was once widely used, it is now becoming a forgotten art which should be reviewed in training programs for physicians and for wider use in hospitals. The section on cardiac arrest due to exsanguination is also especially valuable and is often not addressed as a separate entity, which it certainly is both in humans and experimental animals.

The section on fluid replacement is extensive and well documented. As in other chapters in this volume (for example, see Chs. 32 and 37), deliberate hemodilution is recommended for wider consideration, because of altered flow properties, sludging, increased red cell rigidity, and other factors, which more than compensate for the reduced oxygen content. Repeatedly, Safar asserts that in the young, previously fit patient, adequate oxygen transport can be maintained to at least a hematocrit of 20%. This most common area of acute resuscitation needs thorough consideration by the physician and development of suitable protocols for immediate implementation.

The section on drug therapy is also very thoughtful and Safar takes the conservative view that all drugs considered for use in hemorrhagic shock are only adjuncts to adequate blood volume restoration. The section on cerebral resuscitation is valuable in that there are relatively few discussions of this type available. It is evident that we need much more cell research on the CNS in shock, ischemia, and anoxia. Some of the most penetrating data available are those presented by Mela in Chapter 6.

In his chapter, Shoemaker clearly draws the distinction between simple cardiogenic or hemorrhagic shock and most cases of human septic or traumatic shock. He further stresses that simplistic treatment protocols are inadequate and that proper treatment must be based on a comprehensive understanding of the pathophysiology. Shoemaker and his group have made over 10,000 sequential sets of physiological measurements in 180 patients. Much of his analysis is based on this experience. One of the seminal generalizations that derive from his analysis is that increased O_2 consumption by the tissues correlates with increased survival. However, he does not allow us to forget that blood flow to different parts of the body can also be normal, while at the same time shunting secondary to neurohumoral and metaboic factors results in maldistribution of flow elsewhere. He also reminds us that the critical function of the circulation is oxygen transport. To these thoughts, we would suggest that in addition to humoral and metabolic factors, tissue edema is often forgotten as it relates to oxygen transport.

Transfusion therapy is a keystone in the treatment portfolio of hemorrhagic shock. Sohmer and Dawson extensively review this subject. Erythrocytes stored in the blood bank exhibit gradual energy depletion with time, change shape, and markedly increase in overall rigidity. The energy deficit is exemplified by the ATP depletion, the rigidity by an increased level of ionized calcium with its subsequent effects on the erythrocyte cytoskeleton. Energy-depleted cells are satisfactory for acute resuscitation if anemia can be avoided; if it cannot, better results including improved survival occur with high 2,3-DPG cells. High 2,3-DPG, low HbO_2 affinity cells have been demonstrated to be of particular importance in individuals with significant atherosclerotic heart disease who were subjected to extracorporeal circulation during bypass surgery. Similarly, such cells render an individual more tolerant to severe hemodilution with RBC-free resuscitation solutions, e.g., dextrans, which may be essential in the acute resuscitation phase.

The authors also review some of the major adverse effects of transfusion therapy. These include alterations in acid-base balance, citrate toxicity including hypocalcemia, hypothermia, hyper- or hypokalemia, microembolization, alterations in hemoglobin function, and deficiencies in platelet and other coagulation factors.

Most of the principles reviewed in this chapter are in current use in our unit. In our experience, where we formerly used large quantities of stored blood in hemorrhagic shock, it was observed that numerous coagulation problems arose. After changing to blood component therapy (because of an inability to always obtain sufficient quantities of whole stored blood immediately), the incidence of coagulopathies dramatically decreased. Our present therapy protocol for hypovolemia secondary to hemorrhage is as follows:

Plasma Protein Fraction (Plasmanate) 1000 cc immediately

THEN: O−VE OR O+VE PACKED CELLS
THEN: GROUPED PACKED CELLS
THEN: X MATCHED PACKED CELLS
EVERY 6 UNITS OF PLASMA GIVE 2 UNITS FRESH FROZEN PLASMA
EVERY 6 UNITS OF PLASMA GIVE 6 UNITS PLATELETS

Gelin and Dawidson focus on the rheological properties of blood before and after resuscitation. These considerations especially apply to the microcirculation. The viscosity of blood increases at low flow rates and low pressure heads, with increasing hematocrit and with increasing viscosity of the suspending medium. With very low capillary flow rates, in a branched system, separation of cell and plasma flow can be striking.

With these considerations in mind, the authors review the rationale of infusion therapy in resuscitation. The restoration of volume and flow are priorities. Therapy with colloids has several limitations including the permeability of the glomerular basement membrane. Nevertheless, they conclude that these have many advantages over noncolloidal resuscitation solutions.

Therapeutic hemodilution, therefore, includes three main basic concepts:
1. expanded plasma volume,
2. decreased viscosity of the blood at low flow rates, and
3. dispersed aggregated cells for single file perfusion through capillaries.

The use of colloids versus electrolyte-substrate solutions needs much more investigation (see also Ch. 30). In simple experimental hemorrhagic shock in the rat, there is no difference in survival between colloid-containing solutions, whole blood, Ringer's solution, or isotonic saline. This may be unique for the rat and/or unique for the short-term resuscitation. Clearly, however, more work in this area could be extremely fruitful since adequate amounts of either whole blood or blood components are not likely to be available in any major acute disaster.

The chapter on corticosteroids by Shatney has covered the literature nicely by dividing the areas of corticosteroid investigation into major catagories. The findings of each study have been summarized and an attempt is made to contrast or compare the studies. The reader is taken through years of clinical experimentation smoothly, and the viewpoint of the author is delivered effectively.

Schumer's chapter on the general treatment of septic shock is a very useful and practical guide to the recognition and treatment of this disorder; it includes comments on pathophysiology, diagnosis, and treatment. Schumer has himself accomplished the best clinical studies of the efficacy of glucocorticoids in the treatment of septic shock to date.

Schumer emphasizes the effects of endotoxemia on reduction of gluconeogenesis (see also Ch. 3). He has found a good correlation between BP and the glucose/lactate ratio, indicating that this ratio may be a useful prognostic and therapeutic monitor in septic shock. His discussion on disseminated intravascular coagulation (DIC) effectively complements that of Hardaway's chapter.

The comments on antibiotic therapy are amplified in the chapter by Hruksa and Hornick. Our own experience is similar to theirs. We also find that falling platelet counts and decreased mentation are good indicators. The use of furosemide and other loop diuretics may be very useful in minimizing the possibility of acute renal failure. If such is used, however, it is essential to assure adequate volume status in the patient (see Ch. 24).

Hruska and Hornick provide a detailed and useful review of the microbiologic aspects of septic shock. They stress the need for accurate and early diagnosis and treatment (see also Ch. 16). There has been a shift in the type of gram-negative organism in recent years as well as a realization that gram-positive organisms may also cause septic shock, especially in the elderly, in alcoholics, and in patients without a functional spleen. The latter is, of course, relatively common in shock trauma units.

Synergistic antibiotic therapy is the basis of further treatment. The most common combination is an aminoglycoside and either carbenicillin or ticarcillin. This, however, is a complex subject with numerous potential complications which the authors discuss. The use of specific antibiotics undergoes continual evolution. Current useful classes of antibiotics are discussed in detail.

Corticosteroids have become established in animal models as being protective, especially if given early and if accompanied from the beginning by appropriate antibiotic therapy. Controversy remains, however, concerning their use in humans—mainly because more prospective studies are needed. Much more work is also needed on the nonsteroidal anti-inflammatory agents, which may retain many of the beneficial effects of steroids while not having the harmful complications, including impaired bacterial killing and impaired wound repair.

The authors also review the use of granulocyte transfusions in neutropenic patients; these are most beneficial in patients whose bone marrow has not recovered during the course of the infection.

Finally, progress is being made in prevention of septic shock using both laminar flow rooms and prophylactic antibiotics.

CHAPTER 29

Resuscitation in Hemorrhagic Shock, Coma, and Cardiac Arrest

PETER SAFAR

"Shock" can be defined as the clinical picture of a "reduction in overall tissue perfusion, resulting in vital organ systems malfunction." Shock states may be classified as: 1) hemorrhagic shock (oligemia, hypovolemia); 2) cardiogenic shock (pump failure); 3) obstructive shock (e.g., pulmonary embolism, cardiac tamponade); and 4) distribution shock (e.g., sepsis) (Shubin et al., 1978). In shock types 1, 2, and 3, there is a reduction in oxygen transport (i.e., arterial oxygen content times blood flow). The most common causes for hypovolemic shock are trauma (resulting in external or internal blood or plasma volume loss); burns; severe diarrhea; and inflammatory processes like peritonitis or pancreatitis with internal plasma volume loss.

Hypovolemic shock states range in severity and duration from moderate transient blood loss, which may be quickly terminated by spontaneous or therapeutic blood volume restoration, to severe prolonged hypoperfusion resulting in unresponsiveness to fluid therapy (irreversible shock), death of cells, and secondary cardiac arrest. The term irreversibility is a misnomer, since the type of treatment determines whether organ viability can be maintained and function ultimately restored. For example, early resuscitation in hemorrhagic shock consists primarily of hemostasis and rapid replacement of fluid volume lost (fluid resuscitation). Resuscitation for more advanced or complicated oligemic shock states requires additional measures of multiple organ systems life support (Shoemaker and Thompson, 1980).

Cardiopulmonary resuscitation (CPR) is discussed in this chapter, because it is not covered elsewhere in this book. Moreover, CPR is relevant for exsanguination cardiac arrest and for the patient with a pulse who is in hemorrhagic shock and unconscious, either from the shock state itself or from concomitant cerebral injury or anesthesia. Cardiac arrest can be primary, as in sudden cardiac death; secondary and rapidly developing, as in exsanguination; or secondary and slowly developing, as in pulmonary, renal, and multiple organ failure of "irreversible shock."

The *history* of modern CPR started in the 1950s (Elam et al., 1954; Safar et al., 1958; Kouwenhoven et al., 1960) and its expansion to cardiopulmonary-cerebral resuscitation (CPCR) in 1970 (Safar, 1978b). There were earlier important advances in knowledge, largely unappreciated at the time. They include intermittent positive pressure artificial ventilation (IPPV) by Vesalius in the 1500s; jaw thrust for airway control by Esmarch (1878) and Heiberg (1874); tracheal intubation by Kuhn (1911); open chest CPR by Boehm (1878) and Schiff (1882); closed chest CPR by Maass (1892); drug resuscitation by Crile and Dolley (1908); and internal and external electric defibrillation by Prevost and Battelli (1899) and Gurvitch and Yuniev (1946) in animals. The decisive research and introduction of modern CPR in the 1950s and 1960s were by Beck et al. (1947); Beck and Leighninger (1960); Elam et al. (1954); Gordon et al. (1958); Jude et al. (1961); Kouwenhoven et al. (1960); Safar et al. (1958, 1959, 1961); Zoll et al. (1956); and others.

The history of the modern treatment of shock begins with the work of physiologists (Bernard, 1949; Cournand et al., 1943; Crile, 1947; Wiggers, 1950) and culminated in the studies by Blalock et al. (1932) and Blalock (1940), who clearly showed for the first time that trauma and burns cause shock due to internal blood and plasma volume loss, even when there is no external blood loss. Experiences of recent wars added to present concepts of fluid resuscitation.

After some pathophysiologic considerations, we shall briefly review the phases and steps of CPCR (Fig. 29.1, Table 29.1). We will then examine some underappreciated concepts of airway control (Fig. 29.2), ventilation-oxygenation (Figs. 29.2 and 29.3), CPR (Fig. 29.4), control of hemorrhage (Fig. 29.5), fluid resuscitation (Table 29.2), and drugs in shock. We will conclude with comments on cerebral resuscitation (Tables 29.3 and 29.4).

PATHOPHYSIOLOGIC CONSIDERATIONS

In healthy humans, acute hemorrhage results in the *clinical picture* of overall hypoperfusion—namely, cold, moist skin (compensatory vasoconstriction); oliguria-anuria (renal vasoconstriction); tachycardia (may be absent in infancy, old age, or during general anesthesia); faint peripheral pulses (reduced pulse pressure); arterial hypotension; and abnormal CNS function (delirium-stupor-coma). Hypotension may be absent in fit persons until 20–30% of blood volume has been lost, because of compensatory vasoconstriction. While arterioles and veins constrict in skin, muscles, kidneys, and splanchnic bed, coronary and cerebral vessels dilate.

Severity and duration of hypoperfusion secondary to hypotension determine the outcome. In the fit person, acute *mild* hypovolemia (10–20% of blood volume lost) is usually spontaneously corrected with complete recovery. The hematocrit, which at first remains unchanged, soon begins to decrease due to plasma refill from extravascular fluid compartments over 1–2 days (Moore, 1965). Plasma proteins and clotting factors are diluted but recover rapidly. Spontaneous fluid shift, however, cannot be relied upon for self-resuscitation in previously sick individuals, who may need intravenous fluids even for acute mild hypovolemia.

Uncorrected *moderate* hypovolemia (20–30% of blood volume lost) can lead to vital organ malfunction and, therefore, requires fluid resuscitation. Protracted moderate hypovolemia or acute *severe* hypovolemia (30–50% of blood volume lost), if untreated, leads to loss of cell viability and death.

Rapid loss of 50% of blood volume or more can result in *exsanguination* cardiac arrest (Negovsky, 1974; Kirimli et al., 1969). A "terminal state" with rapidly declining mean arterial pressure and loss of consciousness, leads via an "agonal state" (pulselessness, gasping), to "clinical death" (pulselessness, apnea). This state is often reversible if resuscitation is started earlier than about 10 min of pulselessness (Torpey, 1967; Breivik et al., 1978). Cardiac arrest from exsanguination occurs in the form of electromechanical dissociation (mechanical asystole, electrocardiogram complexes without pulse), which progresses to electric asystole. Ventricular fibrillation can occur, in this situation, in patients with diseased hearts or can be provoked by resuscitation attempts. Cardiac arrest from exsanguination is highly resuscitable, because the heart responds well to volume replacement and because it seems to produce less brain damage than the same duration of arrest with normovolemia (Breivik et al., 1978; Hossmann and Kleihues, 1973). Cardiac arrest can also occur suddenly in mild hemorrhagic shock, when ventricular fibrillation is provoked by underlying heart disease, chest injury (cardiac contusion), massive infusion of cold banked blood (cardiac hypothermia), or drugs.

Events at the *cellular* and organ levels are complex. Anaerobic cellular metabolism increases because of tissue hypoxia. The resulting lactacidemia (Cannon, 1918; Huckabee, 1958; Hardaway et al., 1967) may not lead to reduced pH when there is concomitant hyperventilation. Acidemia is transiently more severe during fluid resuscitation when acids are washed out from tissues. During hemorrhage, catecholamine release results in hyperglycemia, with insulin levels first decreased and later increased (Carey et al., 1970). Also, glucose transport seems to be a problem. Bleeding induces a hypercoagulable state, which is later followed by generalized hypocoagulability, with signs of disseminated intravascular coagulation (Hardaway, 1966; Hardaway et al., 1967).

Functional *renal failure* due to renal vasoconstriction can occur even without hypotension. This is transient if normovolemia is restored within about 1 hr. Otherwise, acute renal tubular necrosis, which can heal itself often only after weeks of expensive care including renal dialysis, may follow. The presence of free plasma hemoglobin from blood tranfusions, or of myoglobin from muscle trauma, enhances the development of acute renal failure.

Lung function (Fig. 29.3) is not altered during acute hemorrhage. Increased dead space, from regional hypoperfusion, requires hyperventilation to occur (Freeman and Nunn, 1963). Pulmonary edema may occur when fluid resuscitation is excessive, when aspiration occurs, or when a combination of hypoperfusion, left heart failure, and decreased plasma oncotic pressure leads to increased extravascular fluid volume in the lungs (Moore et al., 1969; Petty and Ashbaugh, 1971; Safar et al., 1972; Guyton and Lindsey, 1959; Skillman, 1976). Such multifactorial pulmonary edema is common when hypovolemic shock is combined with trauma, sepsis, or cardiac insufficiency (Smith et al., 1968); it is rare after promptly treated hemorrhage without these complications. There may be concomitant miliary atelectasis from absence of normal periodic deep breathing and from surfactant failure due to pulmonary hypoperfusion. These changes may result in progressive pulmonary consolidation (Safar et al., 1972), also called "shock lung" (Moore et al., 1969) or "adult respiratory distress syndrome (ARDS)" (Petty and Ashbaugh, 1971)—the pulmonary equivalent of acute renal tubular necrosis (Safar et al., 1972).

Acutely the organ most vulnerable to shock is the *brain* (Kovach and Sandor, 1976; Safar, 1978a). The "shock brain" has been inadequately studied so far. Prolonged severe hemorrhagic shock can cause coma and irreversible neurologic damage (Kovach and Sandor, 1976). Conversely, CNS failure (brain ischemia or trauma) can augment the shock state (Stone et al., 1965; Kovach and Sandor, 1976) and can cause neurogenic pulmonary edema (Luisada, 1967; Moss, 1974; Overland and Severinghaus, 1978), the mechanism of which is still not clear. Protecting the brain with cerebral perfusion during hemorrhagic shock can increase survival (Kovach and Sandor, 1976; Sanderson et al., 1972).

Cerebral blood flow (CBF) depends primarily on cerebral perfusion pressure (CPP), i.e., mean arterial pressure (MAP) minus intracranial pressure (ICP) or central venous pressure (CVP), whichever is higher, and on cerebrovascular resistance (CVR). In hypotension, CVR is reduced (CBF sustained) by dilation of cerebral arterioles, probably due to brain extracellular fluid (ECF) acidosis. CVR is increased (CBF decreased) by constriction of cerebral arterioles due to hyperventilation in shock, which causes brain ECF alkalosis (Stone et al., 1965). Locally released vasoconstrictor substances, blood sludging or tissue edema compressing vessels, can also decrease CBF. Total CBF is not reduced by a reduction in blood volume or cardiac output per se, unless CVR is increased or hypotension or ICP rise reduces CPP. Regional CBF may be inhomogeneously increased or decreased, depending on local changes in brain tissue.

During hypotension, CBF and consciousness are protected at first by cerebral vasodilation, until CPP (i.e., MAP with usually low ICP) is reduced to about 50 torr (CBF autoregulation). A decrease in CPP or MAP to less than about 50 torr results in a reduction of CBF, which leads to delirium, stupor, and coma. While a CPP of 20–30 torr, even for prolonged periods, can apparently maintain viability of neurons (Steen et al., 1979a), a drop in CPP to about 20 torr or less seems to be as damaging to neurons as cardiac arrest. Actually, a trickle of blood flow seems to cause more brain damage than no flow, perhaps because it produces more brain lactacidosis (Siesjo, 1978).

During resuscitation, when MAP is restored, cerebral autoregulation is paralyzed (due to brain acidosis). Thus, total CBF and intracranial blood volume greatly increase for several minutes (after brief cardiac arrest) or for hours (after prolonged shock) following resuscitation. This may be accompanied by an increase in ICP, probably due to increased intracranial blood volume and cerebral edema. Despite the high CBF, however, there is spotty impaired reperfusion. After the initial hyperemia, total CBF falls to below normal levels for hours following a severe global ischemic insult.

When blood volume restoration is delayed or inadequate, several hours of extracerebral vasoconstriction or depressed CNS function may result in unresponsiveness to fluid therapy ("irreversible shock") (Lillehei et al., 1964) or a variety of secondary complications, including fat embolism in the case of skeletal trauma (Szanto et al., 1973). Rising CVP, anuria, persistent lactacidemia, coma, pulmonary edema-ARDS, cardiac dysrhythmias, and secondary cardiac arrest may follow. However, vigorous titrated combination therapy can sometimes turn the tide, despite the development of some of these signs and symptoms.

Blood loss may be unrecognized or underestimated, especially when *internal losses* are concealed, as in bleeding into fracture sites or surgical wounds and plasma loss from exsudation into the peritoneal cavity or the lumen of the bowel (peritonitis, pancreatitis, bowel infarction). Retroperitoneal hemorrhage can cause a shock state in excess of the amount of blood lost, perhaps due to the involvement of autonomic ganglia and renal vessels. Volume loss in pericardial hemorrhage is self-limiting but can cause cardiac tamponade and an obstructive-type shock.

Intracranial hemorrhage does not produce oligemic shock. Even minimal intracranial blood loss acts as a mass lesion, resulting in increased ICP, resultant systemic hypertension and eventual coma from brain shift, and intractable cardiovascular collapse from herniation of the medulla.

STEPS OF CARDIOPULMONARY-CEREBRAL RESUSCITATION (CPCR)

"Life supporting first aid" (LSFA) includes airway control and mouth-to-mouth breathing for the unconscious patient; control of external hemorrhage; extrication ("rescue pull") to a safe place; and appropriate positioning for shock and for coma. LSFA skills are needed for trauma cases at the scene and occasionally also in the hospital. Ambulance personnel, guided via radio by experienced physicians, must resuscitate while carrying out primary and secondary patient evaluation surveys and while transporting the patient to the most appropriate hospital (American Society of Anesthesiologists, 1968; Cowley, 1975). In the emergency department, it is crucial to mobilize all necessary specialists and skills, but fragmentation of patient care must be avoided. The team should be coordinated by *one* physician who is experienced in the management of multitrauma and who determines priorities of diagnosing and treating.

The initial survey at the scene should include assessment of airway, breathing, pulse, bleeding sites, state of consciousness, shock, and suspected spinal cord injury. Evaluation and resuscitation must be continued in the emergency department. While an adequate airway is established, hemorrhage controlled, and blood volume replenished via rapidly inserted intravenous catheter, a search should be made for signs of internal hemorrhage (chest, abdomen, pelvis, crushed extremity). The history should be obtained from the patient (if conscious) and from bystanders, ambulance personnel, and relatives. Undue patient movements must be avoided. Transfer to other hospital areas, such as x-ray, should be minimized. If necessary, the patient must be accompanied by appropriate personnel who will continue life support. Patients in need of immediate surgery should be taken directly via the emergency department to the operating room.

In 1961 we divided emergency resuscitation into three phases, with *alphabetized steps*, to aid in memorizing (Fig. 29.1, Table 29.1): phase I is for emergency oxygenation. It consists of steps A) airway control, B) breathing support and oxygenation, and C) circulation support. Step A has been subdivided into 10 airway control steps (Table 29.1). Phase II is for restoration of adequate spontaneous circulation. It consists of steps D, drugs and fluids; E, electrocardiography; and F, fibrillation treatment (electrical countershock). Although phases I and II are meant primarily for the unconscious, pulseless patient, steps C and D also are relevant for hemorrhagic-traumatic shock, as they include control of hemorrhage and fluid resuscitation. Phase III is prolonged life support (intensive therapy). It includes determining the underlying problem and the patients salvability; the management of prolonged shock and coma (cerebral resuscitation); as well as the operative and postoperative care of multitrauma cases.

For hemorrhagic-traumatic shock, the CPCR steps need the following *changes* in emphases (Fig. 29.1, Table

29.1): The patient should be placed supine, horizontal. After trauma, the head-neck-chest should be held in the aligned position at all times (including during transportation and when rolled from side to side for examination). Hypovolemic shock may be in part counteracted by raising the legs, but lowering the head is not recommended as it may decrease CBF and increase ICP. In the field, the "stable side position," with the head tilted backward, is recommended for the comatose patient, particularly when an attendant cannot stay with him, e.g., for mass casualties. For steps A and B, oxygen inhalation is more often needed than artificial ventilation, because after trauma, apnea is rare but hypoxemia is common. For step C, cardiac compressions are rarely needed. In cases of pulselessness from suspected intrathoracic hemorrhage, open chest rather than closed chest cardiac massage is indicated. For step D, intravenous fluids have a higher priority than drugs. Steps E and F have low priority, but they should not be neglected, since trauma to chest and abdomen and massive transfusions can cause life-threatening dysrhythmias (Demuth et al., 1967; Boyan and Howland, 1963; Howland et al., 1977).

In the management of shock, treatment by "rounding and prescribing" has no place. Management must be continuously "titrated," with the mutually influential steps of monitoring, diagnosing, and treating often occurring simultaneously.

AIRWAY CONTROL

Airway obstruction must be immediately recognized (no airflow, noisy breathing, suprasternal or intercostal retractions) and corrected. After trauma, hypopharyn-

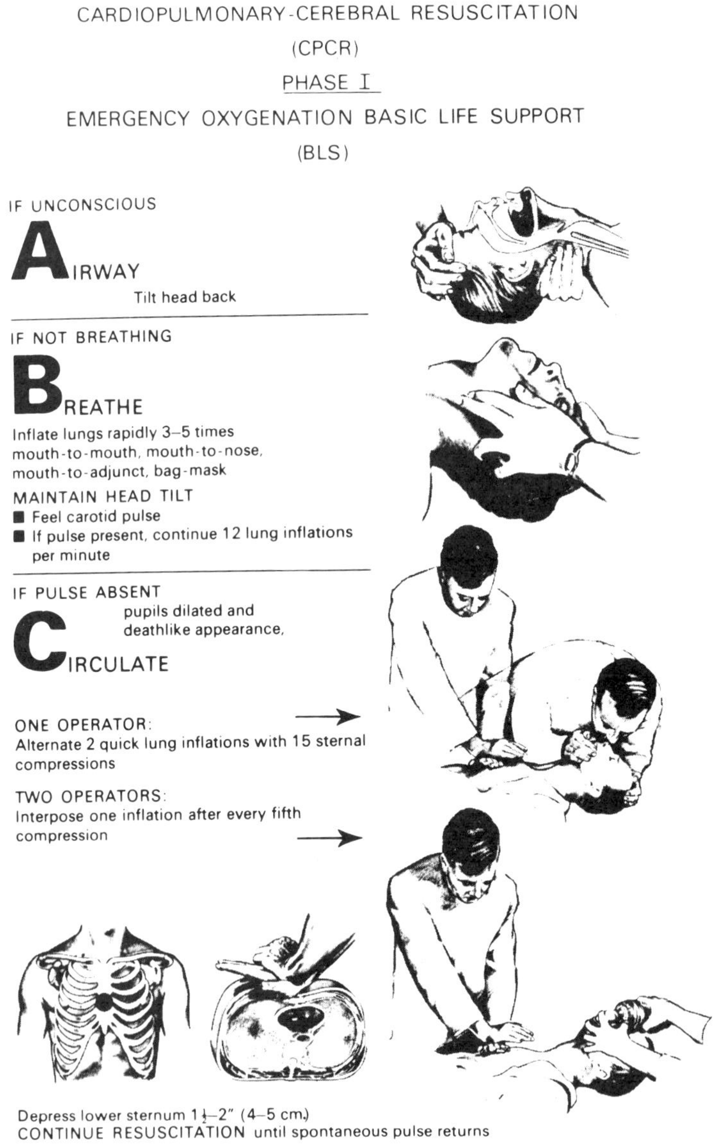

CARDIOPULMONARY-CEREBRAL RESUSCITATION
(CPCR)
PHASE I
EMERGENCY OXYGENATION BASIC LIFE SUPPORT
(BLS)

IF UNCONSCIOUS

AIRWAY
Tilt head back

IF NOT BREATHING

BREATHE
Inflate lungs rapidly 3–5 times mouth-to-mouth, mouth-to-nose, mouth-to-adjunct, bag-mask
MAINTAIN HEAD TILT
■ Feel carotid pulse
■ If pulse present, continue 12 lung inflations per minute

IF PULSE ABSENT

CIRCULATE
pupils dilated and deathlike appearance.

ONE OPERATOR:
Alternate 2 quick lung inflations with 15 sternal compressions

TWO OPERATORS:
Interpose one inflation after every fifth compression

Depress lower sternum 1½–2" (4–5 cm.)
CONTINUE RESUSCITATION until spontaneous pulse returns

Figure 29.1. Phases and steps of cardiopulmonary-cerebral resuscitation. (Reprinted with permission from P. Safar: *Principles and Practice of Emergency Medicine*, edited by G. Schwartz, et al., ch. 9. W. B. Saunders, Philadelphia, 1978.)

CARDIOPULMONARY-CEREBRAL RESUSCITATION

(CPCR)

<u>PHASE II</u>

ESTABLISHMENT OF NORMAL ARTERIAL OXYGEN TRANSPORT

(RESTART SPONTANEOUS CIRCULATION)

ADVANCED LIFE SUPPORT

(ALS)

DO NOT INTERRUPT CARDIAC COMPRESSIONS AND LUNG VENTILATION
INTUBATE TRACHEA WHEN POSSIBLE

DRUGS AND FLUIDS, I.V. LIFELINE
EPINEPHRINE
0.5-1.0 mg IV repeat larger dose as necessary

SODIUM BICARBONATE
1 mEq/kg IV
Repeat dose every 10 minutes until pulse returns.
Monitor and normalize arterial pH

I.V. FLUIDS as indicated

E.K.G. Ventricular fibrillation? Asystole? Bizarre complexes?

FIBRILLATION TREATMENT
EXTERNAL DEFIBRILLATION
D.C. 100-400 W/sec
Repeat shock as necessary
LIDOCAINE
1-2 mg/kg IV if necessary
IF ASYSTOLE
repeat step D - calcium and vasopressors as needed
CONTINUE RESUSCITATION until good pulse
is maintained

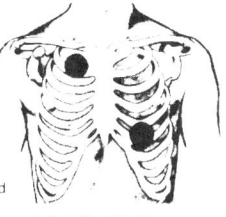

D.C. 100-400 W/sec

<u>PHASE III</u>

POST-RESUSCITATIVE LIFE SUPPORT

(PLS)

GAUGING
Determine and treat cause of demise
Determine salvageability

HUMAN MENTATION -- **C**EREBRAL RESUSCITATION
Support perfusion pressure, oxygenation, ventilation
If arrest > 5 min., coma > 5 min. after reperfusion
---clinical trials (e.g., thiopental)

INTENSIVE CARE

$PaCO_2$ 25-35   Art., CV, (PA) catheters
PaO_2 >100   Temp. Control, EKG
pHa 7.3-7.6   (Curarization)

ICP (osmotherapy, hypothermia)
Suppress convulsions
Steroid, Dextrose 5-10%, electrol., IV Fluids, alimentation
Hct., plasma COP, serum osm.
Outcome

Table 29.1
Steps of Emergency Resuscitation for Shock-Trauma Victims (from CPR Steps A–I); for Use at the Scene, during Transportation, and in the Hospital[a]

Phases I and II—Basic and Advanced Resuscitation
Treat and Diagnose Simultaneously

Diagnosis: Primary Survey (immediately)[b]
    Conscious? Airway? Breathing? Pulse? Bleeding?
  Secondary Survey (as soon as possible)[b]
    Pulse rate. Blood pressure. Respirations. Skin.
    Exam head to toe (wounds, fractures).

Step A: Airway Control—Proceed with sequence 1 through 8 until airway is open; 1–10 suitable for comatose patient; 5, 8, 10 may be needed also by conscious patient.
1. Backward tilt of the head. Position[b]
   Accident victim: moderate tilt, horizontal stable straight position; if unattended, stable side position with head tilted backward
2. IPPV attempt (after each step) (e.g., mouth-mouth or bag-mask)[b]
3. Manual clearing of mouth and throat (crossed-finger, tongue-jaw lift, or finger-behind-teeth maneuver for wiping, finger probe, extraction)[b]
4. Triple airway maneuver (tilt head backward moderately, open mouth, displace mandible forward)[b]
5. Suction (oro- and nasopharyngeal)
6. Pharyngeal tube insertion (oro- or nasopharyngeal)
7. Esophageal obturator airway insertion (not recommended for trauma victim)
8. Tracheal intubation (orotracheal, nasotracheal), tracheobronchial suctioning, drain stomach
9. Alternatives for tracheal intubation
   a. Cricothyroid membrane puncture
   b. Translaryngeal O_2 jet insufflation
10. Special measures
    a. Tracheotomy
    b. Bronchoscopy
    c. Bronchodilation and clearing
    d. Pleural drainage

Step B: Breathing Support—Ventilation and Oxygenation
1. Direct mouth-to-mouth (nose) with triple airway maneuver, IPPV[b]
2. Mouth-to-mask with triple airway maneuver, IPPV
3. Bag-valve-mask (tracheal tube) with O_2, IPPV; PEEP optional
   O_2 hand-triggered ventilator (alternative to bag-valve-O_2)
4. Blood gas monitoring
   Keep $PaCO_2$ 25–35 torr (coma)   ⎫
   Keep $PaCO_2$ 35–45 torr (conscious) ⎬ With step B5
   Keep PaO_2 >100 torr (coma)   ⎫
   Keep PaO_2 >60 torr (conscious) ⎬ With step B6
   Keep pHa 7.3–7.5 with volume ($NaHCO_3$ prn)
   Keep Hct 25–35% with blood or red blood cells
5. Prolonged artificial ventilation via tracheal tube
   IMV with IPPV; or AV with IPPB
   CV with IPPV
6. Prolonged oxygenation with O_2 100% (short term) or 50% (long term)
   SB with atmospheric pressure
   SB with CPAP
   IMV with PEEP
   CV with IPPV plus PEEP. Optimize PEEP (5–20 cm H_2O)
   Diuretic. Colloid osmotic press >15 torr

Step C: Circulation Support (CPR Steps C–F)
1. Positioning: horizontal face up; legs raised[b]
2. Monitoring: feel carotid pulse, radial pulse; EKG; insert catheters into bladder, Sup. V. Cava, artery, pulmonary artery. Temp.
3. Blood volume resuscitation (Table 29.2). Urine flow >0.5 ml/kg/hr
   a. Control of hemorrhage: external (compression, elevation)[b]
                               internal (MAST, operation)
   b. Fluid resuscitation, via IV catheters. MAP >60 torr (conscious), >90 torr (unconscious). CVP 10–20 torr electrol, colloid, blood or red blood cells (fluorocarbons, stroma-free hemoglobin), fresh frozen plasma (Table 29.2)
4. Cardiac resuscitation: cardiac compressions + defibrillation
   Closed chest CPR[b]
   Open chest CPR
5. Drugs in resuscitation from cardiac arrest
   Vasoconstrictor
   Cardiac stimulant
   Sodium bicarbonate

Phase III: Prolonged Life Support

Steps G, H, I: Gauging—Humanizing—Intensive Care
    Cerebral resuscitation (Tables 29.3 and 29.4)
    Intensive care life support; use asepsis
    Definitive therapy (surgical operations); drain pus; drain hematomas

---
[a] Abbreviations: *IPPV*, intermittent positive pressure ventilation; *PEEP*, positive end-expiratory pressure; *IMV*, intermittent mandatory ventilation; *AV*, assisted ventilation; *CV*, controlled ventilation; *CPAP*, continuous positive airway pressure; *SB*, spontaneous breathing.
[b] Education-research and epidemiologic data suggest that these steps should also be taught to lay personnel.

geal obstruction is common, due to coma causing soft tissue obstruction by the tongue (Safar et al., 1959). Obstruction may also be due to aspiration of vomitus, mucus, or blood; laryngospasm; or airway injury. The emergency airway control steps (Table 29.1) should be pursued swiftly and vigorously until the airway is open (Safar, 1980a).

In coma, *jaw thrust* with moderate backward tilt of the head and opening of the mouth (triple airway maneuver) (Fig. 29.2) should be applied. Exaggerated backward tilt of the head and flexion or lateral turning of head and neck may aggravate a cervical spinal cord injury. The "triple airway maneuver" can be learned even by lay personnel (Esposito et al., 1980). Health professionals can replace jaw thrust with an oro- or nasopharyngeal tube. A nasopharyngeal tube is better tolerated and is preferred when there is trismus but is not recommended when a basal skull fracture is suspected.

The esophageal obturator airway is contraindicated in the conscious and the spontaneously breathing unconscious patient, because its insertion can provoke vomiting, regurgitation, aspiration, and laryngospasm. Moreover, it does not permit tracheal suctioning.

Tracheal intubation is indicated when the patient has lost consciousness (unless his upper airway protective reflexes are intact, coma is expected to be brief, and he is attended continuously by experienced personnel) and in the conscious patient with inadequate spontaneous clearing of the tracheobronchial tree, suspected aspiration, upper airway areflexia, or need for prolonged mechanical ventilation. Improved endotracheal tubes and cuffs have minimized laryngotracheal damage (Safar, 1978; Carroll et al., 1969; Lindholm, 1969).

Tracheal intubation, the ultimate step of emergency airway control, does not have first priority in cases of suspected head injury (Safar, 1978, 1979; Bruce et al., 1978). Reflex hypertension and unskilled intubation attempts often accompanied by straining, asphyxia, and aspiration can cause ICP rise and intracranial disaster. To intubate the trachea successfully without causing such complications requires special techniques and an experienced operator (Stept and Safar, 1970). If head injury is suspected and an experienced operator is not available, oxygenation and assisted ventilation by bag-mask-oxygen is safer than attempts at tracheal intubation. For emergency airway control, orotracheal intubation is preferred. Nasotracheal intubation is less predictable, more time consuming, and potentially more traumatic and is contraindicated in suspected basilar fracture. Nasotracheal intubation, however, may be preferable in the spontaneously breathing patient without asphyxia if there is trismus or inability to tilt the head backward (suspected neck fracture).

Cricothyroid membrane puncture (Safar and Penninckx, 1967) or translaryngeal oxygen jet insufflation (Smith, 1974) can be used as an alternative to tracheal intubation but is rarely needed.

Tracheotomy (below the cricoid cartilage) should be considered for long term airway care, after a translaryngeal tube has been in place for several days, or earlier when coma is expected to last longer than about 1 week; and in patients who are conscious and would be more comfortable with a tracheotomy tube, which permits them to talk (Safar, 1978).

Bronchoscopy is indicated in cases of aspiration for clearing solid foreign matter or thick mucus or blood from the tracheobronchial tree. The rigid tube bronchoscope (with ventilation-oxygenation attachment) is more effective than the fiberoptic bronchoscope for clearing such materials.

Pleural drainage is listed under airway control (Table 29.1), because tension pneumothorax kills via lung collapse, bronchial compression, and asphyxia (Safar, 1978). Tension pneumothorax should be supected when chest injury or IPPV is followed by tracheal shift, progressive inability of the chest to deflate, progressive abdominal distension (inversion of the diaphragm and pneumoperitoneum), progressive hypotension, and mediastinal shift to percussion. Proof is by needle puncture via the second intercostal space anteriorly, and treatment is by large tube drainage (Safar, 1978).

VENTILATION AND OXYGENATION

Accidental injury, particularly head trauma, can cause transient sudden coma, breath-holding, and hypoventilation. At the scene, treatment includes moderate head tilt plus jaw thrust, opening of the mouth, and exhaled air ventilation. In case of trismus, mouth-to-nose ventilation may be required. Ambulance and hospital personnel should switch as soon as possible to inhalation of 50–100% oxygen with spontaneous, assisted, or controlled ventilation, for example by pocket mask with oxygen nipple (Fig. 29.2) (Safar, 1974) or a bag-valve-mask unit (Ruben, 1958) with oxygen reservoir.

By the time the patient with hemorrhagic shock arrives in the emergency room, he is usually spontaneously hyperventilating. Nevertheless, he should continue to receive 50–100% oxygen. In cases of severe multitrauma, irrespective of the state of consciousness, controlled ventilation with an inhaled oxygen concentration (FIO_2) of 50–100%, facilitated by mechanical hyperventilation (Moerch et al., 1956) or immobilization with a muscle relaxant, is desirable to stabilize ventilation and oxygenation while control of hemorrhage, fluid resuscitation, and emergency surgery are accomplished. Softening doses of a relaxant (e.g., pancuronium) do not hamper recognition of an intracranial mass lesion. Weaning from controlled ventilation can be accomplished with intermittent mandatory ventilation (IMV; i.e., combination of spontaneous breathing and gradually decreased rate of mechanical lung inflations) or assisted ventilation, gradually progressing to spontaneous breathing.

In the hands of prehospital personnel not trained in anesthesiology, use of the pocket mask is more effective than use of the bag-valve-mask unit, since the former leaves both hands available to provide mask fit and jaw thrust (Fig. 29.2). When the bag-valve-oxygen unit is used with a tracheal tube, a simple modification permits IPPV with positive end-expiratory pressure (PEEP)

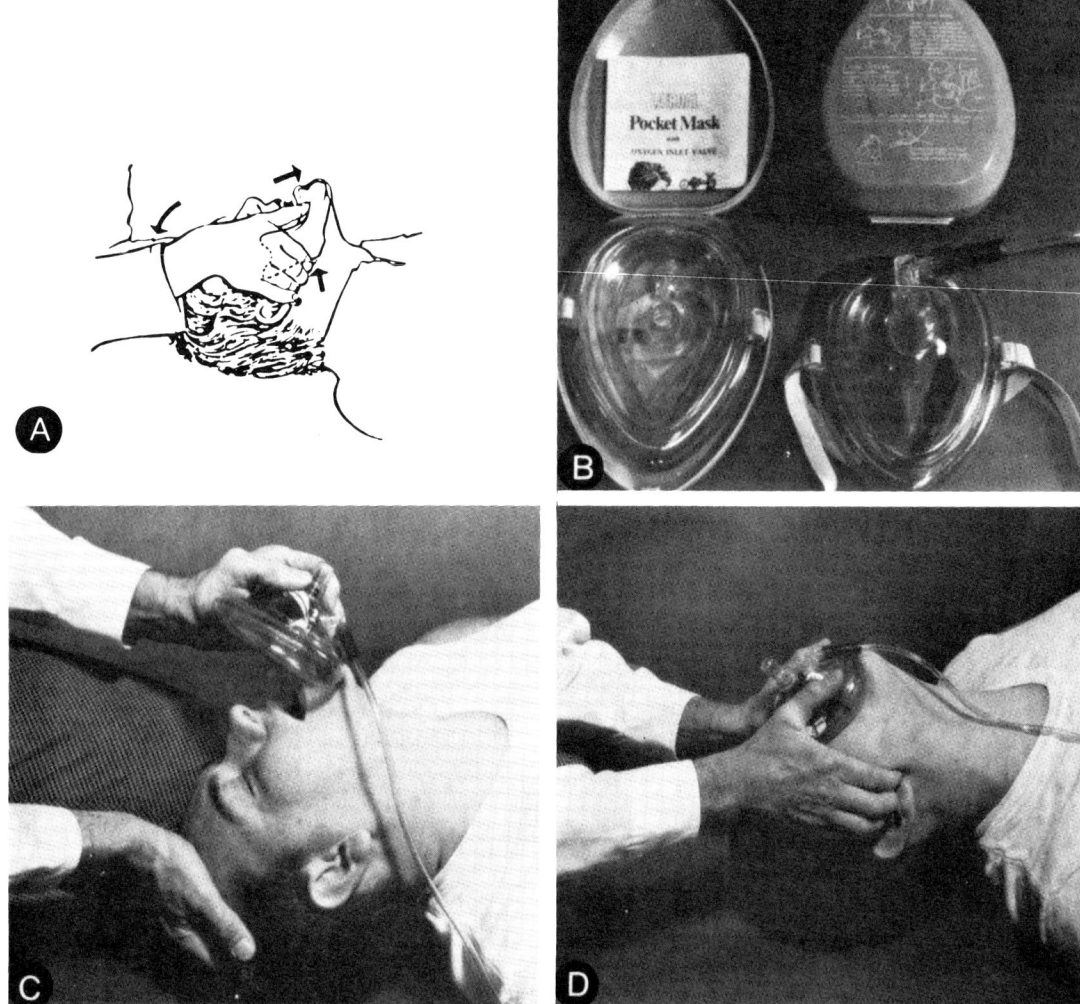

Figure 29.2. Airway control. *A*, without equipment—triple airway maneuver (head tilt, jaw thrust, and open mouth). *B*, with pocket mask—for oxygen inhalation and artificial ventilation by mouth-to-mask. Laerdal transparent folding mask with 15-mm male breathing port and oxygen insufflation nipple, inflated cushion, and head strap. *C*, in comatose patient, tilt head backward; open mouth by retracting lower lip, apply rim of mask over chin to keep mouth open; apply entire mask over mouth and nose. *D*, in comatose patient, clamp mask to face with both thumbs (thenar eminences) on top of mask and fingers 2 to 5 of both hands grasping both ascending rami of mandible in front of earlobes. Pull forcefully upward (forward) so that lower teeth are in front of upper teeth and chin juts out. Mouth must remain open under mask. Front of neck must be maximally stretched. Do not pull on the chin, as this tends to close the mouth. Sustain this maneuver as long as the patient is unconscious or until a pharyngeal or tracheal tube can be inserted. (In infants apply mask upside down and cover the entire face). If patient breathes spontaneously, strap mask to face. If he is apneic or breathing shallowly, take a deep breath, blow into mask until chest moves, take mouth off, and let him exhale passively. When available, deliver oxygen via nipple of mask; 10–15 liters/min flow results in about 50% O_2 inhaled. With higher flows, artificial ventilation with 100% O_2 is possible by intermittently occluding port with tongue and opening it when the chest rises. (Reprinted with permission from P. Safar: Critical Care Medicine 2:273, 1973.)

(Safar and Lind, 1975). Use of a simple portable pressure-set ventilator (e.g., Bird Mark 7) is acceptable in cases with normal lungs. However, if the patient has abnormal lungs, use of a volume-set time-cycled ventilator, with PEEP and IMV attachments, is preferred for controlled ventilation, at least after hospital admission.

Hospitals receiving trauma cases must be equipped for arterial *blood gas* analyses. In cases of moderate shock with prompt resuscitation, intermittent arterial punctures are adequate. In severe or protracted shock, an arterial catheter should be inserted. This also permits continuous arterial pressure monitoring via strain gauge, which in hypotension is more accurate than the Riva-Rocci cuff method. Percutaneous PO_2 (Huch et al., 1973) is even of value in shock, as it decreases not only with decreased arterial PO_2 but also in shock states with normal arterial PO_2, when there is reduced PO_2 in capillaries and venules. Peripheral venous blood gas values are not useful. Changes in central venous (mixed venous) PO_2, however, are valuable, as they reflect oxygen supply-demand relationships (of value during acute hemodilution therapy). Assessment of pulmonary and ventilatory status requires arterial PO_2 (in relation to FIO_2) and arterial PCO_2.

The adequacy of alveolar *ventilation* is determined by arterial PCO_2 (normal $PaCO_2$ values are 35–45 torr). Most spontaneously breathing patients in hemorrhagic shock hyperventilate spontaneously. Since shock can decrease, and trauma as well as resuscitation can increase, oxygen consumption and CO_2 production, ventilation requirements in terms of tidal volumes and rates are unpredictable and should ideally be adjusted according to arterial PCO_2 determinations. During controlled ventilation, moderate hyperventilation to $PaCO_2$ of 25–35 torr is desirable. This can usually, in the patient with normal cardiac output and oxygen consumption, be accomplished by tidal volumes of 15 ml/kg at a rate of 12/min.

The adequacy of arterial blood *oxygenation* (pulmonary status) is determined by arterial PO_2 in relation to inhaled PO_2 or FIO_2. Normal PaO_2 is 75–100 torr with FIO_2 21%; over 250 torr with FIO_2 50%; and over 500 torr with FIO_2 100%. Lower than expected PaO_2 values are caused by ventilation/perfusion mismatching. If these is no significant increase in shunt, hypoxemia is easily corrected by FIO_2 50%. If arterial PO_2 values are considerably lower than 500 torr with FIO_2 100% (increased alveolar-arterial PO_2 gradient with FIO_2 100%), shunting is suspected. This may require FIO_2 100% (short-term) or 50% (long-term) plus some form of continuously increased airway pressure for alveolar recruitment and stabilization (controlled ventilation with the use of PEEP) (Petty and Ashbaugh, 1971). Hypoxemia after shock or cardiac arrest is common (Smith et al., 1968). Shunting may occur due to aspiration, overtransfusion, lack of deep breathing, and pulmonary edema-consolidation (ARDS) (Fig. 29.3).

Arterial PO_2 should be kept at a minimum of 60 torr (the knee of the hemoglobin oxygen dissociation curve) in the conscious patient or at a minimum of 100 torr in the unconscious patient. Pulmonary oxygen toxicity can be prevented by limiting the use of FIO_2 100% to less than 6–12 hours. FIO_2 50% appears safe for unlimited periods. Shunting per se increases the tolerance by the lungs of FIO_2 100% (Winter et al., 1967).

A compromise between intratracheal IPPV with PEEP and spontaneous breathing of oxygen at atmospheric pressure is the technique of spontaneous breathing with continuous positive airway pressure (SB-CPAP) via mouthpiece, mask (strapped on or held on), or tracheal tube, introduced by Gregory into neonatal respiratory care. This technique can also be provided for adults, using easily available supplies, such as elastic reservoir bag, nonrebreathing valve, PEEP valve at the expiratory port, and airway pressure gauge (Safar, 1978). Upper airway pressures over 15 cm H_2O tend to cause gastric insufflation. SB-CPAP by mask, therefore, should stay below this level.

In shock, mean airway pressure should be kept as low as possible, since increased mean intrathoracic pressure tends to reduce further the return of blood to the right heart (Werko, 1947; Brecher, 1956). If spontaneous breathing is inadequate, IPPV is recommended. Positive-negative pressure ventilation (PNPV) enhances venous return, but the negative pressure promotes pulmonary edema and lung collapse. PEEP during IPPV is indicated only when there is increased shunting (reduced compliance); fortunately, in patients with stiff lungs who may need PEEP, hypotension due to PEEP is less likely to develop, because the noncompliant lungs prevent transmission of airway pressure to the venae cavae (Pontoppidan et al., 1972). Optimal PEEP is best established by following changes in pulmonary artery or central venous PO_2, which reflects the relationship between oxygen consumption and delivery, or by minimizing dynamic lung compliance (the airway pressure difference required for a given tidal volume) (Suter et al., 1975).

Sustained increased airway pressure may also cause pulmonary barotrauma (alveolar rupture causing pneumothorax or interstitial emphysema), particularly after lung injury. This is another reason for keeping PEEP as low as possible. Pleural drainage equipment should always be at hand.

High frequency oxygen jet ventilation (Klain and Smith, 1977; Smith and Klain, 1980) is a new, still experimental technique. One hundred percent oxygen is intermittently insufflated via a thin catheter inserted into the tracheal tube or percutaneously through the cricothyroid membrane. Cycling rates of 100–1,000/min, delivering 100% oxygen with tidal volumes smaller than estimated dead space, can restore and maintain normal arterial PO_2 and PCO_2 values in nonbreathing subjects with normal lungs. This technique allows simultaneous spontaneous breathing to occur, lessens the chance for injury to the tracheal mucosa, and lowers mean airway pressure, with less risk of causing barotrauma or reduction in cardiac output. The ability of this technique to recruit alveoli and increase arterial PO_2 in the presence of reversible shunt (e.g., aspiration, pulmonary edema) has not yet been determined.

CARDIOPULMONARY RESUSCITATION

"Cardiac arrest" is defined as "the clinical picture of sudden cessation of circulation in a patient who was not expected to die at that time" (Safar, 1968). Cessation of circulation is verified when *all* the following conditions are present: unconsciousness, apnea or gasps, death-like appearance, and no pulse in the carotid or femoral artery. Absence of heart sounds and presence of dilated pupils are unreliable signs.

Closed Chest CPR

Irrespective of the EKG pattern of cardiac arrest,

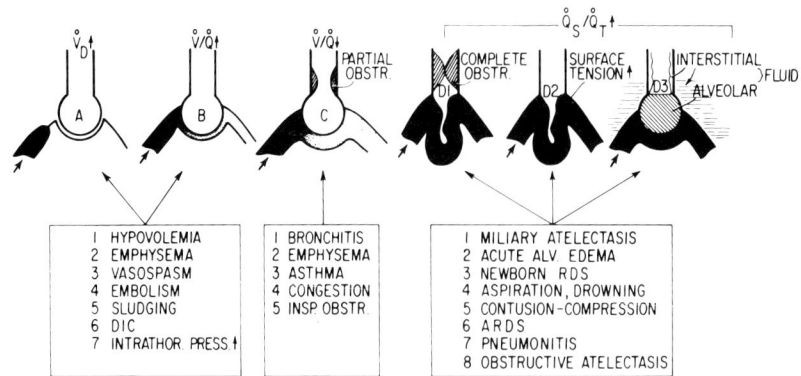

Figure 29.3. Mechanisms of hypoxemia in shock, trauma and sepsis—breathing of air. Variable combinations of the following coexist: A, alveoli ventilated but not perfused (i.e., alveolar dead space); B, alveoli more ventilated than perfused; C, alveoli perfused more than ventilated; D, alveoli perfused but not ventilated at all (right-to-left shunting; "venous admixture"). A does not produce hypoxemia unless during breathing of air ventilation is not increased to compensate for increase in dead space and $PaCO_2$ is increased. B in itself also does not produce hypoxemia. C is reduced ventilation-perfusion ratio, the most common cause of hypoxemia; it is readily correctable by oxygen inhalation. D is hypoxemia due to shunting; it may not be correctable by oxygen inhalation alone, but may yield in part to a continuous increase in airway pressure, which may recruit and stabilize collapsed or fluid-filled alveoli. The 100% oxygen test permits differentiation between C and D. Clinical examples are listed in the figure. Those under D are listed in the order of likelihood of improvement by positive pressure: D2 due to increased surface tension as in newborn respiratory distress syndrome, or D3 due to acute pulmonary edema, permit alveolar re-expansion with positive pressure more likely than (D1) due to complete airway obstruction or (D3) pneumonia. (Reprinted with permission from P. Safar and N. Caroline: *Principles and Practice of Emergency Medicine*, edited by G. Schwartz et al., ch. 3. W. B. Saunders, Philadelphia, 1978.)

pulselessness calls for an immediate start of standard closed chest CPR, i.e., external cardiac compressions at a rate of two successive lung inflations after every 15 sternal compressions at a rate of 80/min for one operator; or 60/min with one interposed lung inflation after every five sternal compressions for two operators (Harris et al., 1976b). This combination of IPPV plus sternal compressions is continued until a spontaneous pulse returns. IPPV should start with FIO_2 100% if available. IPPV via tracheal tube does not have to be synchronized with sternal compressions. Standard closed chest CPR produces borderline blood flow for cerebral viability (Bircher et al., 1980; Alifimoff et al., 1980). Lung inflations simultaneous with sternal compressions result in improved carotid blood flow (Rudikoff et al., 1980; Bircher et al., 1980; Harris et al., 1967a; Wilder et al., 1963), but increased ICP and reduced brain oxygenation (Bircher et al., 1981). "New CPR" (IPPV simultaneous with chest compressions at 40/min, and abdominal binding), based on the "chest-pump" rather than "heart-pump" mechanism of CPR, requires tracheal tube and apparatus (Chandra, 1980) and is still experimental.

Blood volume must be restored and expanded. Electrical asystole and electromechanical dissociation call for epinephrine; ventricular fibrillation and ventricular tachycardia call for electric countershock; and recurrent ventricular fibrillation calls for lidocaine (Carden and Steinhaus, 1956) or bretylium (Koch-Weser, 1979) in addition to countershock. Recommended energy levels for external electric defibrillation start with about 3–5 W sec/kg body wt and increase for repeated shocks. Precordial thumping cannot reliably defibrillate; it actually can cause ventricular fibrillation. During asystole or severe bradycardia due to heart block, however, repetitive precordial thumping in the conscious patient or external cardiac compressions in the unconscious patient (the latter is too painful for the conscious patient) can be effectively used to pace the oxygenated heart, while waiting for infusion of isoproterenol or insertion of a transvenous pacemaker.

Open Chest CPR

Open chest CPR (Fig. 29.4) was widely used in hospitals before the 1960s with good results (Beck, 1947; Dripps et al., 1948; Stephenson, 1974). It is now a forgotten art, but it should be revived to be taught in training programs for physicians and for wider use in hospitals. It produces significantly better perfusion pressures and blood flows than the closed chest CPR technique, since direct heart massage (in contrast to sternal compressions) does not increase venous pressures and, if prolonged, provides a better chance to restart the heart and for the brain to recover (DelGuercio et al., 1963; Bircher et al., 1981; Alifimoff et al., 1980). Other advantages are the ability to feel and visualize the heart, to inject cardiac drugs directly into the heart, and to recognize and treat intrathoracic pathology, such as hemorrhage. It also gives access to a pulmonary embolus.

Resuscitation

Physicians in hospitals should consider an *early* switch from the closed chest to the open chest CPR technique in circumstances for which it may be the only effective method of restoring life, such as: 1) suspected intrathoracic pathology, such as tension pneumothorax or hemorrhage, particularly from penetrating wounds of the chest, crushing chest injury, or following intrathoracic surgery; 2) inability to produce a palpable femoral or carotid pulse with sternal compressions, as is occasionally the case with chest injury, chest or spine deformities, or severe emphysema with barrel chest; 3) intractable ventricular fibrillation or mechanical asystole, as may be the case in severe heart disease or hypothermia.

A *delayed* switch to open chest CPR should be considered in intractable, prolonged electromechanical dissociation or ventricular fibrillation.

The *technique* of open chest CPR is as follows (Fig. 29.4). Cut through skin and muscles under the left breast over approximately the fourth intercostal space. Pierce the intercostal space open with a blunt instrument or your fingers. Insert a rib spreader when available. Compress the heart immediately, before opening the pericardium, by placing the fingers of one hand behind the heart and the thenar and thumb in front of the heart. Use a wringing action with 80–100 compressions per min. Take care not to pierce the atrium with your thumb. Compress large hearts with one hand behind and one hand in front of the heart. If the heart feels empty, speed up intravenous fluids and compress the descending aorta during massage.

When you feel the ventricular fibrillation or see it on the EKG, perform internal defibrillation by placing two paddle electrodes with saline-soaked pads directly on the heart—one behind the left ventricle, the other over the anterior surface of the heart. Start with 0.5 W sec/kg body wt. High energy shocks applied directly to the heart can cause burns. In intractable ventricular fibrillation or when intracardiac drugs are needed, open the pericardium. Inject epinephrine and other cardiac drugs into the cavity of the left ventricle. Do not give norepinephrine or sodium bicarbonate via the intracardiac route.

In suspected cardiac tamponade, if time permits and the patient is not yet pulseless, rapid drainage of the pericardial sac by needle puncture may obviate the need for thoracotomy. This technique should be augmented by closed chest CPR in cases of pulselessness.

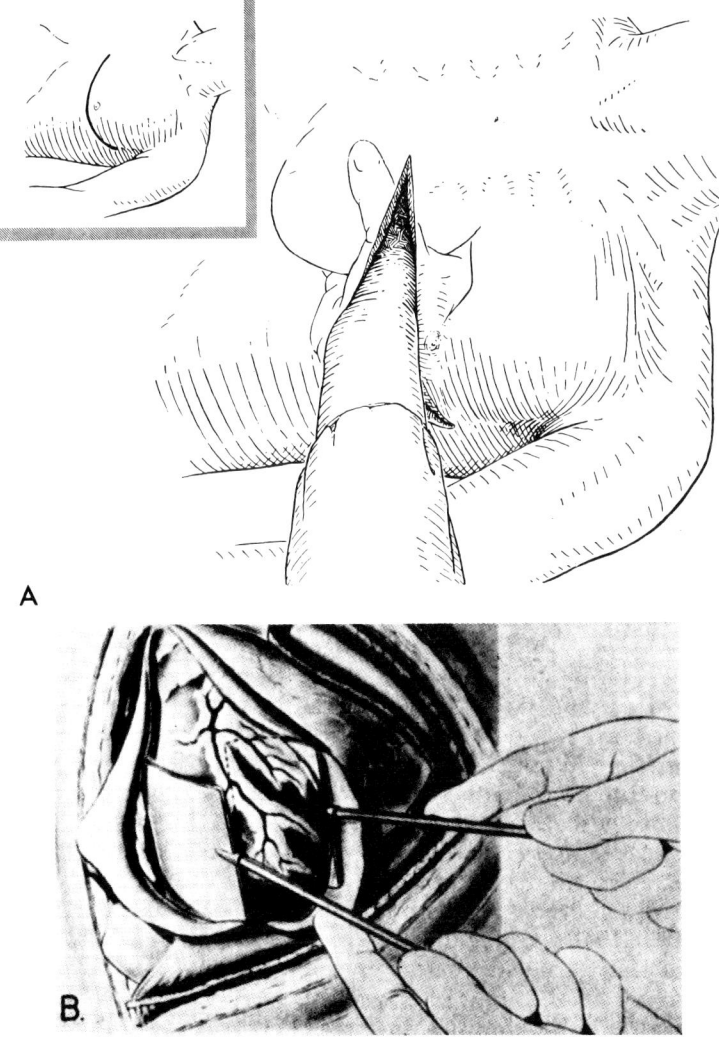

Figure 29.4. Open chest cardiac resuscitation. *A*, open the chest via the fifth left intercostal space (*inset*). Grasp and rhythmically compress the heart as described in the text. (Reprinted with permission from J. Johnson: *Surgery of the Chest.* Year Book Medical Publishers, Chicago, 1952.) *B*, internal direct electric defibrillation. When fibrillation is felt, apply internal electrodes to the pericardium (wearing rubber gloves), as illustrated, and apply countershock. For prolonged massage and repeated countershocks open the pericardial sac. (Reprinted with permission from H. Stephenson: *Cardiac Arrest and Resuscitation.* C. V. Mosby, St. Louis, MO, 1974.)

Drugs for CPR

In sudden primary ventricular fibrillation, no drugs are needed before an initial trial of electric defibrillation. After circulatory arrest of at least 1 min, epinephrine is indicated. After longer periods of arrest and before additional doses of epinephrine, sodium bicarbonate is indicated as well. Drugs given intravenously should be circulated by cardiac massage for about 1 min before countershock is applied.

Epinephrine, 0.5–1 mg in adults, should be given as the first drug (Crile and Dolley, 1906), either intravenously or in 10 ml of water via tracheal tube, without need to wait for EKG diagnosis. Although epinephrine can produce ventricular fibrillation in a nonfibrillating heart, it facilitates defibrillation (Redding, 1977). Epinephrine stimulates sympathetic α- and β-receptors. The α-receptor stimulation increases peripheral vascular resistance without constricting the coronary and cerebral vessels. The resulting increase in diastolic pressure improves myocardial perfusion and makes the heart more resuscitable. The β-receptor stimulation is not important during CPR (Pearson and Redding, 1965), but may be advantageous when spontaneous circulation returns, at which time it enhances cardiac contractility and cardiac output. In aystole and electromechanical dissociation, epinephrine helps restart spontaneous cardiac action by elevating perfusion pressure and increasing myocardial contractility.

Vasoconstrictors, i.e., predominantly α-receptor agonists, are also effective in facilitating restoration of spontaneous circulation but have not been studied and used as extensively as epinephrine. These drugs, which include norepinephrine (Levophed), metaraminol (Aramine), phenylephrine (Neosynephrine), methoxamine (Vasoxyl), and dopamine in high doses, have been used effectively for MAP support after restoration of spontaneous circulation.

Cardiac stimulants, i.e., predominantly β-receptor agonists, when given during cardiac massage, do not enhance restoration of spontaneous circulation but may be useful in intractable electromechanical dissociation and, after restoration of spontaneous circulation, in intractable hypotension. These drugs include isoproterenol (Isuprel), dopamine in low doses, dobutamine, and calcium chloride.

Sodium bicarbonate is the second drug to be given intravenously during cardiac compressions (Stewart, 1964). The recommended initial dose is 1 mEq/kg of body wt. Not more than 0.5 mEq/kg should be repeated every 5–10 min of CPR without arterial pH monitoring, to avoid severe alkalemia and hyperosmolality, which can make the heart nonresuscitable. As soon as possible, bicarbonate administration should be guided by arterial pH values, which should be maintained between 7.3 and 7.6. With near normal arterial pH, there is no evidence that base deficit itself must be normalized. Moderate acidosis may be beneficial (Bing et al., 1973).

Bicarbonate alone does not enhance restoration of spontaneous circulation, but it enhances the effect of epinephrine, which is inactivated by acidosis, when the arrest was prolonged (Kirimli et al., 1966). Immediately after restoration of spontaneous circulation, washout of acids from tissues calls for further bicarbonate administration with careful pH monitoring. Transient hyperventilation is needed to eliminate the CO_2 that has accumulated in tissues and that is being released from the bicarbonate.

Tris buffer (THAM) has been tried in lieu of sodium bicarbonate. While THAM does not increase arterial PCO_2 and blood sodium and has a greater intracellular effect, it carries the disadvantages of enhancing apnea, producing hypoglycemia, and not being available in a usable solution that does not sclerose veins.

Lidocaine (Xylocaine) is a local anesthetic that raises the ventricular fibrillation threshold (Carden and Steinhaus, 1956). It is usually given in individual doses of 1 mg/kg intravenously, which may be repreated as necessary, and as an intravenous infusion of 1–4 mg/70 kg/min. Lidocaine is the drug of choice for the prevention and treatment of ventricular extrasystoles and ventricular tachycardia. In ventricular fibrillation it is not a substitute for electric countershock—nor are other antiarrhythmic agents. In recurrent ventricular fibrillation lidocaine is indicated, in addition to repeated countershocks and control of arterial pH, blood gases, and perfusion pressure. *Bretylium* is a new, promising antiarrhythmic agent that should be considered when lidocaine fails (Koch-Weser, 1979); recommended doses are 5 mg/kg intravenously repeated to a maximum of 30 mg/kg.

Cardiac Arrest Due to Exsanguination

Resuscitation methods for exsanguination cardiac arrest, worked out in the laboratory (Negovsky, 1974; Kirimli et al., 1969), have proven effective in the field (Torpey, 1967). These consist of the simultaneous application of the following:

1. IPPV with FIO_2 50–100%, plus external cardiac compressions.
2. Massive *intravenous* infusion of the most immediately available plasma substitute (e.g., lactated Ringer's in four times volume lost; Dextran, starch, albumin, or plasma in one time volume), with or without "universal donor" (group O, rhesus negative) warmed banked blood or red cells.
3. Epinephrine (1 mg) and sodium bicarbonate (1 mEq/kg) intravenously.
4. Control of hemorrhage (compression; tourniquet; military (medical) antishock trousers; laparotomy; thoracotomy for open chest CPR and hemostasis in intrathoracic exsanguination, or rupture of the abdominal aorta for compression of the descending thoracic aorta).
5. EKG monitoring and defibrillation as indicated.

In experimental animals with exsanguination arrest, spontaneous cardiac activity is usually restored when about 50% of shed blood volume has been replaced. The other 50% of shed blood, plus an additional 10–20% of estimated blood volume (to compensate for vasodilation and capillary leakage) should be restored more slowly, with monitoring to avoid overloading.

Hemoglobin is usually not needed to restart the circulation if the bleeding site is controlled, since rapid exsanguination leaves about 40% of total red cell mass in the body (Kirimli et al., 1969). Continued blood loss accompanied by further washout of hemoglobin with plasma substitutes, however, may reduce hematocrit below 20%, which reduces the chance of successful resuscitation. Where typed and cross matched blood is immediately available, it should be used in conjunction with a plasma substitute. After restoration of spontaneous circulation and control of hemorrhage, the desired hematocrit of 25–35% may be restored and clotting factors replaced. Oxygen carriers (hemoglobin, fluorocarbon) deserve clinical trial in exsanguination cardiac arrest.

Since the speed of infusion is more important than its hemoglobin content, whole blood or packed red cells (which need dilution with saline) have lower priority than colloid plasma substitutes. Massive intravenous infusion of Ringer's solution alone, however, can also restart the heart (Kirimli et al., 1969). However colloid must be added later (Takaori and Safar, 1967a and b; Brinkmeyer et al., 1980). Therefore, priority should be given to dextrans, hydroxyethyl starch, or albumin, at least for part of the initial infusion.

Exsanguination cardiac arrest can be reversed somewhat more rapidly and with less volume when using the *intra-arterial* route of infusion (Negovsky, 1974). Negovsky's animal model of arterial pressure infusion, of the 1940s, however, uses warm oxygenated heparinized blood with epinephrine. This approach can usually restart the arrested heart even without cardiac compressions, apparently by retrograde perfusion of the coronary arteries. When clinically available plasma substitutes or banked blood were used via the arterial route, these impressive results could not be reproduced and the infusion usually failed to restart the heart and sometimes initiated ventricular fibrillation (Kirimli et al., 1969). This probably is due to the fact that these solutions are not oxygenated, are acidic, and are cold. However, when given by the venous route they were effective; they are oxygenated as they pass through the lungs.

Intra-arterial infusion carries with it the hazards of delay due to arterial cutdown; retrograde cerebral gas or thromboembolism (even with use of a peripheral artery); and loss of limb from arterial thrombosis. However, when an artery is readily available, as in a large open wound during a surgical operation, a trial of arterial pressure infusion during cardiac compressions may be justified, at least to get spontaneous circulation restarted. In profound hypovolemic shock without cardiac arrest, arterial transfusion did not prove to be superior to venous infusion (Maloney et al., 1953).

CONTROL OF HEMORRHAGE

External hemorrhage can usually be controlled by the standard first aid procedures of elevating the bleeding site, applying local manual pressure, and applying a pressure bandage. "Tourniquets should be used as a last resort and only in cases of extremely traumatized extremities in which major vessels have been injured. If a tourniquet must be applied to any extremity, it should be maintained until proper provisions have been made to correct shock" (American College of Surgeons). Bleeding arteries should be clamped if possible; however, in traumatic amputation, severed vessels usually retract and do not bleed.

Suspected *internal* hemorrhage below the chest can be treated nonsurgically in the prehospital setting with use of "military (medical) antishock trousers" (MAST) (Fig. 29.5) (Kaplan et al., 1973; Crile, 1947). Recommended inflation to about 100 torr intrasuit pressure can promptly reverse hypotension, presumably by mobilizing blood volume, compressing bleeding vessels, containing a hematoma, and perhaps even compressing the abdominal aorta. Inflation of MAST over legs alone (not abdomen) is useful for hemostasis and splinting of lower extremities and for autotransfusion in shock and during CPR. MAST over the abdomen cause renal ischemia and, therefore, if possible, should be inflated no longer than about 1 hr. However, they should not be removed until fluid resuscitation has started and the team is ready for resuscitative laparotomy. Inflation of MAST, which pushes the diaphragm upward, requires increased FIO_2 and, in the unconscious patient, intratracheal controlled ventilation. Abdominal binding during external CPR enhances the likelihood of liver rupture (Bircher et al., 1980; Alifimoff et al., 1980). For release of the MAST, which should be gradual (abdominal garment first, leg garments last), one must also be prepared with vasopressor and IV sodium bicarbonate to treat the washout of acids.

In cases of intra-abdominal arterial hemorrhage, fist pressure on the aorta may also be life saving. Exsanguinating intra-abdominal hemorrhage, as from ruptured aneurysm, has been controlled effectively by using MAST first, and removing the MAST suit only after thoracotomy and clamping of the thoracic descending aorta (R. Stewart, personal communication).

In severe intrathoracic hemorrhage, when shock continues in spite of drainage of the hemothorax and seemingly adequate blood replacement, thoracotomy should be performed immediately. Suspected intracranial hemorrhage calls for cerebral resuscitation measures, computerized axial tomography (CAT) scan or cerebral arteriography, and immediate craniotomy.

FLUID RESUSCITATION

The objective of fluid resuscitation in hypovolemic shock is the immediate restoration of normal circulatory blood volume with adequate oxygen-carrying capacity (Table 29.2). (Blalock, 1940; Carey et al., 1971; Wiggers, 1940; Hardaway et al., 1967; Dillon et al., 1966; and Weil and Shubin, 1967). Realistic animal models of hemorrhagic shock (Bar-Joseph et al., 1981) and normovolemic hemodilution without shock (Takaori and Safar, 1967b) are needed for controlled comparison of different resuscitation fluids and protocols.

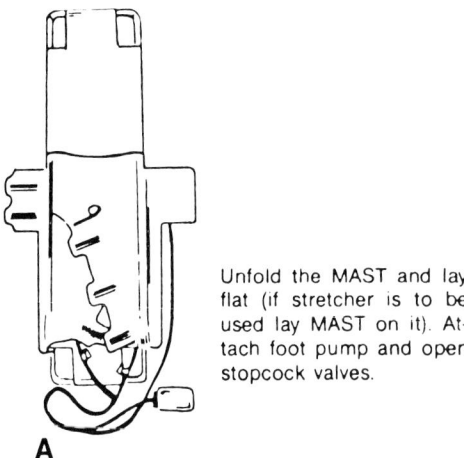
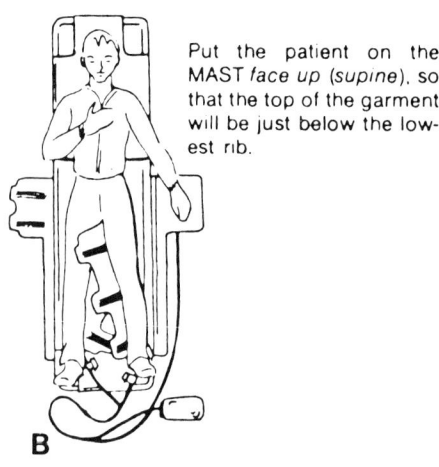
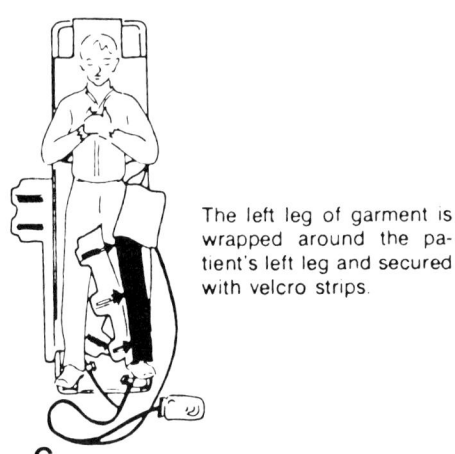
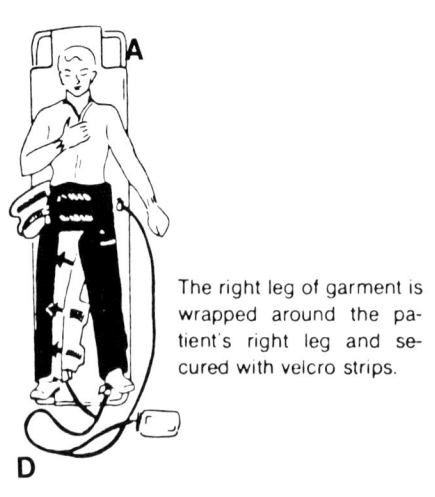
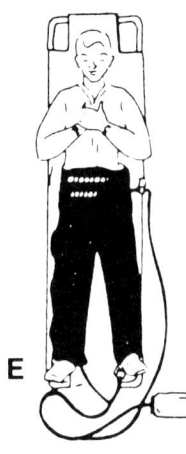

Figure 29.5. Military (medical) antishock trousers, for controlling internal hemorrhage below the diaphragm, for immobilizing fractures, and for autotransfusion in oligemic shock. For application, see text. (Reprinted with permission from N. Caroline: *Emergency Care in the Street.* Little, Brown, Boston, 1980.)

Infusion Strategies

During massive blood loss priority should be given to rapid, titrated venous infusion. Arterial pressure, urine flow, and CVP are reliable clinical parameters of volume replacement, which should be carefully monitored. Heart rate is a less reliable indicator of adequacy of circulating blood volume. EKG and blood gases should be monitored when feasible. Pulmonary edema from overinfusion is detected from changes in breath sounds (via esophageal stethoscope if the patient's trachea is intubated) or arterial PO_2 (with unchanged FIO_2).

Peripheral venous catheter insertion should receive first priority. This is followed as soon as feasible by insertion of a central venous catheter and a bladder catheter. Infusion via metal needles is not recommended because these are easily dislodged, particularly during CPR. The peripheral venous cannula should be a large bore catheter (14-16 gauge in the adult). It should be inserted percutaneously into the following locations in this order of preference: 1) a not injured arm; 2) a not injured foot, provided there is no abdominal or pelvic injury; 3) the external jugular vein; and 4) the femoral vein (located in the inguinal region just medial to the femoral artery). If percutaneous cannulation is not feasible, a quick venous cutdown is recommended, best at the ankle in front of the internal malleolus (saphenous vein) or at the wrist or elbow.

Central venous catheter insertion is not immediately required. It is ill advised in cardiac arrest during cardiac compressions, because it interferes with resuscitation and delays administration of fluids and drugs. Subclavian vein catheterization attempts, particularly during CPR, may result in pneumothorax.

A central venous catheter is indicated, when time permits, to obtain CVP monitoring and an additional route for fluid administration. Insertion of a long central venous catheter (catheter-inside-needle) from the cubita is usually easy; however, when the arm veins are collapsed, the subclavian vein is often chosen. Both routes require check of catheter position by x-ray, since the catheter can pass into the opposite arm or the jugular vein. Superior vena cava catheterization via the *right internal jugular vein* does not require x-ray control, is reliable, and is less likely to produce pneumothorax than subclavian vein catheterization. External jugular vein catheterization is an acceptable compromise. During CVP line insertion, precautions must be taken against air embolization. Manometers or transducers must be zeroed at the level of the right atrium (midaxillary line). During resuscitation, relative changes of CVP (read with airway pressure equal to atmospheric) are more important than absolute values.

Pulmonary artery catheterization is not needed in previously healthy young patients with acute hemorrhagic shock. In these patients, monitoring of right heart filling pressure by CVP line is sufficient. Monitoring of left heart filling pressure (left atrial pressure), as reflected by pulmonary artery wedge pressure or pulmonary artery diastolic pressure, can sometimes be helpful in guiding fluid therapy in patients with protracted treatment-resistant oligemic shock, pre-existing heart disease, or severe lung disease.

Systemic artery catheterization is not essential in acute hemorrhagic shock with mild or moderate hypotension and a rapid response to fluid therapy. Arterial catheterization (radial artery for less than about 24 hr, femoral artery for long-term use), however, is indicated for the same reasons as pulmonary artery catheterization and also in severe shock states with loss of consciousness in order to permit continuous monitoring of arterial pressure and repeated sampling for blood gas and pH determinations. Use of the arterial catheter for pressure infusion of blood or plasma substitutes is controversial.

Infusion techniques for restoration of blood volume must permit administration of large amounts of fluid rapidly. Doubling the height of the infusion bottle doubles the flow rate, but doubling the internal diameter of the catheter increases the flow rate 16 times (Poiseuille's law). Equipment to allow infusion of blood and plasma substitutes under pressure must be available. Unfortunately, most presently available pressure infusion devices are impractical, particularly for massive infusion of red blood cell concentrates, which require dilution with isotonic saline immediately before or during infusion.

In massive blood loss, plasma or plasma substitutes, as well as blood, should be given rapidly by titrated infusion, to restore blood volume, maintain perfusion pressure, and assure a hematocrit of about 25-35%. However, care must be taken to avoid fluid overload resulting in acute pulmonary edema. Therefore, infusion rates should be guided by recovery of arterial pressure, urine flow, and CVP. The latter is a measure of the adequacy of right heart filling and function.

Amount and rate of fluid administration depend on the amount and rate of blood loss and the type of fluid selected. Circulating blood volume normally accounts for 7.5% of body weight in men, 6.5% in women, and 8.5% in the newborn. Normal circulating plasma volume is 4.5% of body weight and red blood cell volume 3%. For rapid estimation of loss and replacement, estimating "normal" blood volume as 10% and plasma volume as 5% of body weight is acceptable.

When blood loss is 10% of total blood volume or less, usually no therapy is required. An acute 20% volume loss produces postural hypotension, vasoconstriction and other signs of hypovolemia; previously healthy persons can recover from it without intravenous fluids, but they should be treated with electrolyte solution intravenously to speed recovery. When 20-50% of blood volume is lost rapidly, shock develops that requires intravenous fluid therapy including a colloid. Loss of 50% blood volume or more can rapidly result in cardiac arrest.

When choosing salt solutions, one must appreciate that intracellular fluid (ICF) and extracellular fluid (ECF) volumes are in equilibrium. Total body water constitutes 70% of lean body mass or 60% (40-68) of total body weight in men and 50% (30-53) in women. ECF volume is 20-25% of body weight; it encompasses the intravascular space (one-fifth) and the interstitial space (four-fifths).

The type of fluid to be given is the source of much controversy. Ideally it seems that lost blood should be replaced by equal volumes of type-specific cross matched fresh blood. However, in most set-ups, this is not immediately available. In severe acute blood loss, blood or colloid plasma substitutes should be given to replace approximately the amount lost. If salt solutions are used, they should be given in volumes up to four times the blood volume lost (ECF space) with additional replacement for urine losses. There is strong evidence that the type of fluid chosen and the replacement of lost hemoglobin are less critical than the immediate restoration of blood volume. The goal is prevention of shock with concurrent treatment of blood loss. This is usually only possible inside the hospital; it results in normovolemic hemodilution if plasma substitutes are used.

Deliberate hemodilution should be considered more widely (Takaori and Safar, 1967b; Messmer, 1976). One reason is that banked blood has certain undesirable characteristics (see below). In addition, the necessary typing and cross matching require 15–45 min, during which time plasma substitutes can be given.

Normally, plasma contributes only minimally to the transport of oxygen (0.3 ml of oxygen per 100 torr PO_2 in 100 ml of blood). Raising FIO_2 to 100%, and thus arterial PO_2 to 600 torr, may be critical in severe hemodilution, because it would add 1.5 ml of oxygen per 100 ml of blood, which can amount to a sizable proportion of total arterial O_2 content in severe anemia. After hemodilution to hematocrit 20–25%, the red blood cell mass is spontaneously partially restored within a few days and fully restored within 1–2 weeks.

Moderate hemodilution actually seems to be desirable, since it results in decreased blood viscosity, which is beneficial in the reperfusion of areas with stasis and blood sludging (Messmer, 1976; Replogle et al., 1965; Dawidson et al., 1979; Knisel et al., 1945) and even in the treatment of cerebral edema (Jurkiewicz, 1977). Furthermore, decreased viscosity results in increased cardiac output and improved tissue blood flow, as evident in improved tissue PO_2 (Messmer, 1976) and cerebral venous PO_2 (Brinkmeyer et al., 1980). This in the young previously fit person can compensate for the reduced O_2 content and maintain adequate O_2 transport to a hematocrit of at least 20%. However, patients with hypovolemia or cardiopulmonary disease may decompensate at hematocrit values above 20% because of inability to increase cardiac output or because of reduced arterial PO_2. The limits of hemodilution can be ascertained in each individual patient from a decrease in mixed venous PO_2 (indicating that arterial oxygen transport no more satisfies oxygen needs) and/or from an increase in blood lactate (reflected in base deficit).

Takaori and Safar (1967a and b, 1976) and Takaori et al. (1970) studied normovolemic hemodilution with colloid plasma substitutes in normal lightly anesthetized dogs. They demonstrated specific responses to progressive levels of hemodilution: 1) complete compensation of arterial oxygen transport through increase in cardiac output and increased oxygen extraction until hemoglobin values reached about 6 g/100 ml (hematocrit 20%); 2) partial compensation at hemoglobin levels of 6–4 g/100 ml (hematocrit 20–15%); 3) reversible decompensation with metabolic acidemia but survival, with hemoglobin of 4–3 g/100 ml (hematocrit 15–10%); 4) irreversible decompensation, resulting in late deaths, when hemoglobin dropped below approximately 3 g/100 ml (hematocrit 10%); 5) early cardiac arrest, when hemoglobin dropped to 1.5–2 g/100 ml (hematocrit 5–10%), when arterial oxygen content was 2–3 ml/100 ml. Oxygen breathing increased slightly the tolerance of lethal normovolemic hemodilution.

When bleeding has been stopped and the patient remains in shock, after "assumed" restoration of blood volume, intermittent fluid challenges with electrolyte or colloid solution in increments of 200 ml/70 kg are appropriate (Weil and Shubin, 1967, 1969). If after a transient rise, CVP (or pulmonary artery wedge pressure, PAWP) returns to prechallenge levels, the fluid challenge is repeated, until CVP (or PAWP) remains 3–5 torr above the prechallenge value. Signs of overinfusion, which include CVP or PAWP rise to values of 20 torr or above, call for blood volume to be withdrawn or for improving cardiac contractility (e.g., by low dose dopamine) and reducing body water with a diuretic (e.g., furosemide).

Parenteral Plasma Substitutes

The distribution of various intravenous fluids is the key to understanding what type and how much of a given plasma substitute should be used. Five percent dextrose in water distributes throughout total body water (60% body wt) so that only $\frac{1}{12}$ remains in plasma volume. Isotonic salt solutions distribute throughout extracellular fluid (20–25% body wt) so that only one-fourth remains in plasma volume. Colloid plasma substitutes remain for hours to days entirely in the intravascular space, provided there is no gross capillary leak.

Dextrose in water is contraindicated in the initial treatment of shock (Carey et al., 1971). The dextrose is metabolized and the large quantities of water may produce water intoxication, including cerebral edema. The calories delivered are minimal (1 liter of dextrose 5% delivers only 200 calories) and not needed since these patients are hyperglycemic. However, the use of hypertonic glucose in the treatment of protracted shock states, when intracellular water is increased, has not been studied in oligemia but has been found useful in septic shock (Hinshaw et al., 1974).

Electrolyte solutions, such as isotonic (0.9%) sodium chloride and lactated Ringer's solution, are widely used as plasma volume expanders (Moyer, 1954; Dillon et al., 1966; Shires et al., 1961; Carey et al., 1971). Intravascular volume can be maintained with these solutions only by first overfilling the interstitial space. This requires up to four times the volume of blood lost. The previously recommended two to three time replacement formula (Moyer, 1954; Moyer et al., 1965) proved inadequate (Takaori and Safar, 1967a and b).

In mild hemorrhage, not exceeding 20% of blood

Table 29.2
Fluid Resuscitation in Hemorrhagic-Traumatic Shock

Agent	Advantages	Disadvantages
Crystalloids—adequate for early transient replacement of moderate plasma volume loss		
Dextrose/water	In renal failure	Hypo-osmolality, edema
5–10% dextrose/0.25–0.5% NaCl	Recommended for hydration	Too hypotonic for plasma replacement
0.9% NaCl	Inexpensive, isotonic	Lost into interstitial space (edema) and urine; needs three to five times volume lost; enhances tissue acidosis
5–10% dextrose[a]/lactated Ringer's (acid)	Inexpensive, composition like ECF	
5–10% dextrose[a]/buffered Ringer's (pH 7.4)	Theoretically ideal	
Colloids—needed for sustained replacement of severe plasma volume loss; remain intravascular		
Albumin, 5%/0.9% NaCl	Physiologic	High cost
Dextran 40, 10%/0.9% NaCl	Reduces sedimentation, aggregation, inexpensive, long shelf life	Reduces clotting,[b] plugs renal tubules in shock and oligemia
Dextran 70, 10%/0.9% NaCl	Inexpensive, long shelf life	Reduces clotting[b]
Hydroxyethyl starch 10%/0.9% NaCL	Inexpensive, long shelf life	Reduces clotting[b]
Pooled human plasma	Physiologic	Hepatitis risk
Fresh frozen single donor human plasma	Clotting factors preserved	High cost, requires cross match
Oxygen Carriers—needed when with IV plasma substitute alone Hct < 30		
Whole blood, CPD stored	Apparently physiologic	High cost, low availability, requires type-cross matching, hepatitis risk, hemolytic reaction risk, cold, acid, high K, low Ca, low platelets
Packed red blood cells, CPD stored	Permits component therapy, more economic than whole blood	Same as whole blood, poor flow (viscous), needs dilution
Fresh blood	Most physiologic; normal pH, electrolytes	As stored blood, except clotting factors normal,
Fluorocarbons	Long shelf life, none of the disadvantages of blood, no cross match	Unphysiologic, storage and elimination unclear, still experimental, needs O_2 breathing
Stroma-free hemoglobin	No crossmatch	Rapidly eliminated, metabolized, vasoactive, possible renal toxicity

[a] Dextrose IV rarely needed in acute shock; should be gauged according to blood sugar in protracted shock (keep BS 100–300 mg/100 ml.

[b] Clotting reduced in excess of degree of hemodilution. All colloids except fresh blood and fresh plasma reduce clotting by dilution of platelets and clotting factors. Hypocoagulability can be advantageous in protracted shock without active bleeding.

volume, salt solution alone is adequate to maintain blood volume and homeostasis. In moderate to severe hemorrhage, however, use of salt solution alone is unphysiologic. Even if continued loss through urine and into tissues and the peritoneal and pleural spaces is also replaced, blood volume and tissue perfusion cannot be maintained (Rush and Eiseman, 1967; Takaori, and Safar, 1967a and b; Brinkmeyer et al., 1980; Shoemaker, 1976).

Shires (1979) and Shires et al. (1961) demonstrated that following trauma or hemorrhagic shock a "third space" loss of extravascular fluid occurs. One can suspect loss into ischemic cells and injured tissue. The need for replenishing interstitial fluid has not been demonstrated. In hypovolemic shock, *small volumes* of Ringer's solution (in addition to colloid) seem indicated to restore interstitial tissue pressure and aid venous return (Guyton, 1981; Takaori and Safar, 1967a, 1976). Shires recommended that lactated Ringer's solution be given *in addition* to blood, as survival rates in laboratory animal models of shock were increased when electrolyte solution was added to blood. He did not recommend that moderate to severe blood loss be replaced by Ringer's solution *only*.

Ideally, salt replacement solutions should resemble extracellular fluid, which has a pH of 7.4, and electrolyte concentrations in mEq/liter of 138 for sodium, 5 for potassium, 108 for chloride, 27 for total base, and 5 for calcium. Normal saline solution has more sodium and chloride and none of the other electrolytes of extracellular fluid and has a pH of 6.0. Lactated Ringer's solution has a pH of 6.5 and electrolyte concentrations resembling those of extracellular fluid. The lactate, however, is inadequate to neutralize fixed acids in shock. Normosol resembles Ringer's solution (except that it lacks calcium) and has its pH buffered to 7.4. There is no evidence, however, that these differences matter in the replacement of mild to moderate blood loss (Weil and Shubin, 1967; Carey et al., 1971).

Colloid plasma substitutes leak through capillary walls very slowly. Intravascular retention is essential for plasma substitution and volume expansion without causing tissue edema.

The normal plasma colloid osmotic pressure (COP), which opposes capillary hydrostatic pressure and interstitial COP, is about 25 torr; it is primarily determined by the serum albumin concentration (normal value 5 g/

dl). A reduction of serum albumin concentration to one-half of normal reduces COP to one-third. This is the level at which tissue edema develops. COP-PAWP levels below 4 torr seem to enhance the development of pulmonary edema. Thus, albumin would seem to be the ideal colloid plasma substitute. However, serum albumin levels are fairly rapidly restored from the total body albumin pool of about 5 g/kg body wt (one-half of this is extravascular). In addition to this albumin refill, resynthesis of albumin occurs within days (Rothschild et al., 1972).

Normal dogs survive acute normovolemic hemodilution with dextran or starch solutions to hematocrit of 10%, but they cannot survive hemodilution with lactated Ringer's solution in two times the volume lost, even to a hematocrit of only 20% (Takaori and Safar, 1967a and b). Acute normovolemic hemodilution with lactated Ringer's solution to 10% hematocrit was possible without causing pulmonary edema (Lowenstein et al., 1968), even when hematocrit was maintained at 10% for 4 hr (Brinkmeyer et al., 1980). This required Ringer's solution infused in seven times the blood volume lost; however, without hypotension, anuria developed (probably triggered by severe acidosis from tissue edema) and was followed by cardiac arrest. Tolerance of severe hemodilution with Ringer's solution was somewhat increased by normalizing arterial pH with sodium bicarbonate, but survival was not improved unless the serum albumin level was increased to at least 2 g/100 ml by intravenous albumin. Lymphatic drainage of the lungs, controlled ventilation, and 100% oxygen may have been responsible for the absence of pulmonary edema. However, Ringer's solution became sequestered in interstitial spaces throughout the body and in the peritoneal cavity (Brinkmeyer et al., 1980). This iatrogenic tissue edema cannot be harmless (Eufinger, 1964; Frey et al., 1974; Horatz and Frey, 1964; Gelin et al., 1961; Brinkmeyer et al., 1980; Dawidson et al., 1979). If severe blood loss is treated with a one time administration of lactated Ringer's solution in two to three times the blood volume lost, blood volume and cardiac output decline toward cardiac arrest within 2–3 hr (Takaori and Safar, 1967a). Normovolemic hemodilution to 10% hematocrit with albumin in dogs does not alter cerebral variables, while the same degree of hemodilution with lactated Ringer's solution results in increased ICP and CSF lactacidosis (Brinkmeyer et al., 1980).

Since in trauma and shock there are increased antidiuretic hormone secretion (augmenting water retention) and increased glucocorticoid and aldosterone (augmenting salt retention), dextrose in water should not be used. Isotonic salt solution should be used only to replace slight to moderate blood loss. Maintenance hydration should include some solute (0.25–0.5% sodium chloride). Maintaining diuresis above 1 ml/kg/hr seems to decrease renal failure after trauma. This can best be accomplished by conservative amounts of salt solutions plus, if necessary, mannitol or furosemide (Powers, 1965).

Differences in price and in physiologic characteristics, such as intravascular persistence (clearance), permanent tissue storage, renal function, microcirculatory changes (viscosity, cell aggregation), clotting changes, and allergenic properties should influence the clinician in his selection of colloid plasma substitutes (Thompson, 1975). Most of these characteristics have not been compared in rigidly controlled experiments.

The most widely used colloid plasma substitute in the United States is human *albumin*. Europe and other parts of the world preferentially use artificial colloid substitutes, such as dextrans and hydroxyethyl starch (HES). All of these support survival equally well and far better than salt solutions.

Dextran 70 (6% in isotonic saline), for example, has an intravascular retention of 30% after 24 hr (Metcalf, et al., 1962). The organism's mobilization of interstitial fluid and albumin compensate thereafter, even if initial hemodilution was to 10% hematocrit (Takaori and Safar, 1967b). Retention of dextran 40 (10% in isotonic saline) is shorter than of dextran 70 but is adequate to sustain survival from 10% hematocrit with 1:1 replacement. *HES* (6% in isotonic saline) has a retention slightly greater than dextran 70 (Thompson et al., 1970; Takaori et al., 1970). The still experimental low molecular weight HES has a retention similar to dextran 40 (Thompson, 1975). Dextrans and HES are cleared by the kidneys, after brief storage in kidney and liver cells and phagocytes, without apparent toxicity (Thompson, et al., 1970; Thompson, 1975). They are eventually metabolized. When used for experimental hemodilution to 10% hematocrit in 1:1 exchange, they attract fluid into the circulation and increase total blood volume to 130–150% of control (Takaori et al., 1970). The return of plasma protein concentrations to normal was not influenced by dextrans and HES (Takaori and Safar, 1967b; Rothschild et al., 1972; Lewis et al., 1966). The persistence of plasma substitutes in the circulation depends upon molecular size, resistance to enzymatic action, quantity administered, and presence or absence of hemorrhage.

The kidneys are not affected by synthetic substitutes, except that during hypotension, dextran 40, due to its renal excretion, increases urine viscosity and may cause renal failure (Matheson and Diomi, 1970). Therefore, it should be used after urine flow has been started with other plasma substitutes. Oliguria during use of dextran 40 should be treated by mannitol or furosemide.

All plasma substitutes improve the microcirculation; they reduce viscosity by reducing red cell and fibrinogen concentrations (Meiselman et al., 1967; Gregersen et al., 1963). Dextran 40 might have an additional beneficial effect on the microcirculation, as it slows sedimentation rate (Thompson, 1966; Lewis et al., 1966: Replogle et al., 1965; Litwin, 1972; Gelin et al., 1961). Dextran 70 with constant hematocrit increases shear stress (Meiselman et al., 1967; Replogle et al., 1965; Collins and Ludbrook, 1966) and increases sedimentation rate (Thompson, 1966). HES has not been adequately studied in this regard.

All plasma substitutes produce hypocoagulability through dilution of clotting factors. Hypocoagulability is undesirable before control of hemorrhage but may be desirable in protracted shock states. Dextran 40, in addition, reduces platelet adhesiveness and aggregation (Lewis et al., 1966). Dextran 40 and dextran 70 result in increased bleeding times (Lewis et al., 1966; Thompson and Gladsden, 1965; Gollub et al., 1967). The ability of dextrans (Sawyer and Moncrief, 1965) and HES (Arrants et al., 1969) to inhibit thrombus formation in thromboembolic disease is still controversial, but dextran 70 seems superior to the others (Litwin, 1972; Gelin et al., 1961). Preliminary studies suggest that bleeding tendency is the same or less with HES (Karlson et al., 1967; Takaori and Safar, 1967b; Thompson, 1975).

Allergenic reactions are rare, so they should not be considered in the choice of substitutes for life-threatening hemorrhage. However, dextrans have caused anaphylactic reactions (Michelson, 1968; Brisman et al., 1968; Thompson, 1975). No such reactions have been reported with HES so far (Maurer and Berardinelli, 1968; Brickman et al., 1966).

Plasma pooled from multiple donors (Hillman, 1964), although theoretically the ideal volume expander, should not be used because of the risk of transmitting hepatitis and other infections (Miller and Tisdall, 1945). Pasteurized plasma (5% plasma protein fraction), which contains mainly albumin and a small amount of globulins is safe, except for occasionally containing vasodilator substances (Bland et al., 1973). Purified human *albumin* 5%, either salt free or in isotonic saline, is the physiologically ideal plasma substitute (Brinkmeyer et al., 1980; Skillman, 1976; Weil and Shubin, 1967). It contains no vasodilator substances and is sterile. Even in experimental normovolemic hemodilution to 10% hematocrit it sustained cardiovascular, pulmonary, and cerebral variables near normal and was followed by long-term survival. Because of its high cost it may be prudent to use electrolyte solutions and synthetic colloids at first and albumin later to maintain a critical serum albumin level of about 2–3 g/100 ml. None of these substances interfere with typing and cross matching of blood. Dextran and starch solutions may hamper the agglutination test of blood group typing; this can be overcome by dilution and washing of cells.

Blood and Blood Components

The advantage of whole blood over plasma substitutes is that it carries 1.34 ml of oxygen per gram of hemoglobin, which results in an arterial oxygen content of about 20 ml/dl when fully saturated with O_2 (PaO_2 over 90 torr) and with a hemoglobin concentration of 15 g/dl. The following disadvantages of banked whole blood, however, make it less than the ideal fluid as the first line of therapy (Boyan and Howland, 1963; Howland and Schweizer, 1965; Bunker, 1974): high price, frequent unavailability, the need for typing and cross matching to prevent hemolytic reaction, increased hematocrit due to fluid leakage when used without additional plasma substitute, low pH, high potassium, low calcium, loss of platelets, risk of hepatitis and bacterial contamination, and the need for warming it on the way into the patient to prevent cardiac arrest from cardiac hypothermia. In addition, microfilters that reduce infusion rate should be used to avoid microembolization and pulmonary failure.

All emergency services should have type O Rh-negative blood available, as fresh as possible, for use in exsanguinating hemorrhage, where the hematocrit cannot be maintained above 20% with plasma substitutes, and where type-specific cross matched blood is not available. This "universal donor blood" is indicated, in spite of the small risk of a hemolytic transfusion reaction, while waiting for cross matched blood, when irreversible shock or cardiac arrest cannot otherwise be prevented.

Citric acid-phosphate-dextrose (CPD) anticoagulant has replaced citric acid-citrate-dextrose (ACD); this has led to banked blood with lower potassium, higher pH, and higher 2,3-diphosphoglycerate (DPG). Reduced DPG shifts the oxygen hemoglobin dissociation curve to the left and thereby reduces release of oxygen in capillaries.

Calcium administration is not needed even during massive replacement (Howland et al., 1977), since serum ionized calcium is depressed only transiently due to administration of citrate, and this does not create hemodynamic effects. The low pH of banked blood however, calls for sodium bicarbonate intravenously but only if the patient has proven metabolic acidemia. The most common cause of cardiac arrest during massive transfusions in past years has been cardiac hypothermia from cold blood, which has been eliminated by the use of blood warmers (Boyan and Howland, 1963).

Packed *red blood cell* solution, which usually has a hematocrit of about 70%, is adequate for increasing oxygen-carrying capacity, while using plasma substitute for volume. Packed cells require dilution with normal saline solution if rapid infusion is needed. The risks are the same as with whole blood, but plasma-related risks are reduced. Packed cells have largely replaced banked whole blood, except for use of fresh whole blood to treat clotting problems.

Red blood cells can be stored for years in the *frozen* state when glycerol is added as a cryoprotective agent (Valeri et al., 1967; Moss et al., 1968). However, they are of little use in the treatment of acute hemorrhage, because of the time required to thaw and wash them. Moreover, frozen blood is expensive.

Coagulation problems are rare during and after acute hemorrhagic shock. However, in protracted shock resistant to fluid resuscitation, disseminated intravascular coagulation (DIC) may be a problem, and after massive infusion of old banked blood dilutional hemorrhagic diathesis can occur. The simplest approach to these problems is use of *fresh blood*. During massive transfusions of banked blood, adding about 250 ml of *fresh frozen plasma* every time about 50% of the estimated blood volume has been replaced with old banked blood has been recommended. Platelet levels below about 50,000/mm^3 may need correction by platelet concentrates, fresh whole blood, platelet-rich packed red blood cells, or platelet-rich plasma. Low platelet count should be suspected when there is increased bleeding time or inadequate clot retraction, even with normal clotting time. Clotting time and clot retraction can be monitored during resuscitation, using the one tube method with constant temperature and predetermined tilt. The sample should clot in less than 4 min.

Oxygen Carriers (Artificial Blood)

A breakthrough in resuscitation is imminent through the clinical availability of stroma-free oxygen-carrying blood substitutes, namely the fluorocarbons (Naito and Yokoyama, 1975; Geyer et al., 1973; and Clark and Gollan, 1966; Sloviter and Kamimoto, 1967; Jamieson and Greenwalt, 1978) and stroma-free hemoglobin solutions (Ambersen et al., 1934; Rabiner et al., 1967; Jamieson and Greenwalt, 1978). These substances may carry as much oxygen as whole blood does, and increase blood volume without increasing viscosity, as plasma substitutes do. However, the oxygen carriers cannot replace coagulation, immune response, and other functions of fresh whole blood.

Animals have survived fluorocarbon breathing (Clark and Gollan, 1966) as well as complete blood replacement with *fluorocarbons* as blood substitutes (Geyer et al., 1973). They sustained arterial oxygen transport for 2–3 days at which time one-third of the circulating red cell mass had recovered spontaneously (Steinmetz and Balko, 1973). They are ready for clinical trials, particularly for use in cases of rare blood types or refusal of blood products.

Fluorocarbons carry oxygen in simple solution, namely 40 ml of oxygen/100 torr PO_2/100 ml—in vitro 2 times the normal fully saturated whole blood. The half-life of perfluoro chemicals in the circulation is 24 hr in the dog (Naito and Yokoyama, 1975). The presently available in vivo O_2 content solutions for clinical trial are Fluosol-43 and Fluosol-DA, which are emulsions made isotonic with Ringer's solution and iso-oncotic with HES.

Some of the technical and physiological obstacles to flurocarbon infusion have not been clarified. Clinicians hesitate to use them because of permanent tissue storage, particularly in liver and kidneys; they fear this might block the reticular endothelial system. Carcinogenic long-term effects cannot be ruled out at this time. The risk of anemia must be weighed against suspected but yet unproven long-term side effects.

Stroma-free hemoglobin is obtained from outdated human red blood cells. A one-time replacement of blood volume with a solution containing 6.6 g of hemoglobin/dl sustained oxygen-carrying capacity in experimental animals for about 3 hr, after which time loss of volume and oxygen-carrying capacity rapidly led to death. By continuing infusion of the hemoglobin solution, however, life could be sustained until the animals regenerated blood cells and proteins. In spite of a leftward shift of the oxygen hemoglobin dissociation curve, oxygen delivery seems adequate. In spite of rapid removal from the circulation of the infused hemoglobin, in part by leakage into tissues and in part via the urine, stroma-free hemoglobin does not irreversibly damage the kidneys.

Enteral Fluid Resuscitation

Oral fluids have a place in the treatment of mild to moderate hypovolemic shock, when IV fluid administration is not possible, as in the extrahospital treatment of mass casualties (Ahnefeld and Doelt, 1973; Doelt and Mehrkens, 1980). Oral fluids offer prophylaxis of heat stroke. For shock due to severe diarrhea (e.g., cholera) oral isotonic salt solutions have been lifesaving if given in amounts in excess of the fluid lost through diarrhea. Where IV therapy is available, oral fluid substitution is only adjunctive and contraindicated in established shock, coma, and abdominal injuries, because of malabsorption and risk of causing aspiration or peritonitis. Where the gastrointestinal tract is intact and active, oral salt solutions can be supplemented with calories, amino acids, fat, vitamins, and selected minerals. There is no evidence that the rectal administration of fluids has an advantage over the orogastric route.

Limitations of oral fluid administration include the inability to infuse colloid solutions via the gastrointestinal tract; tissue edema produced by large amounts of salt solutions; poor gastrointestinal absorption of water and salt in the shock state (splanchnic vasoconstriction, paralytic ileus); and intolerance of isotonic salt solution by mouth.

Field-tested oral replacement fluids are electrolyte-carbohydrate lemonades or orangeades. They are available as solutions or in self-prepared or commercially available powder form. Most reflect electrolyte concentrations in a ratio similar to ECF, such as Ringer's solution, with carbohydrates added and made to taste acceptable. Such powders, diluted in water to a one-half isotonic solution, are better tolerated than isotonic Ringer's solution. Chicken soup which contains ECF-like electrolyte concentrations, has also been effective in shock secondary to starvation, dehydration, or diarrhea (Caroline and Schwartz, 1975). Even in massive diarrhea, giving orally more electrolyte solution than lost can sometimes support life until "healing" occurs.

Hypodermic and intramuscular infusions of salt solutions require sterile infusion equipment that, when available, might as well be used for the more effective IV administration. Absorption of fluids from connective tissue and muscles in shock states is unpredictable.

DRUGS FOR SHOCK

The most important "drugs" in the treatment of hemorrhagic shock are plasma substitutes and blood. In acute hemorrhagic shock all drug therapy is adjunctive.

Metabolic tissue acidosis always accompanies hypovolemic shock in humans (Cannon, 1918). The resulting acidemia is transiently increased during resuscitation, due to washout of acids from tissues. Attempts to correct arterial pH in experimental or clinical hypovolemic shock have failed to consistently improve physiologic variables and survival (Carey et al., 1971). Outcome is more related to prompt restoration of perfusion by IV fluids, which in most cases promptly corrects the acidemia without need for sodium bicarbonate. Lactated Ringer's solution does not seem to be more effective than sodium chloride solution in correcting acidemia (Carey et al., 1971).

Sodium bicarbonate or THAM is indicated if arterial pH decreases below about 7.2, in spite of volume restoration and moderate hyperventilation. Severe hyperventilation in acute shock may worsen cerebral ischemia (Stone et al., 1965). Whether a severe blood base deficit (over 10 mEq/liter) with arterial pH near normal (due to compensatory hyperventilation) requires correction, is not known. If correction of base deficit is decided upon, it can usually be achieved, at least transiently, with a dose of sodium bicarbonate in milliequivalents that equals one-fourth of the body weight in kilograms (extracellular fluid volume in liters) times the base deficit in milliequivalents per liter. One-half of this dose is given first, and the other half is infused slowly according to monitored pH.

Other drug therapy may be indicated, as an act of desperation, when the shock state has become irreversible in spite of overcorrection of hypovolemia (continued lactacidemia, oliguria, hypotension, rising CVP, pulmonary failure, and loss of consciousness) (Lillehei et al., 1964). In such situations, trials with inconclusive or beneficial results have included corticosteroids (Schumer, 1976), vasodilators (Nickerson, 1963), vasoconstrictors (Loeb and Gunnar, 1976), cardiac inotropic drugs (Loeb and Gunnar, 1976), heparinization for disseminated intravascular coagulation (Hardaway, 1966; Stephenson, 1974), and hypertonic glucose intravenously, which improves myocardial function in protracted hemorrhagic shock (Stremple et al., 1976) as it does in septic shock (Hinshaw et al., 1974).

Corticosteroids may or may not have a beneficial effect on cell survival after ischemic injury in shock. They have no place in acute hemorrhagic shock. They exert, however, clearly beneficial effects on cell structure and function in the distributive-type shock of sepsis (Schumer, 1976; Trump et al., 1971), which resembles "irreversible shock" after hemorrhage and trauma. Also, cerebral ischemia, as well as pulmonary aspiration with wheezing, and ARDS might benefit from a trial of steroid therapy. Therefore, in such circumstances, one massive dose (or several pharmacologic doses, short term, for less than 2–7 days) seems justified. Such brief steroid therapy is not known to produce impaired wound healing, infection, or stress ulcers.

Vasodilators are recommended on the basis of animal experiments which show seemingly deleterious pre- and postcapillary vasoconstriction in refractory hemorrhagic shock (Nickerson, 1963). Vasodilators tried in experimental shock include α-receptor blockers such as phenoxybenzamine, phentolamine, and chlorpromazine; ganglionic blockers like trimethaphan (Arfonad); and direct vasodilators like nitroprusside or nitroglycerine. Phenoxybenzamine improves CBF in protracted oligemic shock in monkeys (Kovach and Sandor, 1976). In acute hemorrhage, venodilation can lead to cardiac arrest by further reducing cardiac output, arterial pressure, and coronary perfusion. In any shock state with cerebral ischemia, further reduction in MAP must be avoided. In irreversible hemorrhagic shock with documented increase in peripheral and pulmonary vascular resistances, a trial of vasodilator, in addition to blood volume expansion, may be justified. Occasional observers have reported dramatic improvement with vasodilators when volume replacement alone was inadequate (Hardaway et al., 1967). Vasodilation, without causing a severe decrease in diastolic perfusion pressure and without causing severe tachycardia, may also benefit the ischemic heart by reducing peripheral resistance, cardiac wall tension, and, thereby, myocardial oxygen consumption.

Vasoconstrictors (Loeb and Gunnar 1976) include the α-receptor agonists norepinephrine, phenylephrine, methoxamine, metaraminol, and dopamine in large doses, as well as the nonadrenergic drug angiotensin. Most of these drugs constrict arterioles and tend to slow the heart rate via baroreceptor reflex, particularly if MAP is raised above normal. The naturally occurring transmitter norepinephrine may be the drug of choice if used by meticulous IV titration.

The *prolonged* use of vasoconstrictors in hemorrhagic shock in lieu of blood volume restoration must be *condemned*. However, the *brief* use of a vasoconstrictor to prevent cardiac arrest in severe rapid hemorrhage may be *lifesaving* when used to support MAP while blood volume restoration is being initiated. This increase in extracerebral peripheral resistance is meant to sustain cerebral perfusion pressure, thus protecting the brain, and to sustain diastolic arterial pressure, thus maintaining coronary perfusion and preventing cardiac arrest. This can be of great importance, especially in the elderly atherosclerotic patient with cardiac disease. MAP should only be raised to normal, because excessive vasoconstriction can be arrhythmogenic and cause renal failure.

Inotropic drugs (Loeb and Gunnar, 1976), such as epinephrine, dopamine in low doses, dobutamine, and isoproterenol (the only pure β-receptor agonist) increase the force of cardiac contractions, as well as heart rate and automaticity. They may also, however, cause dysrhythmias. Isoproterenol not only stimulates the heart, but also dilates vessels in skin and muscles and, thereby, has a negative effect on vital organ perfusion. Dobutamine seems to have no advantage over dopamine. Digitalis probably has no place in the treatment of shock states in patients with initially healthy hearts. In patients with pre-existing heart disease, however, rapid digitalization in protracted hemorrhagic shock may be effective in improving the hemodynamic state. Glucagon, a naturally occurring weak cardiac stimulant, seems to improve cardiac contractility by converting ATP to cyclic AMP.

All drugs that are considered for use in hemorrhagic shock are *only adjuncts* to blood volume restoration and should be given in cautiously titrated doses either by continuous IV infusion or by small individual doses, repeated as necessary.

CEREBRAL RESUSCITATION

The therapies recommended for use after complete global brain ischemia (cardiac arrest) (Safar et al., 1976, 1978; Safar, 1978a, 1980a and b) should also be considered after incomplete global brain ischemia (shock), although the conditions are not identical (Siesjo, 1978; Safar, 1979; Kovach and Sandor, 1976). Little is known about the effects of shock states of various severity and duration on the degree and reversibility of brain damage caused by hypotension itself or by accompanying cerebral trauma (Nemoto, 1978; Kovach and Sandor, 1976). Hemorrhagic shock without head injury can cause impaired brain function, and possibly irreversible brain damage, if the patient is pulseless for at least 15 min or if MAP is 30–50 torr for prolonged periods or accompanied by hypoxemia. Such patients may benefit from intensive therapy measures recommended for comatose patients after cardiac arrest (Table 29.3) and from specific, still controversial brain resuscitation measures (Table 29.4).

During shock, severe hyperventilation is probably undesirable (Stone et al., 1965). MAP should not be permitted to drop below about 50 torr, and when hypotension causes stupor or coma, MAP should be raised promptly. If *after* shock, without cerebral trauma, there is depressed consciousness, slight hypertension (by blood volume expansion and vasopressor) may benefit cerebral recovery (Safar et al., 1976; Hossmann and Kleihues, 1973; Ames et al., 1968). However, after cerebral trauma (Bruce et al., 1978), when the blood-brain barrier is grossly damaged, MAP should be maintained at or slightly below normal (e.g., 80–90 torr), because hypertension can provoke vasogenic edema and hemorrhage. After restoration of normotension, the postischemic brain may benefit from mild controlled hyperventilation. Arterial PO_2 should be kept above 100 torr with FIO_2 50–100%. PEEP should be kept at a minimum. Increase in mean intrathoracic pressure can reduce cardiac output further during shock and can increase ICP after shock. General life support, to benefit the brain, should include control of blood variables, temperature, IV fluids, serum electrolytes, blood glucose, alimentation, and drugs (Table 29.3) (Safar, 1979, 1980).

The brain injured by anoxia or trauma may suffer further damage from noxious afferent stimuli and reflexes (Siesjo, 1978). Therefore partial neuromuscular blockade (e.g., pancuronium) (Safar, 1978) and "therapeutic anesthesia" (Laborit and Huguenard, 1954) should be considered throughout postischemic coma, as for example with conventional doses of barbiturates (Safar, 1980b).

In the absence of head injury, ICP monitoring is probably not necessary in stupor or coma following oligemic shock. ICP, however, does transiently increase with fluid resuscitation (Simeone and Witoszka, 1970).

Barbiturates given before cardiac arrest (Goldstein et al., 1966) or shock (Seeley et al., 1936) for protection seem to improve cerebral and overall recovery. Also, conventional and large doses of thiopental or pentobarbital given after focal ischemia (Hoff, 1978), as well as large doses of thiopental given after complete global ischemia (Bleyaert et al., 1978), have been shown to have a brain damage-ameliorating effect. The latter is presently under controlled clinical investigation for cardiac arrest cases (Safar, 1980b; Breivik et al., 1978; Detre et al., 1981). Barbiturates may help the injured brain by reducing its metabolism (Michenfelder and Theye, 1970), improving intracerebral differential perfusion (Feustel et al., 1981), reducing ICP (Shapiro, 1975), preventing convulsions, and possibly stabilizing membranes (Smith et al., 1980).

During hypovolemia, IV barbiturates should not be used at all or only with extreme caution and intensive monitoring, since in such patients they produce profound cardiovascular depression and possibly cardiac arrest (Breivik et al., 1978; Lundy and Adams, 1942). After restoration of normovolemia, however, the person without ischemic heart disease tolerates even large doses of barbiturates well (Papper and Bradley, 1942; Breivik et al., 1978). Large dose barbiturate loading following cerebral ischemia is not recommended at this time for routine clinical use. Conventional doses of thiopental or pentobarbital (1–5 mg/kg intravenously, repeated as needed, with blood levels of 2–4 mg/100 ml) may be justified in coma after brain ischemia for prevention of convulsions, stabilization of the patient on the ventilator, blocking of noxious afferent impulses, and ICP normalization.

Therapeutic *hypothermia* of a few hours' duration, which clearly protects against anoxia (Bigelow et al., 1950) and slows ATP depletion in ischemia (Michenfelder and Theye, 1970), has been shown to ameliorate the results of focal ischemia and brain contusion, even when given early after the insult (Rosomoff et al., 1960). It has not yet been reliably tested after global ischemia. Hypothermia is arrhythmogenic and difficult to manage safely. Prolonged hypothermia can have deleterious effects on the brain, because it increases blood viscosity and depresses cardiovascular function and CBF (Steen, 1979b). Short-term hypothermia deserves investigation as a therapeutic potential.

There are many drugs and physiologic measures that have *brain resuscitation potential*, including anesthetics that depress brain metabolism without increasing CBF and intracranial blood volume and, thereby, ICP (as volatile anesthetics do); anticonvulsants; free radical scavengers; osmotherapy; normalization of cerebral pH; hemodilution; and others. Physicians treating oligemic shock should keep abreast of developments in brain resuscitation for any type of acute cerebral insult, because some of these measures have relevance for the encephalopathy following the incomplete global cerebral ischemia of severe shock (Table 29.4) (Safar, 1978, 1979, 1980b; Kovach and Sandor, 1976).

CONCLUDING COMMENTS

In hemorrhagic shock, immediate correction of hypovolemia-induced hypoperfusion by immediate restoration of circulating blood volume is more important than

Table 29.3
Standard Measures of Life and Brain Support

Guidelines for coma following global ischemia-anoxia (cardiac arrest, severe shock)

Rule Out Intracranial Mass Lesion (history, clinical, angiography, CAT scan)

1. Control mean arterial pressure (MAP); normalize blood volume; expand plasma volume (e.g., 10 ml/kg); vasopressor/vasodilator
   a. Brief mild hypertension (MAP 110–130 torr) for 1–5 min immediately after restoration of circulation (optional)
   b. *Maintain normotension* or slight hypertension throughout coma; (MAP 90–110 torr) (brain trauma MAP 60–90 torr); vascular catheters—CVP, arterial, pulmonary artery (optional)
2. Immobilization—controlled ventilation; softening doses of relaxant (e.g., pancuronium)
3. Anesthesia IV for deafferentation, prevention/control of seizures—e.g., thiopental or pentobarbital 2–5 mg/kg + 1–2 mg/kg/1–2 hr IV; maximum 30 mg/kg (blood level 2–4 mg/dl); or diphenylhydantoin 7 mg/kg IV repeat prn
4. Arterial PCO_2 25–35 torr, controlled ventilation
5. Arterial pH 7.3–7.6
6. Arterial PO_2 over 100 torr, with FIO_2 50% and minimal PEEP
7. Steroid (optional)—methylprednisolone 5 mg/kg followed by 1 mg/kg 6 hr; or dexamethasone 1 mg/kg followed by 0.2 mg/kg/6 hr; short term (1–4 days)
8. Blood variables
   Hematocrit 30–40%; electrolytes normal
   Plasma colloid osmotic pressure over 15 torr (albumin over 3 g/100 ml)
   Serum osmolality 280–330 mOsm/l
   Glucose 100–300 mg/100 ml
9. Fluids—alimentation
   No dextrose in water
   Use dextrose 5–10% in 0.25–0.5% NaCl. IV; 30–50 ml/kg/24 hr (100 ml/kg/24 hr in infants) + potassium
   Calories (2,000–4,000 cal/24 hr/70 kg); amino acids, vitamins
10. Maintain normothermia or mild hypothermia (short-term hypothermia optional; long-term hypothermia contraindicated)
11. Monitor intracranial pressure (only if safe technique established; optional after CPR; recommended after head injury; hollow skull screw (Vries) or ventricular catheter (Lundberg)
12. Control ICP (≤ 15 torr)
    a. Further hyperventilation ($PaCO_2$ 20 torr)
    b. CSF drainage (if ICP catheter)
    c. Mannitol 0.5g/kg; plus 0.3g/kg/hr short term
    d. Diuretic (e.g., furosemide)
    e. Thiopental or pentobarbital 2–5 mg/kg IV, repeat as needed (see 3)
    f. Hypothermia, 30–32°C, short term (relaxant, anesthesia, vasodilation)
13. Evaluate insult, coma score, outcome

Table 29.4
Summary of Present Knowledge of Measures in Brain Resuscitation[a,b]

Treatment	Acute ICP Rise		Cardiac Arrest		Brain Infarct		Trauma, Edema		Toxic-Metabolic, Inflammatory	
	Animal	Man	Animal	Man	Animal	Man	Animal	Man	Animal	Man
Moderate hypertension	?	?	(+)	?	(+)	(+)	−	−	?	?
Severe hypertension	−	−	−	?	?	?	−	−	?	−
Hemodilution (IV)	?	?	0	?	+	(+)	(+)	?	?	?
Heparinization	?	?	0	?	−	−	−	−	?	?
Barbiturate—high dose	+	+	(+)	*	+	?	+	?	?	(+)
Barbiturate—conventional dose	+	+	?	?	+	?	?	?	?	(+)
Immobilization-hypervent.	+	+	(+)	?	+	?	(+)	+	?	?
Osmotherapy	+	+	?	?	(+)	?	+	+	?	(+)
Hypothermia	+	+	?	(+)	+	?	+	(+)	?	(+)

[a] From P. Safar, 1980b.
[b] ?, not known; 0, no effect shown; −, may increase brain damage; (+), possibly reduces brain damage; +, reduces brain damage; *ICP*, intracranial pressure; *, randomized study in progress (1973–1983), University of Pittsburgh.

the type of fluid used. When more than about 20% of estimated blood volume is lost, colloid is needed. Prevention or immediate correction of hypoperfusion seems to reduce the likelihood of complications to develop secondarily, such as intravascular coagulation, fat embolism, renal failure, ARDS, "irreversible shock" that is resistant to fluid therapy, and cerebral failure.

Phases and steps of cardiopulmonary-cerebral resuscitation (CPCR), slightly modified for trauma cases, are a useful guideline also for the management of hemorrhagic shock. Cardiac arrest due to exsanguinating hemorrhage requires an all out resuscitative effort, because it has a good prognosis. In hemorrhage without cardiac arrest, drugs have only adjunctive value. Blood substitutes should be selected on the basis of physiologic and economic considerations. For prolonged fluid resuscitation in severe blood loss, colloids are superior to electrolyte solutions, and mild hemodilution is desirable.

Resuscitative care should start with bystanders at the scene and continue during transportation to the most appropriate hospital, where a team coordinated by a physician experienced in the management of shock and trauma should use common sense, speed, and well monitored titrated support of all vital organ systems.

Acknowledgments. This review is based in part on the author's previous publications including: Safar, P: Chapters 2, 3, 9, and 10, in *Principles and Practice of Emergency Medicine*, edited by G. Schwartz et al., W. B. Saunders, Philadelphia, 1978; and Safar, P: *Cardiopulmonary-Cerebral Resuscitation*, World Federation of Societies of Anesthesiologists, A. Laerdal, Stavanger, Norway, 1981. The author's research on this subject was supported in part by The Surgeon General of the United States Army, The National Institutes of Health, The Pennsylvania State Department of Health, the Asmund Laerdal Company, and Travenol Laboratories. Norman Abramson, M.D., Carmela Falchetti, and Tancy Crawford helped in the preparation of this manuscript.

References

Ahnefeld, F.W., and Doelt, R.: Water and electrolyte solutions for primary substitution. In *Clinical Anesthesiology and Intensive Therapy*, vol. I, p. 202. J. F. Lehmanns, Munich, 1973.

Alifimoff, J.K., Safar, P., Bircher, N., Stezoski, W., and Barbati, R.: Cardiac resuscitability after closed-chest, MAST-augmented, and open-chest cardiopulmonary resuscitation (CPR); Cerebral recovery after prolonged closed-chest, MAST-augmented and open-chest cardiopulmonary resuscitation (CPR). Anesthesiology 53/3:S147 and S151, 1980.

Ambersen, W.R., Flecksner, J., Steggerda, F.R., Mulder, A.G., Tendler, M.J., Pankratz, D.S., and Laug, E.P.: On use of Ringer-Locke solutions containing hemoglobin as substitute for normal blood in mammals. J. Cell Compar. Physiol. 5: 359, 1934.

American Society of Anesthesiologists, Committee on Acute Medicine (P. Safar, Chairman): Community-wide emergency medical services: Recommendations. J.A.M.A. 204: 595, 1968.

Ames, A., III, Wright, R.L., Kowada, M., Thurston, J.M., and Majno, G.: Cerebral ischemia. II. The no-reflow phenomenon. Am. J. Pathol. 52:437, 1968.

Arrants, J.E., Cooper, N., and Lee, W.H.: The effects of a new plasma expander (hydroxyethyl starch) on intravascular clot formation. Am. Surg. 35:465, 1969.

Bar-Joseph, G., Safar, P., and Stezoski, W.: Irreversible hemorrhagic shock model in monkeys. *Disaster and Medicine*, vol. 4. Springer-Verlag, New York, in press, 1981.

Beck, C.F., and Leighninger, D.S.: Death after a clean bill of health. J.A.M.A. 174:133, 1960.

Beck, C.F., Pritchard, H., and Feil, S.H.: Ventricular fibrillation of long duration abolished by electric shock. J.A.M.A. 135:1985, 1947.

Bernard, C.: *An Introduction to the Study of Experimental Medicine*. Schuman, New York, 1949.

Bigelow, W.G., Lindsay, W.K., Harrison, R.C., et al.: Oxygen transport and utilization in dogs at low body temperatures. Am. J. Physiol. 160:125, 1950.

Bing, O.H.L., Brooks, W.W., and Messer, J.V.: Heart muscle viability following hypoxia: Protective effect of acidosis. Science 180:1297, 1973.

Bircher, N., Safar, P., and Stewart, R.: A comparison of standard, "MAST"-augmented, and open-chest CPR in dogs: A preliminary investigation. Crit. Care Med. 8:147, 1980.

Bircher, N., and Safar, P.: Comparison of standard and "new" closed-chest CPR and open-chest CPR in dogs. Crit. Care Med. 9:384, 1981.

Blalock, A.: *Principles of Surgical Care, Shock and Other Problems*. C. V. Mosby, St. Louis, MO, 1940.

Blalock, A., Beard, J.W., and Thuss, C.: Intravenous injections: A study of the effects on the composition of the blood of the injections of various fluids into dogs with normal and low blood pressure. J. Clin. Invest. 11:267, 1932.

Bland, J.H.L., Laver, M.B., and Lowenstein, E.: Vasodilator effect of commercial 5% plasma protein fraction solutions. J.A.M.A. 224:1721, 1973.

Bleyaert, A.L., Nemoto, E.M., Safar, P., Stezoski, S.W., Mickell, J.J., Moossy, J., and Rao, G.R.: Thiopental amelioration of brain damage after global ischemia in monkeys. Anesthesiology 49:390, 1978.

Boehm, R.: Über Wiederbelebung nach Vergiftungen und Asphyxie. Arch. Exp. Pathol. Pharmakol. 8:68, 1878.

Boyan, C.P., and Howland, W.S.: Cardiac arrest and temperature of banked blood. J.A.M.A. 183:144, 1963.

Brecher, G.A.: *Venous Return*. Grune & Stratton, New York, 1956.

Breivik, H., Safar, P., Sands, P., Fabritius, R., Lind, B., Lust, P., Mullie, A., Orr, M., Renck, H., and Snyder, J.V.: Clinical feasibility trials of barbiturate therapy after cardiac arrest. Crit. Care Med. 6:228, 1978.

Brickman, R.D., Murray, G.F., Thompson, W.L., and Ballinger, W.F.: The antigenicity of hydroxyethyl starch in humans: Studies in seven normal volunteers. J.A.M.A. 198: 1277, 1966.

Brinkmeyer, S., Safar, P., Motoyama, E., and Stezoski, W.: Pulmonary and cerebral variables during acute normovolemic hemodilution with lactated Ringer's versus albumin in dogs. Anesthesiology 53/3:S194, 1980 and Crit. Care Med. 9:369, 1981.

Brisman, R., Parks, L.C., and Haller, J.A.: Anaphylactoid reactions associated with the clinical use of dextran-70. J.A.M.A. 204:824, 1968.

Bruce, D.A., Gennarelli, T.A., and Langfitt, T.W.: Resuscitation from coma due to head injury. Crit. Care Med. 6:254, 1978.

Bunker, J.P.: Metabolic effects of blood transfusion. Anesthesiology 27:446, 1974.

Cannon, W.B.: Acidosis in cases of shock, hemorrhage, and gas infection. J.A.M.A. 71:531, 1918.

Carden, H.I., and Steinhaus, J.E.: Lidocaine resuscitation from ventricular fibrillation. Circ. Res. 4:640, 1956.

Carey, L.C., Lowery, N.D., and Cloutier, C.T.: Blood sugar and insulin response of humans in shock. Ann. Surg. 172: 342, 1970.

Carey, L.C., Lowery, N.D., and Cloutier, C.T.: Hemorrhagic shock. Curr. Probl. Surg., pp. 1–48, Jan. 1971.

Caroline, N.L., and Schwartz, H.: Chicken soup rebound and relapse of pneumonia: Report of a case. Chest 67:215, 1975.

Caroline, N.: *Emergency Care In The Streets.* Little, Brown, Boston, 1980.

Carroll, R., Hedden, M., and Safar, P.: Intratracheal cuffs: Performance characteristics. Anesthesiology *31:*275, 1969.

Chandra, N., Rudikoff, M., and Weisfeldt, M.L.: Simultaneous chest compression and ventilation of high airway pressure during CPR. Lancet *1:*175, 1980.

Clark, L.C., and Gollan, F.: Survival of mammals breathing organic liquids equilibrated with oxygen at atmospheric pressure. Science *152:*1755, 1966.

Collins, G.M., and Ludbrook, J.: The rheologic properties of low molecular weight dextrans: Fact or fancy? Am. Heart J. *72:*741, 1966.

Cournand, A., Riley, R.L., Bradley, S.E., Breed, E.S., Noble, R.P., Lauson, H.D., Gregerson, M.I., and Richards, D.W.: Studies of circulation in clinical shock. Surgery *13:*964, 1943.

Cowley, R.A.: A total emergency medical system for the State of Maryland. Md. State Med. J. *24:*37, 1975.

Crile, G.W.: *An Autobiography,* edited by G. Crile. J. B. Lippincott, Philadelphia, 1947.

Crile, G., and Dolley, D.H.: An experimental research into the resuscitation of dogs killed by anesthetics and asphyxia. J. Exp. Med. *8:*713, 1906.

Dawidson, I., Gelin, L.E., and Haglind, E.: Hemodilution and oxygen transport to tissue in shock. Acta Chir. Scand. (Suppl.) *489:*245, 1979.

DelGuercio, L.R.M., Feins, N.R., Cohn, H.D., Coomaraswamy, R., Wollman, S.B., and State, D.: Comparison of blood flow during external and internal cardiac massage in man. Circulation *30:*63, 1964 and (Suppl. 1) *31:*171, 1965.

Demuth, W.E., Baue, A.E., and Odom, J.E.: Contusions of the heart. J. Trauma *7:*443, 1967.

Detre, K., Abramson, N., Safar, P., et al: Collaborative randomized clinical study on cardiopulmonary-cerebral resuscitation. Crit. Care Med. *9:*395, 1981.

Dillon, J., Lynch, L.J., Meyers, R., Butcher, H.R., and Moyer, C.A.: A bioessay of treatment of hemorrhagic shock. Arch. Surg. *83:*537, 1966.

Doelt, R., and Mehrkens, H.H.: Possibilities of oral fluid substitution under disaster conditions. In *Disaster Medicine,* edited by F. Frey and P. Safar, vol. II, p. 46. Springer-Verlag, New York, 1980.

Dripps, R.D., Kirby, C.K., Johnson, J., and Erb, W.H.: Cardiac resuscitation. Ann. Surg. *127:*592, 1948.

Elam, J.O., Brown, E.S., and Elder, J.D., Jr.: Artificial respiration by mouth-to-mask method: A study of the respiratory gas exchange of paralyzed patients ventilated by operator's expired air. N. Engl. J. Med. *250:*749, 1954.

Esmarch, J.R.: *The Surgeons Handbook on the Treatment of Wounded in War.* Schmidt, New York, 1878.

Esposito, G., Safar, P., Medsger, A., and Nesbitt, J.: Life supporting first aid (LSFA) self training for the lay public. Anesthesiology *53/3:*S375 1980 and Crit. Care Med. *9:*403, 1981.

Eufinger, H.: Shock and plasma expander. In *Shock and Plasma Expander,* edited by K. Horatz, and R. Frey, p. 84. Springer-Verlag, Heidelberg, 1964.

Feustel, P. T., Ingvar, M. C., and Severinghaus, T. W.: Cerebral oxygen availability and blood flow during middle cerebral artery occlusion. Personal communication.

Freeman, J., and Nunn, J.F.: Ventilation-perfusion relationships after hemorrhage. Clin. Sci. *24:*135, 1963.

Frey, R., Eyrich, K., Lutz, H., Peter, K., and Weis, K.-H.: *Infusionstherapie.* Aesopus Verlag, Munich, 1974.

Gelin, L.E., Solvell, L., and Zederfeldt, A.: The plasma volume expanding effect of low viscous dextran and macrodex. Acta Chir. Scand. *122:*309, 1961.

Geyer, R.P., Monroe, R.G., and Taylor, K.: Survival of rats having red cells totally replaced with emulsified fluorocarbon. N. Engl. J. Med. *289:*1077, 1973.

Goldstein, A., Wells, B.A., and Keats, A.S.: Increased tolerance to cerebral anoxia by pentobarbital. Arch. Int. Pharmacodyn. Ther. *161:*138, 1966.

Gollub, S., Schaefer, C., and Squitieri, A.: The bleeding tendency associated with plasma expanders. Surg. Gynecol. Obstet. *124:*1203, 1967.

Gordon, A.S., Frye, C.W., Gittelson, L., Sadove, M.S., and Beathe, E.J.: Mouth-to-mouth versus manual artificial respiration for children and adults. J.A.M.A. *167:*320, 1958.

Gregersen, M.I., Usami, S., Peris, B., et al.: Blood viscosity at low shear rates: Effects of low and high molecular dextrans. Biorheology *1:*247, 1963.

Gurvich, N.L., and Yuniev, S.G.: Restoration of a regular rhythm in the mammalian fibrillating heart. Am. Rev. Sov. Med. *3:*236, 1946.

Guyton, AC: *Textbook of Medical Physiology,* ed. 6. W.B. Saunders, Philadelphia, 1981.

Guyton, A.C., and Lindsey, A.W.: Effect of elevated left atrial pressure and decreased plasma protein concentration on the development of pulmonary edema. Circulation *7:*649, 1959.

Hardaway, R.M.: Studies on pH changes in endotoxin and hemorrhagic shock. J. Surg. Res. *1:*278, 1961.

Hardaway, R.M.: *Syndromes of Disseminated Intravascular Coagulation: With Special Reference to Shock and Hemorrhage.* Charles C Thomas, Springfield, IL, 1966.

Hardaway, R.M., James, P.M., Anderson, R.W., Bredenberg, C.E., and West, R.L.: Intensive study and treatment of shock in man. J.A.M.A. *199:*115, 1967.

Harris, L.C., Kirimli, B., and Safar, P.: Augmentation of artificial circulation during cardiopulmonary resuscitation. Anesthesiology *28:*730, 1967a.

Harris, L.C., Kirimli, B., and Safar, P.: Ventilation-cardiac compression rates and ratios in cardiopulmonary resuscitation. Anesthesiology *28:*806, 1967b.

Heiberg, J.: A new expedient in administering chloroform. *Medical Times and Gazette,* January 10, 1874 (abstract from Zentralbl. Chir. *9:*141, 1874).

Hillman, R.S.: Pooled human plasma as a volume expander. N. Engl. J. Med. *271:*1027, 1964.

Hinshaw, L.B., Peyton, M.D., Archer, L.T., Black, M.R., Coalson, J.J., and Greenfield, L.J.: Prevention of death in endotoxin shock by glucose administration. Surg. Gynecol. Obstet. *139:*851, 1974.

Hoff, J.T.: Resuscitation in focal brain ischemia. Crit. Care Med. *6:*245, 1978.

Horatz, K., and Frey, R.: *Schock und Plasmaexpander.* Springer-Verlag, Berlin, 1964.

Hossmann, K.A., and Kleihues, P.: Reversibility of ischemic brain damage. Arch. Neurol. *29:*375, 1973.

Howland, W.S., and Schweizer, O.: Physiologic compensation for storage lesion of banked blood. Anesth. Analg. *44:*8, 1965.

Howland, W.S., Schweizer, O., Carlon, G.C., and Goldiner, P.: Cardiovascular effects of low levels of ionized calcium during massive transfusion. Surg. Gynecol. Obstet. *145:*581, 1977.

Huch, A., Huch, R., and Arner, O.: Continuous transcutaneous oxygen tension measured with a heated electrode. Scand. J. Clin. Lab. Invest. *31:*269, 1973.

Huckabee, W.E.: Relation of pyruvate and lactate during anaerobic metabolism: Effects of infusion of pyruvate or glucose and of hyperventilation. J. Clin. Invest. *37:*244, 1958.

Jamieson, G.A., and Greenwalt, T.J. (Eds.): *Blood Substitutes and Plasma Expanders.* A. R. Liss, New York, 1978.

Jude, J.R., Kouwenhoven, W.B., and Knickerbocker, G.G.: Cardiac arrest: Report of application of external cardiac massage on 118 patients. J.A.M.A. *178:*1063, 1961.

Jurkiewicz, J.: The effect of haemodilution on experimental brain edema. Eur. J. Intensive Care Med. *3:*167, 1977.

Kaplan, B.C., Civetta, J.M., and Nagel, E.L.: The Military Anti-Shock Trouser in civilian pre-hospital emergency care. J. Trauma *13:*843, 1973.

Karlson, K.E., Garzon, A.A., Shaftan, G.W., and Chu, C.: Increased blood loss associated with administration of certain plasma expanders: Dextran-75, dextran-40, and hydroxyethyl starch. Surgery *62:*670, 1967.

Kirimli, B., Harris, L.C., and Safar, P.: Drugs in cardiopulmonary resuscitation. Acta Anaesth. Scand. (Suppl.) *23:*255, 1966.

Kirimli, B., Kampschulte, S., and Safar, P.: Resuscitation from cardiac arrest due to exsanguination. Surg. Gynecol. Obstet. *129:*89, 1969.

Klain, M., and Smith, R.B.: High frequency percutaneous transtracheal jet ventilation. Crit. Care Med. *5:*280, 1977.

Knisely, M.H., Eliot, T.S., and Block, E.H.: Sludged blood in tramatic shock. Arch. Surg. *51:*220, 1945.

Koch-Weser, J.: Drug therapy: Bretylium. N. Engl. J. Med. *300:*473, 1979.

Kouwenhoven, W.B., Jude, J.R., and Knickerbocker, G.G.: Closed chest cardiac massage. J.A.M.A. *173:*1064, 1960.

Kovach, A.G.B., and Sandor, P.: Cerebral blood flow and brain function during hypotension and shock. Ann. Rev. Physiol. *38:*571, 1976.

Kuhn, F.: *Die Perorale Intubation.* Karger, Berlin, 1911.

Laborit, H., and Huguenard, P.: *Practice of Hibernation Therapy in Surgery and Medicine (French).* Masson, Paris, 1954.

Lewis, J.H., Szeto, I.L.F., Bayer, W.L., Takaori, M., and Safar, P.: Severe hemodilution with hydroxylethyl starch and dextrans. Arch. Surg. *93:*941, 1966.

Lillehei, R.C., Longerbeam, J.K., Block, J.H., and Mannax, W.G.: The nature of irreversible shock: Experimental and clinical observations. Ann. Surg. *160:*682, 1964.

Lindholm, C.E.: Prolonged endotracheal intubation. Acta Anaesthiol. Scand. (Suppl.) *33:* 1969.

Litwin, M.S.: Comparison of effects of dextran 70 and dextran 40 on postoperative animals. Ann. Surg. *71:*295, 1972.

Loeb, H.S., and Gunnar, R.M.: Vasoactive agents in the treatment of shock: A review. In *Shock,* edited by I. Ledingham, p. 257. Excerpta Medica, Amsterdam, 1976.

Lowenstein, E., Michalski, A., and Laver, M.B.: Blood volume and circulatory measurements during extreme acute hemodilution. Anesthesiology *29:*203, 1968.

Luisada, A.A.: Mechanism of neurogenic pulmonary edema. Am. J. Cardiol. *20:*66, 1967.

Lundy, J.S., and Adams, R.C.: Thiopental sodium intravenous anesthesia. Army Med. Bull. *63:*90, 1942.

Maas: Die Methode der Wiederbelebung bei Herztod nach chloroformeinathmung. Berl. Klin. Wochenschr. *29:*265, 1892.

Maloney, J.V., Smith, C.M., Gilmore, J.P., and Hundford, S.W.: Intra-arterial and intravenous infusion: A controlled study of their effectiveness in the treatment of experimental hemorrhagic shock. Surg. Gynecol. Obstet. *97:*529, 1953.

Matheson, N.A., and Diomi, P.: Renal failure after the administration of dextran 40. Surg. Gynecol. Obstet. *131:*661, 1970.

Maurer, P.H., and Berardinelli, B.: Immunologic studies with hydroxyethyl starch (HES), a proposed plasma expander. Transfusion *8:*265, 1968.

Meiselman, J.H., Merrill, E.W., Salzman, E.W., Gilliland, E.R., and Pelletier, G.A.: Effect of dextran on rheology of human blood: Low shear viscometery. J. Appl. Physiol. *22:*480, 1967.

Messmer, K. (Ed.): Hemodilution (a symposium). Anaesthesist *25:*123, 1976.

Metcalf, W., Dargan, E.L., Hehre, E.J., Leditsky, S., and DiBuono, T.J.: Clinical physiological characterization of a new dextran. Surg. Gynecol. Obstet. *115:*199, 1962.

Michelson, E.: Anaphylactic reaction to dextrans. N. Engl. J. Med. *278:*552, 1968.

Michenfelder, J.D., and Theye, R.A.: The effects of anesthesia and hypothermia on canine cerebral ATP and lactate during anoxia produced by decapitation. Anesthesiology *33:*430, 1970.

Miller, E.B., and Tisdall, L.H.: Reactions to 10,000 pooled liquid human plasma transfusions. J.A.M.A. *128:*863, 1945.

Moerch, E.T., Avery, E.E., and Benson, D.W.: Hyperventilation in the treatment of crushing injuries of the chest. Surg. Forum *6:*270, 1956.

Moore, F.D.: The effects of hemorrhage on body composition. N. Engl. J. Med. *273:*567, 1965.

Moore, F.D., et al: *Post-traumatic Pulmonary Insufficiency.* W. B. Saunders, Philadelphia, 1969.

Moss, G.: The role of the central nervous system in shock: The centroneurogenic etiology of the respiratory distress syndrome. Crit. Care Med. *2:*131, 1974.

Moss, G.S., Valeri, C.R., and Brodine, C.E.: Clinical experience with the use of frozen blood in combat casualties. N. Engl. J. Med. *278:*747, 1968.

Moyer, C.A.: *Fluid Balance.* Year Book Medical Publishers, Chicago, 1954.

Moyer, C.A., Markraf, H.W., and Monafo, W.W.: Burn shock and extravascular sodium deficiency: Treatment with Ringer's solution with lactate. Arch. Surg. *90:*799, 1965.

Naito, R., and Yokoyama, K.: On the perfluorodecalin/phospholipid emulsion as the red cell substitute. In *Proceedings of the 10th International Nutrition Symposium on PFC Artificial Blood,* p. 55. Kyoto, 1975.

Negovsky, V.A.: Introduction: Reanimatology—the science of resuscitation. In *Cardiac Arrest and Resuscitation,* edited by H. E. Stephenson, ed. 4. C. V. Mosby, St. Louis, MO, 1974.

Nemoto, E.M.: Pathogenesis of cerebral ischemia-anoxia. Crit. Care Med. *6:*203, 1978.

Nickerson, M.: Sympathetic blockade in the therapy of shock. Am. J. Cardiol. *12:*619, 1963.

Overland, E.S., and Severinghaus, J.W.: Noncardiac pulmonary edema. Adv. Intern. Med. *23:*307, 1978.

Papper, E.M., and Bradley, S.E.: Hemodynamic effects of intravenous morphine and pentothal sodium. J. Pharmacol. Exp. Ther. *74:*319, 1942.

Pearson, J.W., and Redding, J.S.: Influence of peripheral vascular tone on cardiac resuscitation. Anesth. Analg. *44:*746, 1965.

Petty, T.L., and Ashbaugh, D.G.: The adult respiratory distress syndrome. Chest *60:*233, 1971.

Pontoppidan, H., Geffin, B., and Lowenstein, E.: Acute respiratory failure in the adult. N. Engl. J. Med. *287:*690, 1972.

Powers, S.: Relation of acute tubular necrosis to shock and the effect of mannitol. Am. J. Surg. *110:*330, 1965.

Prevost, J.L., and Battelli, F.: On some effects of electrical discharges on the hearts of mammals. C. R. Acad. Sci. [Paris] *129:*1267, 1899.

Rabiner, S.F., Helbert, J.R., Lopas, H., and Friedman, L.H.: Evaluation of a stroma-free hemoglobin solution for use as a plasma expander. J. Exp. Med. *126:*1127, 1967.

Redding, J.S.: Drug therapy during cardiac arrest. In *Advances in Cardiopulmonary Resuscitation*, edited by P. Safar, pp. 113–117. Springer-Verlag, New York, 1977.

Replogle, R.L., Kundler, H., and Gross, R.E.: Studies on the hemodynamic importance of blood viscosity. J. Thorac. Cardiovasc. Surg. *50:*658, 1965.

Rosomoff, H.L., Shulman, K., Raynor, R., and Grainger, W.: Experimental brain injury and delayed hypothermia. Surg. Gynecol. Obstet. *110:*27, 1960.

Rothschild, M.A., Oratz, N., and Schreiber, S.S.: Albumin synthesis. N. Engl. J. Med. *286:*748, 1972.

Ruben, H.: Combination resuscitator and aspirator. Anesthesiology *19:*408, 1958.

Rudikoff, M.T., Maughan, W.L., Effron, M., Freund, P., and Weisfeldt, M.L.: Mechanisms of blood flow during cardiopulmonary resuscitation. Circulation *61:*345, 1980.

Rush, B., and Eiseman, B.: Limits of noncolloid solution replacement in experimental hemorrhagic shock. Ann. Surg. *165:*977, 1967.

Safar, P.: Pocket mask for emergency artificial ventilation and oxygen inhalation. Crit. Care Med. *2:*273, 1974.

Safar, P. (Ed.): Brain resuscitation (symposium issue). Crit. Care Med. *6:*199–291, 1978a.

Safar, P.: Mechanisms of dying and their reversal (Ch. 2) and cardiopulmonary cerebral resuscitation (Ch. 9). In *Principles and Practice of Emergency Medicine*, edited by G. Schwartz et al. W. B. Saunders, Philadelphia, 1978b.

Safar, P.: Pathophysiology and resuscitation after global brain ischemia. Int. Anesthesiol. Clin. *17:*239, 1979.

Safar, P.: *Cardiopulmonary-Cerebral Resuscitation: A Manual for Physicians and Instructors*. World Federation of Societies of Anesthesiologists, eds. 1 and 2. A. Laerdal, Stavanger, Norway, 1968 and 1980a.

Safar, P.: Amelioration of postischemic damage with barbiturates. Stroke *15:*1, 1980b.

Safar, P., and Caroline, N.: Acute respiratory insufficiency (ch. 3) and Respiratory care techniques and strategies (ch. 10). In *Principles and Practice of Emergency Medicine*, edited by G. Schwartz et al. W. B. Saunders, Philadelphia, 1978.

Safar, P., and Lind, B.: Triple airway maneuver, artificial ventilation and oxygen inhalation by mouth-to-mask and bag-valve-mask techniques. *Proceedings of a National Conference on Standards for CPR, May 1973*, p. 49. American Heart Association, Dallas, 1975.

Safar, P., and Penninckx, J.: Cricothyroid membrane puncture with special cannula. Anesthesiology *28:*943, 1967.

Safar, P., Escarraga, L., and Elam, J.: A comparison of the mouth-to-mouth and mouth-to-airway methods of artificial respiration with the chest-pressure arm-lift methods. N. Engl. J. Med. *258:*671, 1958.

Safar, P., Aguto-Escarraga, L., and Chang, F.: A study of upper airway obstruction in the unconscious patient. J. Appl. Physiol. *14:*760, 1959.

Safar, P., et al.: Ventilation and circulation with closed chest cardiac massage in man. J.A.M.A. *176:*575, 1961.

Safar, P., Grenvik, A., and Smith, J.: Progressive pulmonary consolidation: Review of cases and pathogenesis. J. Trauma *12:*955, 1972.

Safar, P., Stezoski, S.W., and Nemoto, E.M.: Amelioration of brain damage after 12 minutes' cardiac arrest in dogs. Arch. Neurol. *33:*91, 1976.

Safar, P., Bleyaert, A., Nemoto, E.M., Moossy, J., and Snyder, J.V.: Resuscitation after global brain ischemia-anoxia. Crit. Care Med. *6:*215, 1978.

Sanderson, J.M., Wright, G., and Sims, F.W.: Brain damage in dogs immediately following pulsate and non-pulsate blood flows in extra-corporeal circulation. Thorax *27:*275, 1972.

Sawyer, R.B., and Moncrief, J.A.: Dextran specificity in thrombus inhibition. Arch. Surg. *90:*562, 1965.

Schiff, J.: Über direkte Reizung der Herzoberfläche. Arch. Ges. Physiol. *28:*200, 1882.

Schumer, W.: Steroids in the treatment of clinical septic shock. Ann. Surg. *184:*333, 1976.

Seeley, S.F., Essex, H.E., and Mann, F.C.: Comparative studies on traumatic shock produced experimentally under ether and under sodium amytal anesthesia. Ann. Surg. *105:*332, 1936.

Shapiro, H.M.: Intracranial hypertension: Therapeutic and anesthetic considerations. Anesthesiology *43:*443, 1975.

Shire, G.T.: Management of hypovolemic shock. Bull. N.Y. Acad. Med. *55:*139, 1979.

Shires, G.T., Williams, J., and Brown, F.: Acute change in extracellular fluids associated with major surgical procedures. Ann. Surg. *154:*803, 1961.

Shoemaker, W.C.: Comparison of the relative effectiveness of whole blood transfusions and various types of fluid therapy in resuscitation. Crit. Care Med. *4:*71, 1976.

Shoemaker, W., and Thompson, L. (Eds.): *Critical Care Medicine: State of the Art*. Society of Critical Care Medicine, Los Angeles, 1980.

Shubin, H., Weil, M.H., Carlson, R.W., and Freund, U.: Cardiovascular system failure (ch. 4). In *Principles and Practice of Emergency Medicine*, edited by G. Schwartz et al. W. B. Saunders, Philadelphia, 1978.

Siesjo, B.K.: *Brain Energy Metabolism*. John Wiley & Sons, New York, 1978.

Simeone, F.A., and Witoszka, M.: The central nervous system in experimental hemorrhagic shock: The cerebrospinal fluid pressure. Am. J. Surg. *119:*427, 1970.

Skillman, J.J.: The role of albumin and oncotically active fluids in shock. Crit. Care Med. *4:*55, 1976.

Sloviter, H.A., and Kamimoto, T.: Erythrocyte substitute for perfusion of brains. Nature *216:*458, 1967.

Smith, D.S., Rehncroma, S., and Siesjo, B.K.: Inhibitory effects of different barbiturates on lipid peroxydation in brain tissue in vitro: Comparison with the effects of Promethazine and chlorpromazine. Anesthesiology *53:*186, 1980.

Smith, J., Penninckx, J.J., Kampschulte, S., and Safar, P.: Need for oxygen enrichment in myocardial infarction, shock, and following cardiac arrest. Acta Anaesthesiol. Scand. (Suppl.) *29:*127, 1968.

Smith, R.B.: Transtracheal ventilation during anesthesia. Anesth. Analg. *53:*225, 1974.

Smith, R.B., Klain, M., and Babinski, M.: Limits of high frequency percutaneous transtracheal jet ventilation using a fluidic logic controlled ventilator. Can. Anaesth. Soc. J. *27:*351, 1980.

Steen, P.A., Michenfelder, J.D., and Milde, J.H.: Incomplete versus complete cerebral ischemia: Improved outcome with a minimal blood flow. Ann. Neurol. *6:*389, 1979a.

Steen, P.A., Soule, E.H., and Michenfelder, J.D.: Detrimental effect of prolonged hypothermia in cats and monkeys with and without regional cerebral ischemia. Stroke *10:*522, 1979b.

Steinmetz, T.R., and Balko, C.: Fluorocarbon—polyol artificial blood substitutes. N. Engl. J. Med. *289:*1077, 1973.

Stephenson, H.E. (Ed.): *Cardiac Arrest and Resuscitation*. C. V. Mosby, St. Louis, MO, 1974.

Stept, W.J., and Safar, P.: Rapid induction/intubation for

prevention of gastric content aspiration. Anesth. Analg. *49:* 633, 1970.

Stewart, J.S.: Management of cardiac arrest with special reference to metabolic acidosis. Br. Med. J. *1:*476, 1964.

Stone, H.H., Donnelly, C.C., MacKrell, T.N., et al.: The effect of acute hemorrhagic shock on cerebral circulation and metabolism of man. In *Proceedings of the Hahnemann Medical College Symposium on Shock and Hypotension*, 257 pp. Grune & Stratton, New York, 1965.

Stremple, J.E., Thomas, H., Sakach, V., et al.: Myocardial utilization of hypertonic glucose during hemorrhagic shock. Surgery *80:*4–13, 1976.

Suter, P.M., Fairley, H.B., and Isenberg, M.D.: The optimum end-expiratory airway pressure in patients with acute pulmonary failure. N. Engl. J. Med. *292:*284, 1975.

Szanto, G.Y., Honig, V., and Szekely, O.: *Traumatic Shock*. Akademiai Kiado, Budapest, 1973.

Takaori, M., and Safar, P.: Acute severe hemodilution with lactated Ringer's solution. Arch. Surg. *94:*67, 1967a.

Takaori, M., and Safar, P.: Treatment of massive hemorrhage with colloid and crystalloid solutions. J.A.M.A. *199:*297, 1967b.

Takaori, M., and Safar, P.: Critical point in progressive hemodilution with hydroxyethyl starch. Kawasaki Med. J. *2:* 211, 1976.

Takaori, M., Safar, P., and Galla, S.J.: Changes in body fluid compartments during hemodilution with hydroxyethyl starch and dextran 40. Arch. Surg. *100:*263, 1970.

Thompson, W.L.: Interaction of hydroxyethyl starch and dextran with plasma proteins and erythrocyte envelopes. Biorheology *3:*49, 1966.

Thompson, W.L.: Rational use of albumin and plasma substitutes. Johns Hopkins Med. J. *136:*220, 1975.

Thompson, W.L., and Gladsden, R.H.: Prolonged bleeding times and hypofibrinogenemia in dogs after infusion of hydroxyethyl starch and dextran. Transfusion *5:*440, 1965.

Thompson, W.L., Fukushima, T., Rutherford, R.B., and Walton, R.P.: Intravascular persistence, tissue storage, and excretion of hydroxyethyl starch. Surg. Gynecol. Obstet. *131:* 965, 1970.

Torpey, D.: Resuscitation and anesthetic management of casualties. J.A.M.A. *202:*955, 1967.

Trump, B.F., Croker, B.P., and Mergner, W.J.: *Cell Membranes: Biological and Pathological Aspects*, edited by N. Kaufman and G. W. Richter, p. 84. Williams & Wilkins, Baltimore, 1971.

Valeri, C.R., Runck, A.H., and McCallum, L.E.: Observations on autologous, previously frozen, deglycerolized, agglomerated, resuspended red cells. Transfusion *7:*105, 1967.

Vesalius, A.: *De Corporis Humani Fabrica.* Libri Septem, 1543.

Weil, M.H., and Shubin, H.: VIP approach to the bedside management of shock. J.A.M.A. *207:*337, 1969.

Weil, M.H., and Shubin, H. (Eds.): *Diagnosis and Treatment of Shock.* Williams & Wilkins, Baltimore, 1967.

Werko, L.: The influence of positive pressure breathing on the circulation in man. Acta Med. Scand. Suppl. *193:*1–125, 1947.

Wiggers, C.J.: The physiological bases for cardiac resuscitation from ventricular fibrillation: Method for serial defibrillation. Am. Heart J. *20:*413, 1940.

Wiggers, C.J.: *Physiology of Shock*. Commonwealth Fund, New York, 1950.

Wilder, R.J., Weir, D., Ruch, B.F., and Ravich, M.M.: Methods of coordinating ventilation of closed-chest cardiac massage in the dog. Surgery *53:*186, 1963.

Winter, P.M., Gupta, R.K., Michalski, A.H., and Lanphier, E.H.: Modification of hyperbaric oxygen toxicity by experimental venous admixture. J. Appl. Physiol *23:*954, 1967.

Zoll, P.M., et al.: Termination of ventricular fibrillation in man by externally applied electric countershock. N. Engl. J. Med. *254:*727, 1956.

CHAPTER 30

Pathophysiology and Therapy of Hemorrhage and Trauma States

WILLIAM C. SHOEMAKER

Traditional concepts have considered hemorrhagic and traumatic shock as one entity and characterized it as a low flow syndrome. This is because hemorrhage is usually found with trauma and vice versa, and no distinctions were made between the effects of hemorrhage and those of trauma. Moreover, low cardiac output with high peripheral resistance initially was observed in both hemorrhagic and cardiogenic shock (Courand et al., 1943; Wiggers, 1950). Accordingly, therapy by this concept should be directed toward correction of the low cardiac output. However, subsequent studies have clearly shown that the hemodynamic patterns of the anesthetized, exsanguinated dog and the patient with hypovolemic or myocardial infarction are not representative of most clinical shock syndromes, particularly traumatic and septic shock. Furthermore, shock is not a single entity that may be optimally treated by the principles of an oversimplified experimental model. Moreover, the effects of hemorrhage per se are very different from those of trauma (Shoemaker, 1971, 1973, 1980; Shoemaker et al., 1973).

Shock is best described as a complex group of syndromes produced by a wide variety of etiologic events; it is a stage in the pathways leading toward death from circulatory failure. More importantly, shock states should not be represented as though they were static physiologic states; their alterations vary as the syndromes evolve in time. Therefore, shock states are best described in terms of sequential cardiorespiratory patterns that begin with the onset of the precipitating etiologic event, not when the physician recognizes hypotension or when the patient is unresponsive to therapy. Thus, the simplistic notion that shock states are a single disease entity is incorrect. Moreover, therapy based upon simplistic notions is not likely to be optimally effective.

It is essential to understand the natural history of the various shock syndromes and their pathophysiology in order to provide maximally effective therapy. In an effort to understand the pathophysiology of shock syndromes, the temporal cardiorespiratory patterns of shock following specific etiologic events, i.e., hemorrhage, trauma, and sepsis were described (Shoemaker, 1973, 1980). The monitored cardiorespiratory variables, their abbreviations, units, formulas, normal values, and preferred (optimal) values are listed in Table 30.1.

PATHOPHYSIOLOGY

The natural physiologic history of various shock syndromes was developed from the description of the common cardiorespiratory patterns obtained by serial cardiorespiratory measurements taken remote from therapy, i.e., before the therapy was given or after the immediate direct effects of therapy had worn off (Figs. 30.1–30.3). In this analysis, over 10,000 sequential sets of cardiorespiratory measurements were made in 180 patients (Shoemaker, 1973, 1980).

Sequential Stages

The physiologic alterations were divided into early, middle, and late periods by criteria of time and arterial pressure to analyze data from patients with different etiologic types of shock at comparable time periods. Because some patients go through their circulatory failure more rapidly or more slowly than others, criteria for staging are needed to analyze the data from patients with different etiologic types of shock at comparable time periods.

The stages were defined as follows: stage A, the preillness control period; stage B, the initial period of falling arterial pressure immediately after the etiologic event; stage Low, the lowest initial arterial pressure that separates stage B from stage C, the middle period; stage C was divided into C_1 and C_2 by the point in time when arterial pressure returned halfway to control values; stage D, the late or recovery period for surviving patients, started when arterial pressures had returned to control values; stage E, the preterminal period in patients who subsequently died.

It is obvious from this description that physiologic mechanisms underlying the early cardiorespiratory events may have pathogenic significance. Similarly, physiologic events occurring in the late stage probably reflect only terminal mechanisms. It is evident that shock

Table 30.1
Cardiorespiratory Variables—Abbreviations, Units, Calculations, Normal Values, and Preferred Values

	Abbreviations	Units	Measurements or Derived Calculations	Normal Values	Preferred Values
Volume-related variables					
Mean arterial pressure	MAP	mm Hg	Direct measurement	82–102	>84
Central venous pressure	CVP	cm H_2O	Direct measurement	1–9	<5
Central blood volume	CBV	ml/M^2	CBV = MTT × CI × 16.7	660–1,000	>925
Stroke index	SI	ml/M^2	SI = CI ÷ HR	30–50	>48
Hemoglobin	Hgb	g/dl	Direct measurement	12–16	>12
Mean pulmonary arterial pressure	MPAP	mm Hg	Direct measurement	11–15	<19
Wedge pressure	WP	mm Hg	Direct measurement	0–12	>9.5
Blood volume	BV	ml/M^2	BV = PV ÷ (1-Hct)[a] × surface area	Men 2.74	>3.0
				Women 2.37	>2.7
Red cell mass	RCM	ml/M^2	RCM = BV − PV	Men 1.1	>1.1
				Women 0.95	>0.95
Flow-related variables					
Cardiac index	CI	liter/min·M^2	Direct measurement	2.8–3.6	>4.5
Mean transit time	MTT	sec	Direct measurement	12–18	<13
Left ventricular stroke work	LVSW	g·M/M^2	LVSW = SI × MAP × .0144	44–68	>55
Left cardiac work	LCW	kg·M/M^2	LCW = CI × MAP × .0144	3–4.6	>5
Mean systolic ejection rate	MSER	ml/sec·M^2	MSER = SI ÷ duration of systole	580–980	>1,100
Tension rate index	TTI	mm Hg·sec/cm	TTI = MAP × HR × duration of systole	270–470	>342
Right ventricular stroke work	RVSW	g·M/M^2	RVSW = SI × MPAP × .0144	4–8	>13
Right cardiac work	RCW	kg·M/M^2	RCW = CI × MPAP × .0144	0.4–0.6	>1.1
Stress-related variables					
Systemic vascular resistance	SVR	dyne·sec/cm^5·M^2	SVR = 79.92 (MAP − CVP)[b] ÷ CI	1,760–2,600	<1,450
Pulmonary vascular resistance	PVR	dyne·sec/cm^5·M^2	PVR = 79.92 (MPAP − WP)[b] ÷ CI	45–225	<226
Heart rate	HR	beat/min	Direct measurement	72–88	<100
Rectal temperature	temp	°F	Direct measurement	97.8–98.6	>100.4
Oxygen-related variables					
Arterial hemoglobin saturation	SaO_2	%	Direct measurement	95–99	>95
Arterial CO_2 tension	$PaCO_2$	torr	Direct measurement	36–44	>30
Arterial pH	pH		Direct measurement	7.36–7.44	>7.47
Mixed venous O_2 tension	$P\bar{v}O_2$	torr	Direct measurement	33–53	>36
Arterial-mixed venous O_2 content difference	$a\bar{v}DO_2$	ml/dl	$a\bar{v}DO_2 = CaO_2 − C\bar{v}O_2$	4–5.5	<3.5
O_2 delivery	O_2 deliv	ml/min·M^2	O_2 deliv = CaO_2 × CI × 10	520–720	>550
O_2 consumption	$\dot{V}O_2$	ml/min·M^2	$\dot{V}O_2 = a\bar{v}DO_2$ × CI × 10	100–180	>167
O_2 extraction rate	O_2 ext	%	O_2 ext = $(CaO_2 − C\bar{v}O_2) ÷ CaO_2$	22–30	<31
Perfusion-related variables					
Red cell flow rate	RCFR	liter/min·M^2	RCFR = CI × Hct	0.6–1.8	>1.3
Blood flow/volume ratio	BFVR		BFVR = CI ÷ BV	0.6–1.8	>1.7
O_2 transport/red cell mass ratio	OTRM		OTRM = $\dot{V}O_2$ ÷ RCM	0.06–.18	>0.25
Tissue O_2 extraction ratio	TOE		TOE = $a\bar{v}DO_2$ ÷ RCFR	1.8–6.6	<5.7
Efficiency of tissue O_2 extraction	ETOE		ETOE = $a\bar{v}DO_2$ ÷ RCM	0.06–.18	>1.3
O_2 transport/red cell flow ratio	OTRF		OTRF = $\dot{V}O_2$ ÷ RCFR	1–7	<3

[a] Hct correct for packing fraction and large vessel hematocrit/total body hematocrit ratio.
[b] Venous pressures expressed in mm Hg.

is usually first recognized by hypotension, but by this time the major pathophysiologic reactions have already taken place.

Influence of Therapy

To separate the natural physiologic history from the confounding effects of the therapy, cardiorespiratory measurements were taken before, during, and after therapy. In this way, the effectiveness of each therapeutic intervention could be evaluated on the background of the natural physiologic history of the specific etiologic type of shock. The body's initial responses to different types of stress were quite variable, but within each etiologic category the cardiorespiratory patterns were rather similar. By the same token, there were remarkable similarities in the responses of each of the therapeutic agents (Brown et al., 1966; Carey et al., 1967; Matsuda and Shoemaker, 1974a and b; Mohr et al., 1969; Shoemaker, 1976).

Hemorrhagic Shock

The cardiorespiratory pattern and hemorrhage in the early period consist of decreases in arterial pressure, cardiac output, central venous pressure (CVP), blood volume, stroke index, left ventricular work, O_2 delivery, and O_2 consumption ($\dot{V}O_2$), as well as increases in heart rate, systemic vascular resistance, arteriovenous O_2 content difference ($a\bar{v}DO_2$), and O_2 extraction. The body's compensatory responses to hemorrhage consist of tachycardia, systemic and pulmonary metarteriolar vasoconstriction, and increased myocardial contractility (Shoemaker, 1973).

Pathophysiology and Therapy

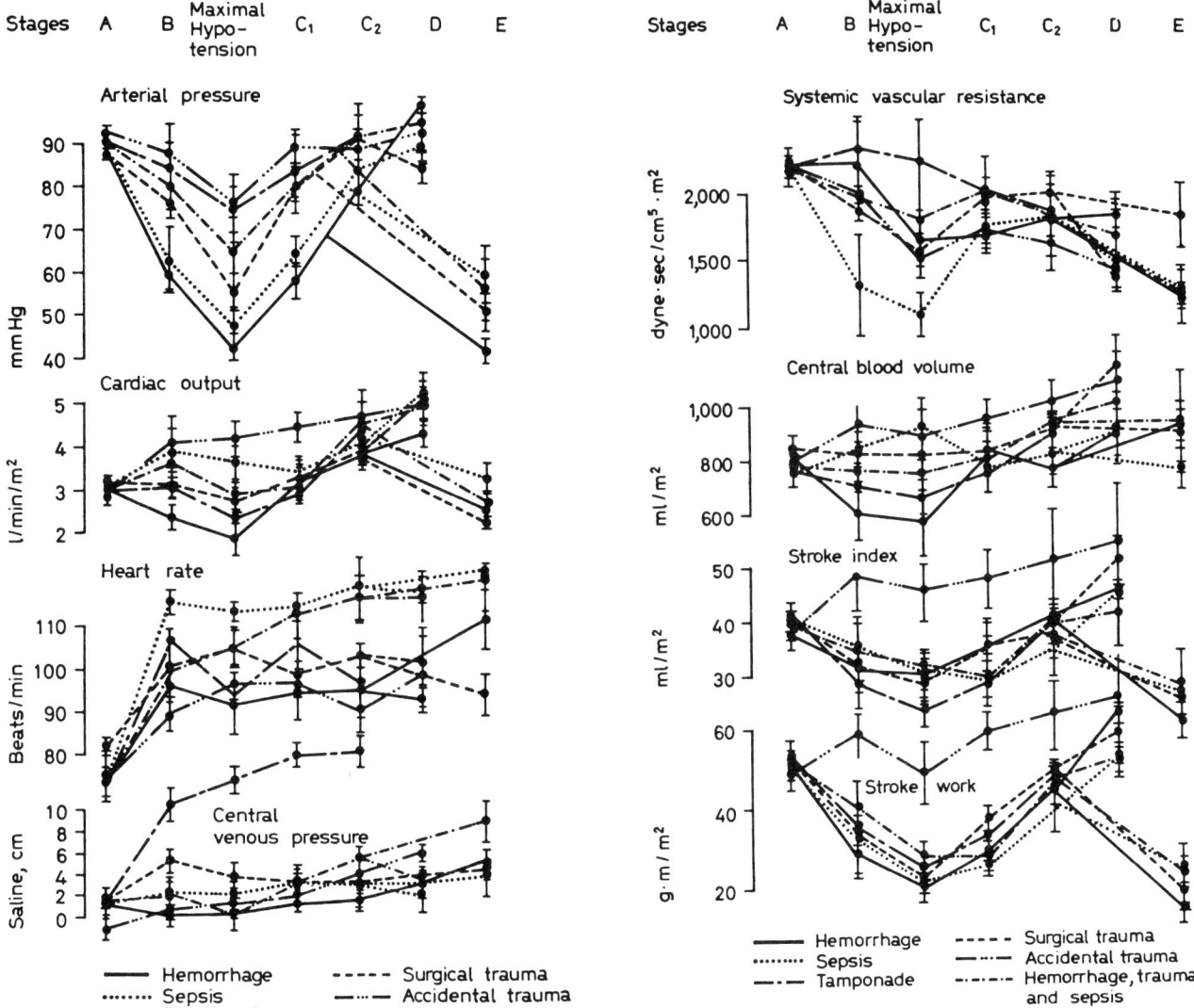

Figure 30.1. Sequential hemodynamic patterns illustrated by mean values (*dots*) and SEM (*vertical bars*) at each temporal stage after various etiologic types of shock for mean arterial pressure, cardiac index, heart rate, and central venous pressure. Note the fall in cardiac index in the B and Low stage with hemorrhagic and cardiogenic shock, but the cardiac index values of septic and traumatic shock were normal or increased. Heart rates increased in all etiologic groups but were greatest in the two types of sepsis. Except for the cardiac patients, venous pressures were within the normal range. (Reprinted with permission from W. C. Shoemaker: Seminars in Drug Treatment 3:211, 1973.)

Increased sympathetic neural activity after hypovolemia and low flow produce metarteriolar vasoconstriction. The vasoconstriction, being uneven, results in relatively greater percentages of blood flow to the heart and brain but lesser flow to the kidney, gut, and skin (Slater et al.,

Figure 30.2. Sequential hemodynamic patterns at each temporal stage after various etiologic types of shock shown by mean values ± SEM (*vertical bars*) for systemic (peripheral) vascular resistance, central blood volume, stroke index, and left ventricular stroke work. Note the slight transient rise in peripheral resistance in the B stage after hemorrhage and cardiogenic shock and the subsequent progressive decrease in resistance with time in all categories. Also, central blood volume values tended to be low in the B and Low stages of hemorrhagic and cardiogenic shock, but the values of the other groups were normal or high. The stroke volume and stroke work were increased in accidental trauma, but these variables decreased in the B, Low, and C_1 stages in the other groups. (Reprinted with permission from W. C. Shoemaker: Seminars in Drug Treatment 3:211, 1973.)

1973). Normally flow in the microcirculation is also redistributed by neural regulatory mechanisms. But when prolonged vasoconstriction occurs, the redistribu-

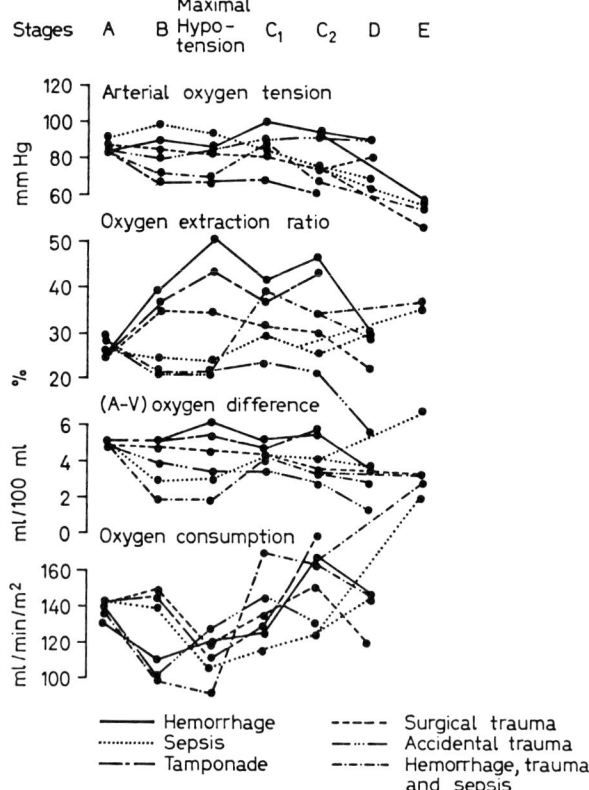

Figure 30.3. Sequential patterns in bulk oxygen movement after various types of shock illustrated by mean values of PaO_2, oxygen extraction ratio, $a\bar{v}DO_2$ (arteriovenous oxygen content differences), and oxygen consumption. Note that PaO_2 values were not appreciably reduced until the late stages. The oxygen extraction ratio and the $a\bar{v}DO_2$ rose in the hemorrhage and cardiogenic patients. The $a\bar{v}DO_2$ fell in the accidental trauma, sepsis, and hemorrhage-trauma-sepsis groups. Oxygen consumption fell in the early (B or Low stage) period in all groups and rose in the middle periods in all etiologic types of shock. (Reprinted with permission from W. C. Shoemaker: Seminars in Drug Treatment 3:211, 1973.)

tions of both flow and volume develop into maldistributions. It is the maldistribution of flow leading to inadequate oxygen transport to the tissues that is the principal physiologic defect of shock states. The tissues extract oxygen more completely, because less blood is flowing more slowly. But despite this compensation, the uneven flow results in inadequate tissue oxygenation and is manifest by reduced $\dot{V}O_2$. Metabolic acidosis occurs with hypovolemia and reduced blood flow; respiratory alkalosis is a compensatory mechanism to acidosis.

Traumatic Shock

Trauma produces an immediate response consisting of increased cardiac output, heart rate, stroke volume, stroke work, and O_2 delivery, as well as reduced arterial pressure, systemic vascular resistance, oxygen extraction, $a\bar{v}DO_2$, and $\dot{V}O_2$. After trauma there is a generalized increase in autonomic neural activity that releases neurohormones and stimulates the cardiac and respiratory centers of the brain to increase heart rates, myocardial contractility, and alveolar ventilation. With normovolemia, the stroke volume increases due to myocardial stimulation; cardiac output then increases because of increased stroke volume and heart rate. Minute ventilation increases without hypovolemia to produce respiratory alkalosis without the antecedent metabolic acidosis seen after hemorrhage (Shoemaker, 1973, 1980; Shoemaker et al., 1967, 1971a and b, 1973).

Physiologic responses to trauma and hemorrhage are primarily mediated by neural mechanisms. The generalized increase in autonomic neural tone stimulates cardiac and respiratory centers of the brain to increase cardiac and ventilatory drives. The duration and magnitude of these autonomic responses depend on many factors; e.g., the increased cardiac output after trauma and sepsis may be limited by hypovolemia and impaired myocardial function. Cellular breakdown products from direct tissue injury and the need for tissue repair increase metabolic requirements. These metabolic influences intensify the high cardiac output and low resistance (Shoemaker, 1973, 1980; Shoemaker et al., 1973).

Septic Shock

Septic shock rarely occurs by itself; usually it occurs as a complication of hemorrhage, trauma, postoperative states, etc. It is the sepsis complicating postoperative states associated with profound hypotension that carries high mortality rates.

Infection may occur with or without systemic manifestations and with or without hypotension. The early cardiorespiratory pattern initially consists of hypotension, tachycardia, normal or high cardiac output, as well as reduced systemic vascular resistance, stroke work, $a\bar{v}DO_2$, and $\dot{V}O_2$. Subsequently, the $\dot{V}O_2$ increases, especially with hyperthermia and hypermetabolism. The body's physiologic responses to sepsis consist of increased heart rate, myocardial contractility, and ventilation by neural mechanisms. When blood volume is not reduced by dehydration, there are marked increases in cardiac index, heart rate, and myocardial contractility. The increased respiratory drive produces hyperpnea, tachypnea, and respiratory alkalosis (Shoemaker, 1971, 1973, 1980).

Physiologic Defects Common to Shock States

The common physiologic denominator in the early period of the various shock states prior to the initial hypotension is not *low flow*, but inadequate oxygen transport from maldistribution of flow. The body's physiologic response to stresses, including the various etiologic types of shock, is increased cardiorespiratory function manifest by increased heart rate, myocardial contractility, and alveolar ventilation. The first two increase cardiac output unless there is reduced blood volume or reduced myocardial function. Metabolic acidosis occurs when hypovolemia and inadequate perfusion are present; this may be compensated by the increased ventilation. Respiratory alkalosis occurs from increased alveolar ventilation in the absence of hypovolemia.

Cardiorespiratory function increases from: 1) stimulation of cardiac centers of the brain stem by a generalized increase in autonomic nervous system activity due to the stress response; 2) cellular breakdown products, hyperthermia, vasoactive peptides, metabolic end products, and endotoxins; and 3) increased metabolic needs of the peripheral tissues. After these physiologic responses appear, many other physiologic changes occur, including cellular aggregation and other microrheologic changes, bradykinin cascade, coagulation cascade, etc. The increased metabolic requirements are reflected by increased oxygen delivery and $\dot{V}O_2$, which are seen in the middle (C_1 and C_2) stages of survivors and nonsurvivors as well as the late (D) stage of survivors.

THERAPEUTIC GOALS

It is axiomatic that shock should be recognized and treated as early as possible. Despite the plethora of therapeutic generalizations and admonitions, the priorities of shock treatment as well as the goals of therapy are controversial. To achieve maximal effectiveness, therapy must be directed toward the underlying pathophysiologic mechanisms. The normal hemodynamic values are not necessarily optimal, because the compensatory bodily responses to stress produce departures from the normal values. The major problem in the therapy of shock states is to define the therapeutic goals in terms of optimal physiologic criteria that result in reduced mortality and morbidity.

The cardiorespiratory patterns of survivors and nonsurvivors were described in a large series of critically ill patients subjected to major surgical procedures for life-threatening conditions. The data obtained remote from therapy were analyzed by the conventional statistical approach (mean ± SE) for each variable and by a nonparametric multivariate method that analyzes differences in the distributions of survivors' and nonsurvivors' values (Fig. 30.4). This was done: 1) to define therapeutic goals from the patterns of the survivors, 2) to provide early warning of circulatory deterioration and death from the pattern of nonsurvivors, 3) to evaluate the usefulness of each variable in terms of its capacity to predict outcome, and 4) to evaluate the severity of illness by means of a predictive index that relates the values of each variable to mortality (Shoemaker et al., 1979).

Despite the wide variety of illnesses and operations, there were marked differences in the patterns of survivors and nonsurvivors. In the early period, cardiac index, left ventricular stroke work, systemic vascular resistance, hematocrit, blood volume, O_2 delivery, and $\dot{V}O_2$ were greater in the survivors. The mean arterial pressures, CVP, heart rate, wedge pressure, PaO_2, and $P\bar{v}O_2$ values of the two groups were not significantly different in the early period; these variables were poor predictors and, therefore, were not very useful except as screening tests.

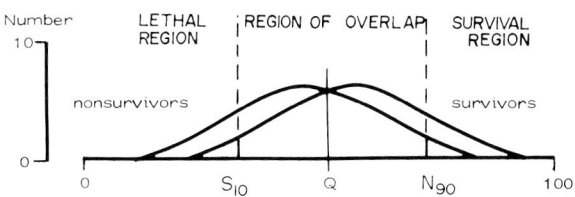

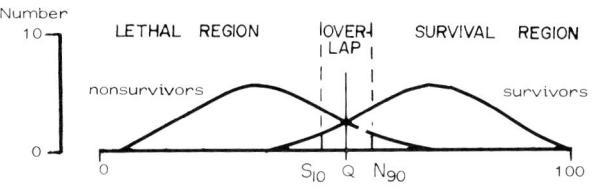

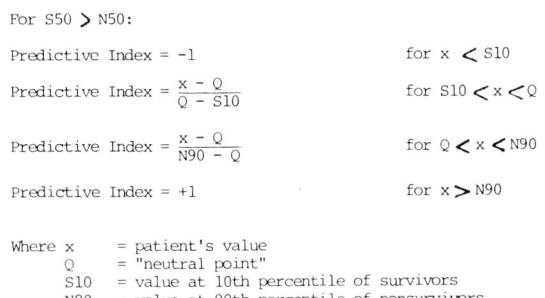

Figure 30.4. Idealized frequency distributions of survivors and nonsurvivors of a variable with wide overlap (*upper figure*) and with good separation (*lower figure*) showing the 10 percentile value of survivors (S_{10}), the 90 percentile value of nonsurvivors (N_{90}), and the classification point, Q, that maximally separates the survivors and nonsurvivors. The algorithm for calculation of the predictive index is given in the lower section of the figure. (Reprinted with permission from W. C. Shoemaker: In *Critical Care: State of the Art*, vol. 1, edited by W. C. Shoemaker and W. L. Thompson. Society of Critical Care Medicine, Fullerton, Calif., 1980.)

In the early period, nonsurvivors had slightly higher pulmonary arterial pressures, markedly higher pulmonary vascular resistance, and lower pH than did survivors. Table 30.1 shows the normal range of values for each variable as well as the preferred or "optimal" values defined as the median values of survivors of life-threatening postoperative conditions (Bland et al., 1978).

Wide differences in the distributions of survivors' and nonsurvivors' values for pulmonary vascular resistance, oxygen delivery, $\dot{V}O_2$, left and right ventricular stroke work, PCO_2, pH, and mean transit time make them useful as outcome predictors. However, no single variable was capable of accurately predicting outcome.

We developed an algorithm from the probability distributions of survivors' and nonsurvivors' values. This algorithm quantified the distance of each observed value of each cardiorespiratory variable from a single classification point that maximally separated the nonsurvivors' and survivors' values. A predictive or severity index was determined as the weighted average of all of these distances for all variables; this was found to be a reasonably sensitive, specific, and accurate predictor of outcome. We have used this index over the past 2 years to assess the severity of illness, to track the patient's cardiorespiratory status, and to evaluate the relative efficacy of alternate types of therapy (Shoemaker et al., 1979).

We also used the capacity of each cardiorespiratory variable to predict outcome correctly as a criterion of its biologic significance as well as its usefulness in clinical management (Shoemaker and Czer, 1979). That is, its usefulness in therapeutic decision making may be measured by its ability to differentiate the dying patient from the patient who survives. The percentage of correct predictions of outcome for each cardiorespiratory variable average over all stages are shown in Table 30.2. Unfortunately, these data showed that the poorest outcome predictors were usually the most commonly used monitoring variables.

The capability of cardiorespiratory variables to predict outcome at each stage may be expressed as the "percent correct predictions." These percentages change from stage to stage, indicating their specificity for early, middle, or late stages. For example, pulmonary vascular resistance (PVR) is a good predictor in the early stages (B, Low), but not in the middle or late stages. Mean arterial pressure (MAP) is a poor predictor in the early stages but is good in the late stages. Obviously, in the late stage, most variables predict outcome with a high degree of probability, but at this time clinical judgment also may be rather good and the need for prediction is less.

No single monitoring variable was entirely accurate as a predictor, because no one problem was responsible for all postoperative deaths; patients may succumb from a wide variety of physiologic conditions including hypovolemic, cardiac, pulmonary, septic, or peripheral perfusion problems. In general, our perfusion-related variables were found to be the best predictors, because they reflect interrelationships of O_2 transport with volume and flow (Tables 30.2 and 30.3). These perfusion variables do not just represent O_2 transport, blood flow, or volume by themselves, as each of these were separately assessed by individual variables. These variables quantify the peripheral perfusion in shock; they express the interactions of O_2 transport per unit of red cell flow or red cell mass. On the basis of these data, we have proposed a tentative list of preferred or "optimal" therapeutic goals in terms of cardiorespiratory variables (Table 30.1).

THERAPY

The therapeutic implications of this multivariate statistical analysis were integrated with cardiorespiratory data comparing the relative effectiveness of various therapeutic agents and with clinical experience in shock and trauma states. A protocol or clinical algorithm was developed for the management of the critically ill postoperative patient (Shoemaker, 1980). The general principles and priorities are briefly described below.

1. Control hemorrhage and restore blood volumes, maintain arterial pressures, and then volume load to about 500–1000 ml in excess of predicted norms unless CVP is greater than 15 cm water or wedge pressure is greater than 18 mm Hg (Shoemaker, 1980).

2. Maintain patent upper airway, and provide adequate ventilation.

3. Respiratory care, including: chest physical therapy, encourage coughing, endotracheal suction, turn patient

Table 30.2
Weights for Each Cardiorespiratory Variable, Averaged over Stages B, Low, C_1, C_2, and D, E, F. The Second Column Indicates the Ranking of the Average Weight from Highest (1) to Lowest (35). The Third Column Indicates the Number of Patients in Whom the Variable Was Measured, Summed over Stages B, Low, C_1, C_2, and D, E, F.

	Weight	Rank	N
Volume-related variables[a]			
MAP	.519	7	270
CVP	.241	32	270
CBV	.220	34	221
SI	.337	30	269
Hgb	.310	26	199
MPAP	.349	19	95
WP	.393	6	95
BV	.520	2	88
RCM	.693		88
Flow-related variables			
CI	.403	17	270
MTT	.418	15	221
LVSW	.474	12	269
LCW	.522	5	269
MSER	.314	29	214
TTI	.464	13	214
RVSW	.398	18	94
RCW	.365	23	94
Stress-related variables			
SVR	.238	33	270
PVR	.527	4	91
HR	.186	35	269
temp	.265	31	168
Oxygen transport-related variables			
SaO_2	.343	27	169
$PaCO_2$	.380	21	179
pH	.474	11	178
$P\bar{v}O_2$	.351	25	175
$a\bar{v}DO_2$	.357	24	174
O_2 deliv	.511	8	178
$\dot{V}O_2$	.383	20	174
O_2 ext	.366	22	174
Perfusion-related variables			
RCFR	.428	14	175
BFVR	.504	9	88
OTRM	.575	3	64
TOE	.498	10	150
ETOE	.819	1	64
OTRF	.415	16	150

[a] See Table 30.1 for abbreviations.

Table 30.3
Cardiorespiratory Variables with Weights Greater Than .50 and Less Than .25, in Each Stage[a,b]

	Stage B	Stage Low	Stage C$_1$	Stage C$_2$	Stages D, E, F
Weight greater than .50	ETOE PVR O$_2$ deliv RCM TOE WP MAP	ETOE ⎤ RCM ⎦ BFVR OTRM OTRF TOE TTI ⎤ pH ⎦ O$_2$ deliv ⎤ O$_2$ ext ⎦ LCW PVR P$\bar{v}$O$_2$	ETOE TOE	ETOE ⎤ OTRM ⎦ RVSW	ETOE ⎤ BV ⎦ RCM ⎤ BFVR ⎦ OTRM MAP LCW TTI LVSW O$_2$ deliv CI pH RVSW RCFR $\dot{V}$O$_2$
Weight less than .25	RCW RVSW CBV P$\bar{v}$O$_2$ SI HR	RVSW CBV CVP SVR HR PM	PaCO$_2$ MPAP LCW SaO$_2$ SVR Hgb temp pH CVP HR CBV	O$_2$ ext ⎤ a$\bar{v}$DO$_2$ ⎦ CVP SI TTI TOE P$\bar{v}$O$_2$ O$_2$ deliv RCFR PaCO$_2$ temp HR SVR	CBV

[a] Brackets indicate variables with the same weight. The largest weights are at the top of each column, and the smallest are at the bottom of each column.
[b] See Table 30.1 for abbreviations.

side to side every 2 hr, postural drainage, humidification of inspired air, avoid salt and water overload, oxygen via mask or nasopharyngeal catheter, tracheal intubation with mechanical ventilation when PaO$_2$ falls below 50–60 torr or PaCO$_2$ rises above 60 torr, enriched concentrations of inspired oxygen as needed to maintain PaO$_2$ above 70 torr but less than 120 torr.

4. Correct acid-base alterations: a) metabolic acidosis with sodium bicarbonate administration, fluids, improvement of blood flow; b) respiratory acidosis with endotracheal suction, bronchodilators, and mechanical ventilation; c) respiratory alkalosis by sedation, proper adjustment of the mechanical ventilation, increase in dead space, and addition of CO$_2$ to the inspired air; and d) metabolic alkalosis (when appreciable) with ammonium chloride or HCl.

5. Use cardiotonic agents for cardiac failure with pulmonary edema: inotropic agents (digitalis, isoproterenol, dolbutamide, calcium, and dopamine); fluid and salt restriction; diuretics; glucagon and glucose; antiarrhythmic agents; blocking agents such as nitroprusside, nitroglycerine, phentolamine, and chlorpromazine when fluid overload occurs; phlebotomy, ultrafiltration, or dialysis for large fluid overloads unresponsive to other therapy.

6. Resort to vasopressors when all other measures to correct hypotension have been tried and found ineffective.

7. Prevent or correct fluid maldistribution (i.e., excess interstitial water with deficient plasma volume) by adequate plasma expansion with oncotically active agents and by avoidance of salt and water overload from excessive volumes of sodium-rich solutions. After hemodynamic stability is achieved, correct extracellular overload by restriction of salt and water and by diuretics, such as furosemide, ethacrynic acid, mannitol, or 50% glucose; if these are ineffective, resort to dialysis.

8. Control infections—culture all potentially infected body fluids, drain abscesses or fluid collections, provide wound care, and give appropriate antibiotics.

9. Use steroids in high doses for septic and traumatic shock.

10. Provide for nutritional needs: 2000 or 3000 calories/day with hypertonic glucose, amino acids, and intravenous fat solution.

11. For coma or semiconsciousness that may be associated with cerebral edema, give high doses of steroids, urea, fluid and salt restriction, diuretics, adequate parenteral alimentation, etc.

12. Provide for psychologic and social needs.

SUMMARY

Understanding the pathophysiology of shock should be based upon descriptions of its natural physiologic history obtained from sequential cardiorespiratory measurements during periods remote from the therapeutic interventions. There are characteristic cardiorespiratory patterns of postoperative survivors and nonsurvivors of life-threatening illness despite the wide variety of illnesses and operations.

The early, common hemodynamic alteration in shock is not low cardiac output and high peripheral resistance; rather, it is inadequate tissue oxygenation due to uneven blood flow. Flow is not necessarily low; it may be normal or high, but it is maldistributed. Moreover, tissue oxygenation measured by $\dot{V}$O$_2$ is not necessarily low except in the early period; it may be normal or high, but it is inadequate for the increased metabolic needs. The most critical circulatory function is the transport of oxygen; therefore, the development of circulatory failure may be viewed in terms of the patterns of oxygen transport variables.

The major factor leading to maldistribution of microcirculatory flow is the imbalance between neurohumoral vasoconstriction and metabolic vasodilation. In high flow areas, more oxygen than needed may be carried through the wide open metarteriolar-capillary networks, but the blood oxygen is less completely extracted. This is because cells adjacent to the wide open capillary channel are able to extract only that amount that they themselves utilize, since oxygen cannot be stored. However, the oxygen supply to cells at a distance from the open capillaries is limited by diffusion of the gas across tissues. The perfusion defect of shock is manifest by low a$\bar{v}$DO$_2$, low oxygen extraction, and low or inadequate oxygen consumption in the presence of normal or high flow with normal or high oxygen delivery.

Tissue perfusion as well as the overall bulk oxygen transport may be adversely affected by hypoxemia from pulmonary insufficiency, anemia, and rheologic abnormalities. The perfusion defect may be self-perpetuating and may develop a negative feedback system; e.g., poor perfusion and oxygen transport to the heart may limit myocardial performance and result in further circulatory deterioration. Thus, the common peripheral perfusion defect arises from combinations of uneven vasoconstriction, metabolic vasodilation, redistribution of blood flow, redistribution of blood volume, and rheologic alterations including cellular aggregation. The net result is inadequate oxygenation relative to tissue requirements, which are often above the normal range. Because inadequate oxygen transport is the major pathophysiologic defect in circulatory shock syndrome, the most important physiologic goal is improved oxygen transport to peripheral tissues.

Cardiorespiratory measurements are also used to evaluate the relative effectiveness of various alternative types of therapy. Frequent intermittent or continuous monitoring of cardiorespiratory variables permits trend analysis and early warning of inadequate responses that may signal impending disaster.

Predictors of death and survival were defined by probability distributions of each variable and of the weighted sum of all variables. The latter overall predictor is used as a quantitative measure of the severity of illness; the outcome of a high percentage of patients may be predicted in the early period. The relative frequency with which each physiologic variable can identify survival or nonsurvival reflects the relevance of each of the variables to the pathophysiology of shock.

When the therapeutic goals are defined appropriately by the cardiorespiratory pattern of survivors, the principles of treatment can be arranged by priorities according to the life-threatening capability of each cardiorespiratory derangement. Furthermore, a well defined protocol may be developed for indications and precisely defined end points so that each therapy may be titrated to optimal goals.

References

Bland, R., Shoemaker, W.C., and Shabot, M.M.: Physiologic monitoring goals for the critically ill patient. Surg. Gynecol. Obstet. *147:*833, 1978.

Brown, R.S., et al.: Comparative evaluation of sympathomimetic amines in clinical shock. Circulation *34:*260, 1966.

Carey, J.S., et al.: Cardiovascular function in shock. Circulation *35:*327, 1967.

Courand, A., et al.; Studies of the circulation in clinical shock. Surgery *13:*964, 1943.

Matsuda, H., and Shoemaker, W.C.: Cardiorespiratory responses to dextran-40. Arch. Surg. *110:*296, 1974a.

Matsuda, H., and Shoemaker, W.C.: Survivors' and nonsurvivors' responses to dextran 40: Hemodynamic and oxygen transport changes in critically ill patients. Arch. Surg. *110:*301, 1974b.

Mohr, P.A., et al.: Sequential cardiorespiratory events during and after dextran-40 infusion in normal and shock patients. Circulation *39:*379, 1969.

Shoemaker, W.C.: Cardiorespiratory patterns in complicated and uncomplicated septic shock. Ann. Surg. *174:*119, 1971.

Shoemaker, W.C.: Pathophysiologic basis of therapy for shock and trauma syndromes. Semin. Drug. Treat. *3:*211, 1973.

Shoemaker, W.C.: Effects of transfusion on surviving and nonsurviving postoperative patients. Surg. Gynecol. Obstet. *142:*33-40, 1976.

Shoemaker, W.C.: Pathophysiology, monitoring and therapy of shock syndromes. In *Critical Care: State of the Art*, vol. 1, edited by W.C. Shoemaker and W.L. Thompson. Society of Critical Care Medicine, Fullerton, CA, 1980.

Shoemaker, W.C., and Czer, L.S.C.: Evaluation of the biologic importance of various hemodynamic and oxygen transport variables. Crit. Care Med. *7:*424, 1979.

Shoemaker, W.C., et al.: Hemodynamic patterns after acute anesthetized and unanesthetized trauma. Arch. Surg. *95:*492, 1967.

Shoemaker, W.C., et al.: Sequential hemodynamic events after trauma to the unanesthetized patient. Surg. Gynecol. Obstet. *132:*651, 1971a.

Shoemaker, W.C., et al.: Sequential oxygen transport and acid-base changes after trauma to the unanesthetized patient. Surg. Gynecol. Obstet. *132:*1023, 1971b.

Shoemaker, W.C., et al.: Physiologic patterns in surviving and nonsurviving shock patients. Arch. Sug. *106:*630, 1973.

Shoemaker, W.C., et al.: Cardiorespiratory monitoring in postoperative patients. Crit. Care Med. *7:*237, 1979.

Slater, G., et al.: Sequential changes in the distribution of cardiac output in various stages of experimental hemorrhagic shock. Surgery *73:*714, 1973.

Wiggers, C.J.: *Physiology of Shock*. Commonwealth Fund, New York, 1950.

CHAPTER 31

Transfusion Therapy in Hemorrhagic Shock

PAUL R. SOHMER
R. BEN DAWSON

The technological advances which have fostered the development of modern hemotherapy have occurred in parallel with or in response to an increased understanding of the treatment requirements of patients in hemorrhagic shock. The discovery of red cell antigenicity and the development of blood preservation strategies have, in fact, made the treatment of shock possible. Therefore, it is appropriate that this text should include a chapter devoted to a description of the characteristics of the primary therapeutic agent of hemorrhagic shock: stored blood.

Rationale for Transfusion: Fick Equation

$$VO_2 = Q \times 1.39 \text{ Hb} \times (SaO_2 - SvO_2)$$

Because the basic underlying pathophysiologic defect of hemorrhagic shock is impaired oxygen transport, the Fick equation, which quantitatively defines oxygen delivery, is readily applied as a guide to the priorities of its treatment. Three principal variables are described that have a direct effect on oxygen delivery: blood flow, hemoglobin concentration, and the fractional unloading of oxygen from hemoglobin.

The first priority of treatment is restoration of blood volume and blood flow. As predicted by the Fick equation, even when commenced with a non-oxygen-carrying solution, volume resuscitation alone will improve oxygen delivery and increase oxygen consumption (Shoemaker and Bryan-Brown, 1973). The second and third variables of the Fick equation describe the "functional" oxygen content of arterial blood—i.e., the concentration of red cell hemoglobin that is available to carry oxygen and the ability of hemoglobin to carry, bind, and release oxygen. This has traditionally been translated to mean that the second priority of resuscitation is restoration of the red cell mass. In the context of the Fick equation, this maxim makes two basic assumptions about the restored red cell mass. First, it should consist of *viable* red cells whose hemoglobin is maintained intact and will circulate for an appropriate length of time; and second, that these red cells are *functional* and will readily release oxygen to body tissues.

Although developed to optimally maintain red cell viability and function, the presently available methodologies for in vitro blood preservation are of a limited capacity. The efficiency of a blood preservation system is best measured by its impact on the patient and his or her response to therapy. This is dependent on the effects of collection and storage, on the viability and function of blood elements, and the presence of potentially toxic, storage-related by-products that accumulate in vitro. The impact is greatest in the patient treated for hemorrhagic shock who has required the transfusion of large volumes of stored blood. In this chapter, we propose to place our present knowledge of the characteristics of stored blood in proper perspective relative to the treatment of hemorrhagic shock. Given the context of shock, anoxia, and ischemia, we will concentrate on the red blood cell.

VIABILITY

Adenosine Triphosphate (ATP)

Having lost its intracellular organelles during maturation, the red cell lacks the capacity for mitochondrial respiration and fatty acid and protein synthesis. Only anaerobic glycolysis and the hexose monophosphate shunt remain to support its metabolic obligations. Approximately 90% of the total glucose consumed is metabolized via the glycolytic pathway (Murphy, 1960). The major products of this metabolic pathway are the organic phosphates, adenosine triphosphate (ATP) and 2,3-diphosphoglycerate (2,3-DPG) (see below).

The anaerobic metabolism of glucose may, of itself, be dependent on the presence of ATP. Since its depletion may inhibit the initial (hexokinase) and rate-limiting (phosphofructokinase) steps of glycolysis, ATP may actually serve as a pH-dependent regulator of glucose metabolism (Rapoport, 1968). A transformation in red cell shape from disc to sphere (Weed and LaCelle, 1969; Weed et al., 1969) and decreased membrane deformability (LaCelle, 1969), which is associated with a reduction in intraerythrocytic ATP, may inhibit the passage of red blood cells through small tortuous vessels and hasten their removal from the circulation. Although there is no clear relationship between these physicostructural changes and diminished red cell survival, it is generally accepted that the intraerythrocytic concentration of ATP is an important determinant of red cell viability (Nakao et al., 1962; Dern et al., 1967). Although at times this relationship may be tenuous, because exceptions are often encountered, blood preservation systems geared to maintain red cell viability for prolonged periods of in vitro storage have traditionally evolved from efforts directed at maintaining red cell ATP.

Blood Preservative Solutions

A blood preservation solution should be nontoxic, relatively inert, have in vitro anticoagulant effects that are rapidly reversed in vivo, sustain red cell viability and function, and minimize the accumulation of toxic storage-related by-products.

Since its introduction by Lewisohn (1915) in 1914, sodium citrate has served as the basic anticoagulant preservative for most liquid blood preservation systems. The utility of this solution is severely limited since after 1 week only 50% of red cells so stored will remain viable (Ross et al., 1947). Rous and Turner (1916) demonstrated that the addition of glucose improves the maintenance of red cell viability. The acidification of this citrate-dextrose solution (acid citrate dextrose (ACD)) by Loutit et al. (Loutit and Mollison, 1943; Loutit et al., 1943) resulted in a preservative solution that could be relied upon to maintain a standard minimum of 70% 24-hr post-transfusion red cell survival for up to 21 days of storage at 4°C.

In an effort to preserve red cell viability for longer storage periods, to reduce the acid load attendant with transfusions of blood stored in ACD, and to minimize the detrimental effects of storage and collection, Gibson et al. (1957) introduced a phosphate-containing, higher pH preservative, citrate phosphate dextrose (CPD) in 1957. In the original report, storage in this preservative resulted in reduced hemolysis, reduced leakage of potassium, and improved red cell survival. Later comparisons of CPD with ACD indicate that viability is only somewhat better preserved in CPD. However, due to its higher pH (Dawson et al., 1970), CPD maintains 2,3-DPG and red cell hemoglobin function far better than does ACD. After 1 week in CPD, 2,3-DPG is nearly normal or only slightly less than normal; whereas, in ACD 2,3-DPG falls to a level that is approximately 40% of control (de Verdier et al., 1972). Due to its better maintenance of red cell function, CPD has displaced ACD as the most widely used blood preservative solution in the United States.

In 1960, Nakao et al. demonstrated that the addition of the purine nucleotides, adenine and inosine, would promote ATP synthesis. Simon (1962) made practical use of this phenomenon when he demonstrated that the addition of adenine to blood stored in ACD preserved red cell viability such that a 24-hr post-transfusion red cell survival of 72% was achieved after 42 days in storage, as compared to 42% in ACD controls. As a result, an ACD-adenine preservative solution has been used in Europe since the mid-1960s. Its acceptance in the United States was delayed in part because of concern regarding the possible nephrotoxic effects of the adenine metabolite, 2,8-dioxyadenine (2,8-DOA) (see below). In 1978 a CPD-adenine solution, CPDA-1, received Food and Drug Administration approval for the in vitro preservation of blood for up to 35 days (Federal Register, 1978).

In Vivo Viability

For practical purposes, viability may be defined in terms of the percent of transfused red cells which survive 24 hr after transfusion. Red cells that survive this initial post-transfusion period exhibit a normal life-span. By convention, a blood preservative solution must ensure a minimum 70% 24-hr post-transfusion survival of red cells. This implies that a minimum 2% increment in hematocrit is expected following the infusion of 1 unit of packed red cells (Hct = 75%) in a 70-kg recipient. When viability is better preserved, as in blood stored for shorter periods or when an improved preservative formulation is utilized, a higher post-transfusion increment and reduced transfusion requirements are anticipated. For example, in general, approximately 75–80% of transfused red cells stored in CPD for 21 days will survive the initial 24 hr after transfusion, whereas approximately 85–90% of those stored for 21 days in CPD-A1 will survive. This average increase of 10% viable red cells suggests that, in practice, a typical major surgery case that requires eight units of blood stored for 21 days in CPD might require only seven units of blood stored in CPD-A1.

The Burden of Preservation: Chemical Changes in Stored Blood

Blood preservative solutions have been developed to maintain red cell viability during blood bank storage as reviewed in the two previous sections. This section will review the other pertinent changes that occur, except for the defect in oxygen transport function that develops as red cell 2,3-DPG levels decrease. Hemoglobin's cofactor for normal red cell function, 2,3-DPG, will be discussed in the final section.

Multiple biochemical changes occur during blood storage. These may alter the response to therapy and add to the risk of transfusion. One must anticipate that the transfusion of large quantities of bank blood will cause significant physiological changes. Applying the mathematics of exchange transfusion (Marsaglia and Thomas, 1971), it is clear that when 50% of the blood volume has been lost and 10 units of bank blood transfused, only 28% of original blood elements and plasma remain; after 20 units of bank blood, only 11% remain; and after 30 units of bank blood, only 4% of original blood elements remain (Collins, 1974; Gill and Champion, 1974).

COAGULATION

After 48 hr of in vitro storage, blood is essentially devoid of functional platelets (Murphy and Gardner, 1969). Regardless of pretransfusion levels, thrombocytopenia accompanies the massive transfusion of bank blood. Platelet deficiencies are common after the infusion of 10 or more units of bank blood. Platelet counts of $40,000/mm^3$–$70,000/mm^3$ are often recorded after the transfusion of 20 units of bank blood. In general, these deficiencies need not be replaced. With normal bone marrow function, the platelet count is restored to normal within 7–10 days. However, in the face of active bleeding it is appropriate to administer platelet concentrates in anticipation of severe thrombocytopenia. In general, 6 units of platelet concentrates given with each 20 units of bank blood are adequate.

Coagulation factors V and VIII are labile in storage. These factor levels deteriorate 50% within 7 days of donation. However, fibrinogen and other stable factors are retained in stored blood. The massive transfusion of stored blood may be associated with a dilutional defect in coagulation due to a deficiency of factors V and VIII. Depression of fibrinogen and other stable factors in association with factors V and VIII suggests the presence of an underlying consumptive process. Transfusion of 2–4 units of fresh frozen plasma given for each 10 units of bank blood usually prevents dilution coagulopathy.

CITRATE TOXICITY

Citrate actively binds ionized calcium. Although ionized calcium levels are reduced in the transfused patient, recovery is rapidly achieved when transfusion is terminated. Citrate is rapidly metabolized and excreted in the urine. Parathyroid hormone is released in response to citrate, causing a rapid mobilization of endogenous calcium (Blum et al., 1974). As a result, toxic levels are attained only when large volumes of citrate are rapidly infused or when impaired liver function, circulation, or hypothermia inhibit citrate metabolism (Howland et al., 1957). Exchange-transfused neonates and adults with impaired liver function are at greatest risk. Skeletal muscle tremors, cardiac arrhythmias, and cardiac arrest have been observed during the exchange transfusion of newborn infants.

The routine administration of calcium at predetermined transfusion intervals is not recommended since it may be associated with iatrogenically induced hypercalcemia and myocardial hyperexcitability (Wolf et al., 1970). If hypotension and cardiac arrythmias occur as the result of low ionized calcium levels, 0.3 g of calcium chloride or 2–10 ml of 10% calcium gluconate solution will adequately replace ionized calcium. The infusion of citrate and its toxic effects are reduced with packed red cells and are avoided when washed, frozen-thawed, or heparinized blood is used.

POTASSIUM

The plasma concentration of potassium in blood stored in CPD at 4°C for 21 days is approximately 20–30 mEg/liter as compared to 5 mEq/liter in fresh donor plasma. This increase in plasma potassium occurs independently of red cell hemolysis. Most of this potassium represents leakage from stored red cells due to depletion of adenosine triphosphate. After the transfusion of viable red cells this lesion is corrected and the ATP-dependent sodium-potassium pump resumes its function, taking in potassium and expelling sodium (Valeri, 1971). Indeed, it is fairly well documented that the majority of massively transfused patients have normal or low plasma potassium levels (Bunker et al., 1955; Schweizer and Howland, 1962; Wilson et al., 1971).

With prolonged storage and decreasing ATP content, the percentage of nonviable red cells will increase. The percentage of nonviable red cells after storage in CPD for 7 days is 3%, at 14 days it is 15%, and at 21 days it is 20–25% (Simon and Bove, 1971). The lysis of these cells in the first 24 hr after transfusion is associated with an increase in plasma potassium.

Although removal of the supernatant plasma reduces the potassium load, one must anticipate a possible increase in the recipient's plasma potassium concentration due to hemolytic release from cells rendered nonviable during storage. As a result, the patient in whom an increased potassium load cannot be tolerated should be transfused with blood that is less than 5 days old. In combination with removal of the supernatant, cell washing, if necessary, should adequately reduce the risk of hyperkalemia.

ACID BASE

The acidity of bank blood (pH = 6.8 at 21 days in CPD) is due to the citrate present and the lactate (5–9 mEq/liter at 21 days) accumulated during storage. These are both rapidly metabolized by the recipient after transfusion. When tissue perfusion is well maintained, alterations in acid-base balance are managed without difficulty. Buffering with 44.6 mEq of sodium bicarbonate for each 5 units of blood has been advocated. However, iatrogenically induced alkalinemia will cause an increase in the patient's hemoglobin-oxygen affinity and a reduction in ionized calcium levels.

AMMONIA

Blood stored for 21 days may have an ammonia content of 900 µg/dl as compared to 100 µg/dl in fresh blood. Therefore, the transfusion of large volumes of stored blood to patients in liver failure may be dangerous. Washed or frozen-thawed red cells are preferred for these patients.

HYPOTHERMIA

The rapid infusion of blood stored at 4°C may cause a sudden drop in the patient's temperature. This is not a problem unless large volumes of stored blood are administered. Even 3 or 4 units are well tolerated when administered at a slow and controlled rate of infusion. Hypothermia may be adversive for the following reasons: it will increase hemoglobin-oxygen affinity, increase potassium leakage from red cells, may cause cardiac arrhythmia, and may inhibit citrate metabolism. Hypothermia may be prevented by warming blood to no more than 37°C by passage through coils immersed in a water bath or a dry incubator. Hemolysis may occur if the blood temperature exceeds 40°C. The warming of blood is required only when large volumes are rapidly infused or when the recipient has a potent cold-reacting antibody.

MICROAGGREGATES

When blood is stored at between 1°C and 6°C for more than 7 days, degradation products consisting of platelets, leukocytes, and fibrin strands precipitate to form microaggregates in the buffy coat layer of blood. Since these microaggregates range in size from 10 to 164 μ, they are not removed by the standard 170-μ blood filter. Transfusion of large volumes of bank blood may be associated with the delivery of large numbers of microaggregates to the circulation. Some studies have attributed post-transfusion pulmonary (Hessen and Swank, 1965; McNamara et al., 1972; Reul et al., 1974; Swank and Porter, 1968), brain (Hirsch et al., 1964), and renal (Jenevein and Weiss, 1964) dysfunction to entrapments of microaggregates. Considering the amount of particulate matter that may be delivered when large volumes of blood are transfused, it may be prudent to pass blood through a microaggregate filter system, although the value of such filtration is still unclear. Because microaggregates are made large enough by "hard centrifugation" to be filtered by the standard blood filter and removal by cell washing (Solis and Gibbs, 1972) techniques, packed or frozen-thawed red cells need not be passed through a microaggregate filter. When a microaggregate filter is used, there is increased resistance to flow after the passage of 2 or more units of stored blood.

ADENINE

Moore et al. (Moore and Ledford, 1977; Moore et al., 1978) have studied the distribution of adenine between plasma and red cells as well as the disappearance kinetics of intra- and extracellular adenine throughout 21–42 days' blood storage in CPDA-1. Less than 30% of the original 17.3 mg of adenine is available after 21 days' whole blood storage. A similar study with whole blood showed that less than 13% of the original adenine preservative content is available after 35 days' and less than 11% after 42 days' storage. Blood stored as concentrated red cells contains less than 50% of the free adenine in whole blood due to the removal of adenine-rich plasma during preparation of concentrated red cell units.

Nephrotoxicity is the principal acute adverse effect in animals and humans resulting from adenine administration (Philips et al., 1952); it is thought to be related to precipitation of the poorly soluble metabolite of adenine, DOA, in the urinary tract.

Only one human case of proven adenine toxicity has been reported (Stone and Spies, 1948). In this patient, approximately 71.4 mg/kg (assumes body weight of 70 kg) per day for 5 days were administered orally in an attempt to treat pernicious anemia. The patient developed severe uremia but recovered almost completely (residual blood urea nitrogen of 38 mg was the only abnormality).

One case of possible toxicity resulting from administration of an adenine-containing blood product has been reported (Falk et al., 1972). One hundred eighteen units of ACD-A (adenine 95 mg/kg) were administered during a 5-day period to a postoperative cardiac surgery patient. Evidence for adenine toxicity included impaired renal function and postmortem demonstration of renal calculi that were morphologically similar to DOA. However, this patient had transient serum creatinine elevations prior to receipt of ACD-A blood and experienced multiple episodes of hypotension and shock in the postoperative period. In spite of the combined effects of shock and possible adenine toxicity, a diuresis was maintained until just before death. Death was attributed to hemorrhagic shock.

Numerous studies attest to the safety of intravenous administration of adenine to humans in doses up to 15 mg/kg (equivalent to 60 units of fresh CPDA-1 whole blood). No immediate or long-term (5-yr follow-up) toxicity has been detected despite extensive renal function tests (Peck et al., 1980). Roth et al. (1975), for example, assessed glomerular function (creatinine clearance, urinary protein excretion), proximal tubular function (urinary excretion of glucose and 15 amino acids), and distal tubular function (maximal urinary acidifying and concentrating ability) and found no adverse effect of intravenous infusion of adenine, 5 and 10 mg/kg in normal volunteers. Complete exchange transfusions with adenine-fortified blood in neonates had no detectable physical, biochemical, or renal effects acutely and up to 5 yr later (Kreuger, 1973).

Consideration of an upper adenine dose limit has relied upon the demonstrated safety of rapid intravenous infusion of 10–15 mg/kg. On this basis, Simon (1977) suggested that up to 30 fresh, 0.5 mM adenine (e.g., ACD-A or CPD-2A) whole blood units or 60 fresh, 0.25 mM adenine (e.g., CPDA-1) whole blood units could be safely transfused. However, it must be recognized that the safety of this dosage was established in healthy adult volunteers. Recipients of adenine blood products who are hypotensive, dehydrated, or have compromised renal function may be at increased risk for precipitation of DOA crystals and subsequent renal parenchymal damage. However, mere demonstration of DOA crystals in the urine of a recipient of adenine blood is not sufficient evidence for "adenine toxicity." Like uric acid crystalluria, DOA crystals may precipitate from a drop of urine placed on a cold microscope slide, although the compound was soluble in urine at body temperature. Peck et al. (1977) suggested that up to 25 fresh CPDA-1 whole blood units can be given over a relatively short period of time without formation of DOA crystals in the urine in vivo.

FUNCTION

2,3-Diphosphoglycerate

The post-transfusion survival of red blood cells determines the transfused red cell mass and hemoglobin concentration and, in part, determines the efficacy of transfusion. However, storage-induced furnctional alterations that impair the oxygen transport and delivery mechanism without affecting red cell survival may limit this therapeutic effect. A functional defect reflected in an increase in hemoglobin oxygen affinity is demonstrable after storage in citrate solutions at 4°C. The transfusion of large volumes of stored blood may cause a "left shift" of the oxygen hemoglobin dissociation curve and a reduction in the volume of oxygen delivered at a given oxygen tension (Valtis and Kennedy, 1954). This phenomenon is closely correlated with the duration of in vitro blood storage and occurs as the result of a storage-related depletion of 2,3-DPG (Akerblom et al., 1968; Bunn et al., 1969). A linear relationship exists between stored red cell 2,3-DPG content and P_{50} (a term of convenience for hemoglobin oxygen affinity that designates the oxygen tension (torr) at which hemoglobin is 50% saturated with oxygen).

Theoretically, acute elevation of hemoglobin oxygen affinity may result in impaired oxygen delivery. However, unless examined under conditions that accurately reflect human pathophysiology, the effect of 2,3-DPG and the oxygen dissociation curve cannot be isolated nor their significance adequately evaluated. Inasmuch as oxygen transport and delivery are accomplished as the result of the cumulative effect of multiple factors, the impact of 2,3-DPG must be defined relative to a complex mechanism. Oxygen transport is dependent on blood flow and hemoglobin concentration as well as the ability of red cells to bind, carry, and release oxygen. In vivo oxygen transport is influenced by numerous factors, including PCO_2, pH, and temperature. These contribute to a compensatory response that may minimize the effects of an acute elevation of hemoglobin oxygen affinity. In addition, the regeneration of 2,3-DPG and correction of the oxygen dissociation curve begin shortly after transfusion (Beutler and Wood, 1969; Valeri and Hirsch, 1969). In fact, recipient hemoglobin oxygen affinity returns to normal 24 hr after transfusion (Valtis and Kennedy, 1954). In the individual who is not otherwise compromised, cardiovascular homeostatic mechanisms appear to compensate for impaired red cell function.

Because of the rate at which the alteration in hemoglobin oxygen affinity due to blood storage is corrected and the adaptive potential of the human body, it would appear that transfused blood, as presently prepared and stored, is adequate for most conditions requiring transfusion. This would include the anemia of chronic renal failure, aplastic anemia, and anemias associated with malignancy. However, in the recipient whose capacity for compensation is limited by an underlying physiologic disturbance, the time required for regeneration of 2,3-DPG and correction of the hemoglobin oxygen affinity lesion of stored blood may not be tolerated.

Because the regulation of cardiac output and blood flow is an important compensatory mechanism, compromised myocardial performance may render impotent the patient's facility for physiologic adaption. In this setting, an acute elevation of hemoglobin oxygen affinity may be detrimental. In fact, when the elasticity of the coronary artery is lost, as in severe atherosclerotic heart disease, a reduction in hemoglobin oxygen affinity will occur as a compensation for reduced blood flow in the face of high oxygen extraction and low coronary sinus oxygen tensions (Shappell et al., 1970). Holsinger et al. (1973) studied the effects of transfusion with high hemoglobin oxygen affinity, low 2,3-DPG blood in dogs that were convalescing several weeks after sustaining anterior myocardial infarctions induced by coronary artery ligation. Immediately following perfusion, the left ventricle of all experimental animals failed. Ischemia and injury were demonstrable by the inversion of electrocardiographic T waves and elevation of the ST segments. This study suggests that an acute elevation of the hemoglobin oxygen affinity due to transfusion with blood depleted of 2,3-DPG may precipitate the decompensation of a borderline heart.

The combined effects of impaired myocardial function and elevated hemoglobin oxygen affinity that are often encountered following cardiopulmonary bypass may be circumvented by transfusion of blood that is rich in 2,3-DPG. Dennis et al. (1975) studied 22 matched patients with severe atherosclerotic heart disease who were subjected to extracorporeal circulation during coronary artery bypass surgery. Postoperative myocardial function was evaluated relative to intra- and preoperative transfusions with blood whose red cell 2,3-DPG content was 70% of normal or red cells that had been chemically rejuvenated to raise their 2,3-DPG content to 150% of normal. Immediately following the termination of cardiopulmonary bypass, those patients who had received high 2,3-DPG, low hemoglobin oxygen affinity blood exhibited a trend toward improved cardiac index and increased oxygen consumption. Myocardial performance as measured by the response to fluid challenge was significantly improved in these patients. This augmented cardiac function was associated with an increase in in vivo P_{50}, red cell 2,3-DPG content, oxygen consumption, and arteriovenous oxygen difference. In addition, morbidity and mortality were reduced in these patients. Although marred by a lack of strict experimental control, this study suggests that the improved oxygen delivery achieved in patients receiving high 2,3-DPG, low hemoglobin oxygen affinity blood transfusions may have clinical significance in patients whose facility for cardiopulmonary compensation is compromised by an underlying disease process.

In resuscitation from hemorrhagic shock, where the restoration of fluid volume and red cell mass are of primary importance, the impact of 2,3-DPG is not well defined. Bowen and Fleming (1974) could not identify a detrimental effect of measured oxygen transport variables in 15 combat casualties resuscitated with large volumes of stored blood. The facility for physiologic adaptation in these patients was such that the detrimental effects of a temporary impairment of red cell function could be tolerated. Rice et al. (1975) observed an improved clinical condition that required less hemodynamic compensation in baboons resuscitated with chemically rejuvenated 2,3-DPG-enriched red blood cells. Resuscitation with red cells depleted of 2,3-DPG placed a greater burden on the cardiorespiratory system as the demands for hemodynamic compensation were increased. This suggests that the patient in whom hemorrhagic shock is complicated by pre-existing heart or lung disease may be at further risk if resuscitation is attempted with 2,3-DPG-depleted, high oxygen affinity blood.

Persistent anemia in the face of hemorrhage may compromise the patient such that an acute elevation of hemoglobin oxygen affinity may be detrimental. Huggins et al. (1971) reported that rats exchange transfused with normal 2,3-DPG red cells tolerated hemodilution to severe anemia with dextran significantly better than those who had been exchange transfused with red cells depleted of 2,3-DPG. Collins (1976) observed an increase in mortality in rats who were exchange transfused with 2,3-DPG-depleted blood if the animal's red cell mass was reduced to 50% of control. Woodson (1976) observed a shortened survival in hypotensive rats treated with 2,3-DPG-depleted red blood cells.

Collins (1978) sought to better define the relationship between hematocrit, 2,3-DPG, P_{50}, and survival by studying the response of rats to exchange transfusion, hemorrhage, and resuscitation with stored (low 2,3-DPG) and fresh (normal 2,3-DPG) blood. At normal hematocrits, depletion of 2,3-DPG had little effect on survival after hemorrhage. However, when animals were hemodiluted to half-normal hematocrits, there was a significant reduction in survival after hemorrhage in rats who had been exchange transfused with low 2,3-DPG blood. Similarly, the ability of low 2,3-DPG blood to rescue rats from anemia and severe hemorrhage was significantly less than that of fresh blood. This study suggests that if anemia is avoided even extensive exchange transfusion with 2,3-DPG-depleted blood is an acceptable treatment for hemorrhage. However, if anemia persists, depletion of 2,3-DPG may adversely affect survival. Alternatively, maintenance and elevation of 2,3-DPG and P_{50} may improve the oxygen delivery capacity of an anemic animal such that transfusion to a normal hematocrit is not required. This suggests that the in vivo maintenance and augmentation of P_{50} and 2,3-DPG may provide a therapeutic adjunct that would decrease or delay the need for blood transfusion.

CONCLUSION

Multiple biochemical changes reflect the "lesion(s) of storage." These may alter the expected response to transfusion and add to the risk of therapy. Because of the frequent requirement for the massive transfusion of stored blood, the patient who is treated for life-threatening hemorrhage is at greatest risk of suffering the adverse effects of transfusion. Alterations in acid-base balance, citrate toxicity, hypothermia, hyperkalemia (or hypokalemia), microembolization, and deficiencies in platelet and coagulation factor activity and hemoglobin function all may have a significant impact on the patient's response to transfusion. A management strategy, then, should be devised so as to minimize adverse effects of transfusion.

The efficacy of transfusion therapy is dependent on the innate characteristics of the blood elements themselves. Rational therapy depends on a clear understanding of the characteristics of the therapeutic agents administered. However, except for the measurement of post-transfusion hematocrit and hemoglobin concentration, the physiologic effects of red cell transfusions are often ignored, particularly in the resuscitation setting. As described in the present chapter, recently acquired knowledge suggests that the impact of blood storage may extend far beyond its effects on red cell mass, hematocrit, and hemoglobin concentration. Although presently available blood preservation methodologies ensure the viability of transfused red blood cells, a functional abnormality of hemoglobin occurs that may significantly alter the response to therapy.

References

Akerblom, O., de Verdier, C.H., Garby, L., and Hogman, C.F.: Restoration of defective oxygen transport function of stored red blood cells by addition of inosine. Scand. J. Clin. Lab. Invest. 21:245, 1968.

Beutler, E., and Wood, L.: The in vivo regeneration of red cell 2,3-diphosphoglycerate acid (DPG) after transfusion of stored blood. J. Lab. Clin. Med. 74:300, 1969.

Blum, J.W., Mayer, G.P., and Potts, J.T.: Parathyroid hormone responses during spontaneous hypocalcemia and induced hypercalcemia in cows. Endocrinology 95:84, 1974.

Bowen, J.C., and Fleming, W.H.: Increased oxyhemoglobin affinity after transfusion. Ann. Surg. 180:760, 1974.

Bunker, J.P., Stetson, J.B., Coe, R.C., et al.: Citric acid intoxication. J.A.M.A. 157:1361, 1955.

Bunn, H.F., May, M.H., Kocholaty, W.F., and Shields, C.F.: Hemoglobin function of stored blood. J. Clin. Invest. 48:311, 1969.

Collins, J.A.: Problems associated with massive transfusion of stored blood. Surgery 75:274, 1974.

Collins, J.A.: Massive transfusion. Clin. Haematol. 5:201, 1976.

Collins, J.A.: The age and hematocrit of stored blood in determining the survival of rats after exchange transfusion and hemorrhage. In *The Red Cell*, edited by G. Brewer, p. 617. Plenum Press, New York, 1978.

Dawson, R.B., Kocholaty, W.F., and Gray, J.L.: Hemoglobin function and 2,3-DPG levels of blood stored at 4°C in ACD and CPD: pH effect. Transfusion 10:299, 1970.

Dennis, R.C., Vito, L., Weisel, R.D., Valeri, C.R., Berger, R.L., and Hectman, H.B.: Improved myocardial performance following high 2,3-diphosphoglycerate red cell transfusions. Surgery 77:41, 1975.

Dern, R.J., Brewer, G.J., and Wirokowski, J.J.: Studies on the preservation of human blood: The relationship of erythrocyte adenosine triphosphate levels and other in vivo measures to red cell storageability. J. Lab. Clin. Med. 69:968, 1967.

de Verdier, C.H., Akerblom, O., Arturson, G., Garby, L., Hogman, C.F., Kreuger, A., and Westman, M.: Maintenance of oxygen transport function of stored blood. In *Communications of the 13th Congress, International Society of Blood Transfusion*, Washington, DC, 1972.

Falk, J.S., Lindblad, T.O., and Westman, B.J.M.: Histopathological studies on kidneys from patients treated with large amounts of blood preserved with ACD adenine. Transfusion 12:376, 1972.

Federal Register, May 26, 1978.

Gibson, J.G., Rees, S.B., McManus, T.J., and Scheitlin, W.A.: A citrate-phosphate-dextrose solution for the preservation of human blood. Am. J. Clin. Pathol. 28:569, 1957.

Gill, W., and Champion, H.R.: Volume resuscitation in critical major trauma. In *Transfusion Therapy*, edited by R. B. Dawson, p. 77. AABB, Washington, DC, 1974.

Hessen, W., and Swank, R.L.: Screen filtration pressure and pulmonary hypertension. Am. J. Physiol. *209*:715, 1965.

Hirsch, H., Swank, R.L., Brener, M., et al.: Screen filtration pressure of homologous and heterologous blood and electroencephalogram. Am. J. Physiol. *206*:811, 1964.

Holsinger, J.W., Salhany, J.M., and Eliot, R.S.: Physiologic observations on the effects of impaired blood oxygen release on the myocardium. Adv. Cardiol. *9*:81, 1973.

Howland, W.S., Bellville, J.W., Zucker, M.B., et al.: Massive blood replacement. V. Failure to observe citrate intoxication. Surg. Gynecol. Obstet. *105*:529, 1957.

Huggins, C.E., Suzuki, H., and Grove-Rasmussen, M.: Life support by liquid and frozen blood. Presented at the 24th Annual Meeting, American Association Blood Banks, Chicago, 1971.

Jenevein, E.P., Jr., and Weiss, D.L.: Platelet microemboli associated with massive blood transfusion. Am. J. Pathol. *45*:313, 1964.

Kreuger, A.O.: Exchange transfusion with ACD-adenine blood: A follow-up study. Transfusion *13*:69, 1973.

LaCelle, P.C.: Alterations of deformability of the erythrocyte in stored blood. Transfusion *9*:238, 1969.

Lewisohn, R.: Blood transfusion by the citrate method. Surg. Gynecol. Obstet. *21*:37, 1915.

Loutit, J.F., and Mollison, P.L.: Advantages of a disodium-citrate-glucose mixture as a blood preservative. Br. Med. J. *2*:744, 1943.

Loutit, J.F., Mollison, P.L. and Young, I. M.: Citric acid-sodium-citrate-glucose mixtures for blood storage. Q. J. Exp. Physiol. *32*:183, 1943.

Marsaglia, G., and Thomas, E.D.: Mathematical consideration of cross circulation and exchange transfusion. Transfusion *11*:216, 1971.

McNamara, J.J., Burran, E.L., and Laeson, E.: Effect of debris in stored blood on pulmonary microvasculature. Ann. Thorac. Surg. *14*:133, 1972.

Moore, G.L., and Ledford, M.E.: The uptake and egress of adenine from human red blood cells in vitro. Transfusion *17*:38, 1977.

Moore, G.L., Ledford, M.E., and Brooks, D.E.: The distribution and utilization of adenine in red blood cells during 42 days of 4°C storage. Transfusion *18*:538, 1978.

Murphy, J.R.: Erythrocyte metabolism. II. The equilibration of glucose-C^{14} between serum and erythrocytes. J. Lab. Clin. Med. *55*:381, 1960.

Murphy, S., and Gardner, F.H.: Platelet preservation: Effects of storage temperature on maintenance of platelet viability—deleterious effect of refrigerated storage. N. Engl. J. Med. *280*:1094, 1969.

Nakao, M., Nakao, T., Arimatsu, Y., and Yoskikawa, H.: A new preservative medium maintaining the level of adenosine triphosphate and the osmotic resistance of erythrocytes. Proc. Jpn. Acad. *36*:43, 1960.

Nakao, K., Wada, T., and Kamiyama, T.: A direct relationship between adenosine triphosphate and in vivo viability of erythrocytes. Nature *194*:877, 1962.

Peck, C.C., Bailey, F.J., and Moore, G.L.: Enhanced solubility of 2,8-dihydroxyadenine (DOA) in human urine. Transfusion *17*:383, 1977.

Peck, C.C., Moore, G.L., and Bolin, R.B.: Adenine in blood preservation. C.R.C. Crit. Rev. Clin. Lab. Sci., *13*:173, 1981.

Philips, F.S., Thiersch, J.B., and Bendich, A.: Adenine intoxication in relation to in vivo formation and deposition of 2,8-dioxyadenine in renal tubules. J. Pharmacol. Exp. Ther. *104*:20, 1952.

Rapoport, S.: Regulation of metabolism in red cells. Proceedings of the 11th Congress of the International Society of Blood Transfusion, Sydney, 1966. Bibl. Haematol. *29*:133, 1968.

Reul, G.T., Solis, T., Greenburg, D., et al.: Experience with autotransfusion in the surgical management of trauma. Surgery *76*:546, 1974.

Rice, C.L., Herman, C.M., and Krekow, L.H.: Benefits from improved oxygen delivery of blood in shock therapy. J. Surg. Res. *19*:193, 1975.

Ross, J.F., Finch, C.A., Peacock, W.C., and Sammons, M.E.: The in vitro preservation and post-transfusion survival of stored blood. J. Clin. Invest. *26*:687, 1947.

Roth, G.J., Moore, G.L., Kline, W.E., and Poskitt, T.R.: The renal effect of intravenous adenine in humans. Transfusion *15*:116, 1975.

Rous, P., and Turner, J.P.: Preservation of living red blood corpuscles in vitro. I. The transfusion of kept cells. J. Exp. Med. *23*:219, 1916.

Schweizer, O., and Howland, W.S.: Potassium levels, acid-base balance and massive blood replacement. Anesthesiology *23*:735, 1962.

Shappell, S.D., Murray, J.A., Nasser, M.G., et al.: Acute change in hemoglobin affinity for oxygen during angina pectoris. N. Engl. J. Med. *282*:1219, 1970.

Shoemaker, W.C., and Bryan-Brown, C.W.: Resuscitation and the immediate care of the critically ill and injured patient. Semin. Drug Treat. *3*:249, 1973.

Simon, E.: Red cell preservation: Further studies with adenine. Blood *20*:495, 1962.

Simon, E.R.: Adenine in blood banking. Transfusion *17*:317, 1977.

Simon, G.E., and Bove, J.R.: The potassium load from blood transfusion. Postgrad. Med. *49*:61, 1971.

Solis, R.T., and Gibbs, M.B.: Filtration of microaggregates in stored blood. Transfusion *12*:245, 1972.

Stone, R.E., and Spies, T.D.: Adenine: Its failure to stimulate hemopoiesis or to produce pellagra in a case of pernicious anemia. Am. J. Med. Sci. *215*:411, 1948.

Swank, R.L., and Porter, G.A.: Microvasculature occlusion by platelet emboli after transfusion and shock. Microvasc. Res. *1*:15, 1968.

Valeri, C.R.: Viability and function of preserved red cells. N. Engl. J. Med. *284*:81, 1971.

Valeri, C.R., and Hirsch, N.M.: Restoration in vivo of erythrocyte adenosine triphosphate 2,3-diphosphoglycerate, potassium ion, and sodium ion concentrations following the transfusion of acid-citrate-dextrose-stored human red blood cells. J. Lab. Clin. Med. *73*:722, 1969.

Valtis, D.J., and Kennedy, A.C.: Defective gas transport function of stored red blood cells. Lancet *1*:119, 1954.

Weed, R.T., and LaCelle, P.C.: ATP dependence of erythrocyte membrane deformability. In *Red Cell Membrane Structure and Function*, edited by T.J. Greenwalt, p. 318. J. B. Lippincott, Philadelphia, 1969.

Weed, R.T., LeCelle, P.C., and Merrill, E.W.: Metabolic dependence of red cell deformability. J. Clin. Invest. *48*:795, 1969.

Wilson, R.F., Mammen, E., and Walt, A.J.: Eight years' experience with massive blood transfusions. J. Trauma *11*:275, 1971.

Wolf, P.C., McCarthy, L.J., and Hafleigh, B.: Extreme hypercalcemia following blood transfusion combined with intravenous calcium. Vox Sang. *19:*544, 1970.

Woodson, R. D., Malmberg, P., and Hlastlia, M.P.: Effect of stored and fresh blood on tolerance of hemorrhagic shock (abstract). *16th International Congress of Hematology,* Kyoto, Japan, September, 1976.

CHAPTER 32

Plasma Expanders and Hemodilution in the Treatment of Hypovolemic Shock

LARS-ERIK GELIN

INGEMAR DAWIDSON

Circulatory shock is defined as a reduction of blood flow to such an extent that tissue cells are being damaged from progressive hypoxia and from the accumulation of waste products. The most obvious form of hypovolemia occurs from hemorrhage. Decreased blood volume leads to a reduction of the supply of oxygen needed for aerobic metabolism and to an impaired off-flow of the waste products, meaning tissue acidosis. The subsequent cell metabolism is characterized by mitochondrial dysfunction (Mela et al., 1971). In shock from trauma, burns, sepsis, toxins, and dehydration the reduced perfusion will appear in a more severe form, where stagnation becomes more marked than the reduction of oxygen supply due to a decreased fluidity of the blood (Gelin, 1970).

In case of hemorrhage, the loss includes all the normal constituents of blood. In other causes of shock, however, the loss is primarily of other constiutents: electrolytes, and proteins, predominantly albumin. The remaining blood volume will then consist of a high concentration of cells and of a plasma of large protein molecules. This will increase the viscosity of blood and decrease the suspension stability, resulting in cellular aggregation that will markedly alter the rheologic properties of blood. This is of special importance for the distribution of flow in the microcirculation and might lead to severe deterioration of vital organs even in case of normovolemia. It then becomes critical to evaluate if oxygen delivery can be maintained to the consuming tissue (Knisely, 1965). The extent of oxygen deficit and the amount of accumulated acid material, which has been built up during shock, correlates to mortality (Crowell and Smith, 1964). A primary goal in the initial resuscitation of shock must, therefore, be to re-establish proper microcirculation.

RHEOLOGY OF BLOOD

The concept of blood viscosity is inseparable from its property of flow. In truly viscous fluids the friction is equal between all laminae provided turbulent flow does not arise. In blood the laminae are multiformed, and the friction between individual laminae will vary widely during flow. In contrast to the flow behavior of truly viscous fluids, there is no proportionality between an increase in pressure head and the increase in flow until a certain critical velocity of flow has been established. Blood is more viscous at low flow rates and low pressure heads than at higher flow rates and higher pressure heads. The most important consequences from changes of the rheologic properties of blood will, therefore, occur in the postcapillary venules and sinusoids. A marked alteration of the viscous properties of blood will occur following various forms of shock-inducing factors. These alterations are more obvious at low shear rates and will decrease the venous return flow. As blood is both a suspension of particles and an emulsion of fat in the plasma, its fluidity will depend both on the concentration of particles and of the property of the suspending medium (Dintenfass, 1976). The inter-relationship between particles and suspending medium on the rheologic properties of red cell suspensions has been elucidated in model experiments showing that the viscosity of a red cell suspension increases with increasing hematocrit, increasing viscosity of the vehicle, and decreasing flow rate. There is, however, an additional increase of the suspension viscosity (a viscosity plus factor) that increases dynamically with increasing hematocrit, increasing viscosity of the suspending medium, and decreasing flow rate (Gelin et al., 1965).

FLOW DISTRIBUTION OF CELLS IN NARROW TUBES

The number of cells decreases during flow in tubes and blood vessels with decreasing diameter (Fåhraeus and Lindqvist, 1931; Lipowsky, 1975). The reduction of cells is due to a more rapid flow rate of cells because of their orientation toward the faster axial stream. This difference in flow rates of cells indicates a separation of cells and of plasma that is exaggerated with aggregation of the formed elements of blood.

A striking microcirculatory event in the critically ill patient is a stagnation of aggregated cells in postcapillary venules and veins indicating that there are different flow characteristics of the *on-flow* side and on the *off-flow* side of the capillary bed. In a branching capillary device, the behavior of such flow disturbances can be determined without the influence of permeability alterations and vasomotor activity (Gelin, 1963). The separation of cell flow and plasma flow is enhanced with decreasing flow rate, decreasing pressure head, increasing viscosity of the suspending medium, and with aggregation of the cells. In the critically ill patient this separation might result in hypostasis of cells, seen as long persisting pale pressure marks in a red cyanotic skin.

HEMODILUTION

Investigations on the factors that influence the fluidity of blood and the distribution of cells and of plasma during flow in narrow tubes show that a high hematocrit and a high plasma viscosity provoke stasis. To break this tendency for stagnation, a decrease of the viscosity of blood and an increase of the flow rate by contributing more pressure head for the venular off-flow must take place. Hemodilution is a rheologic method to overcome this problem (Gelin, 1956; Messmer, 1975; Dawidson, 1980). Infusion therapy for resuscitation has a broad range of practical aims, such as to correct disturbances in water balance, electrolyte balance, and colloid content of the different fluid compartments and thereby to correct hemodynamic disturbances. For resuscitation of shock, the restoration of blood volume and flow has priority. An optimal oxygen transport capacity has been found with a degree of hemodilution at normovolemia corresponding to a hematocrit of 30 (Messmer, 1975; Czer and Shoemaker, 1978).

COLLOID OSMOTIC PRESSURE

A large number of macromolecular substances have been proposed and tested as the osmotic active component in such solutions. At present, blood, plasma, albumin, and dextran are most widely used for this purpose.

The basis for the water-retaining capacity and thereby for a plasma-expanding property depends on the colloid osmotic power of the solution given. The colloid osmotic power depends on the molecular size and shape and diminishes with increasing molecular weight (Ingelman et al., 1969; Tullis, 1977). In vivo this depends on the properties of the membranes against which the colloid osmotic pressure acts. In plasma 80% of the colloid osmotic power is bound to albumin. The glomerular membrane here is of primary importance, as molecules smaller than 50,000 pass through this membrane into the urine (Wallenius, 1954). In different tissues the effect will depend on the permeability of the local capillaries at a given situation (Grotte, 1956; Arturson, 1961). The colloid osmotic pressure is a function of the colloid concentration. Dextran molecules of a mean molecular weight of 70,000 keep a higher colloid osmotic pressure than plasma proteins at equal concentrations (Fig. 32.1) (Ingelman et al., 1969). The concentration of different dextran fractions had to be increased with increasing molecular weights in order to maintain colloid isotonicity

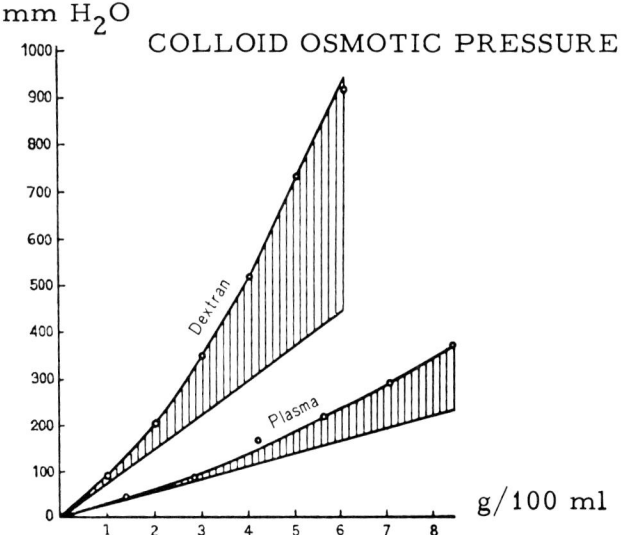

Figure 32.1. Colloid osmotic pressure as a function of protein concentration (g/100 ml) in plasma (*lower curve*) and dextran concentration (*upper curve*). The *straight lines* show the calculated osmotic pressure according to Van't Hoff's law. The *curved lines* represent the measured pressure at different concentrations. The *hatched areas* show the contribution to the pressure due to molecular interactions.

due to the lower water-binding capacity with increasing average molecular weight (as seen from Table 32.1). The plasma-expanding capacities of two different dextran solutions are given in Figure 32.2, from which it is seen that the plasma volume-expanding effect is initially more effective with dextran 40 than with dextran 70 (Gelin et al., 1961). However, this plasma volume-expanding capacity diminishes more rapidly with dextran 40 than with dextran 70 because of a more rapid elimination of the smaller molecules from the plasma into the urine.

Table 32.1
Colloid-isotonic Concentrations and Water-Binding Capacities for Dextrans with different Number Average Molecular Weights (Mn)

Mn of Dextran	Isotonic Concentration	Water-binding Capacity in ml/g Dextran
	g/100 ml	
20,000	2.37	42.2
40,000	3.42	29.2
60,000	3.91	25.6
80,000	4.20	23.8
100,000	4.38	22.8
120,000	4.50	22.2
140,000	4.59	21.8
160,000	4.66	21.4
180,000	4.71	21.2
200,000	4.75	21.0
1,000,000	5.10	19.6

The disappearance rate from the blood after infusion of dextran is given in Figure 32.3. As the loss of the smaller molecules occurs early after infusion, the property of the remaining intravascular colloid will change with time after infusion, as the larger molecules with less water-binding capacity are left within the intravascular volume. To compensate for this loss of the volume-expanding and flow-promoting properties of the smaller molecules, a continuous infusion will be needed (Ingelman et al., 1969).

INTRAVASCULAR PROTEIN LOSS DURING SHOCK

Following hemorrhage, major surgical procedures, burns, and sepsis there is an early and rapid loss of proteins from the plasma, predominantly albumin (Abel 1973; Howland et al., 1976). This protein loss is due to increased venular permeability and can be estimated to be two to four times the normal disappearance rate of radioactive iodinated human serum albumin (RIHSA) (Dawidson, 1980). Hereby the colloid osmotic power and thereby the plasma volume is lost with the albumin disappearing from the intravascular compartment.

PLASMA VOLUME EXPANSION WITH FLUID SUBSTITUTION

In an experimental surgical shock with exteriorization of the small intestine for 3 hr in 60 dogs, the loss of

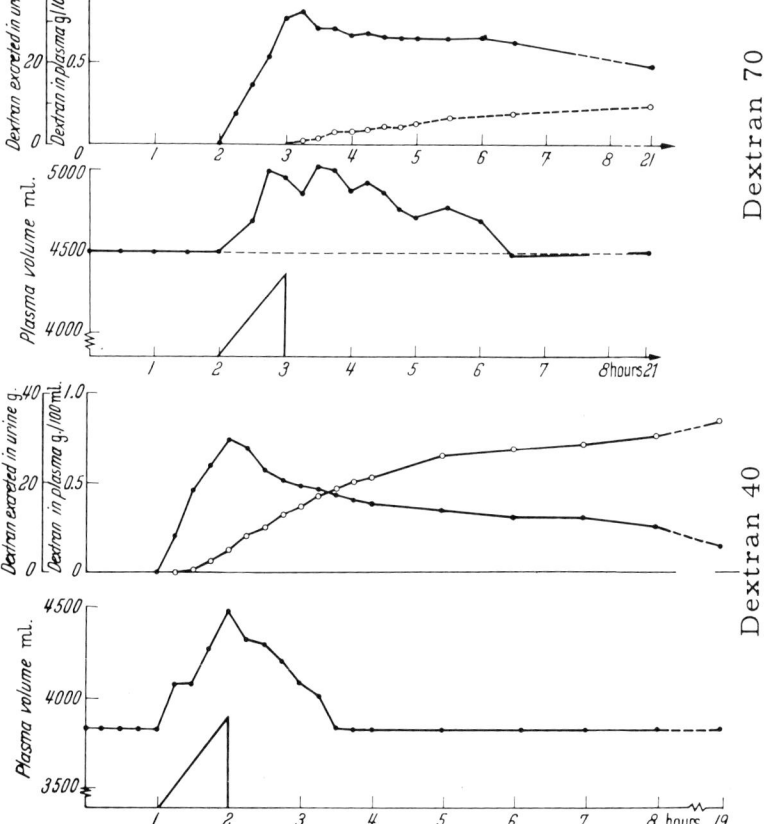

Figure 32.2. Plasma volume-expanding effect of 500 ml dextran 70 and dextran 40 solutions. Dextran concentration in plasma and the cumulative loss in urine are shown.

Plasma Expanders and Hemodilution

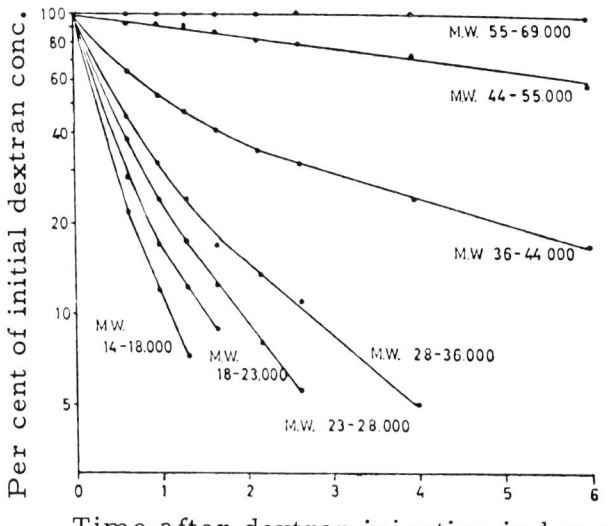

Figure 32.3. The disappearance rate of dextran of different molecular weights from serum.

The Mw is the product of the sum of all molecules of each size and their molecular weights divided by the total weight of all molecules. The Mn is the weight of all molecules divided by the total number of molecules. The duration of plasma volume expansion correlated linearly to the Mn values for colloids, as seen in Figure 32.6.

Table 32.2
Hemodynamic, Intravascular Protein Content, and Metabolic Changes during Shock in Dogs (Mean ± SD)

	Control	Shock	Shock Effect[a]
Mean arterial pressure (mm Hg)	144 ± 16	95 ± 21	−49 ± 22
Plasma volume (ml/kg)	43.7 ± 7.0	29.2 ± 6.3	−14.7 ± 4.3
Oxygen consumption (ml/min/kg)	6.6 ± 0.8	3.9 ± 0.7	−2.7 ± 0.8
Cardiac output (ml/min/kg)	162 ± 34	35 ± 10	−127 ± 30
Hematocrit (%)	50.9 ± 5.7	59.1 ± 5.9	+8.1 ± 4.2
TIA (g/kg)[b]	1.10 ± 0.15	0.67 ± 0.15	−0.43 ± 0.12
TIP (g/kg)[b]	2.73 ± 0.51	1.79 ± 0.46	−0.94 ± 0.28
Q_{Xe} (ml/min/100 g)[b]	15.7 ± 9.3	4.1 ± 4.0	−11.6 ± 10.0
PS_P (ml/min/100 g)[b]	2.1 ± 0.5	0.6 ± 0.2	−1.5 ± 0.5
PmO_2 (mm Hg)[b]	51.1 ± 13.7	18.3 ± 7.9	−32.8 ± 13.7
Base excess (mEq/liter)	−3.3 ± 1.8	−10.8 ± 3.6	−7.5 ± 3.4
Lactate (mg/100 ml of blood)	22.1 ± 12.6	29.9 ± 10.2	+7.8 ± 13.6

[a] $p < 0.001$.
[b] *TIA*, total intravascular albumin; *TIP*, total intravascular protein; Q_{Xe}, skeletal muscle blood flow; PS_P, skeletal muscle capillary permeability surface area; PmO_2, skeletal muscle tissue oxygen tension.

plasma volume was found almost exactly related to the loss of plasma proteins or equal to 40% of their initial albumin content (Dawidson, 1980). Shock was induced in dogs and in rats by laparotomy and exteriorization of small intestine for 3 hr and 1 hr, respectively. The intestinal shock in dogs was mainly due to venular stasis. Complete occlusion of the superior mesenteric vessels was added in rats to obtain a mortality rate of 80% within 24 hr in nontreated animals. This shock in dogs resulted in marked deterioration of central and peripheral circulation, and metabolic acidosis developed (Table 32.2). The total intravascular albumin loss was 13% per hr (Dawidson, 1980). Other characteristics of this shock are given in Table 32.2.

When compensated for this loss of plasma proteins by infusion of different colloidal solutions, albumin was able to restore plasma volume in relation to its intravascular concentration. When other colloidal solutions were given at equal concentrations, the plasma volume increased in proportion to their total colloid content despite the fact that the albumin content remained low (Fig. 32.4).

The plasma volume corresponded with the amount of colloid retained within the circulation. The sum of total intravascular albumin and of total intravascular dextran correlated well with the plasma volume expansion obtained at 1 hr after the infusion (Fig. 32.5), indicating that albumin and dextran had a similar volume expansion per gram of colloid retained. The volume expansion corresponds to approximately 28–35 ml/g of albumin or dextran, as seen from Table 32.3. The plasma volume expansion per gram of retained protein approximated 20 ml/g after infusion of ACD-plasma (Dawidson et al., 1980b). The physicochemical properties of different colloids can be defined by their weight average (Mw) and number average (Mn) molecular weights (Table 32.4).

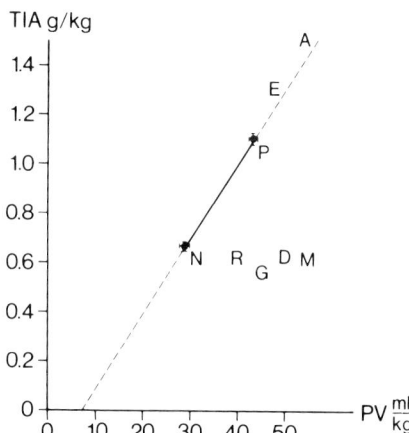

Figure 32.4. Total intravascular albumin (*TIA*) in relation to plasma volume (*PV*) at 1 hr after infusion of different plasma substitutes. The *line with dots* represents 60 dogs in control and after 3 hr of shock. *N*, shocked nontreated; *A*, albumin Cohn; *E*, albumin PEG; *D*, dextran 40; *M*, dextran 70; *G*, gelatin; *P*, ACD plasma; *R*, Ringer's acetate. (Reprinted with permission from I. Dawidson, L.-E. Gelin, and E. Haglind:Critical Care Medicine 8:75, 1980a.)

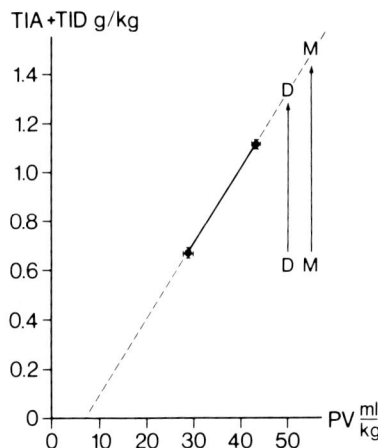

Figure 32.5. The sum of total intravascular albumin (*TIA*) and total intravascular dextran (*TID*) in relation to plasma volume (*PV*) at 1 hr after infusion of dextran 40 (*D*) and dextran 70 (*M*). (Reprinted with permission from I. Dawidson, L.-E. Gelin, and E. Haglind:Critical Care Medicine 8:75, 1980b.)

Table 32.3
Plasma Volume Expansion per Gram of Different Colloids[a]

Minutes after End of Infusion	Plasma Volume Increase	Colloid Change after Infusion	Volume Expansion	
	ml/kg	g/kg	ml/g Colloid	
Albumin (Cohn)		TIA[b]	ml/g TIA	ml/g TIP
40 min	27.2 ± 6.0	0.79 ± 0.17	34.4 ± 7.4	24.3 ± 3.0
100 min	26.1 ± 9.9	0.75 ± 0.27	34.7 ± 3.6	26.3 ± 1.8
Albumin (PEG)		TIA		
40 min	20.7 ± 7.6	0.63 ± 0.22	34.4 ± 6.9	20.7 ± 4.1
100 min	13.4 ± 4.5	0.47 ± 0.08	29.2 ± 9.8	20.6 ± 5.4
ACD plasma		TIP[b]		
40 min	18.3 ± 6.6	1.05 ± 0.41		21.1 ± 11.8
100 min	13.2 ± 3.6	0.83 ± 0.30		17.0 ± 5.3
Dextran 40		TID[b]	ml/g TID	
40 min	20.7 ± 3.5	0.71 ± 0.09	29.4 ± 4.4	
100 min	16.5 ± 3.3	0.57 ± 0.07	30.2 ± 6.6	
Dextran 70		TID		
40 min	24.9 ± 2.3	0.89 ± 0.07	27.8 ± 1.6	
100 min	18.1 ± 5.4	0.79 ± 0.03	23.5 ± 3.8	
Ringer's acetate		TIP		
40 min	10.7 ± 4.9	−0.25 ± 0.27		
100 min	6.0 ± 5.0	−0.24 ± 0.30		

[a] Mean ± SD.
[b] *TIA*, total intravascular albumin; *TIP*, total intravascular protein; *TID*, total intravascular dextran.

EXTRAVASCULAR WATER AFTER SUBSTITUTION

The extravascular water accumulation was calculated from the volume infused minus the sum of plasma volume increase and the accumulated urine volume after infusion. The extravascular water gain was significantly greater after infusion of Ringer's acetate than after colloids (Fig. 32.7). One hour after infusion only 8% of the Ringer's acetate given remained in the circulation, while 73% was found in the extravascular compartment. After 4 hr, Ringer's acetate infusion gave no plasma volume expansion, but 67% of the volume infused was still located in the extravascular space. Of the volumes of colloids infused, 40–63% remained in the circulation 1 hr after infusion and 12–44% was in the extravascular space. After 4 hr, colloids and especially albumin and dextran solutions still gave considerable plasma volume expansion but less extravascular water gain. With albumin (Cohn), water was in fact drawn from the extravascular to the intravascular space at this time, as seen in Figure 32.7 (Dawidson et al., 1980b).

The volume distribution's in the extravascular and intravascular spaces were consistent with changes of the plasma colloid osmotic pressure. Colloid infusions increased and maintained plasma colloid osmotic pressure, while Ringer's acetate infusion was associated with a reduction, as seen in Figure 32.8.

RHEOLOGIC AND MICROCIRCULATORY EFFECTS AFTER INFUSION OF PLASMA EXPANDERS

The differences between various plasma expanders regarding microcirculatory improvements are due to the

Table 32.4
$\bar{M}w$ and $\bar{M}n$ for Various Plasma Expanders

Albumin	69,000	69,000
Dextran 70	70,000	41,000
Dextran 40	40,000	26,000
Gelatin	35,000	6,000
Plasma	119,000	88,000

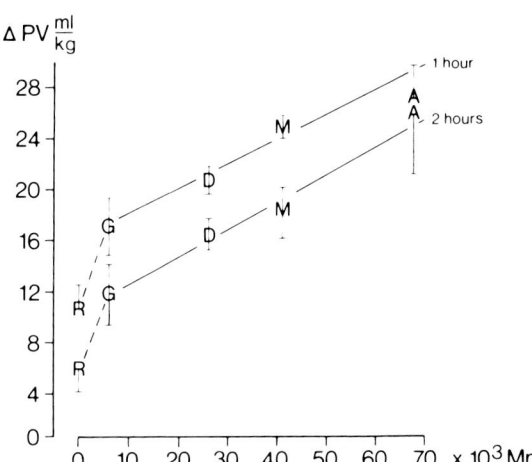

Figure 32.6. The difference between plasma volume (*PV*) after 3 hr of shock and at 1 and 2 hr after infusion of different plasma substitutes in relation to the number average molecular weights (*Mn*) for colloids (mean ± SEM). *A*, albumin Cohn; *D*, dextran 40; *M*, dextran 70; *G*, gelatin; *R*, Ringer's acetate. (Reprinted with permission from I. Dawidson, L.-E. Gelin, and E. Haglind:Critical Care Medicine 8:75, 1980b.)

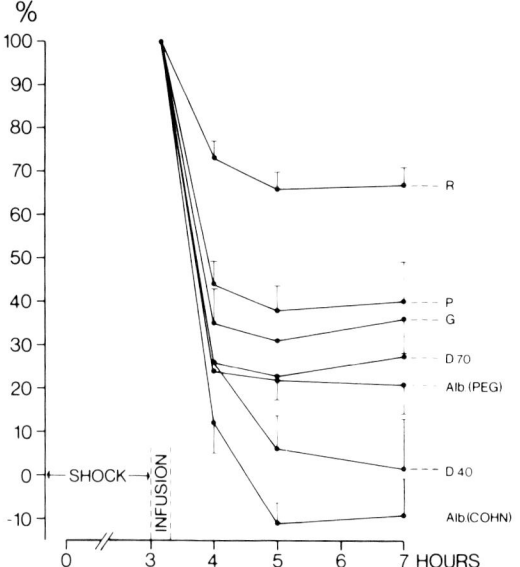

Figure 32.7. Gain or loss of extravascular water as percent of the volume infused, calculated from the volume infused minus the plasma volume increase and the accumulated urine volume at various times after infusion (mean ± SEM). *R*, Ringer's actate; *P*, ACD plasma; *G*, gelation. *D 70*, dextran 70; *Alb. PEG*, albumin PEG; *D 40*, dextran 40; *Alb. Cohn*, albumin Cohn. (Reprinted with permission from I. Dawidson, L.-E. Gelin, and E. Haglind:Critical Care Medicine *8:* 75, 1980b.)

different agents' capacity of plasma volume expansion and flow promotion. Dextran 70 and gelatin caused red cell blood aggregation with increasing colloid concentrations as measured by erythrocyte sedimentation rate (ESR), packed cell viscosity, and number of red cell aggregates (Figs. 32.9–32.11). In clinical concentrations albumin and dextran 40 caused no red blood cell aggregation or increased ESR (Dawidson et al., 1980c).

Both albumin and dextran infusions restored skeletal muscle blood flow and its distribution by increasing capillary blood flow, capillary permeability-surface area (PS), and muscle oxygen tension (Appelgren, 1972; Dawidson et al., 1980a). Such microcirculatory improvements were not seen after infusion of Ringer's acetate, ACD-plasma, or gelatin (Figs. 32.12 and 32.13).

METABOLIC RESPONSES TO INFUSION OF VARIOUS PLASMA EXPANDERS

Oxygen consumption increased after infusion therapy but with varying efficacy. Oxygen consumption was restored and maintained most efficiently after dextran 40 and albumin infusion, as seen in Figure 32.14. Dextran 70, plasma, gelatin, and Ringer's acetate also restored oxygen consumption but less efficiently and in this order (Dawidson et al., 1980b). A marked increase of arterial blood lactate concentration was seen immediately after infusion (Bergentz et al., 1969). This reflects a washout of acidotic products accumulated during shock, which represents a "hidden acidosis" (Litwin et al., 1965). Base excess was restored to control levels after the infusion of albumin and dextran 40. Ringer's acetate, plasma, dextran 70, and gelatin infusion were less able to restore base excess, as seen in Figure 32.15.

OXYGEN CONSUMPTION AND SURVIVAL AFTER SUBSTITUTION WITH DIFFERENT PLASMA EXPANDERS

Regardless of choice of fluid for resuscitation of shock, the initial oxygen consumption increased after the infu-

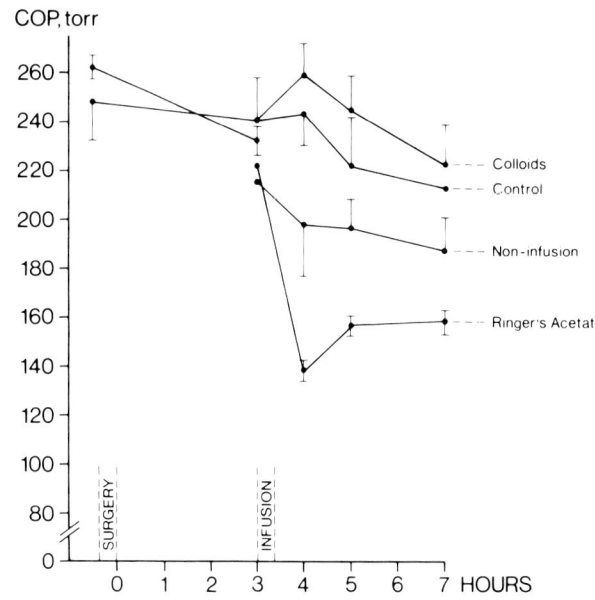

Figure 32.8. Plasma colloid osmotic pressure before and after 3 hr of shock and after infusion of colloids and Ringer's acetate. Noninfused controls are also shown (mean ± SEM).

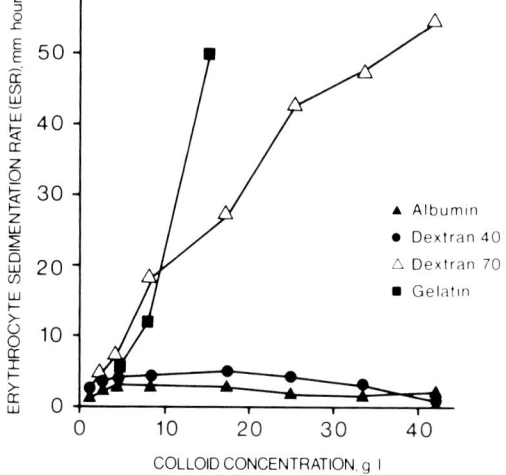

Figure 32.9. Erythrocyte sedimentation rate versus in vitro concentration of different colloidal solutions. (Reprinted with permission from I. Dawidson, L.-E. Gelin, and E. Haglind:Biorheology *17:*9, 1980c.)

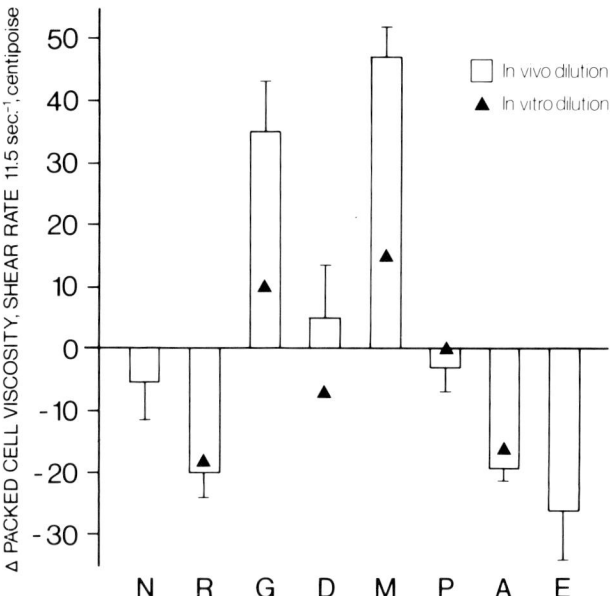

Figure 32.10. Packed cell viscosity change after dilution in vitro and in vivo with 3.5% collodial and Ringer's acetate solutions (mean ± SEM). N, noninfusion; R, Ringer's acetate; G, gelatin; D, dextran 40; M, dextran 70; P, ACD plasma; A, albumin Cohn; E, albumin PEG. (Reprinted with permission from I. Dawidson, L.-E. Gelin, and E. Haglind:Biorheology 17:9, 1980c.)

DOSE VOLUME AND COLLOID CONCENTRATION

Increasing volumes of Ringer's acetate and of colloids at various concentrations were tested on oxygen consumption and survival in intestinal shock in rats. Survival rate increased significantly with increasing volumes and decreasing concentrations of colloids. For each concentration of colloid there seemed to be an optimal effect at a dose of 2 g/kg body wt. Albumin, dextran 40, and dextran 70 given in concentrations of 3, 5, or 6% solutions increased survival rate significantly more than when given in concentrations of 10% solutions, which emphasizes the necessity to maintain water balance in resuscitation and with the use of colloidal infusions. Infusion of Ringer's acetate increased survival rates when large volumes were given (Shires and Canizaro, 1973). Survival was achieved with much smaller volumes of colloids (Fig. 32.18) (Dawidson et al., 1979).

OXYGEN CONSUMPTION AND SURVIVAL

A reduction of oxygen consumption is related to mortality (Crowell and Smith, 1964). An improvement of oxygen consumption is directly related to survival from shock (Shoemaker et al., 1979a and b). The initial therapy should, therefore, aim to restore oxygen consumption. Albumin and dextran solutions increased and maintained oxygen consumption in dogs, rats, and humans subjected to shock (Dawidson, 1980). A similar decrease

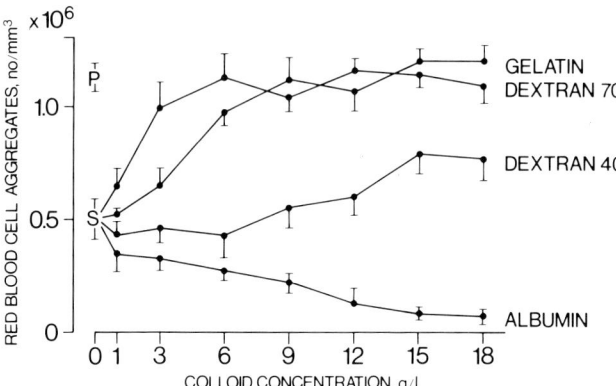

Figure 32.11. Red blood cell aggregate counts versus increasing collodial concentration (mean ± SEM. S, serum; P, plasma. (Reprinted with permission from I. Dawidson, L.-E. Gelin, and E. Haglind:Biorheology 17:9, 1980c.)

sions (Fig. 32.14). This increase of oxygen consumption is strongly correlated to survival in rats subjected to intestinal shock. The increase of oxygen consumption (Fig. 32.16) and survival rate (Fig. 32.17) was significantly greater with albumin, dextran 40, and dextran 70 than with Ringer's acetate or gelatin infusions (Dawidson et al., 1979).

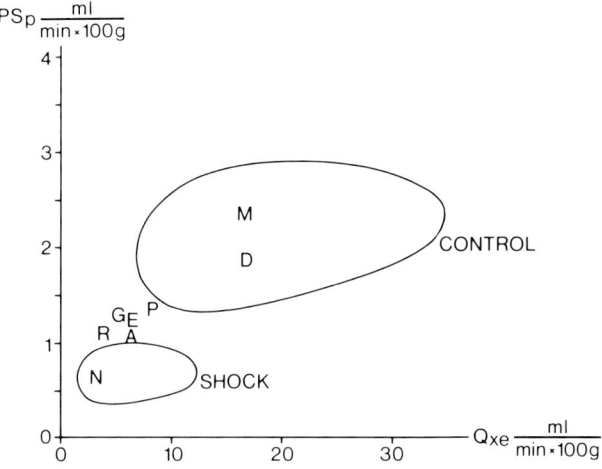

Figure 32.12. Skeletal muscle permeability surface area (PS_p) in relation to skeletal muscle blood flow (Q_{xe}) at 1 hr after start of infusion. The contours represent two standard deviations around the mean values for 60 dogs before and after 3 hr of shock. N, noninfusion; R, Ringer's actate; G, gelatin; D, dextran 40; M, dextran 70; P, ACD plasma; A, albumin Cohn; E, albumin PEG. (Reprinted with permission from I. Dawidson, L.-E. Gelin, E. Hagland, and N. Lund:Circulatory Shock 7:435, 1980a.)

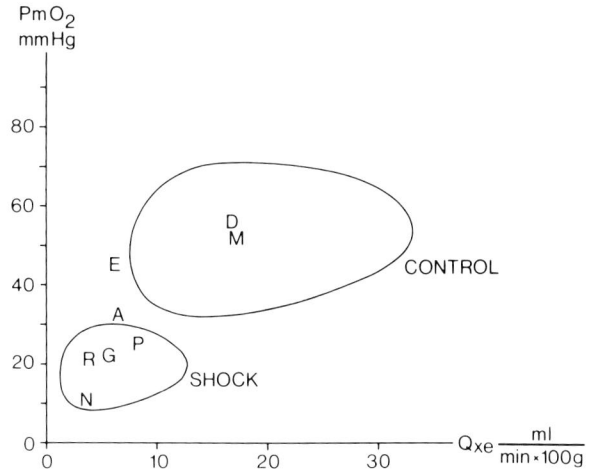

Figure 32.13. Skeletal muscle oxygen tension (PmO_2) in relation to Q_{xe} at 1 hr after infusion. The *capital letters* indicate the mean effect in the different groups. N, noninfusion; R, Ringer's acetate; G, gelatin; D, dextran 40; M, dextran 70; P, ACD plasma; A, albumin Cohn; E, albumin PEG. (Reprinted with permission from I. Dawidson, L. Appelgren, L.-E. Gelin, E. Haglind, and N. Lund: Circulatory Shock 7:435, 1980a.)

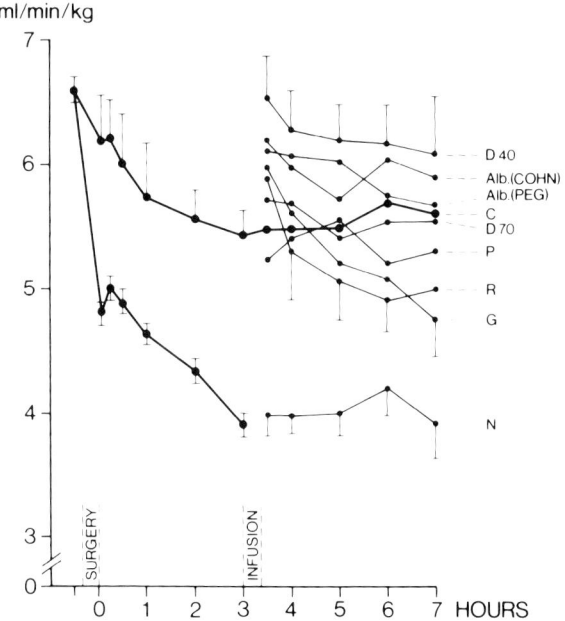

Figure 32.14. Total body oxygen consumption during 3 hr of shock and after infusion of different solutions (mean ± SEM). C, nonshocked control; N, shocked nontreated; Alb. Cohn, albumin Cohn; Alb. PEG, albumin PEG; D 40, dextran 40; D 70, dextran 70; G, gelatin; P, ACD plasma; R, Ringer's acetate. (Reprinted with permission from I. Dawidson, L.-E. Gelin, and E. Haglind: Critical Care Medicine 8:75, 1980b.)

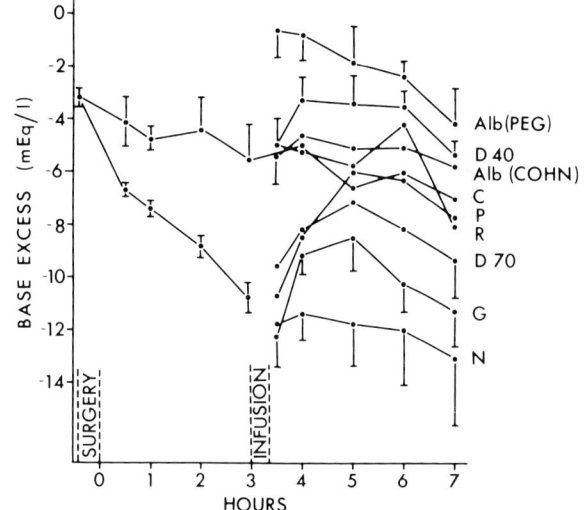

Figure 32.15. Base excess during 3 hr of shock and after infusion of various plasma substitutes (mean ± SEM). C, nonshocked control; N, shocked nontreated; Alb Cohn, albumin Cohn; Alb PEG, albumin PEG; D 40, dextran 40; D 70, dextran 70; G, gelatin; P, ACD plasma; R, Ringer's acetate.

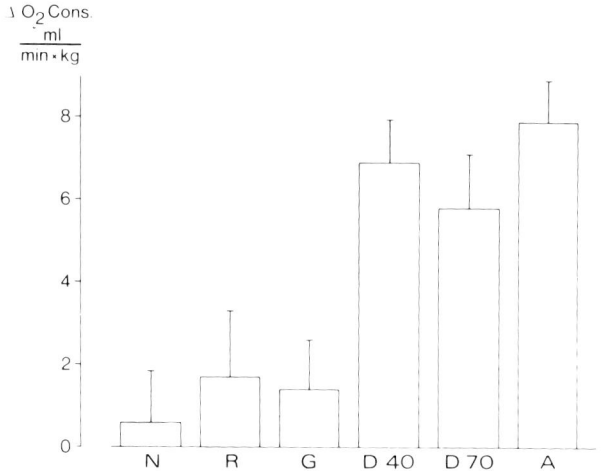

Figure 32.16. The change of oxygen consumption from shock and at 1 hr after infusion of different plasma substitutes in rats subjected to 1 hr of intestinal ischemic shock (mean ± SEM). N, no infusion; R, Ringer's acetate; G, gelatin; D 40, dextran 40; D 70, dextran 70; A, rat albumin PEG. (Reprinted with permission from I. Dawidson, B. Eriksson, L.-E. Gelin, and R. Söderberg: Critical Care Medicine 7:460, 1979.)

of oxygen consumption occurred in patients undergoing major abdominal surgery, but it was restored after infusion of a dextran 40 solution, while an electrolyte solution hardly had any effect on oxygen consumption (Fig. 32.19) (Dawidson et al., 1975).

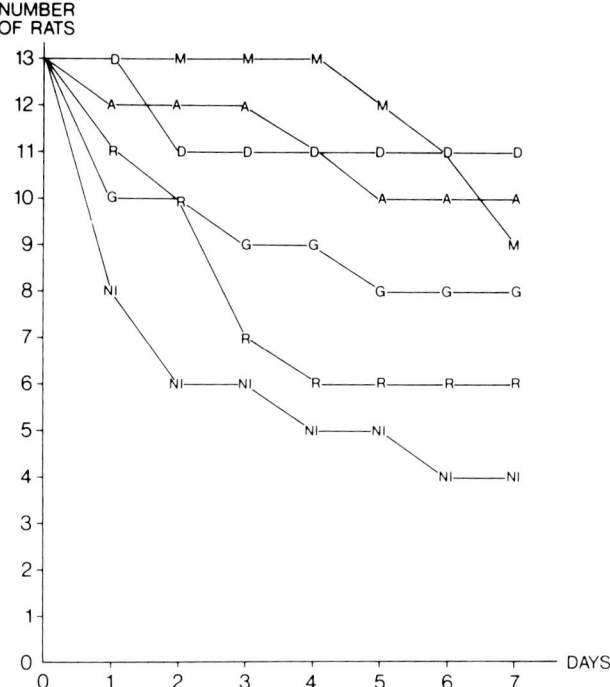

Figure 32.17. The number of surviving rats after infusion of different plasma substitutes. *NI*, noninfusion; *A*, rat albumin PEG; *D*, dextran 40; *M*, dextran 70; *G*, gelatin; *R*, Ringer's acetate.

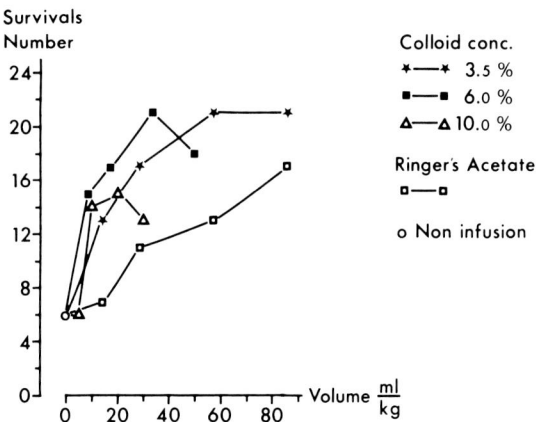

Figure 32.18. Number of rats surviving 24 hr after initial infusion of colloids administered at different concentrations and volumes. Each *point* in the figure represents 27 animals. (Reprinted with permission from I. Dawidson, B. Eriksson, L.-E. Gelin, and R. Söderberg:Critical Care Medicine 7:460, 1979.)

EVALUATION OF VARIOUS PLASMA SUBSTITUTES

Several factors determine the effects of plasma substitutes. Their molecular weight and molecular distribution, the dose, the volume, and the concentration are all of importance. This concentration should be chosen in

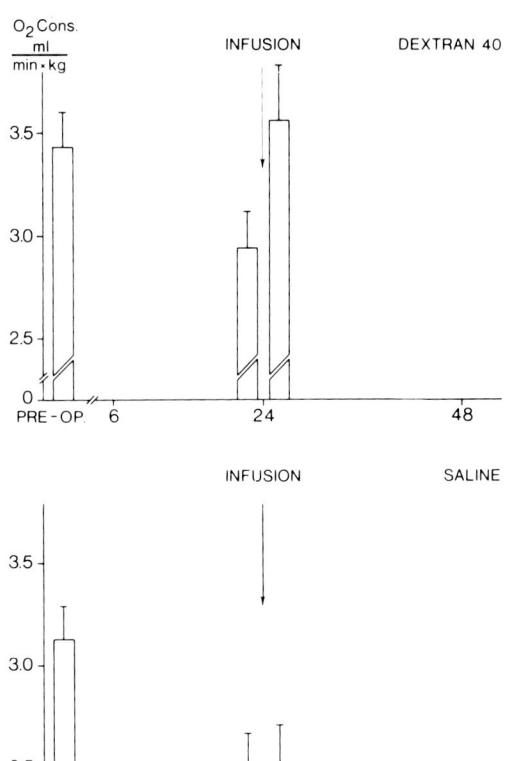

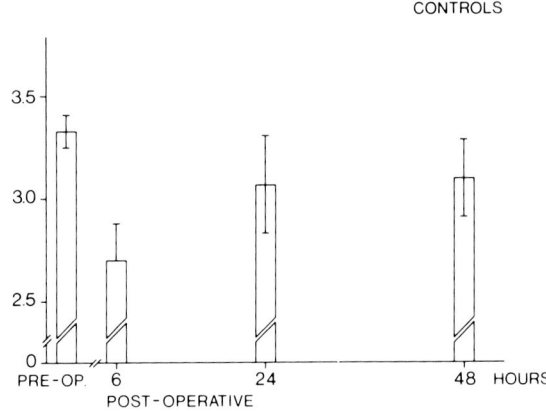

Figure 32.19. Oxygen consumption in pre- and postoperative patients. A uniform reduction of total body oxygen consumption was noted 24 hr and 48 hr after the operation (*bottom*). One thousand milliliters of saline infusion had no effect on oxygen consumption. After 500 ml of dextran 40 infusion oxygen consumption increased to preoperative values. (Modified from I. Dawidson, J. Barrett, E. Miller, and M.S. Litwin:Annals of Surgery 182:776, 1975.)

regard to the hydration status of the recipient. Therapeutic hemodilution includes three basic concepts, namely 1) expansion of plasma volume; 2) decrease of the viscosity of blood at low flow rates, which will enhance venous return flow; and 3) dispersing aggregated cells for single file perfusion of cells through capillaries, thereby making oxygen available to the tissue and releasing venular stasis.

Colloids were more able than electrolyte solutions to increase and maintain plasma volume and oxygen consumption. Among the various colloid solutions tested, albumin and dextran were superior to plasma and gelatin to achieve these effects. The differences are due to a low average molecular weight for gelatin and to less plasma volume expansion per gram of colloid for plasma in comparison to dextran and albumin. Dextran and albumin had similar volume-expanding effects corresponding to their concentration in the plasma. Due to the rheologic properties of plasma and gelatin, these fluids are less effective in improving an impaired microcirculation. Dextran 70 induced red cell aggregation similar to ACD-plasma and gelatin, which explains its decreased ability to restore oxygen consumption and base excess.

Therefore, it is concluded that albumin and dextran 40 are more effective than the other colloids tested in the initial resuscitation of shock.

References

Abel, L.: Increased capillary permeability to ^{125}I-labelled albumin during experimental hemorrhagic shock. Trans. N.Y. Acad. Sci. *35:*243, 1973.

Appelgren, L.: Perfusion and diffusion in shock: A study of disturbed tissue-blood exchange in low flow states in canine skeletal muscle by local clearance technique. Acta Chir. Scand. Suppl. 378, 1972.

Arturson, G.: Pathophysiological aspects of the burn syndrome. Acta Chir. Scand. Suppl. 274, 1961.

Bergentz, S.E., Carlsten, A., Gelin, L.-E., and Krebs, J.: Hidden acidosis in experimental shock. Ann. Surg. *169:*227, 1969.

Crowell, J.W., and Smith, E.E.: Oxygen deficit and irreversible hemorrhagic shock. Am. J. Physiol. *206:*313, 1964.

Czer, L.S.C., and Shoemaker, W.C.: Optimal hematocrit in critically ill postoperative patients. Surgery *147:*363, 1978.

Dawidson, I.: Hemodilution, oxygen consumption, and recovery from shock: An experimental study on the relative effectiveness of various fluid infusions. Ph.D. Dissertation. University of Gothenburg, Sweden, 1980.

Dawidson, I., Barrett, J., Miller, E., and Litwin, M.S.: Effect of intravascular cellular aggregate dissolution in postoperative patients. Ann. Surg. *182:*776, 1975.

Dawidson, I., Eriksson, B., Gelin, L.-E., and Söderberg, R.: Oxygen consumption and recovery from surgical shock in rats: A comparison of the efficacy of different plasma substitutes. Crit. Care Med. *7:*460, 1979.

Dawidson, I., Appelgren, L., Gelin, L.-E., Haglind, E., and Lund, N.: Skeletal muscle microcirculation and oxygenation in experimental intestinal shock: A study on the efficacy of different plasma substitutes. Circ. Shock *7:*435, 1980a.

Dawidson, I., Gelin, L.-E., and Haglind, E.: Plasma volume, intravascular protein content, hemodynamic and oxygen transport changes during intestinal shock in dogs: Comparison of relative effectiveness of various plasma expanders. Crit. Care Med. *8:*75, 1980b.

Dawidson, I., Gelin, L.-E., and Haglind, E.: Blood viscosity and red cell aggregation changes after hemodilution in vivo and in vitro: A comparison between different plasma substitutes. Biorheology *17:*9, 1980c.

Dintenfass, L.: *Rheology of Blood in Diagnostic and Preventive Medicine: An Introduction to Clinical Hemorheology.* Butterworth, Boston, 1976.

Fåhraeus, R., and Lindqvist, T.: The viscosity of blood in narrow capillary tubes. Am. J. Physiol. *96.* 562, 1931.

Gelin, L.-E.: Studies in anemia of injury. Acta Chir. Scand. Suppl. 210, 1956.

Gelin, L.-E.: A method for studies of aggregation of blood cells, erythrostatsis and plasma skimming in branching capillary tubes. Biorheology *1:*119, 1963.

Gelin, L.-E.: Reaction of the body as a whole to injury. J. Trauma *10:*932, 1970.

Gelin, L.-E., Sölvell, L., and Zederfeldt, B.: The plasma volume expanding effect of low viscous dextran and Macrodex. Acta Chir. Scand. *122:*309, 1961.

Gelin, L.-E., Rudenstam, C.-M., and Zederfeldt, B.: The rheology of red cell suspensions. Bibl. Anat. *7:*368, 1965.

Grotte, G.: Passage of dextran molecules across the blood-lymph barrier. Acta Chir. Scand. Suppl. 211, 1956.

Howland, W.S., Schweizer, O., Ragasa, J. and Jascott, D.: Colloid oncotic pressure and levels of albumin and total protein during major surgical procedures. Surg. Gynecol. Obstet. *143:*592, 1976.

Ingelman, B., Grönwall, A., Gelin, L.-E., and Eliasson, R.: Properties and applications of dextrans. Acta Acad. Reg. Sci. Upsaliensis *12:*24, 1969.

Knisely, M.H.: Intravascular erythrocyte aggregation (blood sludge). In *Handbook of Physiology, Section 2: Circulation, Vol. III,* edited by W.F. Hamilton and P. Dow, pp. 2249–2292. American Physiology Society, Washington, DC, 1965.

Lipowsky, H.H.: In vivo studies of the rheology of blood in the microcirculation. Ph.D. Dissertation. University of California, San Diego (University Microfilms No. 75-29446, Ann Arbor, MI 1975).

Litwin, M.S., Bergentz, S.E., Carlsten, A., Gelin, L.-E., Rudenstam, C.-M., and Söderholm, B.: Hidden acidosis following intravascular red blood cell aggregation in dogs: Effects of high and low viscosity dextran. Ann. Surg. *161:*532, 1965.

Mela, L., Bacalzo, L.V., and Miller, L.D.: Defective oxidative metabolism of rat liver mitochondria in hemorrhage and endotoxin shock. Am. J. Physiol. *220:*571, 1971.

Messmer, K.: Hemodilution. Surg. Clin. North Am. *55:*659, 1975.

Shires, G.T., and Canizaro, P.C.: Fluid resuscitation in the severely injured. Surg. Clin. North Am. *53:*1341, 1973.

Shoemaker, W.C., Chang, P., Czer, L., Bland, R., Shabot, M.M., and State, D.: Cardiorespiratory monitoring in postoperative patients. I. Prediction of the outcome and severity of illness. Crit. Care Med. *7:*237, 1979a.

Shoemaker, W.C., Chang, P., Bland, R., Czer, L., Shabot, M.M., and Clifton, J.F.: Cardiorespiratory monitoring in postoperative patients. II. Quantitative therapeutic indices as guides to therapy. Crit. Care Med. *7:*243, 1979b.

Tullis, J.L.: Albumin: Background and use. J.A.M.A. *237:*355, 1977.

Wallenius, G.: Renal clearance of dextran as a measure of glomerular permeability. Acta Soc. Med. Upsaliensis Suppl. 4, 1954.

CHAPTER 33

The Use of Corticosteroids in the Therapy of Hemorrhagic Shock

CLAYTON H. SHATNEY

There is little question that respiratory support and volume replacement with blood and other intravenous fluids constitute the most appropriate initial therapy for hemorrhagic shock. With proper resuscitation, the vast majority of patients will survive the acute shock episode. In fact, patient survival from hemorrhagic shock is better than that from any other form of circulatory collapse. It is interesting, therefore, that there has been so much controversy over the treatment of hemorrhagic shock. Not only has debate been generated regarding the most appropriate fluid to use in resuscitating these patients, but also controversy has continued to exist concerning other modalities of treatment.

The initial impetus for the investigation of pharmacologic agents in the treatment of hemorrhagic shock was the observation that some patients could not be successfully resuscitated with adequate respiratory support and volume replacement. The treatment of this "irreversible" stage of hemorrhagic shock has occupied investigators for several decades. The second major stimulus for pharmacologic research in hemorrhagic shock was the appreciation of the side effects of circulatory collapse, specifically, progressive multiple organ dysfunction. During the last three decades it has become apparent that our increasing success in the resuscitation of patients with hemorrhagic shock has allowed patients to live long enough to develop the complications of shock itself. Hence, there has been considerable interest in developing modes of therapy to prevent the subsequent deterioration in organ function following resuscitation from hemorrhagic shock.

For a number of reasons, corticosteroids have been investigated as possible beneficial agents in the therapy of hemorrhagic shock. As with other forms of circulatory collapse, the use of glucocorticoids during the resuscitation of patients with hemorrhagic shock has generated considerable controversy. Accordingly, it is safe to state that there is no universal agreement on either the desirability or the place of corticosteroid therapy in the treatment of hemorrhagic shock. This paper will review the literature on the subject to determine whether or not these agents are of value in the treatment of hemorrhagic shock.

THE EARLY EXPERIENCE: 1942-1963

The concept of the use of corticosteroids in hemorrhagic shock originated from two observations. First, it had long been known that patients with Addison's disease fared poorly when they developed shock (Lichtman, 1954). Second, experiments in adrenalectomized animals had demonstrated an increased susceptibility to circulatory failure (Selye et al., 1940; Swingle et al., 1943). These observations not only stimulated interest in the use of adrenal cortical compounds in the treatment of shock, but also profoundly influenced the design of experiments with these agents for the next two decades.

The scientific investigation of the effects of steroids in hemorrhagic shock began in 1942 with the publication by Fine et al. of their studies in canine hemorrhagic shock. Prior work on the use of corticosteroids in circulatory collapse had been concerned with traumatic shock not associated with hemorrhage (Selye et al., 1940; Weil et al., 1940). In 1940, Selye and associates demonstrated that physiologic doses of adrenal cortical compounds enhanced survival in traumatic shock in both adrenalectomized and nonadrenalectomized animals. In untreated, intact animals subjected to traumatic shock, the adrenal cortex showed signs of increased hormone production. Since the administration of exogenous adrenal cortical hormones provided protection against shock in intact animals, Selye et al. concluded that the increased endogenous adrenal cortical output during stress was of an insufficient magnitude to confer natural protection on the organism. Hence, the concept of a "relative adrenal cortical deficiency" in shock was proposed.

The generally favorable results following the use of adrenal cortical hormones in traumatic shock stimulated Fine and colleagues (1942) to examine these agents in hemorrhagic shock in intact dogs. Adrenal cortical compounds were studied under two sets of circumstances. In the initial series of experiments, dogs were subjected to massive hemorrhage without shock. Unanesthetized animals were bled 30–40% of their estimated blood volume over a period of 10–20 min. This bleeding produced many physiologic compensatory changes but was not associated with shock. The animals were divided into eight groups, each of which received a different form of therapy. An untreated group was included in the series. The mobilization of fluid and proteins following hemorrhage was measured in all groups. The administration of a solution of adrenal cortical extract following hemorrhage slightly increased the spontaneous mobilization of fluid but not protein. Treatment with either saline or plasma produced a greater mobilization of fluid than either no treatment at all or treatment with cortin. The mobilization of protein was unaffected by fluid alone. However, the combination of cortin plus either plasma or saline substantially increased the mobilization of fluid and of protein, compared to the use of either therapeutic agent by itself. The amount of adrenal cortical extract injected varied from animal to animal, and no dose-response data were presented.

Fine et al. (1942) also studied the effects of 10–15 mg of desoxycorticosterone acetate (DCA) in massive hemorrhage. They noted a slight improvement in the mobilization of fluid, with no effect on mobilization of protein. Animals given both DCA and saline solution mobilized a larger amount of fluid than those given just the steroid, but there was no further enhancement of protein mobilization. Three of the five untreated animals died within 24 hr, whereas all other animals survived. The authors concluded that the administration of corticosteroids alone following massive hemorrhage did not produce significantly favorable effects on compensatory mechanisms. However, the combination of intravenous fluids plus cortin produced beneficial effects on both the measured physiologic parameters and survival. It was also noted that desoxycorticosterone acetate was not as effective as cortin.

Fine et al. (1942) then conducted the same experiments in dogs in shock. In contrast to the relatively mild physiologic consequences in unanesthetized dogs, a loss of 30–40% of blood volume in anesthetized animals uniformly produced shock. Two control animals remained in shock following hemorrhage and died within hours. No beneficial effects were noted in three animals treated with 5 mg of DCA intravenously or in two animals treated with cortin intravenously. In contrast, five dogs treated with 500 ml of saline or 200 ml of plasma survived the shock episode. The combination of cortin and saline or plasma was substantially more beneficial than the administration of fluids alone. There was an almost immediate return of blood pressure to the preshock level in all five dogs so treated.

In 1943, Huizenga et al. evaluated the use of adrenal cortical preparations in canine hemorrhagic shock using a modification of the Wiggers preparation. Animals were subjected to an arterial pressure of 50 mm Hg for 90 min, followed by a subsequent 45-min period of an arterial pressure of 30 mm Hg. Untreated dogs had a 76% mortality rate. Among 20 animals treated in various fashions with physiologic doses of an adrenal cortex preparation, there was a 75% mortality. Huizenga and colleagues concluded that adrenal cortical preparations were ineffective therapeutic agents in the treatment of hemorrhagic shock.

Following this brief flurry of investigative activity in the early 1940s, there was a hiatus in research on the effects of corticosteroids in hemorrhagic shock until the next decade. In 1951, Howard and DeBakey reported the results of their experiments with cortisone and vitamin B_{12} in hemorrhagic shock in the dog. Animals were bled to an arterial pressure of 30 mm Hg. By subsequent bleedings or transfusions, the pressure was maintained at this level until a time when twice within a period of 20 min a small transfusion failed to maintain a pressure at or above 30 mm Hg. At this point the blood remaining in the reservoir was returned to the animal. Dogs were divided into control and treated groups. Among 35 animals in the control series, there was an 86% mortality. Fifty dogs were treated with 50–200 mg of cortisone intramuscularly either before or at variable times during the experiment. The mortality rates among the treated animals varied from 79–86%, depending on the timing of cortisone administration. The authors concluded that cortisone therapy had no beneficial effect on the course of hemorrhagic shock under the conditions of the experiment. However, close examination of their data revealed that, among the treated animals that died, it was necessary to withdraw 25% more blood than in the control group to produce a similar degree of shock.

In 1952, Halpern et al. studied the effects of cortisone and desoxycorticosterone in adrenalectomized rats. Their model of hemorrhagic shock involved the gradual withdrawal of 50% of the blood volume from the animals. The rats were divided into untreated and treated groups. Treated animals received 5 mg of either cortisone acetate or desoxycorticosterone the day before hemorrhage and 4 hr following hemorrhage. When 50% of the calculated blood volume had been withdrawn, the blood that had been removed was reinfused into the animal. Among 10 control animals, only one survived the actual bleeding period. Of 14 rats treated with cortisone, 12 were alive 24 hr after hemorrhage. In animals treated with cortisone the arterial pressure did not fall to the low level seen in untreated rats. Furthermore, following transfusion the arterial pressure returned to normal and was maintained at this level for at least 24 hr. Of the six animals treated with desoxycorticosterone, one died shortly after the conclusion of hemorrhage, and the remaining five animals survived at least 24 hr. Rats receiving desoxycorticosterone maintained a higher blood pressure than control animals but not as high as those receiving cortisone.

The clinical use of adrenal cortical steroids in the treatment of hemorrhagic shock began in 1954 with a report by Lichtman. He administered a "cocktail" of 11 adrenal cortical hormones to 24 patients with postoperative shock that was not reversed by large amounts of intravenous blood and other fluids. One milliliter of the preparation was injected intramuscularly at the start of therapy, followed by repeated doses at 4-hr intervals as indicated. Following steroid therapy all patients were able to maintain a satisfactory blood pressure. Twenty-two of the 24 patients recovered completely. Lichtman observed that the maximum blood pressure effect was seen within 4 hr and lasted approximately 8 hr after steroid administration. All patients showed a definite response to treatment with the adrenal hormone cocktail.

In 1955, Frank and associates presented their results with adrenocorticotropic hormone (ACTH) and cortisone in irreversible canine hemorrhagic shock. Therapy was withheld until the post-transfusion arterial pressure had fallen below 60 mm Hg, which occurred an average of 5½ hr following the onset of bleeding. ACTH was given intravenously in 10- to 50-mg doses until no further pressor response could be elicited. The maximum amount of ACTH administered was 100 mg. Cortisone was given intravenously until a total of 100 mg had been infused. Although ACTH produced an immediate pressor response, this effect was transient. Eventually, the animal became resistant to ACTH. Survival was not improved by ACTH therapy. Cortisone given after transfusion produced no improvement in arterial pressure and no prolongation of survival. Furthermore, the administration of ACTH or cortisone did not improve capillary flow or vascular reactivity as assessed by direct microscopy of the omentum and the mesentery. In a second series of experiments neither cortisone nor ACTH administered prior to bleeding and again before reinfusion influenced the volume of blood removed to produce shock, the duration of hypotension, the blood pressure response to transfusion, or the survival period. Furthermore, both cortisone and ACTH therapy seemed to increase the histologic damage in the adrenal cortex in dogs in irreversible hemorrhagic shock.

The results of Frank and colleagues (1955) were confirmed by Knapp and Howard (1957). These investigators bled mongrel dogs to a mean arterial pressure of 30 mm Hg. When 40% of the blood in the reservoir had been reaccepted, the animals were rapidly transfused and then monitored until death. Six dogs were treated only with retransfusion. Nine dogs received 100 mg of hydrocortisone intravenously in addition to transfusion of the shed blood. No differences were seen between the two groups in the duration of shock, the mean survival time, or the response to transfusion. There were no survivors in either group. Therefore, Knapp and Howard concluded that the administration of hydrocortisone was of no apparent benefit to these animals in irreversible shock and that further study involving the use of adrenal cortical compounds in hemorrhagic shock did not appear justified.

In 1958, Connolly et al. summarized the results of their investigations on the use of hydrocortisone in canine hemorrhagic shock. Animals were bled to a mean arterial pressure of 50 mm Hg. This pressure was maintained for 90 min, when further blood was withdrawn to reduce the systemic blood pressure to 30 mm Hg. This pressure was maintained for an additional 45 min, at which time the shed blood was reinfused. Among 12 control dogs, 11 died of shock within 12 hr. In 37 additional dogs a 100-mg intravenous bolus of hydrocortisone was administered at varying times during the experiment. Additional doses of 100 mg were administered if no blood pressure response was seen following the initial treatment or when the elevation of blood pressure following a dose was lost. It was observed that, if hydrocortisone was given during the first 30 min of hemorrhagic shock, virtually every animal demonstrated an immediate (within 5 min) elevation of the arterial blood pressure to 90–100 mm Hg. In addition, early treatment with hydrocortisone significantly improved the survival rate. Occasionally, hydrocortisone was successful in raising blood pressure if administered as long as 45 min after the onset of hemorrhage. The average amount of hydrocortisone used was 200–300 mg.

Connolly et al. (1958) drew a number of conclusions from these experiments. First, they noted that once hemorrhagic hypotension had persisted longer than 45 min, the administration of hydrocortisone would not affect the eventual outcome of the shock process. Second, they noted that for hydrocortisone to be effective, it must be given intravenously. Third, although the hypertensive effect of hydrocortisone occurred in the absence of fluid administration, blood transfusion was still the most appropriate initial response in clinical hemorrhagic shock. Lastly, it was concluded that at least 100 mg—and probably 200 mg—of hydrocortisone should be administered intravenously to counteract the relative adrenal insufficiency assumed to be present in shock. Extrapolating from these animal data, the authors suggested that 500–1000 mg of hydrocortisone would be an appropriate dose in humans.

In 1959, Bruns and Connolly conducted further experiments with the use of adrenal cortical compounds in canine hemorrhagic shock. They postulated that beneficial effects following hydrocortisone administration were due to a modification by the corticosteroid of the vascular response to endogenous catecholamines, as previously demonstrated by Fritz and Levine (1951). Since the latter investigators had shown a difference between cortisone, a glucocorticoid, and desoxycorticosterone, a potent mineralocorticoid, Bruns and Connolly (1959) investigated the effects of several adrenal cortical compounds on the course of hemorrhagic shock in the dog. Animals were rapidly bled to a mean blood pressure of 50 mm Hg, which was maintained for 20 min. The blood withdrawal cannulas were then occluded, and the blood pressure response was monitored. Sixteen dogs were observed for spontaneous elevation of the blood pressure for a period of 45 min. Forty-nine other animals were given various corticosteroids, including glucocortcoids and mineralocorticoids. In contrast to control animals, in which a minimal spontaneous rise in blood pressure was observed, animals treated with 200–300 mg of hydrocortisone or 120 mg of methylprednisolone intravenously showed a substantial increase in systemic perfusion pressure. The mineralocorticoids, on the other hand, did not effect a substantial increase in blood pressure in the majority of the animals. Hence, Bruns and Connolly concluded that those adrenal cortical compounds that were predominantly glucocorticoid in activity were more effective than agents that were primarily mineralocorticoid. They further concluded that the pressor effect following the administration of glucocorticoids was most likely due to an augmentation of the responsiveness of blood vessels to endogenous circulating vasopressor substances. From a mechanistic standpoint, these results agreed nicely with those of Swingle et al. (1958), who demonstrated that glucocorticoids more readily restored the disturbed fluid and electrolyte balance of adrenalectomized dogs than mineralocorticoids.

The effects of hydrocortisone in canine hemorrhagic shock were further evaluated by Hakstian et al. (1961). Splenectomized mongrel dogs were subjected to blood loss until the arterial pressure reached 40 mm Hg. The pressure was left at this level for 1 hr, following which it was raised to 70 mm Hg for an additional 30 min. The tubing from the reservoir was then clamped, thereby preventing further bleeding or reabsorption of blood from the reservoir. The blood pressure was allowed to remain uncontrolled for the succeeding 90 min. Among 31 control animals the mortality was 100%, with a mean survival time of 13 hr. Thirteen additional animals were treated with 200 mg of intravenous hydrocortisone at the beginning of the clamped period. Eleven animals (85%) survived for at least 2 days. Two animals succumbed during the 48-hr postinfusion interval. Their mean survival time was 38 hr. In the control dogs there was an initial rise in pressure following the clamping, with a subsequent fall until the blood was reinfused. In the steroid-treated dogs, however, the initial rise in pressure after clamping was maintained until reinfusion. Following reinfusion of the shed blood, the dogs receiving hydrocortisone maintained a blood pressure at prehemorrhage levels until cessation of monitoring. In contrast, control animals demonstrated a gradual, progressive decline in blood pressure after reinfusion until death. Although Hakstian et al. demonstrated the effectiveness of hydrocortisone in the therapy of hemorrhagic shock, they were unable to comment on possible mechanisms of action. Since the tubing between the animal and the reservoir was clamped prior to treatment, they did conclude that variations in the uptake of blood did not occur as a result of the pharmacologic intervention. Furthermore, they noted that the mean post-transfusion hematocrit in the treated dogs was lower than that in the control animals. They suggested that perhaps a relative augmentation of plasma volume occurred during the clamped period in the hydrocortisone-treated animals.

In summary, although the early experience with the use of corticosteroids in hemorrhagic shock was filled with controversy, a considerable amount of useful information was generated. It was amply demonstrated that corticosteroids, by themselves, would not significantly improve survival in hemorrhagic shock. Experiments involving the combination of fluids plus corticosteroids reaffirmed the necessity of adequate volume resuscitation as the mainstay of treatment in hemorrhagic shock. These experiments demonstrated, however, the possibility of enhancing the response to fluid therapy by the use of adrenal cortical compounds. The intramuscular route was found to be an unsatisfactory means of delivering these agents. It was also shown that there was an optimal time during shock for the administration of corticosteroids if any benefit was to be obtained. Specifically, only the *early intravenous* administration of hydrocortisone was associated with salutory effects on blood pressure and survival. Delivery of a suprahysiologic dose of glucocorticoids as an intravenous bolus was shown to be more beneficial than the use of lower dosages. Although the mechanism of action of corticosteroids in hemorrhagic shock was not delineated, it was well demonstrated that glucocorticoids were more beneficial than mineralocorticoids. Finally, a most important piece of information derived from these two decades of research was the necessity of consistency in the experimental model of hemorrhagic shock to ensure comparability of data among various investigators.

A NEW ERA—THE PHARMACOLOGIC DOSE: 1964-1973

The concept of the use of pharmacologic (ultraphysiologic) doses of corticosteroids in shock essentially originated with the classic paper of Lillehei et al. in 1964. Although Connolly and associates (1958) had suggested that suprahysiologic doses of hydrocortisone might be beneficial in hemorrhagic shock in humans, the rationale behind their suggestion was erroneous. The dosages that Connolly et al. proposed (500–1,000 mg) were rough approximations derived from the amounts they used in canine hemorrhagic shock to treat what was thought to be a relative adrenal cortical insufficency in shock. Lillehei and colleagues (1964), on the other hand, proposed the use of huge doses of corticosteroids in shock for other reasons. Their animal experiments had demonstrated that progressively larger injections of adrenal cortical compounds were associated with increased survival in shock. In addition, hemodynamic monitoring of animals in shock before and after the administration of glucocorticoids had suggested that large doses of these agents exhibited effects that were totally unrelated to the normal physiologic actions of these compounds. Although the previous work of Lillehei et al. had centered on experimental and clinical cardiogenic and endotoxin shock, they proposed a "unitarian theory" of the pathophysiology and treatment of all types of shock. Consistent with this theory was the idea that high doses of corticosteroids would also be beneficial in hemorrhagic shock—and for reasons unrelated to any possible deficiency in endogenous adrenal cortical secretion during shock.

That pharmacologic dosages of glucocorticoids improve survival in hemorrhagic shock was demonstrated by Nagy et al. in 1964 and by Weil and Whigham in 1965. Using high doses of a synthetic corticosteroid several times more potent than hydrocortisone, Nagy and colleagues (1964) were able to significantly improve the survival rate in canine hemorrhagic shock. Their model involved withdrawing blood into a reservoir until an arterial pressure of 30 mm Hg was reached. This pressure was maintained for 50 min, followed by exposure to an arterial pressure of 60 mm Hg for an additional 20 min. The reservoir tubing was then clamped for 150 min, following which the shed blood was reinfused. In the treated dogs the steroid was administered immediately after the clamping of the reservoir tubing. In animals receiving moderately high and high doses of the synthetic corticosteroid, the survival exceeded 50%. This rate was significantly higher than the 22% survival observed in the untreated group. Animals receiving high doses of steroids during hemorrhagic shock exhibited a significantly lower blood lactic acid level than untreated animals. The plasma glucose concentration in the treated dogs was significantly higher during the initial phases of hemorrhagic shock than that observed in the untreated group. As observed by Hakstian et al. (1961), Nagy and associates (1964) noted that the hematocrit values in the steroid groups were significantly lower after reinfusion than those in the control group. This finding was interpreted by Nagy et al. as a reflection of a relative increase in plasma volume during clamping in the steroid-treated group, perhaps as a result of a reduction in capillary membrane permeability.

The concept of the use of pharmacologic, rather than physiologic, doses of corticosteroids in hemorrhagic shock was firmly entrenched by the publication of Weil and Whigham in 1965. Using an LD_{70} model of hemorrhagic shock in the rat, these investigators demonstrated a significant improvement in survival with massive doses of hydrocortisone, dexamethasone, and methylprednisolone. The best results were obtained with 8 mg/kg of dexamethasone. Aside from substantiating the concept of using pharmacologic doses of corticosteroids in hemorrhagic shock, the authors could shed no light on the mechanism of action of these agents.

Despite the demonstration of the efficacy of high doses of glucocorticoids in hemorrhagic shock, the next two reports in the literature involved the use of physiologic amounts of corticosteroids. These studies were contributory, however, since they demonstrated the positive influence of adrenal corticoid therapy in hemorrhagic shock in two species that had not been previously studied. Telivuo and Louhimo (1965) showed that 10 mg/kg of hydrocortisone was significantly beneficial in hemorrhagic shock in rabbits. Blood was withdrawn until the arterial pressure fell to 20 mm Hg. This pressure was maintained for 20 min by the withdrawal of more blood, as indicated. The tubing was then clamped for an additional 90 min, after which the shed blood was reinfused. Two sets of animals were studied. One group remained untreated during the 90-min clamped interval. The second group received hydrocortisone at the beginning of the 90-min clamped period. There was a 52% mortality in the control population, compared with a 20% mortality in the hydrocortisone-treated group. In contrast to similar studies in dogs by Connolly et al. (1958) and Bruns and Connolly (1959), no appreciable pressor effect was associated with hydrocortisone in the rabbit.

In 1969, Schumer studied the effects of dexamethasone in hemorrhagic shock in the rhesus monkey. Animals were bled at increments of 20%, 40%, and 65% of their blood volume. Two of the animals received 5 mg of dexamethasone intravenously when 40% and 65%, respectively, of the blood volume had been shed. Animals receiving glucocorticoids exhibited lower blood lactate and pyruvate levels than those recorded in the control group. While all five of the control animals died after the loss of 65% of their blood volume, there was only one fatality in eight monkeys treated with corticosteroids. In addition, the treated animals demonstrated better microcirculatory flow at both 40% and 65% of the shed blood volume than was observed in the control group. Schumer attributed the improvement in survival in steroid-treated animals to two actions of these agents. First, as noted by Lillehei et al. (1964) in dogs, Schumer was able to demonstrate a vasodilatory effect of corticosteroids in hemorrhagic shock in the primate. Second, he suggested that these compounds probably exert a gluconeogenic action due to the induction of enzyme systems that direct lactic acid into the glycolytic and tricarboxylic cycles. Schumer's results with dexamethasone in hemorrhagic shock in primates were later confirmed by Rao et al. (1970).

The studies by Lefer and Martin in 1969 shed even more light on the mechanisms of the protective effects of glucocorticoids in hemorrhagic shock. Using a 100% lethal model of hemorrhagic shock in the cat, these investigators demonstrated a significant prolongation of survival following the intravenous administration of pharmacologic doses of both cortisone and dexamethasone prior to the induction of shock. In addition, the plasma activity of a myocardial depressant factor (MDF) was significantly reduced in animals treated with dexamethasone. Thus, in contrast to earlier studies that demonstrated no improvement in survival following pretreatment with low doses of corticosteroids, the use of pharmacologic doses of glucocorticoids prior to the onset of hemorrhage was associated with a significant enhancement of survival.

Encouraged by his experimental results, Schumer and Nyhus (1970) studied the effects of dexamethasone in 50 patients with hemorrhagic shock. Patients were initially treated with blood volume replenishment using whole blood and Ringer's solution. Those who failed to respond to volume replacement were then given either 1 mg/kg of dexamethasone or an equivalent volume of saline in a randomized, double-blind trial. The survival rate was increased from 60% to 80% in the patients receiving glucocorticoid therapy. Although substantial improvement in several metabolic indices was noted in patients receiving corticosteroids, Schumer was unable to determine whether or not this improvement was due to a direct action of the adrenal cortical compound on metabolic pathways or to improved microcirculatory perfusion.

In summary, during the 1960s, several important observations were made on the use of corticosteroids in hemorrhagic shock. The most significant discovery was the necessity of using ultraphysiologic dosages of these agents to achieve a consistent improvement in survival.

Beneficial effects following glucocorticoid therapy were noted in several species, and, most significantly, the potential efficacy of corticosteroids in the treatment of human shock was established. Differences in the reactivity of many species to a given level of hypotension were appreciated, and, likewise, the various responses of several species to a given dose of steroid during hemorrhagic shock were recognized.

THE RECENT EXPERIENCE: 1974-1979

In general, most of the recent studies on the influence of glucocorticoids in hemorrhagic shock have been concerned with the most optimal dose and time of administration of these agents during the shock process. The two exceptions to this trend have been the efforts of Raflo et al. (1975) and Pinilla and Wright (1977). Using a 100% lethal model of hemorrhagic shock in the dog, Raflo and colleagues investigated the effects of 60 mg/kg of methylprednisolone sodium succinate 1 hr prior to hemorrhage. Despite a significant reduction in the total peripheral resistance and transient improvement in the cardiac output in the treated group, there was no difference in the mean survival time for the animals receiving corticosteroids, compared with that in untreated dogs.

In the experiment of Pinilla and Wright (1977), dogs were bled to a mean arterial pressure of 30 mm Hg and maintained at this level for 90 min. Half of the animals were resuscitated by reinfusion of the shed blood plus one and a half times this volume of Ringer's solution. The remaining animals were resuscitated in the same manner, but were also given 30 mg/kg of methylprednisolone prior to reinfusion. Despite a significant enhancement of the mean arterial pressure and a significant reduction of the total peripheral resistance in the group receiving steroids, the mean survival time was similar in both groups. These recent studies are similar in design and results to the investigations by Knapp and Howard (1957) and by Connolly et al. (1958) in the 1950s using physiologic doses of hydrocortisone. It thus appears that neither physiologic nor pharmacologic doses of corticosteroids can improve survival in models of hemorrhagic shock that are so severe as to cause 100% mortality in animals receiving only fluid resuscitation.

The recent studies of Smith and Norman (1979), Altura (1975), and Altura and Altura (1974) represent some of the most thoughtful work that has yet been done on the use of pharmacologic doses of corticosteroids in the treatment of hemorrhagic shock. Smith and Norman evaluated the influence of the timing of glucocorticoid therapy on the course of canine hemorrhagic shock. Dogs were bled to a mean aortic pressure of 40 mm Hg, and this pressure was maintained for 2 hr. Four groups of animals were studied: a control population and three groups receiving 30 mg/kg of methylprednisolone 1) as soon as the blood pressure reached 40 mm Hg, 2) 1 hr after the onset of hypotension, or 3) after 2 hr of hypotension. The hemodynamic and oxygenation indices of the dogs receiving the steroid at the start of hypotension or 1 hr later were significantly better than those in the control group. When steroid administration was delayed until the end of the hypotensive phase, the hemodynamic indices were identical to those of the untreated dogs. Steroid-treated animals required less fluid during the recovery phase to achieve normovolemia. Furthermore, following restoration of normovolemia the hemodynamic indices remained closer to preshock values in the steroid-treated dogs.

Similar results were achieved by Altura (1975) and Altura and Altura (1974) in a sequence of experiments. Initially, the influence of massive doses of hydrocortisone and methylprednisolone on the survival of rats following both graded hemorrhage and hemorrhagic shock were examined (Altura and Altura, 1974). In both instances animals were bled to a mean arterial pressure of 30–40 mm Hg and maintained at this level for 1–2 hr. Corticosteroids were administered prior to reinfusion of the shed blood. In this LD_{50} model of hemorrhagic shock, 300 mg/kg of hydrocortisone and 30 mg/kg of methylprednisolone were significantly more successful in promoting survival than 150 mg/kg of the former or 15 mg/kg of the latter. In a related series of experiments, it was noted that pharmacologic doses of both corticoids failed to alter the microvascular lumen diameters in normal rat arterioles. However, both steroids effectively restored the diameter of constricted arterioles of shocked rats to nearly normal. In addition, pharmacologic doses of both agents inhibited epinephrine, norepinephrine, and vasopressin-induced muscular contractions in a dose-dependent fashion in both in vitro and in vivo preparations. In general, the effects of methylprednisolone were of a greater magnitude than those seen after hydrocortisone administration. Finally, in addition to significantly improving survival rates in hemorrhagic shock, both glucocorticoids effectively restored reticuloendothelial function to normal.

Altura (1975) next investigated the influence of both the timing and the dose of methylprednisolone and hydrocortisone in circulatory collapse. Using a model of graded hemorrhage, varying amounts of hydrocortisone and methylprednisolone were administered both prior to and following the onset of hemorrhage. Rats were bled over a 20- to 30-min interval to a fixed volume representing 3% of body weight. The blood was withheld for a period of 2 hr and then reinfused. Hydrocortisone in doses of 10–300 mg/kg was administered 6 hr prior to hemorrhage, 2 hr prior to hemorrhage, at the onset of hemorrhage, and 2 hr following hemorrhage. A consistent dose-response curve was generated in each instance, such that the optimal dosage at each treatment point was 300 mg/kg. No further improvement in survival was seen with 600 mg/kg. Methylprednisolone in doses of 1–30 mg/kg was administered at the same intervals before or during hemorrhagic shock as in the hydrocortisone experiments. Again, a dose-response curve was generated, such that at each treatment interval the most optimal dose was 30 mg/kg. Altura further observed that the doses of steroid that significantly enhanced survival either prevented or ameliorated the typical reticuloendothelial system (RES) depression seen following shock.

In general, although both corticosteroids improved survival and RES function in hemorrhagic shock, methylprednisolone was considerably more potent than hydrocortisone.

It is of interest that in this study the dosage of hydrocortisone required to approximate the survival rate seen with 30 mg/kg of methylprednisolone was twice the anti-inflammatory equivalent dose. This observation raises the question of whether or not corticosteroids have equivalent dosages in the therapy of shock that are different from those that represent equal anti-inflammatory potency. In this regard, a recent article by Vargish et al. (1977) demonstrated that the most impressive dose of dexamethasone, from the standpoint of maintaining a nearly normal postreinfusion blood pressure, was 15 mg/kg, rather than the customary dosage of 4–6 mg/kg used by Schumer (1976) and Motsay et al. (1970) in clinical septic shock and by Grinstein-Nadler and Bottoms (1976) in canine hemorrhagic shock.

There has been only one recent clinical study on the use of corticosteroids in hemorrhagic shock. This investigation by Lillehei and Shatney (unpublished data) involved a small, noncontrolled series of 15 patients who were resistant to adequate volume replacement and control of blood loss (Table 33.1). These patients were then treated with glucocorticoids. Eleven (73%) were long term survivors. Although this series was uncontrolled, the high rate of survival among patients in apparently irreversible hemorrhagic shock strongly suggests that corticosteroids played a crucial role. In addition to enhancing survival, the patients in this series exhibited significant improvements in the systemic perfusion pressure and cardiac index, as well as substantial reductions in the total peripheral vascular resistance (Fig. 33.1).

In summary, recent experience with the use of glucocorticoids in clinical and experimental hemorrhagic shock has paralleled the findings of the past three decades. The early observation of the inadequacy of late administration of corticosteroids in extremely severe hemorrhagic shock has been further substantiated, in this case with pharmacologic doses. Not only has the necessity of using pharmacologic doses of these agents been confirmed, but also a new concept has emerged concerning the relative potency of the various steroid compounds in shock. Specifically, it seems that equivalent anti-inflammatory doses of the commonly used glucocorticoids may not exert quantitatively similar effects on the outcome of shock.

WHY THEY WORK WHEN THEY WORK

In the preceding sections, several possible mechanisms of action of corticosteroids in hemorrhagic shock have been briefly mentioned. In an effort to identify areas in which these agents may be of potential benefit, this section will summarize the known effects of glucocorticoids in experimental and clinical hemorrhagic shock. It is also hoped that this material will provide the reader with a *reasonable* set of expectations regarding the physiologic actions of adrenal cortical compounds in hemorrhagic shock.

Table 33.1
Refractory[a] Hemorrhagic Shock

Volume—methylprednisolone treatment	
No. patients	15
Survivors[b]	11 (73%)

[a] Failed to respond to volume and control of blood loss.
[b] Thirty-day survival or discharge from hospital.

Investigation into the mechanisms of action of glucocorticoids in hemorrhagic shock really began with Connolly et al. in 1958. This study was probably the first to utilize an easily reproducible model and a reasonable degree of insult to assess adequately any possible salutary effects of steroids in shock. In addition, this study was the first to use a satisfactory dose of corticosteroid as a single injection. Connolly et al. noted a significant increase in the systemic perfusion pressure in animals treated with glucocorticoids early in hemorrhagic shock. They attributed this pressor effect of hydrocortisone to a potentiation of the actions of circulating endogenous catecholamines by the steroid. This effect had been described in 1951 by Fritz and Levine. Subsequent studies by Small et al. (1959) and by Chawla et al. (1968) have shown that under in vivo circumstances the administration of corticosteroids does not potentiate the pressor effects of endogenous catecholamines. Nevertheless, the improvement in arterial blood pressure associated with increased survival, as observed by Connolly and later by Hakstian et al. (1961), ushered in an era of intense investigation into the mechanisms of action of corticosteroids in shock.

Since the diagnosis of shock has always been based on alterations in hemodynamic indices, it was only natural that the hemodynamic effects of corticoids would come under close scrutiny. In 1965, Sambhi and associates reported the pharmacodynamic effects of corticosteroids in nine patients in shock. Three of these patients were suffering primarily from hypovolemic shock. The remainder of the patients, with one exception, were in septic shock. This report confirmed the findings of Lillehei et al. (1964) in endotoxic and cardiogenic shock that glucocorticoids promoted a significant increase in cardiac output and a decrease in total peripheral vascular resistance. These hemodynamic changes were seen not only in patients with circulatory collapse but also in a group of normal subjects given supraphysiologic doses of corticosteroids. As a result of these studies—and later work by Dietzman et al. (1970)—it became generally accepted that the enhancement of survival by corticosteroid therapy was due to the hemodynamic actions of these agents.

In 1971, however, Replogle and associates reported their findings with dexamethasone in canine hemorrhagic shock. Animals were bled 30% of their measured blood volume over a 15-min period, followed by observation without further bleeding or transfusion for 3 hr. The shed blood was then reinfused into the animals. Dogs were randomized into a control group and a group that received 5 mg/kg of dexamethasone after 90 min of

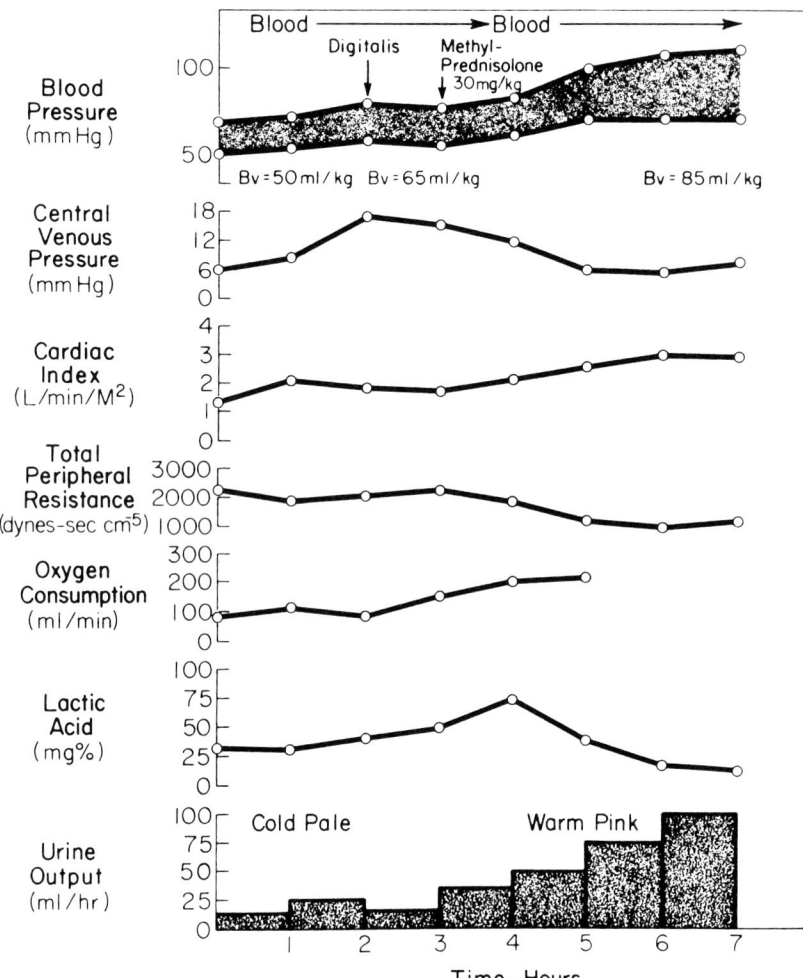

Figure 33.1. Hemodynamic indices in a patient with refractory hemorrhagic shock: The effect of corticosteroid therapy. *Bv,* blood volume.

hypotension. Compared to control animals, there were no significant differences in the hemodynamic or metabolic responses of the dogs treated with dexamethasone during the subsequent 90-min hypotensive period. It was concluded that "while there are indications in the literature that massive doses of adrenal cortical steroids may have a beneficial effect on the outcome of prolonged hemorrhagic shock, the data from this study does not support the concept that these effects are of hemodynamic origin" (Replogle et al., 1971).

Although Replogle was unable to demonstrate significant hemodynamic effects following the administration of corticosteroids in experimental hemorrhagic shock, Nagy and associates (1970), utilizing an equally severe canine model, demonstrated significant improvements in blood pressure, cardiac output, and splanchnic blood flow and in several metabolic parameters. They also noted a significant increase in renal blood flow. Recently, Lozman and associates (1975) reported that the administration of methylprednisolone in shock following trauma in humans was associated with significant increases in the cardiac index and oxygen delivery and significant reductions in the pulmonary vascular resistance, peripheral vascular resistance, and the degree of pulmonary shunting. In contrast, Lefer and Martin (1969) failed to demonstrate significant, consistent hemodynamic effects following corticosteroid administration in experimental hemorrhagic shock.

It is somewhat difficult to reconcile these contrasting findings regarding the hemodynamic actions of corticosteroids in hemorrhagic shock. The most reasonable conclusion is that glucocorticoids, when administered in a sufficient amount and at the appropriate time in the course of hemorrhagic shock, *can* produce beneficial hemodynamic changes. That these effects are not consistently observed in all studies could be explained by the possibility that the observed hemodynamic changes are not due to primary actions on the cardiovascular system but, rather, represent the hemodynamic consequences of the metabolic response to corticosteroid therapy. It is of significance that the improvement in survival that can occur following the use of glucocorticoids in hemorrhagic shock may be seen in the absence of major changes in the hemodynamic status. Hence, it is likely that enhancement of survival is not dependent on any hemodynamic effects of these agents, as suggested by Replogle et al. (1971). As a corollary to these considerations, it should be apparent that the absence of significant hemodynamic alterations following the use of corticosteroids in hemorrhagic shock should not be misconstrued as a failure of response to these agents. In addition, it should be remembered that, although systemic hemodynamic changes may not be seen following the use of steroids in hemorrhagic shock, there do seem to be consistent, salutory actions on the microcirculation (Altura and Altura, 1974).

Another mechanism of action of corticosteroids that has been extensively evaluated is their effect on the cell membrane. In 1969 Lefer and Martin demonstrated that pharmacologic doses of glucocorticoids given before or early in the course of hemorrhagic shock in the cat significantly improved survival. They were unable to demonstrate a significant, consistent hemodynamic action of these agents to explain the enhancement of survival. They did discover, however, that animals receiving corticosteroids had significantly lower circulating blood levels of a myocardial depressant factor (MDF) than the values recorded in untreated animals. Lefer and Martin assumed that the improvement in survival in the treated animals was associated with the reduction in circulating MDF. Further studies demonstrated that, once the serum levels of MDF became elevated, the administration of corticosteroids did not lower MDF concentration. Furthermore, the addition of pharmacologic doses of glucocorticoids to an in vitro preparation containing high amounts of MDF did not reverse the effect of MDF on myocardial contractility. Therefore, Lefer and Martin concluded that corticosteroids decreased the *production* of MDF and through this mechanism reduced the amounts of circulating MDF. Further research in this area, published by Glenn and Lefer in 1971, not only reaffirmed the correlation between an increase in survival time and a reduction in plasma MDF levels but also demonstrated an association between improved survival and a reduction in the circulating levels of the lysosomal enzymes β-glucuronidase and cathepsin. These findings led Glenn and Lefer to conclude that massive doses of corticosteroids exert a protective effect in hemorrhagic shock by preventing the release of lysosomal enzymes, which, in turn, were probably responsible for the formation and/or release of myocardial depressant factor. The concept of cell membrane stabilization or preservation, which they proposed, has subsequently been substantiated by numerous researchers.

Although in their early work, Glenn and Lefer did not specifically study the site of production of MDF, they did suggest that this peptide was most likely of splanchnic origin. That a large portion of the circulating lysosomal enzymes in hemorrhagic shock originates in the splanchnic viscera was demonstrated by the research of Williams and Clermont (1973) and Clermont et al. (1974). Utilizing a 100% lethal model of hemorrhagic shock in the dog, these investigators demonstrated that early treatment with pharmacologic doses of glucocorticoids significantly reduced the plasma and lymph concentrations of lysosomal enzymes, enhanced thoracic duct lymph flow, and improved survival. In addition, animals treated with corticosteroids exhibited a significant reduction in serum lactic acid concentration. These results were interpreted as demonstrating membrane stabilization by glucocorticoids, as well as improvement in peripheral perfusion.

Further evidence of membrane-stabilizing effects of corticosteroids was provided by Fredlund et al. (1974) in pigs. Using a nonlethal model of hemorrhagic shock, these investigators demonstrated that pretreatment with 50 mg/kg of hydrocortisone significantly reduced the plasma activity of β-galactosidase and β-glucosidase, compared with levels seen in the control group. In addition, the steroid-treated group exhibited a reduction in the degree of metabolic acidosis and hyperkalemia seen in the control population. Furthermore, after reinfusion of the shed blood the systemic perfusion pressure was significantly higher in the group treated with steroids. These findings led Fredlund et al. to conclude that the protective effects of corticosteroids in hemorrhagic shock were primarily a result of their actions at the cellular level, rather than any direct effect on the general circulation.

More evidence of a direct membrane-stabilizing influence of glucocorticoids was provided by the studies of Spath et al. (1973) and Jones and associates (1977). Examining the results of multiple experiments in different species utilizing several models of shock, Spath et al. concluded that corticosteroids prevent the release of lysosomal enzymes from the splanchnic viscera, specifically the pancreas. Little evidence could be found that these agents act by inhibiting the synthesis of lysosomal enzymes. Furthermore, pharmacologic doses of adrenal cortical hormones did not antagonize the actions or reduce the circulating levels of lysosomal enzymes once they were released from the pancreas. Hence, high doses of corticosteroids do not increase the clearance of circulating lysosomal enzymes from the plasma of animals in shock. Rather, these agents inhibit the release of lysosomal enzymes from sites of production within the cell. Although Spath et al. did demonstrate a significant increase in superior mesenteric artery blood flow in steroid-treated animals in shock, they felt that this effect was secondary to the cellular actions of the drug in the visceral organs, rather than a primary effect on the vasculature.

More convincing evidence of a direct cell membrane-stabilizing effect of corticosteroids in hemorrhagic shock was presented by Jones et al. (1977). These investigators studied the response of hepatic and intestinal adenyl cyclase activity in dogs in hemorrhagic shock, with and without glucocorticoid therapy. They demonstrated that stimulation of adenyl cyclase activity in the liver is abolished in shocked dogs. Treatment with glucocorticoids, however, restored the adenyl cyclase activity to nearly normal levels. This effect was noted even with corticosteroid administration late in the course of hemorrhagic shock. A similar response was noted in the intestines. Since adenyl cyclase is a membrane-bound enzyme that modulates changes in the intracellular content of cyclic AMP, these findings more clearly demonstrate a direct cellular effect of corticosteroids in hemorrhagic shock.

There is little argument at present that glucocorticoids do exert direct membrane-stabilizing actions. This effect, along with beneficial changes in microcirculatory perfusion, probably accounts for the significant reduction in the levels of circulating lysosomal enzymes in animals in hemorrhagic shock following corticosteroid administration. There is debate, however, as to whether or not the reduction in circulating levels of lysosomal enzymes is responsible for the improvement in survival in animals treated with pharmacologic doses of glucocorticoids. Although Glenn et al. (1972) reported deleterious hemodynamic effects after the administration of a lysosomal preparation to normal dogs, subsequent studies by Mason and Wangensteen (1977) and by Nagasue et al. (1979) have demonstrated little hemodynamic deterioration in normal dogs following the infusion of purified lysosomal enzymes. Nagasue and associates did demonstrate, however, that in normal dogs made acidotic by prior infusion of lactate, purified lysosomal enzyme administration was associated with thrombocytopenia and a decrease in fibrinogen concentration. Since the combination of elevated circulating lysosomal enzymes and acidosis more nearly resembles the state seen in shock, it is likely that increased levels of circulating lysosomal enzymes do contribute to metabolic derangements and, hence, to the mortality of hemorrhagic shock. In this regard it is probable that the reduction in mortality following glucocorticoid administration in hemorrhagic shock is somewhat related to their capacity to decrease the concentration of circulating lysosomal enzymes.

Although the metabolic effects of pharmacologic doses of corticosteroids have been extensively investigated in other forms of shock, relatively little information is available on this subject in hemorrhagic shock. In studies in primates and humans, Schumer and Nyhus (1969) observed significant increases in the blood glucose and lactic acid concentrations following glucocorticoid administration. A decrease in the serum inorganic phosphate concentration was also noticed. Schumer suggested that corticosteroids enhance glucose and lactate metabolism and increase ATP production in hemorrhagic shock. However, Jordan et al. (1972) noted no effect on the blood glucose concentration or the plasma insulin response in four patients in hemorrhagic shock treated with relatively small doses of glucocorticoids. A recent study by Chaudry et al. (1978) demonstrated that during hemorrhagic shock in the rat gluconeogenesis was significantly inhibited by pharmacologic concentrations of steroids. Hence, it seems that the transient increase in circulating blood glucose during hemorrhagic shock following the administration of glucocorticoids may be a reflection of glucose release, rather than an enhancement of glucose production. The apparent lack of a gluconeogenic effect of corticosteroids in hemorrhagic shock is in sharp contradistinction to their influence on glucose metabolism in septic shock.

The reduction in circulating levels of lactic acid seen by Schumer and Nyhus (1969, 1970) was interpreted as an indication of improvement in aerobic metabolism during shock by steroid therapy. Although such an enhancement of aerobic metabolism could be due to direct cellular actions of corticosteroids, a contributing factor may be the effects of steroid therapy on microcirculatory perfusion. In a small series of patients receiving massive blood transfusions, Bryan-Brown et al. (1973) demonstrated that treatment with pharmacologic doses of glucocorticoids moved the characteristic left-shifted oxyhemoglobin dissociation curve toward a more normal position. This effect was observed within 2 hr after administration of the steroid. The net effect of this shift in the oxyhemoglobin dissociation curve would be an increased efficiency of oxygen delivery by reducing the affinity of hemoglobin for oxygen. In addition to this change in the oxyhemoglobin dissociation curve, Bryan-Brown and associates noted increases in the arterial perfusion pressure, cardiac index, left ventricular stroke work, the arteriovenous oxygen difference, and oxygen consumption. Furthermore, preliminary data suggested that corticosteroids also returned the erythrocyte potassium concentration toward a normal level (Bryan-Brown et al., 1974). The influence of glucocorticoids on the oxyhemoglobin dissociation curve noted by Bryan-Brown and associates is remarkably similar to the effect observed by McConn and Del Guercio (1971) in septic patients following the administration of corticosteroids. In summary, although the data are weak and direct proof is lacking, it seems that corticosteroids may enhance cellular metabolism during hemorrhagic shock.

The last major area in which glucocorticoids have been evaluated mechanistically has been their influence on organ function and structure. The first organ to be examined in an isolated fashion was the heart. As part of their assessment of the effects of steroids on the activity of myocardial depressant factor in shock and trauma, Lefer and Martin (1969) examined the possibility that glucocorticoids might be inotropic agents. In several studies utilizing isolated papillary muscle preparations, these investigators were unable to demonstrate an inotropic effect of corticosteroids. In a subsequent extension of this work, Glenn and Lefer (1971) studied the effect of glucocorticoids on myocardial contractility in normal intact cats using a strain gauge attached to the right ventricle. They noted no significant change in contractile force during a 2½-hr observation period following the administration of 20 mg/kg of methylprednisolone. They concluded that pharmacologic doses of corticosteroids did not exert an inotropic effect on the heart. However, a study by Carter and Thomas (1970) in anesthetized mongrel dogs demonstrated a slight, transient improvement in the ventricular function curves in three of four dogs given 50 mg/kg of hydrocortisone. Using a right ventricular strain gauge, they noted a significant increase in the ventricular contractile force for 1 hr following the administration of high doses of corticosteroids. Significant peripheral vasodilatation was also observed following steroid administration. Carter and Thomas concluded that pharmacologic doses of hydrocortisone did exert a *transient* inotropic effect. However, it appeared that any therapeutic value of corticosteroids in low flow states was unrelated to the significant, but therapeutically minimal and transient, hemodynamic effects of these agents.

A more recent study by Abel (1977) directly addressed the issue of the influence of glucocorticoids on ventricular performance during hemorrhagic shock. The effect of 30 mg/kg of methylprednisolone was examined in 14 dogs in severe hemorrhagic shock. The animals were subjected to an arterial pressure of 40 mm Hg for 4 hr. The steroid was administered 1–3 hr after the reinfusion of shed blood. A significant improvement in ventricular performance, as assessed by the maximal dP/dT and the time to peak ventricular pressure, was observed following steroid therapy. The significant improvement in left ventricular performance persisted for 1–2 hr following corticosteroid therapy and gradually diminished during the third and fourth post-treatment hours. Associated with the enhancement of myocardial performance was a significant vasodilatory effect. Thus, it appears that pharmacologic doses of corticosteroids do exert a mild, transient inotropic effect in the intact animal during hemorrhagic shock.

The effects of high doses of glucocorticoids on pulmonary function and structure during hemorrhagic shock have also been examined. Wilson (1972) demonstrated a preservation of the normal architecture of the lung during hemorrhagic shock following either pretreatment or post-treatment with glucocorticoids. These findings were confirmed and extended by the study of Kusajima et al. (1974). These investigators utilized a canine model of hemorrhagic shock in which the animals were maintained at a mean arterial pressure of 40 mm Hg for 2 hr. At the conclusion of the period of hypotension, the shed blood was reinfused. The animals were divided into four groups: a control group and three steroid-treated groups. Corticosteroids were administered at 30 min, 60 min, and 90 min following the onset of hemorrhage. Pulmonary hemodynamic parameters and lung architecture via in vivo microscopy were sequentially examined. Animals treated with methylprednisolone had a significant reduction in the amount of pulmonary venous vasoconstriction and in the histologic damage to the lungs. There was also a significant reduction in pulmonary artery wedge pressure and in the pressure in small pulmonary veins in the groups receiving methylprednisolone. Furthermore, all dogs receiving methylprednisolone had significantly higher systemic perfusion pressures than did control animals. Kusajima and associates (1974) remarked that "a generally normal circulatory pattern is observed."

In a related study Humphrey et al. (1974) measured pulmonary extravascular water in dogs in hemorrhagic shock. Animals were maintained at a mean arterial pressure of 50 mm Hg for 2 hr, at which time the shed blood was reinfused. One group of animals was given 35 mg/kg of methylprednisolone 30 min prior to the reinfusion of shed blood. In comparison to control dogs, animals treated with methylprednisolone maintained a normal percentage of extravascular lung water. Although the findings were discussed in relationship to recruitment of pulmonary capillaries, it is probable that much of the observed effect was due to a preservation of normal capillary integrity by corticosteroid treatment. In this regard, Grinstein-Nadler and Bottoms (1976) recently demonstrated that treatment with dexamethasone during hemorrhagic shock prevented fluid shifts from the extracellular space into the intracellular space by reducing membrane damage and consequent alterations in transport mechanisms. In addition to these direct beneficial effects on pulmonary function and structure, Peer and Schwartz (1975) observed that platelet trapping by the lung following soft tissue trauma was significantly reduced by methylprednisolone administration. Thus, from a number of standpoints glucocorticoid therapy improves pulmonary structure and function in hemorrhagic shock. These salutary effects of corticosteroids on the lung in hemorrhagic shock are the probable basis for the increased survival rate following glucocorticoid therapy in the adult respiratory distress syndrome (Sladen, 1976).

The effects of methylprednisolone on small intestinal mucosal integrity during shock have been extensively evaluated by Haglund et al. (1976a). By controlling perfusion to an isolated small intestinal segment, they created a regional hypotensive preparation that accurately reproduced the intestinal lesions seen during hemorrhagic shock. In comparison to untreated animals, cats given 30 mg/kg of methylprednisolone at the conclusion of a 2-hr ischemic period demonstrated significantly fewer small intestinal mucosal lesions than untreated animals. Since perfusion of the ischemic intestinal segment with oxygenated saline also significantly reduced the number of mucosal lesions, the authors concluded that methylprednisolone probably exerted its protective action by increasing the tolerance of the ischemic mucosa to hypoxia. In a subsequent study utilizing a similar experimental model, further effects of corticosteroids were demonstrated. Methylprednisolone, whether administered early or late during the course of regional small intestinal ischemia, not only reduced the incidence of mucosal lesions but also significantly inhibited the release of cardiotoxic enzymes from the ischemic small bowel into the systemic circulation (Haglund et al., 1976b, 1977). Furthermore, cats treated with glucocorticoids did not manifest systemic hypotension following release of the occlusion of arterial inflow to the isolated segment of small intestine, as occurred in untreated animals. Haglund and associates concluded that there was a causal relationship between the intestinal mucosal injury and the postischemic cardiovascular derangement. They proposed that the cardiovascular collapse was mediated by the release of cardiotoxic material from the hypoxic intestine. They further concluded that corticosteroids prevented the postischemic systemic hemodynamic deterioration by preventing the release of the cardiotoxic material from the hypoxic intestine.

Further evidence of a protective effect of glucocorticoids on the intestine during low flow states was provided by Santiago-Delpin et al. (1978). Using a 1½-hr intestinal arterial occlusion preparation in rats, they demonstrated that the use of methylprednisolone and ampicillin prior to bowel ischemia significantly improved the survival of the animals and prevented the extensive destruction of the intestinal wall seen in the control rats. As with the lung, corticosteroids dramatically alter the pathophysiology of the intestine during experimental hemorrhagic shock. These beneficial changes are associated with an increase in survival.

Two other organs have also been shown to be protected under low flow conditions by high doses of corticosteroids. Ritchie et al. (1978) demonstrated that the systemic administration of 30 mg/kg of methylprednisolone to dogs prior to exposing an isolated segment of gastric mucosa to acid, vasopressin, and sodium taurocholate significantly reduced the number of acute mucosal lesions. Associated with the protection against mucosal alteration was a significant enhancement of mucosal blood flow in the steroid-treated dogs. A clinical correlate to this study is the report by Jama et al. (1975) on the incidence of stress ulcer formation in patients receiving steroid therapy for various types of shock. These investigators found that patients given high doses of corticosteroids as part of their therapy for shock had a significantly lower incidence of stress ulcer formation than patients not receiving steroids.

Attention has also been directed to the influence of glucocorticoids on the liver during low flow states. Figueroa and Santiago-Delpin (1975) studied the effects of methylprednisolone administration on rabbits before and at variable times after hepatic ischemia. The portal triad was occluded for either 30 or 60 min. Methylprednisolone, 30 mg/kg, was administered prior to and at variable times following portal triad occlusion under both experimental conditions. Only two of 19 untreated rabbits survived a 30-min occlusion of the portal triad. In contrast, pretreatment with methylprednisolone produced 100% survival. If methylprednisolone was given after 30 min of hepatic ischemia, the survival rate was 54%. One hour of hepatic ischemia produced a 100% mortality rate in untreated rats. Pretreatment with methylprednisolone, however, increased the survival rate to 50%. In contrast to the marked cytoplasmic disruption of the liver in the control group, animals receiving methylprednisolone prior to occlusion exhibited minimal hepatic congestion and only occasional areas of hemorrhage. No major structural changes and only moderate cellular changes, primarily swelling of the cytoplasm, were noted in the treated animals. The hepatic histology in animals receiving corticosteroids after the ischemic injury was similar to that seen in animals receiving the agent prior to occlusion of the portal triad.

In summary, although a number of beneficial cellular, hemodynamic, and metabolic effects have been observed following the use of pharmacologic doses of glucocorticoids in hemorrhagic shock, (Table 33.2), a satisfactory and generally accepted *primary* mechanism of action of these agents has not been discovered. At present it seems that when these agents are successful in improving survival in hemorrhagic shock, they do so through the combination of a number of different salutory actions in many systems. As indicated, many of the effects of corticosteroids in one system will impinge upon potential effects in other systems. Hence, it is possible to see certain actions of glucocorticoids under one set of experimental circumstances and, yet, not be able to demonstrate these same effects under other experimental circumstances—or in other species. It is probable that a given number or pattern of effects of corticosteroids in many organ systems is necessary to enhance survival. The need for an appropriate combination of effects would explain the variability in survival rates that have occasionally been reported from different laboratories, despite similar models of hemorrhagic shock.

CURRENT STATUS

During the last three decades a great deal has been learned about the usefulness—and limitations—of corticosteroids in the therapy of hemorrhagic shock. It is safe to say that the administration of pharmacologic doses of glucocorticoids during the period from 1 hr prior to the onset of hemorrhage to approximately 1 hr after the initiation of blood loss, in association with adequate volume replacement, will significantly improve the survival of animals in experimental hemorrhagic shock—provided the severity of the experimental preparation is within reason. It is also evident that the administration of corticosteroids late in the course of severe

Table 33.2
Effects of Glucocorticoids in Hemorrhagic Shock

Increases in:
  Survival
  Cardiac output
  Renal blood flow
  Superior mesenteric arterial flow
  Microcirculatory perfusion
  Lactate metabolism
  Oxygen availability
  Adenyl cyclase activity (liver and intestine)
  RES activity
  Blood glucose (transient)
  Systemic perfusion pressure (variable)
  Myocardial contractility (mild, transient)
  Systemic oxygen consumption (variable)
Decreases in:
  Pulmonary vascular resistance
  Vascular membrane permeability
  Gluconeogenesis
  Lactic acid concentration
  MDF
  Actions of epinephrine, norepinephrine, vasopressin
  Pulmonary shunting (after transient increase)
  Total peripheral resistance (variable)
Preservation of:
  Normal cellular architecture (liver, lung, intestine)
  Lysosomal membrane integrity

hemorrhagic shock does not improve survival and is not associated with consistently reproducible hemodynamic or metabolic effects. We have learned that the basis for the beneficial effects of steroids in hemorrhagic shock is not the correction of a relative inadequacy of endogenous circulating adrenal cortical compounds. Rather, the efficacy of glucocorticoids in experimental hemorrhagic shock is based upon a combination of systemic and cellular effects unique to massive doses of these agents. As a corollary, we have also realized that appropriate dosages of these compounds must be presented to the organism as a bolus and that the effects of more frequent administration of smaller than optimal doses are not as substantial. In addition, there is evidence in the recent literature that perhaps the dosages of hydrocortisone and dexamethasone that are the anti-inflammatory equivalents to 30 mg/kg of methylprednisolone are, in fact, inadequate amounts with respect to the treatment of shock. Finally, although a precise primary mechanism of action of glucocorticoids in hemorrhagic shock has not been identified, a sufficient number of beneficial effects in multiple organ systems has been discovered to adequately account for the enhancement in survival following the administration of these agents.

It would be unfair at the present time to make any recommendations regarding the use of corticosteroids in clinical hemorrhagic shock. The few studies that have been conducted in humans have been uncontrolled trials with small numbers of patients and without adequate monitoring of the results of therapy. The only rational conclusion that can be drawn from these studies is that there is a suggestion that glucocorticoids may be of some benefit to patients in irreversible hemorrhagic shock. Furthermore, there does not seem to be any appreciable hazard in the use of corticosteroids in hemorrhagic shock in humans. Although the results in experimental shock are encouraging and suggest that steroids might be of some benefit in human hemorrhagic shock, it must be remembered that the vast majority of patients suffering from hemorrhagic shock can be adequately resuscitated and will be long-term survivors with appropriate fluid administration. Hence, it seems likely that if corticosteroids are ultimately demonstrated to be beneficial in human hemorrhagic shock, they will probably be most useful in patients who are resistant to volume replacement or in whom massive amounts of blood and intravenous fluids are required in the resuscitative process. In summary, at present we can only speculate on the possible usefulness of glucocorticoids in clinical hemorrhagic shock. Specific recommendations must await a properly conducted, controlled clinical study using these agents in a randomized, double-blind fashion in large numbers of patients.

References

Abel, F.L.: Effects of glucocorticoids on ventricular performance and capillary permeability during hemorrhagic shock. Circ. Shock *4*:345, 1977.

Altura, B.M.: Glucocorticoid-induced protection in circulatory shock: Role of reticuloendothelial system function. Proc. Soc. Exp. Biol. Med. *150*:202, 1975.

Altura, B.M., and Altura, B.T.: Peripheral vascular actions of glucocorticoids and their relationship to protection in circulatory shock. J. Pharmacol. Exp. Ther. *190*:300, 1974.

Bruns, D.L., and Connolly, J.E.: A comparative study of the effectiveness of adrenal cortical compounds in hemorrhagic shock. Surg. Forum *10*:382, 1959.

Bryan-Brown, C.W., Baek, S.M., Makabali, G., and Shoemaker, W.C.: Consumable oxygen: Availability of oxygen in relation to oxyhemoglobin dissociation. Crit. Care Med. *1*: 17, 1973.

Bryan-Brown, C.W., Makabali, G., Baek, S.M., and Shoemaker, W.C.: Hemodynamic responses and oxygen delivery after methylprednisolone sodium succinate. In *Steroids and Shock*, edited by T.M. Glenn, pp. 361–375. University Park Press, Baltimore, 1974.

Carter, J.W., and Thomas, C.S., Jr.: The circulatory response to pharmacological levels of hydrocortisone. J. Surg. Res. *10*:437, 1970.

Chaudry, I.H., Adzick, N.S., and Baue, A.E.: Glucocorticoid effects on gluconeogenesis during hemorrhagic shock. J. Surg. Res. *24*:26, 1978.

Chawla, R.C., Seaton, J.F., Robinson, B.H., and Harrison, T.S.: Steroid modifications of alpha adrenergic blockade and catecholamine secretion. Surg. Gynecol. Obstet. *127*:824, 1968.

Clermont, H.G., Williams, J.S., and Adams, J.T.: Steroid effect on the release of the lysosomal enzyme acid phosphatase in shock. Ann. Surg. *179*:917, 1974.

Connolly, J.E., Bruns, D.L., and Stofer, R.C.: The use of intravenous hydrocortisone in hemorrhagic shock. Surg. Forum *9*:17, 1958.

Dietzman, R.H., Castaneda, A., Lillehei, C.W., et al.: Corticosteroids as effective vasodilators in the treatment of low output syndrome. Chest *57*:440, 1970.

Figueroa, I., and Santiago-Delpin, E.A.: Steroid protection of the liver during experimental ischemia. Surg. Gynecol. Obstet. *140*:368, 1975.

Fine, J., Fischmann, J., and Frank, H.A.: The effect of adrenal cortical hormones in hemorrhage and shock. Surgery *12*:1, 1942.

Frank, H. A., Jacob, S., Weizel, H.A.E., et al.: Effects of ACTH and cortisone in experimental hemorrhagic shock. Am. J. Physiol. *180*:282, 1955.

Fredlund, P.E., Kallum, B., Nagasue, N., et al.: Release of acid hydrolases in hemorrhagic shock after pretreatment with hydrocortisone in the pig. Am. J. Surg. *128*:324, 1974.

Fritz, I., and Levine, R.: Action of adrenal cortical steroids and nor-epinephrine on vascular responses of stress in adrenalectomized rats. Am. J. Physiol. *165*:456, 1951.

Glenn, T.M., and Lefer, A.M.: Anti-toxic action of methylprednisolone in hemorrhagic shock. Eur. J. Pharmacol. *13*: 230, 1971.

Glenn, T.M., Lefer, A.M., Beardsley, A.C., et al.: Circulatory responses to splanchic lysosomal hydrolases in the dog. Ann. Surg. *176*:120, 1972.

Grinstein-Nadler, E., and Bottoms, G.D.: Dexamethasone treatment during hemorrhagic shock: Changes in extracellular fluid volume and cell membrane transport. Am. J. Vet. Res. *37*:1337, 1976.

Haglund, U., Abe, T., Ahren, C., et al.: The intestinal mucosal lesions in shock. I. Studies of the pathogensis. Eur. Surg. Res. *8*:435, 1976a.

Haglund, U., Abe, T., Ahren, C., et al.: The intestinal mucosal lesions in shock. II. The relationship between the mucosal lesions and the cardiovascular derangement following regional shock. Eur. Surg. Res. *8*:448, 1976b.

Haglund, U., Lundholm, K., Lundgren, O., and Schersten, T.: Intestinal lysosomal enzyme activity in regional simulated shock: Influence of methylprednisolone and albumin. Circ. Shock 4:27, 1977.

Hakstian, R.W., Hampson, L.G., and Gurd, F.N.: Pharmacological agents in experimental hemorrhagic shock. Arch. Surg. 83:23, 1961.

Halpern, B.N., Bencerraf, B., and Briot, M.: The roles of cortisone, desoxycorticosterone, and adrenaline in protecting adrenalectomized animals against hemorrhagic, traumatic, and histaminic shock. Br. J. Pharmacol. 7:287, 1952.

Howard, J.M., and De Bakey, M.E.: The treatment of hemorrhagic shock with cortisone and Vitamin B-12. Surgery 30:161, 1951.

Huizenga, K.A., Brofman, B.L., and Wiggers, C.J.: Ineffectiveness of adreno-cortical preparations in standardized hemorrhagic shock. Proc. Soc. Exp. Biol. Med. 15:77, 1943.

Humphrey, E.W., Lindsay, W.G., Murphy, W.R., and Schwartz, L.: Determinants in the measurement of pulmonary extravascular water. Bull. Soc. Int. Chir. 2:132, 1974.

Jama, R.H., Perlman, M.H., and Matsumoto, T.: Incidence of stress ulcer formation associated with steroid therapy in various shock states. Am. J. Surg. 130:328, 1975.

Jones, C.A., McArdle, A.H., and Hinchey, E.J.: The enhancement of adenyl cyclase by steroid therapy in shock. Surgery 82:483, 1977.

Jordan, G.L., Jr., Fischer, E.P., and Lefrak, E.A.: Glucose metabolism in traumatic shock in the human. Ann. Surg. 175:685, 1972.

Knapp, R.W., and Howard, J.M.: Studies on the effect of hydrocortisone on irreversible hemorrhagic shock in the dog. Surgery 42:919, 1957.

Kusajima, K., Wax, S.D., and Webb, W.R.: Effects of methylprednisolone on pulmonary microcirculation. Surg. Gynecol. Obstet. 139:1, 1974.

Lefer, A.M., and Martin, J.: Mechanism of the protective effect of corticosteroids in hemorrhagic shock. Am. J. Physiol. 216:314, 1969.

Lichtman, A.L.: Adrenal cortical steroids in the treatment of surgical shock. Exp. Med. Surg. 12:434, 1954.

Lillehei, R.C., Longerbeam, J.K., Bloch, J.H., and Manax, W.G.: The nature of irreversible shock: Experimental and clinical observations. Ann. Surg. 160:682, 1964.

Lozman, J., Dutton, R.E., English, M., and Powers, S.R., Jr.: Cardiopulmonary adjustments following single high dosage administration of methylprednisolone in traumatized man. Ann. Surg. 181:317, 1975.

Mason, M.S., and Wangensteen, S.L.: The effects of purified cathepsin D infusions in intact animals. Am. J. Surg. 134:278, 1977.

McConn, R., and Del Guercio, L.R.M.: Respiratory function of blood in the acutely ill patient and the effect of steroids. Ann. Surg. 174:436, 1971.

Motsay, G.J., Alho, A., Jaeger, T., et al.: Effects of corticosteroids on the circulation in shock: Experimental and clinical results. Fed. Proc. 29:1861, 1970.

Nagasue, N., Kanashima, R., Kobayashi, M., and Inokuchi, K.: Effect of purified beta glucuronidase infusion in normal dogs and dogs with acidosis. Surg. Gynecol. Obstet. 149:173, 1979.

Nagy, S., Tarnoky, K., and Petri, G.: Effect of a water-soluble corticosteroid analogue in experimental hemorrhagic shock. J. Surg. Res. 4:62, 1964.

Nagy, S., Barankay, T., and Horpacsy, G.: Effect of corticosteroid treatment on renal blood flow in hemorrhagic shock. Eur. Surg. Res. 2:333, 1970.

Peer, R.M., and Schwartz, S.I.: Development and treatment of post-traumatic pulmonary platelet trapping. Ann. Surg. 181:447, 1975.

Pinilla, J., and Wright, C.J.: Steroids and severe hemorrhagic shock. Surgery 82:489, 1977.

Raflo, G.T., Jones, R.C.W., Jr., and Wangensteen, S.L.: Inadequacy of steroids in the treatment of severe hemorrhagic shock. Am. J. Surg. 130:321, 1975.

Rao, B.N.B., Dhawan, I.K., and Majumdar, S.: Experimental hemorrhagic hypotension: A study of the influence of dexamethasone in monkeys. Indian J. Med. Res. 58:239, 1970.

Replogle, R.L., Kundler, H., Schottenfeld, M., and Spear, S.: Hemodynamic effects of dexamethasone in experimental hemorrhagic shock—negative results. Ann. Surg. 174:126, 1971.

Ritchie, W.P., Jr., Cherry, K.J., Jr., and Gibb, A.: Influence of methylprednisolone sodium succinate on bile-acid-induced acute gastric mucosal damage. Surgery 84:283, 1978.

Sambhi, M.P., Weil, M.H., and Udhoji, V.N.: Acute pharmacodynamic effects of glucocorticoids. Circulation 31:523, 1965.

Santiago-Delpin, E.A., Vivoni, V., Suarez, A., and Roman-Franco, A.A.: Protection of organs during experimental ischemia. Surg. Gynecol. Obstet. 147:740, 1978.

Schumer, W.: Dexamethasone in oligemic shock. Arch. Surg. 93:259, 1969.

Schumer, W.: Steroids in the treatment of clinical septic shock. Ann. Surg. 184:333, 1976.

Schumer, W., and Nyhus, L.M.: The role of corticoids in the management of shock. Surg. Clin. North Am. 49:147, 1969.

Schumer, W., and Nyhus, L.M.: Corticosteroid effect on biochemical parameters of human oligemic shock. Arch. Surg. 100:405, 1970.

Selye, H., Dosne, C., Bassett, L., and Whittaker, J.: On the therapeutic value of adrenal cortical hormones in traumatic shock and allied conditions. Can. Med. Assoc. J. 43:1, 1940.

Sladen, A.: Methylprednisolone: Pharmacologic doses in shock lung syndrome. J. Thorac. Cardiovasc. Surg. 71:800, 1976.

Small, H.S., Weitzner, S.W., and Nahas, G.G.: Cardiovascular effects of levarterenol, hydrocortisone hemisuccinate and aldosterone in the dog. Am. J. Physiol. 196:1025, 1959.

Smith, J.A.R., and Norman, J.N.: Use of glucocorticoids in refractory shock. Surg. Gynecol. Obstet. 149:369, 1979.

Spath, J.A., Jr., Gorczynski, R.J., and Lefer, A.M.: Possible mechanisms of the beneficial action of glucocorticoids in circulatory shock. Surg. Gynecol. Obstet. 137:597, 1973.

Swingle, W.W., Overman, R.R., Remington, J.W., et al: Ineffectiveness of adrenal cortex preparations in the treatment of experimental shock in non-adrenalectomized dogs. Am. J. Physiol. 139:481, 1943.

Swingle, W.W., DaVanzo, J.P., Crossfield, H.C., et al.: Effect of various adrenal steroids on internal fluid and electrolyte shifts of fasted adrenalectomized dogs. Proc. Soc. Exp. Biol. Med. 99:75, 1958.

Telivuo, L., and Louhimo, I.: Experimental hemorrhagic shock in rabbits. Acta Anaesthesiol. Scand. 10:1, 1965.

Vargish, T., Turner, C.S., Bond, R.F., et al.: Dose-response relationships in steroid therapy for hemorrhagic shock. Am. Surg. 43:30, 1977.

Weil, M.H., and Whigham, H.: Corticosteroids for reversal of hemorrhagic shock in rats. Am. J. Physiol. 209:815, 1965.

Weil, P.G., Rose, B., and Browne, J.S.L.: The reduction of mortality from experimental traumatic shock with adrenal cortical substances. Can. Med. Assoc. J. 43:8, 1940.

Williams, J.S., and Clermont, H.G.: Thoracic duct lymph flow and acid phosphatase response to steroid in experimental shock. Ann. Surg. 178:777, 1973.

Wilson, J.W.: Treatment or prevention of pulmonary cellular damage with pharmacologic doses of corticosteroid. Surg. Gynecol. Obstet. 134:675, 1972.

CHAPTER 34

General Treatment of Septic Shock

WILLIAM SCHUMER

PATHOPHYSIOLOGY

The sequence of events leading to the development of septic shock begins with a bacterial invasion secondary to a major inflammatory process, such as penumonitis, subacute bacterial endocarditis, ruptured or perforated viscus peritonitis, and abdominal abscess. The precipitating agents, either gram-negative or gram-positive bacteria, are first opsonized and then phagocytosed. The opsonization factor is probably derived from the complement cascade. When the activated C3, C3b, and C5 attach themselves to the bacterial cell wall, there is a phagocytic recognition of these bacteria. The phagocyte may be either a macrophage (fixed or mobile) or a polymorphonuclear leucocyte that adsorbs bacteria to its surface and engulfs them. This is accomplished by invagination of the plasma membrane of the cell, then fusion of the membrane with itself to form an intracellular vacuole into which lysosomal enzymes are secreted. These antimicrobial enzymes include acid hydrolases, phosphorylases, highly cationic esterases, lysozymes, and myeloperoxidases. Super radicals such as nascent oxygen, peroxidases, and hydroxyl radicals produced in the presence of the myeloperoxidase halide enzymatic system contribute to the destruction of bacteria. After phagocytosis, bacterial products of either cytoplasmic or membraneous origin escape to the tissues and then enter the microcirculatory capillaries. In gram-negative sepsis it is the outer membrane, the lipopolysaccharide (LPS) or endotoxin, that is released, whereas in gram-positive sepsis a bacterial endoplasmic protein, or exotoxin, is released. This exotoxin may manifest different forms of enzymatically active toxicity as exemplified in clostridial infections. Clostridia may have 12 different exotoxins functioning as proteases, collagenases, hyaluronidases, or hemolytic agents. Streptococcus and Staphylococcus have exotoxins that have functional hemolysins, leucocytins, enterotoxins, coagulases, and hyaluronidases. The more commonly seen gram-negative septic shock is a product of the vascular response to endotoxemia. When endotoxin reaches the reticuloendothelial cells (Kuppfer cells) of the liver and spleen, it is opsonized and then adsorbed and absorbed. The reticuloendothelial system (RES) detoxifies the endotoxin. However, high concentrations of endotoxin innundate the RES, depressing its detoxifying capacity. Studies have indicated that high concentrations of LPS are capable of activating the complement system to form biologically active products. These products generated by the activation of third and fifth components produce factors such as anaphylatoxins, chemotatic factors, and immune adherence factors that cause mast cells, platelets, and leucocytes to release histamine, serotonin, and the lysosomal enzymatic system described previously. These autocoids induce increased vascular permeability, resulting in marked losses of plasma fluid into the interstitial space (third space loss) and leading to inadequate circulatory volume and ultimate circulatory collapse and shock (Müller-Eberhard, 1976; Schumer, 1979).

The hemodynamic pattern during this immunologic reaction is a hyperdynamic phase characterized by decreased peripheral resistance, which is probably secondary to the release of histamine and serotonin, as well as an increase in cardiac output. With the loss of plasma volume, the circulatory response becomes similar to that of hypovolemic shock. There is a release of epinephrine and norepinephrine, producing increased peripheral resistance and cardiac rate. Cardiac output is depressed because of the decreased blood volume and venous return. This is known as the hypodynamic phase of septic shock.

Depressed perfusion of nonvital tissues produces deranged cellular metabolism. The lack of oxygen results in the anaerobic metabolism of glucose with increased production of lactic acid, the main cause of metabolic acidosis in the hypodynamic phase of septic shock. Impaired function of the Krebs cycle depresses ATP, or energy production. This energy deficit probably aids in decreasing membrane ATP and function, allowing further loss of fluid through endothelial cells and resulting in the intracellular edema of shock (Schumer, 1979).

Recent work has indicated that endotoxemia interferes with the production of new glucose from alanine, glycerol, and lactic acid. Apparently this is caused by depression of rate-limiting enzymes, specifically phosphoenolpyruvate kinase and fructose diphosphatase, as well as an energy defect since ATP is necessary for converting gluconeogenic precursors into glucose. Depressed gluconeogenesis may also cause the increase in lactic acid since it is not being used by the liver for new glucose production. Our studies in pigs, rats, and mice have shown a positive correlation between serum endotoxin and lactate and a negative correlation between serum glucose and endotoxin. There was a positive correlation between blood pressure (BP) and the glucose/lactate ratio, indicating that the glucose/lactate ratio may be a useful prognostic and therapeutic monitor in septic shock (Schuler et al., 1976; Schumer, 1979).

New and important therapeutic concepts have been derived from studies of the immunology and molecular pathology of septic shock. In vitro studies of corticosteroids have shown that these agents have an anticomplementary effect. When administered in vivo, they decreased the serum histamine and serotonin levels secondary to complement reaction. They also aided in the induction of gluconeogenic enzymes. Studies of the hypoglycemia secondary to gluconeogenic inhibition have shown the need for an exogenous source of glucose. Therefore, glucose, insulin, and potassium solutions are now advocated as adjunctive resuscitative fluids. Although these studies were supported by noteworthy basic science and clinical data, further investigation is needed for the improvement of present therapeutic concepts and techniques to counteract the devastating effects of the complement reaction, the gluconeogenic block, and the membrane injury of endotoxin (Schumer, 1976, 1979).

Disseminated Intravascular Coagulation

Chapter 14, "Pathology and Pathophysiology of Disseminated Intravascular Coagulation", describes the pathophysiology, diagnosis, and treatment of disseminated intravascular coagulation (DIC).

Adult Respiratory Distress Syndrome

Chapter 27, "Treatment of the Adult Respiratory Distress Syndrome," describes the pathophysiology, diagnosis, and treatment of adult respiratory distress syndrome (ARDS).

Diagnosis

Septic shock can be diagnosed by a history of generalized or localized sepsis characterized by a hyperdynamic phase coinciding with the immunologic reaction to endotoxin. During this phase there are notable increases in BP, cardiac output, and pulse rate, as well as a decrease in urinary output and arterial venous oxygen difference. When this combination of symptoms is present, septic shock must be considered because the prognosis is less favorable when treatment is delayed until the hypodynamic phase. In the hypodynamic phase endothelial cell permeability ensues, there is loss of circulating blood volume, and, consequently, BP decreases, pulse rate increases, and the skin becomes cold and clammy. At this critical point a provisional diagnosis of septic shock must be made and therapy must be begun. Waiting for confirmatory blood culture will jeopardize the patient's life.

TREATMENT

In septic shock, it is essential that the septic and hypovolemic processes be treated concomitantly because preventing the complexing of antigen-antibody and complement will deter vascular permeability and its consequent hypovolemia. Prompt and adequate treatment of hypovolemia prevents the development of attending cellular metabolic derangements. The following specific treatment should be immediately instituted:

1. Cleanse and dress wounds or drain abscesses, while maintaining hemostasis.
2. Give 3 mg/kg of dexamethasone or 30 mg/kg of methylprednisolone in a single bolus as soon as septic shock is diagnosed, and repeat after 4 hr if there is no beneficial response. Do not repeat again, unless the septic shock is episodic.
3. Intravenously infuse gentamicin, 5.0 mg/kg body wt, and clindamycin, 35 mg/kg body wt, daily. Maintain serum gentamicin levels at 8–12 µg/ml by monitoring with serial serum determinations, sensitivities to antibiotic with Kirby-Bauer, and bactericidal assays.
4. Obtain six blood cultures and sensitivity tests. Remember to obtain anaerobic cultures.
5. Treat the hypovolemic phase of septic shock as hypovolemic shock, using only balanced salt solution in the following manner:
    a. Place an intravenous cannula, preferably No. 14, in a peripheral vein.
    b. Place a PAP or CVP catheter in the pulmonary artery or the vena cava, respectively.
    c. Replace lost volume with a balanced salt solution (Ringer's solution or normal saline) and bicarbonate as long as the hematocrit remains above 30%. Give whole blood if the hematocrit falls below 30%.
    d. Maintain blood pressure without decreasing PAP or wedge pressure (WP). If either pressure increases abnormally, cardiotonics must be given to maintain cardiac output, 0.5 mg of digitalis given immediately and followed by 0.25 mg every 6 hr or 5 mg of glucagon at a rate of 3–5 mg/hr. The cardiotonic chosen may be isoproterenol, 2 mg/liter in 5% glucose in water at a rate of 0.5–1.0 ml/min, to maintain systolic pressure above 80 mm Hg, or dopamine at a rate of 10–20 µg/min/kg for no longer than 8 hr, or dobutamine hydrochloride at a rate of 10 µg/min/kg.
    e. Give additional bicarbonate if the pH drops below 7.36.
    f. Maintain a urine output of 50–75 cc/hr.
    g. If the urine output falls below 30 cc/hr and there is no response to an increased infusion of Ringer's bicarbonate solution, infuse 12.5 g of mannitol over a period of 5 min. If mannitol fails to produce diuresis, give 50 mg of furosemide intravenously. If diuresis still does not occur, double the dose every 2 hr up to 400 mg. If

there is no effect, acute renal insufficiency has developed. Treatment of established renal failure should be instituted.

7. After resuscitation has been instituted, infuse the following intravenous hyperalimentation solutions every 8 hr through a PAP catheter:
   a. 1000 cc of 20% glucose plus insulin
   b. 44 mEq of potassium chloride
   c. 250 mg of thiamine hydrochloride
   d. 50 mg of riboflavin
   e. 1000 mg of ascorbic acid
   f. 1250 mg of niacinamide
   g. 50 mg of pyridoxine hydrochloride
   h. 500 mg of sodium pantothenate

8. Provide respiratory care.
   a. If the patient is not dyspneic or cyanotic, give 8–10 liters/min of oxygen by mask.
   b. If there has been injury to the chest or if there is dyspnea or cyanosis, then insert an endotracheal tube and attach it to either a "T" tube or a ventilator.

MONITORING

Monitoring of the shock patient requires continuous evaluation of the status of the following: clinical signs, vital organ function, peripheral perfusion, and volume requirements.

Monitoring of Clinical Signs

The two most important aspects in clinical monitoring are observation of the skin and of the sensorium. When the blood volume of the patient in hypovolemic shock is repleted and adequately perfuses the peripheral tissues, the skin becomes warm and dry and the color changes from grayish-white to pink. During the hyperdynamic phase of septic shock, the skin may become reddened and moist, but this is easily differentiated from the warm, pink skin characteristic of a well perfused periphery.

Although the brain is the last vital organ to experience reduced circulating blood volume, the effect on the sensorium is exhibited early in the shock state by the patient's irritability and restlessness. If the volume is not promptly replenished, coma may ensue.

Monitoring of Vital Organ Function

HEART

To monitor the heart, cardiac output and either central venous pressure (CVP) or pulmonary artery wedge pressure (PAWP) should be measured via a CVP or pulmonary artery pressure (PAP) catheter, respectively. PAWP measurement is more accurate than CVP because the latter may be altered by pulmonary hypertension and severe shunting of blood from arteries to venules; therefore, these factors must be considered before using CVP as a function of left myocardial integrity.

LUNG

PO_2 and PCO_2 measurements differentiate the type and extent of injury inflicted by the shock state on the alveolar-vascular membrane. For example, low PO_2 measurement may indicate adult respiratory distress syndrome, and high PCO_2 and low pH measurements may indicate respiratory acidosis, probably representing an underlying massive atelectasis or ventilatory diffusion problems.

LIVER

Serum glucose and lactate measurements (glucose/lactate ratio) determine the status of liver function. A glucose/lactate ratio of 10 or more indicates adequate liver function (gluconeogenesis and glycolysis); less than 10 to reversal of ratio indicates inadequate liver function due to depressed perfusion and possible hepatocellular damage.

KIDNEY

Function is monitored by measuring urinary output, which is normally 30–70 ml/hr with urine osmolality of 600 mOSM/liter. The kidney responds to depressed circulating volume by retaining water, which increases urine osmolality (antidiuretic hormone effect). The glomerular filtration rate is also depressed, causing oliguria and—as hypoperfusion progresses—nephron cell damage, and inability to retain water; finally, a salt-losing nephritis ensues. This effect is reflected in urinary water and salt losses.

Monitoring of Peripheral Perfusion

If shock is to be overcome, peripheral tissue perfusion must be constantly monitored. Skin color and temperature should be observed.

Peripheral resistance, which is indicative of the status of perfusion rate, can be derived by dividing mean arterial blood pressure by cardiac output. A high peripheral resistance indicates shunting, whereas a normal peripheral resistance indicates adequate perfusion. Another way of determining peripheral perfusion rate is by measuring either lactate or the lactate/pyruvate ratio. High concentrations of lactate indicate increased anaerobiosis produced by decreased perfusion, and low concentrations signify improved or normal perfusion.

It is important to monitor peripheral cell function by measuring the arteriovenous oxygen difference (AVO_2), because the ability of the peripheral tissues to extract oxygen from the blood indicates their viability and also identifies the phase of septic shock. In the hyperdynamic phase of septic shock, the peripheral cells have difficulty in extracting oxygen because of the mitochondrial injury secondary to sepsis or endotoxemia. Later in the hypodynamic phase, oxygen extraction increases the AVO_2 difference, which is similar to what occurs in hypovolemic shock. In hypovolemic shock the peripheral cells extract oxygen at an increased rate until the cells are close to death. Once cell death occurs, oxygen extraction decreases.

Measurement of pH and PCO_2 monitors the acid-base alterations occurring secondary to anaerobic metabolism. These are indirect measurements because the main component of anaerobic metabolic acidosis is lactic acid.

Thus, lactic acid measurements are more current and direct methods of monitoring peripheral perfusion. However, pH and PCO_2 determinations monitor the acid-base compensations of blood buffer, respiration, and kidney. A low pH and PCO_2 (metabolic acidosis) indicate severe metabolic alterations secondary to peripheral cell anaerobiosis. Contrariwise, reparation of acid-base imbalance indicates improved perfusion. Respiratory alkalosis, a commonly occurring acid-base imbalance in the hyperdynamic phase of septic shock, may be due to either a primary renal defect or, secondarily, to the compensation for an underlying metabolic acidosis. Metabolic alkalosis, most commonly occurring in gram-positive septic shock, may be due to an aldosterone effect initiated by the septic stress.

Monitoring of Volume Requirements

Volume is monitored by measuring PAP. The pulmonary vascular system blood volume is proportional to PAP, so that as PAP decreases so does volume. CVP determinations can be used to monitor young patients or those with moderate hypovolemic shock. However, it should be noted that the CVP catheter is capable of monitoring blood volume changes as long as the left myocardium is functioning normally and there is no pulmonary hypotension and no severe shunting.

Volume, being directly proportional to either urinary output or mean arterial pressure (MAP), can be monitored by measuring these two parameters. The pulse rate is inversely proportional to volume. Hematocrit, after transcapillary filling has occurred, is directly proportional to volume.

References

Müller-Eberhard, H.J.: The serum complement system. In *Textbook of Immunopathology*, edited by P.A. Miescher and H.J. Müller-Eberhard, pp. 45–73. Grune & Stratton, New York, 1976.

Schuler, J.J., Erve, P.R., and Schumer, W.: Glucocorticoid effect on hepatic carbohydrate metabolism in endotoxin-shocked monkey. Ann. Surg. *183:*345, 1976.

Schumer, W.: Steroids in the treatment of clinical septic shock. Ann. Surg. *184:*333, 1976.

Schumer, W.: Septic shock. J.A.M.A. *242:*1906, 1979.

CHAPTER 35

Treatment of Infection in Septic Shock

JEROME F. HRUSKA
RICHARD B. HORNICK

Septic shock is a problem of major proportions. It occurs predominantly in cases of gram-negative bacteremia, although septic shock in cases of gram-positive organisms (Guenter and Hinshaw, 1970; Kwaan and Weil, 1969), viruses, fungi (MacLean et al., 1967), rickettsiae, and malaria (Spink, 1971) has also been reported. Since the early reports of the association of gram-negative organisms and acute hypotension and shock (Waisbren, 1951; Borden and Hall, 1951), adequate documentation of both the increasing incidence (Finland, 1970) and the change in clinical setting and type of organism (Myerowitz et al., 1971) has been published. It is estimated that there are between 71,000 and 330,000 cases of gram-negative bacteremia per year (McCabe et al., 1972; Landesman and Gorbach, 1978). Estimates of septic shock and mortality in these cases range from 25–50% (Wolff and Bennett, 1974; Bryant et al., 1971). Numerous reviews of the various aspects of gram negative bacteremia and septic shock have been written but in this chapter we will deal primarily with the bacterial flora and the antibiotics and granulocyte transfusion used to treat these patients (Barnett and Sanford, 1969; Carrizosa, 1976; Christy, 1971; Forgacs, 1979; Lees, 1976; McHenry and Hawk, 1974; Melnick and Litvah, 1966; Shubin et al., 1977; Tramont, 1979; Weil and Shubin, 1967; Young et al., 1977).

MICROBIOLOGY

The identification of the etiological agent is important in the treatment of patients with infection and septic shock because they are caused by both gram-positive and gram-negative organisms with various sensitivities to antibiotics. Gram-negative organisms cause septic shock in more than two-thirds of cases. Since recognition of the problem of gram-negative bacteremia, numerous reports have documented a rising incidence of these infections (Finland, 1970; Altemeier et al., 1967). Some institutions have noted a shift in the relative incidence of the various gram-negative organisms. Pseudomonas have surpassed Proteus in incidence at some hospitals (Hassen, 1973), and others reported an increasing incidence of Klebsiella-Enterobacter infections over a 6-yr study period (Freid and Vosti, 1968). Finland et al. (1959) initially related the increasing numbers of gram-negative bacteremias to the lengthening life-span of the population and changing flora due to use of antimicrobial agents. Myerowitz et al. (1971) reported that hospitalized patients accounted for more than 70% of bacteremias. They attributed the rising incidence of gram-negative bacteremia to the increasing number of susceptible hospitalized patients who were infected with more resistant organisms, thus resulting in a high mortality rate. They also showed that the incidence of gram-negative bacteremias increased with the duration of hospitalization. Finally they reported a higher percentage of infection due to Serratia, Pseudomonas and Klebsiella isolates than had previous authors. Table 35.1 lists the bacterial flora of septic shock reported in four series. Note that *Escherichia coli* is the predominant pathogen in most series followed by the Klebsiella-Enterobacter-Serratia group and then Pseudomonas. In some series Proteus accounts for about 16% of the infections. For comparison purposes the flora of gram-negative bacteremias are also listed in Table 35.1 regardless of whether there is septic shock. It seems that the distribution of bacterial pathogens in septic shock is roughly proportional to their incidence in gram-negative bacteremia.

The sources of the microorganisms found in several studies of gram-negative shock are summarized in Table 35.2. The most common source is the genitourinary tract, which is commonly associated with urologic instrumentation, obstruction (especially prostatic disease in elderly men), and chronic indwelling urinary catheters. The gastrointestinal tract, including gallbladder disease, is next in frequency as a source of gram-negative sepsis. Frequently these infections are associated with gastrointestinal tract surgery, perforation of an abdominal viscus with acute intra-abdominal infection, and complications of abdominal neoplasias. The respiratory tract is often a source of gram negative shock, especially in cases of pneumonia that may develop in association with tracheostomy and aspiration of contaminated aerosols or resistant oropharyngeal flora after treatment with broad spectrum antibiotics. Wound infections, intravenous catheters, and infection of patients with burns or severe dermatitis comprise the next most likely sources of infection. Some series also show a high incidence of gram-negative shock following pelvic surgery and septic abortion (Weil et al., 1964).

Gram-positive organisms cause a small but significant proportion of cases of septic shock. The most common organisms are *Streptococcus pneumoniae* and *Staphylococcus aureus*. The clinical setting for septic shock due to gram-positive organisms includes the elderly, the alcoholic, and patients without a functional spleen, who are uniquely susceptible to shock caused by such bacteria. This latter syndrome of overwhelming postsplenectomy infection (OPSI) is most often due to Pneumococci, but *Haemophilus influenzae* ranks second and *S. aureus*, Group A Streptococcus, and Meningococcus occur in others (Chilcote et al., 1976; Case Records of the Massachusetts General Hospital, 1975; Dickerman, 1976).

Table 35.1
Bacterial Flora Found in Septic Shock and Bacteremia

	Septic Shock				Bacteremia		
	Neeley et al. (1971)	Winslow et al. (1973)	McHenry et al. (1975)	Weil et al. (1964)	Weil et al. (1964)	DuPont and Spink (1969)	McCabe and Jackson (1962)
	%					%	
Gram-positive bacteria							
S. aureus	8	10	ND[a]	ND	ND	ND	ND
Pneumococci	5	18	ND	ND	ND	ND	ND
Streptococci		8	ND	ND	ND	ND	ND
Clostridia		2	ND	ND	ND	ND	ND
Gram-negative bacteria							
E. coli	22	16	24	49	49	29	28
Klebsiella and Enterobacter	23	16	30	24	16	19	28
Pseudomonas	22	4	10	7	17	12	18
Bacteroides	0	0	14			5	
Miscellaneous				15	11	11	8
Polymicrobial		10	11			21	10
Total cases	244	50	285	176	535	860	173

[a] *ND*, not done.

Table 35.2
Source of Infection in Gram-Negative Shock and Bacteremias

	McCabe and Jackson (1962)	Winslow et al. (1973)	Neeley et al. (1971)	Nishijima et al. (1973)	Weil et al. (1964)	Christy (1971)	Gimbrere (1977)	McHenry et al. (1975)
				%				
Genitourinary tract	49	32	40	26	39	27	50	18.9
Respiratory	12	36	17	7				10.8
Gastrointestinal	25	6	15	24	7	20	12	15.1
Biliary tract		4		12		6	12	
Skin and wound	12	12	11	12	8		5	
Intravenous lines					1			15.4
Pelvic infection					43		5	9.8
Unknown								9.5

The presenting signs are those of fulminating septic shock with no focus of infection, disseminated intravascular coagulation, and sudden death. The OPSI syndrome occurs largely in children under 5 years of age, most frequently in the first 2 years postsplenectomy (Shochat, 1980), although reports of OPSI occurring in adults from 10–25 years after splenectomy are well documented (Gopal and Bisno, 1977). In addition to those who have had their spleens removed because of traumatic damage (Robinette and Fraumeni, 1977) or for staging in Hodgkin's disease, children with homozygous sickle cell disease have a high risk of overwhelming sepsis due to gram-positive organisms. The incidence of OPSI in normal hosts postsplenectomy is estimated to be 0.58% (Singer, 1973), although the incidence may be much higher after splenectomy in patients who have depressed reticuloendothelial function (e.g., thalassemia, Wiskott-Aldrich syndrome, and histiocytoses) (Eraklis et al., 1967; Smith et al., 1957).

PROGNOSTIC FACTORS IN GRAM-NEGATIVE BACTEREMIA AND SHOCK

Many studies have compared the mortality rate in gram-negative shock due to different bacterial species. McCabe and Jackson (1962) first observed that no statistically significant differences in fatality rate could be attributed to any single microorganism. Instead they found that patients with a rapidly fatal underlying illness (poor prognosis) had a very high fatality; by contrast, patients with a non fatal underlying illness (good prognosis) had the lowest fatality rate; and patients with an intermediate prognosis or ultimately fatal disease demonstrated intermediate fatality rates. These findings have been confirmed in other studies (Freid and Vosti, 1968; McHenry et al., 1975). Table 35.3 shows a multiple series summary demonstrating that the outcome of gram-negative bacteremia is related to the prognosis of the underlying disease.

McHenry et al. (1975) examined the relationship of mortality in gram-negative bacteremia even more closely on the basis of severity of symptoms due to the infection. They divided their patients into three categories: 1) *mild*—uncomplicated infection and minimal systemic illness; 2) *moderate*—uncomplicated infection and definite systemic illness; and 3) *severe*—complicated illness

Table 35.3
Relationship of Mortality in Gram-Negative Bacteremia to Underlying Disease

	Percent Mortality (Total Number of Cases)				
	McCabe and Jackson (1962)	DuPont and Spink (1969)	Bryant et al. (1971)	Freid and Vosti (1968)	Average
Rapidly fatal	91 (23)	94 (80)	81 (21)	86 (36)	90 (160)
Ultimately fatal	66 (65)	63 (299)	48 (67)	46 (92)	58 (523)
Nonfatal	11 (85)	23 (276)	16 (130)	16 (142)	18 (633)

caused by infection. Examples of complications were hypotension, shock, mental confusion, metastatic abscesses, and disseminated intravascular coagulation. As might be expected, the mortality rate was highest in those with the most severely symptomatic infection. However, regardless of the severity of the infection, patients with nonfatal underlying disease always had a better outcome than patients with either a rapidly or ultimately fatal underlying disease. Thus this more detailed analysis confirms all the other studies, which did *not* grade the severity of the symptoms of the infection, concluding that the mortality rate is more closely related to the underlying disease than to the severity of the infection.

The development of shock in gram-negative bacteremia according to the organism is shown in Table 35.4 in a retrospective study by Altemeier, et al. (1967). Shock developed in approximately 40% of the bacteremic patients regardless of the species of the organism. Moreover, the mortality rate directly attributable to the septic shock averaged 82%. Generally, however, in gram-negative bacteremias, without regard to shock, Pseudomonas has been associated with the highest mortality rates followed by Klebsiella, Proteus, *E. coli*, Serratia, and Enterobacter in descending order (Young, 1979).

Other parameters that several studies have found of prognostic value in septic shock are listed in Table 35.5. MacLean et al. (1967) found the classification of cases by central venous pressure (CVP) and blood pH to be useful. In general, the presence of acidosis was associated with a large proportion of deaths due to the shock. Others reported a poor outcome if a patient exhibited 1) a low or normal temperature during bacteremia, 2) Pseudomonas bacteremia, 3) azotemia, 4) leukopenia, or 5) persistent bacteremia.

On the other hand, factors that did *not* seem to affect the prognosis in the 218 patients with gram-negative rod bacteremia reported by Bryant et al. (1971) were race, hospital service, sex, level of leukocyte count (excluding patients with leukopenia), and portal of entry of hospital-acquired infection. Others have found that the mortality rate of hospital-acquired gram-negative bacteria (McCabe and Jackson, 1962; DuPont and Spink, 1969) is higher than for infections acquired in the community. Since as many as 70% of gram-negative bacteremias occur in the hospital, most of the deaths due to gram-negative bacteremia must be nosocomially acquired.

The incidence of gram-negative bacteremia is high in newborns (Altemeier et al., 1967) and in the elderly (Neely et al., 1971; Altemeier et al., 1967; DuPont and Spink, 1969). There are several series with conflicting conclusions when increasing age was studied for its prognostic significance. Some groups reported a higher mortality rate for the elderly bacteremic patient (Altemeier et al., 1967; DuPont and Spink, 1969), whereas others showed no age difference in mortality rate (Neely et al., 1971; Bryant et al., 1971). Nevertheless, the awareness that these types of patients may have subtle or incipient defects in their immune mechanisms and unique manifestations of gram-negative rod infections should prompt careful attention to all details in managing therapy.

TREATMENT OF SEPTIC SHOCK WITH ANTIBIOTICS

The outcome of septic shock and gram-negative infections is more dependent upon factors involved in host prognosis than whether appropriate antibiotics are used. Table 35.6 summarizes several series that attempted to correlate the survival rate in gram-negative sepsis or

Table 35.4
Relationship of Mortality in Gram-Negative Bacteremia to Bacterial Types and the Incidence of Shock[a]

Organism	Total No. Cases	Overall Mortality	Shock	Mortality in Shock
		%	%	%
E. coli	93	48	44	78
Klebsiella	68	66	38	85
Proteus	42	67	38	88
Pseudomonas	39	77	41	94
Paracolon	17	59	35	83
Mixed gram-positive	20	65	50	80
Mixed gram-negative	16	75	44	100
Bacteroides	10	30	50	60
Others	32	19	25	38
Totals	337	58	40	82

[a] Reprinted with permission from W. A. Altemeier et al.: Annals of Surgery 166:530–542, 1967.

Table 35.5
Prognostic Factors in Septic Shock: Factors Associated with Increased Mortality

Underlying disease (McCabe and Jackson, 1962)
  Rapidly fatal
  Ultimately fatal
  Nonfatal
Pseudomonas bacteremia (Bryant et al., 1971; Neely et al., 1971)
Arterial lactic acidosis and blood pH (MacLean et al., 1967)
Low cardiac output (Weil, 1977)
Low or normal temperature during bacteremia (Bryant et al., 1971)
Azotemia (Bryant et al., 1971)
Leukopenia
Persistent bacteremia (McHenry et al., 1975)

shock with antibiotic therapy. In most of these series the individual antibiotics used were not listed, and, incidentally, these therapeutic regimens in most instances were different than would be ordered today. Nevertheless, in all of these studies, treatment with *appropriate* antibiotics reduced the mortality in comparison to *inappropriate* therapy. However, the importance of the host's immune status is clearly delineated when comparing mortality rates of patients with rapidly fatal diseases who were given appropriate antibiotics for their infectious process with those patients with nonfatal diseases who were treated inappropriately (54% versus 25%). It is those patients with the worst prognosis in whom many attempts have been made to improve the outcome by manipulating the manner in which antibiotics are utilized. Some of these are as follows: 1) *empiric therapy*—treatment is started when the first sign of infection is appreciated. Combinations are used that have a broad spectrum designed to be effective against the organisms likely to be etiologically implicated. 2) *Synergistic combinations of antibiotics*—The combination of two drugs displays more activity against an organism than can be expected from the sum of the activities of each individual drug. 3) *Development of new antibiotics*—Determinations of which antibiotics are more effective. 4) *Prophylactic use of antibiotics*—Reduction of the opportunities for nosocomial infections.

Empiric Synergistic Antibiotic Therapy of Presumptive Septic Shock

Antibiotic therapy is started in most suspected cases of infections and septic shock before the culture results return. The antibiotics prescribed are determined by the microorganism suspected, the source of the organism (hospital-acquired are frequently more resistant), the site of the infection, the antibiotics with which the patient has been recently treated, and the underlying disease of the patient. An additional consideration is the requirement of achieving levels of drugs in the plasma that are bactericidal for the suspected organism. Shown in Table 35.7 are some of the suggested antibiotic regimens in cases of suspected sepsis from various sources.

Table 35.6
Mortality of Patients with Gram-Negative Sepsis with Relation to Antibiotic Treatment

Sensitivity Prognosis	Weil et al. (1964)[a]	DuPont and Spink (1969)[b]	Freid and Vosti (1968)[b]	Bryant et al. (1971)[b]	McHenry et al. (1975)[b]	Myerowitz et al. (1971)[b]	Altemeier et al. (1967)[b]	Summary[c]
				% fatality				
Sensitive								
Nonfatal	77.5	15	13	12	9	0		13
Ultimately fatal		45	42	39		5	28	39
Rapidly fatal		45	84	86	51	21		54
Resistant								
Nonfatal	91.5	22	27	29	31	28		25
Ultimately fatal		70	64	72		48	54	65
Rapidly fatal		88	91	71	67	67		79
Total no. of patients		985	269	218	243	129	175	1844

[a] Cases of septic shock only.
[b] All cases gram-negative bacteremia.
[c] Omits data from Altemeier et al. (1967) and Weil et al. (1964).

Table 35.7
Recommended Antibiotic Regimen for Empiric Therapy in Presumed Gram-Negative Bacteremia[a]

Community-acquired infection in non-neutropenic host (neutrophil count >1000/mm³)

Urinary tract source	Cephalosporin or aminoglycoside or ampicillin
Nonurinary tract source	Penicillinase-resistant penicillin plus aminoglycoside

Hospital-acquired infection

Non-neutropenic host	Cephalosporin plus aminoglycoside
Neutropenic patient with hospital-acquired infection	Ticarcillin or carbenicillin plus aminoglycoside
Thermal injury (>20% body surface)	Ticarcillin or carbenicillin plus aminoglycoside
Pulmonary source associated with inhalation therapy	Ticarcillin or carbenicillin plus aminoglycoside
Suspected gentamicin resistance	Amikacin

[a] Adapted with permission from L. S. Young: In *Principles & Practice of Infectious Diseases*, edited by G. L. Mandell, R. G. Douglas, and J. E. Bennett. John Wiley & Sons, New York, 1979.

One group of patients in whom empiric antibiotic therapy has been shown to be crucial consists of neutropenic patients with fever of unknown origin. Numerous empiric antibiotic regimens have been evaluated prospectively, and their results are summarized in Table 35.8. The authors of these studies have individually made some effort to ensure that their data were matched for age, underlying disease, microorganism ultimately found to be causing the infection, source of infection, and the bone marrow status of their patients. However, comparison of one series with another cannot be done because of the possible inherent differences in the prognostic factors in each study.

Based on the results from these controlled trials, the most common antibiotic regimen chosen for the neutropenic patient suspected of having an infection or septic shock is an aminoglycoside (gentamicin, tobramycin, or amikacin) and either carbenicillin or ticarcillin. The combination of carbenicillin and gentamicin seems to give a better response (83%) than either drug alone (50% and 57%, respectively) (Klastersky et al., 1973a). These two different classes of antimicrobials have been demonstrated to act together synergistically in in vitro and in vivo models against some strains of gram negative bacilli, especially *Pseudomonas aeruginosa*, and would be expected to be effective against most other gram-negative rods (Anderson et al., 1975; Andriole, 1971; Klastersky et al., 1970; Konickova and Prat, 1971; Wald et al., 1975; Smith et al., 1977). Klastersky et al. (1972) and Anderson et al. (1978) have correlated the clinical outcome of 321 episodes of gram-negative bacteremia and infection with in vitro synergy. (Synergy was defined as occurring when the minimum inhibitory concentration of each of the drugs in the combination was one-quarter or less of the minimum inhibitory concentration of each drug alone.) Synergistic combinations of antibiotics were especially associated with better clinical responses in those patients with rapidly fatal or ultimately fatal underlying diseases, neutropenia, and Pseudomonas infections. Recent in vitro studies indicate that synergy may occur in other organisms besides *Pseudomonas aeruginosa*, such as Klebsiella, Proteus, Serratia, Enterobacter, and Staphylococcus (D'Alessandri et al., 1976; Andriole, 1979; Comber et al., 1977; Weinstein et al., 1975; Kaplan and Koch, 1968; Hyams et al., 1974; Klastersky et al., 1973b and c; Farrell et al., 1979; Lin et al., 1979). Although multiple mechanisms of synergy exist, the best described have been the effect of the combination of penicillins and aminoglycosides against the Enterococcus. The penicillins inhibit bacterial cell wall synthesis, allowing the normally excluded aminoglycoside to enter, attach to ribosomes, and inhibit protein synthesis (Moellering, 1979). This mechanism is also operative in other microorganisms, including gram-negative rods, Staphylococci, Streptococci, and Listeria.

Despite the demonstrated advantages of combination chemotherapy, several adverse conditions occur when certain antibiotics are used together. First, carbenicillin or ticarcillin in high concentrations can inactivate aminoglycosides if mixed together before injection (Holt et

Table 35.8
Comparison of Different Antibiotic Regimens in Neutropenic Patients[a]

Study	Drug Regimen[b]	Response %	Continuous or Intermittent	Nephrotoxicity %	Comment
Klastersky et al. (1975)	Ticar and Tobra	60	Int	6	Significantly poorer response and more renal toxicity with Ceph and Tobra
	Ticar and Ceph	63		2	
	Ceph and Tobra	42		21	
Smith et al. (1977)	Amik	77	Int	8	No significant differences in renal or ototoxicity
	Gent	78		11	
Lau et al. (1977)	Amik and Carb	75	Int	8	No significant differences in renal or ototoxicity
	Gent and Carb	75		8.5	
Bodey et al. (1977)	Ceph and Carb	52	Int	8	Response was *poor* with Klebsiella, Serratia, and Enterobacter, especially if neutropenia did not resolve.
	Cef and Carb	49		0	
EORTC (1978)	Ceph and Carb	58	Int	6	Significantly *more* renal dysfunction with Gent and Ceph, especially in group of patients older than 40.
	Gent and Carb	66		3	
	Gent and Ceph	58		16	
Keating et al. (1979)	Gent and Carb	67	Cont Aminoglycoside	15[c]	No significant toxicity differences if comparable serum levels are achieved.
	Amik and Carb	68		8	
	Sis and Carb	67		22	
Love et al. (1979)	Gent and Ticar	97	Int	2	Staph responded to each regimen even before patients switched to penicillinase-resistant penicillin.
	Amik and Ticar	91		6	
	Net and Ticar	95		2	
Gurwith et al. (1978)	Carb and Gent and Meth	70	Int	0	Ototoxicity in 6% of those on Gent.
	Carb and Ceph	54		0	
Klastersky et al. (1973)	Carb and Gent	83	Int		Nephrotoxicity with Gent was 10%; however, most patients had pre-existing renal disease or other reasons for renal impairment
	Carb	50			
	Gent	57			
Schimpff et al. (1976)	Ticar and Gent	63	Int	0	Patients with rise in creatinine due to other potential causes of nephrotoxicity were excluded from side effects data.
	Ticar and Ceph	64		3	
Bodey et al. (1979)	Carb and Cont Tob	54	Cont versus Int	12	Nephrotoxicity occurred more often in documented infections than in presumptive infections.
	Carb and Cont Cef	65		13	
	Carb and Int Cef	57		12	

[a] Comparisons of one study with another should not be done because the patient population of each group may be different in their prognostic features.
[b] *Carb*, carbenicillin; *Tobra*, tobramycin; *Ticar*, ticarcillin; *Amik*, amikacin; *Ceph*, cephalothin; *Sis*, sisomicin; *Cef*, cefamandole; *Net*, netilmicin; *Gent*, gentamicin; *Meth*, methicillin.
[c] Azotemia recorded in infection was higher than that seen in fever of unknown origin.

al., 1976; McLaughlin and Reeves, 1974). The rate of inactivation is dependent upon the concentration of the drugs, the fluid in which they are dissolved, and the temperature. Consequently, it is the practice to administer the drugs at different times. In vivo inactivation of the aminoglycoside by the penicillin does not occur to any clinically significant extent, except in the patient with renal failure (Riff and Jackson, 1972; Davies et al., 1975). In such patients the determination of aminoglycoside levels is recommended to facilitate dosage of drug to ensure an adequate and nontoxic level (Barza and Lauermann, 1978; Murillo et al., 1979).

Second, combination therapy may produce more toxicity than each drug individually. For example, the combination of a cephalosporin and some aminoglycosides is associated with a higher nephrotoxicity than each drug individually (see Table 35.8) (Klastersky et al., 1975; EORTC, 1978; Wade et al., 1978).

In general these randomized, prospective, controlled studies of drug combinations have attempted to answer several questions: 1) Is there any difference in clinical response when various aminoglycosides are used in combination with either ticarcillin or carbenicillin? 2) Is the substitution of a cephalosporin for the aminoglycoside equally efficacious since that combination produces less ototoxicity or nephrotoxicity? From the studies of Keating et al. (1979), Love et al. (1979), and Lau et al. (1977), there were no statistical differences in the rate of response when the aminoglycosides (gentamicin, amikacin, netilmicin, or sisomicin) were compared. When a cephalosporin was substituted for an aminoglycoside in combination therapy with carbenicillin or ticarcillin (Klastersky et al., 1975; EORTC, 1978; Gurwith et al., 1978; Bodey et al., 1979b) there also did *not* seem to be any significant difference in the efficacy over the aminoglycoside control. Thus a cephalosporin plus carbenicillin or ticarcillin seemed to be equally as successful as an aminoglycoside plus carbenicillin or ticarcillin. There are exceptions to this general statement. For instance, Bodey et al. (1977) found that the response rates of patients infected with Serratia or Enterobacter were especially poor when treated with combinations of cephalosporins and carbenicillin because the organisms were often resistant to these drugs. Response rates of patients with Klebsiella infections were even more disappointing because Klebsiella seemed to be sensitive to the cephalosporins in vitro. It should be noted that most authorities have advocated a combination of a cephalosporin and an aminoglycoside for patients with serious Klebsiella infections, such as pneumonia, since synergism may be achieved (D'Alessandri et al., 1976). In addition, few differences in the nephrotoxicities of any of the regimens were observed, although they had been expected in those antibiotic combinations with aminoglycosides (Table 35.8). This suggested that other undefined factors besides the aminoglycoside may be responsible for the nephrotoxicity in sepsis.

Although infections due to gram positive organisms occur with low frequency in neutropenic patients, a genuine concern is raised about whether carbenicillin/ticarcillin plus an aminoglycoside will be effective in those rare cases of Staphylococcus sepsis. Gentamicin, tobramycin, and amikacin all have activity against most *Staphylococcus aureus* strains (Price et al., 1976). Hoeprich (1969) showed that gentamicin inhibited 20 strains that were resistant to methicillin and the cephalosporins. In several studies (Love et al., 1979; EORTC, 1978), patients with *S. aureus* infections were well controlled with an aminoglycoside plus either carbenicillin or ticarcillin. After identification of *S. aureus* was made, the antibiotics were changed to substitute a penicillinase-resistant penicillin, such as nafcillin, for the combination. However, widespread use of aminoglycosides for treating patients with Staphylococcal infections should be avoided because of the toxicity.

Most of these studies have found that, regardless of the antibiotic regimens, the poorest responses were seen in those patients who remained granulocytopenic during the first few days of the infectious process (Schimpff et al., 1976; Love et al., 1979). Some authors have suggested that some antibiotics (such as gentamicin) may not be as efficacious as others (carbenicillin) in the presence of neutropenia (Bodey et al., 1971, 1972). The reasons for this failure to respond to antibiotics alone are not fully understood, but numerous studies have suggested that the persistently neutropenic patient who does not respond to his initial antibiotic therapy will benefit from granulocyte transfusions (see "Granulocyte Transfusions").

Several studies have attempted to measure whether the method of administration of the antibiotic (continuous versus intermittent) had any influence on the outcome of the infection on the hypothesis that part of the failure rate was due to inadequate antibiotic levels during intermittent dosing (Feld et al., 1977, 1979; Bodey et al., 1979b). Although these studies demonstrated a better response rate in the continuous infusion group, the differences were not statistically significant.

The duration of empiric antibiotic therapy in the persistently granulocytopenic patient with a fever of unknown origin who becomes afebrile is unknown. Pizzo et al. (1979) tried to answer this question. They randomized their patients into two groups at 7 days; one group was to continue antibiotics until granulocytopenia resolved, and the other group had antibiotics stopped. Of the patients who were afebrile at 7 days and had their antibiotics stopped despite persistent granulocytopenia, 41% redeveloped a fever or an infection; one patient died. No subsequent infections or superinfections developed in the group who had their antibiotics continued until return of bone marrow function. The median duration of granulocytopenia was 12–14 days with a range of 7–25 days. These authors suggested that empiric antibiotic therapy be continued while the granulocytopenia persists in any neutropenic patient with a fever of unknown origin who becomes afebrile on the antibiotics. Whether this approach represents inadequate treatment of an existing infection or prophylaxis for a newly developing infection is unknown (see "Prophylactic Antibiotics").

In summary, the neutropenic patient with a suspected infection, bacteremia, or episode of septic shock should be covered with a synergistic combination of an aminoglycoside plus either carbenicillin or ticarcillin, pending culture results. When the organism is identified, the antibiotic regimen should be tailored to fit the particular infection using the most efficacious and least toxic drugs.

Use of Specific Antibiotics

AMINOGLYCOSIDES

Four aminoglycosides useful for the treatment of gram-negative infections are currently marketed in the United States: kanamycin, gentamicin, tobramycin, and amikacin. Kanamycin is active against most Enterobacteriaceae including E. coli, Enterobacter, Klebsiella, Proteus, and Serratia. However, with its use, reports of kanamycin-resistant strains of Klebsiella (Eickhoff et al., 1966), Proteus, Serratia (Sabath, 1969), and even *E. coli* (Baker et al., 1974) were published. Therefore, kanamycin should not be considered as a first line drug in any patient placed on empiric antibiotic therapy. Consequently, gentamicin has been used as a primary antibiotic in many hospitals because it is active against all kanamycin-sensitive organisms as well as Pseudomonas and many other kanamycin-resistant strains of Enterobacteriaceae. Once again, following widespread use of the drug, it was recognized that gentamicin resistance occurred in burn units (Shulman et al., 1971) and surgical wards (Falkiner et al., 1977). In one hospital the use of gentamicin for cardiac surgery prophylaxis led to an increase in the incidence of resistant Pseudomonas from 3 to 15% and of resistant Serratia species from 8 to 33%. After gentamicin was eliminated from the prophylactic regimen, resistant isolates decreased (Roberts and Douglas, 1978).

For the problem of resistance, tobramycin, amikacin, netilmicin, and sisomicin were developed (netilmicin and sisomicin are not currently marketed in the United States). Tobramycin is pharmacokinetically identical to gentamicin. Most gentamicin-resistant Enterobacteriaceae are also resistant to tobramycin. Tobramycin's major advantages are its activity against some gentamicin-resistant strains of Pseudomonas, as well as a slightly better minimum inhibitory concentration against Pseudomonas.

The pharmacokinetics of amikacin can be viewed as identical to kanamycin. The main advantage of this drug is its activity against most gentamicin- and tobramycin-resistant strains of Pseudomonas and many Enterobacteriaeceae. Inversely most amikacin resistant organisms are also resistant to the other two aminoglycosides (Valdivieso et al., 1975).

The most common mechanism for bacterial resistance to aminoglycosides is the plasmid-determined modification of the drug that leads to a block in the transport of the drug into the microorganism. These modifications occur by acetylation, adenylation, or phosphorylation of side groups on the aminocyclitol ring structure (Davies and Courvalin, 1977). Kanamycin's antibacterial activity is known to be suppressed by eight bacterial modifying enzymes; tobramycin, gentamicin and sisomicin by seven; and amikacin by only two, one of which is produced by S. aureus and the other by gram-negative organisms (Price et al., 1976). As would be expected logically from these mechanisms of resistance, amikacin is observed to be more active against aminoglycoside-resistant strains of bacteria than either tobramycin or gentamicin.

The side effects of the aminoglycosides as a group are predominantly renal, auditory, and vestibular toxicity (Akiyoshi, 1978; Brummett et al., 1978). Other less frequent reactions include neuromuscular blockade, usually following introduction of the drug intraperitoneally in an anesthetized patient (Finegold, 1966; Fisk, 1961), although occasionally it has occurred following parenteral administration in the postoperative period (Warner and Sanders, 1971).

Nephrotoxicity is reported in 6–12% of the patients studied in the series of antibiotic treatment regimens in neutropenic patients listed in Table 35.8. Comparative studies in animals using large excessive doses of aminoglycosides have found that the most nephrotoxic drug was gentamicin, followed by tobramycin and then amikacin (Reiner et al., 1978; Barza et al., 1978). The incidence of aminoglycoside toxicity in humans also suggests that gentamicin is more nephrotoxic than tobramycin (Fee et al., 1978; Kahlmeter et al., 1978) or amikacin (Lerner et al., 1977), but the numbers are neither statistically significant nor unequivocal. The incidence of toxicity is particularly high in elderly patients (EORTC, 1978) and in patients with pre-existing renal impairment (Klastersky et al., 1973a) or hypotension. Regular monitoring of renal function as well as serum antibiotic levels is recommended (Barza and Lauermann, 1978). Reduction of dose in renal disease can be made using published guidelines (Bennett et al., 1977). Special caution should be taken when using the aminoglycosides with such other drugs as cephalosporins or ethacrynic acid because of the increased nephrotoxicity and ototoxicity, respectively.

In summary, aminoglycosides are useful antibiotics in gram-negative infection because of their broad spectrum activity. Often they are used with carbenicillin, ticarcillin, or cephalosporins to achieve both broader coverage and synergy. Amikacin is frequently active against some gentamicin- or tobramycin-resistant strains and is often started empirically in a hospital-acquired infection in a patient with neutropenia or where resistant organisms are suspected. Fear that amikacin-resistant flora will be selected by excessive use of this drug has prompted many clinicians to restrict its usage to the aforementioned situations and to employ gentamicin or tobramycin for all other appropriate infections.

CARBENICILLIN AND TICARCILLIN

Carbenicillin and ticarcillin are two semisynthetic penicillin derivatives that are commonly used with an aminoglycoside because of the combinations' broad spectrum and synergistic effects (Kucers and Bennett, 1979). By themselves, carbenicillin and ticarcillin are active against most gram-positive organisms (except for *Staphylococcus aureus*), anaerobes, and most gram negative rods except for Klebsiella and some Serratia. Their main advantage over ampicillin is their activity against *Pseudomonas aeruginosa*, indole-positive Proteus species, some strains of Serratia, and Enterobacter. Unfortunately their antibiotic activity against gram-negative organisms is optimal only at high concentrations, necessitating doses of 18–24 g/day for ticarcillin and 24–30 g/day for carbenicillin. The lower dose of ticarcillin will achieve similar antibacterial effects as the larger dose of carbenicillin. The spectrum of activities of both drugs is virtually the same. Clinical use has failed to disclose any differences in efficacy.

Besides the relatively rare side effects that these drugs share with the penicillins as an antibiotic class, three additional major toxicities are reported: 1) hypokalemia and electrolyte abnormalities, 2) bleeding diatheses, and 3) hepatotoxicity. Each gram of these drugs contains 4.7 mEq of sodium. Thus, the recommended 30 g/day dose can become an excessive sodium load in patients with congestive heart disease or renal failure. Hypokalemia sometimes associated with a metabolic alkalosis (Klastersky et al., 1973d) can also be a significant problem. The incidence of hypokalemia is reported to be from 25–50%. One study (EORTC, 1978) reported no difference between the two drugs in their propensity to cause hypokalemia, despite the fact that twice as much carbenicillin was administered per dose. On the other hand, Schimpff et al. (1976) reported only a 20% incidence of hypokalemia with ticarcillin, whereas Bodey et al. (1977) reported a 50% incidence with carbenicillin. Despite the development of this electrolyte abnormality, antibiotic therapy is usually continued with the addition of either oral or intravenous potassium replacement.

The bleeding diathesis is also believed to be dose dependent and to result from a disturbance of platelet function (Brown et al., 1974). Most of the bleeding complications have been reported to occur in patients in renal failure who failed to have their carbenicillin adjusted for decreased renal function.

In summary, carbenicillin/ticarcillin are two drugs of similar antibacterial spectrum with identical toxicities. Since some of the toxicities are probably dose dependent, it may be beneficial to use the drug with the lowest dose.

CEPHALOSPORINS

Cephalosporins are produced by chemical modifications of cephalosporin C, a naturally occurring antibiotic produced by a mold. The nucleus of cephalosporins is closely related to the penicillin nucleus, and the mechanism of action is similar to that of penicillin. Recently many new cephalosporins have been produced and evaluated with the hope that a broad spectrum antibiotic could be produced that would have the antibacterial spectrum of the aminoglycosides without their toxic side effects. Some promising candidates are being tested and evaluated but are not available except for experimental use. Listed in Table 35.9 are the parenteral cephalosporins currently approved for use by the Food and Drug Administration (FDA). The orally administered cephalosporins (cephalexin, cefadroxil, and cefaclor) are not listed, because oral antibiotics have no place in the treatment of severe bacterial sepsis. Of the seven parenteral cephalosporins listed in Table 35.9, cephalothin, cefazolin, cephapirin, and cephradine are remarkably similar in therapeutic effectiveness and toxicity, although more data on clinical efficacy have been accumulated for cephalothin. For that reason cephalothin is often recommended in serious staphylococcal infections when a penicillinase-resistant penicillin cannot be used because of reports that it resists inactivation by staphylococcal β-lactamase better than the other cephalosporins (Fong et al., 1976). In addition, there have been reports of the failure of cefazolin in staphylococcal endocarditis (Bryant and Alford, 1977), although several centers have reported good success at doses of 6 g/day (Kaye et al., 1977); a rabbit endocarditis model showed no differences in cure rate between these two drugs (Carrizosa et al., 1978).

Cefazolin generally has slightly greater antibacterial activity against gram-negative bacteria—particularly *E. coli* and *Klebsiella pneumoniae*—in comparison to cephalothin, cephapirin, or cephradine (DelBusto et al., 1976). It is also better tolerated intramuscularly, has a longer half-life, and achieves higher serum levels than the other cephalosporins. Quintiliani and Nightingale (1978) believed that the choice among cefazolin, cephalothin, cephapirin, and cephradine is dictated by their pharmacokinetics and cost effectiveness rather than their therapeutic value. The Medical Letter (1976) also concurred with that opinion. In addition the authors pointed out that the newer cephalosporins generally have no advantage over the older ones, which have been evaluated over the years and, therefore, carry less risk of unexpected adverse reactions. Certainly, the long half-life and good intramuscular tolerance of cefazolin make it the cephalosporin of choice in the parenteral treatment of a patient with poor venous access. However, cephaloridine, an older cephalosporin for intramuscular use, is no longer recommended because of its inherent nephrotoxicity, which is not found in the newer drugs (Medical Letter, 1976).

Cefamandole and cefoxitin are newer cephalosporins with some unique antibacterial activities that make them more useful than the previously mentioned cephalosporins in certain circumstances. They are more active against some gram-negative bacilli—such as Enterobacter, Citrobacter, Providencia (cefamandole—Moellering, 1978), and Serratia (cefoxitin—Stapley et al., 1979)—than cephalothin. However, a special sensitivity test must be done for each since the cephalothin disc sensitivity test will not predict their activity. The main advantage of these two drugs is that a cephalosporin might be able to be used instead of an aminoglycoside, thus avoiding the toxicity of the latter. In perspective, however, the aminoglycosides still possess a broader spectrum of activity against the gram-negatives than even these newer cephalosporins. An additional advantage of cefamandole is its activity against ampicillin-resistant and sensitive strains of *Haemophilus influenzae*; however, like most of the cephalosporins, it does not penetrate into the cerebral spinal fluid and, therefore, should not be used to treat meningitis. Cefoxitin does *not* have activity against *H. influenzae* but does have an effect against most *but not all* strains of *Bacteroides fragilis*.

The toxicities of cephalosporins are mostly similar to those seen with the penicillins. Anaphylaxis and immediate hypersensitivity reactions have been reported. The degree of cross reaction with penicillin is uncertain, but 90% of patients with a history of a penicillin allergy do not react with cephalosporins (Dash, 1975). Thus, although the risk seems to be slight, special precautions should be taken when giving a cephalosporin to a penicillin-allergic patient, and probably complete avoidance is wise in the patient with a history of an immediate-type penicillin hypersensitivity reaction or anaphylaxis (Petz, 1978).

Except for cephaloridine, which has inherent nephrotoxicity, most of the cephalosporins have minimal effects on renal function when used alone. The reported nephrotoxicity of the combination of cephalothin with an aminoglycoside has already been discussed, although one surveillance program did not support the hypothesis that cephalothin potentiates gentamicin nephrotoxicity (Fanning et al., 1976).

In summary, the four cephalosporins—cephalothin, cefazolin, cephradine, and cephapirin—are similar in their activity against gram-positive organisms and gram-negative organisms such as *E. coli*, *Klebsiella pneumoniae* and *Proteus mirabilis*. Choice of these antibiotics should be made on the basis of relative cost, pharmacokinetics, and mode of administration. Cefamandole and cefoxitin

Table 35.9
Parenteral Cephalosporins

Generic Name	Brand Name	Dosage in Severe Infections	Intramuscular Use
Cephalothin	Keflin	2 g IV every 4 hr	Painful
Cefazolin	Ancef, Kefzol	1–1.5 g IV every 6–8 hr	Acceptable
Cephaloridine	Loridine	Not recommended	Acceptable
Cephapirin	Cefadyl	2 g IV every 4–6 hr	Painful
Cephradine	Velosef	2 g IV every 6 hr	Acceptable
Cefamandole	Mandol	2 g IV every 4–6 hr	Approved
Cefoxitin	Mefoxin	2 g IV every 4–6 hr	Painful

are slightly broader in their coverage of gram-negative bacilli and in special circumstances would be an acceptable alternative to the more toxic aminoglycosides.

USE OF STEROIDS IN SEPTIC SHOCK

The effect of corticosteroids in the treatment of septic shock has been controversial. Although other chapters deal with this subject in more detail (see Ch. 33), it is briefly reviewed here because many series recommend its use in combination with antibiotics (Cavanagh et al., 1968; Rigby and Christy, 1968). Several animal models have shown that early steroid therapy of lethal gram-negative bacteremia in conjunction with appropriate antibiotic therapy markedly reduces the mortality seen in the antibiotic-treated controls, which did not receive steroids (Balis et al., 1979; Greisman et al., 1979; Ashford et al., 1966; Lillehei et al., 1964). Balis et al. showed that steroids alone protected against lethality during the first 15 hr better than gentamicin alone, although with time both eventually displayed the same mortality rate. Greisman et al. also showed that steroids and antibiotics lessened mortality by comparison with gentamicin alone, although large numbers of animals were required to demonstrate statistical significance. Moreover, the protective effect was not seen if either the antibiotic regimen was suboptimal or therapy with steroids and antibiotics was delayed. The mechanism by which corticosteroids are believed to be beneficial in shock includes their inotropic effect on the heart; stabilization of lysosomal membranes; augmentation of microcirculation function by some direct or indirect mechanism, resulting in decreased peripheral vascular resistance and increased perfusion of vital organs; and possibly by direct detoxification of endotoxin. These have been discussed in more detail by Reichgott and Melmon (1973), Rigby and Christy (1968), and O'Flaherty et al. (1977).

Justifiably, there is concern that steroids may *not* be beneficial in humans for the treatment of infections because of their demonstration that they 1) suppress acute and chronic inflammation, 2) alter immunologic response, and 3) impair the normal intracellular mechanism for disposal of ingested foreign material by phagocytic cells (reviewed by Dale and Petersdorf, 1973). McCabe and Jackson (1962) showed that patients being treated with steroids prior to the onset of sepsis had a higher mortality from gram-negative bacteremia. Klastersky et al.'s study (1971) of the use of steroids in the compromised host with suspected infection before the onset of hypotension failed to show any significant difference in mortality or even in the incidence of septic shock. A summary of the relation of steroid treatment to the mortality of patients with gram-negative sepsis is shown in Table 35.10. Most of these studies confirm the findings in the animal studies that large doses of steroids increase survival. The protective effect was seen only if high doses of steroids were given, and little to no effect was seen with low or physiologic doses. Steroids were continued for 48–72 hr in most series, after which they were abruptly discontinued without any adverse reactions.

In summary, steroids seem to confer a protective effect on survival in gram-negative sepsis in both animal models and human studies. The protective effect was seen when high doses of steroids (such as 30 mg/kilo/day of methylprednisolone) were given. Because most of these recommendations have been derived from retrospective studies (except for the 1976 study of Schumer), these results should be considered tentative until confirmed.

GRANULOCYTE TRANSFUSION

The poor prognosis observed in septic patients with leukopenia (see "Prognostic Factors") has led to attempts to assess the role of granulocyte transfusion in the therapy of gram-negative sepsis in the neutropenic patient. Although a multitude of studies have been done, only six controlled studies have been reported (Table 35.11). A review of these studies by Strauss (1978) stated that among these controlled studies there were sufficient numbers in the gram-negative sepsis category to conclude that there is a "role for polymorphonuclear transfusion in the therapy of serious infection caused by gram-negative bacilli in neutropenic patients."

In general, these six controlled studies were performed on neutropenic patients who had a peripheral WBC less than 500 cells/mm^3 and had not responded to appropriate antibiotics (gentamicin and carbenicillin with or without cephalothin in most cases) for anywhere between 1–3 days. The neutrophils were harvested from normal donors by two different methods: 1) continuous flow centrifugation (CFC) and/or 2) filtration leukophoresis (FL), the latter method allowing slightly higher yields (Schiffer et al., 1975). Although the individual doses were extremely variable and not always listed in the six controlled studies, most patients did not receive more than 1.5×10^{10} neutrophils per transfusion when prepared by CFC or more than 5×10^{10} when prepared by FL. Insufficient studies have been performed to determine the optimum granulocyte transfusion dose, but larger numbers are probably more effective.

The neutrophils harvested by both these means have been tested for their immunological functions and have been found to be relatively normal, even if steroids or other compounds have been used to augment yields (Glasser et al., 1977). These neutrophils were examined for bactericidal activity (Glasser et al., 1977; Pole et al., 1976; Graw et al., 1972), phagocytic function (Glasser et al., 1977; Pole et al., 1975), chemotaxis (Glasser et al., 1977; Alavi et al., 1977), quantitative nitroblue tetrazolium test (Fortuny et al., 1975), and the production of colony-stimulating activity (Curtis et al., 1977).

Although five of the six controlled studies of the efficacy of polymorphonuclear transfusion (PMN-Tx) in the infected neutropenic patient demonstrated a significant benefit, the advantages were even more obvious when the subclass of patients without spontaneous bone marrow recovery was examined (Table 35.12). Sixty-six percent versus 0% and 75% versus 20% of the PMN-Tx patients in the controlled studies of Herzig et al. (1977) and Alavi et al. (1977), respectively, survived the septic

Table 35.10
Mortality of Patients with Gram-Negative Sepsis with Relation to Steroid Treatment

Steroids	Percent Mortality (Total No. of Patients)						
	Christy (1971)[a]	Weil et al. (1964)[a]	Schumer (1976)[a]	McCabe and Jackson (1962)[b]	Bennett et al. (1963)[a]	Melnick and Litvah (1966)[a]	Klastersky et al. (1970)[c]
High dose	10% (21)	57% (30)	10% (86)			34% (6)	40% (46)
Intermediate dose	89% (18)	85% (55)		70% (20)	56% (96)	80% (10)	
None	89% (9)	83% (84)	38% (86)	24% (111)	43% (98)	86% (7)	40% (39)
Comment	Uncontrolled	Retro[d]	($p < .001$)	Retro	Pro (not significant)	Retro ($p < .05$)	Pro
Steroid used and dose		Hydrocortisone >300 mg/day or ≤300 mg/day	Methylprednisoline 30 mg/kg/dose	Cortisone 200 mg/day	Hydrocortisone 300 mg/day	Hydrocortisone 100–400 mg/day 400–1000 mg/day	Betamethasone 1 mg/kilo/day

[a] Cases of septic shock only.
[b] All cases gram-negative bacteremia.
[c] Prophylactic before shock occurred.
[d] Retro, retrospective; Pro, prospective.

Table 35.11
Use of Polymorphonuclear Transfusions (PMN-Tx) in Neutropenic Patients with Infection

Treatment	Percent Survival (Total Patients)						
	Graw et al. (1972)	Higby et al. (1975)	Fortuny et al. (1975)	Vogler and Winton (1977)	Herzig et al. (1977)	Alavi et al. (1977)	Total
PMN-Tx and antibiotics	46 (39)	83 (12)	71 (17)	55 (17)	75 (16)	78 (14)	63 (115)
Antibiotics alone	30 (37)	14 (7)	71 (21)	30 (13)	36 (14)	53 (19)	41 (111)
Method of collection	CFC and FL[a]	FL	CFC	CFC	FL or CFC	FL	($p < .02$)[b]

[a] CFC, continuous flow centrifugation; FL, filtration leukophoresis.
[b] Student's t-test.

Table 35.12
Survival from Septicemia in Neutropenic Patients

	Without Bone Marrow Recovery		With Bone Marrow Recovery	
	Herzig et al. (1977)	Alavi et al. (1977)	Herzig et al. (1977)	Alavi et al. (1977)
PMN-Tx and antibiotics	8/12 (66%)	6/8 (75%)	4/4 (100%)	5/6 (83%)
Antibiotics alone	0/8 (0%)	2/10 (20%)	5/6 (83%)	8/9 (89%)

episode, even though their bone marrow had not recovered. By contrast, if bone marrow recovery occurred during the septic episode, then survival of the infection was high regardless of whether PMN-Tx was used (Bucholz et al., 1979).

Thus, the patient who would certainly benefit from a granulocyte transfusion would seem to be the patient with a gram-negative infection who is unlikely to have a return of his bone marrow function during the episode of sepsis.

The duration treatment of total dose of PMN-Tx in gram-negative sepsis is unknown. Most studies treated their patients until the bone marrow recovered, until sterilization of the cultures and loss of the fever, or until antibiotics were stopped. Following administration of 5.6×10^9 PMNs procured by CFC, the corrected PMN increase was 850, whereas 20.4×10^9 PMNs procured by FL gave an increase of only 233 (Graw et al., 1972). The percentage PMN recovery in peripheral blood was related to the degree of matching of (HLA) and ABO types in the donor and recipient. Nevertheless, leukocytes matched only by ABO typing were used in two controlled studies with excellent results (Vogler and Winton, 1977; Herzig et al., 1977; Alavi et al., 1977). Blood of a different HLA type was used as long as no leukoagglutinins were present against the donors cells before transfusion.

The side effects of therapy were more common with granulocytes prepared by FL. Most reactions consisted of fevers and chills (Herzig et al., 1977; Higby et al., 1975) and occasionally chest pain, dyspnea, and cyanosis due to pulmonary leukostasis.

Prophylactic granulocyte transfusion in neutropenic patients has been examined in several studies (Clift et al., 1978; Curtis et al., 1977; Ford and Cullen, 1977). Significant reductions in the number of confirmed infections were seen in the first two studies but not in the third. Several problems exist with granulocyte prophylaxis in the neutropenic patient. First, use of leukocytes routinely will immunize the recipient. Secondly, attempts to reduce immunization by using closely matched HLA typed granulocytes are impractical even if a donor could be found because of the difficulty in performing daily granulocyte collections from a single donor.

In summary, granulocyte transfusions for therapy in the neutropenic patient with gram-negative infection have proven valuable. Although they do not seem to greatly raise the peripheral leukocyte count, they seem to lessen the mortality due to infection, shorten the duration of fever, and, with the help of antibiotics, improve the clinical response to infection. They are *most* beneficial in the patient whose bone marrow has *not* recovered during the course of the infection. Although prophylactic granulocyte transfusions have been shown to lessen the occurrence of infection, alloimmunization and transfusion reactions overshadow their usefulness at present.

PREVENTION OF INFECTION IN THE NEUTROPENIC PATIENT

Granulocytopenic patients become infected with endogenous flora as well as newly acquired hospital flora. Numerous studies have been performed to test whether sterilization of the patient's own flora as well as isolation from the normal hospital environment will decrease the incidence of fever, serious infection, and the mortality rate (Editorial, Lancet, 1978). A combination of a protected environment and prophylactic antibiotics has been shown to significantly lower the risk of fatal infection in patients with leukemia (Levine et al., 1973; Rodriguez et al., 1978; Schimpff et al., 1975), bone marrow transplants (Buckner et al., 1978), and malignant lymphoma (Bodey et al., 1979a). These randomized, prospective studies used laminar flow room isolation of the patient and various combinations of oral nonabsorbable antibiotics, such as mycostatin, gentamicin, vancomycin, paramomycin, and polymyxin. Use of oral nonabsorbable antibiotics alone in the patient in a conventional hospital bed with reverse isolation may be nearly as efficacious (Schimpff et al., 1975; Storring et al., 1977), although controversy still exists (Levine et al., 1973; Rodriguez et al., 1978). Because some of the oral nonabsorbable antibiotic regimens have not been tolerated by the patient, other regimens have been tried (Watson and Jameson, 1979). Sulfamethoxozole-trimethoprim alone or in addition to oral nonabsorbable antibiotics have been shown to reduce the infection rate of leukopenic patients on routine reverse isolation (Gurwith et al., 1979; Enno et al., 1978a and b; Guiot et al., 1978).

In summary, prophylactic antibiotics seem to reduce infection and improve survival in neutropenic hosts. A protective environment, such as a laminar flow room, probably adds to these gains. Only time will tell whether bacteria resistant to the oral prophylactic antibiotic regimens will become a problem and necessitate using antibiotics that are less likely to be used for the treatment of infection.

PREVENTION OF PNEUMOCOCCAL SEPSIS IN THE SPLENECTOMIZED PATIENT

The generally accepted approach to the prevention of overwhelming pneumococcal sepsis in the splenectomized patient or the patient with sickle cell anemia is prophylaxis with penicillin V, 125 mg bid for children and 250 mg bid for adults (Medical Letter, 1977). The duration of prophylaxis is unknown since there are no data on this point. Yeager (1980) recommended administering prophylactic penicillin to children up to the age of 5 and immunizing at age 5 with the pneumococcal vaccine, which has the capsular polysaccharide of the 14 pneumococcal serotypes that cause 85% of pneumococcal disease. Thereafter, routine penicillin prophylaxis would be used only on patients whose underlying disease (such as Hodgkin's disease, sickle cell anemia, etc.) would put them at extremely high risk. Pneumococcal vaccine is protective against systemic pneumococcal infection in the patient with splenectomy or sickle cell disease (Ammann et al., 1977), although failures have occurred due to both poor immunogenic response to the vaccine (Ahonkhai et al., 1979) or to infection with a serotype not included in the vaccine (Appelbaum et al., 1979). It is also generally recommended that these patients be given a supply of oral penicillin or ampicillin to take at the first sign of respiratory illness or high fever if a physician's evaluation cannot be obtained immediately because of the rapid progression of the infection (Medical Letter, 1977; Yeager, 1980).

References

Ahonkhai, V.I., Landesman, S.H., Fikrig, S.M., Schmalzer, E.A., Brown, A.K., Cherubin, C.E., and Schiffman, G.: Failure of pneumococcal vaccine in children with sickle-cell disease. N. Engl. J. Med. *301*:26–27, 1979.

Akiyoshi, M.: Evaluation of ototoxicity of tobramycin in guinea pigs. J. Antimicrob. Chemother. (Suppl. A) *4*:A69–72, 1978.

Alavi, J.B., Root, R.K., Djerassi, I., Evans, A.E., Gluckman, S.J., Mac Gregor, R.R., Guerry, D., Schreiber, A.D., Shaw, J.M., Koch, P., and Cooper, R.A.: A randomized clinical trial of granulocyte transfusions for infection in acute leukemia. N. Engl. J. Med. *296*:706–711, 1977.

Altemeier, W.A., Todd, J.C., and Inge, W.W.: Gram-negative septicemia: A growing threat. Ann. Surg. *166*:530–542, 1967.

Ammann, A.J., Addiego, J., Wara, D.W., Lubin, B., Smith, W.B., and Mentzer, W.C.: Polyvalent pneumococcal-polysaccharide immunization of patients with sickle-cell anemia and patients with splenectomy. N. Engl. J. Med. *297*:897–900, 1977.

Anderson, E.L., Gramling, P.K., Vestal, P.R., and Farrar, W.E.: Susceptibility of *Pseudomonas aeruginosa* to tobramycin or gentamicin alone and combined with carbenicillin. Antimicrob. Agents Chemother. *8*:300–304, 1975.

Anderson, E.T., Young, L.S., and Hewitt, W.L.: Antimicrobial synergism in the therapy of gram-negative rod bacteremia. Chemotherapy *24*:45–54, 1978.

Andriole, V.T.: Synergy of carbenicillin and gentamicin in experimental infection with Pseudomonas. J. Infect. Dis. (Suppl) *124*:446–55, 1971.

Andriole, V.T.: Staphylococci and combination therapy. Arch. Intern. Med. *139*:1090–1091, 1979.

Appelbaum, P.C., Shaikh, B.S., Widome, M.D., Gordon, R.A., and Austrian, R.: Fatal pneumococcal bacteremia in a vaccinated splenectomized child. N. Engl. J. Med. *300*:203–204, 1979.

Ashford, T., Palmerio, C., and Fine, J.: Structural analogue in vascular muscle to the functional disorder in refractory

traumatic shock and reversal by corticosteroid. Ann. Surg. *164:*575–584, 1966.
Baker, C.J., Barrett, F.F., and Clark, D.J.: Incidence of kanamycin resistance among *Escherichia coli* isolates from neonates. J. Pediatr. *84:*126, 1974.
Balis, J.V., Paterson, J.F., Shelley, S.A., Larson, C.H., Fareed, J., and Gerber, L.I.: Glucocorticoid and antibiotic effects on hepatic microcirculation and associated host responses in lethal gram-negative bacteremia. Lab. Invest. *40:*55–65, 1979.
Barnett, J.A., and Sanford, J.P.: Bacterial shock. J.A.M.A. *209:* 1514–1517, 1969.
Barza, M., and Lauermann, M.: Why monitor serum levels of gentamicin? Clin. Pharmacokinetics *3:*202–215, 1978.
Barza, M., Pinn, V., Tanguay, P., and Murray, T.: Nephrotoxicity of newer cephalosporins and aminoglycosides alone and in combination in a rat model. J. Antimicrob. Chemother. (Suppl. A) *4:*A59–68, 1978.
Bennett, I.L., Finland, M., Hamburger, M., Kass, E.H., Lepper, M., and Waisbren, B.A.: The effectiveness of hydrocortisone in the management of severe infections: A double-blind study. J.A.M.A. *183:*462–465, 1963.
Bennett, W.M., Singer, I., Golper, T., Feig, P., and Coggins, C.J.: Guidelines for drug therapy in renal failure. Ann. Intern. Med. *86:*754–783, 1977.
Bodey, G.P., Whitcar, J.P., Middleman, E., et al.: Carbenicillin therapy of Pseudomonas infections. J.A.M.A. *218:*62–77, 1971.
Bodey, G.P., Middleman, E., Umsawasdi, T., et al.: Infections in cancer patients: Results with gentamicin sulfate therapy. Cancer *29:*1697–1701, 1972.
Bodey, G.P., Valdivieso, M., Feld, R., Rodriguez, V., and McCredie, K.: Carbenicillin plus cephalothin or cefazolin as therapy for infections in neutropenic patients. Am. J. Med. Sci. *273:*309–318, 1977.
Bodey, G.P., Rodriguez, V., Cabanillas, F., and Freireich, E.J.: Protected environment-prophylactic antibiotic program for malignant lymphoma: Randomized trial during chemotherapy to induce remission. Am. J. Med. *66:*74–81, 1979a.
Bodey, G.P., Ketchel, S.J., and Rodriguez, V.: A randomized study of carbenicillin plus cefamandole or tobramycin in the treatment of febrile episodes in cancer patients. Am. J. Med. *67:*608–616, 1979b.
Borden, C.W., and Hall, W.H.: Fatal transfusion reactions from massive bacterial contamination of blood. N. Engl.J. Med. *245:*760, 1951.
Brown, C.H., Natelson, E.A., Bradshaw, W., Williams, T.W., and Alfrey, C.P.: The hemostatic defect produced by carbenicillin. N. Engl. J. Med. *291:*265–270, 1974.
Brummett, R.E., Fox, K.E., Bendrick, T.W., and Himes, D.L.: Ototoxicity of tobramycin, gentamicin, amikacin, and sisomicin in the guinea pig. J. Antimicrob. Chemother. (Suppl. A) *4:*A73–83, 1978.
Bryant, R.E., and Alford, R.H.: Unsuccessful treatment of staphylococcal endocarditis with cefazolin. J.A.M.A. *237:* 569–570, 1977.
Bryant, R.E., Hood, A.F., Hood, C.E., and Koenig, M.G.: Factors affecting mortality of gram-negative rod bacteremia. Arch. Intern. Med. *127:*120–128, 1971.
Buchholz, D.H., Blumberg, N., and Bove, J.R.: Long-term granulocyte transfusion in patients with malignant neoplasms. Arch. Intern. Med. *139:*317–320, March, 1979.
Buckner, C.D., Clift, R.A., Sanders, J.E., Meyers, J.D., Counts, G.W., Farewell, V.T., Thomas, D., and the Seattle marrow transplant team: Protective environment for marrow transplant recipients: A prospective study. Ann. Intern. Med. *89:* 893–901, 1978.
Carrizosa, J.: Gram-negative sepsis. J. Am. Med. Wom. Assoc. *31:*354–362, 1976.
Carrizosa, J., Santoro, J., and Kaye, D.: Treatment of experimental *Staphylococcus aureus* endocarditis: Comparison of cephalothin, cefazolin, and methacillin. Antimicrob. Agents Chemother. *13:*74–77, 1978.
Case Records of the Massachusetts General Hospital: Fever and circulatory collapse in an asplenic man. N. Engl. J. Med. *293:*547–553, 1975.
Cavanagh, D., Clark, P.J., and McLeod, A.G.W.: Septic shock of endotoxin type: Some observations based on the management of 50 patients. Am. J. Obstet. Gynecol. *102:*13–20, 1968.
Chilcote, R.R., Bachner, R.L., Hammond, D., and the investigators and special studies committee of the children's cancer study group: Septicemia and meningitis in children splenectomized for Hodgkin's disease. N. Engl. J. Med. *295:*798–800, 1976.
Christy, J.H.: Treatment of gram-negative shock. Am. J. Med. *50:*77–78, 1971.
Clift, R.A., Sanders, J.E., Thomas, E.D., Williams, B., and Buckner, D.C.: Granulocyte transfusions for the prevention of infection in patients receiving bone-marrow transplants. N. Engl. J. Med. *298:*1052–1057, 1978.
Comber, K.R., Basker, M.J., Osborne, C.D., and Sutherland, R.: Synergy between ticarcillin and tobramycin against *Pseudomonas aeruginosa* and Enterobacteriaceae in vitro and in vivo. Antimicrob. Agents Chemother. *11:*956–964, 1977.
Curtis, J.E., Hasselback, R., and Bergsagel, D.E.: Leukocyte transfusion for prophylaxis and treatment of infections associated with granulocytopenia. Can. Med. Assoc. J. *117:* 341–345, 1977.
Dale, D.C., and Petersdorf, R.G.: Corticosteroids and infectious diseases. Med. Clin. North Am. *57:*1277–1288, 1973.
D'Alessandri, R.M., McNeely, D.J., and Kluge, R.M.: Antibiotic synergy and antagonism against clinical isolates of Klebsiella species. Antimicrob. Agents Chemother. *10:*889, 1976.
Dash, C.H.: Penicillin allergy and the cephalosporins. J. Antimicrob. Chemother. (Suppl). *1:*S107, 1975.
Davies, J., and Courvalin, P.: Mechanisms of resistance to aminoglycosides. Am. J. Med. *62:*868–872, 1977.
Davies, M., Morgan, J.R., and Anand, C.: Interactions of carbenicillin and ticarcillin with gentamicin. Antimicrob. Agents Chemother. *7:*431–434, 1975.
DelBusto, R., Haas, E., Madhaven, T., et al.: In vitro and clinical studies of cefatrizine, a new semisynthetic cephalosporin. Antimicrob. Agents Chemother. *9:*397–405, 1976.
Dickerman, J.D.: Bacterial infection and the asplenic host: A review. J. Trauma *16:*662–668, 1976.
DuPont, H.L., and Spink, W.W.: Infections due to gram-negative organisms: An analysis of 860 patients with bacteremia at the University of Minnesota Medical Center, 1958–1966. Medicine *48:*307–332, 1969.
Editorial: Infection prevention in acute leukemia. Lancet *2:* 769–770, 1978.
Eickhoff, T.C., Steinhauer, B.W., and Finland, M.: The Klebsiella-Enterobacter-Serratia division: Biochemical and serological characteristics and susceptibility to antibiotics. Ann. Intern. Med. *65:*1163, 1966.
Enno, A., Catovsky, D., Darrell, J., Goldman, J.M., Hows, J., and Galton, D.A.G.: Co-trimoxazole for prevention of infection in acute leukemia. Lancet *2:*395–397, 1978a.

Enno, A., Catovsky, D., and Darrell, J.: Prophylactic co-trimazole in leukemia. Lancet 2:625, 1978b.

EORTC International Antimicrobial Therapy Project Group: Three antibiotic regimens in the treatment of infection in febrile granulocytopenic patients with cancer. J. Infect. Dis. 137:14–29, 1978.

Eraklis, A.J., Kevy, S.V., Diamond, L.K., et al.: Hazard of overwhelming infection after splenectomy in children. N. Engl. J. Med. 276:1225–1229, 1967.

Falkiner, F.R., Keane, C.T.T., Dalton, M., Clancy, M.T., and Jacoby, G.A.: Cross infection in a surgical ward caused by *Pseudomonas aeruginosa* with transferable resistance to gentamicin and tobramycin. J. Clin. Pathol. 30:731, 1977.

Fanning, W.L., Gump, D., and Jick, H.: Gentamicin and cephalothin associated rises in blood urea nitrogen. Antimicrob. Agents Chemother. 10:80, 1976.

Farrell, W., Wilks, M., and Drasar, F.A.: Synergy between aminoglycosides and semi-synthetic penicillins against gentamicin-resistant gram negative rods. J. Antimicrob. Chemother. 5:23–29, 1979.

Fee, W.E., Vierra, V., and Lathrop, G.R.: Clinical evaluation of aminoglycoside toxicity: Tobramycin versus gentamicin, a preliminary report. J. Antimicrob. Chemother. (Suppl. A)4:31–36, 1978.

Feld, R., Valdivieso, M., Bodey, G.P., and Rodriguez, V.: A comparative trial of sisomicin therapy by intermittent versus continuous infusion. Am. J. Med. Sci. 274:179–188, 1977.

Feld, R., Tuffnell, P.G., Curtis, J.E., Messner, H.A., and Hasselback, R.: Empiric therapy for infections in granulocytopenic cancer patients: Continuous infusion of amikacin plus cephalothin. Arch. Intern. Med. 139:310–314, 1979.

Finegold, S.M.: Toxicity of kanamycin in adults. Ann. N.Y. Acad. Sci. 132:942, 1966.

Finland, M.: Changing ecology of bacterial infections as related to antibiotic therapy. J. Infect. Dis. 122:419, 1970.

Finland, M., Jones, W.F., and Barnes, M.W.: Occurrence of serious bacterial infections since introduction of antibacterial agents. J.A.M.A. 170:2188–2197, 1959.

Fisk, G.C.: Respiratory paralysis after a large dose of streptomycin. Br. Med. J. 1:556, 1961.

Fong, I.W., Engelking, E.R., and Kirby, W.M.M.: Relative inactivation by *Staphylococcus aureus* of eight cephalosporin antibiotics. Antimicrob. Agents Chemother. 9:939–944, 1976.

Ford, J.M., and Cullen, M.H.: Prophylactic granulocyte transfusions. Exp.Hematol. (Suppl. 1)5:65–72, 1977.

Forgacs, P.: Treatment of septic shock. Med. Clin. North Am. 63:465–471, 1979.

Fortuny, I.E., Bloomfield, C.D., Hadlock, D.C., Goldman, A., Kennedy, B.J., and McCullough, J.J.: Granulocyte transfusion: A controlled study in patients with acute nonlymphocytic leukemia. Transfusion 15:548–558, 1975.

Freid, M.A., and Vosti, K.L.: The importance of underlying disease in patients with gram-negative bacteremia. Arch. Intern. Med. 121:418–423, 1968.

Gimbrere, J.S.F.: Septic shock. Neth. J. Med. 20:184–190, 1977.

Glasser, L., Huestis, D.W., and Jones, J.F.: Functional capabilities of steroid-recruited neutrophils harvested for clinical transfusion. N. Engl. J. Med. 297:1033–1036, 1977.

Gopal, V., and Bisno, A.L.: Fulminant pneumococcal infections in "normal" asplenic hosts. Arch. Intern. Med. 137:1526–1530, 1977.

Graw, R.G., Herzig, G., Perry, S., and Henderson, E.S.: Normal granulocyte transfusion therapy: Treatment of septicemia due to gram-negative bacteria. N. Engl. J. Med. 287:367–371, 1972.

Greisman, S.E., DuBuy, J.B., and Woodward, C.L.: Experimental gram-negative bacterial sepsis: Prevention of mortality not preventable by antibiotics alone. Infect. Immun. 25:538–557, 1979.

Guenter, C.A., and Hinshaw, L.B.: Comparison of septic shock due to gram-negative and gram-positive organisms. Proc. Soc. Exp. Biol. Med. 134:780, 1970.

Guiot, H.F.L., Van der Meer, J.W.M., and VanFurth, R.: Prophylactic co-trimoxazole in leukemia. Lancet 2:678, 1978.

Gurwith, M., Brunton, J.L., Lank, B., Ronald, A.R., Harding, G.K.M., and McCullough, D.W.: Granulocytopenia in hospitalized patients. II. A prospective comparison of two antibiotic regimens in the empiric therapy of febrile patients. Am. J. Med. 64:127–132, 1978.

Gurwith, M.J., Brunton, J.L., Lank, B.A., Harding, G.K.M., and Ronald, A.R.: A prospective controlled investigation of prophylactic trimethoprim/sulfamethoxazole in hospitalized granulocytopenic patients. Am. J. Med. 66:248–256, 1979.

Hassen, A.: Gram-negative bacteremic shock. Med. Clin. North Am. 57:1403, 1973.

Hershko, C.: Granulocyte transfusion. Vox Sang. 34:129–135, 1978.

Herzig, R.H., Herzig, G.P., Graw, R.G., Bull, M.I., and Ray, K.K.: Successful granulocyte transfusion therapy for gram-negative septicemia. N. Engl. J. Med. 296:701–705, 1977.

Higby, D.J., Yates, J.W., Henderson, E.S., and Holland, J.F.: Filtration leukapheresis for granulocyte transfusion therapy. N. Engl. J. Med. 292:761–766, 1975.

Hoeprich, P.D.: Gentamicin versus *Staphylococcus aureus*. J. Infect. Dis. 119:391, 1969.

Holt, H.A., Broughall, J.M., McCarthy, M., and Reeves, D.S.: Interactions between aminoglucoside antibiotics and carbenicillin or ticarcillin. Infection 4:107–109, 1976.

Hyams, P.J., Simberkoff, M.S., and Rahal, J.J.: Synergy between cephalosporin and aminoglycoside antibiotics against Providencia and Proteus. Antimicrob. Agents Chemother. 5:571–577, 1974.

Kahlmeter, G., Hallberg, T., and Kamme, C.: Gentamicin and tobramycin in patients with various infections. J. Antimicrob. Chemother. (Suppl. A)4:A47-52, 1978.

Kaplan, D., and Koch, W.: Synergistic effect of combinations of cephalothin and kanamycin on strains of *E. coli*. Nature 218:1165–1168, 1968.

Kaye, D., Hewitt, W., Remington, J.S., and Turck, M.: Cefazolin and *Staphylococcus aureus* endocarditis. J.A.M.A. 237:2601, 1977.

Keating, M.J., Bodey, G.P., Valdivieso, M., and Rodriguez, V.: A randomized comparative trial of three aminoglycosides: Comparison of continuous infusions of gentamicin, amikacin and sisomicin combined with carbenicillin in the treatment of infections in neutropenic patients with malignancies. Medicine 58:159–170, 1979.

Klastersky, J., Swings, G., and Daneau, D.: Antimicrobial activity of the carbenicillin/gentamicin combination against gram-negative bacilli. Am. J. Med. Sci. 260:373–380, 1970.

Klastersky, J., Cappel, R., and Debusscher, L.: Effectiveness of betamethasone in management of severe infections: A double-blind study. N. Engl. J. Med. 284:1248–1250, 1971.

Klastersky, J., Cappel, R., and Daneau, D.: Clinical significance of in vitro synergism between antibiotics in gram-negative infections. Antimicrob. Agents Chemother. 2:470–475, 1972.

Klastersky, J., Cappel, R., and Daneau, D.: Therapy with

carbenicillin and gentamicin for patients with cancer and severe infections caused by gram-negative rods. Cancer *31:* 331–336, 1973a.

Klastersky, J., Henri, A., and Vandenborre, L.: Antimicrobial activity of tobramycin and gentamicin used in combination with cephalothin and carbenicillin. Am. J. Med. Sci. *277:*13–21, 1973b.

Klastersky, J., Swings, G., Vandenborre, L., Weerts, D., and deMaertelaer, V.: Effectiveness of the carbenicillin/cephalothin combination against gram negative bacilli. Am. J. Med. Sci. *265:*45–53, 1973c.

Klastersky, J.B., Vanderkelen, B., Daneau, D., and Mathieu, M.: Carbenicillin and hypokalemia. Ann. Intern. Med. *78:* 774–775, 1973d.

Klastersky, J., Hensgens, C., and Debrusscher, L.: Empiric therapy for cancer patients: Comparative study of ticarcillin-tobramycin, ticarcillin-cephalothin, cephalothin-tobramycin. Antimicrob. Agents Chemother. *7:*640–645, 1975.

Konickova, L., and Prat, W.: Effect of carbenicillin, gentamicin and their combination on experimental *Pseudomonas aeruginosa* urinary tract infection. J. Clin. Pathol. *24:*113–116, 1971.

Kucers, A., and Bennet, N.: *The Use of Antibiotics: A Comprehensive Review with Clinical Emphasis,* ed. 3. J.B. Lippincott, Philadelphia, 1979.

Kwaan, H.M., and Weil, M.H.: Differences in the mechanism of shock caused by bacterial infections. Surg. Gynecol. Obstet. *128:*37, 1969.

Landesman, S.H., and Gorbach, S.L.: Gram negative sepsis and shock. Orthop. Clin. North Am. *9:*611–625, 1978.

Lau, W.K., Young, L.S., Black, R.E., Winston, D.J., Linne, S.R., Weinstein, R.J., and Hewitt, W.L.: Comparative efficacy and toxicity of amikacin/carbenicillin versus gentamicin/carbenicillin in leukopenic patients: A randomized prospective trial. Am. J. Med. *62:*959–966, 1977.

Lees, N.W.: The diagnosis and treatment of endotoxic shock. Anesthesia *31:*897–909, 1976.

Lerner, S.A., Seligsohn, R., and Matz, G.J.: Comparative clinical studies of ototoxicity and nephrotoxicity of amikacin and gentamicin. Am. J. Med. *62:*919–923, 1977.

Levine, A.S., Siegel, S.E., Schreiber, A.D., Hauser, J., Preisler, H., Goldstein, I.M., Seidler, F., Simon, R., Perry, S., Bennett, J.E., and Henderson, E.S.: Protected environments and prophylactic antibiotics: A prospective controlled study of their utility in the therapy of acute leukemia. N. Engl. J. Med. *288:*477, 1973.

Lillehei, R.C., Longerbeam, J.K., Bloch, J.H., and Manax, W.G.: Nature of irreversible shock: Experimental and clinical observations. Ann. Surg. *160:*682, 1964.

Lin, M.Y.C., Tauzon, C.V., and Sheagren, J.N.: Synergism of aminoglycosides and carbenicillin against resistant strains of *Serratia marcescens.* J. Antimicrob. Chemother. *5:*37–44, 1979.

Love, L.J., Schimpff, S.C., Hahn, D.M., Young, V.M., Standiford, H.C., Bender, J.F., Fortner, C.L., and Wiernick, P.H.: Randomized trial of empiric antibiotic therapy with ticarcillin in combination with gentamicin, amikacin, or netilmicin in febrile patients with granulocytopenia and cancer. Am. J. Med. *66:*603–610, 1979.

MacLean, L.D., Mulligan, W.G., McLean, A.P.H., and Duff, J.: Patterns of septic shock in man: A detailed study of 56 patients. Ann. Surg. *166:*543–562, 1967.

McCabe, W.R., and Jackson, G.G.: Gram-negative bacteremia. I and II. Arch. Intern. Med. *110:*847–864, 1962.

McCabe, W.R., Kreger, B.E., and Johns, M.: Type specific and cross-reactive antibodies in gram-negative bacteremia. N. Engl. J. Med. *287:*261–267, 1972.

McHenry, M.C., and Hawk, W.A.: Bacteremia caused by gram-negative bacilli. Med. Clin. North Am. *58:*623, 1974.

McHenry, M.C., Gavan, T.L., Hawk, W.A., et al.: Gram-negative bacteremia: Variable clinical course and useful prognostic factors. Cleve. Clin. Q. *42:*15–32, 1975.

McLaughlin, J.E., and Reeves, D.S.: Clinical and laboratory evidence for inactivation of gentamicin by carbenicillin. Lancet *1:*261–264, 1974.

Medical Letter: The cephalosporins. *18:*33–35, 1976.

Medical Letter: Prevention of serious infections after splenectomy. *19:*2–4, 1977.

Melnick, I., and Litvah, A.S.: Gram-negative bacteremia: An evaluation of fifty-nine cases during 1963. J. Urol. *96:*257–262, 1966.

Moellering, R.C.: Cefamandole: A new member of the cephalosporin family. J. Infect. Dis. (Suppl.)*137:*S2–S9, 1978.

Moellering, R.C.: Antimicrobial synergism: An elusive concept. J. Infect. Dis. *140:*639–641, 1979.

Murillo, J., Standiford, H.C., Schimpff, S.C., and Tatem, B.A.: Gentamicin and ticarcillin serum levels. J.A.M.A. *241:*2401, 1979.

Myerowitz, R.L., Medeiros, A., and O'Brian, T.F.: Recent experience with bacillemia due to gram-negative organisms. J. Infect. Dis. *124:*239–246, 1971.

Neely, W.A., Berry, D.W., Rushton, F.W., et al.: Septic shock: Clinical, physiological and pathological survey of 244 patients. Ann. Surg. *173:*657–666, 1971.

Nishijima, H., Weil, M.H., Shubin, H., and Cavanilles, J. Hemodynamic and metabolic studies on shock associated with gram negative bacteremia. Medicine *52:*287–293, 1973.

O'Flaherty, J.T., Craddock, P.R., and Jacob, H.S: Mechanism of anticomplementary activity of corticosteroids in vivo: Possible relevance in endotoxin shock. Proc. Soc. Exp. Biol. Med. *154:*206–209, 1977.

Petz, L.D.: Immunologic cross-reactivity between penicillins and cephalosporins: A review. J. Infect. Dis. (Suppl.)*137:* S74, 1978.

Pizzo, P.A., Robichaud, F.J., Gill, F.A., Witebsky, F.G., Levine, A.S., Deisseroth, A.B., Glaubiger, D.L.: Maclowry, J.D., Magrath, I.T., Poplack, D.G., and Simon, R.M.: Duration of empiric antibiotic therapy in granulocytopenic patients with cancer. Am. J. Med. *67:*194–200, 1979.

Pole, J.G., Davie, M., Kershaw, I., Barter, D.A.C., and Willoughby, M.L.N.: Granulocyte transfusion in treatment of infected neutropenic children. Arch. Dis. Child. *51:*521–527, 1976.

Price, K.E., Casson, K., DeRigis, R.G., Kresel, P.A., Pursiano, T.A., and Leitner, F.: Amikacin: Antimicrobial properties and resistant mechanisms affecting its activity. U.S. Amikacin Symposium, pp. 14–24. University of California Medical School, Los Angeles, November 9–10, 1976.

Quintiliani, R., and Nightingale, C.H.: Cefazolin. Ann. Intern. Med. *89:*650–656, 1978.

Reichgott, M.J., and Melmon, K.L.: Should corticosteroids be used in shock? Med. Clin. North Am. *57:*1211–1223, 1973.

Reiner, N.E., Bloxham, D.D., and Thompson, W.L.: Nephrotoxicity of gentamicin and tobramycin given once daily or continuously in dogs. J. Antimicrob. Chemother. (Suppl. A)*4:*A85–101, 1978.

Riff, L.J., and Jackson, G.G.: Laboratory and clinical conditions for gentamicin inactivation by carbenicillin. Arch. Intern. Med. *130:*887–891, 1972.

Rigby, R.A., and Christy, J.H.: Recovery following prolonged gram-negative shock and "shock lung." Am.J. Med. 45:959–966, 1968.

Roberts, N.J., and Douglas, R.G.: Gentamicin use and Pseudomonas and Serratia resistance: Effect of a surgical prophylaxis regimen. Antimicrob. Agents Chemother. 13:214–220, 1978.

Robinette, C.D., and Fraumeni, J.F.: Splenectomy and subsequent mortality in veterans of the 1939–45 war. Lancet 2:127–129, 1977.

Rodriguez, V., Bodey, G.P., Freireich, E.J., McCredie, K.B., Gutterman, J.B., Keating, M.J., Smith, T.L., and Gehan, E.A.: Randomized trial of protected environment-prophylactic antibiotics in 145 adults with acute leukemia. Medicine 57:253–266, 1978.

Sabath, L.D.: Current concepts: Drug resistance of bacteria. N. Engl. J. Med. 280:91, 1969.

Schiffer, C.A., Buchholz, D.H., Aisner, J., Betts, S.W., and Wiernik, P.H.: Clinical experience with transfusion of granulocytes obtained by continuous flow filtration leukophoresis. Am. J. Med. 58:373–381, 1975.

Schimpff, S.C., Greene, W.H., Young, V.M., Fortner, C.L., Jepsen, L., Cusack, N., Block, J.B., and Wiernik, P.H.: Infection prevention in acute nonlymphocytic leukemia. Ann. Intern. Med. 82:351, 1975.

Schimpff, S.C., Landesman, S., Hahn, D.M., Standiford, H.C., Fortner, C.L., Young, V.M., and Wiernik, P.H.: Ticarcillin in combination with cephalothin or gentamicin as empiric antibiotic therapy in granulocytopenic cancer patients. Antimicrob. Agents Chemother. 10:837–844, 1976.

Schumer, W.: Steroids in the treatment of clinical septic shock. Ann. Surg. 184:333–341, 1976.

Shochat, S.J.: Splenic trauma in children. West. J. Med. 132:60–61, 1980.

Shubin, H., Weil, M.H., and Carlson, R.W.: Bacterial shock. Am. Heart J. 94:112–114, 1977.

Shulman, J.A., Terry, P.M., and Hough, C.E.: Colonization with gentamicin-resistant *Pseudomonas aeruginosa*, pyocine type 5, in a burn unit. J. Infect. Dis. (Suppl.) 124:S18, 1971.

Singer, D.B.: Post splenectomy sepsis. In *Perspectives in Pediatric Pathology*, vol. 1, pp. 285–311. Year Book Medical Publishers, Chicago, 1973.

Smith, C.H., Erlandson, M.E., Schulman, I., et al.: Hazard of severe infections in splenectomized infants and children. Am. J. Med. 22:390–404, 1957.

Smith, C.R., Baughman, K.L., Edwards, C.Q., Rogers, J.F., and Lietman, P.S.: Controlled comparison of amikacin and gentamicin. N. Engl. J. Med. 296:349–353, 1977.

Spink, W.W.: The ecology of human septic shock. In *Conference on the Dynamics of Septic Shock in Man*, edited by S.G. Hershey, L.R.M. DelGuerico, and R. McConn, p. 3. Little, Brown, Boston, 1971.

Stapley, E.O., Birnbaum, J., Miller, A.K., Wallick, H., Hendlin, D., and Woodruff, H.B.: Cefoxitin and cephamycins: Microbiological studies. Rev. Infect. Dis. 1:73–87, 1979.

Storring, R.A., Jameson, B., McElwain, T.J., and Wiltshaw, E.: Oral non-absorbed antibiotics prevent infection in acute non-lymphoblastic leukemia. Lancet 2:837–840, 1977.

Strauss, R.G.: Therapeutic neutrophil transfusions: Are controlled studies no longer appropriate? Am. J. Med. 65:1001–1006, 1978.

Tramont, E.C.: The diagnosis and treatment of septic shock. Milit. Med. 144:153–157, 1979.

Valdivieso, M., Feld, R., Rodriguez, V., and Bodey, G.P.: Amikacin therapy of infections in neutropenic patients. Am. J. Med. Sci. 270:453, 1975.

Vogler, W.R., and Winton, E.F.: A controlled study of the efficacy of granulocyte transfusions in patients with neutropenia. Am. J. Med. 63:548–555, 1977.

Wade, J.C., Smith, C.R., Petty, B.G., Lipsky, J.J., Conrad, G., Ellner, J., and Lietman, P.S.: Cephalothin plus an aminoglycoside is more nephrotoxic than methicillin plus an aminoglycoside. Lancet 2:604–606, 1978.

Waisbren, B.A.: Bacteremia due to gram-negative bacilli other than the Salmonella: A clinical and therapeutic study. Arch. Intern. Med. 88:467, 1951.

Wald, E.R., Standiford, H.C., Tatem, B.A., Calia, F.M., and Hornick, R.B.: BL-P1654, ticarcillin, and carbenicillin: In vitro comparison alone and in combination with gentamicin against *Pseudomonas aeruginosa*. Antimicrob. Agents Chemother. 7:336–340, 1975.

Warner, W.A., and Sanders, E.: Neuromuscular blockade associated with gentamicin therapy. J.A.M.A. 215:1153, 1971.

Watson, J.G., and Jameson, B.: Antibiotic prophylaxis for patients in protective isolation. Lancet 1:1183, 1979.

Weil, M.: Current understanding of mechanisms and treatment of circulatory shock caused by bacterial infections. Ann. Clin. Res. 9:181–191, 1977.

Weil, M.H., and Shubin, H. (Eds.): *Diagnosis and Treatment of Shock*. Williams & Wilkins, Baltimore, 1967.

Weil, M.H., Shubin, H., and Biddle, M.: Shock caused by gram-negative microorganisms. Ann. Intern. Med. 60:384–400, 1964.

Weinstein, R.J., Young, L.S., and Hewitt, W.L.: Comparison of methods for assessing in vitro antibiotic synergism against Pseudomonas and Serratia. J. Lab. Clin. Med. 86:853–862, 1975.

Winslow, E.J., Loeb, H.S., Rahimtoola, S.H., et al.: Hemodynamic studies and results of therapy in 50 patients with bacteremic shock. Am. J. Med. 54:421–432, 1973.

Wolff, S.M., and Bennett, J.V.: Gram-negative rod bacteremia. N. Engl. J. Med. 291:733–734, 1974.

Yaeger, A.S.: Use of pneumococcal vaccine. West. J. Med. 132:63–64, 1980.

Young, L.S.: Gram-negative sepsis. In *Principles & Practice of Infectious Diseases*, edited by G.L. Mandell, R.G. Douglas, and J.E. Bennett, pp. 571–608. John Wiley & Sons, New York, 1979.

Young, L.S., Martin, W.J., Meyer, R.D., Weinstein, R.J., and Anderson, E.T.: Gram-negative rod bacteremia: Microbiologic, immunologic and therapeutic considerations. Ann. Intern. Med. 86:456–471, 1977.

PART 4

STRATEGIES FOR FUTURE DIAGNOSIS AND THERAPY

EDITORS' SUMMARY

Among the many problems in this area is the very difficult one of forcasting the future. In his chapter, Wilson admirably reviews the present and looks into the future.

His premise involves early diagnosis and early treatment. Although this sounds gratuitous, it is essential, especially in septic shock. Without accurate information on the state of the patient, the physician is working in the dark. Wilson argues, in fact, that such data represent the principal difference between a small rural hospital and a STU in a major metropolitan area.

He goes on to review the major present "state-of-the-art" techniques and concepts. He mentions that many such current techniques should be in routine use in the future. In the future, we must be able to obtain all necessary physiologic parameters instantaneously. The laboratory must truly be at the bedside or inserted into the patient.

Communication will also be a major advance in the future. Physicians anywhere will be able to compare their patients and data with the largest centers in the world. Satellite TV is currently only the "tip of the iceberg." Future diagnosis and treatment of shock will also include much more involvement of nursing, medical technology, and bioengineering. Wilson laments the present circumstance that a physician in a relatively remote community cannot compare his observations with a larger center; the technology to correct this is now available—it only needs to be utilized.

When a patient first comes to a trauma unit, control of bleeding becomes an obvious and critical initial problem. Current methods of diagnosing sites of bleeding are inadequate. Wilson visualizes new systems for rapid and accurate diagnosis—and, therefore, rapid and accurate therapy.

With respect to cardiogenic shock, Wilson visualizes major advances in diagnosis of size and location of infarcts as well as of residual function of the myocardium. Assisted counterpulsation should markedly improve. Mechanical cardiovascular support will revolutionize this area, especially if we can determine methods for intervening in the primary process to facilitate healing.

In the area of septic shock, many advances are badly needed. For example, the enhancement of immunity and prevention of the entire syndrome. Much more immunologic research is, therefore, needed. Nutrition is also a serious problem; the severe protein catabolism cannot be controlled by present techniques. In Chapter 3, Bessman and Renner comment that we must learn to modulate the inappropriate hormonal responses. This is further addressed by Wilson, and he speculates on possible roles of corticosteroids in modulating calcium control by mitochondria.

Many improvements are also needed in the area of acute resuscitation. Among the many areas of possible improvement is that of ventilation. Our studies have shown that the typical traumatized patient loses the ciliated cells in the tracheobronchial epithelium (TBE) and, thus, a major defense system against microorganisms. This particular modulation might be corrected by vitamin A-related retinoid therapy. At the same time, these changes might be trivial though a side effect of current respiratory therapy. Wilson argues that future respiratory therapy could be much better controlled or even monitored through a data processing system. Hyperbaric O_2 may well come back into extensive use. Fluid therapy in the immediate postresuscitation period is extremely important. Wilson predicts that many new types of colloids will be manufactured with a range of molecular weights to compensate for any type of capillary defect.

Fluids superior to blood in O_2 carrying capacity and rheologic properties will be developed. Additionally, improved substrate mixtures will be added to such fluids to improve retrieval of injured cells. New drug carriers (e.g., liposomes) may also be utilized to modify delivery of agents, e.g., ATP or steroids. Further understanding of the inflammatory reaction may lead to better manipulation of and substitution for mediators.

In his chapter, Clark addresses the current state-of-the-art of fluorcarbon emulsions as blood substitutes. These emulsions have a remarkable potential for future therapy; in many ways their characteristics may be better than blood as they have unique physical chemical properties including high solubility for oxygen and CO_2, chemical and biologic inertness, and improved flow properties. Moreover, they can be made economically, can be stored in very large quantities, are free from disease, and can be used without the need for typing and cross matching. In short, they not only can substitute for blood but can do more than such substitution. Much of the future utilization of these emulsions according to Clark will center around the technology of making emulsions of a small particle size, potentially to the point where they could exert oncotic pressure. Clinical trials are in progress in Japan and for use in Jehovah's Witnesses. It would appear that further efforts in this direction may well yield much improved resuscitation fluids in the future and ones which have the capacity for utilization in mass casualty situations.

Bradley, in his chapter on hyperbaric oxygen therapy, has concisely described the mechanism and physiology of hyperbaric oxygen therapy. The physiologic actions of high concentrations of oxygen in the normal situation have been so stated that one cannot automatically infer that the same situation is valid in the ill patient. He has limited his discussion of diseases treatable in a hyperbaric environment to those related to acute shock.

The discussion on acute head injury, cerebral edema, acute spinal cord injury, and stroke is very comprehensive. There is a detailed discussion on carbon monoxide and cyanide poisoning which is appropriate for their importance in terms of morbidity and mortality in fires, etc. His discussion on acute stroke and myocardial infarction is limited to the treatment of these conditions in a hyperbaric environment. Again, it must be stressed that many of these patients can be treated in a monoplace chamber where adequate monitoring may still be undertaken.

Although difficult to follow for those not well versed in mathematical modeling techniques, the chapter on mathematical models presents a good beginning to physiologic modeling. Masaitis should consider writing a text on this subject. By applying modeling laws to specific problems, the reader (the physician) could learn to apply this powerful tool. As we all become further acquainted with modeling systems, especially as they relate to computer techniques, much of the long drawn out animal experimentation used in the past will become obsolete. With a properly designed model, various parameters can be substituted. Once the significant variables have been tested, only a few well defined experiments will be required to verify the facts.

One might wonder why Milholland's chapter should be included in a book on shock. The answer is obvious to the clinician investigating shock as it related to a large set of injuries. Accurate information as to the type of injury, its location, its extent, and its effect on other organ systems makes it imperative that an accurate data storage and retrieval system be used to further identify the shock process, its severity, its prognosis, and its therapy.

In all, Part 4 offers many exciting possibilities for the management of future shock problems as they relate to diagnosis and therapy.

CHAPTER 36

Future Treatment of Shock

ROBERT F. WILSON

It is difficult to estimate what's going to happen to the treatment of shock in the future. Part of the problem is that many physicians are still practicing "past shock," particularly in smaller rural hospitals. To improve shock management in general in the United States, our concern probably should not be so much with performing increasingly sophisticated research in the large medical centers and universities, but rather bringing our current information to the smaller hospitals and physicians who only infrequently see patients with severe shock.

DATA COLLECTION

Most of the advances that we have seen in the treatment of shock have been largely based on advances in obtaining data. However, the main problem I find at smaller hospitals is that of data collection. The physicians are uncertain as to what data they should obtain. In addition, they often have little or no knowledge of how to obtain it. Most physicians, particularly if they go to the literature, have at least some idea of what to do if they are given appropriate data.

The Importance of Trends

Much of the time only static data is available. Biologic systems react primarily to rate of change. Consequently, the dimension of time and rate of change must be correlated with all data. Absolute levels or static numbers have relatively little meaning or importance. Patients may gradually accommodate to chemical abnormalities that would rapidly kill them if they developed suddenly. Optimally we should detect abnormal states as they are developing from the trends that the data is taking. Improvement in trend monitoring may well be the most important factor in providing better treatment of shock in the future.

Earlier Diagnoses are Essential

One of the best ways to improve results with the treatment of shock in the future is to diagnose it or its impending states earlier. For example, much of the success that Schumer's group (Schumer, 1976) had with his massive steroid study was related to aggressive therapy in the very early stages of shock. They did not wait for all of the classic signs, symptoms, and laboratory changes of shock. The low mortality rate of only 40% in the patients with septic shock receiving a placebo (instead of massive steroids) is due to this fact. Now his group is closely following the cardiac output, vascular resistance, and oxygen consumption using pulmonary artery catheters to diagnose septic shock even earlier. If the patients begin to show that they're getting into trouble, i.e., having a rising cardiac output or falling vascular resistance or oxygen consumption, they are treated aggressively *before* shock becomes clinically apparent.

Response to Therapy as a Guide to Further Therapy

Once the treatment of shock begins, the best guide for determining the type or extent of continuing or later therapy is the response of the patient. How much fluid is given to a patient? The answer is that you don't know until you see the reaction to the last bolus of fluid given. The best data is that which provides information on trends and responses. The problem is to determine what should be monitored and the best way to accomplish this in the future.

CURRENT BASES FOR THE TREATMENT OF SHOCK

Clinical Examination

If we look at the ways that patients in shock can be managed, the treatment modalities available are pretty much the same for all physicians. The differences in shock management in a small rural hospital and in a large trauma center are due primarily to differences in monitoring. In many small hospitals the clinical examination, the cuff blood pressure, and the pulse rate provide much of the data used for treating the patient. The clinical examination is important but, unfortunately, is sometimes overlooked when a great deal of other data is available. Nevertheless, it is not adequate for very early diagnosis and accurate monitoring of responses to therapy.

Cardioscopes

Most hospitals now have cardioscopes, particularly in the operating room and postanesthesia recovery room (PAR). In many smaller hospitals the only difference between the ICU and general wards is the presence of a cardioscope in the ICU. Continuous EKG monitoring is particularly important in cardiac patients, where it can be used effectively to warn the personnel of impending dangerous arrhythmias.

Hourly Urine

It is rather easy to measure the hourly urine volume, and this can provide important information concerning organ perfusion. However, many patients do not have Foley catheters inserted unless the bladder does not empty properly or until it becomes obvious that the patient has been oliguric for several hours.

Central Venous Pressure (CVP)

The CVP is now widely used as a guide to fluid therapy. In small rural hospitals, many physicians are not familiar with CVP catheter insertion and have difficulty evaluating the data. Other physicians may use the CVP more frequently but still believe that a CVP exceeding 12–16 cm H_2O indicates that the patient is overloaded with fluid. It is now fairly well known that the CVP level can be extremely deceptive, especially in patients with sepsis or lung disease. In these patients much more accurate information can be obtained by monitoring the CVP response to a fluid challenge (Wilson et al., 1971b) or by inserting a pulmonary wedge pressure catheter. Consequently, CVP are often done late in small hospitals and only on the very sickest patients.

Arterial Blood Gases

Arterial blood gases are essential for following pulmonary function, particularly if oxygen or ventilatory therapy is required. However, in very small hospitals, they may have to call a technologist or even the pathologist to obtain this data at night or on weekends.

Special Laboratory Procedures

Special laboratory procedures such as blood lactate levels may be very helpful. They are of particular benefit in evaluating the adequacy of tissue perfusion and for estimating prognosis. In the future, tremendous amounts of laboratory data from very small blood samples will be obtainable with the use of microtechniques. Indwelling catheters in arteries, veins, and various tissues will also provide almost continuous data.

Many of our best investigators are now providing much information on the chemical abnormalities in the blood of critically ill patients. In the future, they will be providing much the same information about blood from vessels in specific organs.

Flow-Directed Pulmonary Artery Catheter

Flow-directed pulmonary artery catheters, such as the Swan-Ganz catheter, currently provide much of our most useful hemodynamic data. They provide pulmonary artery pressures (to help calculate pulmonary vascular resistance) and pulmonary artery wedge pressures (reflecting filling pressures in the left heart). Some of these catheters can also be used to measure the cardiac output by a thermodilution technique. By regulating fluid or diuretic therapy to obtain pulmonary artery wedge pressures (PAWP) of 15–18 mm Hg, the preload of the heart can be optimized. Occasionally these catheters cause arrhythmias, and balloon hyperinflation may cause pulmonary artery damage or infarction. In the future, I believe we will have better, smaller, safer catheters with more accurate transducers which can be calibrated easily or even automatically.

Cardiac Output Determinations

Cardiac output can now be measured in a variety of ways. The cardiogreen indicator dilution technique is currently the "gold standard," but it is generally used only in research units. Calculations of cardiac output using the Fick technique require assuming (or preferably measuring) the oxygen consumption and obtaining arterial and mixed venous gases to calculate arteriovenous oxygen differences.

At this time, cardiac outputs are measured most frequently with the thermodilution technique. Although thermodilution cardiac output values tend to be higher in critically ill patients than those obtained with cardiogreen, they can provide very helpful trends. Such data is particularly important when using high levels of positive end-expiratory pressure (PEEP). In the future, cardiac outputs will be done noninvasively and almost constantly. Perhaps the principle of impedance plethysmography will be sufficiently improved to obtain accurate information of this kind in the future.

Mixed Venous Gases

True mixed venous blood is available via pulmonary artery catheters. However, the lumen of these catheters is rather small, and it is often difficult to withdraw blood from the catheters intermittently for more than a few hours. Central venous blood, especially from the right atrium, may be a reasonable substitute.

In combination with arterial blood gases, mixed venous gas data allows one to calculate shunting in the lung (pulmonary arteriovenous admixture). If cardiac output is also available, oxygen consumption can be calculated. Oxygen consumption determinations may be the best guide to the adequacy of tissue perfusion and cell metabolism. In the future we will hopefully be able to measure oxygen consumption constantly and easily from the inhaled and exhaled gases.

Computer Data Collection

If you've watched Star Trek, you know that eventually we're going to be able to insert a patient into a machine that looks and acts like a chemical CAT scanner. After we get all this data back, we'll be able to perform exotic therapeutic maneuvers, such as applying electrical charges here and there, to change metabolic and other functions.

Before we get to such an advanced stage, however, it is essential that systems be developed so that all data obtained on patients in shock can be entered into a computer. The responses to therapy will also be included. Consequently, it will be possible to predict, from a relatively small sample of data, the pathophysiologic changes present and the type(s) of therapy most apt to be beneficial. As increasing amounts of data are fed into the on-line computer, increasing accuracy in diagnosis and optimum therapy will be obtained.

Communication

One of the things toward which we must be working very hard is some form of communication between physicians in smaller hospitals and investigators in large centers with large computer banks. The physician in the rural area hopefully will be able to transmit all his available data to the computer and almost instantaneously obtain a list of diagnoses in order of their probability along with a list of recommended steps in treatment or additional data collection. With some problems and when desired, physicians will be able to contact experts to review data and make recommendations. This type of system may be similar to the EKG computers now used. Most EKGs are relatively straight forward and can be read easily. Only about 5–10% require examination by a skilled individual.

TREATMENT OF THE UNDERLYING PROCESS

Hypovolemia and Bleeding

One of the problems, particularly in trauma victims, is diagnosis of the location of bleeding and determination of its severity. If large accessible vessels are bleeding, the surgeon can often control these rapidly. However, in crush victims it may be difficult or almost impossible to know how much bleeding is due to the fractured pelvis and other fractures.

Currently it can be very difficult to clinically determine if there is significant intra-abdominal bleeding and we must often resort to peritoneal lavage or surgical exploration. In the future we will be able to detect bleeding sites more rapidly and accurately. An isotope technique for this seems reasonable. Hopefully, we will also have better ways of continuously evaluating the relationship between blood volume and vascular capacity. With improved engineering we should have smaller and smaller catheters to evaluate many of these hemodynamic changes.

The importance of rapidly restoring blood volume and controlling hemorrhage may be exemplified by some data collected on patients receiving massive transfusion. During the 3-year period, 1975–1977, 368 patients received more than 10 units of blood in a 24-hr period. Most of these patients had trauma or massive gastrointestinal bleeding. As in a previous study (Wilson et al., 1971a), we found that if we were able to correct the hypotension in less than 30 min in previously healthy individuals, the mortality rate was only 12%. If the hypotension (systolic BP < 80 mm Hg) was not corrected within 30 min, the mortality rate rose to 50%. If the patients had pre-existing disease, such as cirrhosis, congestive heart failure, or a malignancy, the mortality rate with massive transfusions and prolonged shock was 93%. Approximately 70% of the mortality occurred within 48 hr of the massive transfusion. Almost all the others died later of multiple organ failure due to sepsis. Even those who survived tended to have multiple complications requiring prolonged hospitalization. The average time in the hospital for the patients who survived was over 25 days.

Cardiogenic Shock

In the future we will be able to rapidly and accurately determine 1) the size and location of myocardial infarctions, 2) the amount of coronary artery disease present, and 3) the function of the remaining myocardium. One of the advantages of the Swan-Ganz catheter is that it has helped document that as many as 20–40% of the patients with acute myocardial infarction have some element of hypovolemia. In such individuals, raising the PAWP between 15 and 18 mm Hg has corrected many of the perfusion problems.

Counterpulsation to mechanically assist a weak or failing left ventricle or improve coronary blood flow is now done most frequently with intra-aortic balloon pumping (IABP). Its main benefit is increased coronary artery blood flow during diastole. In addition, it frequently also reduces systolic pressure, thereby reducing myocardial oxygen requirements. IABP has greatly improved survival in patients with cardiogenic shock and crescendo angina. However, complications do occur. In the future, smaller, more easily inserted and controlled balloon catheters will become available.

We're also going to have better mechanical cardiovascular support and better membranes so that this artificial membrane will not damage blood components. With an improved membrane, we may be able to prevent denaturation of protein (with resultant activation of the complement and coagulation cascade) and thrombocytopenia. Once we can develop membranes that act like endothelium, we'll be a quantum jump ahead in cardiac support by artificial hearts.

Septic Shock

The most important aspect of the management of septic shock is accurate localization and eradication of the septic foci. If there is any pus or nonvariable tissue, it must be drained or debrided as rapidly as possible. Otherwise, all the antibiotics and supportive measures may be to no avail.

Currently the most difficult cases of sepsis are those with intra-abdominal pus, particularly if the patient is immunosuppressed and does not show the usual fever and leukocytosis. Clinical signs including pain or localized tenderness may be absent. X-rays and gallium scans are also usually of little benefit, particularly if the patient cannot be moved from ICU. Hopefully, in the future, improved scanning techniques, possibly with labeled leukocytes or chemicals, will allow us to localize the septic foci accurately and quickly.

Recently, there has been increasing interest in "blind" laparotomies in patients with evidence of sepsis or progressive multiple organ failure but no apparent source, particularly if they have had recent abdominal surgery or trauma. In 50% of these laparotomies pus was found.

Immunity will be enhanced by a wide variety of agents. Various "normal" host defense substances, such as complement and immunoglobulins, will be administered intravenously into the blood or various body cavities. In addition various immunorestorative drugs are being studied. Levamisole has been found to improve neutrophil function in anergic surgical patients (Meakins and Christon, 1978). Thiobendazole has been found to reverse the postoperative suppression of a cell-mediated immunity, (the one way mixed leukocyte culture (MCL) in mice) (Lundy et al., 1978). Lethal peritonitis in rats has been reduced by intraperitoneal injection of thioglycollate (attracts granulocytes and monocytes) (Hau et al., 1978) and formylmethionylphenylalanine (a synthetic polymorphonuclear leukocyte chemoattractant) (Schiffman et al., 1975).

Improved nutrition will also be available. It has been clearly shown that malnutrition is a major cause of immunosuppression. Hopefully we will not only be able to accurately diagnose all nutritional deficiencies, including the micronutrients, but also rapidly correct them. In the future, we will be able to accurately quantitate the size of the protein pool and rate of protein synthesis.

Much improved antibiotics will also become available. It may even be possible to rapidly design and make new antibiotics as needed to handle resistant organisms. It may even be possible to develop phages to seek and destroy particular microorganisms.

RESUSCITATION

Ventilation

The importance of early ventilatory support for critically ill or injured patients cannot be overemphasized. Over a 2-year period, of 1132 patients admitted to Detroit General Hospital with chest trauma about one-fifth (218) had shock or respiratory failure, requiring urgent intubation in the Emergency Department. If they already had evidence of respiratory problems, the mortality rate rose 10-fold to 73%, and no patient past the age of 43 survived (Wilson et al., 1977).

One of the interesting ventilatory techniques that has not been tried in the United States very much is high frequency ventilation (HFV) (Klein et al., 1978). The use of small tidal volumes and respiratory rates of 200/min theoretically should not work, according to what most of us know. Nevertheless, there are increasing testimonials to its clinical benefit.

Indwelling electrodes, particularly for tissue, are going to be a help in determining optimal ventilator settings. By hooking these electrodes to a computer and then to a ventilator, we will have a system that adjusts automatically to the patient's condition.

Hyperbaric oxygen will probably come back into use, particularly to bring oxygen to ischemic tissues. Improved technology will greatly reduce the complications and side effects of this modality.

Fluids

CRYSTALLOIDS

As far as the fluids given, their electrolyte concentrations will be much more easily adjustable. We will probably also be using more and more hyperosmolar solutions. These are currently used primarily in burns (Jelenko et al., 1979) but we will probably find improved uses for them in nonburn situations.

COLLOIDS

We will be able to manufacture almost any type of colloid desired with virtually any molecular weight. With increased data collection, it will become obvious that there are certain instances in which a colloid is very beneficial, particularly with mild to moderate capillary leak problems. Since we will probably be able to determine pore size in capillaries, we will also be able to determine what size particle will remain in the vascular system.

OXYGEN CARRIERS

Hemoglobin

In general, the more oxygen carried to the tissues, the better the oxygen consumption. In the past we attempted to maintain the hematocrit at 30 and 35%. A higher hematocrit was felt to be detrimental because it was likely to cause a rather marked decrease in cardiac output, oxygen transport, and oxygen consumption. However, when this was studied (Wilson and Gibson, 1978), it was found that the patients with hemoglobin levels above 15.0 g/dl did now show the decrease in cardiac output that many physiologists predicted on the basis of their study of normal individuals. In fact, the studies in critically ill patients showed that even with a rather high arterial oxygen content, the percentage of oxygen extraction remained relatively constant at 25–30% and oxygen consumption rose proportional to the increased arterial oxygen content. Raising the hemoglobin from 10.0 to 15.0 g/dl increased oxygen content by 50% but reduced cardiac output by only 10–15%, thereby increasing oxygen transport by about 35%. In a study of 200 critically ill patients, those with a hemoglobin of 15 g/dl or higher had a mortality rate of only 23%, whereas those whose hemoglobin was less than 12.5 g/dl had a mortality rate of 64%.

Consequently, hemoglobin should be maintained at the level which produces the highest oxygen consumption. This level will vary from individual to individual, and it may be difficult to separate the effect of the increased hemoglobin from that of an increased blood volume.

Because of the problems of obtaining adequate quantities of blood and because of blood transfusion complications such as hepatitis, there has been increased interest in other oxygen carriers such as stroma-free hemoglobin and the fluorocarbons. If they replaced even a small percentage of the 10,000,000 units of blood transfused annually, it would be helpful.

Stroma-Free Hemoglobin

Stroma-free hemoglobin (SFH) currently has problems of excess oxygen affinity (i.e., decreased oxygen release to tissues) and rapid excretion (half-life of 2–3 days). Investigators are working to overcome these problems. Pyridoxalating SFH, for example, greatly improves oxygen release at the periphery (Greenberg et al., 1978).

Fluorocarbons

Fluorocarbons are gas-transporting molecules which usually contain about 10 carbon atoms and many fluoride atoms. They are essentially non-toxic, are not metabolized, and are excreted as a vapor from the lungs or skin. Emulsions of perfluorodecalin can almost completely replace the blood of baboons and rats, but much basic research is still required in emulsion formation, stabilization and storage.

There are a number of potential special uses for the fluorocarbons including: 1) replacement for lost blood when adequate bank blood is not available or when isoagglutinins prevent a proper cross-match, 2) improved perfusion in ischemic vascular beds, 3) substitution for blood during extracorporeal circulation (fluorocarbon may tolerate the trauma of cardiopulmonary bypass or prolonged membrane oxygenation much better than red blood cells) and 4) angiography (addition of a bromine or iodine atom may produce a much safer radiopaque emulsion for angiography). New computerized tomography may allow greatly improved examination of small vessels with such agents, thereby permitting non-invasive measurements of regional perfusion.

Acid-Base Correction

Accurate and rapid acid-base correction will be possible because of in-line indwelling electrodes providing information from tissues as well as arterial and mixed venous blood. Minute ventilation and bicarbonate administration could then be adjusted automatically to provide an optimal pH, PCO_2 and bicarbonate level.

Hormonal Manipulation

ADRENAL CORTICOSTEROIDS

Adrenal Insufficiency

The 3–15% of otherwise normal adults who either have or develop a relative adrenal insufficiency during shock (Sibbald et al., 1977) will be detected early by rapid laboratory determinations. The quantity of cortisol-like agents that should be administered to these individuals who otherwise tend to respond poorly to standard shock therapy will also be more apparent.

Massive (Pharmacologic) Doses

In spite of Schumer's large double-blind study (Schumer, 1976), there continue to be controversies concerning the role or benefits of massive steroids in the treatment of shock. The role of these agents in prevention of excess complement activation (Jacob, 1978), lysosomal membrane stabilization (Weissman and Thomas, 1962), oxygen transfer (Bryan-Brown et al., 1973) and many other actions will be clarified by sophisticated monitoring during and following their administration.

One of the newest roles that steroids may play in the treatment of shock is being investigated by White et al. (1980). These workers have found that the reduction in ATP formation that usually occurs when mitochondria pump excess calcium out of the cytoplasm can be reversed by administering large doses of steroids. When calcium is added to an in vitro mitochondrial preparation, ATP production ceases. However, White et al. found that adding massive steroids restores the ATP production to normal. This may be one of the mechanisms involved in the improved energy production that may occur with massive steroids in shock.

Insulin and the Catabolic Hormones

The absolute or relative lack of insulin that occurs in shock will be measured rapidly and accurately in the future so that just the right amount of glucose and insulin can be given to provide optimal cell metabolism. The catabolic hormones will also be analyzed and administered or blocked in an optimal fashion.

Nutrition

In concert with the hormonal manipulation, we are going to find better energy substrates to administer or other ways to improve ATP production. The direct administration of ATP is particularly exciting (Hirasawa et al., 1978). We are also going to be able to interfere with the uncoupling of oxidative phosphorylation, thereby preserving increased energy for useful functions, and to administer these agents into specific vascular beds using new drug carriers.

Vasopressors and Vasodilators

Improved computerized tomography (CT) and scanning techniques will provide exact information about the relative vasoconstriction-vasodilatation present in virtually all vascular beds. In the meantime, pharmacologic manipulation will have provided us with a wide variety of compounds, many of which may well be prostaglandin derivatives, that will have very specific effects on very specific vascular beds.

It is amazing how a simple substitution of a radical on a compound can profoundly alter its activity. Consequently, there is an almost infinite number of compounds that can be made and tested. This may require a great deal of time unless computers can be used to help predict which of the new chemical compounds will be most useful and least toxic.

Coagulation

We are going to have early rapid assay techniques for all of the coagulation and fibrinolytic factors and agents. We will also be able to control these processes by giving specific activating or blocking agents. I think particularly of the management of the patient who has had 35 units of blood, has had massive liver trauma, and is oozing from multiple sites. Hopefully, we will be able to prevent such problems by adequate early monitoring and therapy.

Organ Preservation and Support

We are going to find practical techniques for maintaining hypothermia in critically ill patients. When we find we are not going to be able to rapidly correct the primary problem (such as a large abscess) or institute appropriate resuscitative therapy, we will slow down all cell metabolism to give us the necessary time. Not infrequently, when we lose critically ill or injured patients, it is just because there is not enough time to do everything. We also tend to give "shot-gun" therapy because there is not enough time to adequately note the response to each therapeutic maneuver. If an individual could be safely cooled to 5°C, circulation could be completely stopped for 30 min. In individuals with severe trauma, this might be adequate to control even the most severely bleeding injuries.

One of the most important organs to support in shock is the liver. Once an acceptable endothelial-like substance is developed, circulation will be easily maintained by various pumps. Then the main problem will be maintenance of normal metabolism, for which the liver is essential.

With renal failure, adequate nutrition (including essential amino acids) and early prophylactic dialysis two to three times a week without waiting for chemical changes should improve survival, particularly with improved dialysis techniques and apparatus.

Currently, membrane oxygenators are felt to be of little or no benefit in ARDS. However, this will be dramatically reversed once an adequate endothelial substitute is developed. One example of the need for multiple organ support was a group of 17 trauma patients who had more than 15 units of blood within 24 hr. Four of these patients died, but only after living long enough to develop complications. Of these 17 patients, 16 developed infections, 13 had pulmonary problems, 13 had hepatic problems, 8 had renal problems, 6 had severe GI problems (including prolonged ileus in 3 and stress bleeding in 3), 3 developed postresuscitation hypertension crisis, and 2 had wound or anastamotic disruptions. This is an example of a group of patients in whom organ problems could be anticipated; with this knowledge, better preventive or supportive measures could be instituted earlier.

SOCIOECONOMIC PROBLEMS

It has been estimated that if the cost of medical care continues to increase at the rate it has been for the past decade, by the year 2000 our entire gross national product will be spent on health care. There will be nothing left for food, housing, national defense, or the little pleasures of life. Thus, it seems clear that we will not be able to apply this improved technology to everyone.

Many of the patients that are now treated aggressively in shock units, trauma units, and intensive care units have an extremely poor prognosis and/or no prospects of enjoying life even if they survive. However, for various political or social reasons, it is almost impossible to deny maximal care. There are going to have to be some hard decisions about who can have the very expensive sophisticated care. Who decides? I think that we are going to see a tremendous amount of improvement in medical care in the future, but a lot of very hard decisions will have to be made concerning its application.

Acknowledgment. Supported by the Detroit General Hospital Research Corporation.

References

Bryan-Brown, C.W., Baek, S.M., Makabali, G., et al.: Consumable oxygen: Study of oxygen availability in relation to oxyhemolglobin dissociation. Crit. Care Med. *1:*26, 1973.

Greenberg, A.G., Schooley, M., Ginsburg, K.A., and Pesken, G.W.: Pyridoxylated stroma free hemoglobin in resuscitation of hemorrhagic shock. Surg. Forum *29:*44, 1978.

Hau, T., Hoffman, R., Nelson, R.D., and Simmons, R.L.: Prevention of lethal peritonitis by intraperitoneal chemotactic agents. Surg. Forum *29:*9, 1978.

Hirasawa, H., Chaudry, I.H., and Baue, A.E.: Beneficial effect of ATP-$MgCl_2$-glucose administration on survival following sepsis. Surg. Forum *29:*11, 1978.

Jacob, H.S.: Granulocyte complement interaction—a beneficial antimicrobial mechanism that can cause disease. Arch. Intern. Med. *138:*461, 1978.

Jelenko, C., Williams, J.B., Wheeler, M.L., Callaway, B.D., Fackler, V.K., Albus, C.A., and Barger, A.A.: Studies in shock and resuscitation. Crit. Care Med. *7:*157, 1979.

Klain, M., Smith, B., and Babinki, M.: High frequency ventilation—an alternative to IMV (abstract). Crit. Care Med. *6:* 95, 1978.

Lundy, J., Lovett, E.J., III, and Conran, P.B.: Recovery from postoperative immunosuppression: Efficacy of an immunorestorative drug. Surg. Forum *29:*3, 1978.

Meakins, J.L., and Christon, N.J.: Neutrophil function in anergic surgical patients: Modulation by drugs. Surg. Forum *29:*9, 1978.

Schiffman, E., Corcoran, B.A., and Wahl, S.M.: N-formylmethionyl peptides as chemoattractants for leukocytes. Proc. Natl. Acad. Sci. U.S.A. *72:*1059, 1975.

Schumer, W.: Steroids in the treatment of clinical septic shock. Ann. Surg. *184:*41, 1976.

Sibbald, W.V., Short, A., Cohen, M.P., and Wilson, R.F.: Variations in adrenocortical responsiveness during acute bacterial infections. Ann. Surg. *186:*29, 1977.

Weissman, G., and Thomas, L.: Studies on lysosomes, the effects of endotoxin tolerance and cortisone on the release of acid hydolases from a granular fraction of rabbit liver. J. Exp. Med. *116:*433, 1962.

White, B.C., Hoehner, P., and Wilson, R.F.: Mitochondrial O_2 use and ATP synthesis: Kinetic effects of Ca^{++} and HPO_4^{-2} modulated by glucocorticoids. Ann. Emerg. Med. *9:*396, 1980.

Wilson, R.F., and Gibson, D.: The use of arterio-central venous oxygen differences to calculate cardiac output and oxygen consumption in critically ill surgical patients. Surgery *84:* 362, 1978.

Wilson, R.F., Mammen, E., and Walt, A.J.: Eight years of experience with massive blood transfusions. J. Trauma *11:* 275, 1971a.

Wilson, R.F., Sarver, E., and Birks, R.: Central venous pressure and blood volume determinations in clinical shock. Surg. Gynecol. Obstet. *132:*631, 1971b.

Wilson, R.F., Antonenko, D., and Gibson, D.B.: Shock and acute respiratory failure after chest trauma. J. Trauma *17:* 697, 1977.

CHAPTER 37

Theoretical and Practical Considerations of Fluorocarbon Emulsions in the Treatment of Shock

LELAND C. CLARK, JR.

Fluorocarbon emulsions will have advantages in the treatment of shock which whole blood, or hemoglobin-based substitutes, do not have. These advantages stem from the unique physicochemical properties of exhaustively fluorinated substances. Their high solubility for oxygen and carbon dioxide, together with their chemical and biological inertness, make them impressive agents for use as neat liquids or as emulsions for oxygen transport in biology and medicine.

In this chapter I have tried to distill the essential features of fluorocarbon artificial bloods as they may be applied in transporting oxygen in the vascular system and possibly through tissue as a kind of myoglobin. The application of fluorocarbon emulsions in clinical medicine began in Japan and the United States, largely as a *substitute* for whole blood. The potential utility of fluorocarbon emulsions as a substitute for whole blood lies in the fact that such preparations can be made economically and stored in very large quantities, free from disease and used without the need for typing and cross matching. Present commercially available emulsions have the disadvantage that they must be stored frozen and used shortly after thawing; they have the advantage that they will save lives under conditions where whole blood cannot be used. But fluorocarbons can do more than substitute for blood.

I want to point out some of the unique features of fluoroblood as compared with hemoblood and to emphasize that the future may well see synthetic blood compositions which are specifically tailored to meet special medical needs. Normal blood is for healthy animals. Fluoroblood is for injured and sick animals. The very elements of whole blood—platelets, red cells, fibrinogen—may work to a disadvantage when the animal is sick.

The way in which a fluorocarbon emulsion is made has a pronounced effect on the physiological effects it produces when infused. Not only must particle size be controlled and fluoride generation avoided, but even the timing and order in which the salts and oncotic agents are added previous to the use of the emulsion are important. A minimum description of an emulsion is its appearance after standing undisturbed for a day and its optical density at a specified wavelength (540 nm).

My discovery that animals could survive the breathing of normobarically oxygenated silicone oils and perfluorochemical liquids (Clark and Gollan, 1966)*, led to the use of inert organic substances (Tables 37.1 and 37.3) as artificial blood. The main liquid used for these early experiments (Fig. 37.1) was FC75, perfluorobutyltetrahydrofuran. Later it was found that P12F worked as well or better than FC75.† We have studied a number of highly fluorinated neat liquids for liquid breathing.‡

Gollan and Clark (1966) perfused an isolated heart with neat liquid. The heart behaved as if it were being

---

* Since 1966 a large number of publications have appeared. Particular reference is made to the work of J. Modell and D. J. Sass.

† FC75 is also referred to in the literature as FX80 and FC80. It is probably a mixture of isomers of perfluorobutyl- and perfluoropropyltetrahydrofuran and up until recently was available from the 3M Co. P12F was made in small quantities by Allied Chemical and is no longer available. It is

$$CF_3CF_2CF_2CF_2CF_2CF_2-O-\underset{\underset{CF_3}{|}}{\overset{\overset{CF_3}{|}}{CF}}$$

‡ I found that a cat could survive breathing FC43 liquid if respiration was assisted during the liquid breathing. Liquids with higher vapor pressures such as F-dimethylcyclohexane can be breathed if the PO_2 is increased in a closed chamber, so that the partial pressure of the F-vapor is compensated. Perfluorooctylbromide, which is radiopaque, has been breathed with survival. Dr. Marian Miller is preparing a publication dealing with pulmonary ultrastructure following the breathing of Freon E3 (DuPont) and other liquids.

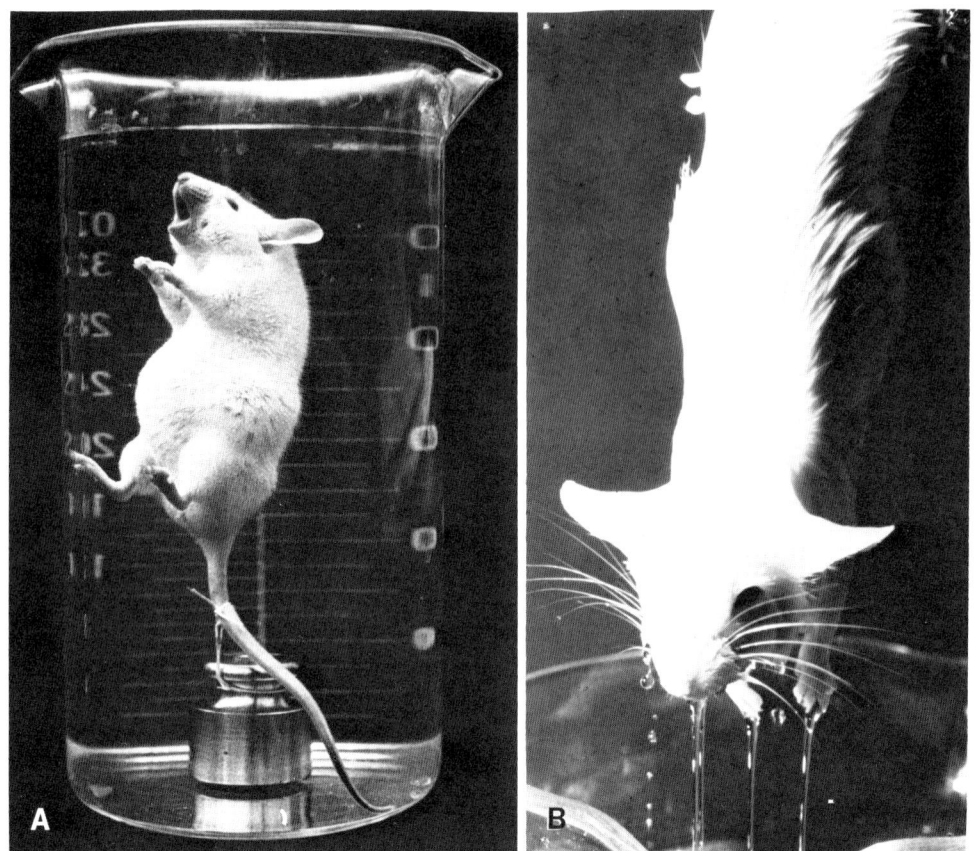

Figure 37.1. Liquid breathing mouse. The mouse is totally immersed in FC75 (FC80, F-butyltetrahydrofuran), which has been saturated with oxygen by bubbling at room temperature. Such a mouse can survive liquid breathing for many hours. After removal (B), the liquid is drained by gravity, the remainder evaporates from its fur and lungs, and the animal returns to a normal life.

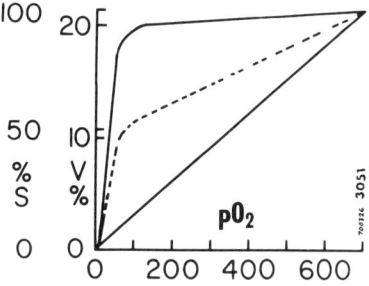

Figure 37.2. Oxygen capacity of blood (*upper solid line*) and F emulsion versus (*lower solid line*) oxygen tension. The *dotted line* represents a 50/50 mixture of the emulsion and blood. Note that F emulsion does not contribute significantly at air PO_2 but is excellent at high PO_2.

Table 37.1
Solubility of Gases

Liquid	O_2	CO_2
	ml/100 ml	*ml/100 ml*
Water	2.4	56
Whole Blood	20.0	50
Blood Plasma	2.4	67
Silicone oil (5CS)	23.7	—
F-Butylfuran (FC75, FC80)	48.5	160
F-Tributylamine (FC43, FC47)	38.9	142
F-Decalin (PP5)	40.3	134
Fluosol-DA (20%)	7.2	60

perfused with oxygen. After a while the heart stopped beating but it could be restarted by perfusion with an oxygenated aqueous solution.

Figure 37.2 shows the way in which fluorocarbon emulsions transport oxygen as a function of oxygen tension as contrasted with natural blood. The familiar S shaped curve is replaced by a straight line. The amount of oxygen carried in the fluorocarbon is a function of the oxygen tension only and is not influenced by the pH or the PCO_2. The classic gas laws of physical chemistry are followed. The amount of carbon dioxide gas carried in the fluorocarbon phase is also a linear function of the carbon dioxide tension. Virtually everything—salts, hydrogen ions, glucose, protein, lipids—in biological systems is *completely insoluble* in fluorocarbon. Only gases, vapors, and certain highly halogenated substances such as carbon tetrachloride or the fluoroanesthetics are soluble. Iodine forms a violet colored solution of the nonionized molecule. The fluorocarbon particle is perhaps easiest to imagine as a nongaseous microbubble of blood gases in instantaneous equilibrium with the dissolved gases in the aqueous phase. Fluorocarbon particles behave as incompressible gas bubbles.

Because fluorocarbons are such excellent solvents for gases, it is possible to *dissolve* enough oxygen in the circulating emulsion to completely meet the oxygen requirements of the body. This can be seen diagrammatically in Figure 37.3 and is easily accomplished in intact animals having partial or total replacement of blood by fluorocarbon emulsion. Figure 37.4A shows mixed venous PO_2 values obtained several years ago in partial replacement experiments in anesthetized dogs. It is quite striking to observe such a completely oxygenated animal. The venous blood samples cannot be distinguished by eye from the arterial samples, and the substance of the liver bleeds bright red when the surface is cut several days later while the animal breathes oxygen. The liver PO_2 is increased this way because of the trapped fluorocarbon particles.

The hypotensive effect of the injection of very small amounts (0.2 cc/kg) of any fluorocarbon emulsion in the dog (shown in Fig. 37.4B) is completely prevented by pretreatment with ephedrine as shown by Suyama et al., (1978). The PO_2 of the arterial blood, of course, can be set by the PO_2 of the inspired gas while the mixed venous PO_2 is a function largely of the cardiac output and oxygen consumption. Hence, tissue PO_2 can be controlled in new ways, ways which resemble those obtained in hyperbaria but which are in fact quite different. The main difference is due to the high solubility of oxygen in fluorocarbon emulsions contrasted with its low solubility in plasma. Extremely high inspired oxygen tensions, with their possible complications, can be avoided and yet hyperbaric-like tissue oxygen levels can be obtained. Of course, a bottle of emulsion is less expensive than a hyperbaric chamber.

It is important to realize that even with the increased oxygen dissolved in the plasma in hyperbaria, the PO_2 drops precipitously as it traverses the capillary, while it drops only slowly when F emulsions* travel through under the same circumstances. This will be of great value in increasing tissue oxygen tensions where circulation is impaired.

Tissue oxygen levels with bare platinum cathodes have been measured and found to be high, as expected (Fig. 37.5). Cole et al. (1978) have measured oxygen consumption at various levels of arterial PO_2 in a fluorocarbon emulsion-perfused heart and found that it is increased as the PO_2 increases, as shown in Figure 37.6. There are many publications,† largely from Japan and the United States (Symposium on Inert Organic Liquids, 1970; Symposium on Artificial Blood, 1975; Proceedings of the IVth International Symposium on Perfluorochemical Blood Substitutes, 1979; Hasegawa and Kishimoto, 1975; Novakova and Plantin, 1978; Riess and LeBlanc, 1978), which sustain the conclusion that venous and tissue PO_2 can be very substantially increased during oxygen breathing while circulating fluorocarbon emulsion in whole animals or isolated organs.

It is surprising that red blood cells with a diameter of about 8 μ so easily travel through 2-μ capillaries. It is

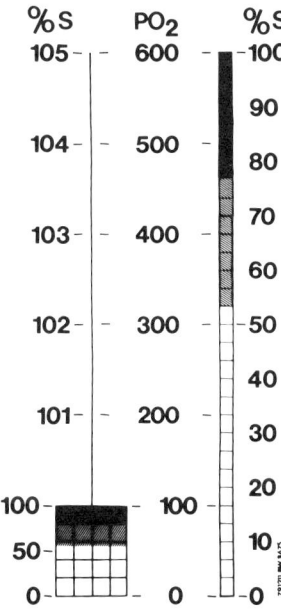

Figure 37.3. In each of the diagrams above, the height represents oxygen tension and the area the oxygen content. The diagram on the *left* is that for whole blood and on the *right* for a fluorocarbon emulsion having the same oxygen capacity as the whole blood. If 5 volume % oxygen is consumed from the whole blood, the tension drops from 600 to 80. The *solid black* area represents the amount consumed. If the same amount (5 volume %) of oxygen is consumed from the emulsion, the PO_2 drops from 600 to 465, again with the *solid black* representing the amount. Doubling the oxygen consumption (*hatched lines*) gives a PO_2 of 55 in whole blood, but 320 in fluorocarbon emulsion.

---

* I am using the term "F emulsion" to designate an emulsion made with a perfluorinated liquid. In this loose way, one could also refer to F blood or F substance. F is a prefix used in chemical publications to designate "perfluoro," hence, FC75 is F-butyltetrahydrofuran. Perfluoro refers to the substitution of H by F in an organic compound (except when H is in a functional group).

† Our laboratory here in Cincinnati has published over 60 papers on all aspects of artifical blood in a continuing program of chemical and biological research. These papers cover detailed considerations of chemical structure, vapor pressure, solubility, membrane permeability, emulsion technology, color tests, infra red analysis, whole body transpiration, blood and organ retention times, electron capture, and sodium combustion analysis of tissues, toxicity measurements of neat liquids and emulsions, and physiological measurements following blood replacement in small animals and nonhuman primates. A bibliography of over 500 publications directly related to fluorocarbon artificial blood is being prepared.

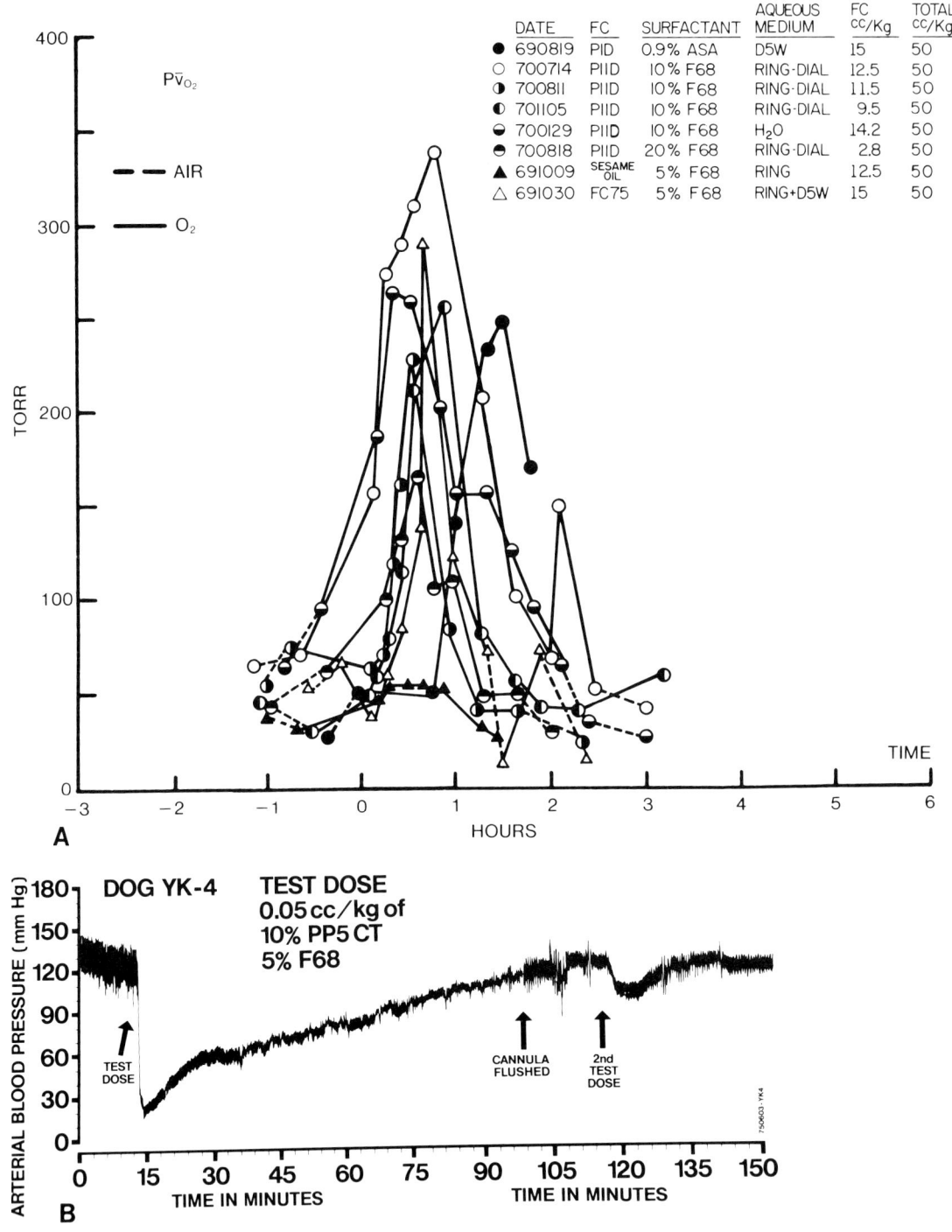

Figure 37.4. A, the effect of the infusion of F emulsion on mixed venous PO_2. Shown are infusions of emulsions of PID, PIID, FC75, and sesame oil in the dog. Emulsion dose was 50 cc/kg in all cases. Doses of the neat liquids (in the emulsion component) ranged from 2.8–15 ml/kg. These experiments, performed a number of years ago, are published here for the first time. B, hypotensive effect of emulsion in the dog.

perhaps more surprising that fluorocarbon particles having a diameter of only 0.4 μ do not travel as well. Injection of a milky appearing F emulsion with particles visible under the phase microscope often results in severe complications in perfused organs and death in animals. On the other hand, infusion of an emulsion with particles below 0.2 μ and having a bluish cast, also often having an orange tinge by transmitted light, results in physiological effects similar to those obtained following infusion of albumin, dextran, hydroxyethyl starch, and the like.

How small should F emulsion particles be? Okamoto

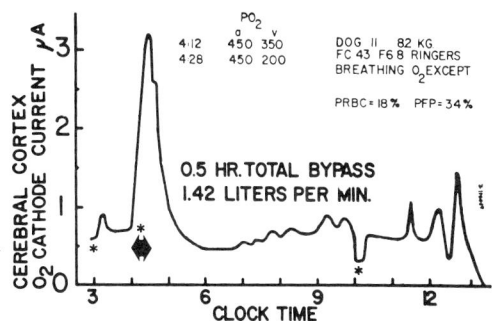

Figure 37.5. Oxygen availability in the dog brain during perfusion with blood containing a large concentration of fluorocarbon. The electrode was an implanted platinum cathode held at 0.6 V. O_2 was breathed except where indicated by asterisks. (Reprinted with permission from L.C. Clark, Jr., S. Kaplan, F. Becattini, and G. Benzing III.: Federation Proceedings 29:141, 1970.)

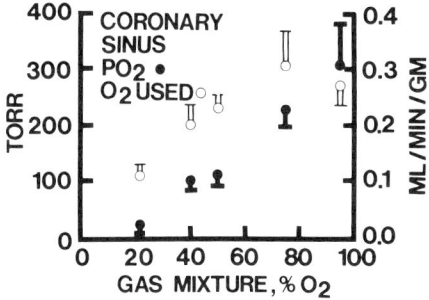

Figure 37.6. Increased oxygen consumption and increased venous PO_2 in the isolated perfused heart. Replotted from the work of Cole et al. (1978)

et al. (1975) have reported that the larger the particle size the shorter the retention time in the blood.

If suitable emulsifying conditions can be found, fluorocarbon emulsion particle size can be completely controlled. Perhaps finer emulsion particles can be used when trying to transport oxygen to ischemic tissues. There is as yet no satisfactory means to measure particle size and particle size distribution in *intact emulsions*. Laser scattering techniques being developed by Nicoli (1978; Nicoli and Benedek, 1976; Jedziniak et al., 1978) and others (Kerker, 1969; McIntyre and Gornick, 1964; Benedek, 1969; Chu, 1974; Cummins and Pike, 1974; Koppel, 1972; Conti and DiGiorgio, 1978) have real potential because the emulsion, hopefully, can be measured as is and not after treatment by centrifugation, chromatography, filtration, significant dilution, or other manipulations which are required by some methods. Such manipulations almost certainly change the mileu of the particle, cause sheer stress, alter the electrical charge, and affect the size and aggregation of the particle. Until better means are found, optical density is monitored (at 540 nm) during mechanical or sonic homogenization until a plateau is reached (Clark et al., 1972), as shown diagrammatically in Figure 37.7. We are satisfied when the optical density is near 1.0. We have made some transparent or nearly transparent emulsions which are remarkably stable and reasonably free from toxicity. Such emulsions have a beautiful blue cast and a rainbow sheen. Similar nearly transparent F emulsions are sometimes seen circulating in the blood of animals after the reticuloendothelial system has removed the population of larger particles and particle aggregates and also perhaps even further emulsification has occurred.

If density gradient beads are added to an emulsion or to plasma removed from an emulsion-treated animal, the beads settle at discrete boundaries not visible to the eye. This is shown in Figure 37.8. We interpret these specific gravity measurements to mean that there are some fluorocarbon particles of such a small size that they could easily exert oncotic pressures both in vitro and in vivo. The future will reveal means to prepare emulsions so that they carry oxygen and yet behave in other ways like plasma.

Much of the future will revolve around the emulsion problem, not gas solubility, toxicity, or even body retention. Oxygen solubility is high in all perfluoro compounds measured, with a tendency to be higher the lower the molecular weight (Fig. 37.9). Fluorination increases the solubility of oxygen in a hydrocarbon (Table 37.2). There are ways to measure and calculate the oxygen solubility (Lawson et al., 1978; Wesseler et al., 1977). Aside from a remote possibility of binding at very low oxygen tensions (Zander, 1974), there is no evidence to suggest that anything except pure solubility and passive diffusion is involved.

The vapor pressure problem is now well understood in the sense that F compounds having vapor pressures found in carbon-8 (or equivalent) molecules or smaller are too high and cause a gas vapor embolism in the lungs (Gollan and Clark, 1967; Sass et al., 1976) when injected

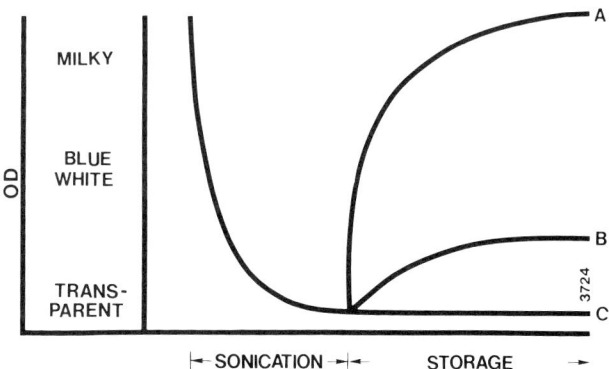

Figure 37.7. Particle size decrease on sonication and increase with time. The vertical axis is optical density (OD). The period indicated by sonication is a matter of minutes. The storage period is a matter of days or weeks. *A*, an unstable emulsion such as F-decalin; *B*, a tolerably stable emulsion; *C*, a perfectly stable emulsion.

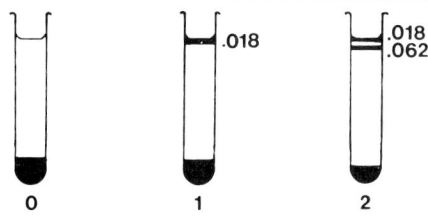

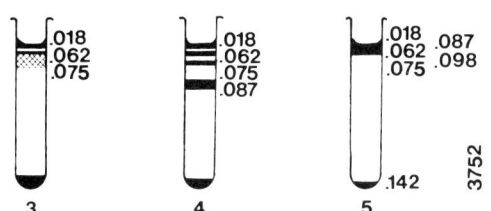

Figure 37.8. The effect of increasing fluorocarbon particle content on the flotation of calibrated specific gravity beads. Before giving emulsion (O, above) all 6 grades of beads sunk. An adult anesthetized cat (4 kg) was given 40 cc/kg of a 15% v/v of a Gaulin-prepared Decamine 60 emulsion and samples were removed 5 min after each 10 cc/kg infusion. Sample number five was removed 20 hr after the infusion. Beads are Sephadex density marker beads (Pharmacia). The numbers refer to the density.

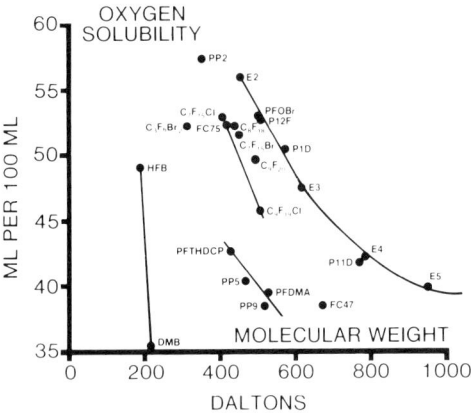

Figure 37.9. Oxygen solubility in a number of F compounds related to molecular weight. (Reprinted with permission from E.P. Wesseler, R. Iltis, and L.C. Clark, Jr.: Journal of Fluorine Chemistry 9:137, 1977.) For identification of compounds see Wesseler et al. (1977).

intravenously or an abdominal gas pocket (Fig. 37.10) when given intraperitoneally as a neat liquid. Obviously, a fluorocarbon particle having a vapor pressure of zero—Teflon is a good example—will remain in the body forever. Indeed, some perfluorochemicals when ingested by macrophages remain for very long times (Miller et

Table 37.2
Oxygen Solubility at 25°C.

	ml/100 ml
Benzene	22.5
Hexafluorobenzene	48.8
Decalin	14.4
Perfluorodecalin	40.3
Octylbromide	18.4
Perfluorooctylbromide	52.7
Tributylamine	23.9
Perfluorotributylamine	38.4
Heptane	33.0
Perfluoroheptane	54.8
Octane	28.6
Pefluorooctane	52.1
Nonane	26.4
Perfluorononane	49.6

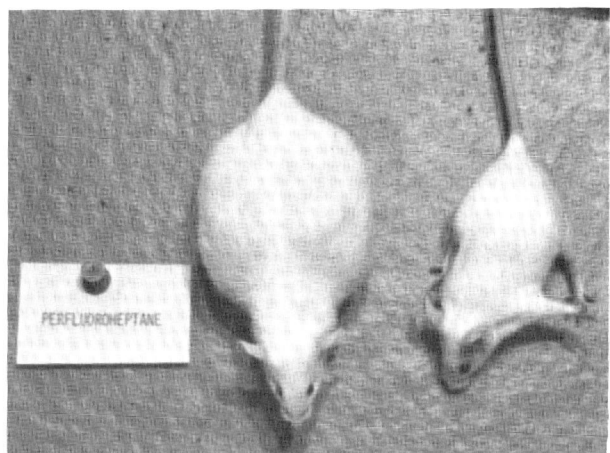

Figure 37.10. Intraperitoneal gas pocket in mouse on *left*, 1 day following injection of 0.2 µl of a neat liquid of F-heptane. The gas vapor appears in a matter of hours and persists for months. Control on *right*. (Reprinted with permission from L.C. Clark, Jr., R.E. Moore, S. Diver, and M.L. Miller: *Proceedings of the IVth International Symposium on Perfluorochemical Blood Substitutes* p. 55–67. Excerpta Medica, Amsterdam, 1978.)

al., 1976). Particles of F-tributylamine, one of the earliest emulsions used (Sloviter and Kamimoto, 1967; Geyer et al., 1968)*, remain in the liver and spleen for the lifetime of the animal. This incredible retention time is found in spite of the fact that F-tributylamine has a vapor pressure of about 2 torr; a drop of the neat liquid spread on a table surface will evaporate before your eyes. Vapor pressure (Table 37.3) is not the only factor, then, in liver retention.

---
* Sloviter was the first to publish the use of an F emulsion to sustain life; he used FC75 and albumin. I prepared Pluronic F68 emulsions of FC75 and FC43 and injected them in rabbits. Geyer was the first to describe the total replacement of the blood in an oxygen-breathing rat with an F emulsion; he used Pluronic F68/FC43.

Table 37.3
Vapor Pressure of Perfluorinated Liquids for Liquid Breathing and Artificial Blood

Designation	Chemical Name or Structural Formula	Vapor Pressure[a]
		torr, at 37.5 C
FC47	Perfluorotributylamine	2.5
PIID	$(CF_3)_2CF-O-(CF_2)_8OCF(CF_3)_2$	3
PP9	Perfluoromethyldecalin	5
EPFO	$F(CF_2)_8CH_2CH_3$	6
PFD	Perfluorodecane	8*
E3	$CF_3CHF[O-CF_2CF(CF_3)]_3F$	10
PID	$(CF_3)_2CF-O-(CF_2)_4OCF(CF_3)_2$	13
1913	Perfluorooctylbromide	14*
PP5	Perfluorodecalin	14
PFN	Perfluorononane	15*
PFO	Perfluorooctane	50*
FC75	Perfluorobutyltetrahydrofuran	51
E2	$CF_3CHF[O-CF_2CF(CF_2)]_2F$	56
PP3	Perfluoro-1,3-dimethylcyclohexane	62
PP2	Perfluoromethylcyclohexane	180
PP1	Perfluorohexane	372

[a] The vapor pressures listed are those reported by the manufacturer, except those indicated by * which are estimated here from the boiling points.

In addition to F-tributylamine, the Freon E series of ethers, and other compounds containing atoms other than carbon and fluorine persist in the body for months or years. Our laboratory (Clark et al., 1973) and Okamoto (Okamoto et al., 1973) reported that the F-decalins (Fig. 37.11) do not persist in the body. Our search for suitable perfluoro components for artificial blood would have been over when we discovered that F-decalin (and other related F cyclic substances) left the body in a reasonable time, except for the fact that, while F-decalin makes a very fine particle emulsion (in Pluronic F68), the optical density increases rapidly, as shown in Figure 37.7. The rate of this increase in optical density is a function of temperature. Surprisingly, and unlike most other emulsions of any kind (e.g., mayonnaise), F-decalin emulsions are stable when frozen and stored in a deep freeze in sealed containers. It can be seen from Figure 37.12 that emulsions of F-tributylamine are stable for a long time, even when stored at 2°C. We found that mixtures of F-decalin and F-tributylamine are also stable. A mixture of neat liquids consisting of six parts of F decalin and four parts of F-tributylamine (which we dub "Decamine 60") has proven to be useful in making stable emulsions for many kinds of perfusion studies.

Naito mixed F-decalin with F-tripropylamine to form the trade named emulsion "Fluosol-DA," the first to be used in humans (Makowski et al., 1979; Maugh, 1979; Ohyanagi et al., 1979) and which is now finding increasing clinical application, particularly in Japan and by Jehovah's Witnesses. The composition of this emulsion is given in Table 37.4. The F-tripropylamine ($C_9F_{21}N$) has a longer body retention time than F-decalin ($C_{10}F_{18}$) but nowhere near as long as the F-tributylamine ($C_{12}F_{27}N$) molecule. Much more is known about F-decalin and F-tributylamine, because of their many uses over the past 10 or 15 years, than F-tripropylamine. F-tripropylamine does not make a particularly stable emulsion by itself, without admixture with F-decalin, but stabilizes F-decalin emulsions when added in the proper amount.

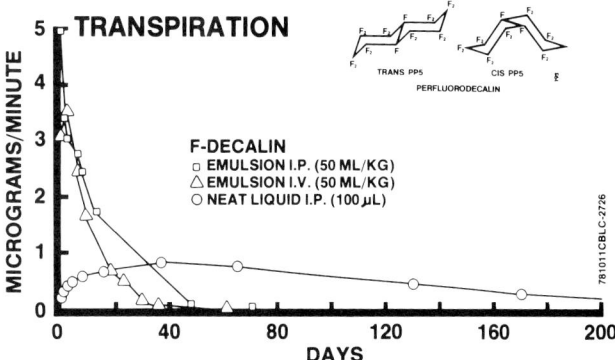

Figure 37.11. Whole body transpiration of F-decalin emulsion and F-decalin neat liquid in the intact awake mouse. (Reprinted with permission from L.C. Clark, Jr., R.E. Moore, S. Diver, and M.L. Miller: *Proceedings of the IVth International Symposium on Perfluorochemical Blood Substitutes* p. 55–67. Excerpta Medica, Amsterdam, 1978.)

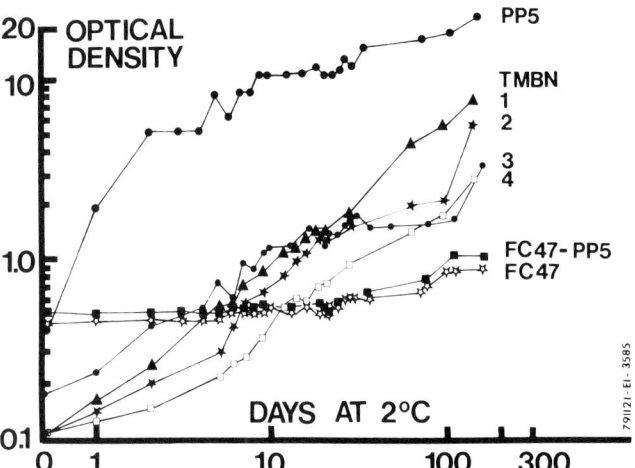

Figure 37.12. Optical density of F emulsions stored in the cold. Note log scales. PP5 is F-decalin. TMBN represents 4 different distillation fractions of trimethyl(3.3.1.)bicyclononane. FC47-PP5 is a 50/50 mixture of the two neat liquids.

Our own work has involved the synthesis of carbon-fluorine compounds, thinking that these structures have a better chance of leaving the body rapidly than do those containing heteroatoms such as nitrogen and oxygen.

We have tested over two dozen specially synthesized paraffinic, monocyclic, alkyl monocyclic, bicyclic, alkyl bicyclic, tricyclic, and alkyl tricyclic fluorocarbons.

A word about synthesis of fluorine organic compounds—such syntheses are difficult and cannot be carried forward on any practical scale in an ordinary laboratory. The reactions are difficult to manage because they are strongly exothermic. It is this loss of energy

Table 37.4
Composition of Fluosol-DA (20%)[a]

	W/V%
Perfluorodecalin	14.0
Perfluorotripropylamine	6.0
Pluronic F-68	2.7
Yolk phospholipids	0.4
Potassium oleate	0.04
Glycerol	0.8
NaCl	0.6
KCl	0.034
$MgCl_2$	0.020
$CaCl_2$	0.028
$NaHCO_3$	0.210
Glucose	0.180
Hydroxyethylstarch	3.0

[a] From Ohyanagi et al., 1979.

which makes the final perfluorinated products so inert. The carbon-fluorine bond is exceedingly strong. Very little progress was made in their synthesis until World War II, when they were prepared as inert media to fractionate corrosive uranium isotopes needed in the Manhattan Project. The four main methods are: 1) electrochemical (Simon's), 2) use of metallic fluorides and high temperatures, 3) telomerization, and 4) direct fluorination at low temperature. The first three methods have been used to make multiton lots for commercial purposes. F-tributylamine is made by the Simon's process. F-decalin is made by the CoF_3 process. The compounds of the Freon E series (DuPont) and the PID series (Allied Chemical) which were extensively studied in our laboratory were made by telomerization. F-tetramethylpentane (see Fig. 37.13) is made by direct fluorination (Shimp and Lagow, 1977). Much of our synthetic work has revolved around polycyclic compounds, notably adamantane (Fig. 37.14) and derivatives. Typically, F-adamantane is prepared by exhaustive fluorination as shown below.

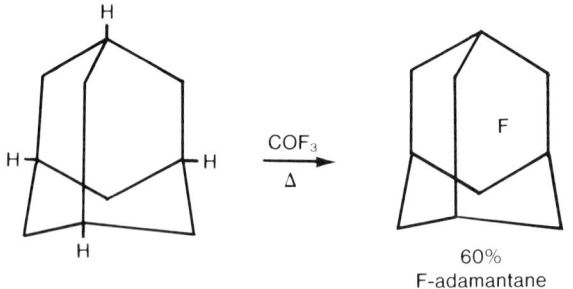

Similar exhaustive fluorination of dimethyladamantane leads to some open ring structures, as shown in Figure 37.15. We have found that some of these F-adamantane derivatives produce stable emulsions, even though not yet stable enough for room temperature storage. None of these carbon-fluorine cyclic compounds persists in the liver as long as comparable amines and ethers, and some leave about as rapidly as F-decalin.

The retention time of a compound in the body can be

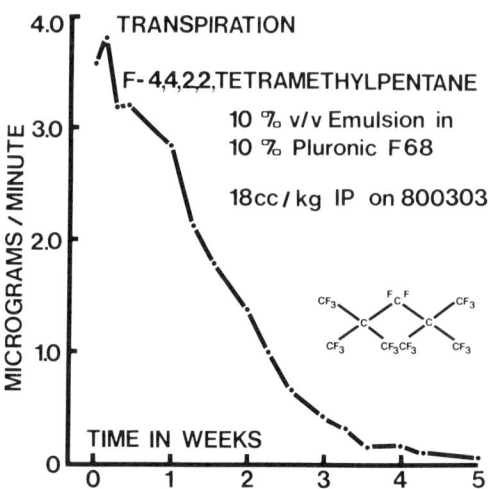

Figure 37.13. Transpiration of F-tetramethylpentane in the intact awake mouse. This preparation of fluorocarbon contained appreciable amounts of CH bonding, as we can show by absorption in the 2800 cm^{-1} region of the infrared in our laboratory.

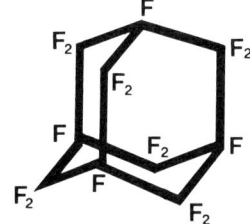

Figure 37.14. Perfluoroadamantane.

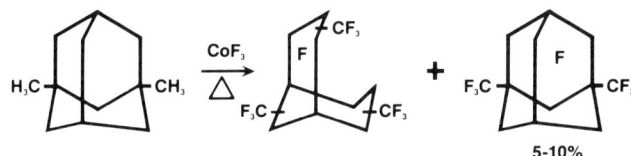

Figure 37.15. Exhaustive fluorination of dimethyladamantane leads to F-dimethyladamantane and F-trimethylbicyclononane. (Reprinted with permission from R.E. Moore, L. C. Clark, Jr., and M.L. Miller: *Proceedings of the IVth International Symposium on Perfluorochemical Blood Substitutes*, p. 69–79. Excerpta Medica, Amsterdam, 1979.)

measured by measuring whole body transpiration, as shown in Figure 37.16. This is the method used for most of our work. Their transpiration is also easily measured (though not quantitatively) by gas chromatography (GC) analysis of subcutaneous gas pockets or cups sealed on the skin. We have also measured thousands of samples by combustion of the liver using sodium biphenyl (or sodium emulsions) followed by direct measurement of the so generated fluoride ion by a lanthanum fluoride potentiometric electrode. Other methods in use are extraction of tissue by organic solvents, such as hexane or

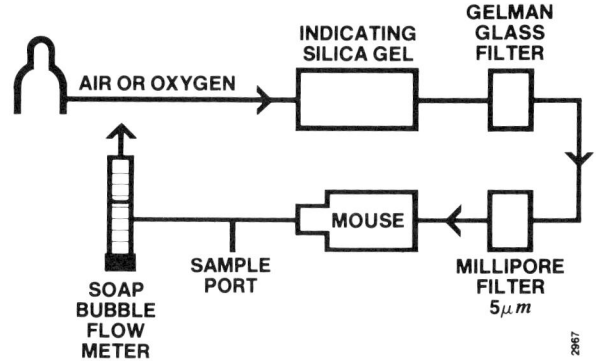

Figure 37.16. Method of measuring transpiration in intact awake animals.

chlorofluoropropanes and the like, followed by GC or infrared analysis. NMR could also be used (if one was lucky enough to have one). In measurement of fluorinated compounds the electron capture detector used routinely in our GC work is orders of magnitude more sensitive than flame ionization, thermal, or other detectors, and together with an SE 30/Chromosorb W column, is used for most of our analytical work. Unfortunately, electron capture detectors and their associated electronics can be frustratingly fickle; great patience with the apparatus and their manufacturers is required. Unknowns must be sandwiched between standards, to obtain accurate data.

Gas chromatography not only yields quantitative data from peak height and/or area computation, but also yields information not obtainable in any other way. Such a murine chromatogram is shown in Figure 37.17. It can be seen that, as time proceeds, there is at first an exodus of compounds, present but not revealed in the chromatogram of the original compound. This is sometimes followed much later by the appearance of a long retention compound, hidden under the major peak, and revealed only when the major compound had largely been transpired.

Besides there being a relationship between emulsion stability and F compound *mixtures* there is also a relationship between transpiration rate and *mixtures* as shown in Figure 37.18. The presence of one fluorochemical can influence the rate at which another leaves. Could this happen because residual particles somehow form "windows" in membranes through which another fluorochemical vapor can diffuse? Could fluorocarbon windows purposely be formed to increase the diffusion of oxygen in the lungs?

F-butylcyclohexane ($C_{10}F_{20}$) and F-diethylcyclohexane ($C_{10}F_{20}$), both having vapor pressures within a torr or so of F-decalin ($C_{10}F_{18}$), leave the liver at a much slower rate than F-decalin (Fig. 37.19). Hence, both vapor pressure *and* structure are involved in transpiration.

In searching for relationships between transpiration rate, or body retention time, and physicochemical properties, we found that critical solution temperature, easily measured with a hydrocarbon solvent, a temperature

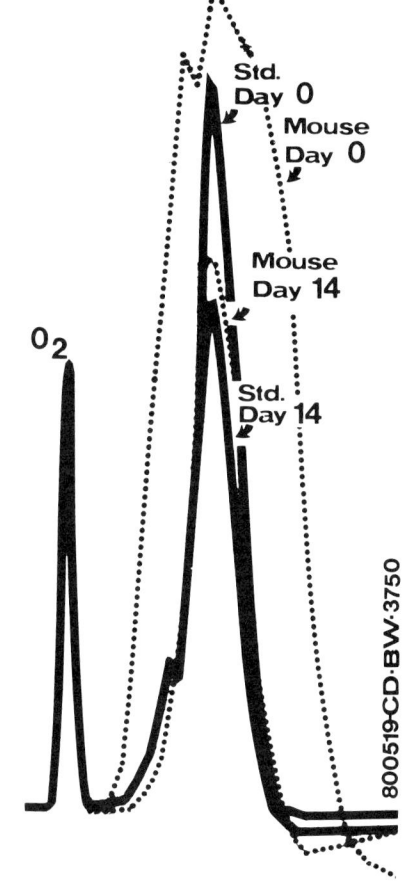

Figure 37.17. Gas chromatogram of samples of transpired gas on day 0 and day 14. The mouse received 50 cc/kg intraperitoneally of a 10% v/v emulsion (800407B) of an experimental F liquid. Column: SE 30/Chromosorb; Electron capture detector. Carrier gas: N_2. Attenuation adjusted to get peaks on scale of chart.

controlling bath, and a thermometer, is related to body retention, as shown in Figure 37.20. Those compounds tending to have long retention times are in the top area and to the left. Cyclic F compounds tend to leave faster than paraffinic F compounds.

And, now, a word about purity and the concept of perfluorination and exhaustive fluorination. The method of synthesis used has a definite bearing on the kind of product obtained. The Simon's and CoF_3 processes tend to yield a number of side products which must be removed before the material can be used for biological purposes. They also can yield a number of products which are so closely related that they probably may just as well be left there. For example, in the manufacture of F-tributylamine, about eight isomers are produced, each one of which seems to have the same biological properties and each one of which is next to impossible to separate from the other by physicochemical means or by passage through an animal. A gas chromatogram of FC47 extracted from the liver of an animal after a residence time

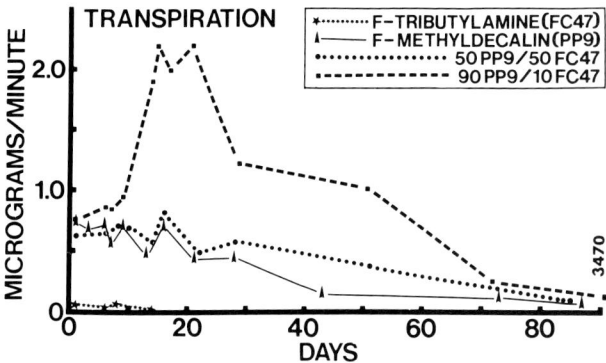

Figure 37.18. Whole body transpiration of F vapors by the intact awake mouse. The fluorochemical was administered intraperitoneally as a 15% v/v emulsion in 10% Pluronic F68. Each group consisted of 10 mice which were sampled at random to give the four curves. The number of determinations in each group were as follows: FC47: $n = 24$; PP9: $n = 84$; 50/50: $n = 72$; 90/10: $n = 102$.

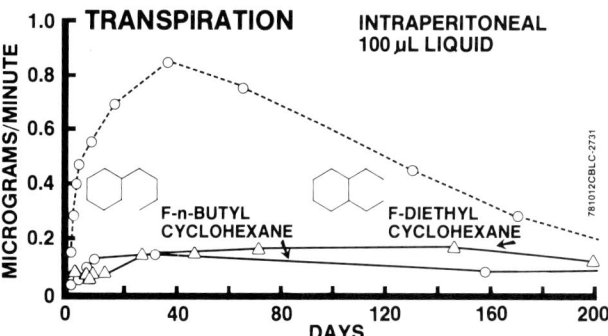

Figure 37.19. Whole body transpiration of intraperitoneal neat liquid in the intact awake mouse. The two substituted F-cyclohexanes are compared with F-decalin (*dotted line* at top). Fifty-six determinations were made of the butyl compound and 96 determinations of the diethyl compound. (Reprinted with permission from R.E. Moore, L.C. Clark, Jr., and M.L. Miller: *Proceedings of the IVth International Symposium on Perfluorochemical Blood Substitutes*, p. 69–79. Excerpta Medica, Amsterdam, 1979).

of several years is no different from the pattern found in the original neat liquid used to make the emulsion. In another example, F-diethylcyclohexane and F-butylcyclohexane are formed as by-products in the exhaustive fluorination of F-decalin (Cottrell, 1978). We have found, as we pointed out earlier, that these compounds are retained longer than the bicyclic compound, F-decalin. But these compounds can be readily removed by spinning band distillation, which we use, or by preparative GC.* Products prepared by telomerization such as

---

* We have separated small amounts of cis- and transdecalin in our laboratory by preparative gas chromatograpy using a ½

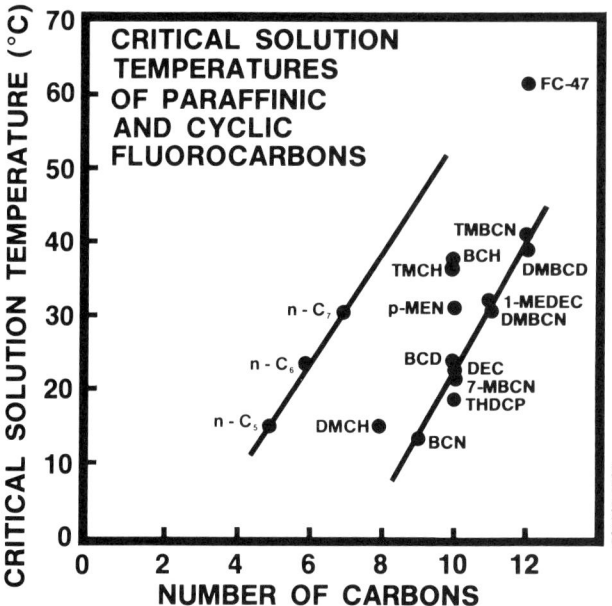

Figure 37.20. Relationships between critical solution temperature and molecular weight of a number of perfluorinates. The perfluorinated derivatives of the following compounds are shown: N—C_7, normal heptane; N—C_6, normal hexane; N—C_5, normal pentane; FC47, tributylamine; TMBCN, trimethylbicyclo-(3.3.1.)nonane; DMBCD, dimethylbicyclo(5.3.0.)-decane; BCH, bicyclohexane; TMCH, trimethylcyclohexane; 1-MEDEC, 1-methyldecalin; P-MEN, P-menthane; DMBCN, dimethylbicyclo(3.3.1.)nonane; BCD, bicyclo(5.3.0.)decane; DEC, decalin; 7-MBCN, 7-methylbicyclo(4.3.0.)nonane; THDCP, tetrahydrodicyclopentadiene; DMCH, dimethylcyclohexane; BCN, bicyclo(4.3.0.)nonane. (Reprinted with permission from R.E. Moore, L.C. Clark, Jr., and M.L. Miller: *Proceedings of the IVth International Symposium on Perfluorochemical Blood Substitutes*, p. 69–79. Excerpta Medica, Amsterdam, 1979.)

PID and E3 (see Table 37.3) can be made very pure. Allied Chemical made batches of PID and PIID for us which we believe may be the purest perfluoro compounds ever made. Unfortunately, both of these perfluoro ether classes of compounds have exceedingly long retention times in the liver and spleen. The fourth process, theoretically, should perhaps be capable of making purer compounds than either of the first two processes because of the low temperatures which can be used: The F-tetramethylpentane, the transpiration of which is reported here for the first time (Fig. 37.13), was prepared by direct fluorination of the corresponding hydrocarbon (Shimp and Lagow, 1977).

---

inch, SE 30/Chromosorb column. The technology of preparative gas chromatography has advanced rapidly so that now columns 1 m in diameter are being used to sparate compounds, e.g., perfume components, in metric ton quantities.

```
         CH₃   CH₃         F₂        CF₃   CF₃
          |  H  |                     |  H  |
   H₃C—C—C—C—CH₃    →   F₃C—C—C—C—CF₃
          |  H  |       −78°          |  H  |
         CH₃   CH₃                   CF₃   CF₃
                                        14%

         CF₃   CF₃                   CF₃   CF₃
          |  F  |                     |  F  |
   + F₃C—C—C—C—CF₃  +  F₃C—C—C—C—CF₃
          |  H  |                     |  F  |
         CF₃   CF₃                   CF₃   CF₃
           66%                         20%
```

The overall yield was about 70% with the ratios as shown above. When the exposure time to fluorine was increased from 36 to 85 hr and the starting material was decreased in half, the overall yield increased to about 95%, but the ratios of the dihydro, monohydro, and perfluoro products were not changed. The dihydro compound could be readily separated from the other two, but it was only on a dinonylphthalate column at 10°C that the perfluoro and 3-hydro compound could be separated. All this indicates that the middle carbon position is hindered by the physical bulk of the F-tertiary butyl groups on either side. Could this proton, so hindered as to be unattacked by fluorine, participate in biological reactions? The evidence so far indicates that it cannot, and that both compounds behave as one.

The possible undesirable effects of a remaining proton cannot yet be ruled out. In industry great pains are taken to remove traces (ppm) of incompletely fluorinated material, largely because their presence causes deleterious effects on electronic circuitry. Such incompletely fluorinated material is monitored by infrared and is removed by proprietary processes which probably include amine extraction.

The general purification process used in the preparation of our exhaustively fluorinated polycyclic derivatives is as follows:

1. aqueous bicarbonate wash to remove hydrofluoric acid;
2. distillation in a 45-plate spinning band column—to remove lower molecular weight species, followed by;
3. distillation in a 75-plate or 200-plate spinning band column, depending on the complexity of the product, to concentrate specific isomers;
4. preparative chromatography over a ½ inch × 42 ft column packed with 15% SE 30 on Chromosorb W to isolate pure isomers;
5. aqueous KOH (4N) reflux for 3 hr to remove partially fluorinated (hydrogen containing) species;
6. extraction with diethylamine to remove olefinic and other similar reactive species; and finally
7. aqueous bicarbonate wash, using phenol red as an indicator.

Even after this, traces of a proton-containing material remain, probably

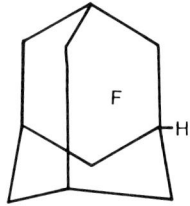

The presence of double bonds in highly fluorinated compounds to be used as oxygen and carbon dioxide carriers in biological systems is generally regarded as undesirable.

We have recently discovered (Clark and Moore, 1979; Clark and Inscho, 1980) a relatively simple and very sensitive test for the presence of protons and/or double bonds remaining on perfluorinated compounds. It is based upon an observation made in 1950 (Pruett et al., 1950) concerning the reaction of organic amines and olefinic fluorocarbons. The equation is:

```
   n-C₄H₉NH₂ + ClCF=CF₂ → [CHClFCF₂NHC₄H₉]
                                          ↓
              NC₄H₉
              ∥          n-C₄H₉NH₂
   CHClFC ←─────────────────── CHClFCF=NC₄H₉
              \
              NHC₄H₉

              O
              ∥              H₂O
   CHClFC—NHC₄H₉ ←────────
```

In our test, 10 μl of the perfluoroliquid are added to 2 ml of pyridine in a tube which is either heated to hasten the reaction, or allowed to stand 24 hr (or more). A standard, such as F-heptene-1 is added, to a pair of tubes. The presence of a double bond or a proton results in an intense yellow color which is read at 380 nm in an ordinary clinical spectrophotometer. It is likely that this same reaction, or one with a similar amine, can also be used to remove such impurities from F liquids since the yellow color is water soluble and can be removed from the fluorocarbon layer in a separatory funnel.

The term "perfluoro" has been generally used in biological and industrial literature to cover the classes of compounds useful as inert gas solvents and x-ray contrast agents. But "perfluoro" properly refers to the replacement of hydrogen atoms by fluorine atoms. Hence, *perfluoro*benzene is hexafluorobenzene, C_6F_6 and, being a powerful anesthetic, is far from inert. But *perfluoro*hexane is C_6F_{12}, completely saturated with fluorine and, at least by comparison, biologically inert. Sooner or later a word must be found which will refer to compounds which can take up no more fluorine, since these completely fluorine-saturated compounds are those desired in biology due to their liklihood of being nonmetabolizable and pharmacologically inactive. "Exhaustively fluorinated" seems to be the best, albeit clumsy, term so far.

Finally, something must be said about fluorocarbon emulsions. First, there is something of a mystery that the best emulsions, those that cause the fewest undersirable reactions, are those having particle sizes below 0.2 μ. Since particle size, or agglomerates of particles, rapidly increase in some emulsions, it is easy to imagine that they could also undergo similar changes in vivo, even though the blood contains many "emulsifying agents" such as the lipoproteins. A knowledge of particle size and particle size distribution patterns in vitro and in vivo is highly desirable. Unfortunately, the two methods available at present, as we said earlier, are tedious and subject to error.

If 15 ml of fluorocarbon liquid is added to 85 ml of saline and sonicated, a milky emulsion is formed which rapidly settles again, as shown in Figure 37.21. If sonication takes place in the presence of an emulsifier, say 10% Pluronic F68, then a stable milky, opalescent, blue-white, or transparent emulsion results. The specific gravity of this emulsion as measured in a pycnometer, where the weight of a known volume is measured, will be the same whether or not the two phases are separate or emulsified. But, if the specific gravity is measured by floating something, like beads, in it, then the specific gravities should reveal the extent to which the particles are broken down to finer particles. Hence, from the pycnometer, one can obtain an exact measurement of the amount of fluorocarbon present and from the distribution of beads an expression of the colloidal state of the fluorocarbon. These concepts are illustrated by the findings shown in Figure 37.8. The bead distribution in samples of plasma removed from a cat after five consecutive doses of a Decamine 60 emulsion (15% v/v in 10% Pluronic F68) is illustrated. It can be seen that more of the heavier beads floated as the circulating fluorocarbon level increased. At the end of the infusion (50 cc/kg) the packed fluorocarbon volume was 64% and the hematocrit was 19%. The flotation gravity, therefore, behaved as if much of the Decamine 60 were *dissolved* in the plasma.

Gelin (1964) and Yen and Fung (1978) have shown that red cells tend to follow the greatest flow. This is shown in Figure 37.22, taken from Yen. We would like it if, in ischemic tissue, the flow of oxygen would go towards the deprived tissue, where the plasma goes. It would appear that the colloidal nature of fluorocarbon emulsions may allow them to carry oxygen where plasma flows in ways not heretofore possible. If one couples the unique oxygen solubility properties (Fig. 37.3) of fluorocarbons and the colloidal aspects of fine particle emulsions with oxygen breathing, new means to treat ischemic heart and brain disease may well be on the horizon.

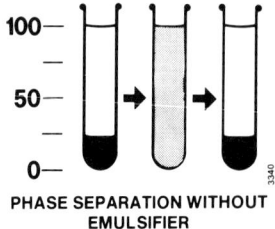

Figure 37.21. Phase separation without emulsifier.

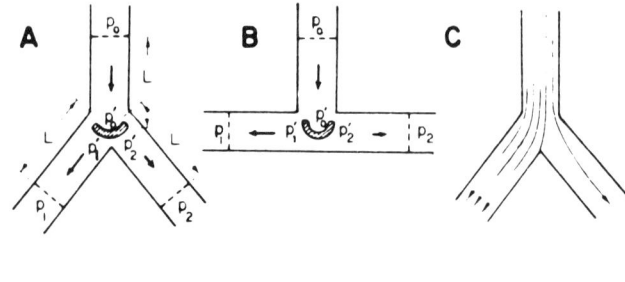

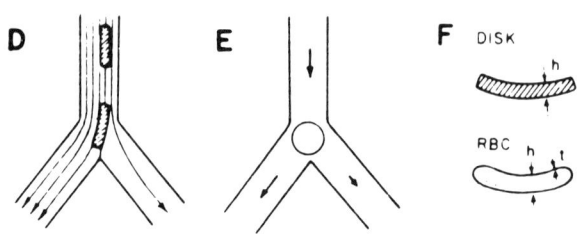

Figure 37.22. The silicone discs follow the lines of greatest flow. Silicone elastomeric discs (designed to mimic erythrocytes) tend to be distributed into the branch having the greatest flow. The studies of Gelin with natural red cells are in accord with the silicone model. (Reprinted with permission from R. T. Yen and Y. C. Fung: American Journal of Physiology 235: H251, 1978.)

In hemorrhagic shock, the PO_2 on the surface of organs decreases. Figure 37.23 shows the dramatic way in which the PO_2 of the brain and the liver decrease as blood is withdrawn and returned. We have observed a decrease of PO_2 to zero on the surface of the rat liver as measured with a transcutaneous ($TCPO_2$) electrode set at 37°C as blood is withdrawn and a return to normal or above as the blood is replaced with F emulsion.

In Figure 37.24, we measured the $TCPO_2$ on the carefully shaved belly skin of a cat as blood was withdrawn and replaced with an emulsion of FC47. The drop in $TCPO_2$ is very rapid after a certain, apparently critical point is reached. In Figure 37.25, blood was removed as shown and replaced. In the first experiment, a cardiac arrest occurred which was reversed by massage through the chest wall and return of the blood. In a second experiment, a few days later, the experiment was repeated but the blood was replaced by an FC47 emulsion, with a return to normal skin PO_2, much the same as when blood was used. We came to believe with these and other experiments on cats, that $TCPO_2$ may be a valuable indicator of circulatory shock; the ratio of the arterial to the skin PO_2 may be useful as a numerical index. In the baboon (Fig. 37.26), blood replacement with F emulsion was followed by a rapid increase in $TCPO_2$. The points indicated by V are PO_2 values obtained as samples of blood removed from the venous catheter (tip in the inferior vena cava). This animal sat up and ate a banana in the early evening of the experiment and by the end of the week had regained his normal hematocrit and macho social position with his female cage mate.

Fluorocarbon Emulsions

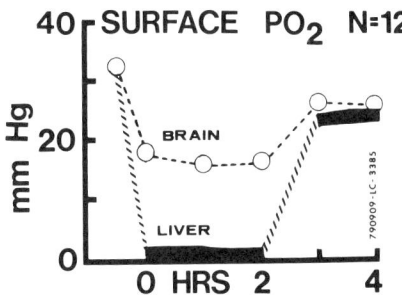

Figure 37.23. Oxygen tension on the surface of the brain and the liver as reported by Miller et al. (1974) and redrawn for use here.

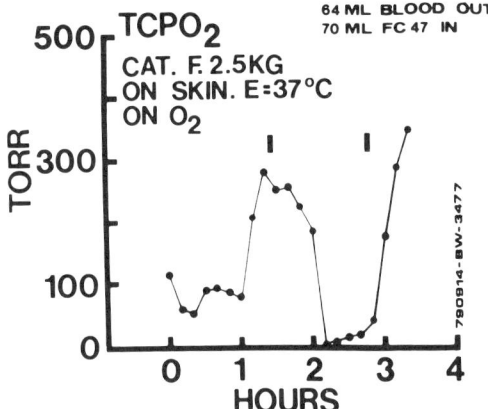

Figure 37.24. The effect of blood withdrawal and replacement by an FC47 emulsion on transcutaneous oxygen tension in a pentobarbital-anesthetized cat. The femoral arterial pressure never fell below 65 mm Hg. Bars indicate point at which blood was withdrawn and at which FC47 was replaced.

CONCLUDING REMARKS

Fluorocarbon emulsions will find wide use as substitutes for whole blood because of their high solubility for blood gases and the ease with which their purity, sterility, buffering capacity, ionic composition, and osmotic and oncotic properties can be controlled.

In general, moderate vapor pressure highly fluorinated compounds containing only carbon and fluorine atoms have a short retention time in the body but are difficult to maintain as stable emulsions without freezing. Highly fluorinated compounds containing nitrogen or oxygen in their structure tend to form more stable emulsions and to stabilize fluorocarbon emulsions, but are apt to persist in the liver and spleen (Fig. 37.27). Clinical success with present formulations should herald only the *beginning* of the fluorocarbon blood substitute era, for much research remains to be done in designing the best highly fluorinated compounds for use in biology and medicine.

More important than their use as substitutes for whole blood, circulating fluorocarbon emulsions, because of their unique capability of being able to transport large *amounts* of oxygen at high oxygen tension, when breath-

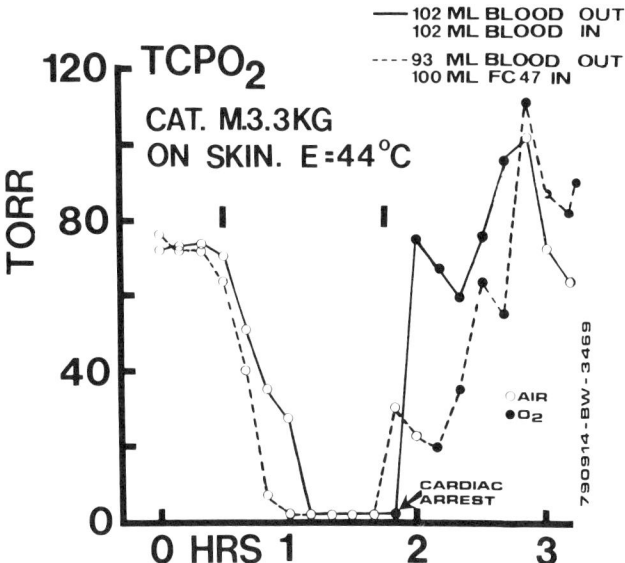

Figure 37.25. The effect of venesection and blood replacement by either blood or an FC47 emulsion on skin oxygen tension as measured by a transcutaneous oxygen electrode at 44°C. The adult male cat was anesthetized with sodium pentobarbital and the electrode was placed on the abdomen where there was no body hair. A cardiac arrest, reversed by blood administration and external massage, occurred in the first experiment. Except for the period of cardiac arrest, the direct mercury (femoral arterial cannula) blood pressure remained above 60 mm.

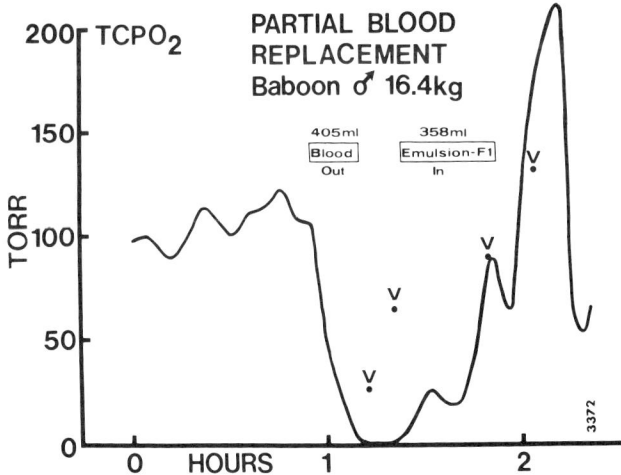

Figure 37.26. Transcutaneous oxygen tension recording from the shaved skin of a pentobarbital-anesthetized normal male baboon during phlebotomy and replacement by an FC47 emulsion. The Vs stand for inferior vena cava PO_2 measurements. The arterial blood pressure never fell below 70 mm.

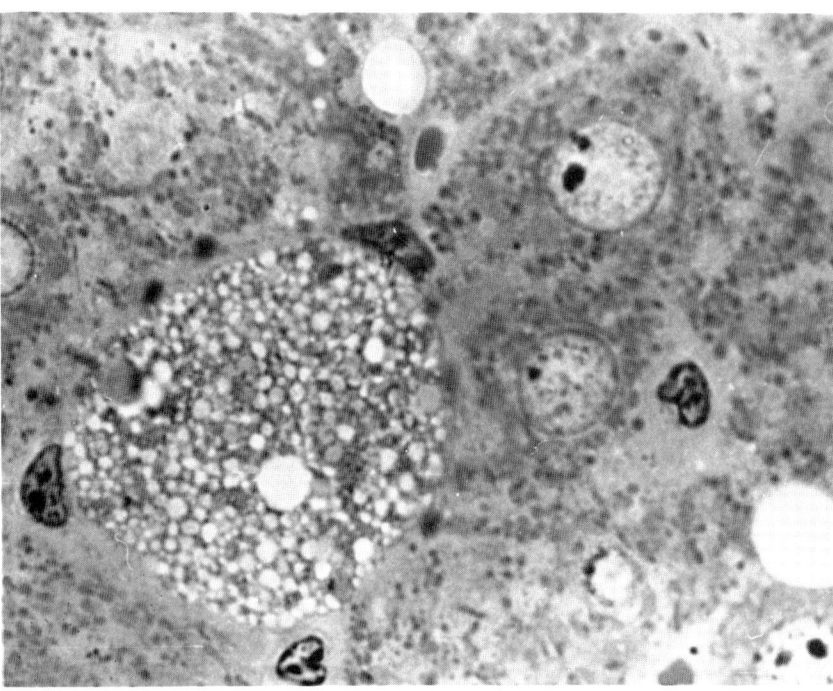

Figure 37.27. Photomicrograph of selected liver section from a mouse which received 50 cc/kg intravenously of Fluosol-DA 570 days previously. Note the large number of perfluorochemical particles, which are presumably F-tripropylamine. Toluidine blue. (Sections prepared by M.L. Miller.) ×1500.

ing oxygen at ambient pressures, offer unusual opportunities to study and possibly treat ischemic diseases such as heart attack and stroke. Further, because of their ability to increase tissue oxygen tensions, to flow where plasma rather than red cells flow, and to circulate as particles of extremely small size, these synthetic emulsions may prove valuable in the salvation of tissues primarily injured by trauma as well as those such as the liver which are metabolically involved in shock. Their low surface tensions, high radiopacity when brominated, unique solubility and diffusion characteristics, and biological inertness add to their potential for diagnosis and treatment of disorders of oxygen transport and delivery.

Addendum. Since preparation of this chapter, a paper describing decreased TCPO$_2$ in rabbits subjected to acute hemorrhage has appeared (F. A. Matsen III, C. R. Wyss, R. V. King, and C. W. Simmons: Effect of acute hemorrhage on transcutaneous, subcutaneous, intramuscular and arterial oxygen tensions. *Pediatrics 65:*881–883, 1980. The authors suggest, as I did, that transcutaneous hypoxia may be a clinically valuable danger signal.

In hypovolemic shock in dogs, the TCPO$_2$ electrode output has been found to "follow oxygen delivery rather than PaPO$_2$" and, hence, may be a continuous noninvasive indicator of shock (K. K. Tremper, K. Waxman, and W. C. Shoemaker: Effects of hypoxia and shock on transcutaneous PO$_2$ values in dogs. *Critical Care Medicine 7:*526–531, 1979).

Recently the fluorocarbon emulsion (Fluosol-DA) prepared by the Green Cross Corporation has found increasing use (150 patients in Japan and 7 in the United States by May, 1980).

D. H. Glogar, R. A. Kloner, L. C. Clark, Jr., J. Muller, L. W. V. DeBoer, and E. Braunwald (Fluorocarbons: Synthetic oxygen carrying compounds with potential for reducing myocardial ischemic damage. *Science 211:*1439–1441, 1981) have recently shown that the ischemic zone in experimental myocardial infarction in dogs can be greatly reduced by fluorocarbon emulsion infusion and oxygen breathing.

Acknowledgments. Thanks are due to many individuals who have over the years contributed to this research: Charlene E. Bostrom, Kathleen A. Chalfin, Eleanor W. Clark, Donald Denson, Carol Duggan, Edward W. Inscho, Susan M. Jacobs, Patricia A. Turner, Lucinda S. Wead, Betsy J. Weiner, Eugene P. Wesseler, Barbara Williams, and Joan Youtsey. Robert E. Moore and his colleagues at Suntech conducted much of the synthetic work on the F-polycyclic compounds. We are grateful to Radiometer and Litton for the TCPO$_2$ measuring instrumentation used in these studies.

This work was supported in part by National Institute of Health (NIH) grants HL23526 and HD05221, and by NIH contract 1-HB6-2927, by a grant from Suntech, Inc., Marcus Hook, Pennsylvania, and by the Children's Hospital Research Foundation, Cincinnati.

Mrs. Elaine Adelburg kept a steady but pleasant pressure, without which this paper might not have been finished. Richard Lagow has been most helpful in theoretical and practical consultation on synthetic work. Christ Tamborski's enthusiasm for applying the knowledge of fluorine organic chemistry in biology and medicine is a sustaining force in our research.

References

Benedek, G.B.: Optical mixing spectroscopy with applications to problems in physics, chemistry, biology and engineering. In *Polarization, Matter, and Radiation.* Presses Universitaire de France, Paris, 1969.

Chu, B.: *Laser Light Scattering.* Academic Press, New York, 1974.

Clark, L.C., Jr., and Gollan, F.: Survival of mammals breathing organic liquids equilibrated with oxygen at atmospheric pressure. *Science 152:*1755, 1966.

Clark, L.C., Jr., and Inscho, E.W., Jr.: A simple colorimetric test for protons and double bonds in perfluorinated compounds. In preparation, 1980.

Clark, L.C., Jr., and Moore, R.E.: Diethyl amine purification of perfluorochemicals for biological use (abstract). American Chemical Society, Fourth Winter Fluorine Conference, Daytona, Florida, January 1979.

Clark, L.C., Jr., Becattini, F., and Kaplan, S.: Can fluorocarbon emulsions be used as artificial blood? Triangle *11:*115, 1972.

Clark, L.C., Jr., Becattini, F., Kaplan, S., Obrock, V., Cohen, D., and Becker, C.: Perfluorocarbons having a short dwell time in the liver. Science *181:*680, 1973.

Cole, R.P., Wittenberg, B.A., and Caldwell, P.R.B.: Myoglobin function in the isolated fluorocarbon-perfused dog heart. Am. J. Physiol. *234:*H567, 1978.

Conti, M., and DiGiorgio, V.: Laser-light-scattering investigation on the size, shape and polydispersity of ionic micelles. Ann. Phys. *3:*303, 1978.

Cottrell, D.W.: The production, purity and some properties of fluorocarbon liquids. In *HS Symposium, Research on Perfluorochemicals in Medicine and Biology*, edited by V. Novakova and L-O. Plantin, pp. 32–41. Karolinska Institute Research Center, Huddinge University Hospital, Huddinge, Sweden, 1978.

Cummins, H.Z., and Pike, E.R.: (Eds.): *Photon Correlation and Light Beading Spectroscopy*, 504 pp. Plenum Press, New York, 1974.

Gelin, L-E.: A method for studying the aggregation of blood cells, erythrostatis and plasma skimming in branching capillary tubes. Bibl. Anat. *4:*362, 1964.

Geyer, R.P., Monroe, R.G., Taylor, K.: Survival of rats having red cells totally replaced with emulsified fluorocarbon. Fed. Proc. *27:*384, 1968.

Gollan, F., and Clark, L.C., Jr.: Organ perfusion with fluorocarbon fluid. Physiologist *9:*191, 1966.

Gollan, F., and Clark, L.C., Jr.: Rapid decompression of mice breathing fluorocarbon liquid at 500 psi. Ala. J. Med. Sci. *4:*336, 1967.

Hasegawa, E., and Kishimoto, I. (Eds.): *Proceedings of the Xth International Congress for Nutrition: Symposium on Perfluorochemical Artificial Blood*, Kyoto, Japan, August 1975, 294 pp. Igakushobo, Osaka, Japan, 1975.

Jedziniak, J.A., Nicoli, D.F., Baram, H., and Benedek, G.B.: Quantitative verification of the existence of high molecular weight protein aggregates in the intact normal human lens by light-scattering spectroscopy. Invest. Opthalmol. Vis. Sci. *17:*51, 1978.

Kerker, M.: *The Scattering of Light and Other Electromagnetic Radiation*, 666 pp. Academic Press, New York, 1969.

Koppel, D.F.: Analysis of macromolecular polydispersity in intensity correlation spectroscopy: The method of cumulants. J. Chem. Phys. *57:*4814, 1972.

Lawson, D.D., Moacanin, J., Scherer, K.V., Jr., Terranova, T.F., and Ingham, J.D.: Methods for the estimation of vapor pressures and oxygen solubilities of fluorochemicals for possible applications in artificial blood formulations. J. Fluorine Chem. *12:*221, 1978.

Makowski, H., Tentschev, P., Frey, R., Necek, S., Bergmann, H., and Blauhut, B.: Tolerance of an oxygen-carrying colloidal plasma substitute in human being. In *Proceedings of the IVth International Symposium on Perfluorochemical Blood Substitutes*, pp. 47–54. Excerpta Medica, Amsterdam, 1979.

Maugh, T.H., II.: Blood substitute passes its first test. Science *206:*205, 1979.

McIntyre, D., and Gornick, F. (Eds.): *Light Scattering From Dilute Polymer Solutions*, 318 pp. Gordon and Breach, New York, 1964.

Miller, M.L., Wesseler, E.P., Jones, S.C., Clark, L.C., Jr.: Some morphologic effects of "inert" particulate loading on hemopoietic elements in mice. J. Reticuloendothel. Soc. *20:*385–398, 1976.

Miller, A.F., Jr., Shen, A.L., and Bonner, F.B.: Hemorrhagic shock in the rat: Metabolic changes in brain and liver. Arch. Int. Physiol. Biochem. *82:*69, 1974.

Modell, J.H., Calderwood, H.W., Ruiz, B.C., Tham, M.K., and Hood, C.I.: Liquid ventiliation of primates. Chest *69:*79. 1976.

Nicoli, D.F.: Computerized molecular size measurement using light scattering spectroscopy. Proceedings of the 17th Annual San Diego Biomedical Symposium, 1978.

Nicoli, D.F., and Benedek, G.B.: Study of thermal denaturation of lysosome and other globular proteins by light scattering spectroscopy. Bipolymers *15:*2421, 1976.

Novakova, V., and Plantin, L-O. (Eds.): HS Symposium, *Research on Perfluorochemicals in Medicine and Biology*, Huddinge, Sweden, April 1977, 373 pp. Karolinska Institute Research Center, Huddinge University Hospital, Huddinge, Sweden, 1978.

Ohyanagi, H., Toshima, K., Sekita, M., Okamoto, M., Itoh, T., Mitsuno, T., Naito, R., Suyama, T., and Yokoyama, K.: Clinical studies of perfluorochemical whole blood substitutes: Safety of Fluosol-DA (20%) in normal human volunteers. Clin. Therap. *2:*306, 1979.

Okamoto, H., Yamanouchi, K., Imagawa, T., Murashima, R., Yokoyama, K., Watanabe, R., and Naito, R.: Persistence of fluorocarbons in circulating blood and organs. In *Proceedings of the Second Intercompany Conference on Fluorocarbon*, Osaka, Japan, April 1973, pp. 169–180.

Okamoto, H., Yamanouchi, K., and Yokoyama, K.: Retention of perfluorochemicals in circulating blood and organs of animals after intravenous injection of their emulsions. Chem. Pharm. Bull. *23:*1452, 1975.

Proceedings of the IVth International Symposium on Perfluorochemical Blood Substitutes, Kyoto, Japan, October 1978, 460 pp. Excerpta Medica, Amsterdam, 1979.

Pruett, R.L., Barr, J.T., Rapp, K.E., Bahner, C.T., Gibson, J.D., and Lafferty, R.H., Jr.: Reactions of polyfluoro olefins. II. Reactions with primary and secondary amines. J. Am. Chem. Soc. *72:*3646, 1950.

Riess, J.G., and LeBlanc, M.: Perfluoro compounds as blood substitutes. Angewandte Chemie *17:*621, 1978.

Sass, D.J., VanDyke, R.A., Wood, E.H., Johnson, S.A., and Didisheim, P.E.: Gas embolism due to intravenous FC80 liquid fluorocarbon. J. Appl. Physiol. *40:*745, 1976.

Sass, D.J., Wood, E.H., Greenleaf, J.F., Ritman, E.L., and Smith, H.C.: Study of effect of breathing liquid fluorocarbons on regional differences in pleural pressures and other physiological parameters. SAM-TR-72-15, DOD-318. pp. 1–173, December 1972. U.S.A.F. School of Aerospace Medicine, Aerospace Medical Division (AFSC), Brooks Air Force Base, San Antonio, TX.

Shimp, L.A., and Lagow, R.J.: Direct fluorination of 2,2,4,4 tetramethylpentane. Sterically protected residual protons? J. Org. Chem. *42:*3437, 1977.

Symposium on Inert Organic Liquids for Biological Oxygen Transport, Atlantic City, New Jersey, April 13, 1969. Fed. Proc. *29:*1695, 1970.

Symposium on Artificial Blood, Bethesda, Maryland, April 5–6, 1974. Fed. Proc. *34:*1429, 1975.

Suyama, T., Watanabe, M., Hanada, S., Yano, K., Yokoyama, K., and Naito, R.: Pharmacological analysis on the mode of transient hypotensive action of Fluosol-DA found in dog. In *Proceedings of the IVth International Symposium on Perfluorochemical Blood Substitutes*, p. 257. Excerpta Medica, Amsterdam, 1979.

Sloviter, H., and Kamimoto, T.: Erythrocyte substite for perfusion of brain. Nature *216:*458, 1967.

Wesseler, E.P., Iltis, R., and Clark, L.C., Jr.: The solubility of

oxygen in highly fluorinated liquids. J. Fluorine Chem. 9: 137, 1977.
Yen, R.T., and Fung, Y.C.: Effect of velocity distribution on red cell distribution in capillary blood vessels. Am. J. Physiol. 235:H251, 1978.
Zander, R.: Oxygen solubility in fluorocarbon liquids. Res. Exp. Med. 164:97, 1974.

Note Added in Galley. Since this paper was delivered, the following works dealing with fluorocarbon emulsions as artificial blood have been published:

Ciccolello, R., Nicoli, D., and Clark, L.C., Jr.: Perfluorochemical artificial blood particle size determination by dynamic light scattering. In preparation.
Clark, L.C., Jr.: Basic and experimental aspects of oxygen transport by highly fluorinated organic compounds. In *ACS Symposium on Biomedicinal Aspects of Fluorine Chemistry*, edited by R. Filler and Y. Kobayashi. Kodansha-Scientific, Japan, 1981.
Clark, L.C., Jr.: Acellular oxygen delivering resuscitation fluids: perfluorocarbons. In *Proceedings of Symposium on Current Concepts of Combat Casualties*, September 15–19, 1980. American Institute of Biological Sciences, Arlington, VA, 1981.
Clark, L.C., Jr, and Moore, R.: Replacement of red cell function by cyclic fluorocarbon emulsions. In *The Red Cell: Fifth International Conference on Red Cell Metabolism and Function*, edited by G.J. Brewer. Alan R. Liss, New York, 1981.
Clark, L.C., Jr., Moore, R.E., Diver, S., and Miller, M.L.: A new look at the vapor pressure problem in red cell substitutes. In *Proceedings of the IVth International Symposium on Perfluorochemical Blood Substitutes*, p. 55. Excerpta Medica, Amsterdam, 1979.
Glogar, D.H., Kloner, R.A., Muller, J.E., DeBoer, L.W.V., Braunwald, E., and Clark L.C., Jr.: The use of fluorocarbons in reducing myocardial ischemic damage following coronary occlusion. Science 211:1439, 1981.
Miller, M.L., Moore, R.E., and Clark, L.C., Jr.: Morphology and morphometry of the liver after infusion of perfluorochemical emulsions. In *Proceedings of the IVth International Symposium on Perfluorochemical Blood Substitutes*, p. 81. Excerpta Medica, Amsterdam, 1979.
Moore, R.E., Clark, L.C., Jr., and Miller, M.L.: Synthesis and biological activity of perfluoroadamantane and some closely related compounds. In *Proceedings of the IVth International Symposium on Perfluorochemical Blood Substitutes*, p. 69. Excerpta Medica, Amsterdam, 1979.
Rude, R.E., Glogar, D.H., Khuri, S., Karaffa, S., Kloner, R.A., Clark, L.C., Jr., Muller, J.E., and Braunwald, E.: Effects of Fluorocarbons and supplemental oxygen on acute myocardial ischemia assessed by intramyocardial gas tension measurement. Paper presented at the American Cardiologists Society Meeting, San Franciso, March 15–19, 1981.

CHAPTER 38

Hyperbaric Oxygen Therapy

MARK E. BRADLEY

Discussing the applications of hyperbaric oxygen therapy is akin to discussing the merits of vitamin C. Both are topics that have generated fierce loyalties and irrational hatreds. There are valid reasons for the antipathy. The history of hyperbaric therapy has often been marred by unscientific studies and indiscriminate application.

There are, however, sound, rational physiologic bases for the application of hyperbaric oxygen therapy. My purpose is to delineate the state of the art of hyperbaric oxygenation as it bears on the scope of this book.

Hyperbaric therapy involves the use of barometric pressures greater than those present at the earth's surface. The units commonly used to express barometric pressure include atmospheres absolute (ATA), millimeters of mercury (mm Hg), and feet of sea water (fsw) (Table 38.1).

Both the tension and concentration of oxygen will rise almost five-fold in alveolar gas when 100% oxygen is breathed. When atmospheric pressure is increased, there is an additional proportional rise in tension. If respiratory gas exchange is efficient, similar tensions can be attained in blood perfusing the pulmonary capillaries. As a result, at three atmospheres of absolute pressure the measured tension of oxygen in the arterial blood of normal animals and man approaches 2000 mm Hg.

Hemoglobin becomes almost fully saturated when exposed to an oxygen tension of 100 mm Hg during passage through the pulmonary circulation. For this reason, additional oxygen, forced into blood at high tensions, enters solution in the aqueous compartment. Because oxygen is a relatively insoluble gas, the content increases only 3 volumes percent (vol%) in the aqueous compartment of blood with each 1000 mm Hg rise pressure of the dissolved gas.

The quantity of dissolved oxygen achieved by breathing 100% oxygen at 3 atmospheres ideally would be equal to 6.2 vol%. This quantity is about 30% of that normally carried by hemoglobin at an arterial partial pressure of oxygen (PO_2) of 100 mm Hg; a fact that underscores the relative inefficiency of physical solution as a means of transporting oxygen. However, 6 vol% of oxygen is at least equal to the normal blood oxygen extraction, or arteriovenous differences of the body as a whole (Fig. 38.1).

Two apparent theoretical advantages are derived from hyperbaric oxygen at the tissue level: 1) the absolute number of oxygen molecules delivered in each unit of blood should increase; and 2) the higher PO_2 should increase the extravascular penetration of oxygen and enlarge the volume of tissue protected from hypoxia by diffusion from a single capillary (Brown et al., 1965). When perfusion of a tissue is normal or moderately reduced, substantial improvement in oxygen delivery may occur during hyperbaric exposure. Where perfusion is very low and the extraction of oxygen is very great, or where blood flow to a tissue is virtually absent, one would expect little improvement of oxygenation at the cellular level despite very high oxygen tensions in arterial blood.

Oxygen at increased pressure is a potent pharmacologic agent, which produces marked physiologic and biochemical alterations. During hyperoxygenation, cardiac output and heart rate decrease and peripheral vascular resistance increases (Whalen et al., 1965). Regional blood flow, as measured in muscle, brain, and kidney, also falls (Hahnlosu et al., 1966). Direct observation reveals vasoconstriction when the PO_2 arises in arterial blood (Saltzman et al., 1965). In normal man, these changes have been quantitated in the retinal blood vessels. Here, the decrease in vessel diameter is roughly proportional to the rise in oxygen tension and is independent of barometric pressure or hypocapnia. The most important biochemical effects of hyperbaric oxygenation are those on acid-base status. Increased blood oxygen concentrations impair carbon dioxide transport. As a consequence, a tissue acidosis and hypercarbia develops concomitantly in the presence of an arterial alkalosis and hypocarbia (Lambertsen et al., 1953).

I would like to review in broad compass some of the applications of hyperbaric oxygen in shock, anoxia, and ischemia.

APPLICATIONS OF HYPERBARIC OXYGEN

There are a number of conditions in which anoxia and ischemia are present and hyperbaric oxygen is either the primary mode of treatment or an important therapeutic adjunct: decompression sickness, gas embolism, gas gangrene, compromised skin grafts, and Meleney ulcer. There are other disorders in which there are experimental data or clinical experience suggesting that hyperbaric oxygen therapy is useful, but additional data are needed to delineate the usefulness of this therapeutic modality. These additional disorders in which hyperbaric oxygen therapy is useful are: actinomycosis (refractory); acute, peripheral, arterial insufficiency; bacteriodes infection (refractory); cord injury; osteomyelitis (refractory); osteoradionecrosis; radionecrosis (soft tissue); thermal burns; chronic skin ulcer, secondary to arterial insufficiency; and stasis ulcer. A detailed discussion of the physiologic rationale for hyperbaric oxygen therapy in these disorders is beyond the scope of this book.

Table 38.1
Comparison of Pressure Units Used in Hyperbaric Therapy

Atmospheres Absolute	Millimeters of Mercury	Feet of Sea Water
1	760	0
2	1520	33
3	2280	66
4	3040	99
6	4560	165

Figure 38.1. Blood oxygen content relative to arterial oxygen partial pressure.

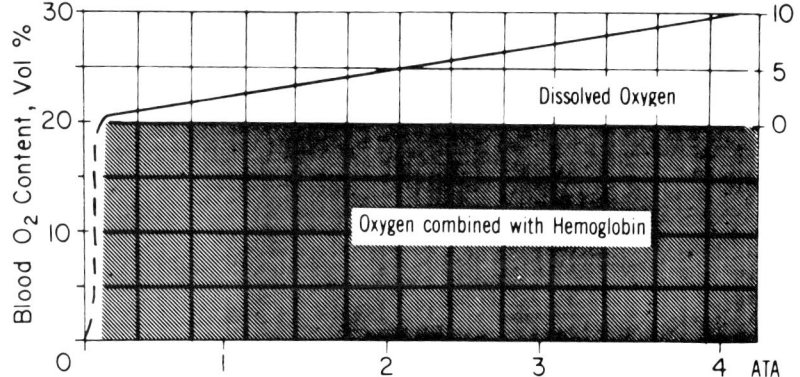

Hemorrhagic and Septic Shock

Cowley et al. (1964, 1965) have provided guidelines for the effective use of hyperbaric oxygenation in the therapy of hemorrhagic shock. Experimentally, in hemorrhagic shock, hyperbaric oxygen is useful if administered early but not during the refractory period (Attar et al., 1966). During the administration of hyperbaric oxygen, animals have markedly better tissue oxygen tensions and improved cardiovascular performance and metabolic status than do nontreated animals. Cowley et al. (1964, 1965) found that hyperbaric oxygen therapy reduced the mortality rate of the shocked animals almost two-fold. The beneficial effects of this treatment are primarily the result of improved tissue oxygenation and hemodynamic status.

Clinically, hyperbaric oxygen has not been widely used as a therapeutic adjunct in the treatment of hemorrhagic shock. The reasons for this are obvious. Transfusion, fluid replacement, and surgery are primary therapeutic modalities in treatment of hemorrhagic shock. Additionally, one must have the fortuitous availability of a large hyperbaric chamber. Nonetheless, hyperbaric oxygen can be employed beneficially when one is unable to provide transfusion or control bleeding (Amonic et al., 1969).

The role of hyperbaric oxygen in the treatment of septic shock is unclear. Cowley et al. (1964) showed that survival time of dogs with fecal peritonitis was increased by exposing the animals to hyperbaric oxygen at 3 ATA with the abdomen vented and the peritoneum directly exposed to oxygen. However, Filler et al. (1966) reported that hyperbaric oxygen failed to reduce mortality in rats with *Escherichia coli* peritonitis and may, in fact, have been detrimental. It is apparent that the pressure level used is important. Accompanying small increases in oxygen tension, there is an enhancement in growth of both pseudomonas and *E. coli*. Inhibition of growth is accomplished only when the pressure of oxygen is raised above 2 ATA. At higher pressures, benefits derived from hyperbaric oxygenation may be secondary to signs of oxygen poisoning. Therefore, at present, hyperbaric oxygen is not considered to be a useful therapeutic modality in treatment of septic shock.

Head Injury

Experimental studies have demonstrated the value of hyperbaric oxygenation in the treatment of head trauma. The psychophysiologic performance of animals that had cerebral concussion followed by hyperbaric oxygenation improved at a significantly faster rate than did the psychophysiologic performance of control animals (Coe and Angyan, 1971). The mortality rates of animals with experimentally produced cerebral edema and compression have been substantially reduced by application of hyperbaric oxygenation (Sukoff et al., 1967). Hemodilution coupled with oxygen at high pressures has been reported to produce even greater reductions in mortality; these reductions probably resulted from lowered blood viscosity and improved perfusion (Mead et al., 1970; Moody et al., 1970).

The mechanisms underlying these beneficial actions of hyperbaric oxygen appear clear and are well supported. Cerebral edema is a frequent result of head injury. Hyperbaric oxygen acts directly on autoregulated small arteries and causes reduction in blood flow and intracranial pressure. Vasogenic edema may be decreased. Additionally, cytotoxic brain edema is reduced because this therapy can improve substantially oxygen delivery to hypoxic tissue.

In clinical studies, the responses to treatment of head injury with hyperbaric oxygen have been variable (Holbach and Gott, 1970; Mogami et al., 1969). Patients with autoregulatory paralysis, shown by lack of responsiveness to carbon dioxide, are not likely to benefit from hyperbaric oxygen treatment. The current consensus of clinical studies is that the earlier the patient is treated, the greater the therapeutic effect of hyperoxygenation, and that the beneficial effects are most impressive in patients with mild rather than severe cerebral damage (Hayakawa, 1974).

Hyperbaric oxygen therapy for head injury must be considered an adjunct rather than a replacement for other methods of treatment. This treatment should be recommended for patients who are responsive to standard therapeutic measures but who are still critically ill because of cerebral hypoxia, brain edema, or increased intracranial pressure.

Spinal Cord Injury

Recent experimental studies in animals have reported a beneficial effect of hyperbaric oxygen on nondisruptive spinal cord trauma (Hartzog et al., 1969; Yeo et al., 1977). The rationale for hyperoxygenation of tissue damaged in cord trauma is the reoxygenation of those cells that are rendered hypoxic by vascular insufficiency from capillary or large vessel damage and edema. If these neurons, which are in a critical state of survival, are reoxygenated and cellular acidosis is alleviated, the chance for survival may be increased and the long-term neurologic deficit may be reduced.

These studies (Kelley et al., 1972) have shown the presence of a profound hypoxia in the injured cord, which could be raised to normal levels by the administration of 100% oxygen at 2 ATA. Preliminary experimental work has shown that with hyperbaric oxygen, there is some return of the spinal evoked response in animals with acute cord compression. No return of evoked response is seen in the control group (D.E. Evans, personal communication).

In animals treated with hyperbaric oxygen, the degree of functional recovery was significantly better and there was less histologic evidence of damage. These differences were seen only if the animals were treated with hyperbaric oxygen within a few hours of injury.

Only a few small clinical trials (Jones et al., 1978; Yeo et al., 1978) of hyperbaric oxygen therapy in spinal cord injury have been reported. The investigators reporting these trials believe that the treatment played a beneficial role in the return of functional improvement of some of their patients. Presently, however, the data supporting a beneficial role of hyperbaric oxygen in spinal cord trauma must be considered promising but inconclusive.

The hyperbaric oxygen therapy protocol used at the Maryland Institute for Emergency Medical Services (R. Myers, personal communication) is suggested as a reasonable therapeutic schema. Patients with acute cord injury are initially taken to 2 ATA for a period of 2 hr every 8 hr for a total of 3 dives. Thereafter, they breathe 100% oxygen for 90 min at 2 ATA twice a day for 14 days. If there is no improvement in the patient's condition after the first 72 hr of hyperbaric oxygen therapy, the treatments are stopped.

Stroke

Treatment of acute cerebral vascular insufficiency with hyperbaric oxygen has, for the most part, produced variable and generally disappointing results (Heyman et al., 1966; Saltzman et al., 1966). An occasional patient with acute cerebral ischemia of a few hours' duration will improve dramatically when exposed to hyperbaric oxygen. Unfortunately, this improvement frequently persists for only an hour or so after the termination of the hyperbaric exposure with subsequent relapse. Subsequent exposure to hyperbaric oxygen may again temporarily restore neurological function.

Although hyperbaric oxygenation may not provide appreciable therapeutic benefit in the treatment of acute cerebral vascular insufficiency, it may be a useful diagnostic tool in the selection of patients for cerebral revascularization procedures. Holbach et al. (1977) have reported that patients with chronic stroke (of 9–10 weeks duration) who showed significant improvement in neurologic function during a course of hyperbaric oxygenation (10–15 daily treatments at 1.5 ATA for 40-min treatment) benefited most from anastomosis of the temporal artery to a cortical branch of the middle cerebral artery. Saltzman's statement some 13 years ago (Saltzman, 1967, p. 1311) may indeed be correct: "This form of treatment (OHP) [oxygen at high pressure] may have greater value, however, if hyperoxygenation is combined with methods for restoring the patency of the involved cerebral blood vessel."

Myocardial Infarction

The application of hyperbaric oxygenation in the therapy of acute myocardial infarction remains an extremely controversial area. The response of animals with experimental myocardial ischemia to hyperbaric oxygenation has generally shown reduction of arrhythmias and enhanced survival (Gage et al., 1965; Van Elk, 1964). Ordinarily, the animals were hyperoxygenated before the experimental production of myocardial ischemia. This factor makes extrapolation of experimental findings to the clinical setting difficult unless one has the extraordinary good luck to have an infarct while breathing hyperbaric oxygen. Additionally, other experimental work has demonstrated that hyperbaric oxygen administered shortly after coronary artery ligation does not appear to improve oxygenation of the ischemia area. In fact, this treatment may worsen the ischemia because of a potent vasoconstrictive effect on the coronary vessels (Marshall et al., 1974).

Clinical experience with hyperbaric oxygenation in the treatment of myocardial infarction is inconclusive. Although one series of studies has shown an appreciable reduction in mortality (Thurston et al., 1973), other series (Cameron et al., 1965) have not demonstrated any significant effect. Patients with uncomplicated myocardial infarction have comprised the majority of persons included in these studies, and the results are difficult to evaluate in these low risk populations. For this reason, selected high risk patients will be needed in a carefully controlled and monitored study to evaluate hyperbaric oxygenation.

Carbon Monoxide and Cyanide Poisoning

Carbon monoxide is a gas that is toxic in even very low concentrations. It seems probable that carbon monoxide exerts its toxic action by causing tissue hypoxia. This hypoxia is the result of several actions by which carbon monoxide operates (Root, 1965): 1) carbon monoxide interferes with the function of oxygen transport in blood by combining with hemoglobin; 2) the presence of carboxyhemoglobin (HbCO) impedes the dissociation of that oxyhemoglobin (HbO_2) that can still be utilized for oxygen transport; and 3) carbon monoxide combines with certain intracellular respiratory enzyme systems. It is probably because of this third mode of action that clinically one frequently does not find good correlation between the severity of symptoms and the level of HbCO. Because of the discrepancies between the apparent clinical condition of the patient and absolute level of HbCO in the blood, some groups have employed psychometric tests, in addition to HbCO levels, to assess the severity of carbon monoxide poisoning and the need for hyperbaric oxygen therapy.

The efficacy of hyperbaric oxygen in the treatment of carbon monoxide poisoning has been recognized for many years. Oxygen under high pressure can be forced into physical solution in blood to maintain viability of hypoxia tissues despite the absence of sufficient functioning hemoglobin. In a classic experiment, Haldane (1927) showed that mice in 2 atmospheres of oxygen could not be killed even though all the circulating hemoglobin was combined with carbon monoxide.

Additionally, increasing the oxygen tension in blood has the salutary effect of accelerating the washout of carbon monoxide. The half-time for carbon monoxide elimination in resting men breathing air at sea level is 320 min. Breathing 100% oxygen at 2 and 3 atmospheres yields half-times of 80 and 23 min, respectively (Peterson and Stewart, 1970). Thus, the duration of central nervous system hypoxia can be abbreviated by exposure to hyperbaric oxygen.

Hyperemia and edema of the brain are frequent pathologic accompaniments of carbon monoxide intoxication. One benefit of hyperbaric oxygenation therapy in carbon monoxide poisoning is that the treatment decreases cerebral blood volume and intracranial pressure as well as counteracts cytotoxic brain edema. Of course, this form of therapy does not obviate the requirement to use conventional methods and/or hyperosmolar agents and steroids for control of increased intracranial pressure.

There is abundant experimental work which clearly demonstrates that hyperbaric oxygenation improves or even eliminates mortality in animals poisoned by carbon monoxide. These studies (Pierce et al., 1972; Takeya et al., 1970) have shown that metabolic acidosis, cardiovascular dynamics, and electrocardiographic changes are quickly improved by the application of hyperbaric oxygen. Many clinical series, some of which have been very large (~400 patients), have reported rapid recovery in patients critically ill with carbon monoxide intoxication when the patients were treated with hyperbaric oxygen. Unfortunately, there is not a single controlled clinical study of the effects of hyperbaric oxygen on morbidity and mortality in this form of poisoning. At present, one can only say that it is unclear whether hyperbaric oxygenation appreciably reduces mortality in carbon monoxide intoxication. Available evidence strongly suggests that the treatment considerably reduces morbidity and that it may be of great value in allaying the development of late sequelae of carbon monoxide poisoning.

A number of combinations of pressure and time have been employed to treat carbon monoxide intoxication with hyperbaric oxygen. One protocol that seems sensible is that employed at the Maryland Institute for Emergency Medical Services (R. Myers, personal communication). There, the patient is taken to 3 ATA (66 feet) and breathes 100% oxygen for 46 min, which is 2 half-times for the elimination of carbon monoxide at this pressure. The pressure is then reduced to 2 ATA, where the patient breathes oxygen for 120 min. Six hrs thereafter, this therapeutic schema may be repeated if there is residual neurologic impairment.

Oxygen at high pressure antagonizes the toxic action of cyanide. Experimentally, it has been shown that the mortality of animals poisoned with cyanide is reduced from 96% to 20% when treated with hyperbaric oxygenation (Skene et al., 1966). Neurologic sequelae in these animals treated with oxygen at high pressure was markedly decreased. Clinical reports of cyanide-poisoned patients successfully treated with hyperbaric oxygen are available. These reports range to the extreme of a patient presenting with massive cyanide poisoning—the result of falling into a vat of silver and potassium cyanide (Trapp, 1970).

The primary therapy for cyanide poisoning is chemical. The therapy, which consists of amyl nitrite inhalation and/or injection of a sodium nitrite and sodium thiosulfate, converts cyanide to cyanmethemoglobin and, ultimately, to thiocyanate. Hyperbaric oxygen does not replace the chemical treatment for cyanide poisoning; however, it is supplemental and should, where possible, be administered in conjunction with chemical therapy. The same sort of protocol for administration of hyperbaric oxygen that is employed for carbon monoxide intoxication can be used here.

Increasingly, we live in a plastic world. The combustion of plastics liberates generous amounts of carbon monoxide, hydrofluoric acid (HF), hydrochloric acid (HCl), and cyanides. Patients presenting with smoke inhalation may therefore be suffering not only from carbon monoxide intoxication but also from cyanide poisoning and tracheobronchitis, resulting from HF and HCl inhalation. Although hyperbaric oxygenation will not help tracheobronchitis, it usually helps carbon monoxide and cyanide intoxication.

OXYGEN TOXICITY

Of course, oxygen, itself, is a toxic agent and in excessive doses can cause serious damage or death (Wood, 1975). However, untoward effects from hyperbaric oxygen therapy are relatively rare and almost never serious. Two major forms of oxygen toxicity afflict the central nervous system and the lung. Central nervous system toxicity is characterized by nausea, muscular twitching, nervousness, and finally convulsions. Recovery is prompt when the patient is removed from the hyperoxic environment. Susceptibility to this form of toxicity varies widely from individual to individual and in the same individual from one day to the next. This form of toxicity can be minimized by limiting the hyperoxic exposure to 3 ATA or preferably less. Periodic interruption of 100% oxygen breathing with air breathing also helps to retard the rate of development of toxicity.

Pulmonary oxygen toxicity develops upon prolonged exposure to one or more atmospheres of oxygen. Serious pulmonary oxygen toxicity can be avoided by limiting the length of exposure to no more than 6 hr in every 24 and by periodic interruption with short (about 5 min) periods of air breathing.

Other organ systems may be poisoned by high oxygen concentrations. These systems include blood where there may be hemolysis and decreased erythropoiesis, and the eye, where long-term hyperbaric oxygen therapy has been shown to cause nuclear sclerosis. One curious phenomenon that has been noted during hyperbaric oxygen administration is a change in refraction; for example, over a course of 8 weeks of daily therapy, patients may become more myopic by as much as −2.5 dioptera. Upon cessation of hyperbaric oxygen therapy, this refractive change usually reverts to what it was pretreatment.

Deliberately, I have been cautionary and circumspect in this discussion of hyperbaric oxygen therapy. Without this treatment, management of decompression sickness, gas embolism, and gas gangrene would be very difficult, if not impossible. But, like many other therapeutic modalities, the appropriate role of hyperbaric oxygen in the clinical management of many disorders of shock, anoxia, and ischemia remains to be clearly defined. Only rational application in controlled, well designed studies will provide this definition.

Acknowledgments. Naval Medical Research and Development Command, Research Task M0099PN002.7062. The opinions and assertions contained herein are the private ones of the writer and are not to be construed as official or reflecting the views of the Navy Department or the Naval Service at large.

The author gratefully acknowledges the advice and superb editorial assistance of Ms. M. Matzen and Mrs. R. Balenger.

References

Amonic, R.S., Cockett, A.T.K., Lorhan, P.H., and Thompson, F.C.: Hyperbaric oxygen therapy in chronic hemorrhagic shock. J.A.M.A. *208:*2051, 1969.

Attar, S., Esmond, W.G., and Cowley, R.A.: Hyperbaric oxygenation in vascular collapse. J. Thorac. Cardiovasc. Surg. *44(6):*759, 1962.

Attar, S., Scanlan, E., and Cowley, R.A.: Further evaluation of hyperbaric oxygen in hemorrhagic shock. In *Proceedings of the Third International Conference on Hyperbaric Medicine*, edited by I.W. Brown, Jr., and B. G. Cox, p. 417. National Academy of Science, Washington, DC, 1966.

Brown, I.W., Jr., Fuson, R.L., Mauney, F.M., and Smith, W.W.: Hyperbaric oxygenation (hybaroxia): current status, possibilities and limitations. In *Advances in Surgery*, p. 285. Year Book Medical Publishing, Chicago, 1965.

Cameron, A.J.V., Gibb, B.H., Ledingham, I. McA., and McGuiness, J.B.: A controlled clinical trial of hyperbaric oxygen in the treatment of acute myocardial infarction in hyperbaric oxygenation. In *Hyperbaric Oxygenation: Proceedings of the Second International Congress*, edited by I. M. Ledingham, p. 277. E. and S. Livingstone, Edinburgh, 1965.

Coe, J.E., and Angyan, A.V.: The effect of hyperbaric oxygenation upon recovery of maze performance after experimental concussion. J. Trauma *11:*436, 1971.

Cowley, R.A., Attar, S., Esmond, W., and Blair, E.: The utilization of hyperbaric oxygenation in hemorrhagic shock in dogs. In *Clinical Application of Hyperbaric Oxygen*, edited by I. Boerema, W. H. Brummelkamp, and N. G. Meijne, p. 177. North-Holland, Amsterdam, 1964.

Cowley, R.A., Attar, S., Blair, E., Esmond, W.G., Ollodart, R., and Hashimoto, S.: Hyperbaric oxygenation in hypoxic shock states. In *Hyperbaric Oxygenation: Proceedings of the Second International Congress*, edited by I. M. Ledingham, p. 333. E. and S. Livingstone, Edinburgh, 1965.

Filler, R.M., Reeves, E., and Sherman, H.K.: Effect of hyperbaric oxygen on experimental peritonitis. In *Proceedings of the Third International Conference on Hyperbaric Medicine*, edited by I. W. Brown and B. G. Cox, p. 593. National Academy of Science, Washington, DC, 1966.

Gage, A.A., Federico, A.J., Lamphier, E.H., and Chardock, W.M.: The effect of hyperbaric oxygenation on the mortality from ventricular fibrillation following coronary artery ligation. In *Hyperbaric Oxygenation: Proceedings of the Second International Congress*, edited by I. M. Ledingham, p. 288. E. and S. Livingstone, Edinburgh, 1965.

Hahnlosu, P.B., Domanig, E., Lamphier, E.H., and Schenk, W.A.: Hyperbaric oxygenation: alterations in cardiac output and regional blood flow. J. Thorac. Cardiovasc. Surg. *52:*223, 1966.

Haldane, J.B.S.: Carbon monoxide as tissue poison. Biochem. J. *21:*1068, 1927.

Hartzog, J.T., Fisher, R.G., and Snow, C.: Spinal cord trauma: effect of hyperbaric oxygen therapy. Proc. Veterans Adm. Spinal Cord Inj. Conf. *17:*70, 1969.

Hayakawa, T.: Hyperbaric oxygen treatment in neurology and neurosurgery. TIT. J. Life Sci. *4:*1, 1974.

Heyman, A., Saltzman, H.A., and Whalen, K.E.: The use of hyperbaric oxygenation in the treatment of cerebral ischemia and infarction. Circulation (Suppl. 2) *33–34:*20, 1966.

Holbach, K.H., and Gott, U.: Effect of hyperbaric oxygenation therapy on neurosurgical patients. In *Proceedings of the Fourth International Congress on Hyperbaric Medicine*, edited by J. Wada and T. Iwa, p. 441. Williams & Wilkins, Baltimore, 1970.

Holbach, K.H., Wasserman, H., Hoheluchter, K.L., and Jain, K.K.: Differentiation between reversible and irreversible post-stroke changes in brain tissue: its relevance for cerebrovascular surgery. Surg. Neurol. *7:*325, 1977.

Jones, R.F., Unsworth, I.P., and Marosszeky, J.E.: Hyperbaric oxygen and acute spinal cord injuries in humans. Med. J. Aust. *2:*573, 1978.

Kelley, D.L., Lassiter, K.R.L., Vongsvivat, A., and Smith, J.M.: Effects of hyperbaric oxygenation and tissue oxygen studies in experimental paraplegia. J. Neurosurg. *36:*425, 1972.

Lambertsen, C.J., Kough, R.H., Cooper, D.Y., Emmel, G.L., Loeschke, H.H., and Schmidt, C.F.: Oxygen toxicity: effects in man of oxygen inhalation at 1 and 3.5 atmospheres upon blood gas transport, cerebral circulation and cerebral metabolism. J. Appl. Physiol. *5:*471, 1953.

Marshall, R.J., Parrott, J.R., and Ledingham, I.M.: The effect of hyperbaric oxygen (2 ATA) on myocardial blood flow and oxygen consumption in normal and ischemic areas of myocardium after acute coronary artery ligation in the dog. In *Fifth International Congress on Hyperbaric Medicine*, edited by W. G. Trapp, E. W. Banister, A. V. Davison, and P. A. Trapp, p. 699. S. Fraser University, Burnaby, Australia, 1974.

Mead, C.O., Moody, R.A., Ruamsuke, S., and Mullan, S.: Effect of isovolumic hemodilution on cerebral blood flow following experimental head injury. J. Neurosurg. *32:*40, 1970.

Mogami, H., Hayakawa, T., Kanai, N., Kuroda, R., Yamada, R., Ikeda, T., Katsukada, K., and Sugimota, T.: Clinical application of hyperbaric oxygenation in the treatment of acute cerebral damage. J. Neurosurg. *31:*636, 1969.

Moody, R.A., Mead, C.O., Ruamsuke, S., and Mullan, S.: Therapeutic value of oxygen at normal and hyperbaric pressure in experimental head injury. J. Neurosurg. *32:*51, 1970.

Peterson, J.E., and Stewart, R.D.: Absorption and elimination of carbon monoxide by inactive young men. Arch. Environ. Health *21:*165, 1970.

Pierce, E.C., II., Zacharias, A., Alday, J.M., Hoffman, B.A., and Jacobson, J.H., II.: Carbon monoxide poisoning: experimental hypothermia and hyperbaric studies. Surgery *72:*229, 1972.

Root, W.S. Carbon monoxide. In *Handbook of Physiology, Section 3: Respiration, vol. 2*, edited by W. O. Fenn and H. Rohn, p. 1087. American Physiological Society, Washington, DC, 1965.

Saltzman, H.A.: Hyperbaric oxygen. Med. Clin. North Am. *51:*1311, 1967.

Saltzman, H.A., Hart, L., Sieker, H.O., and Duffy, E.J.: Retinal vascular response to hyperbaric oxygenation. J.A.M.A. *191:*114, 1965.

Saltzman, H.A., Anderson, B., Whalen, R.E., Heyman, A., and Sieker, H.O.: Hyperbaric oxygen therapy of acute cerebral vascular insufficiency. In *Proceedings of the Third International Conference on Hyperbaric Medicine*, edited by I. W. Brown, Jr., and B. G. Cox, p. 440. National Academy of Science, Washington, DC, 1966.

Skene, W.G., Norman, J.N., and Smith, G.: Effects of hyperbaric oxygen on cyanide poisoning. In *Proceedings of the Third International Congress on Hyperbaric Medicine*, edited by I. W. Brown, Jr., and B. G. Cox, p. 705. National Academy of Science, Washington, DC, 1966.

Sukoff, M.H., Hollin, S.A., and Jacobson, J.H.: The protective effect of hyperbaric oxygenation in experimentally produced cerebral edema and compression. Surgery *62:*40, 1967.

Takeya, H., Suzuki, K., Yoshida, T., and Furukawa, K.: Hyperbaric oxygen therapy in carbon monoxide poisoning and experimental study. In *Proceedings of the Fourth International Congress on Hyperbaric Medicine*, edited by J. Wada and T. Iwa, p. 297. Williams & Wilkins, Baltimore, 1970.

Thurston, J.G.B., Greenwood, T.W., Bending, M.R., Connor, H., and Curren, M.P.: A controlled investigation into the effects of hyperbaric oxygen on mortality following acute myocardial infarction. Q. J. Med. *168:*751, 1973.

Trapp, W.: Massive cyanide poisoning with recovery: a Boxing Day story. Can. Med. Assoc. J. *102:*517, 1970.

Van Elk, J.: Ventricular fibrillation following coronary occlusion in the dog heart and the possible protective effect of high pressure oxygen. In *Clinical Application of Hyperbaric Oxygen*, edited by I. Boerema, W. H. Brummelkamp, and N. G. Meijne, p. 116. North-Holland, Amsterdam, 1964.

Whalen, R.E., Saltzman, H.A., Holloway, D.H., Jr., McIntosh, D.D., Sieker, H.O., and Brown, I.W., Jr.: Cardiovascular and blood gas responses to hyperbaric oxygenation. Am. J. Cardiol. *15:*638, 1965.

Wood, J.D.: Oxygen toxicity. In *The Physiology and Medicine of Diving and Compressed Air Work*, edited by P. Bennett and D. Elliott, p. 166. Williams & Wilkins, Baltimore, 1975.

Yeo, J.D., Starback, S., and McKenzie, B.: A study of the effects of hyperbaric oxygen on the experimental spinal cord injury. Med. J. Aust. *2:*145, 1977.

Yeo, J.D., Lowry, C., and McKenzie, B.: Preliminary report on ten patients with spinal cord injuries treated with hyperbaric oxygen. Med. J. Aust. *2:*572, 1978.

CHAPTER 39

Mathematical Models

ČESLOVAS MASAITIS

Mathematical models date as far back as the Ptolemaic planetary system. For a long time they were used to describe various physical systems. However, recently computational power of electronic computers made it possible to manipulate, at least numerically, very complex mathematical problems. This produced an explosive proliferation of mathematical models in fields as diverse as transportation and socioeconomics, war gaming, and physiological control systems. Modeling became an indispensable tool almost in every research field, and, thus, familiarity with what such models can accomplish, as well as with their limitations, is very useful to every researcher.

The purpose of this chapter is to introduce basic principles of model construction to researchers in the field of shock and ischemia. These principles and basic steps in constructing a mathematical model are described in the first part of the chapter. In the second part, several physiological models developed by various researchers are described to illustrate the procedure which is further elucidated by synthesizing the models of various physiological subsystems into a model for studying complexity of a hypovolemic shock.

CONSTRUCTING A MATHEMATICAL MODEL

Usually construction of a mathematical model begins with a definition of a model system and its purpose. A model system is simply a collection of abstract concepts of physical reality, each concept consisting of a limited number of attributes and representing only certain as-

Mathematical Models

pects of the corresponding physical phenomenon. These attributes are selected according to the purpose of the model. Concepts in a mathematical model must be defined precisely with no ambiguity left as to their meaning and scope. This is attained by including only the attributes that are either explicitly stated or formally implied by explicit assumptions of a model. For instance, blood circulation is a very complex phenomenon that includes cardiac output, vascular resistance, blood viscosity pulsatile waves, and elasticity of blood vessels, to name just a few. However, in a mathematical model such as, for instance, the cardiovascular model developed by Grodins (1959) blood circulation is described by cardiac output Q, arteriovenous pressure difference ΔP, and vascular resistance R and is modeled by the relation $Q = \Delta P/R$, which ignores all other features of this phenomenon that are not included in the relation representing circulation.

Since mathematical relations are always exact, a model system usually differs substantially from the corresponding physical or physiological system. This is amply illustrated by examples described below in this section.

Exactness of mathematical relations requires that a model system be complete in a sense that there is nothing else that affects or is affected by the system and is not a part of it. This is to say, the system must be closed. A phenomenon selected for modeling may interact with other phenomena in a significant manner and these may in their turn be related to still other variables and so on. Thus, it may be impossible to cut off the phenomenon from the rest of the world and to treat it as a closed system. Yet this is done when constructing a mathematical model by reducing interaction of a selected phenomenon with the rest of the world to inputs and outputs or sources and sinks. For instance, in a mathematical model of heart rate control illustrated schematically in Figure 39.1 (Warner and Cox, 1961), frequency of electric pulse applied to the right and left vagus nerves is the input to a model system that consists of a generator of norepinephrine (efferent nerve endings), a carrier of norepinephrine (diffusion medium) to sinoatrial node, and the heart, which produces heart frequency (the output of the model). There is nothing in the model that relates frequency of stimulation to blood pressure or anything else. Thus, the frequency is the input to the model.

The choice of a system to be modeled depends on the purpose for which a model is constructed and the purpose depends how a system is selected. Thus, the system and the purpose are usually selected simultaneously by an interaction that successively modifies the system and the purpose until a compatibility of the two is obtained, as shown in Figure 39.2.

The purpose of a model may be one of five types described below or any mixture of these. Some models are constructed to summarize empirical data. We call these epigrammatic models. Others are developed to provide a detailed description of the system behavior. These are interpretative models. The purpose of comparative models is to determine relative importance of various system variables and inputs. The models may

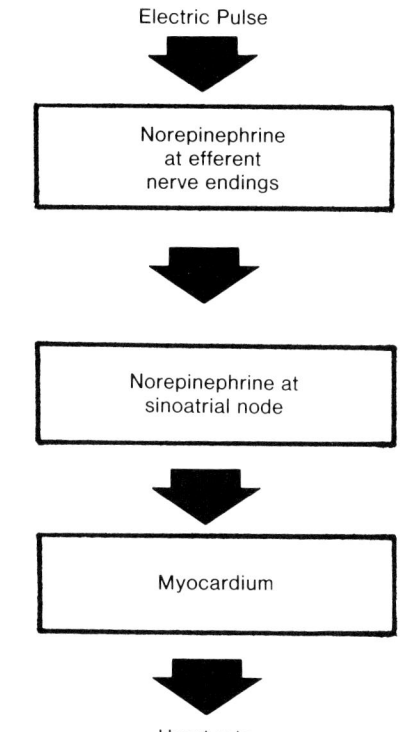

Figure 39.1. Closing of a system by input and output variables.

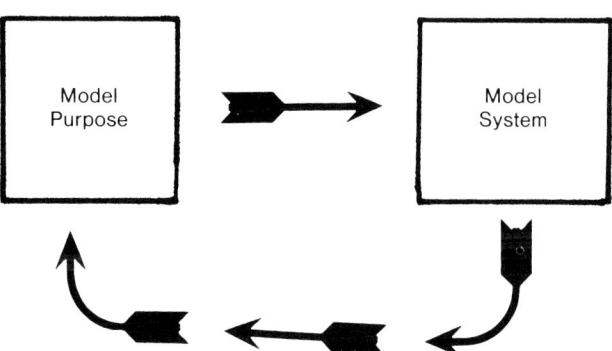

Figure 39.2. Interpretative selection of a model.

also be constructed to determine the input values or model parameters that produce a desired response of the system. These are called here eclectic models. We may also construct predictive models with the goal of estimating the behavior of a system under specified conditions (inputs).

An example of a simple epigrammatic model is a normal range of a physiological variable, such as pH, since a statement of a normal range summarizes a large number of individual observations of this variable. Estimates of the mean and standard deviation of a physiological variable together with an assumption of Gaussian distribution of this variable is also an epigrammatic model.

The respiratory model (Milhorn and Guyton, 1965) depicted in Figure 39.3 can be used to examine a detailed behavior of the modeled system, such as determination of minimum and maximum of respiration rate, change of tidal volume, variation of CO_2 concentration in arterial blood, and so on. Thus, it is an interpretative model. Such models allow us to compute rates, accumulated values of variables, oscillatory periods, limiting values, and other information about system behavior. They are also very useful as generalized interpolating devices that allow us to compute values of physiological variables between those obtained by observation and those employed to construct the models. Such an interpolation is straightforward in a case of deterministic models such as the relation (Grodins, 1963) $V_m = Q_0 + Q_1(pH) + Q_2 P_c + Q_3(c - P_0)^d$ between minute respiratory volume V_m and arterial gas tensions of CO_2 (P_c) and O_2 (P_0) and hydrogen ion (pH). Here the model parameters Q_0, Q_1, Q_2, Q_3, c, and d are obtained from a finite set of observed values of gas tensions corresponding to observed ventilation rate. The equation can readily be applied to compute minute volume V_m corresponding to any values of blood gas tensions within certain range. These are interpolated values of minute volume. More complicated models constructed for a study of detailed behavior of a system can be used also for such an interpolation since they allow us to compute intermediate values of dependent variables.

An example of a comparative model is provided by the relation defining probability of congenital heart disease developed by Warner et al. (1961). This model expresses probability of heart disease in terms of observed frequencies of various symptoms. The model considers 33 different conditions (diseases) and 50 symptoms. A conditional probability $P(S_i/D_j)$ of a symptom S_i, $i = 1, 2, \ldots, 50$, given a disease D_j, $j = 1, 2, \ldots, 33$ is obtained from clinical data. Also a priori probabilities $P(D_j)$ of the diseases are estimated from available information on the frequency of occurrence of various diseases. Then, given a set of symptoms $S_{i1}, S_{i2}, \ldots, S_{ik}$ of a new patient, conditional probability $P(D_j/S_{i1}, S_{i2}, \ldots, S_{ik})$ that he suffers from the disease D_j is obtained from the Bayes' rule: $P(D_j/S_{i1}, S_{i2}, \ldots, S_{ik}) = P(D_j)P(S/D_j)/\sum_{j=1}^{33} P(D_j)P(S/D_j)$ where $P(S/D_j) = P(S_{i1}/D_j) P(S_{i2}/D_j) \ldots P(S_{ik}/D_j)$ by assuming that the symptoms $S_{i1}, S_{i2}, \ldots, S_{ik}$ are statistically independent.

When many physiological variables are included in a model system, it is easier to derive required mathematical relations by dividing the variables into groups according to expected or postulated relations between the variables. Although such a grouping is somewhat arbitrary, frequently the groups consist of variables that describe physiological subsystems or components. Hence, we call these groups model components or compartments, although sometimes the variables of a group need not describe a state of a clearly identifiable physiological component, i.e., model components may be just a collection of mathematically related variables.

Variables of a model system must be defined precisely either in terms of operational procedures that assign

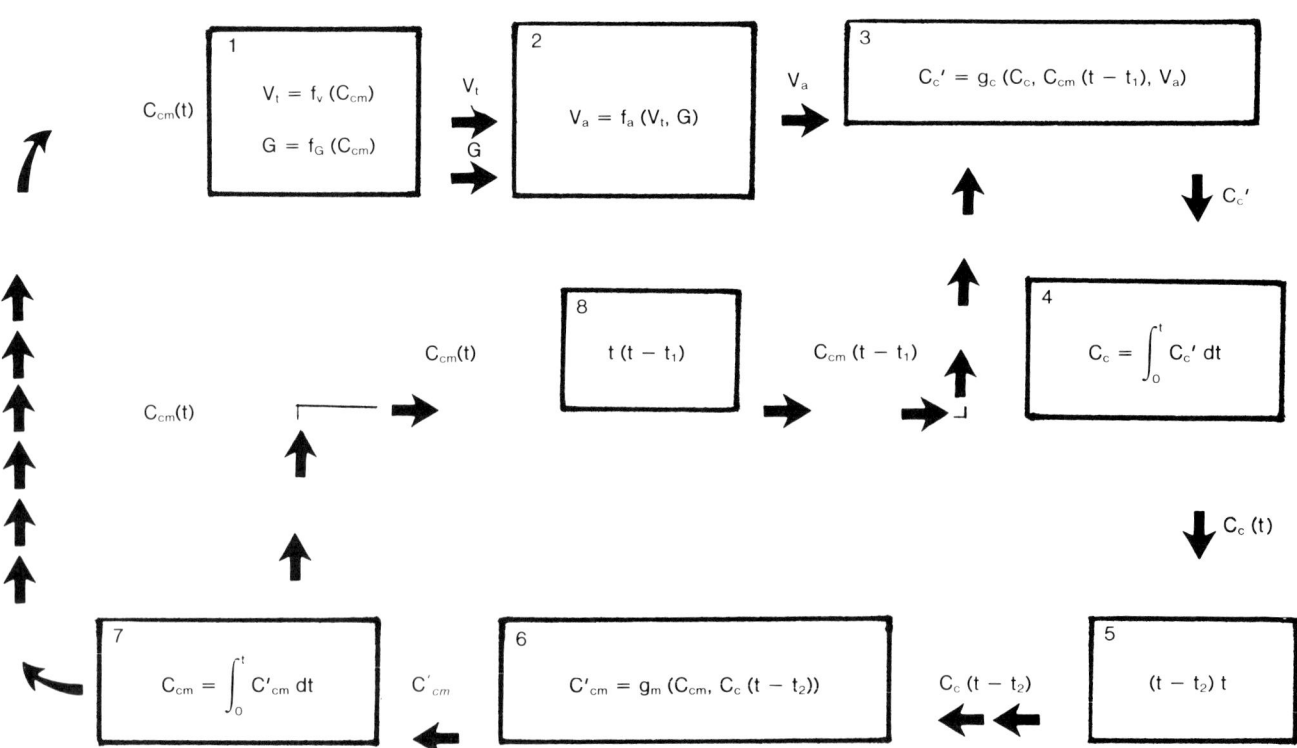

Figure 39.3. Respiratory model.

certain values to the parameters or by their mutual relations. The assigned values need not quantify the variables in a strict sense, i.e., the assigned values need not be measured on a ratio scale, although a quantification on this scale provides the greatest flexibility in selecting mathematical relations that represent the system. Blood pressure, cardiac output, and O_2 concentration in blood are examples of ratio scale variables. The ratio scale quantities can be compared by their ratio, i.e., how many times one of them exceeds the other; also by their difference, measuring by how many units one exceeds the other; and finally by their order, which says which of them is greater. Interval scales allow the comparison of the variables in the last two ways but not by their ratio. Temperature is, perhaps, the only physiological variable measured on an interval scale. The weakest type of quantification is provided by ordinal scale that allows only the third type comparison, i.e., which of the two is greater, but not by how many units or how many times. An example of a physiological variable measured on an ordinal scale is the degree of consciousness such as euesthesia, dull sensorium, stupor, coma, and unconsciousness. System components may also contain physiological variables of a taxonomic nature such as shock, peritonitis, or myocardial infarction. Of course, these variables can be assigned some order relations such as mild or severe shock, but they can be considered in a model only as present or absent.

Many physiological variables may have different values at different anatomical sites. For instance, blood pressure varies from point to point in blood vessels. This can be accounted for by considering blood pressure as a so called distributed variable, i.e., a variable dependent on position specified by a properly chosen coordinate system.

Defining a system, its purpose, and its components are the basic steps in constructing a mathematical model. Another phase of model construction is development of mathematical relations between selected physiological variables, and this phase is also carried out simultaneously with a refinement, modification, and expansion of system variables and components. The system and its components frequently do not remain fixed even during the last phase of model development, namely, during an analysis of developed relations. As analysis proceeds, further modifications of the model system and the mathematical relations may be required to achieve the goal for which the model is being constructed. Nevertheless, the formulation of mathematical relations begins with most of the model system defined. The discussion of model construction is continued with a description of how mathematical relations are formulated.

Unlike most of physical systems such as the solar system, fluid flow, or nuclear reactions, physiological structures exist with a purpose to perform certain functions. Very frequently a function of a physiological system is to maintain status quo. For instance, the purpose of the respiratory system represented in Figure 39.3 is to maintain carbon dioxide concentration at a certain level.

Such a function is accomplished by reaction to a change from a desired state, i.e., by a feedback mechanism. Feedback can be defined as a circular relation such as: A affects B, and B affects A. This circular relation may be direct or indirect, i.e., with a direct mutual response of two variables or by action propagating through several intermediate variables. In any case, mathematical representation of a feedback relation is a system of simultaneous equations, some or all of which may be differential equations. Thus, mathematical formulation of a feedback system proceeds the same way as of any other set of relations. However, interpretation of such simultaneous equations in terms of feedback relations, when appropriate, is very helpful in understanding logical structure of the model system. Thinking in terms of feedback relations also helps to select proper mathematical representation as well as to define a model system and its components, since feedback relations are a consequence of the purpose of a physiological system.

Model components consist of closely related variables. Hence, mathematical representation is obtained by first examining these relations. It is helpful to list first the variables that are assumed to vary with time and to examine which component variables affect the rate of this variation. Next, we look at stationary relations between component variables. In the example of a cardiovascular system (Grodins, 1959) we have five components. The left heart is one of these consisting of four variables, V_{sl}, V_{dl}, V_{rl}, and Q_1, systolic, diastolic and residual volumes, and cardiac output. It is assumed that this component does not change with time unless it is influenced by other components. Thus, we have only static relations between component variables. Definition of residual volume yields the first relation:

$$V_{rl} = V_{dl} - V_{sl}. \quad (1)$$

Also, by definition of systolic volume, we have:

$$Q_1 = V_{sl}F, \quad (2)$$

a relation involving the variable F (heart rate), which constitutes a separate component. Similarly, we have for the right heart

$$V_{rr} = V_{dr} - V_{sr} \quad (3)$$

and

$$Q_r = V_{sr}F. \quad (4)$$

A relation between variables of systemic circuit is obtained by assuming that arterial blood pressure is proportional to blood volume:

$$P_{as} = V_{as}/C_{as}, \quad (5)$$

where the constant of proportionality is denoted by $1/C_{as}$ and C_{as} is called systemic arterial compliance.

Similar relations are obtained for the remaining variables:

$$P_{ap} = V_{ap}/C_{as}, \quad (6)$$

$$P_{vs} = V_{vs}/C_{vs}, \qquad (7)$$

$$P_{vp} = V_{vp}/C_{vp}. \qquad (8)$$

Equations 1–8 provide eight relations between 17 system variables. There are four model parameters, namely, compliances of blood vessels. The first four of these equations are definitions of the system variables and the last four are linear relations. These are quite common types of relations in mathematical modeling. Linear relations are a special case of fitting experimental, laboratory, and clinical data and, thus, obtaining empirical formulas. The equations 5–8 may be interpreted as definitions of compliances. However, these can be obtained only by measuring respective volumes and pressures repeatedly and then by averaging the computed values of compliances. This is equivalent to fitting the corresponding equations to the measured data by the least squares method.

Another example of an empirical relation obtained by the least squares method is the first equation quoted in this section that expressed minute volume as a sum of a linear function of CO_2 and H^- tensions and of exponential function of O_2 tension. Still another example is the equation (Martin, 1970) between left ventricular blood pressure P_{as} and activity levels s and v of sympathetic and vagal nerves.

$$P_{as} = b_1 s + b_2 v + b_3 s^2 + b_4 v^2 + b_5 sv. \qquad (9)$$

Here pressure P_{as} is expressed as a quadratic polynomial of activity levels s and v. The coefficients of this polynomial are obtained by the least squares method applied to experimental data.

The equation for minute volume and equations 5–8 assume linear relationship between variables. This is a very common assumption which is frequently quite satisfactory, since every sufficiently smooth function can be approximated by a linear relation, at least in a limited range of independent variable. Equation 9 also illustrates a rather common practice of choosing a polynomial, usually of a relatively low degree, to approximate a function that cannot be adequately represented by a linear relation. Other common choices for deterministic relations are rational, exponential, logarithmic and trigonometric functions, and their linear combinations.

Some knowledge of how a dependent variable changes as an independent argument is changed is necessary to make a proper selection of an analytical representation. For instance, we may know that a dependent variable increases or decreases as an independent variable grows. If a dependent variable tends to a limiting value as an independent variable becomes large, a negative exponential, logarithmic, or rational representation may be in order. For instance, if the rate of excretion of an injected substance such as radioactive tracer is proportional to its concentration, then its concentration decreases asymptotically to zero and can be represented by an exponential function with negative exponent such as $c \exp(-t/t_0)$, where c is the initial concentration and t_0 is the so called time constant.

If a dependent variable attains its maximum for a certain value of an independent variable, an approximation by a properly selected polynomial or by a certain exponential function may be chosen. If, for instance, our dependent variable is the frequency of different values of a physiological variable, say, systolic blood pressure, and the independent variable is the systolic pressure, we may expect that maximum frequency is near the average value, and an exponential function of Gaussian probability distribution may be an appropriate approximation.

If the dependent variable oscillates between its extremal values as the independent variable changes, an approximation by a sine function or by a linear combination of several such functions may be selected. If we know that for a certain value of the independent variable x the dependent variable vanishes, we may consider a representation $(x - x_0) f(x)$, where $f(x)$ is a function to be selected on the basis of other available information.

If we have no information about the relation, then we choose either a polynomial or a linear combination of certain functions such as exponential, trigonometric, Chebyshev polynomials (Pearson, 1974), and others.

When all the variables are ratio scale variables, dimensional analysis may be very helpful in selecting a proper mathematical form of a postulated relation. We illustrate this procedure by the following example. Suppose we want to determine a mathematical relation between diastolic blood volume V_{dl} of the left ventricle and the following variables: residual volume V_{rl}, filling pressure P_{vp}, filling resistance R_1, compliance of the left ventricle C_1 and duration of the filling cycle t_0. We form the product $\prod = V_{dl}^{d_1} V_{rl}^{d_2} P_{vp}^{d_3} R_1^{d_4} C_1^{d_5} t_0^{d_6}$. The dimensions of these variables are as follow: $[V_{dl}] = [V_{rl}] = [L^3]$, $[P_{vp}] = [ML^{-1}T^{-2}]$, $[R_1] = [ML^{-4}T^{-1}]$, $[C_1] = [M^{-1}L^4T^{-2}]$, and $[t_0] = [T]$. Dimensions of R_1 and C_1 reflect here the fact that we consider resistance and compliance with respect to flow of volume instead of mass. By substituting these dimensions in the product $\prod$ above, we get $[\prod] = [M^{d_3+d_4-d_5} L^{3d_1+3d_2-d_3-4d_4+4d_5} T^{-2d_3-d_4+2d_5+d_6}]$. By equating the exponents of each dimension to zero, we obtain:

$$d_3 + d_4 - d_5 = 0, \qquad (10)$$

$$3d_1 + 3d_2 - d_3 - 4d_4 + 4d_5 = 0, \qquad (11)$$

$$-2d_3 - d_4 + 2d_5 + d_6 = 0 \qquad (12)$$

By solving these equations in terms of d_1, d_2, and d_4, we get:

$$d_6 = d_4 - d_1 - d_2, \qquad (13)$$

$$d_5 = d_4, \qquad (14)$$

$$d_3 = -d_1 - d_2. \qquad (15)$$

Thus all three equations (10–12) are linearly independent. Since we have six variables, the Buckingham theorem implies that there are three independent dimensionless products. These can be selected in many ways by choosing various values of d_1, d_2, and d_4. We make the following choice: (a) $d_1 = 1$, $d_2 = d_4 = 0$; (b) $d_1 =$

$d_4 = 0$, $d_2 = 1$; (c) $d_1 = d_2 = 0$, $d_4 = 1$. The corresponding values of d_6, d_5, and d_3 are obtained from equations 13–15. This yields the following dimensionless products:

$$\tilde{t} = t_0/R_1C_1, \tag{16}$$

$$\tilde{V}_{dl} = V_{dl}/P_{vp}C_1, \tag{17}$$

$$\tilde{V}_{rl} = V_{rl}/P_{vp}C_1, \tag{18}$$

i.e., nondimensional time and nondimensional diastolic and residual volumes. A relation between the six original variables must be a relation between these three nondimensional quantities. A rather general relation is an expression of $\tilde{V}_{dl}$ as a bilinear function of arbitrary functions of the other two variables:

$$\tilde{V}_{dl} = k_1 + k_2 f(\tilde{V}_{rl}) + k_3 g(\tilde{t}) + k_4 f(\tilde{V}_{rl})g(\tilde{t}), \tag{19}$$

where $k_1 - k_4$ are some constants. Since this is a relation between nondimensional quantities, it is not affected by a change of units. Hence, we can normalize the units of volume in such a manner that the maximum of residual volume is unity. This corresponds to a completely filled ventricle with V_{dl} also equaling unity in this case. Thus, we get from equation 19:

$$1 = k_1 + k_2 f(1) + k_3 g(\tilde{t}) + k_4 f(1)g(\tilde{t}). \tag{20}$$

Since $\tilde{t}$ is arbitrary and $g(\tilde{t})$ is not a constant, equation 20 implies the following:

$$k_3 = 0, \tag{21}$$

$$k_4 f(1) = 0, \tag{22}$$

$$k_1 + k_2 f(1) = 1. \tag{23}$$

If the filling time $\tilde{t} = 0$, then $\tilde{V}_{dl} = \tilde{V}_{rl}$ and, hence, we have from equations 20 and 21: $\tilde{V}_{rl} = k_1 + [k_2 + k_4 g(0)] f(\tilde{V}_{rl})$. This relation holds for every value $\tilde{V}_{rl}$. Hence, the right hand side must be linear in $\tilde{V}_{rl}$. Therefore, we have

$$f(\tilde{V}_{rl}) = a + b\tilde{V}_{rl}. \tag{24}$$

By substituting this in the preceding relation, we get: $\tilde{V}_{rl} = k_1 + ak_2 + ak_4 g(0) + [k_2 + k_4 g(0)] b\tilde{V}_{rl}$, or

$$k_1 + ak_2 + ak_4 g(0) = 0, \tag{25}$$

$$[k_2 + k_4 g(0)]b = 1. \tag{26}$$

Equations 21 and 24 yield $(a + b) k_4 = 0$. Suppose $a + b \neq 0$. Then $k_4 = 0$ and consequently equation 19 is independent of $\tilde{t}$. But this implies that $\tilde{V}_{dl} = \tilde{V}_{rl}$, since this is true for $\tilde{t} = 0$.

Therefore, we must have:

$$a + b = 0 \tag{27}$$

But then by equation 22,

$$k_1 = 1. \tag{28}$$

Substitution of equations 21, 26, 27, and 28 in 19 yields:

$$\tilde{V}_{dl} = 1 + ak_2(1 - \tilde{V}_{rl}) + ak_4(1 - \tilde{V}_{rl})g(\tilde{t}). \tag{29}$$

We denote $ak_2 + ak_4 g(\tilde{t})$ by $h(\tilde{t})$ and write equation 29 in the form:

$$V_{dl} = 1 + (1 - \tilde{V}_{rl})h(\tilde{t}). \tag{30}$$

Thus we have for $\tilde{t} = 0$: $\tilde{V}_{rl} = 1 + (1 - \tilde{V}_{rl})h(0)$ or

$$h(0) = -1. \tag{31}$$

If the filling time $\tilde{t}$ is very long, $\tilde{V}_{dl}$ reaches its maximum of unity irrespective of the value of $\tilde{V}_{rl}$. Therefore, we have from equation 30: $1 = 1 + (1 - \tilde{V}_{rl})h(\infty)$ or,

$$h(\infty) = 0. \tag{32}$$

A simple function that satisfies equations 31 and 32 is $h(\tilde{t}) = -\exp(-k\tilde{t})$, where k is an arbitrary constant. Thus, we get from equation 30:

$$\tilde{V}_{dl} = 1 - (1 - \tilde{V}_{rl})e^{-k\tilde{t}}. \tag{33}$$

The constant k must be determined by fitting equation 33 to empirical data. Below we compare equation 33 with the expression derived from different assumptions (Grodins, 1959).

Whichever way the mathematical expressions are selected to represent physiological relations, these expressions usually contain parameters which are determined by fitting the data. The least squares method is most frequently applied to obtain the values of the parameters. This method produces the most likely values of the parameters provided the following conditions hold. First, the selected function with proper values of parameters must represent the relation between dependent and independent variables exactly. Secondly, differences between the data values and the values of the function are due to random measurement errors that are independently normally distributed with zero means. The second condition is quite plausible in many cases because of the central limit theorem which asserts that the errors are normally distributed, provided they are a result of many independent causes, each contributing a random component from a distribution satisfying certain conditions. The first condition on selected function is satisfied only in special cases. Therefore, the root mean square error of a fit and other statistical tests such as the Student t-value applicable in a linear case are not absolute criteria for how well a mathematical formula represents the corresponding physiological relation. Frequently, the dependent variable may be affected by other physiological factors not included in equation. This effect can be represented by a dependence of model parameters on these additional factors. Therefore, a well formulated mathematical model should include a degree of uncertainty of the values of model parameters. This uncertainty can be represented by confidence intervals of the dependent variable corresponding to each choice of independent variables or, better yet, by confidence intervals of model parameters, and still better by probability distribution of these parameters. Thus, a mathematical model of a physiological system is only a first approximation if it consists of deterministic relations, even if these relations are derived from certain laws instead of fitting data as discussed above.

The laws employed in deriving a mathematical representation of physiological relations include the laws of mechanics, various conservation laws, chemical kinetics, and others such as Starling's law of heart, Fick's law of diffusion across a membrane, Poiseuille's law of fluid flow in pipes, etc. Conservation laws and laws of Newtonian mechanics are most universal and exact. However, even these laws are only approximations when applied to a physiological phenomenon or even to a physical system. They provide a very close approximation when applied to a closed system. However, no real system can be completely isolated from the rest of the world. Even conservation laws hold only approximately since a physical or a physiological system usually contains many sources and sinks of a secondary importance that are not included in the mathematical formulation of the laws. For example, irregular variation of friction provide unaccounted sinks of kinetic energy. An unexpected exchange of fluid and gas across a postulated boundary of the system affects the accuracy of a relation derived from mass conservation law. Physiological models usually consider lumped variables which are certain abstractions, as noted earlier. Obviously, the laws of physics need not apply to such abstractions exactly. Application of chemical kinetics laws also need not produce very accurate results if there exist minor secondary chemical reactions not included in the model system or if the concentration of some catalysts varies. The Starling's law of heart is just a definition of the strength of the heart that is assumed to be constant in the expression of this law but hardly ever is. Thus, this law does not represent the relations exactly. The same can be said about other laws such as Fick's diffusion law, etc. Thus, mathematical relations obtained by applying various laws to a physiological system do not necessarily provide a much better representation than do empirical formulas. In either case, it is highly desirable to add to a developed model a description of an associated uncertainty. Complete description of uncertainty requires probability distributions that are relatively simple, when physiological variables can be treated as random variables. It is much more complicated when these variables are stochastic processes. Much more empirical data are needed in either case to characterize corresponding distributions than is required for deriving deterministic representation of physiological relations. Also, mathematical analysis of stochastic relations is much more complex.

Preceding remarks on methods for selecting mathematical expressions are illustrated by returning to the description of Grodins' (1959) cardiovascular model. As already stated, this is a model system of 17 variables divided into five components with a goal to derive an interpretative model. The relations of the variables of individual components are represented by equations 1, 3, and 5–8, with 2 and 4 relating the variables of different components. The remaining relations between variables of different components are examined, beginning with systemic blood circulation, and it is observed that blood volume V_{as} is changed by the input Q_1 from the left ventricle and by the flow to systemic veins through the connecting vessels at the rate, say F_s. Thus, if V'_{as} denotes the rate of change of V_{as}, the volume conservation law implies:

$$V'_{as} = Q_1 F - F_s. \qquad (34)$$

We assume that blood flows according to Poiseuille's law, i.e., that the drop in pressure is proportional to the flow rate F_s:

$$P_{as} - P_{vs} = R_s F_s. \qquad (35)$$

The constant of proportionality R_s is called resistance, which is the lumped systemic resistance in this case. By eliminating F_s from equations 34 and 35 we obtain:

$$V'_{as} = Q_1 F - (P_{as} - P_{vs})/R_s, \qquad (36)$$

a differential equation which defines V_{as} in terms of other variables. In a similar manner, we obtain the following differential equations:

$$V'_{vs} = -Q_r F + (P_{as} - P_{vs})/R_s, \qquad (37)$$

$$V'_{ap} = Q_r F - (P_{ap} - P_{vp})/R_p, \qquad (38)$$

$$V'_{vp} = -Q_1 F + (P_{ap} - P_{vp})/R_p, \qquad (39)$$

where R_p is the lumped pulmonary vascular resistance. Since equations 36–39 are differential equations, initial values of V_{as}, V_{ap}, V_{vs}, and V_{vp} must be specified to complete a mathematical representation of these variables. These relations provide a generalization of the model (Grodins, 1959) by expressing the relation between blood volume and flow rate in terms of differential equations. Thus, the model containing equations 36–39 is a dynamic model, while the model of the reference (Grodins, 1959) is static.

Next, we examine left heart component, i.e., the dependence of the variables V_{sl}, V_{dl}, and V_{rl} on the variables of the other components. We note that the rate of filling V'_{dl} of the left auricle is affected by filling pressure P_{vp} and by the volume of blood V_{dl} already contained in the auricle. The simplest form of this relation is a linear equation $V'_{dl} = aV_{dl} + bP_{vp}$. If we define $R_l = 1/b$ and $C_l = -b/a$, we can write the last relation in the form

$$R_l C_l V'_{dl} + V_{dl} = C_l P_{vp}, \qquad (40)$$

where R_l is called filling resistance and C_l compliance. Thus we have a differential equation that defines V_{dl}. Obviously, the initial condition is $V_{dl} = V_{rl}$ at $t = 0$, i.e., at the beginning of diastole. Equation 40, together with the initial condition, defines the value V_{dl} at all times for which the equation is valid, i.e., during the time of diastole. The required value is the value of V_{dl} at the end of diastole. If we assume that duration of a systole is 0.2 sec, then the time at the end of diastole is $(60/F) - 0.2$. Thus, we obtain V_{dl} by solving equation 40 with the specified initial condition and by evaluating the solution at $t = (60/F) - 0.2$. If we assume that the filling pressure P_{vp} remains constant we obtain

$$V_{dl} = C_l P_{vp} + (V_{rl} - C_l P_{vp}) \cdot \exp\left[-\left(\frac{60}{F} - 0.2\right) \Big/ R_l C_l\right]. \quad (41)$$

We compare this formula with equation 33 derived by the method of dimensional analysis. For this end we let the undetermined constant k in equation 33 equal unity. If we substitute equations 16–18 in 33 and multiply both sides by $C_l P_{vp}$, we get

$$V_{dl} = C_l P_{vp} - (C_l P_{vp} - V_{rl}) e^{-t_0/R_l C_l}. \quad (42)$$

Under present assumption the filling time $t_0 = (60/F) - 0.2$. The substitution of this in equation 42 yields equation 41; i.e, dimensional analysis gave the same expression for V_{dl} as the simplifying assumptions from which equation 41 was derived.

The systolic volume of the left heart is affected by systemic arterial pressure. Hence, we need the relation between V_{sl} and P_{as}. Such a relation is provided by Starling's heart law:

$$W_l = S_l V_{dl} \quad (43)$$

and energy conservation equation

$$W_l = V_{sl} P_{as}, \quad (44)$$

which is obtained by neglecting inertia of blood and change of systemic blood pressure during systole. From equations 43 and 44,

$$V_{sl} = \begin{cases} V_{dl} S_l / P_{as}, & \text{if } S_l \leq P_{as} \\ V_{dl} & \text{otherwise.} \end{cases} \quad (45)$$

Similarly, we get for the right heart:

$$V_{dr} = C_r P_{vs} + (V_{rs} - C_r P_{vs}) \cdot \exp\left[-\left(\frac{60}{F} - 0.2\right) \Big/ R_r C_r\right], \quad (46)$$

and

$$V_{sr} = \begin{cases} V_{dr} S_r / P_{ap}, & \text{if } S_r \leq P_{ap} \\ V_{dr} & \text{otherwise.} \end{cases} \quad (47)$$

Equations 36–39, 41, 45–47 together with 1–8 provide 16 relations between 17 system variables; consequently one variable, say, the heart rate F can be assigned an arbitrary value, i.e., F can be considered as a system input.

The model described above can be used for a study of how its variables change as F is changed. The model system can be readily modified to accommodate other inputs such as bleeding and blood infusion. If blood is infused, say, at the rate $-B_{ap}$ into systemic arteries instead of equation 36 we have

$$V'_{as} = Q_l - (P_{as} - P_{vs})/R_s - B_{ap} \quad (48)$$

In case of bleeding the sign of the last term is negative, i.e., the quantity $-B_{ap}$ is assigned negative value. Similarly, equations 37–39 can be modified to account for bleeding from or infusion into other parts of the blood circuit. The additional terms are system inputs (forcing functions) that can be chosen at will to investigate the corresponding system response. Of course, the range of the input variables is restricted since the validity of the equations of the model is restricted by not including dependence of heart rate and vascular resistance on blood pressure and by ignoring the dependence of the strength of the heart on the rate of perfusion as well as the dependence of arterial and venous compliance on vascular tone and many others. In order to study a wider range of responses, additional physiological variables and relations and, thus, additional system components should be introduced. Such an expansion of a model associated with its analysis yields significant conclusions that are implied by the model. The simplest procedure for obtaining model implications is to examine individual relations. If such a relation contains only two variables, we may treat one of them as an independent variable and investigate its effect on the other. An example of this kind is equation 6, which expresses a linear relation between pulmonary arterial blood volume and pressure. When a relation contains more than two variables, its analysis may be conducted by fixing all but two of them and then examining how one of these is affected by a change of the other. This is usually done for several values of the fixed variables. For instance, equation 9 contains three variables: blood pressure and activity levels of sympathetic and vagal nerves. The author of this equation investigates the effect of activity by vagal nerves on blood pressure while sympathetic activity level remains fixed. He observes that the resulting relation is almost linear with a slope dependent on the fixed value of sympathetic activity, a straightforward implication of equation 9.

Such a procedure of analysis is equivalent to an assumption that the variables of a relation constitute a system, with fixed variables being system inputs. Similarly, several equations of the model can be combined into a "system." For instance, equations 1, 2, 41, and 45, provide relations among the following seven variables: V_{dl}, V_{rl}, V_{sl}, F, Q_l, P_{as}, and P_{vp}. By eliminating V_{rl}, V_{cl}, and V_{sl} from these equations, we obtained a relation between F, Q_l, P_{as}, and P_{vs}. Now we may consider P_{as} and P_{vs} as system inputs and F with Q_l as system variables; i.e., we can examine the effect of heart rate F on cardiac output Q_l. This is the subsystem examined in the reference (Grodins, 1959). It is concluded that Q_l increases to its maximum as F grows to its optimal value dependent on P_{as} and P_{vs} and then Q_l decreases as F moves further up.

A subsystem consisting of a subset of a model equation can also be studied by manipulating two inputs while holding other inputs fixed in such a manner that certain variables of the system remain unchanged. Such a simultaneous manipulation defines a relation between the respective inputs. This again can be illustrated by another subsystem considered in the reference (Grodins, 1959). In this subsystem the relation is examined between P_{vs} and P_{as} for fixed cardiac output Q_l and heart rate F. The corresponding system is obtained by taking equations 1–4, 38, 42, and 45–47. The variables in these equations are: V_{rl}, V_{dl}, V_{sl}, Q_l, F, V_{rr}, V_{dr}, V_{sr}, Q_r, V'_{ap}, P_{ap}, P_{vp}, P_{as}, and P_{vs}. In a static model we set $V'_{ap} = 0$ and $Q_r = Q_l = Q$. Thus, we have 12 variables and 9 equations. We can eliminate eight variables and obtain one equation that relates the remaining four variables, namely, Q, F, P_{as}, and P_{vs}. By solving this equation for P_{vs}, we express the variable by a linear function of P_{as} with coefficients dependent on Q, F, and model parameters R_p, C_l, R_l, C_r, S_l, R_r, and S_r. Of course, this linear relation between P_{as} and P_{vs} is incompatible with equation 36, since now P_{as} and P_{vs} are not system variables but rather its inputs. This subsystem involves equation 47, which has two forms dependent on the ratio S_r/P_{ap}. But P_{ap} affects P_{as} via equations 38, 41, and 45. Hence, the resulting linear relation between P_{vs} and P_{as} is valid only if P_{as} is sufficiently large. When P_{as} is below a certain value and decreases still further, P_{vs} remains constant.

Other subsystems can be constructed from the equations of the cardiovascular system described above. The model parameters such as systemic and pulmonary resistance R_s and R_p, various compliances, etc., have a physiological interpretation. Hence, instead of treating these as model parameters, we can interpret them as system inputs or as system variables by formulating additional equations in the latter case. This way the system can be incorporated into a larger system.

Choice of the subsets of system variables and equations illustrated above depends on the purpose of the model as well as on available and feasible experimental and clinical data that can be compared with conclusions derived from a submodel, such as optimal heart rate mentioned earlier. Subsets of system variables and equations can also be used to select observations and experiments designed for gathering new type of data.

Besides an investigation of submodels as illustrated above, model analysis may consist of other mathematical transformations of its equations that produce new relations suitable for physiological interpretation and, thus, provide new conclusions. However, the most common transformations are those illustrated by the preceding examples. They consist of elimination of dependent variables from a subset of a model equations. A special case of such an elimination is the solution of model equations, since this can be interpreted as elimination of all but one dependent variable. Such a solution is obtained by constructing mathematical expressions that define an algorithm for computing values of dependent variables which correspond to specified values of independent variables.

A method for eliminating dependent variables is contingent upon the structure of equations. If all the relations between dependent variables are linear, the elimination (solution) can be obtained by Cramer's rule. If relations are linear differential equations with constant coefficients, a closed form solution is also readily obtainable. If, however, the system of equations is large, closed form solutions are impractical. Instead, numerical methods must be used to obtain a complete solution of the system. A general solution of a model consisting of linear differential equations can be completely characterized by obtaining particular solutions corresponding to the inputs equal to unit step function and sine functions. Any piecewise continuous function defined on a finite interval and bounded can be approximated by a sum of step functions and sine terms. On the other hand, the response of a linear model to a sum of inputs equals to the sum of responses to the summands. Hence, by examining the response of the model to unit step function and to periodic functions a complete characterization of the model can be obtained. This is the procedure commonly used in engineering design problems.

Physiological models are mostly nonlinear. Hence, neither an analytic solution can be obtained nor an engineering type study of response applied. Therefore, physiological models are studied either by simulating them on an analog computer that yields varying voltage representing a dependent variable or by solving the equations on a digital computer that produces numerical approximations of dependent variables corresponding to specified values of independent variables.

In any case, a properly selected complete or partial solution provides the desired inferences from the model, such as the values of the independent variables and inputs that produce optimal response or a response to selected inputs at some future time.

MODELING HYPOVOLEMIC SHOCK

A complex interaction of many physiological variables in a hypovolemic shock can be better understood if the variables are defined precisely and their relations analyzed in detail. This can be best accomplished by constructing a mathematical model. However, a large number of variables and relations make construction of such a model a rather difficult task. Since shock conditions either deteriorate or improve with time, a dynamic model is needed. A change of physiological variables in response to almost identical injury varies from case to case in a rather unpredictable fashion. Thus, we deal here with a stochastic multidimensional dynamic process— the most difficult kind to model. This section does not provide such a model. It only discusses an outline of a synthesis of several submodels derived by various authors, namely, the cardiovascular model (Grodins, 1959), the heart rate control (Warner and Cox, 1961), the cardiorespiratory model (Farell and Siegel, 1973), the respiratory model (Milhorn, 1966), and the baroreceptor model (Poitras et al., 1966).

The only parallel blood circuits considered here are coronary, systemic, and pulmonary. The latter consists of 10 parallel segments as described in the reference (Farell and Siegel, 1973). Systemic circuit includes all other circuits except pulmonary and coronary, i.e., cerebral, hepatic, renal, etc. Only a few variables describing blood chemistry and hematology are included. Yet we have a model system that consists of 279 variables. Six of these are inputs (exogeneous variables) such as barometric pressure, CO_2 concentration in inhaled air, rate of blood transfusion, and others listed in the Table 39.1. Fifty-six physiological and anatomical variables are left as independent variables (endogenous model variables). Examples of these variables are blood temperature, oxygen consumption rate, heart strength in Starling's heart law, and others. The number of the independent variables can be reduced by postulating additional relations between physiological variables. The remaining 217 variables are dependent variables defined by a set of 217 simultaneous algebraic, transcendental, and differential equations. Some of these relations are definitions, others are various conservation laws, and still others are empirical relations taken from the models quoted above. The values of the model parameters in the empirical relations can be readily obtained from the corresponding parameters of the references by transforming the equations of these references to the equivalent form used below.

All the variables of the model system are listed in Table 39.1. The variables that are selected as dependent system variables are numbered by arabic numerals. The endogenous independent variables are numbered by Roman numerals and the exogenous variables are labeled by the lower case letters. The choice of dependent and independent (endogenous) variables is somewhat arbitrary and is made according to interest and convenience. For instance, Starling's heart law used below relates heart strength cardiac output and mean arterial pressure. We assume that heart strength is an independent variable, i.e., that heart strength and arterial blood pressure define the cardiac output. If desired, we could assume that cardiac output is independent and that Starling's law defines heart strength in terms of cardiac output and blood pressure. The choice depends on the purpose of the model, i.e., on the relations that we wish to study.

Since many model relations are differential equations with time as the independent variable, the system variables vary with time. Besides, both algebraic and differential equations should be interpreted as stochastic with random coefficients distributed according to certain probability distributions instead of assumed being constants as in various models of the references mentioned above.

The model system is specified by listing the variables in Table 39.1.

Exact definition of some of these variables, such as heart rate or oxygen tension, is quite obvious, implied by simple operations that determine their values. The meaning of many other variables is implied by their mutual relations given on the following pages. Most of these relations are taken from the references mentioned above. Since most of the models in the references are static, some algebraic equations of these models have been modified into a differential form representing a dynamic character of the system. Furthermore, dynamic character of the system requires that many model parameters of the referenced submodels be treated as physiological variables requiring additional equations to describe their behavior.

For convenience of analysis the system variables are divided into 28 groups. Thus, our model consists of 28 components as indicated in Table 39.1 and also in Figure 39.4, where we have eight boxes representing various components. Two boxes, namely "Pulmonary Circuit" and "Lungs," represent 11 components each. The remaining boxes are in 1-1 correspondence with the respective components. In each box, arabic and roman numerals and lower case letters indicate the variables comprising the components, just as in Table 39.1. The *arrows* connecting various boxes indicate the feedback relations, with the numbers along the *arrows* showing the number of dependent variables in the exit component that affect the variables in the entrance box. *Arrows* pointing to various boxes with no origin indicate that respective components are affected by a number of independent variables, as indicated along these arrows.

Solid short arrows correspond to endogenous variables and *dashed arrows* to exogenous ones.

The first component contains six variables that describe the metabolic bed. The second and the third components consist of five variables each. These variables describe the functions of the left and right heart. The fourth component includes 11 variables of the state of myocardium. There are seven variables that describe the combined state of the lung segments. We call this collection of variables "lungs." Next, we have seven variables of each of the 10 lung segments, i.e., 10 more components, each consisting of seven variables. The following 12 variables describe coronary blood circulation and then 31 variables constitute the systemic circuit component. Pulmonary circulation is described in a similar fashion as respiratory function, namely, by 11 variables common to all 10 lung segments and by the variables specific to each segment. These constitute the remaining 10 components with identical sets of variables that describe circulation in each segment.

The system can be expanded by including additional variables. For instance, instead of considering lumped variables of the systemic circulation, we can introduce the variables of the cerebral, splanchnic, renal, skin, and other blood circuits in a similar fashion as the variables for lung segments are specified. However instead of trying to expand the model, we mention here a simple method of reducing the system by eliminating some of the variables. The relations of the reduced system implied by the relations of the original model can be derived from suitable empirical data as new empirical formulas instead of the relations constructed from model equations; i.e., the model equations can be referred to only to determine which variables are interdependent according to the original model, with the form of dependence to be derived from the relevant data. A reduced model can again be expanded by gradual inclusion of the eliminated variables as enough information to establish desired relations becomes available.

The third column of Table 39.1 contains mnemonic symbols of the variables described in the second column and numbered in the first. The symbols are selected to simplify the notation. A few of them are adopted from

Table 39.1
Variables and Components of a Model

No. 1	Variable 2	Symbol 3	Defining Relation 4	Related Variables 5
	Metabolic Bed			
1	Volume of O_2	O_m	49	I, 92, 96, 102
2	Volume of CO_2	C_m	50	5, 92, 98, 103
3	O_2 tension	P_{om}	51	1
4	CO_2 tension	P_{cm}	52	2
5	CO_2 production rate	C_{rm}	53	I
I	Oxygen consumption rate	O_{rm}		
	Left Heart			
6	Diastolic volume	V_{dl}	38	3, 18, 114
7	Systolic volume	V_{sl}	42	6, 90, II
8	Residual volume	V_{rl}	1	7, 6
9	Left heart output	Q_l	2	6, 18
II	Strength of the ventricle	S_l		
	Right Heart			
10	Diastolic volume	V_{dr}	40	12, 18, 91
11	Systolic volume	V_{sr}	47	6, 10, 90, III
12	Residual volume	V_{rr}	3	10, 11
13	Right heart output	Q_r	4	11, 18
III	Strength of the ventricle	S_r		
	Myocardium			
14	Sympathetic nerve activity	f_1	54	90
15	Vagus nerve activity	f_2	55	90
16	Concentration of norepinephrine at the site of pacemaker	A_2	56	14
17	Concentration of acetylcholine	C_2	57	15
18	Heart rate	F	58	16, 17
19	O_2 content	O_h	59	78, 102
20	CO_2 content	C_h	60	21, 78, 84, 103
21	CO_2 production rate	C_{hr}	61	IV
22	O_2 tension	P_{oh}	62	19
23	CO_2 tension	P_{ch}	63	20
IV	Oxygen consumption rate	O_{hr}		
	Lungs			
25	Minute volume	V_m	64	105, 107, 108
26	Total tidal volume	V_t	66	V–XXIV, XXXV
27	Respiration rate	G	67	25, 26
28–37	Tidal volume of a lung segment	V_{tj}	77	
38–47	Alveolar O_2 concentration in a segment	C_{oej}	78, 87	27–47, 116–125, 156–165, 216, XXV–XXXIV, a
48–57	Alveolar CO_2 concentration in a segment	C_{clj}	88, 97	27–57, 116–125, 175–184, XXV-XXXIV, b
58–67	Alveolar O_2 tension	P_{opj}	98–107	38–57, c
68–77	Alveolar CO_2 tension	P_{cpj}	108–117	
V–XIV	Compliance of a lung segment	C_{pj}		
XV–XXIV	Air flow resistance in a lung segment	R_{aj}		
XXV–XXXIV	Dead volume of a segment	V_{dj}		
XXXV	Peak air driving pressure	P_o		
a	Inhaled air O_2 concentration	C_{oi}		
b	Inhaled air CO_2 concentration	C_{ci}		
c	Barometric pressure	P_b		
	Coronary Circuit			
78	Coronary blood flow	Q_c	118	90, 91, XXXV
79	O_2 tension in coronary venous blood	P_{oc}	119	22
80	CO_2 tension in coronary venous blood	P_{cc}	120	23
81	Oxyhemoglobin concentration in coronary blood	S_c	121	79, 80, 85, XXXVII
82	O_2 concentration in coronary venous blood	C_{oc}	123	79, 81, XLII, XXXVII
83	CO_2 concentration in coronary venous plasma	C_{cpc}	125	80, 85, 87, XXXVII
84	CO_2 concentration in blood	C_{cc}	124	81, 83, 85, XXXVII
85	pH in coronary venous blood	pH_c	126	80, 86, 87, XXXVII
86	CHO_3 concentration in coronary blood	D_c	127	81, 85, XXXVII
87	pK in coronary venous blood	pK_c	125	85, XXXVII
XXXVI	Coronary vascular resistance	R_c		
XXXVII	Blood temperature	T		
	Systemic Circuit			
88	Arterial blood volume	V_{as}	129	9, 78, 92, d
89	Venous blood volume	V_{vs}	130	13, 78, 92, XL, XLI, e, f
90	Arterial blood pressure	P_{as}	5	88, 90
91	Venous blood pressure	P_{vs}	7	89, XXXIX
92	Blood flow rate	Q_s	131	90, 91, XXXVIII
93	O_2 tension in end-capillaries	P_{os}	132	3

Mathematical Models

Table 39.1—Continued

No. 1	Variable 2	Symbol 3	Defining Relation 4	Related Variables 5
	Systemic Circuit			
94	CO_2 tension in end-capillaries	P_{cs}	133	4
95	Oxyhemoglobin concentr.	S_s	134	93, 94, XXXVII
96	O_2 concentration in end-capillaries	C_{os}	135	93, 95, XLIII
97	CO_2 concentration in end-capillaries	C_{cps}	136	94, 99, 100, XXXVII
98	CO_2 concentration in end-capillary blood	C_{cs}	146	95, 97, 99, XLIII
99	pH in end-capillary blood	pH_s	138	94, 100, 101, XXXVII
100	pH in end-capillary blood	pK_s	139	99, XXXVII
101	CHO_3 concentration in end-capillary blood	D_s	140	95, 99, XLII
102	O_2 concentration in mixed arterial blood	C_{oa}	141	115–125, 156–165, 216
103	CO_2 concentration in mixed arterial blood	C_{ca}	142	116–125, 176–185, 217
104	Oxyhemoglobin concentration in mixed arterial blood	S_a	143	
105	O_2 tension in mixed arterial blood	P_{oa}	149	102, 103, XXXII, XLII, XLIII
106	CO_2 concentration in plasma	C_{cpa}		
107	CO_2 concentration in mixed arterial blood	P_{ca}		
108	pH in mixed arterial blood	pHa	143–158	102, 103, XXXII, XLII, XLIII
109	pK in mixed arterial blood	pKa		
110	CHO_3 in mixed arterial blood	D_a		
XXXVIII	Systemic vascular resistance	R_s		
XXXIX	Venous compliance	C_{vs}		
XL	Interstitial vascular fluid exchange rate	F_{es}		
XLI	Rate of blood sequestration	B_s		
XLII	Hemoglobin	H		
XLIII	Hematocrit	H_t		
d	Arterial blood loss	B_{as}		
e	Venous blood loss	B_{vs}		
	Pulmonary Circuit			
111	Arterial blood volume	V_{ap}	150	13, 115–125, LVI, g
112	Venous blood volume	V_{vp}	151	5, 115–125, LVII
113	Arterial blood pressure	P_{ap}	6	111
114	Venous blood pressure	P_{vp}	8	112, LV
115	Shunt flow rate	Q_b	162	113, 114, LIV
116–125	Blood flow rate through a segment	Q_{pj}	152–161	113, 114, XLIV-LIII
126–135	O_2 tension in end-capillaries of a segment	P_{opj}	163–172	58–67
136–145	CO_2 tension in end-capillaries of a segment	P_{cpj}	173–182	68–77
146–155	Oxyhemoglobin concentration in end-capillaries of a segment	S_{pj}	183–192	126–145, XXXVII
156–165	O_2 concentration in end-capillaries of a segment	C_{opj}	193–202	126–135, 146–155, XLII, XLIII
166–175	CO_2 concentration in end-capillary plasma of a lung segment	C_{cppj}	203–212	136–145, 186–205, XXXVII
176–185	CO_2 concentration in end-capillary blood of a lung segment	C_{cpj}	213–222	146–155, 166–175, 186–195, XLII
186–195	pH in end capillaries of a lung segment	pH_{pj}	223–232	136–145, 196–215, XXXVII
196–205	pK in end-capillaries of a lung segment	pK_{pj}	233–242	186–195, XLVII
206–215	CHO_3 concentration in end-capillaries of a segment	D_{pj}	243–252	146–155, 186–195, XLII
216	O_2 concentration in mixed venous blood	C_{ov}	253	78, 82, 92, 96
217	CO_2 concentration in mixed venous blood	C_{cv}	254	78, 84, 92, 98
XLIV-LIII	Vascular resistance of a lung segment	R_{pj}		
LIV	By pass (shunting) resistance	R_b		
LV	Venous compliance	C_{vp}		
LVI	Interstitial-vascular fluid exchange rate	F_{ep}		
g	Arterial blood loss	B_{ap}		

the references but most are somewhat simplified. In many cases a capital letter is the first letter in the principal word of the descriptive name of the variable such as "concentration," etc. The first subscript usually indicates the principal modifier of the main term and the second subscript indicates the component of the corresponding variable. Of course, there are several deviations from this rule, yet the rule is helpful in identifying the symbols.

Various relations are listed below, and they may be considered as equations defining certain variables in terms of the others. Thus, each relation can be associated with a system variable as indicated in the fourth column of the Table 39.1. Here we have a number of an equation appearing somewhere in this chapter and selected to define the respective variable in terms of the other variables appearing in the equation. The numbers of these variables were listed in the last column of table.

All model parameters in the formulas discussed in this section are denoted by the symbol "a" with successive subscripts. Besides these, the parameters in the equations of the preceding sections referenced in the table are additional model parameters. These are also assigned a new symbol "a" with a proper subscript for the uniformity of notation. Normal values of certain physiological variables also appear as model parameters in the equations of this section. They are denoted by the same symbol as the corresponding variables with a bar over the symbol as well as by a letter "a" with a subscript. This provides a simple count of the total number of model parameters.

The first model component is a metabolic bed de-

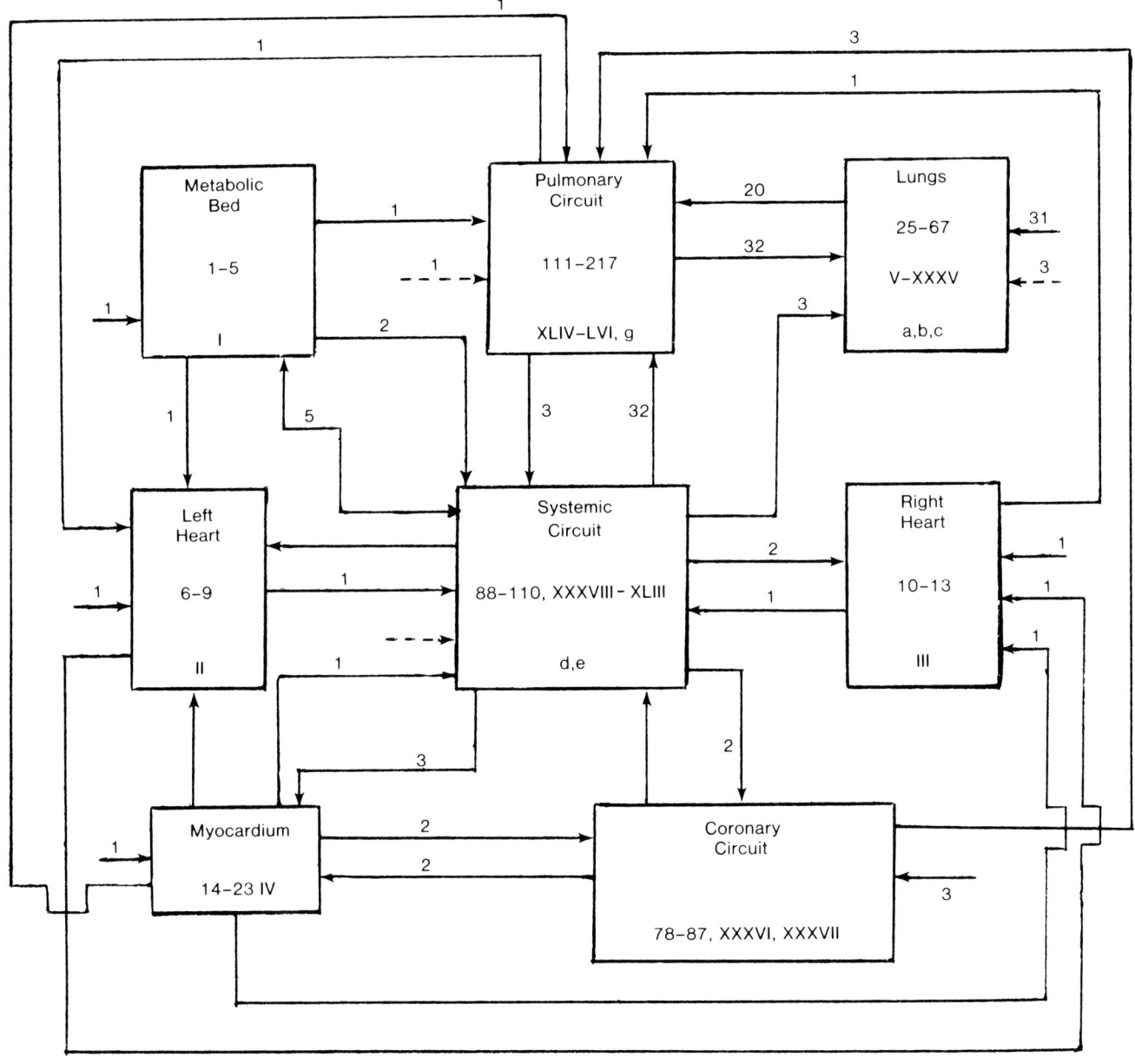

Figure 39.4. Diagram of the hypovalemic shock model.

scribed by six variables. A conservation law defines amount of oxygen in the metabolic bed by the following relation:

$$O'_m = Q_s(C_{oa} - C_{os}) - O_{rm}, \quad (49)$$

where prime denotes the derivative with respect to time. This equation says that the rate of change of the amount of oxygen is equal to the amount extracted from the passing blood per unit time minus the rate of oxygen consumption. Similarly, the rate of change of CO_2 in the metabolic bed is given by:

$$C'_m = C_{rm} - Q_s(C_{cs} - C_{ca}). \quad (50)$$

Gas concentration in the metabolic bed is proportional to gas volume. Therefore, by assuming that gas tension in tissue is proportional to gas concentration we get:

$$P_{om} = a_1 O_m \quad \text{and} \quad (51)$$

$$P_{cm} = a_2 C_m. \quad (52)$$

Production rate of CO_2 is assumed to be proportional to the rate of consumption of O_2 in the metabolic bed:

$$C_{rm} = a_3 O_{rm}. \quad (53)$$

The rate of oxygen consumption O_{rm} depends on physiological activity and is left here as an independent endogeneous variable. This completes the description of the metabolic bed. Systemic blood flow rate Q_s and gas concentrations C_{oa}, C_{os}, C_{cs}, and C_{ca} are included in this description. These variables belong to systemic and pulmonary circuit components.

The left heart component consists of five variables, four of which are treated as dependent variables, and they are specified by equations 41, 45, 1 and 2; this is indicated in column 4 of the table. We recall that the last two equations are definitions and the first two involve a model parameter, compliance of the left ventricle C_l which is assigned here the symbol a_4. The fifth variable, the strength of the left ventricle, is left as an independent (endogenous) variable.

The right heart is described in analogous fashion by equations 3, 4, 46, and 48. This introduces an additional model parameter, the compliance of the right ventricle C_r, which is assigned here the symbol a_5.

The first variable in the myocardium component is activity of sympathetic nerves. According to (Poitras et al., 1966) this activity is determined by blood pressure at the site of carotid sinuses. For simplicity we assume that this pressure equals the average systemic arterial pressure P_{as}. Consequently, the equation for f_1 of the reference is:

$$f_1'' + a_6 f_1' + a_7 f_1 = a_8 P_{as} + a_9 P_{as}' + a_{10} P_{as}'', \quad (54)$$

provided P_{as} is within certain limits, say, P_1 and P_2. For $P_{as} < P_1$, $f_1 = 0$ and for $P_{as} > P_2$, f_1 is the maximum possible value, i.e., $P_{as} = P_2$. Equation 55, defining vagus nerve activity, f_2 is the same as in equation 54, only the coefficients have different values, say, a_{11}, a_{12}, a_{13}, a_{14}, and a_{15}.

The form of the relation defining the next variable, A_2 (norepinephrine concentration), can be obtained by eliminating intermediate variables A_1, B, and AB from equations (Warner and Cox, 1961). The result is a third order nonlinear differential equation in A_2, depending on f_1 and f_1'. Symbolically:

$$A_2''' = f(A_2'', A_2', A_2, f_1, f_1'). \quad (56)$$

This expression contains five model parameters $k_1 - k_5$ of the equations in the reference which are denoted here by $a_{16} - a_{20}$. This equation can be written in an explicit form but it cannot be solved analytically. Thus, analog or numerical methods are needed to obtain a solution. The explicit form of (54) is not convenient in either case. Instead, some auxiliary variables must be introduced and equation 54 replaced by a set of three equations of the first order. However auxiliary variables are just a part of a numerical algorithm or an analog representation. There is no need to include them in a model, especially when they have no physical interpretation. Therefore, the relation expressed by equation 54 is represented here only symbolically, although its explicit form is available in terms of equations of the reference.

Similarly, an expression defining concentration of acetylcholine C_2 in terms of vagal nerve activity f_2 is obtained by eliminating the intermediate variables C_1 and N from equations shown in Figure 8 of the reference (Warner and Cox, 1961). After simplifying the notation of constants, the result is the following second order differential equation:

$$a_{21} f_2 C_1'' + (a_{22} f_2 - a_{23} f_2') C_2' \quad (57)$$
$$+ (a_{24} f_2 - a_{25} f_2') C_2 + a_{26} f_2^3 + a_{27} f_2^2 = 0.$$

According to this reference, heart rate F is a linear function of epinephrine concentration A_2 and is also a linear function of the reciprocal of C_2. This together with a relation for systemic blood pressure (Martin, 1970) suggests the following empirical formula for heart rate.

$$F = a_{28} + a_{29} A_2 + a_{30} A_2^2 \quad (58)$$
$$+ a_{31}/C_2 + a_{32}/C_2^2 + a_{33} A_2 / C_2.$$

The expressions for O_2 and CO_2 contents in myocardial tissue are analogous to those for metabolic bed (e.g., equations 49 and 50):

$$O_h' = Q_c(C_{oa} - C_{oc}) - O_{rh}, \quad (59)$$

$$C_h' = C_{rh} - Q_c(C_{cc} - C_{ca}). \quad (60)$$

The expression for CO_2 production rate in myocardium and for gas tensions are analogous to the corresponding expressions for metabolic bed:

$$C_{rh} = a_{34} O_{rh}, \quad (61)$$

$$P_{oh} = a_{35} O_h, \quad (62)$$

$$P_{ch} = a_{36} C_h. \quad (63)$$

Oxygen consumption rate by myocardium is chosen as an independent variable. It can be expressed as a function of work performed.

Next we list the relations for lung component. According to Grodins (1959) and Farrell and Siegel (1973), minute volume is determined by O_2, CO_2, and H^- tensions in arterial blood. The formulas expressing this relation are essentially different in these references. The formula of the second reference is:

$$V_m = a_{37} \left(1 + \frac{a_{38}}{P_{oa} - a_{39}}\right)(P_{ca} - X) \quad (64)$$

where

$$X = \begin{cases} a_{40}[(\text{pH}_a) - a_{41}] + a_{42} & \text{if pH} \leq a_{41} \\ \tfrac{1}{2} a_{40}[(\text{pH}_a) - a_{41}] + a_{42} & \text{otherwise.} \end{cases} \quad (65)$$

The last equation in the appendix of the work by Farrell and Siegel (1973) can be written as follows:

$$V_t = P_o \left\{ \left[\sum_{0=1}^{10} C_{pj}/(2\prod GR_{pj}C_{pj} + 1)\right]^2 \right.$$
$$\left. + \left[\sum_{j=1}^{10} C_{pj}\sqrt{2\prod GR_{pj}C_{pj}}/(2\prod GR_{pj}C_{pj} + 1)\right]^2 \right\} \quad (66)$$

where R_{pj} is the resistance to the airflow in the jth lung segment and C_{pj} is compliance of the segment.

The expression for the respiration rate G follows from the definition of the minute volume:

$$G = V_m/V_t. \quad (67)$$

Tidal volume in a segment is expressed by,

$$V_{tj} = P_o C_{pj} / \sqrt{2\prod G C_{pj} R_{pj} + 1}, \quad (68\text{-}77)$$
$$j = 1, 2, \ldots, 10$$

We designate this equation by 10 different numbers to indicate that one such equation corresponds to each lung segment.

Expressions for O_2 and CO_2 concentrations in alveoli are obtained from conservation laws assuming perfect gas mixing in each segment. O_2 concentration in blood entering and leaving a lung segment are C_{ov} and C_{op}, respectively. Thus, it carries away from alveoli $Q_p(C_{ov} - C_{op})$ volume units per minute. Oxygen is inhaled at the rate of $GV_t C_{oi}$ and exhaled at the rate $GV_t C_{ol}$. Consequently, the rate of change of O_2 volume in a segment is $GV_t(C_{oi} - C_{ol}) - Q_p(C_{ov} - C_{op})$. We divide this by the volume $V_{tj} + V_{dj}$ of a lung segment and obtain the rate of change of O_2 concentration in a segment:

$$C'_{olj} = [GV_{tj}(C_{oi} - C_{olj}) - Q_{pj} \quad (78\text{-}87)$$
$$\cdot (C_{ov} - C_{opj})]/(V_{tj} + V_{dj}).$$

Since $j = 1, 2, \ldots, 10$ in this equation, we again assign 10 numbers to the equation and also do the same with the equations below that describe individual lung segments.

Similar expressions are obtained for the rate of change of alveolar CO_2 concentration:

$$C'_{clj} = [GV_{tj}(C_{ci} - C_{clj}) - Q_{pj} \quad (88\text{-}97)$$
$$\cdot (C_{cv} - C_{cpj})]/(V_{tj} + V_{dj}).$$

O_2 and CO_2 tensions in lung segments are obtained from their concentrations and barometric pressure P_b:

$$P_{alj} = P_b C_{olj}, \quad (98\text{-}107)$$

$$P_{clj} = P_b C_{clj}. \quad (108\text{-}117)$$

This completes the list of relations for lung segments. The remaining variables of these components are independent (endogenous) variables. Besides these, we have here three input (exogenous) variables, O_2 and CO_2 concentrations in inhaled air and atmospheric pressure.

The first variable of the coronary circuit, the rate of the blood flow is given by Poisseuille's law:

$$Q_c = (P_{as} - P_{vs})/R_c. \quad (118)$$

O_2 and CO_2 tensions in coronary end-capillary blood are assumed to differ by constant amounts from the respective tensions in myocardial tissue. Thus, we write:

$$P_{oc} = P_{oh} + a_{37}, \quad (119)$$

$$P_{cc} = P_{ch} - a_{38}. \quad (120)$$

According to Farrell and Siegel (1973) oxyhemoglobin saturation $S_c(\%)$ is approximated in terms of O_2, CO_2, and H^- tensions and blood temperature T by the following relation:

$$S_c = 100 \, (a_{39}y + a_{40}y^2 + a_{41}y^3 + y^4)/ \quad (121)$$
$$(a_{42} + a_{43}y + a_{44}y^2 + a_{45}y^3 + y^4),$$

where y is an abbreviation for the following:

$$y = P_{oc}[a_{46} \exp(a_{47}T + a_{48}(pH_c)) + a_{49}P_{cc}]. \quad (122)$$

This together with hemoglobin H and hematocrit H_t is used (Farrell and Siegel, 1973) to express oxygen concentration by an empiricial formula which is adopted here for oxygen concentration O_{vc} in venous coronary blood:

$$C_{oc} = a_{50}HS_c + a_{51}P_{oc} + a_{52}P_{oc}H_t. \quad (123)$$

CO_2 concentration in coronary venous blood is obtained by adopting the corresponding equation in the reference:

$$C_{cc} = [(a_{53} + a_{54}S_c + a_{55}(pH_c)$$
$$+ a_{56}(pH_c)^2 + a_{57}(pH_c)S_c + a_{58}(pH_c)^2 S_c)H_t \quad (124)$$
$$+ a_{59}H_t + a_{60}]C_{cpc},$$

where C_{cpc} is CO_2 concentration in coronary blood plasma given by the Henderson-Hasselbach relation:

$$C_{cpc} = (a_{61} + a_{62}T + a_{63}T^2) \quad (125)$$
$$\cdot \{1 + \exp[a_{64} ((pH_c) - (pK_c))]\} P_{cc}.$$

By adapting the corresponding equations of the reference to coronary venous blood, we obtain:

$$pH_c = pK_c + \log D_c - \log(a_{61} + a_{62}T \quad (126)$$
$$+ a_{63}T^2) - \log P_{cc},$$

where D_c is the concentration of carbonic acid and is given by:

$$D_c = a_{64} + a_{65}H + a_{66}(pH_c) \quad (127)$$
$$+ a_{67}H(pH_c) + a_{68}HS_c.$$

We also have in the reference:

$$pK_c = a_{69} + a_{70}(pH_c) + a_{71}T + a_{72}(pH_c)T. \quad (128)$$

Simultaneous solution of equations 126–128 defines pH_c, pK_c, and D_c.

The remaining two variables of this component, namely, vascular resistance R_c and blood temperature T, are independent variables.

Systemic venous and arterial blood volumes are defined by the conservation law:

$$V'_{as} = Q_l F - Q_c - Q_s - B_{as}. \quad (129)$$

$$V'_{vs} = -Q_r F + Q_c + Q_s \quad (130)$$
$$- B_{vs} + F_{es} + B_s + B_r.$$

Equation 129 states that the rate of change of systemic arterial blood volume is equal to cardiac output $Q_l F$, less the coronary and systemic flow rates Q_c and Q_s, and less arterial bleeding rate B_{as}. The rate of change of the venous blood volume is expressed in a similar fashion with three additional terms: rate of blood sequestration B_s, interstitial fluid exchange rate, and blood replacement rate B_r.

Systemic blood flow rate is obtained from Poisseuille law:

$$Q_s = (P_{as} - P_{vs})/R_s. \qquad (131)$$

Equations for the variables 93–101 are analogous to the representation of the corresponding variables of the coronary circuit. Thus, we have:

$$P_{os} = P_{om} + a_{73}, \qquad (132)$$

$$P_{cs} = P_{cm} - a_{74}, \qquad (133)$$

analogous to equations 119 and 120.

Equation 134 for S_s has the same form as 121 with the same coefficients and with P_{oc}, P_{cc}, and pH_c replaced by P_{os}, P_{cs}, and pH_s.

Similarly, equations defining C_{os}, C_{cps}, C_{cs}, pH_s, pK_s, and D_s labeled 135–140 are the same as 123–128 with the variables of the coronary circuit replaced by the corresponding variables of systemic circuit.

O_2 and CO_2 concentrations in mixed arterial blood are obtained from conservation laws. The total amount of O_2 entering the systemic circuit per unit time is $\Sigma Q_{pj} \cdot C_{opj} + Q_b C_{ov}$, where the sum represents the rate of oxygen coming from the lungs and the second term represents the oxygen obtained from admixture of venous blood. Thus we have:

$$C_{oa} = \left(\sum_{j=1}^{10} Q_{pj} C_{opj} + Q_b C_{ov} \right) \bigg/ \left(\sum_{j=1}^{10} Q_{pj} + Q_b \right). \quad (141)$$

Conservation equation 142 for concentration of CO_2 in systemic arterial blood is obtained from 141 by replacing everywhere the subscript o by c.

The variables 104–110 in Table 39.1 are defined by equations 143–149 which are obtained from 121, and 123–128 by replacing the variables of the coronary circuit by the corresponding variables of the systemic circuit. This yields seven simultaneous equations. The solution of these equations expresses the variables 104–110 in terms of the following: 102, 103, XXXII, XLII, and XLIII, as indicated in the table.

The simple representation of the systemic circuit can be readily refined by introducing several parallel circuits, as mentioned previously. All that is needed for such a refinement is to add component subscripts to the appropriate variables as in pulmonary circuit, which is divided into 10 parallel segments. The relations for each segment are essentially the same as for systemic circuit, i.e., each variable and the corresponding equations are repeated 10 times with the subscripts added. Of course, variables such as pulmonary arterial and venous blood volumes are not repeated. These are expressed by formulas similar to the formulas for systemic circuit:

$$V'_{ap} = Q_r F - \sum Q_{pj} - Q_b - B_{ap}; \qquad (150)$$

i.e., the rate of change of arterial blood volume is equal to the output of the right ventricle minus total pulmonary flow rate including the bypass rate Q_b and minus pulmonary arterial bleeding B_{ap}, if any. Similarly, the conservation law yields:

$$V'_{vp} = -Q_l F + \sum Q_{pj} + Q_b - F_{ep}, \qquad (151)$$

an expression in terms of the output by the left ventricle, total pulmonary flow rate, and interstitial fluid exchange rate in pulmonary circuit.

Pulmonary arterial and venous blood pressures are given by equations 1 and 8 and the flow rate in a lung segment is:

$$Q_{pj} = (P_{ap} - P_{vp})/R_{pj}. \qquad (152\text{–}161)$$

The rate of admixture of venous blood is:

$$Q_b = (P_{ap} - P_{vp})/R_b. \qquad (162)$$

Variables 116–215 are in groups of 10 with a total of nine groups, each corresponding to a respective variable of the systemic circuit numbered 93–101. The equations expressing the variables in a group are analogous to the equation for the corresponding variable of systemic circuit. Thus, O_2 and CO_2 tensions P_{op} and P_{cp} in end capillaries are expressed by equations 163–172 and 173–182 with additional model parameters a_{75} and a_{76}. These equations are analogous to 132 and 133.

The equations for the remaining seven types of variables are labeled 183–252, as indicated in Table 39.1. These are obtained from 134–140 by substituting variables of lung segments for those of systemic circuits.

Expressions for the last two variables of the pulmonary circuit are obtained from a conservation law in the same way as equations 141 and 142 for the corresponding systemic variables:

$$C_{ov} = (Q_c C_{oc} + Q_s C_{os})/(Q_c + Q_s), \qquad (253)$$

$$C_{cv} = (Q_c C_{cc} + Q_s C_{cs})/(Q_c + Q_s). \qquad (254)$$

These complete the set of equations defining the dependent variables. The endogenous independent variables R_{pj} and C_{pj} can be manipulated to represent various degrees of embolism and pulmonary edema. Their dependence on other factors such as anoxia, lung congestion, etc., can be introduced by extending and refining the model.

Testing the adequacy of the model equations and determining the values of model parameters require extensive data. However, each equation can be tested separately by fixing all but two variables of the equation and by comparing interdependence of these two variables with respective observations. Also, partial solutions obtained from a small set of selected equations can be used and tested against available data.

A system of simultaneous equations can be interpreted as a feedback model. One can select many subsets of equations from those listed above to define various feedback loops. Such feedback loops may represent known physiological control systems or just a logical structure.

For instance, in isolation from other equations, formula 64 can be interpreted as a feedback equation. Indeed, we can say that here we have a feedback loop that controls minute volume as indicated in Figure 39.5. Here V_{mi} is the desired minute ventilation (input) that is compared with the observed minute ventilation (output) V_{mo}. The tidal volume is adjusted according to equation 64, as shown in the left box of the figure. The system is disturbed by a random change ΔG of respiration rate. The result is the disturbed rate G_d and the output ventilation rate V_{mo} as shown in Figure 39.5 and implied by equation 64. This interpretation of equation 64 implies that the system attempts to maintain minute volume while the respiration rate is changed, which is obviously not the case of the physiological system. However, we selected one of the simplest equations to illustrate how various possibilities of feedback control can be constructed and examined.

A physiologically meaningful feedback control submodel is obtained by beginning with equation 64, which expresses minute volume as a function of O_2, CO_2, and H^- tensions in arterial blood. The feedback model with these four variables is obtained by including equations that define the effect of minute volume on gas tensions. By referring to the last two columns of Table 39.1, we find that the variables pH_a, P_{oa}, and P_{ca} are determined by equations 143–149 in terms of O_2 and CO_2 concentrations in arterial blood, hemoglobin, hematocrit, and blood temperature. The last three variables can be treated as model parameters. Thus, we need two additional equations to define O_2 and CO_2 concentrations. We find in column 4 of the table that the corresponding equations are 141 and 142. By continuing in this fashion we select equations that relate gas concentrations to minute volume. Next we eliminate the variables that are of no interest in this case while holding certain other variables fixed, i.e., treating them as model parameters in the selected set of equations and, thus, arriving at feedback model. This model differs quite considerably from one described by Grodins (1963) because the equations listed above of the venilation process are different from those in this reference. First, the system described here is much larger, consisting of 10 pulmonary circuits instead of only 1. Second, the model described here contains differential equations for gas volumes instead of gas tensions. Third, the dissociation relations adopted here from Farrell and Siegel (1973) are much more complex. Fourthly, we assume that the differences of O_2 and CO_2 tensions across the walls of blood vessels are not zeros.

The model outlined above consists of equations developed by various authors and tested against data of specific experiments. A few of these equations have been somewhat modified here and also a few new relations have been incorporated. These should be tested against appropriate experimental and clinical data. Various conclusions in terms of new hypotheses can be derived from the model by obtaining either closed form or numerical solutions of a selected set of model equations with certain variables kept at some constant values.

Since any system of simultaneous equations can be interpreted as a feedback model, a large variety of such models, besides those described above, can be constructed from the equations of the model in Figure 39.4. A subset of components of this figure, whose interconnecting arrows form a closed loop, provides a collection of feedback models consisting either of all the equations of the selected components or of a part of these equations. For instance, "Systemic Circuit," "Left Heart," and "Right Heart" can be selected as a feedback submodel. In this case the arrows incoming from other components represent inputs to the feedback model and can be interpreted either as control or exogeneous variables, depending on the aspect to be studied.

Thus, the model of Figure 39.4 can be used to study a behavior of numerous subsystems represented by var-

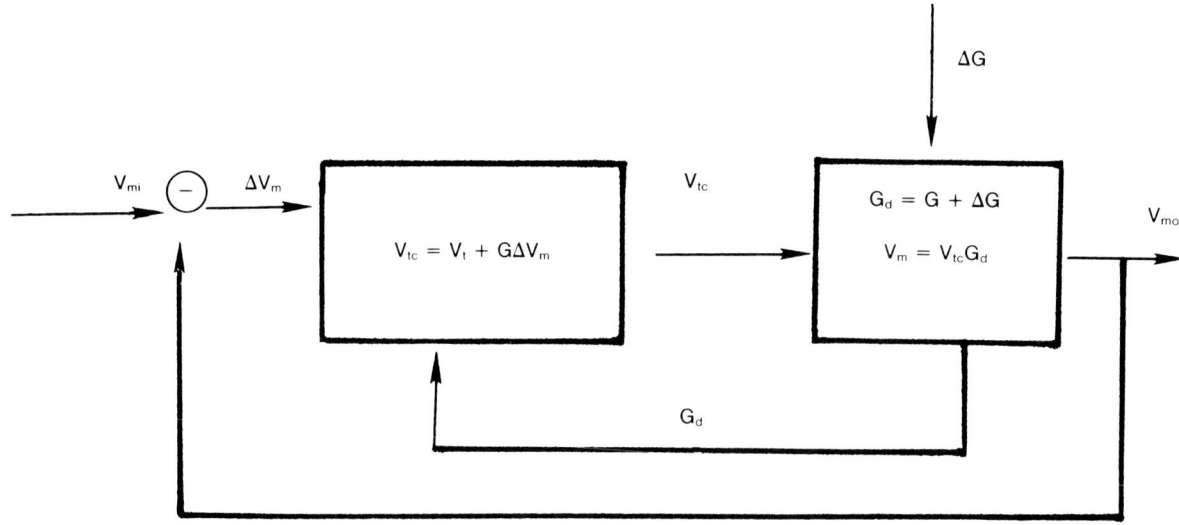

Figure 39.5. Respiration model.

ious subsets of equations. Conclusions obtained from analysis of these subsets of equations provide a description of a system behavior as well as new hypotheses to be tested by further observations and experiment.

The model contains 56 endogenous independent variables. These can be investigated further and additional equations can be derived relating them to other variables of the model.

The submodels from which the model was synthesized contain no relations with time delay. Thus, the synthesized model has no such relations either. Time delay can be readily introduced by inserting a delay operator in any relation represented by a feedback arrow in Figure 39.4. Similarly, a variable may be replaced by the same variable evaluated at a previous time in an algebriac or differential relation, if available information shows a corresponding delay effect. In short, the model outlined in this section provides a large number of topics for clinical and laboratory investigation as well as for mathematical analysis, including numerical solutions of equations under various conditions, i.e., simulation of hypovolemic shock. Such an analysis may provide a useful insight into complexity of hypovolemic shock.

References

Farrell, E.J., and Siegal, J.H.: Investigation of cardiorespiratory abnormalities through computer simulation. Comput. Biomed. Res. *5:*161, 1973.

Grodins, F.S.: Integrative cardiovascular physiology: a mathematical synthesis of cardiac and blood vessel hemodynamics. Q. Rev. Biol. *34:*93, 1959.

Grodins, F.S.: *Control Theory and Biological Systems*, p. 105. Columbia University Press, New York, 1963.

Martin, P.J.: Analysis of myocardial performance in the blood pressure control system. Automatica *6:*175, 1970.

Milhorn, H.T., Jr.: *The Application of Control Theory to Physiological Systems*. W. B. Saunders, Philadelphia, 1966.

Milhorn, H.T., Jr., and Guyton, A.C.: An analog computer analysis of Cheyne-Stokes breathing. J. Appl. Physiol. *20:* 328, 1965.

Pearson, G.E. (Ed.): *Handbook of Applied Mathematics. Selected Results and Methods*, p. 961. Van Nostrand Reinhold Co., New York, 1974.

Poitras, J.W., Pantelakis, N., Marble, C.W., Dwyer, K.R., Barnett, G.O., and Kantona, P.G.: Analysis of blood pressure-baroreceptor nerve firing relationship. *Proceedings of the 19th Annual Conference of English Medical Biologists*, p. 105, 1966.

Warner, H.R., and Cox, A.: A mathematical model of heart rate control by sympathetic and vagus efferent information. J. Appl. Physiol. *17:*349, 1961.

Warner, H.R., Toronto, A.F., Veasay, L.G., and Stephenson, R.: A mathematical approach to medical diagnosis. J.A.M.A., p. 177, 1961.

CHAPTER 40

Design Principles and Objectives for Medical Registries and Other Computer Systems

ARTHUR V. MILHOLLAND

PERSPECTIVE

"Throughout history men have employed elaborate rituals to help them reach a decision. They have poured libations, sacrificed animals, read the stars, and watched the flight of birds. They have put their faith in proverbs and rules of thumb have been devised to take some of the guesswork out of living. Today's management of decision making employs a new and perhaps more scientific ritual, the use of the computer. Unaided, the human mind cannot possibly weigh the complexities involved in the operation of a business enterprise, the design of a missile, or the routing of traffic" (Himmelblau, 1972).

Medicine has not gotten the message, if one may judge from the paucity of rituals that depend upon the nature of the computer for their existence. Except for the CAT scan, the computer's developing role is to improve administrative efficiency and to cut costs. Its place in the art and science of medicine itself is elusive.

The problem certainly is not resistance to new rituals per se—it must run much deeper. Maybe doctors are not very good at quantifying all the ingredients that go into the medical process. Perhaps the process itself defies a systems approach which tries to break the whole into a series of independent subparts. Maybe computer science has not developed the proper tools to fit whatever the problem really is.

Indeed, there often seems to be a mismatch of medicine to computer programming as it has developed so far today. It cannot be expected to yield to the dedicated efforts of either side, totally separate from the other. Nor is it merely a matter of altering a point of view.

Whatever the answer, it seems that a period of uncomfortable growth, side by side, must be experienced before the two accommodate and support one another. The present stage is a shotgun courtship for medicine and computer science.

Until recently, physicians never had the time it takes to make the considerable effort necessary to keep the relationship a healthy one. Many efforts and purchases have been dominated by the instincts, advice, and dictates of a computer system vendor. A large number of unhappy medical buyers now know the "optimistic ostrich" approach does not work.

Of course, it is now common practice to call upon individual doctors and research scientists to draw up needs and specifications whenever a new computer installation is contemplated. They should be provided with an approach, an attitude, to complement their clinical expertise and to guide their actions from the beginning.

For that purpose, let us present the design and implementation of an Emergency Medical Systems (EMS) data registry to serve as a model to develop general principles. Moreover, this particular topic to pertinent to the needs of clinicians and laboratory scientists for collecting their work in a mutually accessible and useful system.

The process begins with a definition of what a registry is and some of the broad purposes for it. Important general issues arise and are presented subsequently.

REGISTRY DEFINITION

From a most basic point of view, a registry consists of 1) the data base itself; 2) ways to enter data; and 3) ways to access the date.

REGISTRY PURPOSE

The purposes of the registry are to:
1. find patients with predefined characteristics (e.g., all with aortic tears):
    a. do some basic comparisons of survival rate and antibiotic usage without revisiting chart
    b. serve as a guide to medical records for data not in registry; and
2. define groups of interest (e.g., what injuries have high reoperation rates?)

DATA BASE DEFINITION

There are several types of data that should be included in a registry:
1. demographic;
2. nature of illness/injury;
3. cause of illness/injury;
4. description of injuries;
5. procedures performed (operations, x-ray, invasive studies, etc.);
6. complications; and
7. outcome data (including stay, survival, disposition)

The form of data which will be coded must be decided upon. In the case of injuries, for example, one might be tempted to develop a new and definitive coding scheme, which has the advantages of being tailor-made for the application.

The alternative is to adapt and extend a coding system

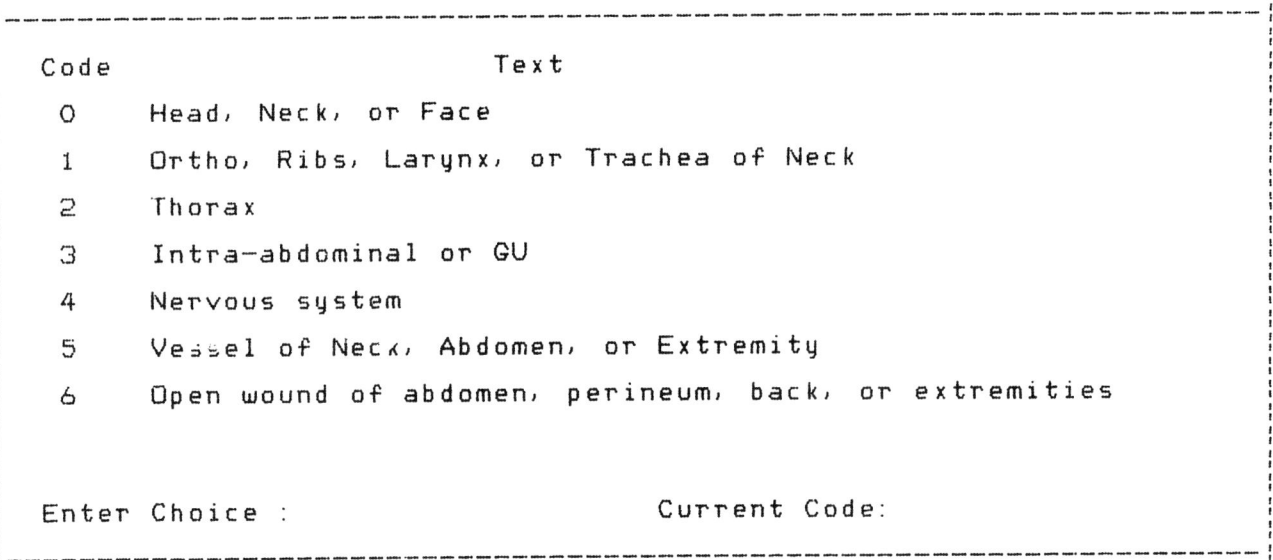

Figure 40.1. Screen 1. General choice screen, does not produce any code. Choose #2 and get next screen.

Design Principles and Objectives

which is standard. This approach may entail some inconvenience but it means: the code-book is available and familiar to many people; widespread data compatibility is possible; and committees already exist to formulate revisions and to distribute them.

Each of the three standard candidates for coded data has its pros and cons:

1. International Classification of Diseases, 9th edition, Clinical Modification (ICD-9-CM) (1979):
   a. categories provided include illness, injuries, causes of injury, complications, and procedures;
   b. limited injury specificity/detail;
   c. moderately awkward logical structure;
   d. requirement of many government agencies.
2. Current Procedural Terminology (CPT) (1979)
   a. categories provided—procedures only;
   b. very awkward logical structure of the numeric codes;
   c. requirement of most third-party payers.
3. Standard Nomenclature of Medicine (SNOMED) (1976)
   a. categories provided (as titled by SNOMED) are: morphology, etiology, function, diseases and syndromes, and procedures;
   b. orderly structure;
   c. provision for user to add categories;
   d. very limited prevalence.

A consideration of scientific, economic, and regulatory requirements may lead to the adoption of a particular system or of some mix of them.

```
Code                Text
 0      (862)   Diaphragm, T Esophagus, T Nerves, T trachea, Bronchi
 1      (901)   Thoracic Blood Vessel
 2      (861)   Heart or Lung
 3      (860)   Traumatic Pneumothorax or Hemothorax
 4      (875)   Open wound of Chest Wall




Enter Choice :                      Current Code:
```

Figure 40.2. Screen 2. This will get a major ICD number, shown in parentheses. Choose #0 and get next screen.

```
Code                Text
 0      Closed  - Diaphragm
 1      Open    - Diaphragm
 2      Closed  - esophagus, nerves, trachea, or bronchus
 3      Open    - esophagus, nerves, trachea, or bronchus




Enter Choice :                      Current Code: 862.
```

Figure 40.3. Screen 3. Note that 862 is shown as "Current Code." Choose #3.

ADOPT AND ADAPT

Whichever is selected, the process of developing a coding system for local use will follow these steps:
1. adopt standard(s);
2. add details by extending the standard (but remain completely compatible with it); and
3. provide for categories of local interest (e.g., county of origin, was patient in the steroid study?).

This process of complete and precise definition cannot be underestimated in either its difficulty or importance. Projects have been known to fail because consideration of some factors was ignored in the planning stages and could not be rectified later on.

For the Maryland Institute for Emergency Medical Services System (MIEMSS) the H-ICDA code (Commission on Professional and Hospital Activities, 1972) was chosen as the basis for all data except procedures and extended to provide increased precision (Milholland and Cowley, 1979); subsequently, this was converted to make it compatible with ICD-9-CM. CPT was chosen for procedures.

ERRORS

Loss of accuracy and precision may occur wherever there is a data transfer. An example of the path from real primary data source, the patient, to the chart, can illustrate this point.

```
Code                Text
 1      Bronchus or Thoracic Trachea
 2      Intrathoracic Esophagus
 3      Nerve of Thorax




Enter Choice :              Current Code: 862.3
```

Figure 40.4. Screen 4. Now the current code is 862.3. Choose #1.

```
Code                Text
 1      Thoracic Trachea
 2      Carina
 3      Main Stem Bronchus
 4      Lobar/Segmental bronchus




Enter Choice :              Current Code: 862.31
```

Figure 40.5. Screen 5.

Design Principles and Objectives

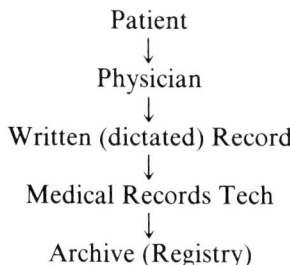

Obviously, each step can introduce error. The physician may overlook some details. The technician may have difficulty in deciphering the written or spoken record. What the technician abstracts must be fitted into the available coding scheme and arbitrarily assigned if no exact category is found.

The magnitude of the final error will be influenced by such factors as: 1) the size of each step or transfer; 2) complexity of transfer methodology; 3) the number of steps; 4) amount of data; 5) elapsed time since occurrence of last transfer (memory decay) (including loss of significance of abbreviated descriptions); 6) perceived purpose of data; 7) personal interest in data accuracy and completeness (motivation); 8) degree of standardization (less imagination); 9) timing of data correction; and 10) degree of data importance (is it operational?).

PROTOTYPE EXAMPLE

The improvement and widespread distribution of digital technology now make it realistic to use computers to

```
Code            Text
  1    Left
  2    Right




Enter Choice :              Current Code: 862.314
```

Figure 40.6. Screen 6.

```
Code            Text
  1    Upper Lobe
  2    Middle Lobe
  3    Lower Lobe




Enter Choice :              Current Code: 862.3142
```

Figure 40.7. Screen 7.

affect almost every aspect in a positive manner. To carry on the injury example, a prototype system does exist at the MIEMSS in which: 1) immediately after an operation (short memory decay time), 2) the surgeon enters injuries directly into a computer terminal (no intermediates) 3) according to a sequence of menu choices (standardization). 4) ICD-9-CM compatible codes are built automatically (no extra step for coding). 5) The compatible codes are extended to include all details that might be of interest for documentation or retrieval (standardization). 6) This constitutes the primary data source during the patient's hospital stay, through a cathode ray tube (CRT). Since it is precisely the data used for care, it is subject to review for completeness and accuracy as part of the care process (operational data). 7) At discharge, transfer to the archival registry is entirely electronic (standardization).

Other systems will be instituted with different emphasis and details, but this should convey the central roles of standardization and the use of operational data, with as few data transfers as possible.

DATA INPUT

Excluding data that comes automatically via automated measuring devices, several types of input modes are available:

1. numeric key pad,
2. standard typewriter keyboard,
3. light pen,
4. touch screen terminal, and
5. voice input.

The device type(s) will be implemented in a system that provides for some combination of: interactive prompting (for physicians and nurses) and straight key-in (for technicians). No one type is "a priori" superior to any other, nor do they all necessarily preclude the others from consideration. The choice will be made in accordance with principles already stated, given goals, and resource constraints.

MAN-COMPUTER INTERACTION

It must be emphasized that the design of the man-machine interaction aspect of data collection is of critical importance. This is widely recognized in the computer industry but, particularly in medical systems, widely ignored. There has been a classic and traditional lack of communication in this matter, with the medical people pretty much taking what they are told they will get.

Computers are too important to be left to the computer scientists, one might say. If the use of a computer terminal is cumbersome or awkward, the system will cause more problems than it solves. It is a great mistake for the "noncomputer" person to leave such matters to the computer programmer or to assume that a proprietary product has addressed these issues successfully. Users must face them directly, in the beginning, before too much money and time are invested. Realistically, there is no formula for success available except for dogged persistence and constant testing, re-evaluation, and revision until the product is satisfactory.

A method of data entry that works well at MIEMSS is representative of techniques that use sequential menu trees for computer interaction. This can be illustrated with a few screens for entry of the injury codes (Figs. 40.1–40–11). The example will indicate some of the detail that can be achieved through this process.

Each figure is a screen on a computer terminal. Choices are selected by striking the number on the terminal key-pad, as indicated under "Code." The ICD-9-CM (extended) that has been generated so far is shown in the lower right corner, and the English translation of it is available at any time by typing "?" (not shown, but similar to last screen) (Fig. 40.11).

Special features to be noted are:

```
Code                Text

  1     Right upper Lobar Bronchus

  2     R upper APICAL segmental

  3     R upper POSTERIOR

  4     R upper ANTERIOR

  9     segmental bronchi, unspecified




  Enter Choice :                    Current Code: 862.31421
```

Figure 40.8. Screen 8.

1. codes develop as the tree is followed;
2. the completed code is displayed in English for confirmation before storage; and
3. the physician can control the registry data, making it as complete and detailed as desired, without intermediate error.

USER MODIFICATIONS

The prospective user must find out how to modify the system to add new features or to remove unsatisfactory ones. This can be done at any level from the source program to the terminals. How much the user can do will depend upon the number and quality of programmers, how often changes are required, and the speed with which changes must be incorporated.

In the EMS registry shown, the user defines the codes and menus that he wants without doing any computer programming at all. The content and presentation are readily tailor-made for each application, either from scratch or beginning with a prototype.

Such a system typically has a rather general purpose program that is individualized by defining a group of tables that control what happens (a "table-driven" system). Obviously, this allows flexibility and independence from the vendor, without requiring an in-house programming staff. Customization that depends upon the continued good will and availability of the seller may be somewhat risky.

DATA RETRIEVAL

The types of data retrieval that are required will be set out at the time of system design and supplemented as

```
Code                 Text
 1      contusion only
 2      laceration w/o loss of a segment
 3      laceration with segmental loss
 4      transection w/o segmental loss
 5      transection with segmental loss
 0      unspecified injury type



Enter Choice :                    Current Code: 862.314212
```

Figure 40.9. Screen 9.

```
Code                 Text
 1      bronchoscopy done -- no mucosal damage
 2      mucosal damage seen by bronchoscopy
 0      unspecified result or not done





Enter Choice :                    Current Code: 862.3142122
```

Figure 40.10. Screen 10.

```
You have entered the following code:   862.31421220

    Thorax
    (862) Diaphragm, T Esophagus, T Nerves, T Trachea, Bronchi
    Open - esophagus, nerves, trachea, or bronchus
    Bronchus or Thoracic Trachea
    Lobar/Segmental bronchus
    Right
    Upper Lobe
    R upper APICAL segmental
    laceration w/o loss of a segment
    unspecified result or not done




Do you want to save this code?
```

Figure 40.11. Screen 11. The injury code is displayed for confirmation, with the English translation of the choices. The user must say whether to save it or not.

time goes by. They are a function of the particular computer system and the user needs.

For example, registry style data banks should provide at least the following basic features:
1. a list of all data for a specified patient—
   a. provide numeric codes, and
   b. English translation;
2. arbitrary unions and intersections—
   a. within and across categories (combinations of injuries, procedures, causes, outcomes);
   b. examples include:
      1) motorcycle and head injury,
      2) gunshot and left or right ventricle, and
      3) colostomy or resection and right colon injury;
   c. survival rates; and
   d. creation of data subsets for further processing and analysis.

SUMMARY

Computer hardware, programs, and medical research and clinical needs are beginning to come together in some very useful and promising ways. Particular care must be exercised in defining system goals and design from the user point of view to ensure that effort and money are well spent. If this is done, it is possible to improve data quality and quantity, to reduce man hours expended, and to improve data retrieval functions.

References

American Medical Association (Monroe, WI, 1977): *Current Procedural Terminology* (CPT), 4th ed. Edwards Brothers, Inc., Ann Arbor, MI, 1979.

Commission on Professional and Hospital Activities: *Hospital Adaptation of ICDA*. Edward Brothers, Ann Arbor, MI, 1972.

Commission on Professional and Hospital Activities: *International Classification of Diseases, 9th Revision, Clinical Modification* (ICD-9-CM). Edward Brothers, Ann Arbor, MI, 1979.

Himmelblau, D.: *Applied Nonlinear Programming*. McGraw-Hill, New York, 1972.

Milholland, A.V., and Cowley, R.A.: Anatomical injury code. Am. Surg. *45*:93–100, 1979.

Systematized Nomenclature of Medicine (SNOMED). College of American Pathologists, Skokie, IL, 1976.

Section 3

Injury of the Central Nervous System

EDITORS' SUMMARY

The chapter by Lindenberg provides a comprehensive overview of the pathology and pathophysiology of head injury and its complications including edema, anoxia and ischemia. For those who do not deal with the myriad of details concerning these phenomena, this provides very important background material. It is evident that although the brain is very susceptible to shock, ischemia, and anoxia, we know very little about the details at the cell level, some of which may differ from those that occur in other organs. In particular, the brain is absolutely dependent on a supply of glucose which rapidly becomes limiting following ischemia. Because of alterations in the cerebral circulation following manifold head injuries, many secondary changes occur due to diminished blood flow. These rapidly complicate many severe kinds of head, as well as spinal cord injury. Still unexplained are the observations reported by Lindenberg which suggest that previously hypoxic portions of the CNS are more resistant to acute ischemia than previously normal areas. The explanation for this is still not apparent. However, our laboratory has repeatedly emphasized the protective effects of reduced extracellular pH. It is interesting to compare the descriptions of Lindenberg on the cell basis of anoxia and ischemia on the brain with the electron microscopic findings in cerebral ischemia mentioned in the next section by Garcia.

Tyson and Jane thoroughly review the pathophysiology of head injury. Head injury defies orderly classification as a single disease entity because of the numerous interacting pathophysiological responses. The authors have primarily reviewed those aspects that are relevant to treatment at the present time. They conceive of head injury from the standpoint of therapy in two stages: 1) the primary biomechanical injury that imposes a degree of reversible and irreversible loss of neural function, and 2) the secondary assault of systemic and intracerebral pathophysiological processes at the cell level.

The authors provide an excellent discussion of the cellular and subcellular factors in cerebral edema and distinguish between the so called vasogenic and cytotoxic forms. The vasogenic type implies a change in the blood-brain barrier while the cytotoxic type results from an increase in cell water due to defective cell volume regulation. Both types occur following head injury; the first is more often due to the mechanical effects than the second which is usually due to ischemia and/or anoxia. These two types of edema may develop simultaneously or in succession in a real patient.

Much more needs to be learned about the characteristics of the normal and abnormal blood-brain barrier. The cerebral capillaries are "tight" but may interact with surrounding astrocytes through their endothelium. The relative roles of vesicular derived intracellular channels versus leaks through abnormal gap or tight junctions remain to be established. Alteration of endothelial cell shape through changes in the cytoskeleton may also prove to be a more important factor in the future than we have previously thought. Following ischemia or anoxia astrocytes and probably later neurons undergo cellular swelling probably due to de-energization of the sodium-potassium ATPase and the Gibbs Donnan effect. This sequence is similar to that occurring in other organs; the exception is the confinement of the CNS within a nonexpansile cranial cavity. This has subsequent and marked effects on cerebral blood flow and other intercerebral dynamics.

The CNS is somewhat uniquely susceptible to ischemia, as it is dependent on oxidative metabolism and specifically on glucose as a substrate. Reduction of oxygenation quickly results in unconsciousness, probably because of limitation on mitochondrial ATP synthesis. Interestingly, an alternate hypothesis for ischemic damage has been mentioned by Demopoulos (1973); this involves membrane lipid peroxidation resulting from free radical reactions which proceed in the absence of molecular oxygen. These may be abetted by phospholipase induced release of polyunsaturated free fatty acids. Along these same lines is the hypothesis that the beneficial effects of barbiturates involve scavenging such free radicals and, accordingly, minimizing cellular damage.

Ransohoff's chapter addresses the problem of spinal cord injury from a pathophysiological point of view. The many important differences from injury to the brain are discussed. Notable among these is the simple principle that since their tracts are gathered into a small space, even a small lesion can be very significant; this is compared to small damage in a cable versus a command post—not to mention the many "silent" areas in the brain. The spinal cord is, moreover, especially susceptible because of the nature of its microvasculature.

Cellular swelling appears to represent a major factor in the damage that results. This usually implies membrane damage, and Ransohoff reviews the role of calcium in this context. Calcium-induced phospholipase attack on cellular membranes can induce loss of phospholipids and release of fatty acids which can undergo lipid peroxidation resulting in accentuation of cell injury. Heme and other iron-containing proteins may catalyze this sequence of events. Ethanol appears to magnify the extent of the lesions.

Therapeutic intervention continues to be a dilemma, in spite of the fact that we know the final lesions develop over a period of many hours following injury. Among the many unsolved problems is the question of delivery of pharmacological agents to the injured area.

The treatment section represents an excellent coverage of the fundamental aspects. Possible new developments include the use of "loop" diuretics to minimize cell swelling, antioxidants to decrease lipid peroxidation, barbiturates which may act as free-radical "sinks," anticonvulsants that may stimulate the sodium-potassium dependent ATPase, and glucocorticoids that may modulate hydrophobic interactions in the cell membrane.

The surgical treatment is also reviewed (see also Ch.

45). In general, the neurosurgeon's role is to minimize the secondary changes that result from hypoxia, ischemia shock, and intracranial hypertension.

It is noted that the Cushing reflex is not always an inevitable sign of increased intracranial pressure (ICP). This is an important point which has also been the experience of others (Nakatani and Ommaya, 1972; Rottenberg and Posner, 1980). Furthermore, it has been shown that there is not absolute correlation between CAT scan findings and levels of ICP (Auer et al., 1980; Harr et al., 1980). These facts strongly support the need for ICP monitoring in order to accurately establish the nature of intracranial pathophysiology and, therefore, to obtain a rational guide to therapy.

The Glasgow coma scale was the first formal attempt to clinically categorize these patients for the purpose of comparing treatment from various centers and to attempt the prediction of outcome based on the score. Since 1974, it has been the most widely used system. It should be mentioned, however, that the scale has certain limitations.

It has been our experience at the Maryland Institute that although the Glasgow scale is good for identifying acute severe outcomes, it is too limited to measure daily variations in neurological functions on which to base immediate changes in therapy. Subsequently, we have developed an expanded Maryland coma scale that contains more neurological parameters and takes account of lateralizing signs and associated injuries (Salcman et al., 1980). Other neurotraumatologists have also expressed concern over the limitations of the Glasgow scale, and ours is not the only center that has attempted to develop an expanded scale (Yen et al., 1978; Obrist et al., 1979).

The initial evaluation of the head injured patient must include a lateral cervical spine film. This is of utmost importance. At out center, the incidence of associated spinal injury with severe head injury is approximately 5%; if the head injury proves fatal, the incidence is near 20%. Some reports show as high as a 24% incidence of occult spine injuries in the fatal multiple injure population (Bucholz et al., 1979).

The medical management outlined by Ransohoff is consistent with most neurotraumatologists thinking. Appropriate emphasis has been placed upon techniques to control intracranial pressure, respiratory status, and biochemical homeostasis. The use of glucocorticoids remains a controversial issue. However, the majority of centers continue the use of these agents. Recently, we advocated the initiation of steroid therapy on all significant head injuries at the time of admission. Continuation after 3 days is dictated by the patient's clinical response to the overall therapeutic regimen. If the patient has shown neurological improvement within 3 days, the steroids are continued for 7–10 days. If there is not improvement, the steroids are discontinued after 3 days. This is based on a previous randomized clinical trial of 100 patients in which there was a statistical trend that implied that patients who responded within the first 3 days were associated with a better outcome if they received steroids; the patients who did not respond in that time were associated with a worse outcome if they were on steroids. In other words, the data suggested that the response to steroids may be different for different patient groups (Saul et al., 1980).

High dose barbiturate therapy for control of elevated intracranial pressure is a promising adjunct to head injury management. At the present time, several randomized clinical trials are being conducted at multiple centers. The true efficacy of this modality remains to be proven. Caution should be exercised in using this technique until the question is answered (see also Ch. 29). This is mainly due to the potential cardiopulmonary complications and the need for advanced physiological monitoring associated with this therapy.

The levels at which ICP is treated vary from center to center. If the ICP is 16–24 mm Hg at rest, the patient is given mannitol therapy and cerebrospinal fluid is drained from the ventricles if an intraventricular catheter is in place. If ICP is greater than 25 mm Hg, the patient is entered into our randomized barbiturate study. As noted in this chapter, some people will begin treating increased ICP at 20 mm Hg.

The surgical treatment of head injuries is quite accurately described in this chapter. We agree emphatically with the need to replace bone flaps in craniotomies for trauma. Recently, Cooper et al. (1980) have shown evidence that large decompressive craniotomies actually enhance edema formation.

A final word should be given to the importance of controlling all other body systems in patients with severe head injury. A deterioration in *any other system* (vascular, infectious, metabolic, etc.) can worsen the outcome or impede the recovery of these patients.

Young and Becker present a thorough summary of the pathophysiology of acute spinal cord injury. Their description of the histopathological, vascular, metabolic, and biochemical changes that occur following cord injury is both clear and representative of the current thoughts on this subject.

Of particular importance is the concept of changes in spinal cord blood flow and the time interval in which these take place. The implications are that if we are to have any beneficial effect on the recovery of spinal cord injury, it will be by intervening during this acute phase with appropriate therapeutic endeavors aimed at the pathophysiology. Our agreement with this will become obvious in the following chapter.

Damage to the microvascular occurs easily after injury. This includes separation of endothelial junctions, platelet aggregates, and small thrombi. Early metabolic changes are similar to those described in other organs, and elevations of calcium is also described here. Alteration of sodium-potassium ATPase has been described and membrane peroxidation suggested. Ischemia is also supported by newer methods for assessing blood flow.

Finally, it is necessary to address the role of biogenic amines in spinal cord injury. As pointed out by the authors, there is not definite agreement in regards to the

Osterholm et al. opinion that the excessive accumulation of certain catacholamines at the injury site contributes to the pathological process. If anything, the majority of investigators refute this. Recently Alderman et al. (1980) reassessed this issue with refined assay techniques. Replication of the experiment has demonstrated a net depression in local tissue norepinephrine after injury with essentially no change in dopamine levels. They conclude that "the results of earlier studies ... were apparently artifactual presumably due to the nonselective nature of the biochemical assay used at that time." Dr. Osterholm's publication of his reanalysis is to be commended.

Saul and Ducker have provided us with the pathophysiology of spinal cord injury. This field has been generally the domain of the neurosurgeon or orthopedic surgeon. Both agree that the area of spinal injury should be immediately immobilized. When problems occur, both specialties have, in the case of multiple injury, tended to ignore related problems as they approach their own special concerns. For example, the neurosurgeon might be so interested in getting a myelogram performed that he does not realize the patient may be dying from a ruptured spleen or lacerated liver.

We have managed this problem by insisting that the trauma team leader, as the member responsible for the patient's total welfare, insist first on a neurological survey by the neurosurgeon, at the same time bringing in the orthopedic surgeon as a consultant. Thus, both services work together to provide expeditious evaluation and management of a patient's sustaining spinal column and/or spinal cord injuries. The two services pool their experience and expedite in order to provide optimal management of the victim.

References

Alderman, J.L., Osterholm, J.L., DeAmore, B.R., Williams, H.D., et al: Catecholamine alterations attending spinal cord injury: A reanalysis. Neurosurgery 6:412–417, 1980.

Auer, L., Oberbuer, R., Tritthart, H., et al.: Relevance of CAT-SCAN for the level of ICP in patients with severe head injury. In *Intracranial Pressure IV*, pp. 45–47. Springer-Verlag, Berlin, 1980.

Bucholz, R., Burkhead, W.Z., Graham, W., Petty, C., et al.: Occult cervical spine injuries in fatal traffic accidents. J. Trauma 19:768–771, 1979.

Cooper, P.R., Hagler, H., and Clark, W.: Decompressive craniotomy, ICP and brain edema. In *Intracranial Pressure IV*. Springer-Verlag, Berlin, 1980.

Demopoulos, H.B.: The basis of free radical pathology. Fed. Proc. 32: 1859–1861, 1979.

Harr, F.L., Sadhu, V.K., Pinto, R.S., et al.: Can CAT SCAN findings predict intracranial pressure in closed head injury patients? In *Intracranial Pressure IV*, pp. 48–53. Springer-Verlag, Berlin, 1980.

Jennett, B., Teasdale, G., Braakman, R., Minderhoud, J., Heiden, J., Kreize, T.: Prognosis of patients with severe head injury. Neurosurgery 4:283–289, 1979.

Nakatani, S., and Ommaya, A.K.: A critical rate of cerebral compression. In *Intracranial Pressure*, edited by M. Brock. Springer-Verlag, Berlin, 1972.

Obrist, W.D., Gennarelli, T.A., Segawa, H., Dolinskas, C.A., and Langfitt, T.W.: Relation of cerebral blood flow to neurological status and outcome in head-injured patients. J. Neurosurg. 51(3): 292–300, 1979.

Rottenberg, D.A., and Posner, J.B.: Intracranial pressure control. In *Anesthesia and Neurosurgery*, edited by J.E. Cottrell and H. Turndoff. C.V. Mosby, St. Louis, 1980.

Salcman, M., Shepp, R.S., and Ducker, T.B.: Calculated recovery rates in severe head injury. J. Neurosurg., submitted, 1980.

Saul, T.G., Ducker, T.B., Salcman, M., et al.: Steroids in severe head injury: A prospective randomized clinical trial. J. Neurosurg., submitted, 1980.

Yen, J.K., Bourke, R.S., Nelson, L.R., Popp, A.J., et al.: Numerical grading of clinical neurological status after serious head injury. J. Neurol. Neurosurg. Psychiat. 41:1125–1130, 1978.

CHAPTER 41

Pathology of Head Injury

RICHARD LINDENBERG

In accordance with the purpose of this book, the present chapter deals chiefly with those aspects of the pathology of craniocerebral injury that may be of practical value to the clinician at the bedside. Information on pathological details, not included in the text, is available elsewhere (Lindenberg, 1971, 1977, 1980).

GENERAL CONSIDERATIONS

In persons who survive a head injury for an hour or longer, three different types of lesions may be encountered: 1) pretraumatic alterations, 2) primary traumatic lesions, and 3) post-traumatic or secondary changes.

Pretraumatic Alterations

These alterations consist of natural diseases or old traumatic lesions. In some of our cases a small angioma or an incipient glioma in an epileptogenic area, such as the limbic brain, precipitated the accident by triggering a psychomotor or generalized epileptic attack. Lesions involving the central visual pathways have contributed to fatal accidents (Freytag and Sacks, 1968). More importantly, a pre-existing disease and not an assumed traumatic damage of the brain may be the true cause of a patient's critical condition and death. This is exemplified by the case of a man who was unconscious when admitted to a hospital and had an external injury of the head. The brain was found to be swollen upon craniotomy. Probing for a hematoma was negative. In spite of all efforts the patient died on the 4th day. As cause of his condition and death we found a bilateral temporal lobe encephalitis indicative of herpes simplex infection. He had no intracranial traumatic lesions.

Primary Traumatic Lesions

The word primary signifies that these lesions originate from mechanical stress at the very moment of injury. They consist of cutaneous injuries, skull fractures, intracranial but extracerebral bleedings, brain lacerations or wounds, brain contusions, and indirect circulatory lesions. More precisely, they consist of various subclassifications of each of the lesions listed.

CUTANEOUS INJURIES

The external lesions are to be divided into four categories: 1) wounds caused by penetrating or perforating force; 2) lacerated wounds from blunt force; 3) abrasions of the epidermis, also called brush burns; and 4) bruises or contusions signifying subcutaneous hemorrhage and/or edema. The lesions of each category can be differentiated again according to the specifics of their pattern. How analysis of the pattern permits one to arrive at conclusions regarding the manner in which the person was injured has been described in detail by Spitz (1980).

SKULL FRACTURES

They result from tearing rather than from compression of the bone during sudden deformation of the skull. Fractures restricted to the area of skull depression by the impact are called *direct* fractures. Linear fractures usually converging to the area of impact and those involving the base of the skull are referred to as *indirect* fractures. They are caused by an outbending of the skull peripheral to the area depressed or flattened by the impact. The fractures commence distant to the site of impact and burst open to the outside. The dura may separate from the bone and thus create the condition for the development of an extradural hematoma. It may tear and permit arachnoidal tissue and even an artery as large as the basilar artery (Loop et al., 1964) or a vertebral artery (Lindenberg, 1966) to slip into the gaping fracture and be trapped. Fracturing consumes energy and often protects the brain from being seriously damaged.

INTRACRANIAL EXTRACEREBRAL BLEEDINGS

These lesions include extradural (epidural), subdural, subarachnoid, and intraventricular hemorrhages and hematomas. The word hemorrhage denotes minor bleeding. Hematomas of these types of bleeding are more frequent in injuries from blunt force than from penetrating force.

BRAIN WOUNDS OR LACERATIONS

These lesions are caused by penetrating or perforating objects. They are called open injuries, because the dura, a natural barrier against intracranial invasion of infective agents, is lacerated. Usually skin and skull are penetrated. However, a seemingly closed injury may actually be open if one of the cranial sinuses is fractured and a bone fragment has lacerated the dura, the arachnoid, and perhaps the brain. Escape of CSF from nose, mouth, or ear and an aerocele indicate that the injury is open.

BRAIN CONTUSIONS

The term contusion stands for all those traumatic lesions that occur while the dura and often the skull remain intact. They dominate the pathologic scene in injuries from blunt force but also occur in open injuries at a distance from wounds. Their cause is local mechanical stress, most often from shearing, that exceeded the cohesive strength of vessel walls, of cells and their processes, or of the tissue as a whole. Accordingly, contusions consist of three separate entities: hemorrhages, necroses, and tears. Contusion hemorrhages may enlarge to hematomas, but contusion necroses and tears reach their ultimate size at the moment of injury.

INDIRECT CIRCULATORY NECROSES

In contrast to secondary post-traumatic necroses, these lesions originate at the time of injury when blood flow through a traumatized artery, vein, or dural sinus is instantaneously interrupted.

Secondary Post-Traumatic Changes

Most of these changes are the result of systemic and/or focal circulatory deficiencies. They are of foremost importance and may develop within minutes after the injury but often commence while the patient is already under the care of a physician. Other secondary alterations are post-traumatic hydrocephalus of various causes and inflammatory conditions due to infection.

These brief outlines illustrate the complexity of the pathology of craniocerebral injury. The subsequent text provides more detailed information, first on each of the intracranial primary lesions in the order in which they were mentioned above. Thereafter, the secondary alterations of circulatory origin will be the principal topic of discussion.

INTRACRANIAL PRIMARY LESIONS

Extradural Hematoma

Extradural hemorrhage does occur but is of interest only to the pathologist. Of clinical importance are the extradural hematomas. They can be expected in 2% of all patients hospitalized because of head injury (Hooper, 1954; Gurdjian and Webster, 1958). They are more frequent in medicolegal autopsies because many patients die without having been admitted to a hospital. Freytag (1963a) found them in 15% of 1367 casualties from head injury by blunt force. What is more significant, they were present in 22% of all cases that had skull fracture and only in 1% (four cases) of all those without a fracture.

The fractures are almost always indirect and linear. By bursting open to the outside, the bone pulls away from the dura, creating an extradural space. This space is requisite for the development of a hematoma. In rare instances the dura may separate without fracture if the skull is very resilient or if dehiscence of a suture has occurred (Mealey, 1960). The hematoma may derive from an injured meningeal artery, as is often the case, or from a lacerated dural sinus. Additional bleeding may be from small meningeal vessels ripped out of the bone. How fast a hematoma enlarges depends, among other factors, on the size of the traumatic extradural space. The fact that some hematomas are fatal within an hour or two after the injury—the shortest interval in our cases was 30 min—suggests that the extradural space was rather large and that the accumulating mass of blood did not have to separate much additional dura by its own pressure to reach its ultimate size.

Approximately 70% of all hematomas originate from branches of a middle meningeal artery, and most of them are located over the middle third of the convexity of the underlying hemisphere (Lewin, 1953). If the stem of the artery is injured, most of the blood accumulates beneath the anterior temporal lobe before it reaches the lower temporal convexity. A hematoma deriving from the ethmoidal artery extends over frontal pole and beneath adjacent orbital convolutions. A rent in a dural sinus may be responsible for a hematoma over the posterior part of a hemisphere and is often the source of a posterior fossa hematoma. The latter hematomas represent approximately 2–3% of all extradural hematomas.

Most hematomas are unilateral. Crossing of the midline requires separation of the superior or occipital sinus. Separation of one or both transverse sinuses and of the torcular herophili is not rare with posterior fossa hematomas because they often extend above the level of the tentorium and compress one or both occipital poles.

Almost all extradural hematomas occur in blunt force injuries. The force of impact is often moderately severe and produces only a few small coup or contrecoup contusions, if any at all. Sometimes the impact is not even concussive. Occasionally, however, it may have caused a second, usually ipsilateral extradural or a contralateral subdural hematoma or both.

As with all unilateral space-occupying lesions above the tentorium, herniation of the uncus occurs and is known to produce the lateralizing sign of a dilated pupil not reacting to light and accommodation by exerting pressure on the parasympathetic fibers in the oculomotor nerve. Laterally located extradural hematomas produce the herniation more readily than those over the frontal region. Herniation may come late with posteriorly located hematomas and is absent or insignificant with posterior fossa hematomas. This is the reason why the latter hematomas may produce pupillary changes but never the lateralizing sign. If it is present it is indicative of an additional lesion above the tentorium.

Dysfunction of the midbrain is the most dangerous consequence, as it is with any other supratentorial space-taking process. It is responsible for coma and decerebration and leads to depression of respiration, the most frequent cause of death. It may be brought on by the herniating hippocampal gyrus pressing on the midbrain and pushing it across the midline against the contralateral margin of the tentorium. The margin may injure the peduncle and thus produce Kernohan's crus syndrome. Hematomas depressing the upper hemispheric convexity tend to cause an early caudal shift of the ipsilateral half of the midbrain, distorting its symmetry. If the midbrain is not relieved early from these stresses it may rather rapidly be damaged by secondary circulatory alterations (to be discussed later). In cases of posterior fossa hematomas, the tegmentum of the midbrain may also be pressed upon by rostral cerebellum becoming wedged into the posterior opening of the tentorium. This may affect the level of consciousness but rarely causes other midbrain signs. Life is endangered in these cases by pressure exerted on the medulla oblongate by displaced cerebellum. Arrest of respiration is sometimes unexpectedly sudden. Signs of upper motor neuron dysfunction in these cases may be attributable to one or both pyramids being pressed against lower clivus or ventral rim of the foramen magnum. Obliteration of the exits of the fourth ventricle causes internal hypertensive hydrocephalus. Removal of CSF by ventricular or lumbar puncture proved to be catastrophic in our cases.

In rare instances the onset of signs and symptoms is delayed for 1 week or more (Turnbull, 1944; Rowbotham and Whalley, 1952; Irsigler, 1958). This chronic form of the hematoma may be caused by a temporary cessation of the bleeding or by a late enlargement of an existing lesion secondary to disintegration of the clot.

Subdural Hematoma

It is not unusual to find a sheet of fresh blood in the subdural space. When old, it constitutes a thin, brownish membrane. Because it contains numerous sinusoidal blood vessels, it is a potential source of a spontaneous, otherwise unexplainable subdural hematoma.

Subdural hematomas can be expected to be present in 5% of all patients hospitalized because of head injury. Most of them occur in injuries from blunt force. At autopsy they have been found as the sole traumatic lesion in 7% of such injuries. In 79% of these hematomas, the skull remained intact (Freytag, 1963a).

The cause of a subdural hematoma may be a blow or a fall on head or face or even a step into an unsuspected hole or a fall on the buttocks. The force of impact may be so mild that it produces no external injury. It may enlarge and produce stupor and unconsciousness as fast as the average extradural hematoma. If the bleeding is less acute and the pressure on the brain less severe, there may be only mental changes, among them loss of spontaneity, forgetfulness, hallucinations, and confusion. The patient is still able to answer questions, but his answers should not be taken seriously, particularly those regarding the traumatic event.

In impacts not deforming the head, the source of the hematoma is most likely a tear in a bridging vein, i.e., in a cerebral vein as it traverses the subdural space on its way to a sinus. The tear is brought on by a brief oscillation of the cerebral hemispheres within their compartments upon sudden acceleration or deceleration of the skull. Pudenz and Shelden (1946) were the first to observe these brain movements through lucid calvaria implanted in monkeys. They used nonconcussive blows to the movable head. One of the animals developed subdural bleeding from an injured bridging vein. Congenital ectopic bridging veins of the convexity leaving the subarachnoid space at a distance from a sinus are particularly vulnerable. The bleeding may be in part arterial because these veins are often accompanied by an anastomosis between a cerebral and a dural artery.

If the impact causes skull deformation or fracture, the hematoma often derives from other sources. Krauland (1961) could attribute the bleeding to tears in the dura in 26.4% of his cases, to a rent in a dural sinus in 11.3%, to hemorrhage from cerebral contusion in 4%, and to small holes in superficial cerebral arteries in 6%. Branches of the middle cerebral artery emerging from the sylvian fissure seem to be particularly vulnerable to be so injured when intimately attached to the arachnoid proper. The hole extents through the arachnid so that the blood spurts like a fountain into the subdural space, as Drake (1961) observed during operation in 11 of 100 cases of subdural hematoma. The bleeding is usually contralateral to the side of impact.

With rare exceptions the subdural hematomas are supratentorial lesions and are usually situated over the convexity of one and occasionally of both cerebral hemispheres. Their distribution over various parts of the convexity is practically the same as that described for extradural hematomas. The site of a hematoma is, however, not dependent on the location of the fracture. In rare instances the blood accumulates paramedially along one or both sides of the falx and extends beneath an orbital or temporal lobe.

Brain displacement, herniation of uncus and hippocampal gyrus, and midbrain involvement from acute hematomas are the same as with extradural hematomas. A slowly developing hematoma depresses the underlying hemisphere but may not force it across the midline or in caudal direction. Herniation of the uncus may be insignificant. Absence of midline shift in the presence of signs of uncal herniation and midbrain involvement is suggestive of bilateral hematomas.

Organization of the subdural blood is accomplished by cells lining the dura and perivascular cells of nearby dural vessels. These cells sprout first into the adjacent layer of blood and soon also along the outer surface of the hematoma facing the arachnoid. After a few weeks the hematoma is encapsulated by a connective tissue membrane that thickens with time and becomes collagenous and sometimes calcified. However, in many instances it remains relatively thin. The enclosed dead blood is initially friable, then paste-like, and eventually liquified. It does not enlarge by taking up fluid, as has been postulated to explain the phenomenon of chronic subdural hematoma. It is now accepted that an enlargement of an older hematoma is caused by spontaneous or again traumatically induced bleeding into the capsule from sinusoidal blood vessels that were formed in great number during the early process of organization. The bleeding may be so severe that the capsule ruptures. The fresh blood filling the residual subdural space often obscures its origin.

Old subdural membranes or capsules are adherent to the arachnoid only if this membrane was torn and mesodermal cells of the subarachnoid space participated in the organization of the blood. The resulting dural adhesions are known to be one of the causes of post-traumatic epilepsy. Since the arachnoid, when intact, is not permeable for dyes, xanthochromia of the CSF is not caused by subdural but by subarachnoid bleeding.

Subdural bleeding is not always traumatic. Even hematomas may be from nontraumatic causes, such as ruptured angiomas and aneurysms (Freytag, 1966).

Subarachnoid Hemorrhage and Hematoma

Subarachnoid hemorrhage occurs in many nontraumatic conditions but not as often as in head injury. It derives from injured external blood vessels, mostly from small veins, or is part of cortical contusion. It may be localized or diffuse anywhere at the surface of the brain. The blood may soon be carried by CSF to other areas of the subarachnoid space. Where it becomes clotted, adhesions of the subarachnoid space may develop. Adhesions around cranial nerves or roots of spinal nerves may adversely affect their function. Widespread adhesions in basal cistern and around the brainstem may be one of the causes of post-traumatic hydocephalus, another cause being an impaction of villi of Pacchionian granulations with blood, as will be described later.

As a rule, subarachnoid blood dissolves rather fast by lysis. Phagocytosis is usually moderate. Hemosiderin is formed not only in phagocytes but also in marginal astrocytes (marginal hemosiderosis). It may still be visible in these glial cells long after all traces of the hemorrhage have disappeared in the leptomeninges.

More massive subarachnoid bleeding is often related to severe underlying contusion of cortex and white matter. In the absence of such contusion, hematomas are occasionally seen at the cerebral convexity but more often at the base of the brain occupying the basal cistern and its adjacent subarachnoid spaces, an area they have in common with bleedings from ruptured aneurysms of the circle of Willis. The traumatic hematomas originate from injured arteries. Tears in arteries of the base of the brain have been identified at various occasions (Krauland and Stögbauer, 1961; Simonsen, 1963; Tatsuno and Lindenberg, 1974). It is remarkable that almost all basal subarachnoid hematomas are caused by a blow of moderate severity (fist blow, kicking) to the movable head and that the areas of impact are almost invariably the face and the lateral aspect of head and neck. One of three mechanisms may be responsible: 1) oscillation of the brain as a result of rotational acceleration of the head, 2) stretching of the vertebral-basilar system in hyperextension of the head, and 3) a sudden increase in intra-arterial pressure by a blow to the carotid artery in the neck. Fifty percent of our cases (total of 34) died within the first 30 min after the injury, 35% lived for up to 6 hr, and 15% for up to 3 days.

Intraventricular Hematoma

A bloody CSF is not an uncommon finding in more severe injuries. A massive bleeding into the ventricles is rare. It may be caused by a contusion hematoma perforating the ventricle wall. The outcome of such an event is a traumatic porencephaly. The source of the bleeding may also be a tear in the choroid plexus or its affixing membrane, a rent in the ventricle wall, a tear in the ventral corpus callosum, or a rupture of the septum pellucidum. The ventricles may be distended by the amount of blood. In our few cases the hematoma resulted from the head striking a firm object, and the impact area was located above the level of the corpus callosum. The skull was not fractured. The impact need not be concussive, but unconsciousness may develop fast and survival time may be short. Additional traumatic lesions may be absent or consist of minor cortical contusions.

Brain Wounds

Most brain wounds are inflicted by an object striking the head. Others are caused by the head striking a protruding object or by fragments of bone. Their morphologic features vary as much as the shape and size of the objects. Nevertheless, one may categorize them in three major groups: lacerated, incised, and punctured wounds.

Lacerated wounds are usually large and of odd shape. Their margin is very irregular and torn up, in part by bone fragments driven into the brain. In contrast, incised wounds are more or less linear and their margin is sharp and cut-like because they are caused by edged objects, such as a hatchet. Punctured wounds are round or slit-like. The usually small entrance wound leads into a wound canal of the same dimension. Only two varieties of punctured wounds are discussed: stab wounds inflicted by an icepick, screwdriver, or knife, and wounds by bullets fired from rifled firearms. They are selected because some of their features may be of value for clinical considerations.

The stab wounds have several traits in common. The skin wounds are small, look innocuous and may be misjudged in their significance or even be overlooked in the presence of other injuries or when covered by hair. The wound canals extend far deeper than is usually anticipated because once the weapon has overcome the resistance of skin, bone, and dura it needs not much energy for penetrating the soft brain tissue. This is particularly true for stab wounds of the orbit. A wound caused by a thin longer butcher knife extended in one of our cases from an eyelid to the rostral surface of a cerebellar hemisphere. The wound canal being small in diameter may pass through the brain without damaging a neurologically important structure. Bleeding into the wound canal is usually the cause of a deterioration of the patient's condition. Unconsciousness persisting since the moment of injury suggests penetration of the midbrain. This occurred in the above case. If only half of the midbrain's tegmentum is injured and no hematoma develops, the lesion need not be fatal by itself. Brain damage is not always limited to a single wound canal. Occasionally the weapon was wiggled upon retraction and produced multiple cuts or cut-like injuries extending from the original wound in various directions. Characteristically, the cuts are most extensive distant to the entrance wound. Most of these patients die before reaching a hospital.

In gunshot injuries the bullets are usually of small caliber and low velocity. If fired from a distance such bullets may only injure the skin or cause a fracture of the skull without damage to the dura. However, such seemingly inconsequential injury may contuse the underlying cortex and, by injuring a vessel, produce a subdural or intracerebral hematoma (Noetzel, 1956). By bouncing off the skull the bullet may produce an exit wound that may give the false impression of the person having been struck by two bullets. If the bullet passed tangentially through the skull without touching the brain, the underlying hemisphere is usually severely damaged by indirect infarction from injury of superficial vessels by bone fragments.

Most bullets penetrate bone and dura. Depending on its residual energy, the bullet may be arrested on its way through the brain or reach the opposite side. Here it may rest, may bounce back into the canal, or may take any of the courses shown in Figure 41.1. The drawing also shows that right from the beginning the bullet may glide along the inner surface of the skull (inner tangential course) instead of entering the brain. Freytag (1963b) found these variations of bullet courses in 38% of autopsied gunshot cases in which the bullet had remained in the cranium. With its residual kinetic energy still greater, the bullet may fracture the contralateral skull or may produce an exit hole and thus create a perforating injury.

Depending on the velocity with which the bullet passes through the brain, it may push the tissue so much aside that the wound canal expands momentarily. The degree of this so called cavitation is determined by the velocity rather than by the caliber of the bullet. High velocity bullets, although rather small in diameter, may explode the skull by cavitation. The effect of cavitation from regular ammunition is often a shifting of the brain toward the foramen magnum. The shifting is sudden because the cavitation from beginning to end takes place in approximately 4 msec. It often results in contusion hemorrhages in or near cerebellar tonsils and in the tegmentum of the adjacent medulla oblongata (cerebellar or tonsilar herniation contusions), although the bullet wound may involve the faraway frontal lobes. The medullary hemorrhages are not always fatal. They only evidence that the medulla was exposed to mechanical stress. With greater cavitation of a frontal or central area wound canal, additional contusion hemorrhages may be seen in cerebral structures situated above the tentorial opening and the tentorial margin. Interestingly, the distribution pattern of these contusions is the same as that of those resulting from forehead or convexity of head striking a firm object. Tonsilar herniation contusions are rare in this type of injury from blunt force. They occur, however, in injuries from a blow to the head.

Cavitation is indirectly also responsible for fractures of the orbital roofs and/or of the lamina cribrosa. These fractures are not uncommon in gunshot injuries above the tentorium. At autopsy, fragments of the orbital roofs are often found in the orbit, proving that sudden pressure by the brain caused the fracture. The optic nerves may be injured in this process.

Concussive unconsciousness and depression or transient arrest of respiration is probably in most cases also related to cavitation because these signs are often absent when the bullet was unable to produce a longer wound canal. If consciousness is lost soon after the injury it is most likely due to shock rather than to intracranial bleeding. The bleeding is often delayed and not as massive as may be assumed.

Brain Contusions

Contusions consisting of hemorrhages, necroses, and tissue tears are the hallmark of injuries from blunt force and the result of local shearing and/or stretching force.

Hemorrhages are the most frequent contusions. The extravasation of blood into the perivascular space is immediate. With survival many hemorrhages enlarge insignificantly. When occurring in great number

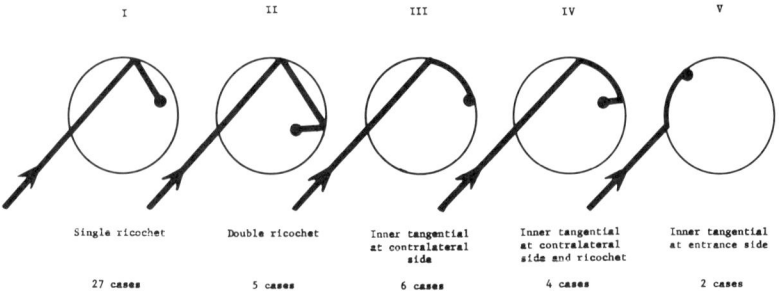

Figure 41.1. Five variations of internal ricochet and tangential course of a bullet. (Reprinted with permission from E. Freytag: Archives of Pathology 76:215–225, 1963.)

throughout an area of contusion necrosis, they may give it the appearance of a hematoma. Hemorrhages from larger veins usually involve white matter, most often that of frontal lobes. They may form composite hematomas by confluence. Arterial bleeding usually forms solid hematomas with the devastating power of an apoplectic hematoma. The temporal lobes are sites of predilection.

Contusion necroses are caused by shearing and not by a circulatory disorder or by the often present contusion hemorrhages. They involve almost exclusively the cerebral cortex at the crest of the convolutions pointing wedge-like toward or into the white matter. They signify that a forceful collision of cortex and dura took place during which displacement on the cellular level proceeded through the tissue with lightning speed and necrotized all cellular elements at once. The necrosis is of the coagulative type. It has other characteristic features that cannot be discussed here. It terminates in crater- and furrow-like defects of the visible surface of the brain, often stained by hemosiderin. Hence their French names: plaques jaunes and état vermoulu.

Contusion tears are rare in the mature brain. They may involve the corpus callosum if forehead or vertex strikes a firm object. Tears of the rostral pyramids at the pontomedullary junction are pathognomonic for hyperextension of the head (Lindenberg and Freytag, 1970). In the immature brains of infants up to the age of 5 months, contusion tears are the principal traumatic lesions. They involve the cerebrum and may be so long that they extend from the subarachnoid space through cortex and white matter and connect with the lateral ventricles. Significant bleeding is rare. They occur in falls as well as in blows on the head. The main reasons for them being limited to early infancy are the soft consistency of the not fully myelinated brain and the great pliancy of the skull. Contusion hemorrhages and necroses are rare at this young age (Lindenberg and Freytag, 1969).

Contusions underlying the area of impact have always been called *coup contusions*, and those occurring at the opposite side of the brain are *countrecoup contusions*. The location of the latter is determined by the direction of the impact relative to the head. Contusions found in between the two are referred to as *intermediary coup contusions*. Additional contusions not related to site and direction of impact are designated according to their own cause. *Tonsilar herniation contusions* were already mentioned under gunshot wounds. Those produced by indirect fractures at a distance from the area of impact are *fracture contusions*. Rotational movement of the brain in the undeformed skull may result in *gliding contusions* along the upper margin of the hemispheres. In the same area *stretching contusions* may occur when the brain abruptly moves against the base of the skull as it does, for example, upon stepping into an unsuspected hole. Stretching is also the cause of indirect trauma of the optic nerves because in arrest of forward movement of the head the eyes tend to continue moving out of the orbit (Walsh and Lindenberg, 1963).

Regarding coup and contrecoup contusions, the following empirical facts are important. An impact of contusing force, if caused by an object striking the unrestrained head (blow), always produces a coup contusion, while a contrecoup contusion is absent or smaller than the coup contusion. Conversely, if such impact is caused by the head striking a blunt object (fall), the contusion is always a contrecoup contusion, while a coup contusion is absent or smaller than the contrecoup damage. Only if the object struck by the head is small and protruding may the finding be the same as that produced by a blow. Finally, if a blunt object strikes a head that is firmly supported, neither coup nor contrecoup contusions occur.

These facts are obviously as significant for a clinical evaluation of a case as they are for a postmortem analysis. Contrecoup and intermediary coup contusions caused by the head striking a blunt object deserve additional comment because they are often responsible for clinical symptomatology seen particularly in patients who survived the injury.

The most extensive contrecoup damage is usually caused by a fall on an area between the temple and the occipital protuberance. A fall on the protuberance may result in destruction of both frontal poles, orbital lobes, olfactory bulbs and tracts, and temporal poles. The clinical signs indicative of this pattern of contrecoup lesions are anosmia and an orbital lobe behavioral change characterized by a lack of inhibition in dealing with others, a morbid tendency to joke and to be prankish, and a lack of being concerned about oneself. With a slight deviation of the impact direction, contusion of the above mentioned structures may be limited to one or the other hemisphere. If the site of impact is lateral from the protuberance, orbital lobes and olfactory nerves may remain intact, and the convexity of the contralateral inferior frontal and central region and that of the anterior temporal lobe may be contused instead. If the dominant hemisphere is so damaged, the patient may have a motor aphasia. An impact to the lower occiput may produce contusion hemorrhages or hematomas solely in the base of the pons, causing signs similar to those produced by pontine infarction or apoplectic bleeding. If such impact was directed toward the tentorium and its opening, the cerebellum, pons, midbrain, and thalami may be interspersed with intermediary coup contusions. A fall on the side of the head may produce a few contrecoup contusions in convolutions facing the falx and its free margin. Since in most of these cases the main force of impact is directed through the opening of the falx, contrecoup damage is by far more severe at the contralateral convexity and may involve the posterior second and third frontal convolutions, the inferior central convolutions, the inferior parietal lobe, and/or any portion of the temporal lobe. Clinical signs may include facial palsy ipsilateral to the side of impact, motor aphasia, and/or sensory aphasia.

It is remarkable that even the most pronounced contrecoup lesions in the cortical areas mentioned are rarely accompanied by intermediary coup contusions. The situation is different, however, if the forehead or convexity of the head above the level of the corpus callosum struck an object and if the impact was directed toward the tentorium and its opening. In injuries of this type, intermediary coup contusions dominate the pathologic scene. They may involve any of the following structures: corpus callosum, adjacent caudate nucleus, septum pellucidum, base of pallidum and putamen, the vicinity of the mamillary bodies including the lower internal capsules, dorsal and ventral thalami, midbrain, and brachia conjunctiva of the upper pons and their adjacent cerebellar cortex as well as the trochlear nerves in between them. Coup contusions may be absent or are small and usually occupy one or both first frontal convolutions. Contrecoup contusions are also small and characteristically involve uncus and/or hippocampal gyrus and its vicinity. This pattern of contusions is most frequently seen in occupants of a motor vehicle who were thrown foreward at the moment of collision, striking the windshield or its frame with their head, and in pedestrians who, being struck by a vehicle, were lifted into the air and landed with forehead or vertex on the windshield or the ground. Thirty-five of 51 cases with corpus callosum lesions described by Lindenberg et al. (1955) were injured in traffic accidents. It is of interest that a blunt force injury to forehead or vertex inflicted by a blow does not produce the deep seated intermediary coup contusions.

In general, the intermediary coup contusions retain their original, often small size and leave focal areas of atrophy (corpus callosum and brachium conjunctivum) and faintly yellow spots without obvious loss of tissue. Only occasionally a contusion hemorrhage may enlarge to a hematoma of moderate size. The clinical sequelae of this type of head injury may be rather severe. The concussive unconsciousness may last unusually long and may be followed by a prolonged period of post-traumatic confusion and delirium. Aside from forgetfulness and emotional lability there may be signs of ataxia and extrapyramidal motor disorder, including parkinsonism (Lindenberg, 1964). These and other signs can only in part be attributed to the grossly visible contusions. As was first shown by Strich (1961), there is usually also widespread microscopic injury of nerve fibers from shearing, particularly in the overall area where the intermediary coup contusions tend to occur.

In regard to the mechanism of coup, intermediary coup, and contrecoup contusions, all theories brought forward so far have been concerned with solving the problem of contrecoup. Already in 1767 the Royal Academy of Surgeons in Paris had offered a price for the best solution of this problem. However, none of the solutions proposed then or later yielded an answer satisfactory to the pathologist familiar with the great variety of the actual lesions. This led us to approach the problem on the basis of the above mentioned empirical facts gathered at autopsy (Lindenberg and Freytag, 1960). Our conclusions are briefly the following.

1. Presence, as well as absence, of any of the three coup-related types of contusion is related to the interplay of two different, impulse-like pressure changes within the cranium at the time of impact. One of them is caused by the initial deformation of the skull (depression or flattening) and the other by acceleration of the head. The pressure from skull deformation is positive and most severe beneath the area of impact where the skull pushes the brain predominantly in the direction of the impact force. In sudden acceleration of the head, however, the inertia of the brain causes a positive pressure where the skull pushes the brain to participate in the acceleration and a negative pressure contralaterally where the skull attempts to pull away from the brain.

2. In a contusing blow to the unrestrained head, skull deformation and head acceleration occur practically simultaneously. Therefore, two positive pressures act on the convolutions underlying the area of impact; but, contralaterally, the negative acceleration pressure reduces any positive pressure that may arrive here from the sudden shifting of the brain along the line of impact force. This is the essential reason why in a blow to the head there is always a coup contusion and often no contrecoup contusion.

3. In a fall, the head is acutely accelerated just prior to impact. Therefore, there is negative pressure between skull and brain in the area of impending impact and a positive pressure contralaterally. At the moment of impact the negative pressure reduces the positive pressure exerted on the brain by the deforming skull, and the contralateral positive pressure is enhanced by the positive pressure from the brain shifting along the line of force. This explains why in a fall contrecoup contusions prevail and coup contusions are often absent.

The rate of acceleration prior to impact has to be greater than that occurring in a free fall because if the fall was from great height (10th floor of a building) and head and brain accelerated at the same rate, producing no intracranial pressure changes, coup-related contusions are often minimal or may be absent, although the skull may be severely fractured.

4. If the forehead or the vertical area of the head strikes a firm object, the flattening of the skull is associated with an outbending of its lateral portions. The flattening of the skull pushes the cerebral hemispheres against the tentorium and the core of the cerebrum into the relatively small opening of the tentorium. This produces shearing forces within the central portions of the hemispheres. Because of outbending of the lateral portions of the skull, the corpus callosum is exposed to stretching at the same time. This explains the high incidence of intermediary coup contusions in this type of injury. However, it is necessary that the head was accelerated prior to impact. If there is no acceleration prior to impact, as in a blow to the top of the head, often caused by a falling object, deep seated intermediary coup contusions rarely occur.

5. A blow to the firmly supported head produces no acceleration and no shifting of the brain because with flattening of the skull in the area of impact there is

simultaneous flattening of the contralateral area of support. This is the reason why coup-related contusions are absent as a rule.

Indirect Circulatory Necroses

These relatively rare lesions are mainly seen in open injuries (Lindenberg, 1948). The ischemia responsible for them commences at the time of injury and may be caused by transection and/or spasm of an artery or by an instantaneous thrombosis of an injured artery, large vein, or dural sinus.

Incomplete as well as complete laceration of cerebral arteries may trigger immediate spastic contraction, as is evidenced by larger wounds showing no trace of bleeding for up to 2 hr after the injury. Under such circumstances, the tissue supplied by distal branches of the injured artery or arteries is in a state of sudden ischemia and undergoes infarction, particularly if spasm is followed by thrombosis. Infarcted tissue swells, and this may complicate the intracranial pressure situation or be the cause of death, although the wound may have been superficial. An outer tangential gunshot, for example, caused laceration of several superficial arteries by bone fragments. In spite of debridement, the large infarct continued to swell and led to fatal pressure on the midbrain 17 hr after the injury.

The brain may not be injured at all if one of the internal carotid arteries was lacerated and thrombosed. One of our patients was shot in the tip of the nose, immediately developed a hemiparalysis, became unconscious, and died 24 hr later. The bullet was not in the cranium as had been suggested by x-rays but in the sphenoid sinus. By fracturing the lateral wall of the sinus it had injured and thrombosed the adjacent internal carotid. The infarcted hemisphere was severely swollen, simulating unilateral cerebral edema. Midbrain compression was the cause of death.

SECONDARY ALTERATIONS

As was mentioned earlier in the text, most of these post-traumatic alterations are the result of deficiencies in circulation. Others consist of internal hydrocephalus and of various types of infection.

Circulatory Alterations

These alterations are known to be the most perilous complications of head injury. They encompass a variety of sometimes inter-related changes consisting of several types of generalized swelling of the brain, of localized, often perifocal edema, and of areas of predominantly gray matter necrosis varying in extent and location and ranging in intensity from selective loss of tissue components to complete infarction.

None of these alterations is specific for head injury. The changes occur just as well in nontraumatic space-occupying conditions and, with the exception of perifocal edema, also in cases of an acute failure of the systemic circulation, irrespective of its cause. Therefore, observations made in such nontraumatic cases are included in the subsequent discussion.

GENERALIZED SWELLING OF THE BRAIN

The word *swelling* simply signifies that the brain is enlarged and that the enlargement is not due to an increase in the number of its cells. The swelling may have one of three causes: 1) global hyperemia, 2) systemic arterial oligemia, and 3) arterial oligemia combined with systemic passive venous congestion.

The *hyperemic swelling* is occasionally seen at autopsy in persons who had died suddenly while in a state of hypercapnia. Because of the engorgement of all capillaries, the brain is heavier than normal and of dark color, the gray matter being darker than the white matter. Sulci and ventricles are narrow. Although the convolutions may not be flattened, the unci are protruding and the cerebellar tonsils may be sufficiently herniated to produce a tent-like deformation of the tegmentum of the medulla oblongata. Microscopic changes in neurons and glia are uncommon. Since hypercapnic vasodilatation occurs fast and simultaneously throughout the brain, it is conceivable that acute deformation of the medulla oblongata by herniating tonsils may occasionally be the cause of sudden, unsuspected arrest of respiration.

The *oligemic swelling* is a common finding in persons who died after acute shock, regardless of its cause. The convolutions of the heavy brain are flattened and its ventricles are compressed. Characteristically it is the white matter that is swollen. It is pale and anemic, as if the brain had been embalmed. The cortex often retains its color, but the basal ganglia are somewhat pale and the thalami may be almost as white as the adjacent internal capsules. The midbrain, bilaterally under pressure by the hippocampal gyri, may be just as white. The unci are symmetrically protruding, and the cerebellar tonsils are often herniated.

The enlargement of the white matter is not caused by edema but by a swelling of the glia, predominantly of astrocytes. Its paleness is due to the capillaries being either compressed or containing only blood fluid and an occasional red blood cell. Myelin sheaths and axons do not participate in the early swelling.

It is little known that this type of swelling, sometimes referred to as dry swelling, may develop rapidly and be fatal within 15–20 min after the onset of unconsciousness from shock. Children and adolescents are particularly vulnerable.

In contrast to hyperemic swelling, the oligemic swelling usually does not involve all of the white matter simultaneously. Our cases suggest that it starts in the white matter of the posterior half of the cerebrum, that it may remain limited to this area or spread, as it most often does, throughout the cerebral white matter and ultimately involve the white matter of brain stem and cerebellum. It is a reversible process, but it may take several days to regress once the systemic circulation is up to par again. It usually leaves no more than a fibrosis of the astrocytes of the white matter. Focal areas of necrosis, mostly in gray matter, are usually secondary to vascular compression, as will be discussed later. Some findings suggest that hyperemic swelling may occasionally have preceded the pale, oligemic swelling.

It is important to note that oligemic swelling develops only if the decrease in cardiac output is acute. If it proceeds slowly the white matter does not swell. The astrocytes remain normal or may be slightly shrunken. This has been observed in persons who had died slowly from exsanguination, from gradually progressing tamponade of the heart, or from gradual obstruction of the airways.

The third type of brain enlargement may be called *edematous swelling*. It also involves the white matter, which is often not as pale and swollen as in oligemic swelling and is moist on cut sections due to the accumulation of fluid in the extracellular spaces. There is reason to assume that the edematous swelling is caused by two factors: some decrease in the output of the left heart and an increase in venous pressure, usually caused by a failure of the right heart. Individually each factor may have no morphologic consequences; but, when combined, the capillary circulation will be significantly retarded and the scene is set for extravasation of blood fluids and sometimes of blood cells, usually taking place on the venous side of the capillaries.

The white, rather than the gray, matter is the site of edematous swelling for two reasons: 1) the capillary bed of the white matter is more distal to the heart than that of the gray matter and is, therefore, prone to show a decrease in supply early; 2) the route of its venous drainage is longer and more complicated than that of the gray matter. The blood of the latter is drained immediately to the outside, whereas that of the bulk of the white matter is collected by the largest and longest intracerebral veins, which converge toward the lateral ventricles, run within the ventricle wall, and then connect with the internal cerebral veins before draining into the great vein of Galen. This explains why, of all intracerebral veins, those of the white matter are sometimes still visibly distended in edematous swelling.

In most instances the edematous swelling recedes after a while. Residual changes may consist only of fibrosis of the wall of small blood vessels and of perivascular astrocytes. A few phagocytes containing lipids or hemosiderin may be present in perivascular spaces. In other cases the edema may be accompanied by necrosis. Incomplete necrosis selectively damaging oligodendroglia leads to loss of myelin and some axons. Complete necrosis destroying almost all tissue components terminates in tissue defects. Both alterations are usually limited to the cerebral white matter and tend to occupy the border areas of white matter supplied by the three large cerebral arteries, most often the parieto-occipital white matter.

LOCALIZED EDEMA

As with generalized edematous swelling, edema occurs locally where arterial supply is somewhat decreased and venous drainage is impeded. This is brought about when blood vessels are under pressure by a space-occupying lesion and the systemic arterial pressure dips to a normally still harmless level. In the area of such a lesion, however, it will result in the retardation of circulation that is required for the development of edema.

The edema may be perifocal, involving the white matter surrounding a larger cortical contusion or a contusion hematoma. More important is the edema of a hemisphere under pressure by an extradural or subdural hematoma. It may be just as space-occupying as the hematoma. It may occasionally be responsible for a contralateral hemiparesis or paralysis. It accounts for a fast postoperative expansion of the hemisphere and its subsequent swelling. Edema of cerebral gray structures is rare except for the striatum, the putamen in particular. Swelling of this griseum may be unilateral or bilateral and may also involve the internal capsule passing through it. The edema occurs when the anterior sylvian fissure is severely compressed, reducing blood supply via the striate body branches of the middle cerebral artery and drainage via veins connecting with the basal vein of Rosenthal.

Clinically most important is an edema of the tegmentum of midbrain and upper pons. It is a not infrequent finding and is characterized by a pale swelling and a glassy appearance of the somewhat moist tissue. It occurs when pressure by the hippocampal gyri interferes with the tegmental circulation while there is little or no caudal displacement of midbrain and pons. The veins involved are the lateral veins running along the lateral sulci of midbrain and upper pons and those leaving the midbrain in the interpeduncular fossa narrowed by the pressure on the peduncles. If compression of the midbrain is associated with caudal shifting of midbrain and pons, the edema extends into the base of the pons and is often accompanied by hemorrhage and focal necrosis. The hemorrhages are due to small amounts of blood entering the leaky vasculature and are not the result of venous engorgement. They are erroneously called Duret hemorrhages. What Duret (1878) had produced by impacts to the unprotected dura in animal experiments were contusion hemorrhages and tears around the floor of the fourth ventricle and the central canal of the upper cervical cord.

NECROSES PREDOMINANTLY OF GRAY MATTER

All lesions falling under this category are the result of an acute deficiency in arterial supply in the absence of thrombosis or embolism. Because such obstructions are missing, some of the lesions, among them neuronal loss in Ammon's horns and symmetrical infarctions in pallida, were and are still believed to be caused by a particular vulnerability of such grisea to oxygen deficiency. The fact is that anoxia as such produces no morphologic changes and that all "anoxic" lesions are the result of a circulatory disorder. The disorder is caused either by compression of blood vessels, mainly of arteries, or by cardiac arrest. Since both causes are transient, the necrotic changes are usually limited to gray matter.

Arterial compression requires the presence of generalized oligemic or edematous brain swelling or of a space-occupying mass and also an at least transient lowering of the systemic blood pressure, if only to a level that would have no clinical consequence under normal intracranial conditions. Veins are more easily compressed than arteries, but venous compression cannot be the essential cause of the lesions because the areas involved by most of them correspond to areas of arterial supply (Lindenberg, 1955).

The arteries most vulnerable to local compression are those crossing directly or at a short distance the almost unyielding margin of the tentorium. These are the posterior cerebral arteries and their cortical branches, the branches of the superior cerebellar arteries, and the pallidum branches of the anterior choroidal arteries. Compression of stem or branches of the posterior cerebral artery adjacent to the tentorium usually causes hemorrhagic cortical necrosis, which may be bilateral and involve the calcarina cortex. These infarcts occur most often in patients with supratentorial mass lesions. In the Ammon's horn, for the most part also supplied by the posterior cerebral artery, the damage consists of selective neuronal loss terminating in Ammon's horn sclerosis, known to be the most frequent trigger of temporal lobe epilepsy. Compression of the pallidum branches of the anterior choroidal arteries explains why neuronal loss or infarction is always located in the medial two-thirds of these grisea, the supply territory of these branches. The lateral thirds belong to the territories supplied by the striate body branches of the middle cerebral arteries. The lesions are most often bilateral in cases of generalized brain swelling. They are not specific for carbon monoxide poisoning. They can be seen in various types of shock, including shock from blood loss. Branches of the superior cerebellar arteries may be pressed against the tentorial margin because the culmen usually extends through the posterior tentorial opening. Thus, a unilateral, supratentorial mass may push the culmen against the contralateral margin of the tentorium, causing neuronal loss in the rostral cortex of the contralateral cerebellum that extends laterally from the notching caused by the tentorium. A swelling of the cerebellum may produce the same bilaterally. Involvement of the rostral vermis in this manner would be the cause of cerebellar ataxia of the lower extremities, often seen in alcoholics. With shifting of a cerebral hemisphere across the midline, branches of the ipsilateral anterior cerebral artery may be compressed by the margin of the falx, resulting in infarction of paramedical cortex, including that of the paracentral lobulus. At the anterior base of the brain, a herniation of the gyri recti into the prechiasmatic cistern may bring about infarction of the cortex of adjacent orbital and parolfactory convolutions by pressing on the respective arteries as they emerge from the anterior cerebral arteries. By being pressed against the sella and its tentorium, the chiasm may suffer central necrosis that extends into optic nerves and tracts. Also pituitary stalk, tuber cinereum, and supraoptic nuclei may be damaged. It is noteworthy that pressure exerted by herniated gyri recti and chiasm on the tentorium sellae often causes necrosis of the anterior lobe of the pituitary.

Necrosis from pressure also occurs without arteries being pressed against a firm structure. Wedging of the mamillary bodies into the interpeduncular fossa may result in necrosis of their neurons and in a tissue syndrome similar to that of Wernicke's encephalopathy. The wedging may also interfere with the arterial supply of the thalami, causing widespread neuronal loss and, occasionally, infarction. These thalamic lesions are more frequently encountered than is generally known and may be responsible for post-traumatic changes in mentation and emotions. Pressure is also responsible for cortical necrosis along the depth of cerebral and cerebellar sulci. Finally, the entire area of cerebral cortex depressed by an extradural or subdural hematoma may occasionally become infarcted due to vascular compression.

These lesions occur often in combination. In trauma they may be so numerous that they are sometimes more destructive than wounds or contusions, particularly when accompanied by white matter damage from edematous swelling. In shock, when occurring in early infancy, they are often the substrate of cerebral palsy. Their occurrence in the locations mentioned above is rather characteristic. This helps in differentiating the lesions from areas of gray matter necrosis of other origin, among them those caused by transient cardiac arrest.

The so-called "anoxic" brain damage resulting from cardiac arrest has a distribution pattern of its own. It is determined by the law of hydrodynamics in an open supply system. As the pressure falls in such a piping system, the supply of fluid dwindles first at outlets most peripheral to the pressure source. In the brain the arteries supplying the parieto-occipital areas are most distant to the heart. Therefore, these areas are the first to be in stasis as cardiac output fails and are the last of all areas to be supplied again as the blood pressure recovers. Consequently, if necrosis develops at all, it is first seen in the parieto-occiptal cortex of both hemispheres and in symmetrical distribution. Depending on the duration of the stasis, further spreading of the damage takes place rostrally along the border zones of supply by anterior, middle, and posterior cerebral arteries and at the same time toward the stems of these arteries. When the necrosis reaches the precentral cortex, the striate bodies become involved. If the necrosis reaches into the anterior frontal and temporal cortex, pallida, thalami, and cortex of the peripheral portions of the cerebellum show neuronal loss, whereas the Ammon's horns may still be preserved. Only if the damage is still more extensive do they participate in the necrosis, as do the remainder of the cerebellar cortex, the dentate nuclei, and many nuclei in the tegmentum of the brainstem. Well before this stage is reached there may already be neuronal loss in the spinal cord, starting in lower thoracic and in lumbar segments.

We mentioned earlier in the text that oligemic swelling of the brain does not develop in subacute shock. The same can be observed in regard to ischemic necrosis. The lesions described above occur only if the ischemia was of acute onset. Necrotic changes do not develop if blood supply ceased gradually and ischemia lasted for hours. This observation was born out by animal experiments designed to shed light on the morphologic behavior of neurons and glia during continuous global ischemia (Lindenberg and Noell, 1952; Lindenberg, 1956). The two most significant results of this study were as follows:

1. In acute ischemia (onset within 10 min) the cells swell at first, the astrocytes in 10 min, and the neurons in 20–30 min. Thereafter they develop progressive destructive changes, seen first in neurons and later in astrocytes. After 12 and more hr of uninterrupted ischemia, the astrocytes are disintegrated (clasmatodendrosis) and the neurons show alterations identical to those seen in fresh embolic infarcts (ischemic alterations).

2. In subacute ischemia, i.e., an ischemia that was preceded by a critical hypoxemia for periods of 1–6 hr, all cells remain structurally normal during 24 hr of uninterrupted ischemia. Changes developing during the subsequent 48 hr are totally different from those seen in acute ischemia.

How can this seemingly paradoxical phenomenon be explained? In view of the second finding, the prevailing concept of anoxia and the subsequent breakdown of energy metabolism being the cause of necrotic cellular changes is not tenable any longer. Instead, the finding suggests that a factor is essential that is present and pathogenetic in acute ischemia and absent or pathogenetically ineffective in subacute ischemia.

This variable factor is, in our opinion, lactic acid or, generally speaking, the intracellular pH. It is known that in acute ischemia the tissue pH rapidly falls below a physiologically tolerable level because ischemia causes not only anoxia but also an end to removal of metabolites. The acidosis provides an optimal environment for an unrestrained activity of certain lysosomal proteolytic enzymes. By splitting large molecules they create an intracellular hyperosmosis. This hyperosmosis seems to be the most significant factor in the development of necrotic changes. In subacute ischemia, lactic acid is also produced during the period of critical hypoxemia preceding the ischemia, but much of it leaves the tissue while perfusion is still active. After the onset of ischemia there may be some tissue acidosis but not exceeding physiological limits. Therefore, the cells retain their normal structure for some time during ischemia.

Whether or not this explanation has to be changed, the above findings are facts that must be taken into consideration when the effect of anoxia and ischemia is the topic of research and discussion.

Post-Traumatic Internal Hydrocephalus

Both hypertensive hydrocephalus and hydrocephalus ex vacuo are seen after head injury. Only the hypertensive hydrocephalus is discussed briefly, since it may be one of the early post-traumatic complications.

It occurs if the circulation of cerebrospinal fluid is obstructed somewhere between the rostral choroid plexuses and the villi of the Pacchionian granulations. If the obstruction lies within the ventricles or at their exits, the hydrocephalus is called noncommunicating; if it occurs outside the ventricles, one speaks of communicating hydrocephalus. Once the passage of CSF is blocked, the ventricles may enlarge in an hour or two, as is known from autopsies and from experiments performed on dogs and monkeys (Milhorat et al., 1970). However, if the brain is swollen prior to blockage, the ventricles cannot distend, although the pressure of the CSF may be considerable.

In general, acute post-traumatic hydrocephalus is not a frequent finding at autopsy and seldom exceeds a moderately severe degree. It may be limited to one lateral ventricle or involve both lateral and third ventricles. Aqueduct and fourth ventricle are usually not or only slightly enlarged.

An enlargement and some distortion of one lateral ventricle and narrowing of the other is the result of an extradural, subdural, or intracerebral hematoma shifting the hemisphere across the midline and thereby bending and compressing the third ventricle. This occurs more readily with a lateral location of such lesion. A large contusion hematoma of one temporal lobe, for example, produced a rather large hydrocephalus of the contralateral ventricle during not more than 4 hr of survival. It is possible that CSF in the ipsilateral ventricle was squeezed via the still open foramina of Monro into the other ventricle and contributed to its fast distention. A unilateral hematoma in the vicinity of the pallidum may compress the foramina of Monro instead of the third ventricle. This may result in some widening of the ipsilateral ventricle and more severe distention of the contralateral ventricle (Mosberg and Lindenberg, 1959).

Symmetrical hydrocephalus of lateral and third ventricles has several causes. One of them is intraventricular hemorrhage and subsequent obstruction of the entrance of the aqueduct by a blood clot or by a piece of septum pellucidum torn off by the hemorrhage. Since clotted blood produces an ependymitis, a post-traumatic aqueductal stenosis may explain why the hydrocephalus enlarged and continued to exist. If the intraventricular bleeding amounts to a hematoma, clotting is even more likely to occur. In such a case, the distention of the ventricles is due to a combination of hematocephalus and hydrocephalus. Sometimes the acute symmetrical hydrocephalus is brought on by an extradural hematoma of the posterior fossa or by a cerebellar contusion hematoma obliterating the exits of the fourth ventricle. The hydrocephalus may be communicating, and acute obstruction of CSF flow may be due to a subarachnoid hematoma collecting in the cisterna magna, around medulla oblongata and pons, and/or in the cisterns at the base of the cerebrum. The organization of the blood may result in dense fibrosis and adhesions throughout the subarachnoid space. This may continue to impede circulation of CSF and maintain the hydrocephalus. Finally, impaction of the villi of Pacchionian granulations by blood from subarachnoid hemorrhage may affect the absorption of CSF, and this may be the cause of a communicating hydrocephalus (Ellington and Margolis, 1969).

Infective Lesions

Post-traumatic infection, formerly a frequent and dreaded complication, has become a rarity among autopsy findings since the advent of antibiotics. It would exceed the scope of this presentation to elaborate on the pathology of the various types of infective lesions. Only the observation is mentioned that it is occasionally the infection and not the injury that precipitates the emergency requiring hospitalization.

It occurs when a person considered his injury to be too trivial to require medical attention and developed the first signs of intracranial infection days later. If admitted in already critical condition there may be no history of trauma. Since the external injury may raise no suspicion, being small or already healing, diagnosis may be a problem.

This is illustrated by the case of a hunter who had injured the upper lid of one eye when falling into a shrub. Feeling no alarming discomfort, he disregarded the injury and did not mention it to others. Two days later he became acutely ill with headaches and was unconscious when admitted to a hospital. A history of trauma being absent and the lid laceration looking insignificant, an acute, nontraumatic space-occupying lesion was suspected. The patient died before further diagnostic tests could be performed. The autopsy revealed a severe swelling of the brain secondary to a necrotizing fungal encephalitis of the frontal lobes. It had been caused by a dead branch of the shrub into which the person had fallen. The stick had pierced the lamina cribrosa.

References

Drake, C.C.: Subdural hematoma from arterial rupture. J. Neurosurg. *18*:597–601, 1961.

Duret, H.: *Études experimentales et cliniques sur les traumatismes cérébraux.* Thèses de Paris, 1878.

Ellington, E., and Margolis, G.: Block of arachnoid villus by subarachnoid hemorrhage. J. Neurosurg. *30*:651–657, 1969.

Freytag, E.: Autopsy findings in head injuries from blunt forces: Statistical evaluation of 1,367 cases. Arch. Pathol. *75*: 402–413, 1963a.

Freytag, E.: Autopsy findings in head injuries from firearms: Statistical evaluation of 254 cases. Arch. Pathol. *76*:215–225, 1963b.

Freytag, E.: Fatal rupture of intracranial aneurysms: Survey of 250 medicolegal cases. Arch. Pathol. *81*:418–424, 1966.

Freytag, E., and Sacks, J.G.: Abnormalities of the central visual pathways contributing to traffic accidents. J.A.M.A. *204*: 871–873, 1968.

Gurdjian, E.S., and Webster, J.E.: *Head injuries: Mechanisms, Diagnosis, and Management.* Little, Brown, Boston, 1958.

Hooper, R.S.: Extradural haemorrhages of posterior fossa. Br. J. Surg. *42*:19–26, 1954.

Irsigler, F.J.: Recent experiences with extradural hemorrhage. S. Afr. Med. J. *32*:187–190, 1958.

Krauland, W.: *Ueber die Quellen des akuten and chronischen subduralen Hämatoms. Abhandlungen aus dem Gebiet der normalen und pathologischen Anatomie*, vol. 10. Georg Thieme Verlag, Stuttgart, 1961.

Krauland, W., and Stögbauer, R.: Zur Kenntnis der Schlagaderverletzungen am Hirngrund bei gedeckten stumpfen Gewalteinwirkungen. Beitr. Gerichtl. Med. *21*:171–180, 1961.

Lewin, W.: Factors in the mortality of closed head injuries. Br. Med. J. *1*:1239–1244, 1953.

Lindenberg, R.: Ueber Erweichungen nach Gefässdurchtrennung bei offenen Verletzungen des Grosshirns und ihre Bedeutung für den Krankheitsverlauf. Arch. Psychiatr. Z. Neur. *179*:483–501, 1948.

Lindenberg, R.: Compression of brain arteries as pathogenetic factor for tissue necroses and their areas of predilection. J. Neurosurg. Exp. Neurol. *14*:223–243, 1955.

Lindenberg, R.: Morphotropic and morphostatic necrobiosis: Investigations on nerve cells of the brain. Am. J. Pathol. *32*: 1147–1177, 1956.

Lindenberg, R.: Die Schädigungsmechanismen der Substantia nigra bei Hirntraumen und das Problem des posttraumatischen Parkinsonismus. Dtsch. Z. Nervenheilk. *185*:637–663, 1964.

Lindenberg, R.: Incarceration of a vertebral artery in the cleft of a longitudinal fracture of the skull: Case report. J. Neurosurg. *24*:908–910, 1966.

Lindenberg, R.: Trauma of meninges and brain. In *Pathology of the Nervous System*, edited by J. Minckler, vol. 2, Ch. 133. McGraw-Hill, New York, 1971.

Lindenberg, R.: Mechanical injuries of brain and meninges. In *Medicolegal Investigation of Death*, edited by W. U. Spitz and R. S. Fisher, ch. 17, ed. 2. Charles C Thomas, Springfield, IL, 1980.

Lindenberg, R.: Pathology of craniocerebral injuries. In *Radiology of the Skull and Brain: Anatomy and Pathology*, edited by T. H. Newton and D. G. Potts, ch. 94. C. V. Mosby, St. Louis, 1977.

Lindenberg, R., and Freytag, E.: The mechanism of cerebral contusions: A pathologic-anatomic study. Arch. Pathol. *69*: 440–469, 1960.

Lindenberg, R., and Freytag, E.: Morphology of brain lesions from blunt trauma in early infancy. Arch. Pathol. *87*:298–305, 1969.

Lindenberg, R., and Freytag, E.: Brainstem lesions characteristic of traumatic hyperextension of the head. Arch. Pathol. *90*:509–515, 1970.

Lindenberg, R., and Noell, W.: Ueber die Abhängigkeit der postmortalen Gestalt der Astrocyten von praemortalem, bioelektrisch kontrolliertem Sauerstoffmangel. Dtsch. Z. Nervenheilk. *168*:499–517, 1952.

Lindenberg, R., Fisher, R.S., Durlacher, S.H., Lovitt, W.V., and Freytag, E.: Lesions of the corpus callosum following blunt mechanical trauma to the head. Am. J. Pathol. *31*:297–317, 1955.

Loop, J.W., White, L.E., and Shaw, C.M.: Traumatic occlusion of the basilar artery within a clivus fracture. Radiology *83*: 36–40, 1964.

Mealey, J., Jr.: Acute extradural hematomas without demonstrable skull fractures. J. Neurosurg. *17*:27–34, 1960.

Milhorat, T.H., Clark, R.G., and Hammock, M.K.: Experimental hydrocephalus. II. Gross pathologic findings in acute and subacute obstructive hydrocephalus in the dog and monkey. J. Neurosurg. *32*:390–399, 1970.

Mosberg, W.H., Jr., and Lindenberg, R.: Traumatic hemorrhage from the anterior choroidal artery. J. Neurosurg. *16*: 209–221, 1959.

Noetzel, H.: Anatomische Veränderungen beim äusseren Schädelprellschuss. In *Das Hirntrauma, Beiträge zur Behandlung, Begutachtung und Betreuung Hirnverletzter*, edited by E. Rehwald, pp. 124–137, Georg Thieme Verlag, Stuttgart, 1956.

Pudenz, R.H., and Shelden, C.H.: The lucite calvarium—a

method for direct observation of the brain. II. Cranial trauma and brain movement. J. Neurosurg. *3:*487–505, 1946.

Rowbotham, G.F., and Whalley, N.: Prolonged compression of the brain resulting from an extradural hemorrhage. J. Neurol. Neurosurg. Psychiat. *15:*64–65, 1952.

Simonsen, J.: Traumatic subarachnoid hemorrhage in alcohol intoxication. J. Forensic Sci. *8:*97–116, 1963.

Spitz, W.U.: Blunt force injury. In *Medicolegal Investigation of Death*, edited by W. U. Spitz and R. S. Fisher, ch. 7. Charles C Thomas, Springfield, IL, 1980.

Strich, S.: Shearing of nerve fibers as a cause of brain damage due to head injury: A pathologic study of 20 cases. Lancet *2:* 443–448, 1961.

Tatsuno, Y., and Lindenberg, R.: Basal subarachnoid hematomas as sole intracranial traumatic lesion. Arch. Pathol. *97:* 211–215, 1974.

Turnbull, F.: Extradural cerebellar hematoma: a case report. J. Neurosurg. *1:*321–324, 1944.

Walsh, F.B., and Lindenberg, R.: Die Veränderungen des Sehnerven bei indirektem Trauma. In *Entwicklung und Fortschritt in der Augenheilkunde*, edited by H. Sautter, pp. 83–107. Ferdinand Enke, Stuttgart, 1963.

CHAPTER 42

Pathophysiology of Head Injury

GEORGE W. TYSON
JOHN A. JANE

More than any other affliction of the nervous system, head injury resists classification as a single disease entity. This is because brain trauma initiates an unprecedented "avalanche" of interacting pathophysiological responses (Ommaya and Gennarelli, 1976). The fact that all of these responses are ultimately expressed through the same limited repertoire of clinical signs belies the variability and complexity of the interactions. It is thus impossible to review all aspects of the pathophysiology of head injury in a single chapter. We have chosen to restrict our review to those aspects of the pathophysiology that are relevant to rational treatment. Our reason for selecting this particular perspective is elucidated below. However, we are aware that we have omitted many aspects of the pathophysiology of head injury that are of scientific interest, direct diagnostic significance, or perhaps even potential therapeutic importance.

In developing a therapeutic strategy, it is useful to conceive of head injury as occurring in two stages. The first consists of the primary biomechanical injury that disrupts the structural integrity of the nervous system and thus imposes a degree of irremediable loss of neural function. However, the mechanically injured brain is almost immediately assaulted by systemic and intracerebral pathophysiological processes that may further reduce brain function. It is this "second injury" that is the proper object of treatment since its deleterious effects on the brain can often be avoided (Rose et al., 1977). For this reason, the pathophysiology of these secondary insults is reviewed in this chapter.

CEREBRAL EDEMA

Edema formation is a basic response of many organs and tissues to injury. The term "edema" connotes a net increase in tissue water content. Although cerebral edema produces volumetric enlargement of the brain, it is only one cause of "cerebral swelling." Therefore, these two terms should not be used interchangably. Furthermore, cerebral edema is not a single pathological entity. Although it may be classified according to the type of injury that produces it (Langfitt and Bruce, 1975), it is most often classified in terms of the pathological mechanism (Klatzo, 1967). The latter classification distinguishes between "vasogenic" and "cytotoxic" forms of cerebral edema. The former involves an injury to the blood-brain barrier (BBB) that permits a plasma filtrate to extravasate into the cerebral extracellular space (ECS). Mechanical trauma primarily produces this type of brain edema (Klatzo, 1967; Reulen, 1976), and it is thus discussed in detail below. Cytotoxic edema involves an increase in intracellular water due to defective osmoregulation. This results from a disturbance in cellular metabolism and/or maintenance of normal transmembrane ionic gradients. This is the form of edema that is produced (at least initially) by cerebral ischemia, which is a common complication of clinical head injury.

These two types of cerebral edema are not mutually exclusive. They may develop simultaneously or in succession after head injury and may be produced by the same injury agent, e.g., ischemia. Furthermore, there is evidence that either type of edema can itself induce development of the other (Fujimoto et al., 1976; Baethmann et al., 1979). Thus, the classification of a particular case of cerebral edema as either vasogenic or cytotoxic is potentially misleading, except in the case of experimental models.

Vasogenic Edema

A wide variety of physical, chemical, infective, allergic, and neoplastic insults may increase the permeability of the BBB and produce vasogenic edema. After head injury, vasogenic edema commonly occurs in the vicinity of cerebral hemorrhages or contusions but may also occur diffusely with minimal gross evidence of structural brain damage. In addition, this form of edema may be exacerbated by hypoxemia, hypercapnia, and epileptic seizures, all of which may occur after a head injury.

Only a minority of what is known of the pathophysiology of post-traumatic cerebral edema has been derived from models of mechanical brain injury. The majority of studies of "traumatic" edema have actually involved a cryogenic insult. In most cases, a low temperature probe has been applied to the skull or exposed dura. The cortex actually frozen becomes necrotic, but the tissue around and beneath it becomes edematous within 24 hr (Klatzo et al., 1965). The advantage of this model is that the experimental conditions can be well controlled and, as a result, the manifestations of this type of injury are reasonably consistent. The obvious disadvantage of this model is the absence of any definitive study demonstrating that the dynamics of cryogenic edema are similar to those of the edema produced by mechanical trauma (Ommaya and Gennarelli, 1975). The analogy to clinical post-traumatic edema is made still more tenuous by the fact that most experimental injuries are largely confined to the cortex. Although the capillary surface area per unit volume of white matter is only 20% of that in gray, there is evidence that white matter vascular injury may be an important determinant of the magnitude of edema produced by cerebral contusion (Tornheim and McLaurin, 1976). Furthermore, experimental injury differs from clinical head trauma in that the former almost invariably utilizes a transient injury of a single type. In contrast, clinical head injuries are usually produced by multiple injury agents, some of which may be momentary (impact damage) while others may be more protracted (cerebral compression by a hematoma). Clinical head injury has seldom, if ever, been simulated by any experimental model (Langfitt and Bruce, 1975).

Further methodological difficulties arise from the fact that most demonstrations of altered cerebrovascular permeability have utilized macromolecular tracers such as horseradish peroxidase (HRP) or protein-bound markers such as fluorescein-labeled albumin. This would pose no limitation if translocations of water—the most important index of edema production—were invariably reflected by alterations in BBB permeability to protein. However, newer experimental techniques have suggested both a spatial and a temporal discrepancy between the efflux of water from the cerebral microvasculature and the entry of circulating protein-bound markers into the brain ECS (Garcia et al., 1979). Indeed, opening of the BBB to protein molecules as a result of arterial hypertension (Johansson, 1976) or as a result of experimental seizures (Petito et al., 1976) is not invariably accompanied by a measurable increase in brain water content.

THE NORMAL BLOOD-BRAIN BARRIER

In capillary beds outside of the central nervous system, polar substances which are not readily soluble in the lipid membranes of the endothelial cells traverse the capillary wall via water-filled channels. These "pores" have a diameter of approximately 8 nm in skeletal muscle capillaries and are represented by interendothelial cell clefts (Karnovsky, 1967) or perhaps by transcellular tubules formed by temporary coalescence of cytoplasmic vesicles (Simionescu et al., 1975). Transcellular transport of high molecular weight compounds in these extracerebral capillaries is by pinocytosis (Palade, 1961).

In contrast, cerebral capillaries restrict the entry of intravascular proteins, ions, and many water soluble nonelectrolytes into the brain. According to Ohno et al. (1978), cerebrovascular permeability coefficients for water soluble nonelectrolytes are 1000 times less than at porous muscle capillaries. Although the existence of very small (8Å radius) cerebral capillary pores has been suggested by osmotic studies (Fenstermacher and Johnson, 1966), the fact that these permeability coefficients are of the same order of magnitude as those of cell membranes and aporous lipid bilayers casts doubt on this hypothesis. Thus, the BBB has the general properties of a cell membrane, with permeability largely determined by lipid solubility. For highly soluble compounds (including oxygen and carbon dioxide), the rate of entry and exit from the brain is limited mainly by the rate of cerebral blood flow (CBF). However, as lipid solubility decreases, the rate of entry becomes more dependent on the permeability of the capillary endothelium. This, in turn, is determined mainly by the solubility of the nonionized fraction of the compound (or the fraction that is not protein-bound). Even the diffusion of water is restricted to a very small but measurable extent. Unlike capillaries in extraneural tissues (for example, skeletal and cardiac muscle), extraction of labeled water during a single pass through cerebral capillaries is not entirely flow-limited at normal and high blood flow rates (Eichling et al., 1974). As a result, a finite permeability constant can be calculated for water. In this respect, the BBB is equivalent to a high resistance epithelium (Bradbury, 1979).

The ultrastructural basis of these physiological properties is provided by the pentalaminar tight junctions (zonula occludens), which obliterate the extracellular clefts between adjacent endothelial cells and which thus interpose a continuous layer of plasma membrane between blood and extracellular fluid (ECF). Furthermore, cerebral capillary endothelium normally contains relatively few pinocytotic vesicles and there is no evidence that these cells normally ferry protein between blood and the pericapillary ECF (Reese and Karnovsky, 1967; Klatzo, 1972). With other routes for transfer between blood and brain effectively blocked, most hydrophilic compounds are transported by carrier-mediated mechanisms. These may be passive (along a concentration gradient), as in the case of glucose, or active (against a concentration gradient, and thus requiring energy expenditure), as in the case of sodium and potassium. These transport mechanisms are saturable and usually stereospecific (at least for the structural class of a compound) and follow Michaelis-Menton kinetics (Sokoloff et al., 1977).

Raichle and his colleagues (1978) have reported evidence that the cerebral capillaries may be under the control of a central neuroendocrine system that regulates their permeability to water so as to maintain brain volume homeostasis. Capillary water permeability is increased by stimulation of noradrenergic neurons in the locus coeruleus (Raichle et al., 1975) which project, at least in part, to cerebral capillaries (Rennels and Nelson, 1975). This effect is inhibited by intraventricular administration of phentolamine, an α-adrenergic blocking agent. Raichle and others (1978) have also demonstrated that cerebrovascular permeability is influenced by centrally-released vasopressin. It is possible that this central neuroendocrine regulatory system maintains normal cerebral water permeability under conditions that might otherwise promote net capillary filtration.

THE NORMAL EXTRACELLULAR SPACE

Water constitutes 80% of gray matter and 70% of white matter, which has a higher lipid content. The majority of this water is intracellular. However, tracer methods (for example, sucrose and inulin distribution) suggest that extracellular water accounts for 15–20% of cortical wet weight (Levin et al., 1970). The histological manifestations of edema produced by microvascular injury (e.g., tissue freezing) differ considerably in gray and white matter. In the former, there is cellular swelling, which involves mainly astrocytes and dendritic processes (Klatzo, 1967). In contrast, fluid accumulates primarily in the ECS in white matter. These differences can be explained in terms of the particular architectural and biochemical traits of each tissue. Gray matter has high tissue turgor and resists intercellular dissection by water because of its dense neuropil, which consists of intertwined cell processes. The bundles of similarly oriented fibers in white matter create "tissue planes," which pose less resistance to edema fluid and give a directional quality to its spread through the ECS. Nevertheless, the intercellular clefts in white matter probably provide sufficient resistance to bulk flow of fluid to render it insignificant under normal conditions (Fenstermacher and Patlak, 1976). In addition to these structural differences, gray and white matter differ in the concentration of ground substance, which consists largely of the fuzz coat that projects from cell membranes. In gray matter, the density of this polyanionic mucopolysaccharide is sufficient to impede the spread of the protein component of edema fluid (Guyton et al., 1971).

Several factors normally protect the brain against edema formation. The cerebral capillaries not only restrict the transport of protein but are also relatively impermeable to salts and many polar nonelectrolytes. These ions and molecules contribute to the plasma osmotic pressure which opposes the efflux of water from plasma into the cerebral ECS (Rapoport, 1976). Therefore, filtration of plasma water would immediately decrease the osmolarity of the ECF, which normally is isosmotic with plasma. The resultant osmotic gradient would oppose further plasma filtration. In addition, brain ECF pressure differs from that of several other tissues in that it is normally positive (Shulman et al., 1976). On this basis, Taylor and Granger (1976) have calculated that cerebral capillary pressure could vary from moment to moment without causing hydrostatic pressure gradients sufficient to produce tissue edema. Even if a relatively large gradient were created, the extremely low filtration coefficient of cerebral capillaries would tend to minimize water efflux. Because of considerations such as these, some investigators have concluded that a Starling-type of transcapillary water filtration does not exist in the brain under normal conditions, and that diffusion alone accounts for normal water movement into and out of the brain (Bradbury, 1979).

Even under pathological conditions that alter BBB permeability, the brain is at least partially protected against edema formation. The very low compliance of gray matter that was referred to above severely limits the volume of water that can accumulate in the cortical ECS (Rapoport, 1978). In addition, the low hydraulic conductivity of gray matter means that the BBB must remain abnormally permeable for an extended period before fluid is transferred from the injured cortex to the more compliant white matter (Reulen et al., 1976). Thus, opening of the BBB does not invariably cause edema formation. Edema occurs only after a barrier injury of sufficient intensity and duration (Klatzo, 1972; Rapoport et al., 1976).

COMPOSITION OF EDEMA FLUID

The fluid that extravasates into the brain ECS after BBB injury is a plasma filtrate (Bakay and Hague, 1964; Clausen et al., 1967). Its sodium content is slightly lower than that of plasma and the potassium content is slightly higher, at least initially (Go et al., 1976). The latter reflects admixture with intracellular fluid released as a result of the tissue injury (Gazendam et al., 1979). In samples not contaminated by tissue injury, the oncotic pressure of edema fluid is the same as or slightly less than that of plasma (Go et al., 1976). Although the protein content of edema fluid and plasma is approximately the same, the injured BBB displays features of "selective vulnerability" in regard to penetration by some substances, including albumin and globulin (Steinwall and Klatzo, 1966). Rasmussen and Klatzo (1969) demonstrated a particularly high albumin content in edema fluid during the first 24–48 hr after cryogenic injury. This was followed by a marked increase in gamma globulin 3–4 days later. In addition, the temporal profile of sucrose passage through the BBB injured by ischemia may vary from that of inulin and albumin (Spatz et al., 1976). Such observations indicate that under some circumstances the composition of edema fluid may differ from that of a plasma filtrate. It is possible that this variation depends upon the intensity of BBB injury (Klatzo, 1979).

PHYSIOLOGICAL ASPECTS OF EDEMA FORMATION

The basic pathophysiological stimulus for opening of the BBB remains undefined. However, an increase in circumferential vessel wall tension has been noted to be a common factor among such disparate causes of reversible barrier opening as topical or intravascular administration of hyperosmotic solutions (Rapoport et al., 1971), acute hypertension (Johansson, 1976), and repeated seizures and hypercapnia (Johansson and Nilsson, 1977). All except the first of these models produce vasodilatation and/or increased intravascular pressure. According to Laplace's relation, these factors cause increased tension in the vessel wall. In the case of BBB opening by hyperosmolar solutions, it is postulated that circumferential wall tension is increased as a result of osmotic shrinkage of the endothelial cells (Bradbury, 1979). Although such a unifying concept is obviously attractive, there is only circumstantial evidence to support it at present.

The dynamics of cerebral vasogenic edema are frequently explained in terms of Starling's hypothesis regarding the forces that govern transcapillary fluid movements (Fenstermacher and Patlak, 1976; Go et al., 1976; Rapoport, 1976, 1979). This hypothesis relates volume flow across the capillary wall to the product of 1) the capillary hydraulic conductance and 2) the difference between the net hydrostatic and osmotic pressure gradients across the wall. Capillary hydraulic conductance is a measure of the permeability of the capillary wall to the bulk flow of water. It is expressed in terms of the rate of flow across a unit cross sectional area that is induced by a unit hydrostatic or osmotic pressure gradient. Barrier opening of sufficient intensity and duration increases capillary hydraulic conductance. As a result, the capillary hydrostatic pressure is more directly transmitted to the brain ECS (Rapoport, 1979).

The importance of the capillary hydrostatic pressure as the driving force for edema development is illustrated by the fact that the rate and extent of cryogenic edema formation varies directly with the direction of large changes in arterial blood pressure (Klatzo et al., 1967). However, the precise impact of a given change in systemic arterial pressure on capillary hydrostatic pressure—and thus on edema formation—is determined by the tone of the intervening vessels. For example, dilatation of the precapillary resistance vessels (due to inhalation of carbon dioxide) increases the amount of extravasation of Evans blue dye across the BBB at a given level of arterial hypertension (Johansson and Nilsson, 1977). As will be discussed in the next section, cerebral resistance vessels normally constrict in response to increases in arterial pressure in order to prevent an increase in cerebral blood flow (CBF). However, this autoregulation at high perfusion pressures also prevents transmission of a proportion of the arterial pressure increase to the capillary bed and in so doing helps protect the brain against edema formation. It is, therefore, not surprising that the upper pressure limit for autoregulation of CBF approximates the pressure threshold for opening of the BBB to Evans blue (Bradbury, 1979). In addition, barrier permeability—like CBF—can be increased by elevating the arterial pressure at a rate that exceeds the temporal latency of autoregulation. As a result, the pressure threshold for BBB opening is lower for abrupt (as opposed to stepwise) blood pressure increases (Häggendal and Johansson, 1972). Impairment of autoregulation after head injury is thus a major factor in the exacerbation of post-traumatic edema by systemic hypertension (Schutta et al., 1968; Marshall et al., 1969). It is of potential therapeutic significance that, in experimental animals, the restoration of normal vasomotor reactivity may also restore the functional integrity of the BBB (Rapoport, 1976).

Capillary hydrostatic pressure may also increase as a result of elevated cerebral venous pressure. Using serial fluorescein angiography, Soejima and colleagues (1979) observed almost complete arrest of the pial venous microcirculation after cryogenic cortical injury. At one stage, the arterial microcirculation was still patent, creating a condition that might well predispose to vasogenic edema. Marshall et al. (1969) concluded that changes in the caliber of both resistance and capacitance vessels may occur simultaneously or sequentially after head injury and, depending upon the pattern of changes, may either aggravate or attenuate edema formation. For example, cerebral veins may become compressed as intracranial pressure increases. However, precapillary resistance vessels may simultaneously dilate in order to maintain CBF despite the fall in perfusion pressure. The resultant shift in the site of resistance from precapillary to postcapillary vessels increases capillary hydrostatic pressure and may thus predispose to edema formation.

Although the poise of the Starling forces clearly influences the rate and extent of edema formation *after* BBB injury, it remains unclear whether increased capillary hydrostatic pressure itself causes edema in the *absence* of antecedent or concomitant BBB injury. The controversy depends, at least in part, on whether factors that increase cerebral capillary hydraulic conductance also injure the BBB. The validity of the theoretical physiological defenses against edema that were referred to above is also at issue. Pure "filtration edema" would presumably have a low protein content if the BBB otherwise remained intact. This form of vasogenic edema has been postulated to occur in head-injured patients as a result of paralytic dilatation of resistance vessels (Langfitt and Bruce, 1975).

Osmotic forces are generally less significant than hydrostatic pressure gradients in determining the severity of post-traumatic edema. Once the BBB has been opened, plasma electrolytes no longer contribute to the net osmotic pressure that opposes water efflux from the capillaries. However, manipulation of the osmotic gradient may be used to treat cerebral edema. Intravenous infusion of hyperosmotic solutions that do not readily penetrate the intact BBB (e.g., 20% mannitol) creates an osmotic gradient that favors absorption of water from the ECS. This gradient is maintained only across intact portions of the BBB. Where the BBB is disrupted, the osmotically active agent readily enters the ECS. Furthermore, even the low permeability of the intact BBB may fail to prevent significant accumulation of the agent in the ECS if therapy is protracted. Under these circumstances, sudden discontinuation of therapy may transiently produce a reversal in the direction of the osmotic gradient that exacerbates the edema.

A final, very speculative facet of the pathophysiology of post-traumatic edema concerns the possibility that the brain loses its ability to regulate its own water volume as a result of disruption of the central noradrenergic fiber system referred to above. Povlishock and his colleagues (1979) have reported that axon terminals are sensitive to even minimal brain trauma. Clumping of synaptic vesicles was occasionally observed in terminals that were apparently related to capillaries. Whether any of the involved fibers correspond to the dopamine-beta-hydroxylase containing terminals that have been implicated in regulation of microvascular water permeability remains to be determined.

In summary, vasogenic edema is initiated by a vascular insult that increases capillary hydraulic conductance. The amount of edema that results is influenced by the surface area, duration, and severity of the BBB injury. In addition, capillary hydrostatic pressure—which is largely dependent upon the systemic arterial pressure and the tone of cerebral resistance vessels—is a major determinant of the severity of edema. Therefore, even transient hypertension or even focal loss of autoregulation may exacerbate cerebral edema after head injury.

MORPHOLOGICAL ASPECTS OF EDEMA FORMATION

Except in cases in which severe vascular injury actually disrupts the endothelium, the structural basis of BBB opening remains controversial. Initial electron microscopic studies seemed to indicate that protein is transported interendothelially through opened tight junctions (Blakemore, 1969; Hirano et al., 1969; Baker et al., 1971). However, according to Klatzo (1979), this mechanism of barrier opening has been convincingly demonstrated only in edema models that utilize topical or intravascular administration of hyperosmolar solutions (Rapoport et al., 1971; Brightman et al., 1973). There is now considerable evidence that vascular injury induces intraendothelial transport of protein via micropinocytosis, a process that is inconspicuous or absent in normal cerebral vessels. This mechanism has been implicated in BBB opening following experimental seizures (Petito et al., 1976), pharmacologically induced hypertension (Westergaard, 1979) and prolonged ischemia (Fujimoto et al., 1976). In addition, transport of horseradish peroxidase (HRP) within transendothelial tubules has been reported in a post-ischemic model of BBB opening (Garcia et al., 1977, 1979). There have been relatively few careful studies of the mechanism of protein transport after mechanical brain injury. However, Povlishock and others (1979) have studied BBB changes after "minimal intensity" fluid percussion brain injury. This injury produces a physiological response but no intraparenchymal hemorrhage or other structural damage discernible by light microscopy. Intravascular HRP extravasated from arterioles, capillaries, and venules within the ventromedial brainstem. There was no ultrastructural evidence of opening of the tight junctions nor was there HRP within them. However, HRP was clearly observed within cytoplasmic vesicles.

Nevertheless, it is far from certain that tight junction opening has no role in clinical conditions associated with vasogenic edema. Resolution of the controversy is complicated by occasional reports of simultaneous marker transport via tight junctions and cytoplasmic vesicles (Lorenzo et al., 1975). In this regard, it has been suggested that pericapillary astrocytes may have some role in the maintenance of capillary tight junctions and in the normal suppression of pinocytotic activity (Davson and Oldendorf, 1967; Bradbury, 1979). If this were true, astrocytic injury might predispose to either (or both) of the reported mechanisms of barrier opening. There are theoretical difficulties with this hypothesis, not the least of which is the fact that only 80% of the capillary surface area is invested by astrocytic foot processes. Although some investigators have noted a close correspondence between sites of increased barrier permeability and foci of swollen astrocytic foot processes (Nag et al., 1976), it is difficult to determine which alteration constitutes the initial pathologic event. It is possible that different transport mechanisms may be induced by different modes of vascular injury. However, Bradbury (1979) has cautioned that much of the reported variation in mechanisms of BBB opening may be due to differences in tissue processing and in selection and interpretation of electron micrographs.

Finally, there is evidence that formation of edema does not occur exclusively in the capillary bed. Pinocytotic transport of peroxidase across arteriolar and venular endothelium has been reported in a variety of models of BBB injury (Lorenzo et al., 1975; Westergaard, 1975; Petito et al., 1976; Westergaard, 1979), including concussive brain injury (Povlishock et al., 1979). More direct evidence has been provided by Soejima and others (1979) who observed extravasation of fluorescein from capillaries, arterioles, and eventually even from pial arteries following cryogenic cortical injury.

BIOCHEMICAL ASPECTS OF EDEMA FORMATION

Despite experimental scrutiny of a wide variety of endogenous compounds, relatively little is known about the possible role of plasma and tissue factors in the pathogenesis of post-traumatic vasogenic edema. Monoamines have received particular attention. For example, intracerebral injection of serotonin has been reported to increase cerebral water content (Osterholm et al., 1969), and intraventricular administration has been associated with increased cerebrovascular permeability to HRP (Westergaard, 1975). In addition, Costa and colleagues (1974) found a high concentration of serotonin in vessels situated within cortical cryogenic lesions. Nevertheless, Fenske and his associates (1976) have reported that ventriculocisternal perfusion with high concentrations of serotonin not only failed to induce edema, but also failed to exacerbate pre-existent cryogenic edema.

Conflicting evidence has also been gathered with regard to a possible role of prostaglandins in the pathogenesis of vasogenic edema. However, initial attempts to reduce the extent of cryogenic edema by administering indomethacin in doses sufficient to suppress brain prostaglandin synthesis have been unsuccessful (Pappius and Wolfe, 1976).

A set of experiments by Aarabi and Long (1979) casts some doubt on the importance of tissue humoral factors in vasogenic edema formation. Immediate excision of a cryogenic cortical lesion prevented edema formation in the subjacent white matter. In a subsequent experiment, the excised tissue block was immediately replaced in its bed, but edema still was not produced. This observation supports the theory that the capillary hydrostatic pressure is the driving force for edema formation. However, it does not support the hypothesis that a factor that diffuses from the injured tissue is critically involved.

SPREAD OF EDEMA FLUID

Vasogenic edema preferentially involves the white matter (Bakay and Haque, 1964; Klatzo et al., 1967) and spreads along the planes of association and projection fibers, as well as through perivascular spaces which provide a relatively low resistance pathway (Reulen et al., 1976). Extensive spread occurs despite the fact that vessels that lie within the edema territory but outside the area of injury have normal permeability (Hirano et al., 1969; Baker et al., 1971; Blasberg et al., 1979).

There is now considerable evidence that edema fluid spreads through the white matter ECS as a result of tissue pressure gradients generated at the site of BBB disruption. Evidence for this bulk flow theory includes the following:

1. Double-tracer techniques have shown that substances with very different diffusion coefficients migrate centrifugally from the injury site at similar rates (Steinwall and Klatzo, 1966).

2. Migration distances are considerably greater than predicted for migration by diffusion alone (Reulen et al., 1976).

3. The rapidity and extent of edema spread is dependent upon factors that influence the capillary hydrostatic pressure (Klatzo, 1972).

4. As noted above, excision of the injured capillary bed prevents edema formation (Aarabi and Long, 1979).

5. Use of a cotton wick technique to measure interstitual fluid pressure (IFP) at varying distances from a cryogenic lesion has confirmed the existence of tissue hydrostatic pressure gradients during edema formation (Reulen et al., 1976). The highest tissue pressures are found adjacent to the lesion and the pressures decrease progressively along the edema path toward normal white matter. The decreasing tissue pressure gradient is closely correlated with a progressive decrease in tissue water content and with the direction of migration of extracellular markers.

The increase in local IFP and the development of tissue pressure gradients is the result of the fact that the capillary hydrostatic pressure is transmitted to the ECS, but fluid transmission is resisted by the relatively narrow extracellular channels (Reulen et al., 1976). As a result of these two opposing forces, local IFP rapidly rises above cerebrospinal fluid (CSF) pressure. The degree of IFP elevation is dependent upon the tissue compliance and the CSF pressure (Shulman et al., 1976).

Because normal tissue compliance is relatively low, the increase in IFP initially produces little change in the volume of the ECS. This particular pressure-volume relationship has been defined as a "safety factor" that protects against edema formation after minor injuries of the BBB (Guyton et al., 1971). However, once the IFP exceeds the resistance posed by structural forces, tissue compliance rapidly increases. The pressure-volume relationship then changes so that further small increases in IFP are associated with progressively greater expansion of the ECS (Go et al., 1976). This increase in the size of the ECS in turn increases the hydraulic conductance of white matter (Rapoport, 1978). The increased tissue compliance and hydraulic conductance operate as a positive feedback system so that within 24–48 hr after experimental BBB injury the volume of the white matter ECS may increase by 30% (Fenske et al., 1973) and total brain water content may increase by 8–10% (Go et al., 1976). These pathophysiological mechanisms explain why removal of a large portion of the cranial vault has been found to increase the extent of edema formation in experimental animals (Cooper et al., 1979). Decompressive craniectomy increases tissue compliance and decreases CSF pressure. Both of these factors decrease the IFP threshold at which increasingly large volumes of edema fluid can begin to enter the ECS.

In experiments conducted by Marmarou and his colleagues (1976b) tissue pressure gradients dissipated (and bulk movement of edema fluid ceased) within 6 hr after cortical injury. Bruce found that extracellular water content was maximal at 6 hr after injury and then gradually declined (Bruce et al., 1979b). Others have reported a considerably longer time course for edema propagation (Klatzo et al., 1967; Maxwell, et al., 1971). These differences may be explicable in terms of variations in the severity and duration of BBB opening, and the lack of standardization of systemic arterial pressure and of the size of the craniectomy.

MECHANISMS OF EDEMA RESOLUTION

According to Bruce et al.(1979b), repair of the BBB begins within 15–24 hr after injury. Clearance of edema fluid from the ECS begins within this same time interval. Clearance is particularly rapid during the first 48 hr after cryogenic injury, and then continues at a slower rate for the next week. At the end of 7 days, extravasation of fluorescein is limited to the rim of the cortical lesion. At this time capillary hydraulic conductance is almost normal (Marmarou et al., 1976b). This is probably due to the fact that the damaged vessels have become occluded. However, several weeks must elapse before they are replaced by capillaries with normal barrier properties (Björklund et al., 1969).

Bulk flow across the ventricular ependyma into the CSF is apparently the main mechanism for removal of edema fluid from the ECS (Reulen et al., 1976). The importance of the hydrostatic pressure gradient between the edematous area of brain and the CSF has been clearly demonstrated by Reulen and his colleagues (1977). They measured the rate of clearance of marker molecules from the ECS while performing ventriculocisternal perfusion at varying perfusion pressures. At high CSF pressures, which decreased the magnitude of the pressure gradient between the ECS and the CSF, the rate of clearance of the markers decreased. Low CSF pressure—which can be produced by ventricular drainage—had the opposite effect. Since even large molecules can pass between ependymal cell clefts, edema fluid solutes may also be cleared into the ventricular CSF during bulk fluid flow (Bruce et al., 1979b). An alternate pathway may involve diffusion back into the vascular system through the fenestrated epithelium of choroid plexus capillaries (Cserr et al., 1976). Edema fluid and solutes might reach these capillaries via subependymal channels and the spaces between the capillaries and the ependymal lining of the choroid plexus.

After dissipation of tissue pressure gradients, small molecules (e.g., sucrose) continue to be cleared into the ventricles by diffusion. These molecules are then rapidly removed from the CSF, creating large concentration gradients between the ECS and the ventricles (Bruce et al., 1976). Some investigators believe that this "sink action" of the CSF also contributes to the clearance of protein molecules from the ECS (Reulen et al., 1977). However, others believe that once bulk fluid flow ceases, large molecules are removed by local mechanisms. It is possible that some of the capillary pinocytotic activity observed in edematous tissue represents transport of edema fluid protein back into the vascular system (Fujimoto et al., 1976; Bruce et al., 1979b). This hypothesis is difficult to reconcile with the observations that resolution of edema proceeds from the periphery toward the injury site (Klatzo et al., 1979) and that there is little pinocytotic activity in vessels outside of the locus of injury (Hirano et al., 1969). Klatzo and his colleagues (1979) have used an immunohistochemial method to demonstrate uptake of extravascular serum proteins by astrocytes following cryogenic cortical injury. In the later stages of edema resolution, protein was also identified within pericytes and, to a lesser extent, within microglia. These investigators suggested that reduction of ECF osmolarity by phagocytosis of osmotically active substances may be an important mechanism for edema fluid clearance. Even neurons have been implicated in the resolution of edema. Blasberg (1976) has suggested that albumin may be taken up by axon terminals and transported in a retrograde direction to the perikaryon where it is catabolized. At present it seems reasonable to conclude that bulk flow and diffusion into the CSF are the only well established mechanisms for clearance of edema fluid solutes from the ECS. The nature and role of local mechanisms for clearance of large molecules is more controversial.

PHYSIOLOGICAL CONSEQUENCES OF VASOGENIC EDEMA

Cerebral edema may indirectly affect neurological function by inducing ischemia. For example, the ECF volume of white matter may be increased to such a degree that the intracranial pressure (ICP) becomes greatly elevated and the perfusion pressure critically reduced. However, it remains unclear whether edema fluid itself has any deleterious effect. Computed axial tomographic (CAT) scans that clearly demonstrate extensive white matter edema have been obtained in patients with no signs of neurological dysfunction (Penn, 1979). Furthermore, spontaneous (Schaul et al., 1976) and evoked (Bruce et al., 1979a) electrocortical activity is often relatively normal in experimental vasogenic edema. The possible direct and indirect effects of edema fluid on a wide variety of physiological processes have been investigated, but many of the conclusions remain tentative or frankly speculative. The following review deals with 1) the effects of edema on CBF and metabolism, and 2) possible direct cytotoxic effects:

1. Many investigators have documented a significant decrease in regional cerebral blood flow (rCBF) in edematous areas of brain (Poll et al., 1972; Frei et al., 1973; Meinig et al., 1973; Marmarou et al., 1976a; Marshall et al., 1976; Reilly et al., 1977; Blasberg, 1979). This decrease in flow is not always attributable to a reduction in perfusion pressure since the effect has regularly been observed with a normal ICP (Poll et al., 1972; Meinig et al., 1973; Reilly et al., 1977; Marmarou et al., 1976a). Microvascular compression has been proposed as the cause of the rCBF reduction in the absence of a generalized increase in ICP. The normal pressure gradient across the venous end of the capillary is relatively small. Therefore, this portion of the capillary is liable to be compressed as edema fluid dissects into the ECS and local IFP rises. This compression of the venous end of

the capillary reduces capillary blood flow, since capillary resistance is increased and the normally low capillary perfusion pressure is further decreased (Marmarou et al., 1976a; Reulen, 1976). Indirect support for this hypothesis has been provided by demonstrations that the extent of the decrease in rCBF is closely correlated with the extent of the increase in regional tissue water content (Frei et al., 1973; Meinig et al., 1973). The presence of "false autoregulation" within edematous regions (see following section) has also been cited as further evidence of microvascular compression.

Nevertheless, this hypothesis has not been universally accepted. Bruce (1976) has argued that the mechanical support provided by the pericapillary glial "tunnel" should render cerebral capillaries no more compressible than the surrounding parenchyma. Furthermore, in the cryogenic edema model utilized by Marmarou, decreased blood flow was found in regions in which the intersitial fluid pressure was considered insufficient to cause microvascular compression (Marmarou et al., 1976b). In addition, no consistent correlation could be found between the magnitude of the regional blood flow reduction and the regional white matter water content. Blasberg (1979) has reported flow reductions not only in edematous regions, but also in more remote areas that remain impermeable to vital dyes and which have a normal histological appearance.

Marmarou and his colleagues (1976a, 1979) have measured rCBF in animal brains that were made edematous by slow infusion of fluid into hemispheric white matter. The white matter water content was increased by 8–10% and the ultrastructure of the ECS was similar to that observed after cryogenic cortical injury. Despite these changes, both rCBF and autoregulation remained normal. The investigators concluded that in areas remote from the site of BBB injury, the passage of fluid through the ECS was without hemodynamic consequence.

One alternative explanation for the reductions in blood flow that have been observed in some models of vasogenic edema is that the cortical injury itself directly affects blood flow by altering vasomotor tone (Bruce et al., 1973). Several investigators have reported that a standard edematogenic injury produces dysautoregulation even in the occasional animal in which edema fails to form (Reivich et al., 1969; Miller et al., 1976). Another hypothesis is that the decreased flow in edematous areas is a reflection of local metabolic depression. Studies of this hypothesis have thus far raised more questions than they have answered. Using quantitative autoradiography, Pappius (1979) first noted a decrease in glucose utilization within edematous areas approximately 4 hr after a cryogenic or coagulative cortical injury. However, the degree of metabolic depression reached statistical significance only after 24 hr. At this time, rCBF was reduced only in the area adjacent to the lesion. This apparent uncoupling of the blood flow and metabolic rates was even more dramatic after osmotic opening of the BBB (Pappius et al., 1979). In this model, some areas of increased permeability to a vital dye demonstated both enhanced glucose utilization and decreased blood flow. It thus seems reasonable to conclude that the mechanism of any putative reduction in rCBF in the presence of vasogenic edema remains unclear.

Cellular swelling that primarily affects astroglia may occur in vasogenic edema (Hirano, 1979), although it is seldom clear whether the cellular changes are a direct consequence of the presence of a plasma filtrate in the ECS or instead represent a separate response to the injury agent (e.g., ischemia). It has been suggested that tissue oxygen delivery is impaired in vasogenic edema as a result of microvascular compression or interference with normal oxygen diffusion through the ECS (Bruce et al., 1979a). Expansion of the ECS increases the length of the diffusion path between capillaries and cells. In addition, in vitro studies have indicated that the rate of oxygen diffusion is reduced by 50% when albumin and globulin are added to the diffusion medium in concentrations well within the normal plasma range (Navarri et al., 1971). Nevertheless, profound disturbances in oxidative metabolism must be exceptional since several investigators have found normal lactate and high energy phosphate levels in edematous white matter (Nelson and Mantz, 1971; Bruce et al., 1979a). However, maintenance of the tissue energy state during impaired oxygen diffusion may simply be the result of a reduction in the local metabolic rate or an increase in the number of open capillaries (Bruce, 1976).

2. Alterations in cellular function might also be produced by a direct toxic effect of edema fluid constituents (Baethmann et al., 1979). The concentrations of many potentially damaging substances (certain proteins, amino acids, fatty acids, and electrolytes) are higher in a plasma filtrate than in normal extracellular fluid. However, no specific constituent of edema fluid has yet been proven to have a clinically significant pathophysiological effect on neuronal function (at least not in the concentration normally found in edema fluid). Nevertheless, such an effect might be mediated through the astroglia. The anatomic relation of glial processes to synaptic complexes and capillary basement membranes suggests a role in the regulation of the microenvironment of the neuronal surface (Peters and Palay, 1965). In vasogenic edema, astrocytes may not only swell but also alter shape. As a result the astrocytic surface may separate from its normal satellite position at certain synapses (Hirano, 1979). Others have reported fragmentation of glial processes (Feigin and Popoff, 1962) or even total astrocytic disruption (Budzilovich, 1976), although it is possible that these extreme changes represent experimental artifacts. In this regard, it may be significant that Grossman and Seregin (1976) demonstrated that the presence of edema fluid in the cortical extracellular clefts does not injure glia to the extent that their membrane potentials are reduced.

Perhaps the most important test of whether or not vasogenic edema is noxious to the brain is if it alters the outcome of head injury. Miller and his colleagues (1979) recently correlated the presence of cerebral edema (as diagnosed by CAT scan) with the outcome of closed head injury and concluded that post-traumatic edema increases mortality only if it is associated with a contusion or hematoma. Indeed, the importance of cerebral edema in the pathophysiology of the immediate posttraumatic period is far from established in clinical head injury. One can tentatively conclude that vasogenic edema fluid does not exert a direct pathophysiological effect following head injury and that the rationale for antiedema therapy is thus based on the prevention of such secondary effects as intracranial hypertension and cerebral ischemia.

CHANGES IN CEREBRAL METABOLISM AND BLOOD FLOW

Although an entire chapter in this volume is devoted to cerebral ischemia, there is a compelling reason for also dealing with this topic in the context of head injury. In the final analysis most—and perhaps all—secondary insults that further damage the mechanically injured brain do so by causing tissue ischemia and hypoxia.

Cerebral Energy Metabolism
NORMAL METABOLISM

Although the average 1400-g adult brain represents only 2% of the total body weight, it consumes 20% of the oxygen and 25% of the glucose used by the body. This prodigious amount of substrate is required chiefly for transport and biosynthetic work. The former is involved in the maintenance of the electrochemical gradients responsible for membrane excitablity and conductivity and accounts for the majority of the cerebral energy expenditure of 0.25 Kcal/min (Sokoloff, 1976).

Under normal circumstances, glucose is the only energy substrate consumed by the brain. This is indicated by the fact that the cerebral respiratory quotient is unity, by the almost stoichiometric relationship between oxygen and glucose consumption, and by the absence of a significant cerebral arteriovenous difference for any other potential substrate. The brain consumes approximately 77 mg of glucose/min (5.5 mg/100 g brain tissue/min). Glucose crosses the blood-brain barrier by facilitated diffusion which involves a hexose specific carrier. The rate of glucose transport across the barrier is almost never a limiting factor in cerebral glucose utilization, since the transport capacity easily exceeds even maximal metabolic demand. The only exception occurs when transport is itself limited by insufficient glucose delivery to the brain (e.g., hypoglycemia or ischemia).

The brain consumes oxygen at an average rate of approximately 50 ml/min (3.5 ml/100 g/min). This cerebral metabolic rate ($CMRO_2$) is usually calculated from the product of the cerebral blood flow rate (CBF) and the cerebral arteriovenous oxygen content difference (A-VDO_2). Under normal conditions, the $CMRO_2$ is determined by the level of cerebral functional activity. Although the $CMRO_2$ is usually derived for the brain as a whole, it is important to note that it varies (like neural activity) from region to region. It increases during epileptic seizures and decreases during coma (but is unchanged during normal sleep). It is probably not determined by oxygen availability except perhaps during severe hypoxemia (Siesjö, 1978). It is less clear whether $CMRO_2$ decreases as CBF falls below normal levels. Since the brain normally extracts only ⅓ of the oxygen available in arterial blood, a reduction in CBF can be at least partially compensated by an increase in the cerebral A-VDO_2 (normal = 6.7 ml/100 ml blood).

METABOLIC EFFECTS OF HYPOXEMIA

The energy requirements of the brain can be met only by the complete oxidation of glucose in the tricarboxylic acid (Krebs) cycle. Glycolysis, which is the compulsory initial step, provides only 5% of the energy produced during complete oxidative metabolism. Despite the fact that the rate of glycolysis can increase by 5–7 times during hypoxemia, anaerobic metabolism falls very far short of meeting cerebral energy requirements. (MacMillan and Siesjö, 1972).

If oxygen delivery to the brain ceases abruptly, the 7–10 ml of oxygen remaining in the blood and tissue is consumed in less than 12 sec (Rossen et al., 1943). A rapid reduction of the mitochondrial redox systems ensues, with resultant cessation of mitochondrial ATP formation. Increasing anaerobic metabolism is indicated by a progressive increase in the $NADH/NAD^+$ and lactate/pyruvate ratios. The lactic acidosis is the principal cause of the fall in intracellular pH, unless the anoxemia is caused by circulatory arrest. In the latter case, the increase in tissue carbon dioxide tension (to as high as 200–300 mm Hg) significantly exacerbates the acidosis. Despite production of an intracellular pH as low as 6.5, there is no evidence that a transient intracellular acidosis itself diminishes the energy state of the tissue (MacMillan and Siesjö, 1972). Measurable depletion of high energy phosphates is delayed by the fact that ATP formation is favored by shifts in the equilibria of the creatine phosphokinase (CPK) and adenylate kinase (myokinase) reactions. As a result, tissue phosphocreatine levels fall and AMP levels rise. However, after no more than 3 min of anoxemia, the labile phosphate pool is largely depleted and the cerebral energy state consequently declines. Nevertheless, if oxygen delivery is restored at this point, all of these biochemical changes are rapidly reversed (Kaasik et al., 1970).

Theoretical models of tissue diffusion have been used to predict that cerebral mitochondria will be inadequately supplied with oxygen when the venous PO_2 declines below 20 mm Hg (Thews, 1963). Although this level does correspond to the level of hypoxemia that produces loss of consciousness and slowing of the electroencephalogram (EEG), there is evidence that hypoxic thresholds calculated from diffusion models correlate poorly with actual tissue events (Siesjö, 1978). Indeed, in preparations of isolated mitochondria, measurable changes in oxygen consumption occur only when the oxygen tension in the suspension medium is below 1 mm Hg (Starlinger and Lübbers, 1973). The nature of the link between the level of neuronal function and the degree of tissue oxygen availability thus remains unclear.

Oxygen tension normally varies considerably within the brain, and the tension within some areas of rat cortex may normally be lower than 5 mm Hg (Lübbers, 1974). One can speculate that during even moderate hypoxemia, the oxygen tension becomes low enough in scattered neurons or synaptic areas to cause reduction of some mitochondrial redox systems. Another possible link is provided by the fact that oxygen is required for the rate-limiting step in the biosynthesis of certain monoaminergic neurotransmitters. The "mixed function" oxidases that catalyze these steps demonstrate a 50% reduction in oxygen utilization at a PO_2 of 5–10 mm Hg (Fisher and Kaufman, 1972; Friedman et al., 1972), which is a considerably higher oxygen tension than the tension at which the electron transfer system oxidases become unsaturated.

In normal human subjects, pulmonary ventilation is stimulated (via carotid chemoreceptors) when the arterial PO_2 falls to approximately 65 mm Hg. At a PO_2 of 50 mm Hg, CBF begins to increase as does the lactate/pyruvate ratio (Siesjö et al., 1975). As the PO_2 drops below 35 mm Hg, tissue phosphocreatine becomes progressively depleted. [The lactate/pyruvate ratio and the phosphocreatine content have sometimes been used to quantitate the severity of tissue hypoxia. However, the lactate dehydrogenase (LDH) and creatine phosphokinase (CPK) equilibria are both pH-dependent. Therefore, the intracellular pH must be known if these parameters are to be used as indices of tissue hypoxia.] Consciousness is normally lost at an arterial PO_2 below 30 mm Hg. However, at least in rats, the $CMRO_2$ and the phosphorylation state of the adenine nucleotide pool remain nearly normal until the arterial and venous oxygen tensions are reduced below 20 mm Hg and 10 mm Hg, respectively (MacMillan and Siesjö, 1972). At these minimal oxygen tensions, there is a five-fold increase in CBF (Johannsson and Siesjö, 1975).

Because increased CBF is the main physiological mechanism that prevents energy failure during hypoxemia, the brain is profoundly affected by the concurrent status of the cardiovascular system. Indeed, the capacity of the brain to endure hypoxemia without irreversible damage seems to be limited principally by the sensitivity of the cardiovascular system to this insult. For this reason, and because of the frequency of multiple organ system trauma, cerebral ischemia is often superimposed on the hypoxemic complications of clinical head injury. The metabolic effects of these combined insults have been elucidated by Salford et al. (1973) using a modification of the preparation developed by Levine (1960). In this model, rats underwent clamping of one carotid artery before being subjected to graded degrees of hypoxemia. At an arterial PO_2 of 21 mm Hg, the metabolic response in the hemisphere ipsilateral to the clamp was more typical of hypoxemia than ischemia: normal substrate levels, relatively high levels of glycolytic intermediates, and an increase in hemispheric blood flow. However, there was an irreversible decrease in the cerebral energy state which was not anticipated with hypoxemia of this degree. Further studies demonstrated that the threshold for permanent tissue damage in this model occurred at an arterial PO_2 of 28 mm Hg, which is considerably higher than the threshold in uncomplicated hypoxemia. This difference is attributable to the fact that although blood flow in the hypoxic-oligemic hemisphere increased to 120–130% of the control value, the increase was considerably greater in the hemisphere which was only hypoxic. Thus, cerebral hypoperfusion, which is not severe enough to cause metabolic derangements characteristic of ischemia, may nevertheless exacerbate the effects of a given degree of hypoxemia. The reason for this is that compensatory increases in CBF are attenuated.

Normal Cerebral Blood Flow (CBF)

The course of evolution has left the human brain curiously vulnerable to perturbations in the function of other organ systems. Despite its high metabolic rate, the brain has a relatively low capillary density, virtually no capacity to store oxygen, and only meager reserves of carbohydrate substrate and high energy phosphate compounds. The brain is thus vitally dependent upon the cardiovascular system for uninterrupted delivery of energy substrate. For this reason, the brain receives approximately 15% of the cardiac output or approximately 800 ml/min (50–60 ml/100 g/min). As we shall see, CBF is precisely regulated so that the metabolic demands of the brain can still be met during relatively minor disturbances in cardiorespiratory homeostasis.

REGULATION OF CBF

As in all vascular beds, CBF is directly proportional to the cerebral perfusion pressure (CPP) and inversely proportional to the cerebrovascular resistance (CVR). The former represents the difference between the arterial inflow pressure [mean systemic arterial pressure (MAP)] and the outflow pressure in the large cerebral veins that drain directly into the dural venous sinuses. Because the pressure in these veins is practically the same as the intracranial pressure (ICP) (and because the latter is more readily measured), CPP is usually expressed as MAP-ICP. Although neural modulation of the cardiovascular system permits the brain to maintain CBF by modifying the CPP under certain pathological conditions (e.g., the pressor response to severe elevation of the ICP), regulation of CBF is generally achieved by alteration of the CVR. It is important to note that changes in the caliber of cerebral vessels not only alter CBF but alter cerebral blood volume (CBV) as well. Under normal circumstances, the increase or decrease in CBV produced by vasodilatation or vasoconstriction is clinically inconsequential. However, pathological processes (e.g., intracranial hematomas) may exhaust the capacity of the craniospinal compartments to compensate for increases in intracranial volume. Under such circumstances, changes in CBV may have an important impact on ICP. This topic is discussed in more detail in the last section of this chapter.

The most important factor in the normal control of CBF is the level of cerebral metabolic activity. This, in turn, is related to the level of neuronal functional activity. Thus, the fact that cortical blood flow (77–138 ml/100 g/min in conscious cats) is considerably higher than hemispheric white matter blood flow (23 ml/100 g/min) is attributable, at least in part, to the higher neuronal and synaptic density of the cortex (Sokoloff et al., 1977). Although global increases or decreases in $CMRO_2$, and thus CBF, may be produced, for example, by epileptic seizures or by barbiturate administration, metabolic control of CBF is generally a local or regional phenomenon (Gross et al., 1980). After cerebral injury, the regional pattern of blood flow is much less predictable and regional cerebral blood flow (rCBF) may actually become uncoupled from the level of regional metabolic activity.

Superimposed on this metabolic regulation is a regulatory mechanism that keeps CBF constant during changes in CPP. As a result of this pressure "autoregulation," CVR normally varies directly with the CPP. Regardless of whether a given change in CPP is produced by altering the MAP, ICP, or venous pressure, the dynamics of autoregulation are basically the same (Symon et al., 1973; Raisis et al., 1975). Thus, during a fall in CPP (decreased MAP or increased ICP), CBF is maintained as a result of a compensatory decrease in CVR (vasodilatation). Conversely, CBF does not normally increase during elevations of CPP because compensatory vasoconstriction occurs. However, there is a finite range of perfusion pressures over which autoregulation can keep CBF constant. Although pial arteries do not become maximally dilated until MAP has fallen to approximately 35 mm Hg, vasodilation becomes insufficient to prevent a decrease in CBF once the MAP has been reduced below 65 mm Hg (MacKenzie et al., 1979). Assuming a normal ICP (up to 10 mm Hg), this corresponds to a CPP of approximately 55–60 mm Hg. However, this lower limit for autoregulation was obtained in a model that utilized hemorrhagic hypotension to reduce the CPP. There is evidence that when the CPP is reduced by elevating the ICP, CBF is still maintained at a CPP as low as 45 mm Hg (Miller et al., 1971; Grubb et al., 1975). This discrepancy is apparently due to the fact that during hypovolemic hypotension increased sympathetic output causes constriction of cerebral inflow vessels which attenuates the effects of autoregulation (Fitch et al., 1975). It is important to note that although CBF begins to fall once the CPP is reduced below 45–50 mm Hg, this does not mean that symptomatic ischemia immediately supervenes. In normal subjects, symptoms of ischemia emerge only when CBF has decreased to less than 50% of control values (Williams, 1968), which ordinarily occurs at a CPP of less than 25–30 mm Hg.

The upper limit for autoregulation normally occurs at a CPP of approximately 160 mm Hg. This threshold is shifted upward (as is the lower limit for autoregulation) as a result of acute sympathetic stimulation (MacKenzie et al., 1977; Gross et al., 1979) or chronic hypertension. Above this threshold, vasoconstriction is no longer sufficient to prevent an increase in CBF. Furthermore, an increasing proportion of the arterial pressure head will be transmitted to the capillary bed. This may increase the formation of vasogenic edema if the BBB has previously been opened (or may itself disrupt the barrier if capillary pressure becomes high enough.)

Outside of a CPP range of approximately 50–160 mm Hg, CBF varies linearly with the CPP. This relationship also obtains within the normal autoregulatory range if the CPP is changed very rapidly. The latency of autoregulation has variously been reported as 30–120 sec (Harper, 1972). However, recent reports have suggested that compensatory changes in CVR occur within 10–15 sec after abrupt changes in CPP (Kontos et al., 1978; Busija et al., 1979). This latency accounts for the fact that stepwise changes in CPP are better tolerated than abrupt alterations of similar or even lesser magnitude (Häggendal and Johansson, 1972).

The arterial carbon dioxide tension also exerts a profound—and therapeutically important—influence on CBF and CBV. This relationship between the principal end product of cerebral metabolism and CBF apparently subserves homeostasis of brain pH. Hypercapnia causes vasodilatation (decreased CVR) and thus increases CBF and CBV. Hypocapnia has the opposite effect. Blood flow normally changes 2–4% for each 1 mm Hg change in arterial PCO_2, within a CO_2 tension range of 20–60 mm Hg (Gennarelli et al., 1979). Since induction of hypocapnia by controlled hyperventilation is often used in the treatment of increased ICP, it is important to know the level at which hypocapnic vasoconstriction itself causes ischemic cell damage. In a critical review of this subject, Harp and Wollman (1973) found no experimental evidence that an arterial PCO_2 as low as 10 mm Hg produces structural brain damage. However, MacMillan and Siesjö (1973) have reported a progressive increase in cerebral anaerobic metabolism as the arterial PCO_2 of experimental animals is reduced below 25 mm Hg. Because of the paucity of relevant clinical studies and because a decrease in arterial PCO_2 to a level below 20–25 mm Hg further reduces intracranial blood volume to only a minimal extent, few if any neurosurgeons advocate reducing the PCO_2 below this level.

The vasomotor effects of the arterial carbon dioxide tension are mediated by changes in the hydrogen ion (H+) concentration of the extracellular fluid (ECF) (Kontos et al., 1977a and b). As a result, the reduction in CBV that can be obtained by inducing hypocapnia is limited in duration by the ECF bicarbonate-carbon dioxide buffer system. The efficiency of this buffer system is so great that during hyperventilation of stroke patients, the pH of the ECF returns to nearly normal within a matter of hours (Christensen et al., 1973). The experience of many neurosurgeons, including ourselves, indicates that the favorable impact of induced hypocapnia on increased ICP following head injury is more prolonged than this study would indicate. Nevertheless, it remains clear that the efficacy of hyperventilation is transient. Another important point is that sudden normalization of the arterial PCO_2 after hypocapnia of several hours duration may cause a temporary ECF acidosis. In a head-injured patient with increased ICP, the consequent increase in CBV may increase ICP still further.

Alterations in the arterial oxygen tension also affect CBF and CBV. As the arterial PO_2 falls below 50 mm Hg, cerebral resistance vessels progressively dilate. As noted previously, CBF may increase to 4–5 times normal as a result of a reduction in the arterial PO_2 to 15–20 mm Hg. Above a PO_2 of 50 mm Hg, changes in arterial oxygen tension have no effect on CBF unless hyperbaric oxygenation is employed. The latter produces vasoconstriction and thus reduces CBF and CBV. However, this technique is not presently used in the clinical treatment of head injuries, since a similar therapeutic effect can be produced, and at less expense, by inducing hypocapnia.

With the possible exception of pressure autoregulation, which may be an intrinsic response of cerebrovascular smooth muscle to alteration of transmural pressure (Folkow, 1964), changes in CVR are probably mediated by local vasoactive substances. In the past, such substances as hydrogen, potassium, and calcium ions have received particular scrutiny (Purves, 1978). After head injury, abnormal concentrations of these or other substances (eg, certain monoamines or prostaglandins) may be responsible for the alterations in vasomotor activity that have been reported. Recently, adenosine, an adenine nucleoside, has been implicated in the metabolic regulation of CBF (Berne et al., 1974). Dramatic increases in brain adenosine occur very rapidly after the onset of ischemia or hypoxia (Winn et al., 1979a and b). Moreover, recent work has suggested that adenosine may even be critically involved in autoregulation (Winn et al., 1980). It is also quite possible that no single chemical factor is responsible for the control of CVR. Instead, several local chemical regulators may collaborate, with each making a different quantitative or temporal contribution (Rubio et al., 1975; Kuschinsky and Wahl, 1978).

In concluding this discussion of the normal control of CBF, a word should be said about the nature of cerebral "resistance" vessels. Micropuncture techniques have demonstrated that under normal physiological conditions, the total CVR is derived from almost equal contributions by the large basal arteries, large pial arterioles, small pial and parenchymal arterioles, and capillaries and venules (Shapiro et al., 1971; Stromberg and Fox, 1972). However, the contribution of each of these segments of the cerebrovascular bed may vary from moment to moment because each may respond differently to changes in the ambient conditions that determine vascular diameter. For example, small pial and penetrating arterioles may be more sensitive than large pial arterioles to changes in arterial PCO_2 (Kontos et al., 1977a) while the opposite relationship may obtain for pressure autoregulation (Kontos et al., 1977b). Because of these "gradients of responsivity" (Rosenblum and Commonwealth, 1977), it may be misleading to restrict the term "resistance vessels" to only one segment of the cerebrovascular bed. On the other hand, MacKenzie and his colleagues (1979) have demonstrated that the most dynamic segment of the cerebrovascular bed is comprised of arterioles with a diameter of less than 50 μm. This corresponds to the class of vessels generally responsible for regulation of resistance in vascular beds outside of the central nervous system. In any case, it is important to appreciate that under pathological conditions the relative contribution of each vascular segment to the total CVR may be altered, and indeed any segment of the cerebrovascular bed may become the critical determinant of the CVR.

Post-Traumatic Disorders of Cerebrovascular Reactivity

DYSAUTOREGULATION

Disorders in autoregulation are relatively common during the 1st week after a coma-producing head injury. Despite occasional reports to the contrary (Bruce et al., 1973), most investigators have found that autoregulation is rarely abolished throughout an entire hemisphere. Thus, Cold and Jensen (1978) have reported focal or multifocal impairment of autoregulation in 83% of patients in coma after head injury. In this context, it is important to note that impairment of autoregulation (and also chemical reactivity) may not be confined to the regions that demonstrate structural signs of injury.

Impaired autoregulation may be the earliest detectable disturbance in blood flow following focal cortical injury (Reivich et al., 1969; Miller et al., 1976). However, dysautoregulation may also be produced by common complications of clinical head injury including cerebral compression (Reilly et al., 1975), ischemia (Paulson, 1971), hypercapnia (Harper, 1965), acute hypoxia (Häggendal, 1968), posthypoxic states (Freeman and Ingvar, 1968), and perhaps by the presence of intracranial pressure gradients (Symon et al., 1974). Cerebral lactic acidosis is common to several of the above conditions. Because this tissue acidosis abolishes the normal resting cerebrovascular tone, loss of normal cerebrovascular reactivity usually occurs in the setting of paretic vasodilatation (Langfitt and Bruce, 1975). The resulting hyperemia has been termed "luxury perfusion" (Lassen, 1966) since the level of rCBF is greater than the level needed to meet regional tissue substrate requirements. Under these circumstances autoregulation can sometimes be restored or at least improved by hyperventilation, since the respiratory alkalosis attenuates the local tissue acidosis (Paulson et al., 1972; Hadjidimos et al., 1975).

Dysautoregulation causes CBF to vary passively with CPP. Impairment of autoregulation may therefore result in a critical decrease in rCBF at a level of CPP that would otherwise be tolerated. Furthermore, elevations of the systemic arterial pressure that might otherwise be clinically acceptable may increase the severity of cerebral edema and intracranial hypertension because of a passive increase in CBF and CBV. For these reasons, the CPP (or at least MAP if ICP is not monitored) should ordinarily be maintained within a clearly normal range in patients who have suffered a severe head injury.

Finally, in some patients with head injuries, CBF remains relatively constant as the MAP is increased but falls passively as the MAP is decreased. This phenomenon of "false autoregulation" is largely confined to the most severely injured patients. Many of these patients demonstrate a pronounced cerebrospinal fluid (CSF) lactic acidosis and impaired cerebrovascular reactivity to changes in arterial PCO_2 (Enevoldsen and Jensen, 1977). Clinical improvement may coincide with a phase in which CBF varies passively with both increases and decreases in MAP. These observations support the view that "false autoregulation" has no relation at all to true autoregulation and is certainly not a favorable sign. The explanation that has been advanced for apparent preservation of only the hypertensive phase of autoregulation is microvascular compression (Marshall et al., 1969; Reilly et al., 1975). Elevation of the MAP in the setting of dysautoregulation and blood-brain barrier injury causes extravasation of a plasma filtrate into the pericapillary extracellular space. The consequent increase in perivascular tissue pressure allegedly causes local distortion of the vascular bed and thus an increase in the CVR. However, "false autoregulation" may simply be an experimental artifact attributable to disruption of the blood-brain barrier. In both experimental (Reilly et al., 1975) and clinical (Enevoldsen and Jensen, 1977) demonstrations of this phenomenon, the MAP has been elevated by pharmacological agents, such as angiotensin, which cause vasoconstriction when topically applied to pial vessels. Although administered intravascularly, these agents may gain access to the abluminal vessel surface by crossing the damaged blood-brain barrier. In tests of autoregulation using other agents, such as norepinephrine, the direct effect of the drug on vascular smooth muscle may be overshadowed by its effect on cerebral metabolism. After experimental opening of the blood-brain barrier with hypertonic urea, MacKenzie and his colleagues (1976) found that intracarotid infusion of norepinephrine caused an increase in CBF which was apparently secondary to stimulation of cerebral metabolism. A similar phenomenon has been reported in tests of high pressure autoregulation in head-injured patients (Griffith et al., 1972). It is apparent that pharmacological tests of autoregulation in injured brain are difficult to interpret.

IMPAIRED CHEMICAL REGULATION

It is not clear how readily CO_2 reactivity is impaired after head injury. Some studies have demonstrated that chemical regulation may initially be relatively normal, even in patients who ultimately die as a result of their head injury (Gennarelli et al., 1979). Other studies have demonstrated absent reactivity to changes in arterial PCO_2 in almost half of patients who were tested within 4 days of injury (Cold et al., 1977). At present, the weight of experimental and clinical evidence seems to favor the following hypotheses. First, although some degree of chemical reactivity can often be demonstrated in patients who have lost the capacity to autoregulate (Bruce et al., 1978a), these two forms of flow regulation are often impaired concomitantly after severe head injury. Indeed, chemical reactivity is impaired by the same physiological disturbances (e.g. mechanical injury, hypoxia, ischemia, hypertension) that alter autoregulation. Reports of impaired chemical regulation in the presence of intact autoregulation should be examined critically (they may represent examples of "false autoregulation") although an experimental model of this type of dissociated response has been developed (Fenske et al., 1975). Second, even if chemical reactivity is not readily abolished as a result of cerebral trauma, there is convincing experimental evidence that it is readily diminished. In a careful study that eliminated metabolic and hemodynamic causes of hyporeactivity, Saunders and his colleagues (1979) demonstrated that even mild mechanical trauma decreases vascular reactivity to changes in arterial PCO_2 by an average of 40%.

INTRACEREBRAL STEALS

Because cerebrovascular reactivity is often altered in a focal or multifocal pattern after head injury, vasodilating or vasoconstricting stimuli may produce a variable or even paradoxic regional blood flow response. For example, a vasodilator stimulus (e.g., hypercapnia) may actually cause a significant decrease in blood flow and blood volume in some regions of the cerebrovascular bed (Teasdale et al., 1975). Because the decrease in resistance is relatively greater in normally reactive vessels, flow may be diverted away from hyporeactive vessels (intracerebral steal). Conversely, a strong vasoconstrictor stimulus may increase blood flow in poorly reactive portions of the vascular bed (inverse steal). Thus, the salutary effect of controlled hyperventilation on increased ICP is based (at least in part) on the reduction of blood volume in cerebral regions with a normally reactive vascular bed. Local blood volume (and perhaps edema formation) may actually increase in injured regions with a poorly reactive vasculature. In most cases, the blood volume changes in reactive portions of the vascular bed apparently have a greater effect on the ICP than the presumably opposite volume changes in hyporeactive regions.

Post-Traumatic Changes in Metabolism and Blood Flow

METABOLIC DEPRESSION

Although changes in blood flow after head injury are quite variable, the $CMRO_2$ is almost always reduced in post-traumatic coma. Values that are 50% or less of normal are relatively common among severely injured patients (Shalit et al., 1972; Bruce et al., 1973; Brodersen and Jørgensen, 1974; Gennarelli et al., 1979). The lowest values have generally been reported in patients with clinical sings of brainstem injury (Bruce and Langfitt, 1976). On the basis of a series of 45 patients who were studied an average of 7 days after head injury, Hass (1976) concluded that brainstem injury alone consistently diminishes the $CMRO_2$ by at least 40%. This concept is supported by a canine model that involves bilateral electrolytic lesions in the midbrain reticular formation (Hawkins et al., 1979) and by well documented reports of a persistent reduction in $CMRO_2$ in vegetative survivors of brainstem infarcts (Ingvar and Sourander, 1970). Nevertheless, a causal relationship between brainstem injury and cerebral metabolic depression is difficult to document in clinical head injury. Careful autopsy studies have demonstrated that isolated brainstem lesions are distinctly uncommon among patients who initially survive a head injury and that most patients with clinical signs of brainstem injury also have diffuse forebrain injuries (Adams et al., 1977). Thus, the reduced $CMRO_2$ in these patients may represent merely the sum of local energy derangements that are disseminated throughout the cerebrum.

Despite the fact that the extent of the reduction in the cerebral metabolic rate generally parallels the depth of post-traumatic coma (Griffith et al., 1972), the $CMRO_2$ has not proven useful in the prediction of outcome after severe head injury. Cold (1978) could not identify a value below which survival was invariably precluded and reported that a $CMRO_2$ as low as 0.4 ml/100 g/min is compatible with survival. However, Hass (1976) was able to conclude that patients with a $CMRO_2$ less than one-third normal (<1.2 ml/100 g/min) approximately 1 week after injury are unlikely to survive. In his own series there were no deaths directly attributable to head injury among patients with a $CMRO_2$ greater than 75% of normal (>2.7 ml/100 g/min). However, between these extremes, the $CMRO_2$ had little predictive value in individual patients.

One reason that the $CMRO_2$ is such an unsatisfactory prognostic indicator is that it does not reflect the cause— and thus the potential reversibility—of the decrease in metabolism. The $A\text{-}VDO_2$ (= $CMRO_2/CBF$) may provide some indication of whether the decrease in $CMRO_2$ is a primary effect of the injury or is instead secondary to potentially reversible hypoperfusion. A low $A\text{-}VDO_2$ indicates that CBF (even if it too is decreased) is at least adequate relative to the metabolic demand. Under this circumstance, induced increases in CBF usually have no effect on $CMRO_2$ (Hass, 1976). A high $A\text{-}VDO_2$ in the presence of a subnormal $CMRO_2$ indicates that the level of CBF is insufficient to support normal metabolic activity. In these cases, an increase in CBF may produce an improvement in the $CMRO_2$. For example, restoration of a normal CPP accounts, at least in part, for the salutary effect of mannitol on the $CMRO_2$ in some patients with greatly elevated ICP (Bruce and Langfitt, 1976). Mismatch between blood flow and metabolic rate may also occur on a regional basis due to inhomogeneity of tissue perfusion (see below). For example, improvement in the distribution of flow to ischemic regions may explain why hypocapnia apparently improves the hemispheric $CMRO_2$ in some head injury patients despite the fact that it reduces hemispheric blood flow (Gennarelli et al., 1979). A relatively normal $A\text{-}VDO_2$ in comatose patients is more difficult to interpret. An $A\text{-}VDO_2$ greater than 50% of normal is characteristic of survivors of head injury but has also been reported in patients with deep midline lesions (Bruce and Langfitt, 1976). In the latter case, it remains debatable whether the primary derangement is in the control of metabolism or in the regulation of blood flow.

CHANGES IN CBF

The level of CBF is much more variable than the $CMRO_2$ in patients in post-traumatic coma. Obrist and his colleagues (1979b) reported a range of 20–100 ml/ 100 g/min among comatose patients who were studied within a week of injury. Because of this variability, CBF measurements have proven to be unreliable prognostic indicators (Bruce et al., 1973; Enevoldsen et al., 1976; Obrist et al., 1979b). Although Overgaard (1976) found that CBFs less than 20 ml/100 g/min or greater than 65 ml/100 g/min had an equally grave prognosis, there was little correlation between outcome and CBF values within this range. Although mild disturbances in consciousness produce mild reductions in CBF which are distributed over a narrow range of values, it is clear that, unlike the $CMRO_2$, the level of CBF correlates poorly with the neurological status of patients with more serious injuries (Obrist et al., 1979b). As has already been indicated, normal or even supranormal CBF may be found in some comatose patients, indicating an uncoupling between metabolism and blood flow. Conversely, relatively low CBF values have occasionally been reported in noncomatose patients. For example, Enevoldsen and colleagues (1975) have reported that most of their patients who recovered from post-traumatic coma had a CBF less than 25 ml/100 g/min at the time they first became alert.

Early studies with intracarotid injection of Xenon-133 demonstrated that up to 90% of adult patients in post-traumatic coma have an abnormally low CBF at some point in their early hospital course (Bruce et al., 1973; Fieschi et al., 1974; Overgaard and Tweed, 1974; Enevoldsen et al., 1976). More recent techniques that employ intravenous injection of the tracer have not only confirmed these original observations but have also permitted serial measurements as well as simultaneous determination of blood flow in each hemisphere (Obrist et al., 1977). It is now apparent that even when a clinical examination or a computed tomographic (CT) scan indicates injury of only one hemisphere, blood flow reductions (or increases) are almost invariably generalized and bilateral in comatose patients (Obrist et al., 1979b). This finding is analogous to the "diaschisis" observed after acute unilateral cerebral infarction. Although CBF may be decreased homogeneously in comatose patients with no radiographic evidence of focal injury (Obrist et al., 1979a), up to 75% of patients in post-traumatic coma demonstrate significant intra- or interhemispheric blood flow heterogeneity superimposed on the more general pattern of global blood flow reduction (Obrist et al., 1979b). For example, the tissue immediately adjacent to an intracerebral or extracerebral hematoma is often hyperemic (increased local cerebral blood volume) despite the fact that rCBF may be decreased by more than 50% in the tissue contiguous to this hyperemic margin (Obrist et al., 1979a; Kuhl et al., 1980). Despite this heterogeneity, blood flow values for the hemisphere as a whole are consistently lower on the side of the hematoma, as are blood volume measurements (Kuhl et al., 1980). Patients who recover consciousness demonstrate a progressive improvement in CBF. Since the hemisphere contralateral to the hematoma regains normal blood flow more rapidly than the ipsilateral hemisphere, the period of clinical recovery is marked by a transient increase in the flow asymmetry between the two hemispheres (Kuhl et al., 1980). In patients who do not recover, CBF remains depressed or declines still further following evacuation of the hematoma (Obrist et al., 1979b). This probably reflects rather than causes the deterioration in cerebral functional activity. This finding also indicates that blood flow reductions associated with intracranial hematomas are not necessarily due to a decrease in CPP or to vascular compression. Indeed, virtual cessation of CBF has been reported in the presence of normal MAP, ICP, and CPP (Overgaard and Tweed, 1975; Obrist et al., 1979b). In the past, such a finding was sometimes explained in terms of the "no reflow" phenomenon (Ames et al., 1968). In the original studies of the "no reflow" phenomenon, transient total cerebral ischemia produced microvascular occlusion due to swelling of perivascular glia and capillary endothelial cells. As a result, perfusion defects remained even after the cerebral circulation was restored. However, further studies have indicated that "no reflow" is an uncommon sequel to ischemia (Levy et al., 1975a) and that it is neither a necessary nor frequent precursor to experimental infarction (Caronna and Plum, 1976). Indeed, irreversible ischemic neuronal damage becomes evident before "no reflow" is observed and it would thus seem that the latter occurs only after recovery has already been precluded by the duration of the ischemia (Levy et al., 1975a and b; Fraser et al., 1977).

There is conflicting evidence regarding the incidence of cerebral ischemia following head injury. This is due, in part, to variability in the choice of parameters used to define ischemia. For example, certain electrophysiological parameters such as the response of the cortex to direct electrical stimulation become altered as soon as CBF begins to decline from normal levels (Teasdale et al., 1977). Reversible metabolic changes indicative of increasing anaerobic metabolism also occur with relatively mild degrees of ischemia (Welsh et al., 1977). However, other parameters of electrocortical function (such as the EEG) remain relatively normal until CBF is less than 50% of control levels (Gregory et al., 1979), at which time clinical signs of ischemia become prominent (Williams, 1968). Complete cessation of all forms of electrocortical activity occurs only when cortical blood flow has been reduced to 15–20% of control values in anesthetized cats (Gregory et al., 1979). At this level, histological evidence of ischemic cell damage is regularly obtained (Graham et al., 1979). It would appear that a reduction of CBF up to 50% is well tolerated and that cerebral energy production does not begin to fail until CBF has declined to 35–45% of normal (Eklöf and Siesjö, 1972; Marshall et al., 1975). Thus, irreversible structural and biochemical changes probably do not occur until CBF falls below 15–20 ml/100 g/min (Branston et al., 1974), and, indeed, Overgaard (1976) has stated that he has not observed recovery of cortical function in head-injured patients with CBF values below 20 ml/100 g/min.

Several investigators have reported that oligemia of this severity is unusual among head-injured patients and that CBF is seldom less than 50% of normal (Bruce et al., 1973; Fieschi et al., 1974; Bruce et al., 1978a), unless the ICP is severely elevated (Enevoldsen et al., 1976). It has also been observed that even when CBF is markedly reduced, the $CMRO_2$ is often reduced to a proportionately greater extent, thus indicating that the low CBF is adequate relative to the metabolic rate (Bruce et al., 1973). Contrary to what might be expected on the basis of these clinical studies, Graham et al. (1978) found evidence of ischemic damage in more than 90% of a consecutive series of patients who died after head injury. Ischemic changes were localized to arterial boundary zones in more than 20% (Graham et al., 1975). Brierley and his colleagues (1969) found that CPP must be reduced below 25 mm Hg for at least 15 min before histological evidence of boundary zone ischemia can be observed in experimental animals.

This discrepancy between clinical and pathological studies is probably due to the methodological limitations of the former. First, CBF has seldom, if ever, been measured in head-injured patients prior to resuscitation. Second, most of the clinical data presently available was derived by techniques that have a very limited capacity to detect areas of hypoperfusion if they are adjacent to regions with a more normal flow rate (Teasdale et al., 1975). Thus, although hemispheric blood flow may be only moderately decreased and hemispheric flow and metabolism may remain well matched, significant regional ischemia (for example, of the boundary-zone type) may still be present (Welsh et al., 1977). Although newer techniques (e.g., emission computed tomography) can detect macroscopic flow heterogeneity in head injury patients, clinical documentation of microheterogeneity remains elusive. Experimental studies by Welsh and his colleagues (1977, 1979) have demonstrated a microheterogeneous pattern of metabolic failure in gray matter during diffuse cerebral oligemia and have suggested that this pattern is due to inhomogeneous tissue perfusion. They have also obtained some evidence that cortical high energy phosphate content does not decline gradually as the CPP is lowered but is instead affected in an "all or nothing" fashion at a CPP threshold of approximately 30 mm Hg (Welsh et al., 1977). On the basis of these observations, they have suggested that relatively minor microregional differences in blood flow may produce striking heterogeneity in the pattern of tissue metabolic failure.

Although the above observations need further elaboration and confirmation, they illustrate the limitations of current clinically applicable techniques in diagnosing the presence of cerebral ischemia following head injury. Determinations of CBF do occasionally indicate that measures should be instituted to augment local blood flow, particularly in cases in which a mass lesion is present (Bruce et al., 1978a). However, it has not been demonstrated that the outcome of severe head injury can be improved by routinely monitoring CBF. In addition, the expense of this technique presently precludes its widespread use. Many neurosurgical intensive care units are equipped to monitor CPP. Unfortunately, this parameter is of even more limited use in diagnosing regional or even global ischemia. Although there has been a close correspondence between CBF and CPP in some studies of experimental brain compression (Miller et al., 1973), there is no consistent relationship between these two factors in comatose head injury patients (Bruce et al., 1973). Miller (1979) has pointed out that in the presence of dysautoregulation, increased sympathetic tone, vasospasm, and brain edema—all of which are consequences of severe head injury—CBF may be subnormal at a CPP as high as 90 mm Hg and electrocortical function may fail at a CPP as high as 60 mm Hg. Indeed, these thresholds vary from patient to patient. Theoretically, a CPP that is insufficient to correct regional ischemia in one patient may be high enough to aggravate brain edema in another. The inconsistent relationship between CPP and CBF is due to the fact that CBF is also determined by the state of the active component of cerebrovascular resistance that normally compensates for changes in the level of perfusion pressure and by the passive component imposed on the vascular bed by vasospasm, tissue distortion, and perhaps by brain edema (Miller, 1979). Unfortunately, these "resistance" factors cannot be determined as readily as the CPP. In the absence of definite information concerning the state of the cerebral vasculature in a given patient, it is probably wise to maintain the CPP within a normal range (60–100 mm Hg). In some patients even this modest goal may prove elusive, in which case continuous maintenance of even a marginal level of perfusion may be important. A recent study demonstrated that retention of a CBF level less than 10% of normal produces a better neurological outcome in experimental animals than a comparable period of complete ischemia (Steen et al., 1970). However, the authors confined this study to a duration of ischemia that is consistent with meaningful neurological recovery in otherwise normal animals. Although a similar time interval has not been determined for patients with major head injuries, it is likely that this interval is comparatively short.

CEREBRAL HYPEREMIA

The $CMRO_2$ in most comatose head injury patients with a normal or even supranormal CBF is essentially the same as the $CMRO_2$ in comatose patients with subnormal CBF (Obrist et al., 1979b). Thus, CBF in the former group is excessive relative to tissue metabolic demand (as indicated by the low $A-VDO_2$). According to some investigators, this hyperemia is the most common focal abnormality of CBF in head injury patients (Overgaard and Tweed, 1974; Enevoldsen et al., 1976; Enevoldsen and Jensen, 1978). Enevoldsen and his colleagues (1975) found that tracer clearance curves from areas of severe cortical injury had very fast initial components (equivalent to a rCBF greater than 170 ml/100 g/min) which contained up to 40% of the regional distribution of the tracer bolus. The percentage of regional tracer bolus contained within this "tissue peak" varied directly with the severity of the cortical injury and changed with its clinical evolution. These peaks were often succeeded by an abnormally low level of rCBF after several days (Enevoldsen et al., 1976).

In these studies, early draining veins were sometimes seen on angiograms in the area of the tissue peak. This was interpreted as indicative of focally increased blood flow secondary to local tissue acidosis rather than actual arteriovenous shunting. Overgaard and Tweed (1974) found a close correlation between the time course of CSF lactic acidosis and this cerebral hyperemia. In further support of this interpretation are the observations that hyperemia is exacerbated or even provoked by arterial hypertension and is diminished by hyperventilation (Enevoldsen et al., 1976; Enevoldsen and Jensen, 1978). These findings also suggest that dysautoregulation is involved (Obrist et al., 1979a).

Although Enevoldsen (1976) did not observe focal hyperemia in the absence of cortical lacerations or contusions, regional hyperemia has since been reported in association with post-traumatic seizures and intracranial hematomas (Obrist et al., 1979b). Using emission computed tomography, Kuhl and colleagues (1980) demonstrated a 20–50% increase in local blood volume in the displaced cortex subjacent to acute subdural hematomas. This perifocal hyperemia often persisted after the hematoma was evacuated but disappeared as cerebral displacement resolved. According to some reports, local hyperemia may become evident only after the hematoma has been evacuated (Bruce et al., 1978a).

A more generalized form of hyperemia may occur in the absence of focal cerebral lesions. In an early study of this phenomenon, Langfitt et al. (1966) noted an immediate increase in ICP following blunt occipital injury in cats. The immediate appearance and rapid resolution of the increase in ICP made edema an unlikely cause. The fact that the time course of the ICP elevation paralleled that of reflex systemic hypertension suggested that cerebral swelling might be due to traumatically induced cerebrovascular dilatation and a consequent increase in cerebral blood volume. More recently, Saunders and his colleagues (1979) corroborated this view by documenting a transient decrease in CVR after severe concussive injury in cats. Indeed, there is considerable evidence that the initial response of the cerebral circulation to cerebral concussive injury is vasodilatation and increased blood flow, although this may be succeeded by vasospasm and subnormal flow.

Clinically, diffuse cerebral hyperemia has been observed within 24 hr after resuscitation from hypovolemic shock (Obrist et al., 1979b). However, considerable attention has recently been directed to a syndrome of bilateral (occasionally unilateral) cerebral hyperemia that is apparently a primary manifestation of head injury, particularly in children and adolescents. In some series, up to 50% of pediatric patients in post-traumatic coma have demonstrated ventricular compression and obliteration of the perimesencephalic subarachnoid cisterns on CT scan but have no evidence of a focal mass lesion (Zimmerman et al., 1978). Higher than normal Hounsfield numbers on CT scan have been interpreted as indicative of tissue hyperemia, and an analogy has been made to the experimental studies cited above. Although normal or supranormal blood flow has been documented in some patients with these CT scan signs of diffuse swelling (Obrist et al., 1979a), CBF and cerebral blood volume have been found to be normal in others (Kuhl et al., 1980). This discrepancy may be due, at least in part, to an overlap between the CT scan findings in cerebral swelling due to hyperemia and swelling associated with diffuse white matter injury. Nevertheless, these two pathological entities should be separable on the basis of the clinical course. Although both syndromes may initially produce signs indistinguishable from those of brainstem injury, patients with cerebral hyperemia often regain consciousness or at least improve in the hours immediately following the injury. In contrast, patients with diffuse white matter disruption are almost invariably comatose from the moment of impact, since the structural injury is immediate. Unlike patients with swelling secondary to hyperemia, these patients seldom make a satisfactory recovery.

The clinical significance of diffuse cerebral hyperemia lies in the tendency of these patients to develop increased ICP (Brodersen and Jørgensen, 1974; Fieschi et al., 1974; Obrist et al., 1979b). Although distention of the cerebrovascular system decreases cerebral compliance (see following section) it is unclear how often the increase in blood volume is itself the cause of the elevated ICP. Obrist et al. (1979a) reported that the ICP in these patients is usually normal initially but that it increases within 24–36 hr (if the hyperemia does not resolve) due to formation of vasogenic edema. Presumably the paretic vasodilatation causes an increase in capillary hydrostatic pressure which then causes "filtration" edema. It should be stressed that this hypothesis—like many other aspects of the syndrome—is still the subject of lively debate. Nevertheless, Bruce and his associates (1978a and b) recently advocated restraint in the use of mannitol in head-injured children because of concern that the transient expansion of plasma volume will further increase CBV, ICP, and capillary hydrostatic pressure. The same group of investigators also documented that hyperventilation may decrease the cerebral blood volume in patients with cerebral hyperemia and often reduces ICP (Gennarelli et al., 1979). This, too, is consistent with the hypothesis that diffuse hyperemia is due to paretic vasodilatation and impairment of autoregulation.

OTHER EFFECTS OF ISCHEMIA

EDEMA

Although the neurons are the cellular element of the central nervous system most vulnerable to ischemic injury, cellular swelling characteristically involves the glia (Klatzo, 1979). Following ischemic injury, there is a rapid shift of water from the extracellular into the intracellular fluid compartment, as indicated by a decrease in the volume of the inulin and sucrose spaces. However, this fluid translocation does not itself constitute edema since it may occur in the absence of an increase in the total cerebral water content. Indeed, severe hypoxemia may produce just this condition. It has been argued that ischemia does not produce true edema unless the duration of the insult is sufficient to cause tissue necrosis (Plum et al., 1963). However, by applying the sensitive specific gravity technique of Nelson et al. (1971), Fujimoto and colleagues (1976) demonstrated an increase in cerebral water content in the gerbil after only 5 min of bilateral carotid artery occlusion. Such observations imply that cytotoxic edema involves a general disturbance in the regulation of brain volume as well as a specific defect in cellular osmoregulation (Klatzo, 1979). But even if BBB permeability to water is increased, this does not mean that permeability to proteins must also be altered. Indeed, the BBB initially remains impermeable to vital dyes and high molecular weight proteins in experimental models of cytotoxic edema.

Ischemic injury does eventually cause vasogenic edema, even in the absence of tissue necrosis or an increase in CBF (Fujimoto et al., 1976). In early studies, increased BBB permeability was not striking until 18 hr after induction of ischemia (Hossman and Olsson, 1972). However, subsequent reports have demonstrated that the latency of barrier opening varies with the duration of ischemia and with the adequacy of reperfusion. Working with a carotid occlusion model in gerbils, Ito and colleagues (1976) found that increased permeability could not be consistently demonstrated until blood flow had been restored for 5–29 hr. Barrier breakdown following reperfusion was more rapid after longer periods of ischemia.

MEMBRANE LIPID PEROXIDATION

The destructive effects of tissue hypoxia may also be mediated by free radical formation and peroxidation of biomembrane lipids. Free radicals are formed by fission of covalent bonds, which results in a single electron occupying an outer shell of an atom. As a result of this unpaired electron, free radicals are unusually reactive. Because they characteristically react with carbon atoms adjacent to double bonds, the polyunsaturated fatty acids of membrane phospholipids are particularly vulnerable to attack (Demopoulos, 1973). Free radical reactions are not necessarily pathological. For example, free radicals are normal intermediates in the respiratory chain. However, these reactions do not usually lead to net production of free radicals since the transport factors remain tightly associated with electrons as long as oxygen is available to terminate the reactions. In addition, these reactions occur in the hydrophilic phase of the cell, away from the vulnerable fatty acid tails of phospholipid molecules. Furthermore, natural free radical scavengers (e.g., ascorbic acid, alpha-tocopherol, and glutathione) and enzymatic defense systems normally protect the cell membranes.

Demopoulos and his colleagues (1979) have postulated that ischemia initiates free radical reactions by depriving a certain proportion of electron transport chains of the molecular oxygen needed to maintain a continuous flow of electrons. As a result, the free radical forms of certain transport factors accumulate in sufficient quantities to peroxidize the unsaturated lipid groups of biomembranes, particularly those of mitochondria and endoplasmic reticula (Demopoulos et al., 1979). These reactions may be abetted by the fact that polyunsaturated free fatty acids (particularly arachidonic acid) may be released from membrane phospholipids during ischemia (Bazan, 1979). Free radical attack may also be exacerbated by cerebral hemorrhage, since the copper and iron contained in serum and erythrocytes are powerful catalysts of these reactions (Demopoulos, 1973). Although reduced in the process of peroxidation, free radicals are regenerated in the presence of even minimal amounts of oxygen. The superoxide ($\cdot O_2^-$) radical is generated in the process. Barbiturates reportedly interrupt these self-perpetuating cycles of reduction and auto-oxidation by complexing with the oxidized form of these molecules (Siesjö et al., 1977; Nordström et al., 1978).

Since free radicals are reactive transients, they do not accumulate in sufficient steady state concentrations to be readily detected. Thus the evidence for free radical reactions after cerebral injury or ischemia is largely indirect: destructive loss of polyunsaturated fatty acids from gray and white matter, consumption of nervous system antioxidants, and detection of meta-stable or final compounds such as malonaldehyde (Demopoulos et al., 1979; Flamm et al., 1979). The potential consequences of free radical reactions include the loss of normal excitability and fluidity (synaptosome formation) of neuronal membranes and loss of the barrier and compartmentalization functions of other cells of the central nervous system. In addition, certain membrane enzymes, including sodium-potassium ATPase and cytochrome oxidase derive their active tertiary structures from the interaction between their hydrophobic portions and the fatty acid tails of certain membrane phospholipids. These enzymes are thus secondarily inhibited by lipid peroxidation (Schaefer et al., 1975). Demopoulos (1979) has even suggested that the decrease in oxidative metabolism and the increase in glycolysis observed after cerebral injury may be due, in part, to lipid free radical reactions involving the inner mitochondrial membrane.

It should be pointed out, however, that some investigators have not found any correlation between the protection afforded by barbiturates during cerebral ischemia and free radical scavenging (Steen and Michenfelder, 1978). Indeed these investigators have recently questioned the importance of free radical damage during ischemia (Steen et al., 1979).

CHANGES IN INTRACRANIAL VOLUME AND PRESSURE

Many of the pathological processes that are set in motion by head injury directly or indirectly increase intracranial volume. This is reflected in the fact that at least 75% of patients in post-traumatic coma have some degree of elevation of ICP at the time that pressure monitoring is initiated (Langfitt, 1976a; Miller et al., 1977). The potential importance of this high incidence is indicated by the fact that almost half of the patients who died in one major series had severe, uncontrollable intracranial hypertension (Miller et al., 1977). Furthermore, several recent reports have suggested that continuous monitoring and aggressive control of ICP may reduce the mortality of severe head injury (Becker et al., 1977; Bruce et al., 1978b; Marshall et al., 1979).

Despite this strong circumstantial evidence that increased ICP can contribute significantly to the morbidity and mortality of head injury, the responsible pathophysiological mechanisms remain the subject of much debate. It is becoming increasingly clear that post-traumatic intracranial hypertension is not a single disease entity, but instead varies considerably in cause, effect, clinical course, and response to particular therapeutic modalities.

The Pressure-Volume Relationship

VOLUMETRIC COMPENSATION

The brain is unique in that it is the only major organ that is encased in bone. As a result, the total intracranial volume is fixed (at approximately 1900 ml in adults). Thus, an increase in the volume of a normal intracranial compartment (brain, blood, or CSF) or the creation of an abnormal one (e.g. a hematoma) must be compensated for by an equivalent reduction in the volume of another compartment or the ICP will rise. This relationship between intracranial volume and pressure was first appreciated in the 18th century (Monro, 1783). Subsequent investigators have found that intracranial volumetric compensation involves the entire craniospinal axis and that small changes can occur in the intradural volume (Weed, 1929; Pollock and Boshes, 1936).

As much as 70% of volumetric compensation (or "spatial buffering") is provided by the CSF compartment, which normally occupies approximately 10% of the total intracranial volume (Löfgren and Zwetnow, 1973). Volumetric expansion within the craniospinal CSF spaces is compensated for by a number of interacting regulatory mechanisms, which include compliance mechanisms (Löfgren et al., 1973; Löfgren and Zwetnow, 1973; Marmarou et al., 1975, 1978) that are functionally related to the elastic properties of the spinal meninges and craniospinal blood vessels. In addition, there is a nonlinear outflow resistance mechanism which modulates CSF volume by venting fluid into the venous circulation (Johnson et al., 1978; Mann et al., 1978). Within the CSF system, the immediate response to volumetric increments involves fluid shifts from the intracranial to the spinal cavity in combination with compensatory spinal meningeal distention (Langfitt et al., 1964; Martins et al., 1972; Löfgren and Zwetnow, 1973). It should be stressed that compliance mechanisms are important only in the initial, transient response to intracranial volume expansion. During steady state elevations of ICP, the pressure-sensitive outflow resistance to CSF absorption modulates large volume increments (Mann et al., 1978). The role of the CSF system in intracranial spatial compensation is thus dependent upon its capacity to translocate fluid out of the cranial cavity. The effectiveness of this mechanism is dependent on an unimpeded flow of CSF throughout the CSF space and on the functional state (resistance) of the outflow pathways through which CSF is vented into the venous circulation. Arachnoid villi are generally considered to function as a major outflow pathway for CSF. Recent evidence suggests that alterations in the size and shape of vesicles within the arachnoid villus endothelium occur in association with increasing levels of steady state CSF pressure. These changes may represent the structural basis for changes in CSF outflow resistance (Butler et al., 1980). At resting CSF pressures, fluid is transported across the endothelium by micropinocytotic vesicles (and occasionally through open interendothelial clefts). At sustained, elevated pressures, enhanced CSF transport through arachnoid villi is mediated by transendothelial channels formed by either single, enlarged pinocytotic vesicles or chains of fused vesicles. The response of arachnoid villi under conditions of elevated CSF pressure can be interpreted as a valvular mechanism whereby increases in CSF volume, pressure, and flow are modulated by the transport of proportionately greater quantities of fluid out of the CSF compartment. Thus, nonlinear changes in CSF outflow resistance allow the CSF system to achieve stable equilibrium pressures.

The intracranial blood volume accounts for approximately 3–7% of the volume of the cranial cavity. Perhaps 80% is contained in the dural venous sinuses and cerebral veins (Langfitt and Bruce, 1975). Blood can be readily displaced from these low pressure capacitance vessels into the extracranial venous circulation as the ICP increases. This is a further example of an intracranial compliance mechanism. However, it is unclear whether this phenomenon causes a net decrease in intracranial blood volume, since resistance vessels may concurrently dilate (Löfgren and Zwetnow, 1976). As was noted in the previous section of this chapter, this vasodilatation initially maintains CBF in the face of the decline in CPP. The net effect of these changes in vessel caliber obscures the distinction that is normally made between arterial resistance vessels and venous capacitance vessels (Langfitt and Bruce, 1975). Grubb and his colleagues (1975) found that the cerbral blood volume is actually increased at ICP levels of 50–90 mm Hg (which corresponded in their experiments to a CPP of 80–40 mm Hg). However, at still higher levels of ICP, the blood volume as well as CBF began to decrease significantly. Presumably the pressure forces generated by progressive increases in intracranial volume eventually exhaust the capacity of autoregulation to maintain normal blood blow. It would thus appear that the relative contribution of intravascular blood to the total intracranial volume may vary as the ICP rises and that physiological changes that promote flow homeostasis may compete with those that promote volumetric compensation. Once the spatial buffering capacity of the CSF and intravascular compartments has been exhausted, any further volumetric compensation is provided by the viscoelastic properties of the subpial tissues (Schettini and Walsh, 1974). This compensation is very limited since the brain has little, if any, capacity to undergo an acute reduction in volume, although it can be mechanically distorted and displaced.

INTRACRANIAL ELASTANCE

When alterations in intracranial volume involve changes in the volume of the CSF space, the fluid pressure of the CSF is changed as well (Marmarou and Shulman, 1976). The magnitude of the pressure change is dependent upon the magnitude and rate of the volume change and upon the "extensibility" of the CSF space. The latter is determined by the elastic properties of the walls of the CSF space which, broadly considered, includes all of the tissues from the ependyma to the skull (Sullivan et al., 1977). It is also dependent upon the physical properties of any pathological intracranial mass. The intracranial elastance is the net result of the complex interaction of the elastic properties of these individual structures. Changes in the volume or composition of any normal or abnormal structure will potentially alter intracranial elastance.

The elastance represents the relationship between changes in CSF volume and CSF pressure (Löfgren et al., 1973) and is expressed as $\Delta P/\Delta V$ (the ratio of the change in pressure associated with a given change in volume). In containers with "ideal" elastic properties, changes in volume and pressure are linearly related. In other words, the elastance does not vary with the degree of expansion or contraction of the contents of the container. However, in the case of the CSF compartment, volume and pressure are exponentially related. As a result, the elastance is dependent upon the ICP at which it is measured. The elastance (or relative rigidity of the intracranial contents) increases with the ICP. This is reflected by the plot of the ICPs that exist over a continuum of intracranial volumes (Fig. 42.1). Inspection of this idealized pressure-volume curve discloses that it is essentially biphasic. At a "low" initial ICP (A) a unit increase in intracranial volume is associated with a relatively minor increase in ICP. However, at a "high" initial ICP (B), the same unit volume increase produces a relatively large increase in ICP. The initial portion of the curve is associated with a relatively high spatial buffering capacity: increases in intracranial volume are well compensated and thus produce relatively small increases in ICP. This portion of the curve probably represents spatial buffering by the CSF. As volume continues to be added, CSF buffering capacity is diminished and the curve becomes steeper. Further volume increments are less effectively compensated and once the spatial buffering provided by the elastic properties of the blood vessels and the brain are exhausted, otherwise trivial increases in intracranial volume may cause massive increases in ICP.

Although the intracranial elastance varies with the ICP, the elastance is also dependent upon other factors (see below) and thus cannot be inferred from the ICP level alone. However, some notion of the elastance (and of the functional state of the spatial buffering system) can be obtained from inspection of the ICP tracing. A

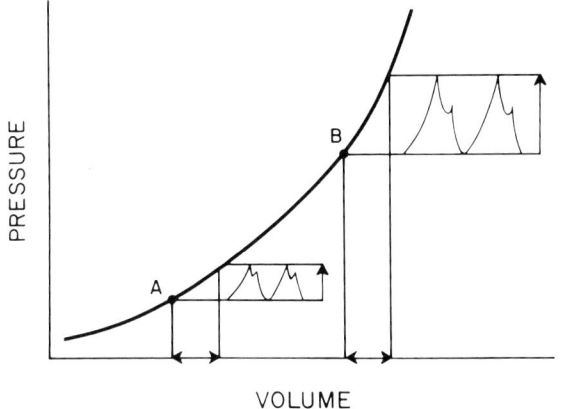

Figure 42.1. Idealized intracranial pressure-volume curve. (See text.)

spontaneous increase in the cerebral blood volume occurs during each cardiac systole. This oscillation in intracranial volume is accompanied by a similar oscillation in ICP. The magnitude of the latter is determined by the intracranial elastance. The amplitude of the ICP wave form is thus a reflection of the elastance (Fig. 42.1). Another qualitative estimate of the elastance can be obtained by observing the change in the level of ICP that is produced by spontaneous increases in intracranial venous volume. The latter occur when the patient coughs during inadequately controlled artificial ventilation or during endotracheal suctioning. A precipitous rise in ICP indicates impending spatial decompensation and thus represents a potentially dangerous situation, even if the ICP subsequently returns to a more acceptable level.

Elastance may be quantified in head-injured patients by determining the volume-pressure response (VPR) (Miller and Pickard, 1974). Ventricular fluid pressure is measured before and after infusion (or withdrawal) of 1 ml of saline over 1 sec. Since the volume change is unity, the change in ventricular fluid pressure is equal to the elastance. A VPR of 2 mm Hg or less is considered normal. There is both experimental and clinical evidence that determination of the volume-pressure respnse may be of value in the management of selected head-injured patients. Sullivan and his colleagues (1977) have studied the temporal relationship between changes in the VPR, the ICP, and clinical neurological signs during progressive inflation of an epidural balloon. They found that the VPR became abnormal (indicating incipient volumetric decompensation) at a balloon volume that was only 64% of that at which signs of uncal herniation first appeared. The mean ICP was 24 mm Hg at the time that the VPR changed. Although this level of ICP is clearly elevated, it is still below some commonly accepted clinical thresholds for vigorous treatment of intracranial hypertension (Miller et al., 1977). In clinical studies, an abnormal VPR has occasionally heralded an unsuspected intracranial hematoma prior to any major rise in the ICP (Miller and Pickard, 1974; Miller et al., 1977). In this context, it appears that the magnitude of the VPR correlates better with the degree of brain displacement than with the level of the ICP (Miller, 1976).

CHANGES IN ELASTANCE

Based on what has thus far been presented, one would expect that the magnitude of the VPR should increase with the ICP as a consequence of the exponential nature of the pressure-volume relationship. Unfortunately, there is ample evidence that the relationship between elastance and ICP is more complicated than this. For example, high levels of ICP are not necessarily associated with a large VPR when the CSF space is greatly enlarged (Leech and Miller, 1974a). Furthermore, in Miller's series of patients in post-traumatic coma, the VPR was relatively normal in many patients with severely elevated ICP (Miller et al., 1977). In fact, elastance does vary predictably with the ICP but only as long as the shape and origin of the pressure-volume curve remain constant (Marmarou and Shulman, 1976). A new pressure-volume curve may be produced if ICP is increased by adding to an intracranial compartment other than the CSF space (Sullivan et al., 1977). In addition, each volume increment may further modify the pressure-volume curve.

There is some evidence that changes in cerebral blood volume produced by altering the arterial PCO_2 do not necessarily change the pressure-volume curve (Leech and Miller, 1974c). Thus, the improvement (decrease) in intracranial elastance that occurs with hypocapnia may be solely a function of the decrease in ICP. Therefore, if the decrease in intracranial blood volume is balanced exactly by an increase in the volume of another intracranial compartment, then the ICP will return to its original level (Miller, 1976). The situation may be different when ICP is reduced by intravenous mannitol infusion. In some experimental studies, the reduction in the VPR was proportionately greater than the reduction in ICP (Miller and Leech, 1975), indicating that the improvement in elastance was due to actual alteration of the pressure-volume curve as well as to the decrease in ICP. Under this circumstance the ICP would not return to its original level if a volume equivalent to that of the lost brain water were added to the intracranial contents. Thus, even if an intracranial hematoma expanded to consume the volume vacated by the dehydrated brain, there would still be a net decrease in ICP because of a favorable change in the pressure-volume relationship. It should be stressed that this has not been clearly demonstrated by any clinical study, so at present it remains a clinical hypothesis. Changes in systemic arterial pressure (SAP) have a more complex effect on intracranial elastance. Leech and Miller (1974b) found that changes in the SAP do not alter elastance at a normal level of ICP. However, when ICP is elevated (>20 mm Hg), elastance varies directly with the SAP. Finally, intracranial elastance rises sharply if the intracranial CSF spaces become isolated from the spinal subarachnoid space (Löfgren and Zwetnow, 1973). Again this is an experimental observation that is difficult to confirm clinically. However, isolation of the cranial and spinal (or supratentorial and infratentorial) CSF compartments from each other may occur as a result of brain herniation through the foramen magnum (or tentorial incisura). The sudden deterioration in intracranial elastance is probably due to the fact that the spinal compartment accounts for at least one-third of the compliance (the reciprocal of elastance) of the CSF space in man (Marmarou and Shulman, 1976).

The concept of elastance is important in the clinical management of head-injured patients because the volume of normal and abnormal intracranial compartments is in dynamic equilibrium. Appreciation of what intracranial elastance is likely to be in a given patient allows the surgeon or anesthesiologist to predict how vulnerable the patient is to sudden, dramatic increases in ICP during coughing, states of relative arousal, fever, temporary loss of control of posttraumatic hypertension, etc. It allows selective use of measures to *prevent* ICP elevation (Bedford et al., 1980), which may produce a more favorable outcome than successful treatment "after the fact" (Miller et al., 1977). This does not mean that routine testing of the VPR should be advocated. However, the significance of a pronounced rise in ICP when a head-injured patient coughs should not escape the surgeon, nor should he be lulled into complacency if the ICP quickly returns to the more acceptable baseline level. It is also important to realize that pathological processes and therapeutic measures that alter the physical properties (particularly the volume) of intracranial compartments do more than simply raise or lower the ICP: they may also have a "prospective" effect, in that they alter the magnitude of the pressure response to subsequent changes in intracranial volume.

Increased Intracranial Pressure

VOLUMETRIC DECOMPENSATION

A sustained elevation of ICP indicates that intracranial spatial buffering mechanisms have become exhausted. As we have seen, these mechanisms involve the compliance properties of the intracranial contents and the capacitance of the spinal subarachnoid space. The adequacy of spatial buffering mechanisms is obviously related to the volume that must be compensated for. In head-injured patients, the most labile contribution to intracranial volume is that of the cerebral blood volume. Stimuli which cause active vasodilatation (hypercapnia, severe hypoxemia, hyperpyrexia, inhalation anesthetics, and some sedatives) deplete spatial buffering capacity, as do factors which cause passive distention of the cerebral arteries (systemic hypertension, post-traumatic cerebral acidosis and vasoparalysis) or veins (compression of jugular veins by tracheostomy tube tape, coughing during intubation). These factors may also increase intracranial volume by exacerbating vasogenic edema. Conversely, the potent cerebral vasoconstrictive effect of hypocapnia will rapidly reduce the ICP, provided that a sufficient portion of the cerebrovascular bed retains normal chemical reactivity. These changes in cerebral blood volume obviously represent a very small percentage change in the total intracranial volume. Therefore, blood volume changes will have a clinically significant effect on ICP only when intracranial elastance is abnormally high. Thus, blood volume changes are particularly important in patients who already have intracranial hypertension.

The adequacy of spatial buffering is also related to the rate at which intracranial volume increases occur. Below a threshold rate of expansion of an epidural balloon implanted in a monkey, little increase in ICP occurs prior to herniation (Nakatani and Ommaya, 1972). The rate of expansion of most acute traumatic intracranial hematomas apparently exceeds this "critical rate of compression," since the ICP is almost invariably elevated with clinically significant masses (Miller et al., 1977). Even so, Miller (1977) has stated that the degree of shift of midline cerebral structures may be a more important indicator of the clinical significance of an acute hematoma than the level of the ICP. The issue is not settled, however, since Teasdale et al. (1980) demonstrated that the level of ICP during the first 6 hr after radiological diagnosis of a clinically silent hematoma will accurately predict whether the patient will later deteriorate neurologically as a result of the hematoma.

PRESSURE WAVES

In addition to sustained elevation of the ICP, volumetric decompensation may be associated with transient but characteristic waves of pressure elevation (Lundberg, 1960). The most important of these are "A" or "plateau" waves. These waves consist of an abrupt increase in ICP to a level of 50 mm Hg or more, which is followed, after an interval of 5–20 min, by a precipitous fall in pressure to the original level. They may occur spontaneously or may be precipitated by hypercapnia or arousal of the patient. The physiological substrate of plateau waves remains unclear, but they are apparently accompanied by cerebral vasomotor paralysis and increased cerebral blood volume (Risberg, et al. 1969). Plateau waves may be accompanied by transient or permanent neurological deterioration. However, they may also occur in the absence of an immediate change in neurological function. In the latter case they are a clear warning that deterioration may be imminent if measures are not undertaken to reduce the ICP and enhance spatial buffering capacity. It should be noted that plateau waves are relatively uncommon in some series of head-injured patients, perhaps because some centers routinely use such prophylactic measures as controlled hyperventilation and ventricular drainage (Miller, 1976).

Other waves of shorter duration and lesser amplitude may also be observed in head-injured patients, but these have a less sinister significance. "B" waves are rhythmic, peaked pressure oscillations that occur at 30–120 sec intervals. Their amplitude is less than that of plateau waves. Although they are not accompanied by neurological deterioration, they nevertheless indicate impending failure of volumetric compensation. Because they are often related to periodic breathing patterns, they are infrequent in patients who are being artificially ventilated (Miller et al., 1977).

TREATMENT THRESHOLDS

Although an ICP that is persistently above 10–15 mm Hg should be regarded as elevated (Miller et al., 1977; Bruce et al., 1978a), this has little practical significance. Few, if any, neurosurgeons would argue that an ICP of 10–15 mm Hg in a patient with a severe head injury demands more than a review of the patient's vital signs, arterial blood gases, serum electrolytes, and position in bed. Johnston and his colleagues have advocated a standardized classification of post-traumatic intracranial hypertension in order to facilitate comparisons among studies (Johnston et al., 1970). They have suggested that an ICP that consistently exceeds 20 mm Hg should be considered "unequivocally elevated" and that a pressure above 40 mm Hg should be classified as "severely elevated." Several published thresholds for vigorous treatment of increased ICP fall between these two levels (Becker et al., 1977; Marshall et al., 1979). However, it is impossible to define a point at which the ICP first becomes "dangerously" elevated for all head injury patients. As we have already seen, there is no level of ICP that invariably marks the onset of spatial decompensation. In the final section of this chapter we will also see that there is no consistent relationship between ICP and CBF or between ICP and brain shift and herniation. Thus, a single ICP value is relatively meaningless when viewed in isolation. It must be considered in the context of the ICP trend, estimates of intracranial elastance, changes in the results of sequential neurological and radiological examinations, and parameters of cardiorespiratory function.

Consequences of Intracranial Hypertension

Increased ICP following head injury may simply reflect a relatively severe degree of impact damage to the brain and its vasculature. This is more likely to be the case when there is no discrete hematoma. Thus, Miller (1977) found a significant correlation between outcome and the magnitude of the elevation of the initial ICP reading in patients with diffuse cerebral injuries but not in patients with hematomas. When intracranial hypertension is largely an epiphenomenon, reduction of the ICP cannot be expected to improve the prognosis. The outcome in these cases is determined by the degree and distribution of biomechanical injury. This fact may account, at least in part, for Miller's observation (1977) that patients whose elevated ICP is readily and scrupulously controlled still have a less favorable outcome than patients whose ICP spontaneously remains normal. Nevertheless, the level of ICP is only one of several parameters of the severity of the parenchymal injury, and thus a normal ICP does not guarantee a favorable outcome (Johnston and Jennett, 1973).

There are also cases in which there appears to be a clear relationship between an increasing ICP and neurological deterioration. However, there is little evidence that intracranial hypertension per se has a direct effect on the function or structural integrity of the cerebrum. For example, patients with the syndrome of "benign intracranial hypertension" (pseudotumor cerebri) tolerate extremely elevated levels of ICP without apparent cerebral dysfunction (although optic nerve damage may occur). Instead, the deleterious effects of increased ICP are mediated by impairment of cerebral perfusion and by distortion and displacement of the neuraxis and its vasculature. Even so, the relationship between the level of ICP and the rate of CBF or the presence and magnitude of brain displacement is complex.

CHANGES IN CBF

The importance of ischemia in mediating the adverse effect of elevated ICP on neural function has been corroborated by Teasdale and his colleagues (1977), who demonstrated that progressive increases in ICP have no effect on electrocortical activity until the decrease in CPP is sufficient to cause a reduction in CBF. Unfortunately, prevention of secondary ischemic damage in patients with brain injuries is not as simple as maintaining the CPP above the lower limit of autoregulation. As was discussed in the preceding section of this chapter, the CPP is only one of several factors that interact to determine the flow through an injured cerebral vascular bed. As a result, the relationship between ICP and CBF has been reported to be inconsistent in head-injured patients, except when the ICP is severely elevated (Bruce et al., 1973; Enevoldsen et al., 1976). However, Teasdale (personal communication, 1980) recently reanalyzed Bruce's data (1973) and demonstrated a positive correlation between CPP and CBF in the subgroup of patients who have an extracerebral hematoma. One explanation for this may be that in this group of patients the brain itself often sustains only minor primary impact damage. As a result, the changes in CBF that occur as the hematoma expands may resemble the rather predictable changes that occur in experimental models of compression of otherwise uninjured brain.

As we have already noted, the early stages of expansion of an extracerebral balloon are marked by compression of the subjacent veins and dilatation of the local resistance vessels (Weinstein and Langfitt, 1967). The latter is tantamount to autoregulation, which initially maintains local CBF despite the reduction in local perfusion pressure. As the balloon is further inflated, vasodilatation becomes insufficient to maintain local blood flow. Flow is further reduced when the forces generated by the balloon become great enough to cause arterial compression (Langfitt and Bruce, 1975). If the balloon is suddenly deflated, the local vascular bed may become hyperemic as the vessels dilate passively under the full force of the restored perfusion pressure. If autoregulation is intact, the tone of the resistance vessels will rapidly adjust so as to normalize the level of flow. If autoregulation has been impaired, the hyperemia will persist. The increase in local tissue blood volume as well as the increase in plasma filtration across a damaged blood-brain barrier may cause brain swelling. If these changes involve a sufficiently large volume of brain, they may cause a "rebound" increase in the ICP. These phenomena probably contribute to the high rate of recurrence

(52%) of intracranial hypertension following evacuation of acute intracranial hematomas (Miller et al., 1977).

As balloon expansion begins to exhaust spatial buffering capacity, pressure rises diffusely within the cranial cavity. This results in generalized vasodilatation, indicating that maintenance of CBF takes precedence over intracranial volume homeostasis. Ischemia eventually supervenes when the reduction in CPP can no longer be compensated by vasodilatation. At that point a state of vasomotor paralysis is induced, probably as a result of the increasing cerebral lactic acidosis (Langfitt et al., 1965). Once this occurs, the cerebral vessels will remain dilated even if the ICP is subsequently reduced. This stage of paretic vasodilatation represents exhaustion of the vascular component of intracranial compliance (Symon, 1976) and thus indicates an advanced stage of volumetric decompensation. As a result of this vasomotor paralysis, a large proportion of the intravascular pressure is transmitted to the brain. Once the ICP increases to the level of the systemic arterial pressure (SAP), diffuse collapse of the cerebral vascular bed occurs (Langfitt and Bruce, 1975). The reactive increase in SAP that is sometimes observed with severe intracranial hypertension was never followed by neurological improvement in Miller's series (1977) and, in fact, was invariably associated with a poor outcome. In that series, a rather constant sequence of signs of terminal deterioration (loss of motor activity, bilateral pupillary dilatation, and finally loss of electrocortical activity) was observed as the ICP approached within 20 mm Hg of the mean arterial pressure.

BRAIN DISPLACEMENT

It is common knowledge that intracranial masses can displace the brain from its normal relationship to the skull and the dural septa that compartmentalize the cranial cavity. Indeed, compression or distortion of the neuraxis (and its vascular supply) may account for the majority of deaths among patients with untreated intracranial mass lesions (Symon, 1976). However, it is not clear what relation these brain shifts have to the level of the ICP or to the development of intracranial pressure gradients.

Despite occasional reports of substantial brain displacement in the presence of a normal ICP (Johnston et al., 1970; Johnston and Jennett, 1973), Miller (1977) found that the ICP was invariably greater than 10 mm Hg in head-injured patients with at least 5 mm displacement of midline cerebral structures. However, there was no significant correlation between higher levels of ICP and greater degrees of brain shift. Langfitt (1976b) has suggested that the magnitude of the brain shift is a function of the volume of the mass that must be compensated and is independent of ICP. This hypothesis is consistent with the clinical observation that temporal lobe masses may locally expand the middle cranial fossa and even cause uncal herniation without causing a generalized increase in ICP. However, this observation applies more readily to long standing lesions than to acutely expanding masses. Although Miller (1976) has expressed the view that some degree of brain compression probably precedes the first major elevation of ICP, it seems unlikely that frank uncal or tonsillar herniation can be caused by an acutely expanding mass without its also exceeding the capacity of spatial buffer mechanisms to maintain a normal ICP. Beyond this, it is impossible to predict the precise level of elevated ICP at which herniation will occur in a given patient. As we have already noted, this depends on the elastic properties, volume, rate of expansion, and intracranial location of the mass itself, as well as on the elastic properties of the structures that are compressed. The importance of the last factor is illustrated by the fact that when an intracranial mass has almost exhausted spatial buffer capacity, a very small further load on the vascular compartment (such as the vasodilatation produced by halothane) may suddenly create a marked pressure gradient across the tentorium (Fitch and McDowell, 1971).

The relationship between pressure gradients within the cranial cavity and brain displacement is even more complex than the relationship between the latter and the level of the ICP. CSF pressure gradients can be created between the supratentorial and infratentorial compartments or between the posterior fossa and the spinal canal (Kaufmann and Clark, 1970; Johnston and Rowan, 1974). The traditional understanding has been that occlusion of the CSF pathways between these compartments is a prerequisite for establishment of the pressure differential (Rowan and Johnston, 1975). Once the subarachnoid cisterns within the tentorial incisura or foramen magnum are obstructed by displaced brain, each compartment establishes its own separate pressure-volume equilibrium, and pressure differences between the compartments are readily created. Brain tissue then migrates further in the direction of the gradient. It is important to note that, according to this hypothesis, intercompartmental pressure gradients are the result of—rather than the cause of—the initial brain displacement. However, this conception has been challenged by Soni (1974), who presented evidence that transtentorial pressure gradients of up to 12 mm Hg can precede brain displacement and occlusion of the CSF pathways.

Although intracompartmental pressure gradients (e.g., between hemispheres or between different regions of the same hemisphere) cannot be documented by measurements made within the unobstructed subarachnoid space (Johnston and Rowan, 1974), such gradients can be recorded from direct measurements of brain tissue pressure. (Symon et al., 1974; Brock et al., 1975; Reulen et al., 1975). Interhemispheric gradients of up to 13 mm Hg have been recorded during the acute expansion phase of unilateral white matter edema (Brock, et al., 1975; Reulen et al., 1975), and even larger gradients have been produced in experimental focal intracerebral hemorrhage (Brock et al., 1975). The magnitude of the gradient is dependent on the volume of the lesion, the rate at which it expands, and the rate at which local tissue compliance factors can adapt to the volume changes (Symon et al., 1974; Brock et al., 1975; Symon and Dorsch, 1975). In regard to the latter, Brock and his colleagues (1975) believe that local tissue pressure is strongly influenced by the vascular component of tissue compliance and that focal abnormalities of vascular tone and reactivity may contribute to focal elevations of brain tissue pressure after head injury.

Brain tissue pressure gradients rapidly dissipate once expansion of an intracranial mass ceases (Brock et al., 1975). In addition, pressure differentials diminish as expansion of the mass exhausts the spatial buffering capacity and causes a diffuse increase in pressure within the cranium. But perhaps the most important means by which tissue pressure gradients are dissipated is by "plastic creep" of the vascoelastic brain away from the area of highest pressure, which is adjacent to the expanding mass (Langfitt, 1975). This is the basis of brain distortion and displacement by intracranial masses. As noted previously, Langfitt (1976b) believes that the amount of brain displacement is dependent upon the volume of the mass. However, the rate at which the brain shifts may be related to the magnitude of the tissue pressure gradient.

CONCLUSION

There is a therapeutic imperative that is implicit in each of the sections of this chapter. It derives from the fact that the mechanically injured brain is exquisitely sensitive to secondary physiological insults and has little or no capacity to undergo functionally significant repair. Therefore, under certain circumstances, a single episode of arterial hypertension, systemic hypotension, cerebral venous hypertension, hypercapnia, hypoxemia, hyperpyrexia, or a major disturbance in serum osmolarity can permanently reduce the patient's level of residual brain function. This imposes an extraordinary burden on those who care for patients with acute head injuries: it requires them to prevent what are often considered to be "unavoidable" complications of multiple organ system trauma and coma (including fever, coughing during endotracheal suctioning, or even sliding down in bed). Yet we are becoming increasingly convinced that rigid "quality control" in patient care is at least as important as any of the newer pharmacological advances in the treatment of patients with severe head injuries. Indeed, it can be argued that until avoidable factors that increase morbidity and mortality are truly minimized, the benefits to be gained from genuine therapeutic innovations will not be maximized.

References

Aarabi, B., and Long, D.M.: Dynamics of cerebral edema. The role of an intact vascular bed in the production and propagation of vasogenic brain edema. J. Neurosurg. *51:*779, 1979.

Adams, J.H., Mitchell, D.E., Graham, D.I., and Doyle, D.: Diffuse brain damage of the immediate impact type. Brain *100:*489, 1977.

Ames, A., Wright, R.L., Kowada, M., Thurston, J.M., and Majno, G.: Cerebral ischemia. II. The no-reflow phenomenon. Am. J. Pathol. *52:*437, 1968.

Baethmann, A., Ottinger, W., Rothenfusser, W., Kempski, O., and Unterberg, A.: Current state of plasma compounds and glutamate as brain edema factors. 1st International Ernst Reuter Symposium: Brain Edema, Berlin, September, 1979.

Bakay, L., and Haque, I.U.: Morphological and chemical studies in cerebral edema. I. Cold induced edema. J. Neuropathol. Exp. Neurol. *23:*393, 1964.

Baker, R.N., Cancilla, P.A., Pollock, P.S., and Frommes, S.P.: The movement of exogenous protein in experimental cerebral edema. An electron microscopic study of freeze-injury. J. Neuropathol. Exp. Neurol. *30:*668, 1971.

Bazan, N.G.: Membrane lipids in the pathogenesis of brain edema; phospholipids and arachidonic acid are the earliest membrane components changed at the onset of ischemia. 1st International Ernst Reuter Symposium: Brain Edema, Berlin, September, 1979.

Becker, D.P., Miller, J.D., Ward, J.D., Greenberg, R.P., Young, H.F., and Sakalas, R.: The outcome from severe head injury with early diagnosis and intensive management. J. Neurosurg. *47:*491, 1977.

Bedford, R.F., Winn, H.R., Tyson, G., Park, T.S., and Jane, J.A.: Lidocaine prevents increased ICP after endotracheal intubation. In *Intracranial Pressure IV*, edited by K. Shulman, A. Marmarou, J.D. Miller, D.P. Becker, G.M. Hochwald, and M. Brock, p. 595. Springer-Verlag, New York, 1980.

Berne, R.M., Rubio, R., and Curnish, R.R.: Release of adenosine from ischemic brain. Effect on cerebral vascular resistance and incorporation into cerebral adenine nucleotides. Circ. Res. *35:*262, 1974.

Björklund, A., Falck, B., Hromek, F., and Owman, Ch.: An enzymatic barrier mechanism for monamine precursors in the newly-forming brain capillaries following elecrtolytic or mechanical lesions. J. Neurochem. *16:*1605, 1969.

Blakemore, W.F.: The fate of escaped plasma protein after thermal necrosis of the rat brain. J. Neuropathol. Exp. Neurol. *28:*139, 1969.

Blasberg, R.G.: Clearance of serum albumin from brain extracellular fluid: a possible role in cerebral edema. In *Dynamics of Brain Edema*, edited by H.M. Pappius and W. Feindel, p. 98. Springer-Verlag, New York, 1976.

Blasberg, R.G., Gazendam, J., Patlak, C.S., and Fenstermacher, J.D.: Quantitative autoradiographic studies of brain edema. 1st International Ernst Reuter Symposium: Brain Edema, Berlin, September, 1979.

Bradbury, M.: *The Concept of a Blood-Brain Barrier*, 465 pp. John Wiley & Sons, New York, 1979.

Branston, N.M., Symon, L., Crockard, H.A., and Pasztor, E.: Relationship between the cortical evoked potential and focal cortical blood flow following acute middle cerebral artery occlusion in the baboon. Exp. Neurol. *45:*195, 1974.

Brierley, J.B., Brown, A.W., Excell, B.J., and Meldrum, B.S.: Brain damage in the rhesus monkey resulting from profound arterial hypotension. I. Its nature, distribution and general physiological correlates. Brain Res. *13:*68, 1969.

Brightman, M.W., Hori, M., Rapoport, S.I., Reese, T.S., and Westergaard, E.: Osmotic opening of tight junctions in cerebral endothelium. J. Comp. Neurol. *152:*317, 1973.

Brock, M., Furuse, M., Weber, R., Hasuo, M., and Dietz, H.: Brain tissue pressure gradients. In *Intracranial Pressure II*, edited by N. Lundberg, U. Ponten, and M. Brock, p. 215. Springer-Verlag, New York, 1975.

Brodersen, P., and Jørgensen, E.O.: Cerebral blood flow and oxygen uptake, and cerebrospinal fluid biochemistry in severe coma. J. Neurol. Neurosurg. Psychiatry *37:*384, 1974.

Bruce, D.A.: Cerebral microcirculation assessed by regional blood flow alterations in damaged brain. In *Head Injuries*, edited by R.L. McLaurin, p. 201. Grune & Stratton, New York, 1976.

Bruce, D.A., and Langfitt, T.W.: The prognostic value of ICP,

CPP, CBF, and $CMRO_2$ in head injury. In *Head Injuries*, edited by R.L. McLaurin, p. 23. Grune & Stratton, New York, 1976.

Bruce, D.A., Langfitt, T.W., Miller, J.D., Schutz, H., Vapalahti, M.P., Stanek, A., and Goldberg, H.I.: Regional cerebral blood flow, intracranial pressure and brain metabolism in comatose patients. J. Neurosurg. *38:*131, 1973.

Bruce, D.A., Ter Weeme, C., Kaiser, G., and Langfitt, T.W.: The dynamics of small and large molecules in the extracellular space and cerebrospinal fluid following local cold injury of the cortex. In *Dynamics of Brain Edema*, edited by H.M. Pappius and W. Feindel, p. 122. Springer-Verlag, New York, 1976.

Bruce, D.A., Gennarelli, T.A., and Langfitt, T.W.: Resuscitation from coma due to head injury. Crit. Care Med. *6:*254, 1978a.

Bruce, D.A., Schut, L., Bruno, L.A., Wood, J.H., and Sutton, L.N.: Outcome following severe head injuries in children. J. Neurosurg. *48:*679, 1978b.

Bruce, D.A., Sutton, L., McHarg, M., and Welsh, F.: Acute effects of vasogenic edema on somatosensory evoked responses and white matter bioenergetics. 1st International Ernst Reuter Symposium: Brain Edema, Berlin, September, 1979a.

Bruce, D.A., Ter Weeme, C., Kaiser, G., and Ghostine, S.: Mechanisms and time course for clearance of vasogenic cerebral edema. In *Neural Trauma*, edited by A.J. Popp, R.S. Bourke, L.R. Nelson, and H.K. Kimelberg, p. 155. Raven Press, New York, 1979b.

Budzilovich, G.N.: On pathogenesis of primary lesions in blunt head trauma with special reference to brain stem injuries. In *Head Injuries*, edited by R.L. McLaurin, p. 39. Grune & Stratton, New York, 1976.

Busija, D.W., Heistad, D.D., and Marcus, M.L.: Temporal response of cerebral vessels during autoregulation (abstract). Fed. Proc. *38:*954, 1979.

Butler, A.B., Mann, J.D., Falk, P.M., Johnson, R.N., Bass, N.H.: Pressure-sensitive vesicular transport of cerebrospinal fluid through the arachnoid villus endothelium. Submitted for publication, 1980.

Caronna, J.J., and Plum, F.: Prognosis and medical coma. In *Head Injuries*, edited by R.L. McLaurin, p. 3. Grune & Stratton, New York, 1976.

Christensen, M.S., Brodersen, P., Olesen, J., and Paulson, O.B.: Cerebral apoplexy (stroke) treated with or without prolonged, artificial hyperventilation. II. Cerebrospinal fluid acid-base balance and intracranial pressure. Stroke *4:*620, 1973.

Clausen, R.A., Sky-Peck, H.H., Pandolfi, S., Laing, I., and Hass, G.M.: The chemistry of isolated edema fluid in experimental cerebral injury. In *Brain Edema*, edited by I. Klatzo, p. 536. Springer-Verlag, New York, 1967.

Cold, G.E.: Cerebral metabolic rate of oxygen ($CMRO_2$) in the acute phase of brain injury. Acta Anaesth. Scand. *22:*249, 1978.

Cold, G.E., and Jensen, F.T.: Cerebral autoregulation in unconscious patients with brain injury. Acta Anaesth. Scand. *22:*270, 1978.

Cold, G.E., Jensen, F.T., and Malmros, R.: The cerebrovascular CO_2 reactivity during the acute phase of head injury. Acta Anaesth. Scand. *21:*222, 1977.

Cooper, P.R., Hagler, H., Clark, W.K., and Barnett, P.: Enhancement of experimental cerebral edema after decompressive craniectomy: Implications for the management of severe head injuries. Neurosurgery *4:*296, 1979.

Costa, J.L., Ito, U., Spatz, M., Klatzo, I., and Demirjian, C.: 5-hydroxytryptamine accumulation in cerebrovascular injury. Nature *248:*135, 1974.

Cserr, H.F., Cooper, D.N., and Milhorat, T.H.: Production, circulation, and absorption of brain interstitial fluid. In *Dynamics of Brain Edema*, edited by H.M. Pappius and W. Feindel, p. 95. Springer-Verlag, New York, 1976.

Davson, H., and Oldendorf, W.H.: Transport in the central nervous system. Proc. Roy. Soc. Med. *60:*326, 1967.

Demopoulos, H.B.: The basis of free radical pathology. Fed. Proc. *32:*1859, 1973.

Demopoulos, H.B., Flamm, E.S., Seligman, M.L., Mitamura, J.A., and Ransohoff, J.: Membrane perturbations in central nervous system injury: Theoretical basis for free radical damage and a review of the experimental data. In *Neural Trauma*, edited by A.J. Popp, R.S. Bourke, L.R. Nelson, and H.K. Kimelberg, p. 63. Raven Press, New York, 1979.

Eichling, J.O., Raichle, M.E., Grubb, R.L., Jr., and Ter-Pogossian, M.M.: Evidence of the limitations of water as a freely diffusible tracer in the brain of the rhesus monkey. Circ. Res. *35:*358, 1974.

Eklöf, B., and Siesjö, B.K.: The effect of bilateral carotid artery ligation upon the blood flow and the energy state of the rat brain. Acta Physiol. Scand. *86:*155, 1972.

Enevoldsen, E.M., and Jensen, F.T.: "False" autoregulation of cerebral blood flow in patients with acute severe head injury. In *Cerebral Function, Metabolism, and Circulation*, edited by D.H. Ingvar and N.A. Lassen, p. 514. Munksgaard, Copenhagen, 1977.

Enevoldsen, E.M., and Jensen, F.T.: Autoregulation and CO_2 response of cerebral blood flow in patients with acute severe head injury. J. Neurosurg. *48:*689, 1978.

Enevoldsen, E.M., Cold, G., Jensen, F.T., and Malmros, R.: Regional cerebral blood flow in brain contusion: Clinical studies. In *Blood Flow and Metabolism in the Brain*, edited by A.M. Harper, W.B. Jennett, J.D. Miller, and J.O. Rowan, p. 13.24. Churchill Livingstone, Edinburgh, 1975.

Enevoldsen, E.M., Cold, G., Jensen, F.T., and Malmros, R.: Dynamic changes in regional CBF, intraventricular pressure, CSF pH and lactate levels during the acute phase of head injury. J. Neurosurg. *44:*191, 1976.

Feigin, I., and Popoff, N.: Neuropathological observations on cerebral edema. Arch. Neurol. *6:*151, 1962.

Fenske, A., Hey, O., Theiss, R., Reulen, H.J., and Schürmann, K.: Regional cortical blood flow in the early stage of brainstem edema. In *Blood Flow and Metabolism in the Brain*, edited by A.M. Harper, W.B. Jennett, J.D. Miller, and J.O. Rowan, p. 1.12. Churchill Livingstone, Edinburgh, 1975.

Fenske, A., Samii, M., Reulen, H.J., and Hey, O.: Extracellular space and electrolye distribution in cortex and white matter of dog brain in cold induced edema. Acta Neurochir. (Wien) *28:*81, 1973.

Fenske, A., Sinterhauf, K., and Reulen, H.J.: The role of monoamines in the development of cold-induced edema. In *Dynamics of Brain Edema*, edited by H.M. Pappius and W. Feindel, p. 150. Springer-Verlag, New York, 1976.

Fenstermacher, J.D., and Johnson, J.A.: Filtration and reflection coefficients of the rabbit blood-brain barrier. Am. J. Physiol. *211:*341, 1966.

Fenstermacher, J.D., and Patlak, C.S.: The movements of water and solutes in the brains of mammals. In *Dynamics of Brain Edema*, edited by H.M. Pappius and W. Feindel, p. 87. Springer-Verlag, New York, 1976.

Fieschi, C., Battistini, N., Beduschi, A., Boselli, L. and Rossanda, M.: Regional cerebral blood flow and intraventricular pressure in acute head injuries. J. Neurol. Neurosurg. Psychiat. 37:1378, 1974.

Fisher, D.B., and Kaufman, S.: The inhibition of phenylalanine and tyrosine hydroxylases by high oxygen levels. J. Neurochem. 19:1359, 1972.

Fitch, W., and McDowell, D.G.: Effect of halothane on intracranial pressure gradients in the presence of intracranial space-occupying lesions. Br. J. Anaesth. 43:904, 1971.

Fitch, W., MacKenzie, E.T., and Harper, A.M.: Effects of decreasing arterial blood pressure on cerebral blood flow in the baboon. Influence of the sympathetic nervous system. Circ. Res. 37:550, 1975.

Flamm, E.S., Demopoulos, H.B., Seligman, M.L., Mitamura, J.A., and Ransohoff, J.: Barbiturates and free radicals. In *Neural Trauma*, edited by A.J. Popp, R.S. Bourke, L.R. Nelson, and H.K. Kimelberg, p. 289. Raven Press, New York, 1979.

Folkow, B.: Descriptions of the myogenic hypothesis. Circ. Res. (Suppl. I) 15:279, 1964.

Fraser, R.A.R., Yoshida, S., and Patterson, R.H.: Focal cerebral ischemia and the "no-reflow" phenomenon. In *Cerebral Function, Metabolism and Circulation*, edited by D.H. Ingvar and N.A. Lassen, p. 120. Munksgaard, Copenhagen, 1977.

Freeman, J., and Ingvar, D.H.: Elimination by hypoxia of cerebral blood flow autoregulation and EEG relationship. Exp. Brain Res. 5:61, 1968.

Frei, H., Wallenfang, T., Pöll, W., Reulen, H.J., Schubert, R., and Brock, M.: Regional cerebral blood flow and regional metabolism in cold induced edema. Acta Neurochir. (Wien) 29:15, 1973.

Friedman, P.A., Kappelman, A.H., and Kaufman, S.: Partial purification and characterization of tryptophane hydroxylase from rabbit hind brain. J. Biol. Chem. 247:4165, 1972.

Fujimoto, T., Walker, J.T., Jr., Spatz, M., and Klatzo, I.: Pathophysiologic aspects of ischemic edema. In *Dynamics of Brain Edema*, edited by H.M. Pappius and W. Feindel, p. 171. Springer-Verlag, New York, 1976.

Garcia, J.H., Kalimo, H., Kamijyo, Y., and Trump, B.F.: Cellular events during partial cerebral ischemia. I. Electron microscopy of feline cerebral cortex after middle-cerebral-artery occlusion. Virchows Arch. (Cell Pathol.) 25:191, 1977.

Garcia, J.H., Conger, K.A., Halsey, J.H., and Lossinsky, A.S.: Post-ischemic brain edema: quantitation and evolution. 1st International Ernst Reuter Symposium: Brain Edema, Berlin, September, 1979.

Gazendam, J., Go, K.G., and van Zanten, A.K.: Composition of isolated edema fluid in cold-induced brain edema. J. Neurosurg. 51:70, 1979.

Gennarelli, T.A., Obrist, W.D., Langfitt, T.W., and Segawa, H.: Vascular and metabolic reactivity to changes in PCO_2 in head injured patients. In *Neural Trauma*, edited by A.J. Popp, R.S. Bourke, L.R. Nelson, and H.K. Kimelberg, p. 1. Raven Press, New York, 1979.

Go, K.G., Patberg, W.R., Teelken, A.W., and Gazendam, J.: The Starling hypothesis of capillary fluid exchange in relation to brain edema. In *Dynamics of Brain Edema*, edited by H.M. Pappius and W. Feindel, p. 63. Springer-Verlag, New York, 1976.

Graham, D.I., Adams, J.H., and Doyle, D.: Ischaemic brain damage in arterial boundary zones in non-missile head injuries. In *Blood Flow and Metabolism in the Brain*, edited by A.M. Harper, W.B. Jennett, J.D. Miller, and J.O. Rowan, p. 13.29. Churchill Livingstone, Edinburgh, 1975.

Graham, D.I., Adams, J.H., and Doyle, D.: Ischaemic brain damage in fatal non-missile head injuries. J. Neurol. Sci. 39:213, 1978.

Graham, D.I., Fitch, W., MacKenzie, E.T., and Harper, A.M.: Effects of hemorrhagic hypotension on the cerebral circulation. III. Neuropathology. Stroke 10:724, 1979.

Gragory, P.C., McGeorge, A.P., Fitch, W., Graham, D. I., MacKenzie, E.T., and Harper, A.M.: Effects of hemorrhagic hypotension on the cerebral circulation. II. Electrocortical function. Stroke 10:719, 1979.

Griffith, R. P., Tindall, G.T., Iwata, K., McGraw, C.P., and Vanderveer, R.W.: Response of cerebral metabolic rate of oxygen to use of norepinephrine in head-injured patients. Surg. Forum 21:415, 1972.

Gross, P.M., Heistad, D.D., Strait, M.T., Marcus, M.L., and Brody, M.J.: Cerebral vascular responses to physiological stimulation of sympathetic pathways in cats. Circ. Res. 44:288, 1979.

Gross, P.M., Marcus, M.L., and Heistad, D.D.: Regional distribution of cerebral blood flow during exercise in dogs. J. Appl. Physiol. 48:213, 1980.

Grossman, R.G., and Seregin, A.I.: Effects of traumatically induced edema on membrane potentials of cortical glial cells and neurons. In *Head Injuries*, edited by R.L. McLaurin, p. 273. Grune & Stratton, New York, 1976.

Grubb, R.L., Raichle, M.E., Phelps, M.E., and Ratcheson, R.A.: Effects of increased intracranial pressure on cerebral blood volume, blood flow and oxygen utilization in monkeys. J. Neurosurg. 43:385, 1975.

Guyton, A.C., Granger, H.J., and Taylor, A.E.: Interstitial fluid pressure. Physiol. Rev. 51:527, 1971.

Hadjidimos, A., Fischer, F., and Reulen, H.J.: Restitution of vasomotor autoregulation by hypocapnia in brain tumors. In *Advances in Neurosurgery*, edited by H. Penzholz, M. Brock, J. Hamer, M. Klinger, and O. Spoerri, vol. 3, p. 92. Springer-Verlag, New York, 1975.

Häggendal, E.: Elimination of autoregulation during arterial and cerebral hypoxia. Scand. J. Clin. Lab. Invest. Suppl. 102:V:D, 1968.

Häggendal, E., and Johansson, B.: On the pathophysiology of the increased cerebrovascular permeability in acute arterial hypertension in cats. Acta Neurol. Scand. 48:265, 1972.

Harp, J.R., and Wollman, H.: Cerebral metabolic effects of hyperventilation and deliberate hypotension. Br. J. Anaesth. 45:256, 1973.

Harper, A.M.: The inter-relationship between $PaCO_2$ and blood pressure in the regulation of blood flow through the cerebral cortex. Acta Neurol. Scand. (Suppl. 14) 41:94, 1965.

Harper, A.M.: Control of the cerebral circulation. In *Scientific Foundations of Neurology*, edited by M. Critchley, J.L. O'Leary, and B. Jennett, p. 235. Heinemann, London, 1972.

Hass, W.K.: Prognostic value of cerebral oxidative metabolism in head trauma. In *Head Injury*, edited by R.L. McLaurin, p. 35. Grune & Stratton, New York, 1976.

Hawkins, R.A., Hass, W.K., and Ransohoff, J.: Cerebral blood flow, glucose utilization, oxidative metabolism, and plasticity after mesencephalic reticular formation lesions. In *Neural Trauma*, edited by A.J. Popp, R.S. Bourke, L.R. Nelson, and H.K. Kimelberg, p. 9. Raven Press, New York, 1979.

Hirano, A.: A possible mechanism of dysfunction as the result of brain edema. 1st International Ernst Reuter Symposium: Brain Edema, Berlin, September, 1979.

Hirano, A., Becker, N.H., and Zimmerman, H.M.: Pathological alterations in the cerebral endothelial cell barrier to peroxidase. Arch. Neurol. 20:300, 1969.

Hossman, K.A., and Olsson, Y.: Functional aspects of abnormal protein passage across the blood-brain barrier. In *Steroids and Brain Edema*, edited by H.J. Reulen and K. Schurmann, p. 9. Springer-Verlag, New York, 1972.

Ingvar, D.H., and Sourander, P.: Destruction of the reticular core of the brainstem: A patho-anatomical follow-up of a case of coma of three years' duration. Arch. Neurol. 23:1, 1970.

Ito, U., Go, K.G., Walker, J.T., Spatz, M., and Klatzo, I.: Experimental cerebral ischemia in Mongolian gerbils. III. Behavior of the blood-brain barrier. Acta Neuropathol. 34:1, 1976.

Johannsson, H., and Siesjö, B.K.: Cerebral blood flow and oxygen consumption in the rat in hypoxic hypoxia. Acta Physiol. Scand. 93:269, 1975.

Johansson, B.: Blood-brain barrier pathology in acute arterial hypertension. Adv. Exp. Med. Biol., 69:517, 1976.

Johansson, B., and Nilsson, B.: The pathophysiology of the blood-brain barrier dysfunction induced by severe hypercapnia and by epileptic brain activity. Acta Neuropathol. 38:153, 1977.

Johnson, R.N., Maffeo, C.J., Mann, J. D., Butler, A.B., Bass, N.H.: A comparative model of cerebrospinal fluid systems. J. Life Sci. 8:79, 1978.

Johnston, I.H., and Jennett, B.: The place of continuous intracranial pressure monitoring in neurosurgical practice. Acta Neurochir. 29:53, 1973.

Johnston, I.H., and Rowan, J.O.: Raised intracranial pressure and cerebral blood flow: 4. Intracranial pressure gradients and regional cerebral blood flow. J. Neurol. Neurosurg. Psychiatry 37:585, 1974.

Johnston, I.H., Johnston, J.A., and Jennett, B.: Intracranial pressure changes following head injury. Lancet 2:433, 1970.

Kaasik, A.E., Nilsson, L., and Siesjö, B.K.: The effect of asphyxia upon the lactate, pyruvate and bicarbonate concentration of brain tissue and cisternal CSF, and upon the tissue concentrations of phosphocreatine and adenine nucleotides in anesthetized rats. Acta Physiol. Scand. 78:433, 1970.

Karnovsky, M.J.: The ultrastructural basis of capillary permeability studied with peroxidase as a tracer. J. Cell. Biol. 35:213, 1967.

Kaufmann, G.E., and Clark, K.: Continuous simultaneous monitoring of intraventricular and cervical subarachnoid cerebrospinal fluid pressure to indicate development of cerebral or tonsillar herniation. J. Neurosurg. 33:145, 1970.

Klatzo, I.: Neuropathological aspects of brain edema. J. Neuropathol. Exp. Neurol. 26:1, 1967.

Klatzo, I. Pathophysiological aspects of brain edema. In *Steroids and Brain Edema*, edited by H. J. Reulen and K. Schürmann, p. 1. Springer-Verlag, New York, 1972.

Klatzo, I.: Cerebral edema and ischemia. In *Recent Advances in Neuropathology*, edited by W.T. Smith and J.B. Cavanagh, p. 27. Churchhill Livingstone, Edinburgh, 1979.

Klatzo, I., Wiśniewski, H., and Smith, D.E.: Observations on penetration of serum proteins into the central nervous system. Prog. Brain Res. 15:73, 1965.

Klatzo, I. Wiśniewski, H., Steinwall, O., and Streicher, E.: Dynamics of cold injury edema. In *Brain Edema*, edited by I. Klatzo and F. Seitelberger, p. 554. Springer-Verlag, New York, 1967.

Klatzo, I., Spatz, M., Chui, E., and Fujiwara, K.: Dynamics and resolution of vasogenic brain edema. 1st International Ernst Reuter Symposium: Brain Edema, Berlin, September, 1979.

Kontos, H.A., Raper, A.J., and Patterson, J.L.: Analysis of vasoactivity of local pH, PCO_2, and bicarbonate on pial vessels. Stroke 8:358, 1977a.

Kontos, H.A., Wei, E.P., Raper, A.J., and Patterson, J.L.: Local mechanism of CO_2 action on cat pial arterioles. Stroke 8:226, 1977b.

Kontos, H.A., Wei, E.P., Navari, R.M., Levasseur, J.E., Rosenblum, W.I., and Patterson, J.L. Responses of cerebral arteries and arterioles to acute hypotension and hypertension. Am. J. Physiol. 234:H371, 1978.

Kuhl, D.E., Alavi, A., Hoffman, E.J., Phelps, M.E., Zimmerman, R.A., Obrist, W.D., Bruce, D.A., Greenberg, J.H., and Uzzell, B.: Local cerebral blood volume in head injured patients. Determination by emission computed tomography of Tc-99m-labeled red cells. J. Neurosurg. 52:309, 1980.

Kuschinsky, W., and Wahl, M.: Local chemical and neurogenic regulation of cerebral vascular resistance. Physiol. Rev. 58:656, 1978.

Langfitt, T.W.: Intracranial volume-pressure relationship. In *Intracranial Pressure II*, edited by N. Lundberg, U. Ponten, and M. Brock, p. 69. Springer-Verlag, New York, 1975.

Langfitt, T.W.: Incidence and importance of intracranial hypertension in head injured patients. In *Intracranial Pressure III*, edited by J.W.F. Beks, D.A. Bosch, and M. Brock, p. 67. Springer-Verlag, Berlin, 1976a.

Langfitt, T.W.: In *Head Injuries*, edited by R.L. McLaurin, p. 263. Grune & Stratton, New York, 1976b.

Langfitt, T.W., and Bruce, D.A.: Microcirculation and brain edema in head injury. In *Handbook of Clinical Neurology, Injuries of the Brain and Skull*, vol. 23, part I, edited by P.J. Vinken and G.W. Bruyn, p. 133. Elsevier, New York, 1975.

Langfitt, T.W., Weinstein, J.D., Kassell, N.F., and Simeone, F.A.: Transmission of increased intracranial pressure. I. Within the craniospinal axis. J. Neurosurg. 21:989, 1964.

Langfitt, T.W., Weinstein, J.D., and Kassell, N.F.: Cerebral vasomotor paralysis produced by intracranial hypertension. Neurology 15:622, 1965.

Langfitt, T.W., Tannenbaum, H.M., and Kassell, N.F.: The etiology of acute brain swelling following experimental head injury. J. Neurosurg. 24:47, 1966.

Lassen, N.A.: The luxury perfusion syndrome and its possible relation to acute metabolic acidosis localized within the brain. Lancet 2:1113, 1966.

Leech, P.J., and Miller, J.D.: Intracranial volume-pressure relationships during experimental brain compression in primates. I. Pressure response to changes in ventricular volume. J. Neurol. Neurosurg. Psychiatry 37:1092, 1974a.

Leech, P.J., and Miller, J.D.: Intracranial volume-pressure relationships during experimental brain compression in primates. II. Effects of induced changes in arterial pressure. J. Neurol. Neurosurg. Psychiatry 37:1099, 1974b.

Leech, P.J., and Miller, J.D.: Intracranial volume-pressure relationships during experimental brain compression in primates. III. The effect of mannitol and hypocapnia. J. Neurol. Neurosurg. Psychiatry 37:1105, 1974c.

Levin, V.A., Fenstermacher, J.D., and Patlak, C.S.: Sucrose and inulin space measurements of cerebral cortex in four mammalian species. Am. J. Physiol. 219:1528, 1970.

Levine, S.: Anoxic-ischemic encephalopathy in rats. Am. J. Pathol. 36:1, 1960.

Levy, D.E., Brierley, J.B., and Plum, F.: Absence of no-reflow after unilateral carotid artery occlusion in the gerbil. In *Blood Flow and Metabolism in the Brain*, edited by A.M. Harper, W.B. Jennett, J.D. Miller, and J.O. Rowan, p. 12.28. Churchill Livingstone, Edinburgh, 1975a.

Levy, D.E., Brierley, J.B., Silverman, D.G., and Plum, F.: Brief hypoxia-ischemia initially damages cerebral neurons. Arch. Neurol. 32:450, 1975b.

Löfgren, J.: Effects of variations in arterial pressure and arterial carbon dioxide tension on the cerebrospinal fluid pressure-volume relationship. Acta Neurol. Scand. 49:586, 1973.

Löfgren, J., and Zwetnow, N.N.: Cranial and spinal components of the cerebrospinal fluid pressure-volume curve. Acta Neurol. Scand. 49:575, 1973.

Löfgren, J., and Zwetnow, N.N.: Intracranial blood volume and its variation with changes in intracranial pressure. In *Intracranial Pressure III*, edited by J.W.F. Beks, D.A. Bosch, and M. Brock, p. 25. Springer-Verlag, New York, 1976.

Löfgren, J., VonEssen, C., and Zwetnow, N.N.: The pressure-volume curve of the cerebrospinal fluid space in dogs. Acta Neurol. Scand. 49:557, 1973.

Lorenzo, A.V., Hedley-White, E.T., Eisenberg, H.M., and Hsu, D.W.: Increased penetration of horseradish peroxidase across the blood-brain barrier induced by metrazol seizures. Brain Res. 88:136, 1975.

Lübbers, D.W.: Das O_2-Versorgungssystem der Warmblüterorgane. In *Jahrbuch der Max-Planck-Gesellschaft zur Förderung der Wissenschaften* E.V., p. 87. 1974.

Lundberg, N.: Continuous recording and control of ventricular fluid pressure in neurosurgical practice. Acta Psychiatr. Neurol. Scand. (Suppl. 149) 36:1, 1960.

MacKenzie, E.T., Farrar, J.D., Fitch, W., Graham, D.I., Gregory, P.C., and Harper, A.M.: Effects of hemorrhagic hypotension on the cerebral circulation. I. Cerebral blood flow and pial arteriolar caliber. Stroke 10:711, 1979.

MacKenzie, E.T., McCulloch, J., O'Keane, M., Pickard, J.D., and Harper, A.M.: Cerebral circulation and norepinephrine: Relevance of the blood-brain barrier. Am. J. Physiol. 231: 483, 1976.

MacKenzie, E.T., McGeorge, A.P., Graham, D.I., Fitch, W., Edvinsson, L., and Harper, A.M.: Breakthrough of cerebral autoregulation and the sympathetic nervous system. In *Cerebral Function, Metabolism and Circulation*, edited by D.H. Ingvar and N.A. Lassen, p. 48. Munksgaard, Copenhagen, 1977.

MacMillan, V., and Siesjö, B.K.: Brain energy metabolism in hypoxemia. Scand. J. Clin. Lab. Invest. 30:127, 1972.

MacMillan, V., and Siesjö, B.K.: The influence of hypocapnia upon intracellular pH and upon some carbohydrate substrates, amino acids, and organic phosphates in the brain. J. Neurochem. 21:1283, 1973.

Mann, J.D., Butler, A.B., Rosenthal, J., Maffeo, C.J., Johnson, R.N., and Bass, N.H.: Regulation of intracranial pressure in rat, dog, and man. Ann. Neurol. 3:156, 1978.

Marmarou, A., and Shulman, K.: Pressure-volume relationships: Basic aspects. In *Head Injuries*, edited by R.L. McLaurin, p. 233. Grune & Stratton, New York, 1976.

Marmarou, A., Shulman, K., and LaMorgese, J.: Compartmental analysis of compliance and outflow resistance of the cerebrospinal fluid system. J. Neurosurg. 43:523, 1975.

Marmarou, A., Poll, W., Shapiro, K., and Shulman, K.: The influence of brain tissue pressure upon local cerebral blood flow in vasogenic edema. In *Intracranial Pressure III*, edited by J.W.F. Beks, D.A. Bosch, and M. Brock, p. 10. Springer-Verlag, New York, 1976a.

Marmarou, A., Shulman, K., Shapiro, K., and Poll, W.: The time course of brain tissue pressure and local CBF in vasogenic edema. In *Dynamics of Brain Edema*, edited by H.M. Pappius and W. Feindel, p. 112. Springer-Verlag, New York, 1976b.

Marmarou, A., Shulman, K., and Rosende, R.M.: A non-linear analysis of the cerebrospinal fluid system and intracranial pressure dynamics. J. Neurosurg. 48:332, 1978.

Marmarou, A., Takagi, H., and Shulman, K.: The biomechanics of cerebral edema and effects upon local CBF. 1st International Ernst Reuter Symposium: Brain Edema, Berlin, September, 1979.

Marshall, L.F., Welsh, F., Durity, F., Lounsbury, R., Graham, D.I., and Langfitt, T.W.: Experimental cerebral oligemia and ischemia produced by intracranial hypertension. Part 3: Brain energy metabolism. J. Neurosurg. 43:323, 1975.

Marshall, L. F., Bruce, D.A., Graham, D.I., and Langfitt, T.W.: Triethyl tin-induced cerebral edema: Implications for determination of cerebral blood flow in edematous tissue. In *Dynamics of Brain Edema*, edited by H.M. Pappius and W. Feindel, p. 83. Springer-Verlag, New York, 1976.

Marshall, L.F., Smith, R.W., and Shapiro, H.M.: The outcome with aggressive treatment in severe head injuries. I. The significance of intracranial pressure monitoring. J. Neurosurg. 50:20, 1979.

Marshall, W.J.S., Jackson, J.L.F., and Langfitt, T.W.: Brain swelling caused by trauma and arterial hypertension: Hemodynamic aspects. Arch. Neurol. 21:545, 1969.

Martins, A.N., Wiley, J.K., and Myers, P.W.: Dynamics of the cerebrospinal fluid and the spinal dura mater. J. Neurol. Neurosurg. Psychiatry 35:468, 1972.

Maxwell, R.E., Long, D.M., and French, L.A.: The effects of glucocorticoids on experimental cold-induced brain edema: Gross morphological alterations and vascular permeability changes. J. Neurosurg. 34:477, 1971.

Meinig, J.S., Reulen, H.J., and Magavly, C.: Regional cerebral blood flow and cerebral perfusion pressure in global brain edema induced by water intoxication. Acta Neurochir. (Wein) 29:1, 1973.

Miller, J.D.: Clinical aspects of intracranial volume-pressure relationships. In *Head Injuries*, edited by R.L. McLaurin, p. 239, Grune & Stratton, New York, 1976.

Miller, J.D.: Barbiturates and raised intracranial pressure. Ann. Neurol. 6:189, 1979.

Miller, J.D., and Leech, P.J.: Effects of mannitol and steroid therapy on intracranial volume-pressure relationships. J. Neurosurg. 42:274, 1975.

Miller, J.D., and Pickard, J.D.: Intracranial volume-pressure studies in patients with head injury. Injury 5:265, 1974.

Miller, J.D., Stanek, A., and Langfitt, T.W.: Concepts of cerebral perfusion pressure and vascular compression during intracranial hypertension. In *Cerebral Blood Flow*, edited by J.S. Meyer and J.P. Schadé, p. 411, Elsevier, Amsterdam, 1971.

Miller, J.D., Reilly, P.L., Farrar, J.K., and Rowan, J.O.: Cerebrovascular reactivity related to focal brain edema in the primate. In *Dynamics of Brain Edema*, edited by H.M. Pappius and W. Feindel, p. 68. Springer-Verlag, New York, 1976.

Miller, J.D., Becker, D.P., Ward, J.D., Sullivan, H.G., Adams, W.E., and Rosner, M.J. Significance of intracranial hypertension in severe head injury. J. Neurosurg. 47:501, 1977.

Miller, J.D., Gudeman, S.K., Kishore, P.R.S., and Becker, D.P.: Relation between radiographic evidence of edema and the outcome of head injury. 1st International Ernst Reuter Symposium: Brain Edema, Berlin, September, 1979.

Miller, J.D., Stanek, A.E., and Langfitt, T.W.: Cerebral blood flow regulation during experimental brain compression. J. Neurosurg. 39:186, 1973.

Monro, A.: *Observations on the Structure and Function of the Nervous System.* Creech and Johnson, Edinburgh, 1783.

Nag, S., Robertson, D.M., Dinsdale, H.B., and Haas, R.A.: Determination of cerebral edema by quantitative morphometry. In *Dynamics of Brain Edema*, edited by H.M. Pappius and W. Feindel, p. 32. Springer-Verlag, New York, 1976.

Nakatani, S., and Ommaya, A.K.: A critical rate of cerebral compression. In *Intracranial Pressure*, edited by M. Brock and H. Dietz, p. 144. Springer-Verlag, New York, 1972.

Navarri, R.M., Gainer, J.L., and Hall, K.R.: A predictive

theory for diffusion in polymer and protein solution. A.I.Ch.E.J. *17:*1028, 1971.
Nelson, S.R., and Mantz, M.: Energy reserve levels in edematous mouse brain. Exp. Neurol. *31:*53, 1971.
Nelson, S.R., Mantz, M.L., and Maxwell, J.A.: Use of specific gravity in the measurement of cerebral edema. J. App. Physiol. *30:*268, 1971.
Nordström, C.H., Rehncrona, S., and Siesjö, B.K.: Effects of phenobarbital in cerebral ischemia. Part II. Restitution of cerebral energy state, as well as of glycolytic metabolites, citric acid cyle intermediates and associated amino acids after pronounced incomplete ischemia. Stroke *9:*335, 1978.
Obrist, W.D., Langfitt, T.W., ter Weeme, C.A., O'Connor, M.J., Gennarelli, T.A., Zimmerman, R.A., and Kuhl, D.E.: Non-invasive, long-term, serial studies of CBF in acute head injury. In *Cerebral Function, Metabolism, and Circulation,* edited by D.H. Ingvar and N.A. Lassen, p. 178. Munksgaard, Copenhagen, 1977.
Obrist, W.D., Dolinskas, C.A., Gennarelli, T.A., and Zimmerman, R.A.: Relation of cerebral blood flow to CT scan in acute head injury. In *Neural Trauma,* edited by A.J. Popp, R.S. Bourke, L.R. Nelson, and H.K. Kimelberg, p. 41. Raven Press, New York, 1979a.
Obrist, W.D., Gennarelli, T.A., Segawa, H., Dolinskas, C.A., and Langfitt, T.W.: Relation of cerebral blood flow to neurological status and outcome in head-injured patients. J. Neurosurg. *51:*292, 1979b.
Ohno, K., Pettigrew, K.D., and Rapoport, S.I.: Lower limits of cerebrovascular permeability to nonelectrolytes in the conscious rat. Am. J. Physiol. *235:*299, 1978.
Ommaya, A.K., and Gennarelli, T.A.: Experimental head injury. In *Handbook of Clinical Neurology, Injuries of the Brain and Skull,* vol. 23, part I, edited by P.J. Vinken and G.W. Bruyn, p. 67, Elsevier, New York, 1975.
Ommaya, A.K., and Gennarelli, T.A.: A physiopathologic basis for noninvasive diagnosis and prognosis of head injury severity. In *Head Injuries,* edited by R.L. McLaurin, p. 49. Grune & Stratton, New York, 1976.
Osterholm, J.L., Bell, J., Myer, R., and Pyenson, J.: Experimental effects of free serotonin on the brain and its relation to brain injury. Part 1: The neurological consequences of intracerebral serotonin injections. J. Neurosurg. *31:*408, 1969.
Overgaard, J.: Reflections on prognostic determinants in acute severe head injury. In *Head Injuries,* edited by R.L. McLaurin, p. 11. Grune & Stratton, New York, 1976.
Overgaard, J., and Tweed, W.A.: Cerebral circulation after head injury. Part 1: Cerebral blood flow and its regulation after closed head injury with emphasis on clinical correlations. J. Neurosurg. *41:*531, 1974.
Overgaard, J., and Tweed, W.A.: rCBF in impending brain death. Acta Neurochir. *31:*167, 1975.
Palade, G.E.: Blood capillaries of the heart and other organs. Circulation *24:*368, 1961.
Pappius, H.M.: Local cerebral glucose utilization in edematous brain. 1st International Ernst Reuter Symposium: Brain Edema, Berlin, September, 1979.
Pappius, H.M., and Wolfe, L.S.: Some further studies on vasogenic edema. In *Dynamics of Brain Edema,* edited by H.M. Pappius and W. Feindel, p. 138. Springer-Verlag, New York, 1976.
Pappius, H.M., Savaki, H.E., Fieschi, C., Rapoport, S.I., and Sokoloff, L.: Osmotic opening of the blood-brain barrier and local cerebral glucose utilization. Ann. Neurol. *5:*211, 1979.
Paulson, O.B.: Cerebral apoplexy (stroke): Pathogenesis, pathophysiology and therapy as illustrated by regional blood flow measurements in the brain. Stroke *2:*327, 1971.
Paulson, O.B., Olesen, J., and Christensen, M.S.: Restoration of autoregulation of cerebral blood flow by hypocapnia. Neurology *22:*286, 1972.
Paulson, O.B., Hertz, M.M., Bolwig, T.G., and Lassen, N.A.: Water filtration and diffusion across the blood-brain barrier. Acta Physiol. Scand. (Suppl.) *440:*85, 1976.
Penn, R.D.: Quantitating focal edema in computed tomography. 1st International Ernst Reuter Symposium: Brain Edema, Berlin, September, 1979.
Peters, A., and Palay, S.L.: An electron microscope study of the distribution and patterns of astroglial processes in the central nervous system. J. Anat. *99:*419, 1965.
Petito, C.K., Schaefer, J.A., and Plum, F.: The blood-brain barrier in experimental seizures. In *Dynamics of Brain Edema,* edited by H.M. Pappius and W. Feindel, p. 38. Springer-Verlag, New York, 1976.
Plum, F., Posner, J.B., and Alvord, E.C.: Edema and necrosis in experimental cerebral infarction. Arch. Neurol. *9:*563, 1963.
Poll, W., Brock, M., Markakis, E., Winkelmuller, W., and Dietz, H.: Brain tissue pressure. In *Intracranial Pressure,* edited by M. Brock and H. Dietz, p. 188. Springer-Verlag, New York, 1972.
Pollock, L.J., and Boshes, B.: Cerebrospinal fluid pressure. Arch. Neurol. Psychiatry *36:*931, 1936.
Povlishock, J.T., Becker, D.P., Kontos, H.A., and Jenkins, L.W.: Neural and vascular alterations in brain injury. In *Neural Trauma,* edited by A.J. Popp, R.S. Bourke, L.R. Nelson, and H.K. Kimelberg, p. 79. Raven Press, New York, 1979.
Purves, M.J.: Control of cerebral blood vessels: Present state of the art. Ann. Neurol. *3:*377, 1978.
Raichle, M.E., Hartman, B.K., Eichling, J.O., and Sharpe, L.G.: Central noradrenergic regulation of cerebral blood flow and vascular permeability. Proc. Natl. Acad. Sci. U.S.A. *72:*3726, 1975.
Raichle, M.E., Grubb, R.L., and Eichling, J.O.: Central neuroendocrine regulation of brain water permeability. In *Cerebral Vascular Smooth Muscle and Its Control,* edited by M.J. Purves, p. 219. Elsevier, Amsterdam, 1978.
Raisis, J.E., Kindt, G.W., and McGillicuddy, J.E.: The effects of elevated cerebral venous pressure on cerebral blood flow and intracranial pressure. In *Blood Flow and Metabolism in the Brain,* edited by A.M. Harper, W.B. Jennett, J.D. Miller, and J.O. Rowan, p. 6.17. Churchill Livingstone, Edinburgh, 1975.
Rapoport, S.I.: Blood-brain barrier permeability, autoregulation of cerebral blood flow, and brain edema. In *Head Injuries,* edited by R.L. McLaurin, p. 115. Grune & Stratton, New York, 1976.
Rapoport, S.I.: A mathematical model for vasogenic brain edema. J. Theor. Biol. *74:*439, 1978.
Rapoport, S.I.: Roles of cerebrovascular permeability, brain compliance, and brain hydraulic conductivity in vasogenic brain edema. In *Neural Trauma,* edited by A.J. Popp, R.S. Bourke, L.R. Nelson, and H.K. Kimelberg, p. 51. Raven Press, New York, 1979.
Rapoport, S.I., Hori, M., and Klatzo, I.: Reversible osmotic opening of the blood-brain barrier. Science *173:*1026, 1971.
Rapoport, S.I., Matthews, K., and Thompson, H.K.: Absence of brain edema after reversible opening of the blood-brain barrier. In *Dynamics of Brain Edema,* edited by H.M. Pappius and W. Feindel, p. 18. Springer-Verlag, New York, 1976.

Rasmussen, L.W., and Klatzo, I.: Protein and enzyme changes in cold injury edema. Acta Neuropathol. *13:*12, 1969.

Reese, T.S., and Karnovsky, M.J.: Fine structural localization of a blood-brain barrier for exogenous peroxidase. J. Cell Biol. *34:*207, 1967.

Reilly, P.L., Farrar, J.K., and Miller, J.D.: Apparent autoregulation in damaged brain. In *Blood Flow and Metabolism in the Brain,* edited by A.M. Harper, W.B. Jennett, J.D. Miller, and J.O. Rowan, p. 6.21. Churchill Livingstone, Edinburgh, 1975.

Reilly, P.L., Miller, J.D., Rowan, J.O., and Farrar, J.K.: Cerebrovascular responses in focal brain edema. In *Cerebral Function, Metabolism, and Circulation,* edited by D.H. Ingvar, and N.A. Lassen, p. 512. Munksgaard, Copenhagen, 1977.

Reivich, M., Marshall, W.J.S., and Kassell, N.F.: Loss of autoregulation produced by cerebral trauma. In *Cerebral Blood Flow,* edited by M. Brock, C. Fieschi, D.H. Ingvar, N.A. Lassen, and K. Schürmann, p. 205. Springer-Verlag, New York, 1969.

Rennels, M.L., and Nelson, E.: Capillary innervation in the mammalian central nervous system: an electron microscopic demonstration. Am. J. Anat. *144:*233, 1975.

Reulen, H.J.: Vasogenic brain edema. Br. J. Anaesth. *48:*741, 1976.

Reulen, H.J., Graham, R., and Klatzo, I.: Development of pressure gradients within brain tissue during the formation of vasogenic brain edema. In *Intracranial Pressure II,* edited by N. Lundberg, V. Pontén, and M. Brock, p. 233. Springer-Verlag, New York, 1975.

Reulen, H.J., Graham, R., Fenske, A., Tsuyumu, M., and Klatzo, I.: The role of tissue pressure and bulk flow in the formation and resolution of cold-induced edema. In *Dynamics of Brain Edema,* edited by H.M. Pappius and W. Feindel, p. 103. Springer-Verlag, New York, 1976.

Reulen, H.J., Graham, R., Spatz, M., and Klatzo, I.: Role of pressure gradients and bulk flow in dynamics of vasogenic edema. J. Neurosurg. *46:*24, 1977.

Risberg, J., Lundberg, N., and Ingvar, D.H.: Regional cerebral blood volume during acute transient rises of the intracranial pressure (plateau waves). J. Neurosurg. *31:*303, 1969.

Rose, J., Valtonen, S., and Jennett, B.: Avoidable factors contributing to death after head injury. Br. Med. J. *2:*615, 1977.

Rosenblum, W.I., and Commonwealth, V.: Vascular resistance in the cerebral circulation: location and potential consequences with respect to the effect of neurogenic stimuli on flow. In *Neurogenic Control of the Brain Circulation,* edited by C. Owman and L. Edvinsson, p. 221. Pergamon Press, Oxford, 1977.

Rossen, R., Kabat, H., and Anderson, J.P.: Acute arrest of cerebral circulation in man. Arch. Neurol. Psychiatry *50:*510, 1943.

Rowan, J.O., and Johnston, I.H.: Intracranial pressure gradients—do they exist? In *Intracranial Pressure II,* edited by N. Lundberg, U. Ponten, and M. Brock, p. 239. Springer-Verlag, New York, 1975.

Rubio, R., Berne, R.M., Bockman, E.L., and Curnish, R.R.: Relationship between adenosine concentration and oxygen supply in rat brain. Am. J. Physiol. *228:*1896, 1975.

Salford, L.G., Plum, F., and Siesjö, B.K.: Graded hypoxia-oligemia in rat brain. I. Biochemical alterations and their implications. Arch. Neurol. *29:*227, 1973.

Saunders, M.L., Miller, J.D., Stablein, D., and Allen, G.: The effects of graded experimental trauma on cerebral blood flow and responsiveness to CO_2. J. Neurosurg. *51:*18, 1979.

Schaefer, A., Komlos, M., and Seregi, A. Lipid peroxidation as the cause of the ascorbic acid induced decrease of ATPase activities of rat brain microsomes and its inhibition by biogenic amines and psychotropic drugs. Biochem. Pharmacol. *24:*1781, 1975.

Schaul, N., Ball, G., Gloor, P., and Pappius, H.M.: The EEG in cerebral edema. In *Dynamics of Brain Edema,* edited by H.M. Pappius and W. Feindel, p. 144. Springer-Verlag, New York, 1976.

Schettini, A., and Walsh, E.K.: Experimental identification of the subarachnoid and subpial compartments by intracranial pressure measurements. J. Neurosurg. *40:*609, 1974.

Schutta, H.S., Kassell, N.F., and Langfitt, T.W.: Brain swelling produced by injury and aggravated by arterial hypertension. Brain *91:*281, 1968.

Shalit, M.N., Beller, A.J., and Feinsod, M.: Clinical equivalents of cerebral oxygen consumption in coma. Neurology *22:*155, 1972.

Shapiro, H.M., Stromberg, D.D., Lee, D.R., and Wiederhielm, C.A.: Dynamic pressures in the pial arterial microcirculation. Am. J. Physiol. *221:*279, 1971.

Shulman, K., Marmarou, A., and Shapiro, K.: Brain tissue pressure and focal pressure gradients. In *Head Injuries,* edited by R.L. McLaurin, p. 279. Grune & Stratton, New York, 1976.

Siesjö, B.K.: *Brain Energy Metabolism,* 607 pp. John Wiley & Sons, New York, 1978.

Siesjö, B.K., Johannsson, H., Norberg, K., and Salford, L.G.: Brain function, metabolism, and blood flow in moderate and severe arterial hypoxia. In *Brain Work, Alfred Benzon Symposium VIII,* p. 101. Munksgaard, Copenhagen, 1975.

Siesjö, B.K., Nordström, C.H., Rehncrona, S.: Metabolic aspects of cerebral hypoxia-ischemia. Adv. Exp. Med. Biol. *78:*261, 1977.

Simionescu, N., Simionescu, M., and Palade, G.E.: Permeability of muscle capillaries to small heme-peptides. Evidence for the existence of patent transendothelial channels. J. Cell. Biol. *64:*586, 1975.

Soejima, T., Yamamoto, Y.L., Meyer, E., Feindel, W., and Hodge, C.P.: Protective effects of steroids on the cortico-microcirculation injured by cold. J. Neurosurg. *51:*188, 1979.

Sokoloff, L.: Circulation and energy metabolism of the brain. In *Basic Neurochemistry,* ed. 2, edited by G.J. Siegel, R.W. Albers, R. Katzman, and B.W. Agranoff, p. 388. Little, Brown, Boston, 1976.

Sokoloff, L., Fitzgerald, G.G., and Kaufman, E.E.: Cerebral nutrition and energy metabolism. In *Nutrition and the Brain,* vol. 1, edited by R.J. Wurtwan and J.J. Wurtman, p. 87. Raven Press, New York, 1977.

Soni, S.R.: Continuous measurement of differential CSF pressures across the tentorium (abstract). J. Neurol. Neurosurg. Psychiatry *37:*1283, 1974.

Spatz, M., Fujimoto, T., and Go, K.: Transport studies in ischemic cerebral edema. In *Dynamics of Brain Edema,* edited by H.M. Pappius and W. Feindel, p. 181. Springer-Verlag, New York, 1976.

Starlinger, H., and Lübbers, D.W.: Polarographic measurements of the oxygen pressure performed simultaneously with optical measurements of the redox state of the respiratory chain in suspensions of mitochondria under steady-state conditions of low oxygen tensions. Pflügers Arch. Ges. Physiol. *341:*15, 1973.

Steen, P.A., and Michenfelder, J.D.: Cerebral protection with barbiturates. Relation to anesthetic effect. Stroke *9:*140, 1978.

Steen, P.A., Michenfelder, J.D., and Milde, J.H.: Incomplete versus complete cerebral ischemia: improved outcome with a minimal blood flow. Ann. Neurol. 6:389, 1979.

Steinwall, O., and Klatzo, I.: Selective vulnerability of the blood-brain barrier in chemically induced lesions. J. Neuropathol. Exp. Neurol. 25:542, 1966.

Stromberg, D.D., and Fox, J.R.: Pressures in the pial arterial microcirculation of the cat during changes in systemic arterial blood pressure. Circ. Res. 31:229, 1972.

Sullivan, H.G., Miller, J.D., Becker, D.P., Flora, R.E., and Allen, G.A.: The physiological basis of intracranial pressure change with progressive epidural brain compression. J. Neurosurg. 47:532, 1977.

Symon, L.: Distribution of pressure within the cranial cavity and its significance. In *Head Injuries*, edited by R.L. McLaurin, p. 249. Grune & Stratton, New York, 1976.

Symon, L., and Dorsch, N.W.C.: The distribution of pressures within the intracranial cavity. In *Intracranial Pressure II*, edited by N. Lundberg, U. Ponten, and M. Brock, p. 203. Springer-Verlag, New York, 1975.

Symon, L., Pásztor, E., Dorsch, N.W.C., and Branston, N.M.: Physiological responses of local areas of the cerebral circulation in experimental primates determined by the method of hydrogen clearance. Stroke 4:632, 1973.

Symon, L, Pásztor, E., Branston, N.M., and Dorsch, N.W.C.: The effect of supratentorial space-occupying lesions on regional intracranial pressure and local cerebral blood flow. An experimental study in baboons. J. Neurol. Neurosurg. Psychiatry 37:617, 1974.

Taylor, A.E., and Granger, H.J.: Interstitial fluid pressure—basic concepts. In *Head Injuries*, edited by R.L. McLaurin, p. 265. Grune & Stratton, New York, 1976.

Teasdale, G.M., Lennox, G., and Harper, A.M.: rCBF measurement in focal ischaemia and the response to hypercapnia. In *Blood Flow and Metabolism in the Brain*, edited by A.M. Harper, W.B. Jennett, J.D. Miller, and J.O. Rowan, p. 12.15. Churchill Livingstone, Edinburgh, 1975.

Teasdale, G., Rowan, J.O., Turner, J.W., Grossman, R., and Miller, J.D.: Cerebral perfusion failure and cortical electrical activity. In *Cerebral Function, Metabolism, and Circulation*, edited by D.H. Ingvar and N.A. Lassen, p. 23.14. Munksgaard, Copenhagen, 1977.

Teasdale, G., Galbraith, S., and Jennett, B.: Operate or observe? ICP and the management of the "silent" traumatic intracranial hematoma. In *Intracranial Pressure IV*, edited by K. Shulman, A. Marmarou, J.D. Miller, D.P. Becker, G.M. Hochwald, and M. Brock, p. 36. Springer-Verlag, New York, 1980.

Thews, G.: Implications to physiology and pathology of oxygen diffusion at the capillary level. In *Selective Vulnerability of the Brain in Hypoxemia*, edited by J.P. Schadé and W.H. McMenemey, p. 27. Blackwell, Oxford, 1963.

Tornheim, P., and McLaurin, R.L.: Traumatic cerebral edema: an experimental model. In *Head Injuries*, edited by R.L. McLaurin, p. 123. Grune & Stratton, New York, 1976.

Weed, L.H.: Some limitations of the Monro-Kellie hypothesis. Arch. Surg. 18:1049, 1929.

Weinstein, J.D., and Langfitt, T.W.: Responses of cortical vessels to brain compression: observations through a transparent calvarium. Surg. Forum 18:430, 1967.

Welsh, F.A., Durity, F., and Langfitt, T.W.: The appearance of regional variations in metabolism at a critical level of diffuse cerebral oligemia. J. Neurochem. 28:71, 1977.

Welsh, F.A., Johns, R.L., and Williams, M.J.: Inhomogeneous perfusion. In *Neural Trauma*, edited by A.J. Popp, R.S. Bourke, L.R. Nelson, and H.K. Kimelberg, p. 27. Raven Press, New York, 1979.

Westergaard, E.: Enhanced vesicular transport of exogenous peroxidase across cerebral vessels induced by serotonin. Acta Neuropath. (Berlin) 32:27, 1975.

Westergaard, E.: The permeability properties of cerebral microvasculature under normal and experimental conditions, studied ultrastructurally. 1st International Ernst Reuter Symposium: Brain Edema, Berlin, September, 1979.

Williams, L.F., Jr.: Hemorrhagic shock as a source of unconsciousness. Surg. Clin. N. Am. 48:263, 1968.

Winn, H.R., Bowe, A.B., Welsh, J.E., Rubio, R., and Berne, R.M.: Changes in adenosine during sustained hypoxia. Acta Neurol. Scand. (Supp. 72) 60:330, 1979a.

Winn, H.R., Rubio, R., and Berne, R.M.: Brain adenosine production in the rat during 60 seconds of ischemia. Circ. Res. 45:485, 1979b.

Winn, H.R., Welsh, J.E., Rubio, R., and Berne, R.M. Brain adenosine production in rat during sustained alteration in systemic blood pressure. Am. J. Physiol. 239:636, 1980.

Zimmerman, R.A., Bilaniuk, L.T., Bruce, D., Dolinskas, C., Obrist, W.D., and Kuhl, D.: Computed tomography of pediatric head trauma: acute general cerebral swelling. Radiology 126:403, 1978.

… CHAPTER 43

Treatment of Head Injury

JOSEPH RANSOHOFF

The response of the central nervous system (CNS) to trauma is unique among all body systems with regard to its lack of resilience and limited regenerative capacity and the devastating effects that permanent CNS dysfunction may have on the entire organism. CNS tissue of semisolid consistency is easily deformed by stress and is subject to serious compromise from shearing forces. Brain stem damage, leading to coma vigil, or high cervical injury, leading to permanent quadriplegia and a respirator dependent life, are striking examples which serve to highlight the critical role of the CNS in the body's economy. To date, whereas isolated fragments as in tissue culture show capacities for regeneration, no evidence has been forthcoming to suggest that the CNS tissue in humans has the capacity for regeneration with the recovery of useful functions following actual disruption of physical continuity. Thus, brain lacerations and spinal cord lacerations produce irreversible deficits. Whereas major laboratory efforts are underway to study the problem of mammalian CNS regeneration, the most promising clinical and laboratory efforts are currently directed towards a better understanding of the phenomenon of ischemia and edema of CNS tissue with emphasis directed towards the control of these secondary phenomena which, in and of themselves, can lead to irreversible damage and death.

In recent years, the most dramatic model of the capacity of the CNS to self-destruct has been seen in the experimental model of spinal cord injury. Here, a known force impacting the spinal cord can produce permanent and irreversible paraplegia if untreated; yet, immediately after the injury, little or no pathological change can be seen. The relentless progression of this process is initiated by the appearance of petechial hemorrhages in the central gray matter, progressing over hours to complete the dissolution of the central cord and spreading edema into the surrounding white matter long pathways to the point of complete necrosis of the spinal cord within 24 hr. This progressive, self-destructing process evolving over time in an animal who is rendered immediately and permanently paraplegic has led to a great flurry of laboratory investigations in an attempt to arrest these pathological events with the hope of preserving anatomical continuity and physiological function.

There are, however, constraining anatomical differences between the spinal cord and the brain which tend to protect the latter against the forces of edema, if not ischemia, and give rise to the well documented difference in prognosis in a patient with an immediate paraplegia with little likelihood of recovery, as against the very real possibility of the patient in coma following head injury having a reasonable chance for significant improvement, if not total recovery. The anatomical configuration of the spinal cord is encased by intimately applied, relatively inelastic pial membranes contained within, which are the closely packed pathways supplied by a longitudinally oriented arterial circulation and a small blood volume. No significant amount of intramedullary spinal fluid allows this structure much possibility of escaping from the effects of hemorrhage, ischemia, and the inevitable edema that represents the response of the CNS to any type of injury. Even a small lesion in the spinal cord will produce a neurological deficit. In contradistinction, the brain contains within itself a significant spinal fluid reservoir and an equally significant circulating blood volume, both of which provide for considerable capacitance for adjustment to the effects of post-traumatic swelling. Furthermore, there are large areas of cerebral tissue which can be permanently destroyed without producing clinically significant neurological deficits. Irrespective of these gross anatomical variances, there is no question that the pathophysiological processes in both brain and spinal cord which develop as sequelae of trauma are identical, according to the studies of the basic cellular and membrane changes which follow. CNS trauma research must direct itself towards these basic phenomena if further significant advances are to be expected.

Traumatic CNS edema is now generally accepted to be of vasogenic origin, based on a breakdown of the tight junctions in the CNS capillary bed as well as alterations in glial membrane structure. This pertubation of membrane function results in a disturbance of the sodium-potassium pump mechanism and a disruption of the membrane bound enzyme systems, which account for the critical preservation of energy metabolism and transport functions without which CNS tissue becomes rapidly and irreversibly damaged. Changes in the calcium ion concentrations are most likely the initial phenomena occurring in milliseconds after injury.

The role of the brain stem reticular activating system appears to be the site of key processes, and not just for the maintenance of consciousness in terms of its upstream or cephalad function of this key brain stem area. Recently, experimental studies documenting the effect of brain stem lesions on cerebral metabolic rate and cerebral blood flow have also shown serious effects upon pulmonary, cardiac, and renal systems, mimicking the dysfunction in these organs often seen in humans following a serious head injury. Our research laboratories have demonstrated not only the cerebral effect of brain stem reticular lesions in animals but also systemic sequelae including pulmonary edema and necrosis, cardiac ischemia and endothelial necrosis, and renal tubular dysfunction. These phenomena occur in the absence of increased intracranial pressure.

In an effort to study the effects of trauma on CNS membrane function, laboratory efforts have been directed towards the hypothesis that lipid peroxidation by the release of free radicals may account for many of the disturbances in energy metabolism and membrane permeability seen after trauma leading to experimental edema. The limiting membrane of CNS cells, the plasma membrane, while differing in quantitative ways among different cell types, is a bimolecular leaflet of phospholipid and other amphipathic substances like cholesterol. The hydrophilic ends of these lipid molecules are directed to the outer surface of the membrane where they are in contact with aqueous millieu. The hydrophobic ends of these amphipathic lipid molecules are directed towards each other in a double layer to form the hydrophobic midzone of the membrane. The fatty acid tails of phospholipids which form this hydrophobic zone are in the Cis configuration, the chain bending at 123° at every double bonded site. This important characteristic of CNS membranes accounts for the interstices within this hydrophobic zone. Membrane-bound molecules are inserted into the archways, including the membrane-bound enzyme and protein molecules responsible for the maintenance of the internal environment of the cell and continued function. Free radical processes catalyzed by the presence of heme rapidly destroy the structural continuity of the hydrophobic membrane zone and may well account for membrane dysfunction and subsequent edema in response to trauma. Glucocorticosteroids are known to insert physically into the hydrophobic midzone of plasma membranes and may protect against the effect of lipid peroxidation. Indeed, considerable experimental evidence is accumulating to indicate that steroids protect membrane function rather than directly effecting edema per se and that once membrane stabilization has occurred, the edema fluid is removed by the normal physiological processes. For example, cats treated with dexamethasone before or shortly after spinal cord injury have significantly better recovery and less histological abnormality in the spinal cord than do untreated cats. The course of posttraumatic edema is similar. Electrophysiological studies measuring spinal cord conductivity show recovery of evoked responses in the corticosteroid-treated animals independent of the degree of edema. In a similar fashion, dexamethasone drastically diminishes the EEG abnormalities which develop in response to a standard cold lesion applied to the brain. This effect also does not appear to be mediated by the dexamethasone diminution of edema.

An interesting by-product of this research has been the demonstration of the effect of ethanol on the response of the CNS to trauma. In an effort to develop a model of CNS trauma in both brain and spinal cord which would minimize the physical effects of energy expended to the CNS tissue, animals were pretreated with intravenous ethanol. The degree of membrane breakdown and subsequent edema was greatly magnified by the exposure to ethanol, a substance which is known to potentiate the breakdown of lipid cell membranes.

A number of therapeutic regimens other than steroids are under intense investigation in various experimental laboratories relative to the protection of the CNS following trauma. The barbiturates have been shown to have a protective function in ischemic hypoxia of CNS tissue, and the role of these agents in trauma is just entering a new phase. Other areas under investigation include: the use of dimethylsulphoxide (DMSO) both as a therapeutic agent itself and as a carrier for other substances; the use of hypothermia, both naturally occurring and artifically induced; the use of antioxidants; and the role of experimental surgical procedures.

Finally, in both experimental animals and in human subjects following trauma, the use of physiological monitoring of CNS conductivity is a burgeoning area of research. Both evoked cortical potentials for evaluating spinal cord function; evoked potential studies involving input via various cranial nerves may well serve to document the site of physiological dysfunction, if not anatomical lesion sites hopefully, will also serve as a method of distinguishing the primary effects of injury versus the secondary effects of edema, herniation, and compression which so often confuse the pathological findings seen after death.

INITIAL EVALUATION

Many factors converge in the individual patient relative to the issue of survival and the quality of life following recovery. Age, pre-existing disease, head trauma, associated injuries, delay in management, as well as the severity of the injury to the brain, must all be considered in evaluating the efficacy of treatment.

The brain is bathed and cushioned by cerebrospinal fluid wrapped in durable meninges and enclosed by the thick bones of the skull. Despite this anatomical protection, automobile accidents, accidents at work and at home, and man's inhumanity to man are responsible for a high and costly incidence of craniocerebral trauma. In 1970, there were an estimated 50,320,000 injuries of all varieties in the United States, with 114,000 accidental deaths. These fatalities exceed the 10-year total for the Vietnam War, and head injury follows only heart disease, neoplasm, and stroke as a leading cause of death. CNS injuries account for 50% of the total of accidental deaths.

Accident prevention is clearly the long-term solution to the devastating problem of craniocerebral trauma. In the individual patient, however, the severity of the injury and the interval prior to adequate medical attention are factors that determine outcome.

Well trained ambulance crews, rendering initial therapy with particular attention to airway clearance, and rapid triage to adequately equipped hospitals, are obviously of great importance. Once a patient has reached an emergency room, the following evaluation should be promptly performed.

Airway

Adequate ventilation is essential for the preservation of cerebral function in the severely injured patient. The nose and mouth should be cleared of blood, mucous, and any foreign bodies. Any clinical signs of upper airway obstruction or abnormality of arterial blood gas determinations should prompt immediate endotracheal intubation with mechanical ventilatory support if required. All conscious patients should be intubated. Tracheostomy should be done if the patient cannot be intubated.

Vital Signs and Associated Injuries

Blood pressure, pulse, and respiration should be recorded immediately and frequently. Hypotension is a terminal event in the pure head injury. Accordingly, an associated intraabdominal, chest, or long bone injury should be suspected in the hypotensive patient. The cervical spine may be unstable, and the patient who appears awake but bradycardic, hypotensive, and flaccid may likely have high spinal cord injury. The Cushing reflex (hypertension, bradycardia, and irregular respiration) is most often but not always an inevitable sign of increased intracranial pressure. Chest and cardiovascular injuries should be ruled out promptly, and abdominal and urinary injuries also should be eliminated by appropriate methods. Long bone injuries may be palpated and confirmed by x-ray. Inspection should include the head—searching for otorrhea, rhinorrhea, scalp lacerations, and compound fractures. Basal skull fractures may leave defects where cranial contents can exit, and nasogastric or endotracheal tubes may be inadvertently inserted.

State of Consciousness

The level of consciousness is the most important indication of the severity of the head injury. Precise, frequent appraisals are necessary to detect any deterioration that heralds an expanding intracranial hematoma or progressive brain swelling.

Consciousness is best defined by describing the patient's response to external stimuli rather than by vague terms such as stupor or coma. The classification in Table 43.1 is based on the patient's response to verbal and noxious stimuli. Any patient categorized at level III or below should be suspected at once of having sustained life-threatening intracranial trauma, and further diagnostic evaluation and therapeutic measures should be instituted immediately. *This pertains especially to any patient manifesting deterioration in level of consciousness.*

Progressive restlessness and agitation should not be confused with improvement in the level of consciousness but may be indicative of increasing intracranial pressure. Sedation for restless agitation must, therefore, be avoided. Headache is rarely complained of early after head injury, and when severe (as the dura is being stripped), it is often a sign of epidural hematoma, particularly when associated with agitation.

Neurological Examination

Following the observation of the level of consciousness, any signs of focal CNS damage should be searched for. The head should again be inspected for evidence of compound or depressed fractures. Otorrhea, rhinorrhea, and mastoid or upper eyelid ecchymosis suggest an accompanying basal skull fracture.

The position of the eyes at rest is noted, with attention focused on abnormalities such as forced gaze or skew deviations, nystagmus, or ocular bobbing. Mydriatic drugs must not be used, as these will confuse pupillary responses for many hours. Unilateral pupillary dilatation or poor responsiveness to light generally indicates brain stem or oculomotor nerve compression by a herniating temporal lobe, secondary to a unilateral expanding intracranial mass which is almost always ipsilateral to the abnormal pupil. This may progress rapidly to bilateral pupillary dilatation, an extremely ominous sign. Tentorial herniation is frequently accompanied by contralateral hemiparesis or decerebration. However, a falsely lateralizing homolateral hemiplegia may occur with compression of the contralateral cerebral peduncle against the tentorium.

The extremities should be evaluated for weakness, flaccidity, spasticity, and rigidity. Bilateral reflexes should be rapidly compared and plantar responses tested. The sensory evaluation is usually of little value; however, the lack of response to a pinprick in a less than comatose patient should raise suspicion of an accompanying spinal cord injury.

Table 43.1
Stages of CNS Response After Head Injury

1. Alert, responds immediately to questions; may be disoriented and confused; follows complex commands.
2. Drowsy, confused, uninterested, does not lapse into sleep when undisturbed; follows simple commands only.
3. Stuporous, sleeps when not disturbed, responds briskly and appropriately to mildly noxious stimuli.
4. Deep stupor, responds defensively to prolonged noxious stimuli.
5. Coma, no appropriate response to any stimuli, includes decorticate and decerebrate responses.
6. Deep coma, flaccidity, no response to any stimuli.

History

A description of the accident is frequently a good indicator of the energy transmitted to the brain and, hence, the severity of the injury. Thus, a patient struck by a rapidly moving vehicle or one who has fallen a good distance must be regarded with concern despite the neurological evaluation, which may be relatively normal early after the trauma. If the patient can be questioned, the degree of amnesia both preceding and following the injury also provides a measure of the severity of the injury.

Recent studies in our experimental laboratories have demonstrated an increased sensitivity of the nervous system to trauma associated with elevated blood alcohol, gainsaying the old adage that "God protects the drunkard."

Fluid Management

In the acute phase, it is important not to over infuse a crystalloid solution into the patient with a head injury. It is preferable to use an isotonic solution of two and one-half dextrose in a one-half normal saline. In the multiple system, the injured patient with head injury and hypotension, colloid or plasma expanders should be used until blood is available. In the head injured patient who is decompensating rapidly or who is in extremis on admission, intravenous diuretics such as furosemide or mannitol can produce a rapid decrease in intracranial pressure with arrest of the deteriorating state or even a transient improvement, thus allowing time for further diagnostic measures to be undertaken.

Summary of Initial Evaluation

Rapid attention to the following items as defined previously will serve as a guide to further treatment: provision for adequate airway and ventilation; observation of vital signs, search for associated injuries; state of consciousness; neurological examination; history of trauma; and fluid management.

CLASSIFICATION OF NEUROLOGICAL STATUS

Clinical examination alone, however, leaves something to be desired in prognostic capability. For one thing, it does not take into account the mode of injury and the energy expended intracranially, each of which can have a great bearing on the ultimate outcome. Pure translational-acceleration forces, leading to localized hematomas and focal tissue destruction, offer on the whole a better prognosis than do rotational-acceleration forces that produce shearing stresses with diffuse white matter and possibly vascular damage. They may, however, have similar initial clinical presentations.

One must at first define the deficit in the traumatized patient in order to localize it functionally and investigate it for reversibility. As is often the case, semantics present the initial difficulty in even communicating about the subject matter at hand. The efforts of Teasdale and Jenett (1974) to provide a clinical scale for describing the head injury victim stand out in this respect. The parameters of best verbal and motor response, eye opening, oculocephalic and oculovestibular response, and respiratory pattern provide a practical scheme for initial evaluation of the patient and continued in-hospital monitoring. They also assist in an initial localization of neural dysfunction within the CNS axis. The formalization of these observations into the Glasgow coma scale has provided us with a vehicle to measure objectively on an interinstitutional basis the results of various treatment regimes. Jennett's outcome scale is of similar importance. It consists of the following categories: 1) death; 2) persistent vegetative state; 3) severe disability; 4) moderate disability; and 5) good recovery.

DIAGNOSTIC STUDIES

Following the initial evaluation, further diagnostic studies are usually indicated. Skull radiography should be obtained routinely to determine the presence of possible fractures, especially those extending across the meningeal arterial channels which are frequently associated with epidural hematomas (Fig. 43.1). A shift of midline structures such as a calcified pineal, if present, is indicative of an intracranial mass. X-rays of the cervical spine should be obtained, since unsuspected fractures in association with severe head injuries are frequently overlooked, particularly at the C_{6-7} level.

Whereas echoencephalography is useful in detecting a shift of midline structures, ventriculography demonstrates unilateral mass lesions, and cerebral angiography distinguish extracerebral hematomas from intracerebral mass lesions, *computerized tomography (CT) has become the most valuable and most reliable diagnostic tool in the management of head trauma.* CT scanning clearly identifies both intra- and extracerebral hematoma in all skull compartments. CT scanning is the only examination which distinguishes brain edema from hemorrhagic contusions and pure hematomas as well as identifies combinations of these pathological processes. Serial CT scanning is critical in evaluating the efficacy of therapy and in revealing delayed complications such as hydrocephalus and late hematomas. Except in critically ill patients who are deteriorating under one's eyes and whose condition justifies burr holes in the emergency room, CT scanning should be carried out as soon as possible in all patients who are deteriorating. If CT scanning is not available, cerebral angiography or ventriculography must be used.

The importance of recording pressure directly from the intracranial cavity has recently been generally recognized. This serves as an adjunctive diagnostic study as well as a means of evaluating the efficacy of both medical and surgical therapy. Several devices are available that allow for epidural, subdural, or intraventricular pressure monitoring. Simple intraventricular monitoring via an indwelling catheter attached to an appropriate pressure transducer is probably the easiest and most reliable method. This can be done immediately on admission to

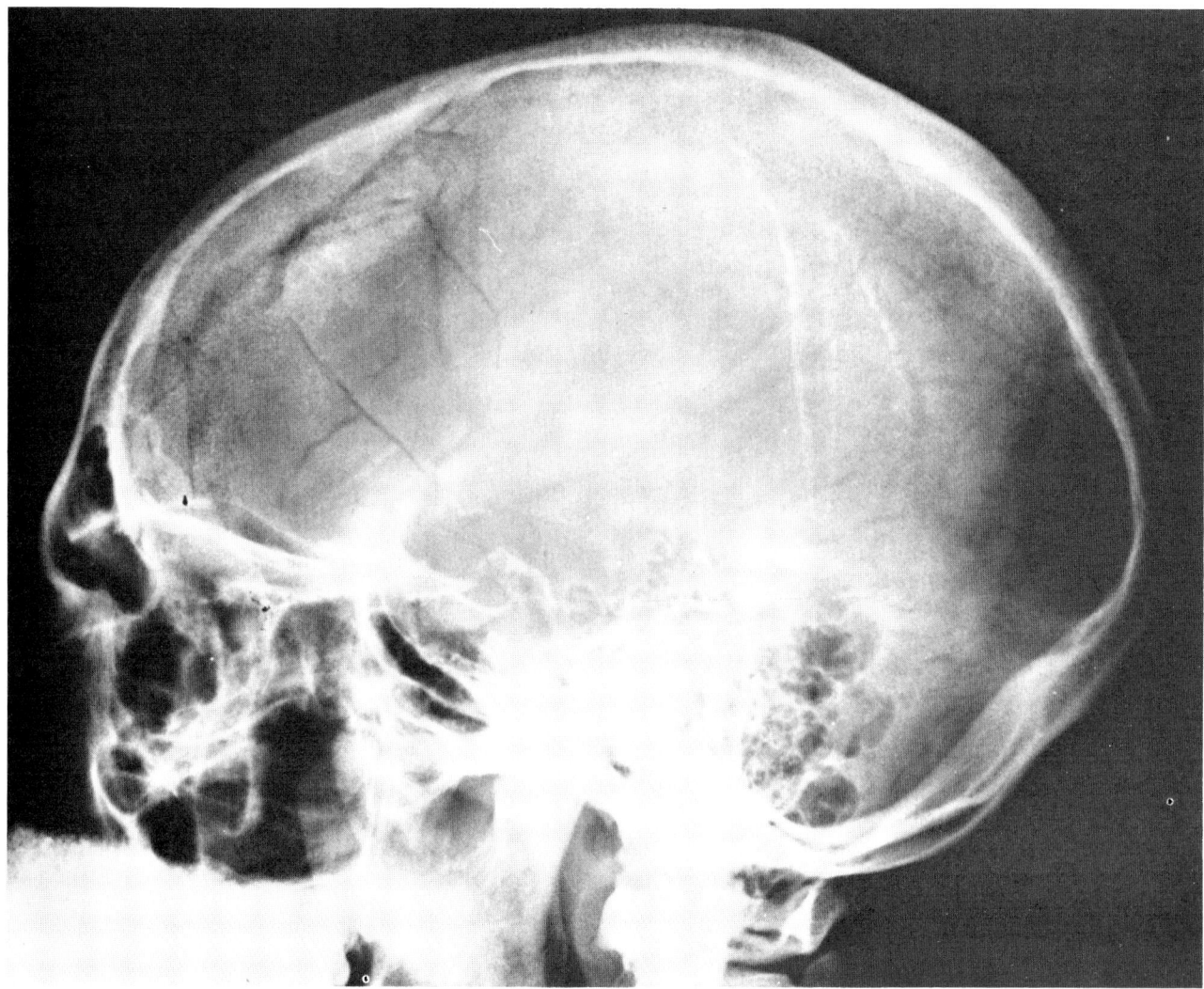

Figure 43.1. A skull fracture crossing the middle meningeal artery groove requires close observation and CT scan to rule out epidural hematoma.

the emergency room. After draining the ventricular fluid, 5 ml of metrizamide and 5 ml of air can be injected into the ventricular system. An anteroposterior and lateral skull x-ray will demonstrate any shift of midline structure including the fourth ventricle (Fig. 43.2a and b).

Lumbar puncture is not indicated in evaluating a patient with acute head trauma unless there is a suspicion of meningitis. Persistent leakage of CSF from the dural puncture site may allow downward herniation of the brain.

MEDICAL THERAPY

Medical therapy is indicated in all seriously injured patients whether or not surgical intervention is carried out. Surgery is indicated for the removal of blood clots, foreign bodies, depressed bone fragments, and irreversibly damaged brain. Surgery is not the management of choice in the treatment of brain edema, a concomitant of all serious brain injuries, hence the need for medical therapy.

Arterial blood gases are monitored to keep the brain well oxygenated. The optimal $PaCO_2$ from 28 to 30 torr keeps down intracranial pressure by intracranial vasoconstriction. Intubation and a volume respirator are usually required.

The seriously injured or rapidly deteriorating patient should receive 500 cc of 20% mannitol as rapidly as possible while awaiting diagnostic studies. The chronic administration of mannitol can be considered for several days, however, careful monitoring of BUN, electrolytes, and serum osmolality is required. More recently, the use of loop diuretics, furosemide, and ethacrynic acid appear to have distinct advantages over the osmotic diuretics. In our clinic, furosemide has been shown to lessen increased intracranial pressure based not only on its diuretic effect but also on its direct cerebral effects, with inhibition of chloride cellular transport preventing astroglial swelling. These effects improve microcirculatory impedence, allowing for easier access of oxygen and nutrients to the brain. All modalities should be utilized on a chronic

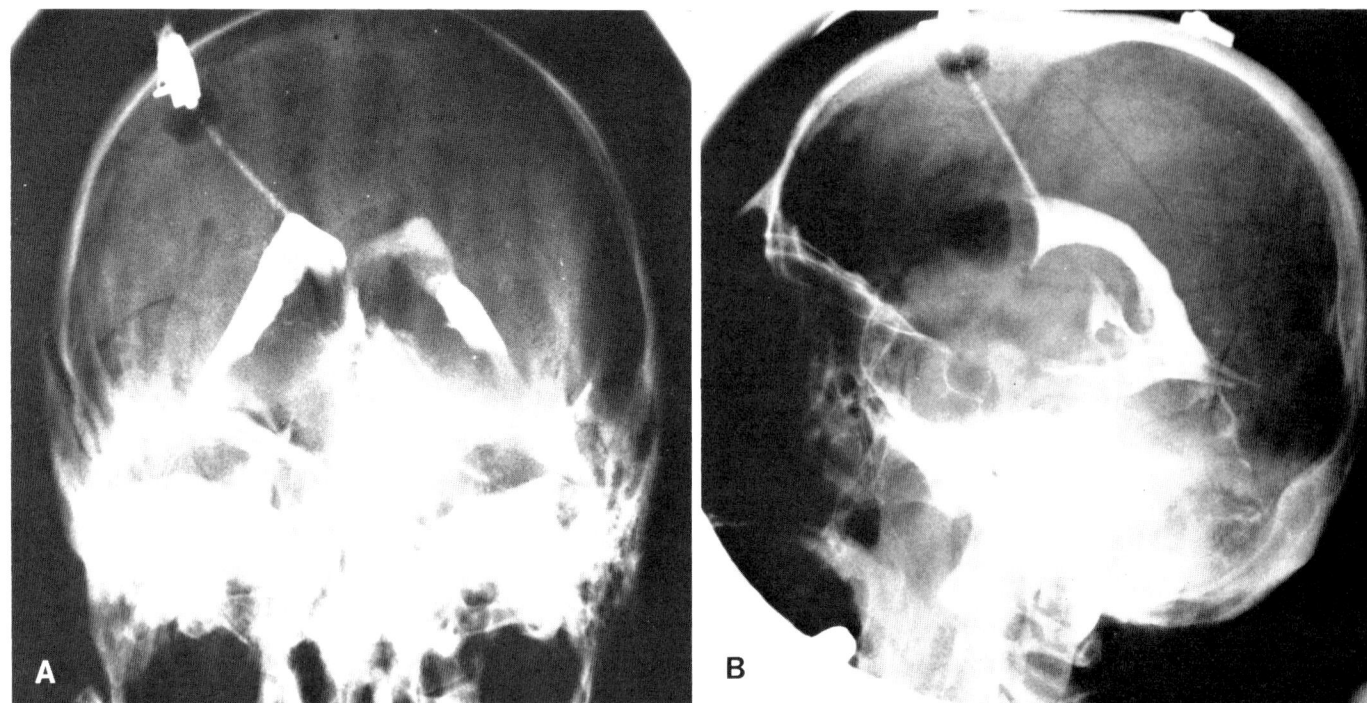

Figure 43.2. The air is in the frontal horns and the metrizamide is in the rest of the ventricular system.

basis in conjunction with monitoring of intracranial pressure (ICP), with the goal of a pressure of 20 torr or lower. Adrenocorticosteroids exert their beneficial effect on injured brain via their capacity to stabilize endothelial and glial membranes. Stabilization of membranes will reduce edema formation and improve the function of all membrane-bound enzymatic activity; methylprednisolone (Solu-Medrol) at the level of 1-2 g per day or equivalent doses of other glucocorticoids should be initiated early and maintained for a period of 7–10 days. Cimetidine and antacids are administered in conjunction with steroid therapy in an attempt to reduce bleeding from "stress" ulcers, although there is no evidence that steroids in and of themselves produce gastrointestinal bleeding. Corticosteroids are not effective in salvaging patients with brain lacerations, and recent random studies have indicated their ineffectiveness in this context.

The use of barbiturates in the management of very severe head injuries with uncontrollable increased intracranial pressure has been a recent development. Patients are carried on short-acting lipid soluble barbiturates (pentobarbitol) to the level of an isolectric EEG. A very rapid reduction in ICP is usually achieved, thus maintaining cerebral perfusion pressure. These patients are obviously intubated and respirator-dependent and require careful monitoring of all vital functions by a team of neurosurgeons, anesthesiologists, and specialized nurses. In about 50% of the patients with an ICP above 40 torr, barbiturates will effectively reduce the intracranial pressure and salvage some of these individuals. The mechanisms whereby barbiturates protect against the effect of brain ischemia, lower ICP, and improve cerebral circulation are matters of intense laboratory investigations. The effect of barbiturates is not only that of reduced metabolic need but appears to have an effect on cerebrovascular microcirculation.

Prophylactic anticonvulsants are administered at least initially to all patients experiencing severe head trauma. Dilantin at the level of 200 mg twice daily and/or phenobarbital at 30–45 mg three or four times daily are utilized. Additional doses of phenobarbital or valium are administered to control seizures if they occur. Any hyperthermia is treated with acetaminophen or hypothermia blankets. Urinary catheter drainage is monitored.

SURGICAL THERAPY

Acute Epidural Hematomas (Fig. 43.3)

These are among the few surgical lesions which are potentially completely salvageable. The brain itself is not injured permanently. Speed is of the essence in their diagnosis and treatment to prevent secondary brain injury. They are largely a disease of the young, and the trauma may appear to have been insignificant. There may or may not have been a transient period of loss of consciousness, the so called "lucid" period. The patient who comes to the emergency room awake, who rapidly becomes agitated, and progresses to coma with or without pupillary dilatation, and hemiparesis despite steroids and diuretics is the prime suspect. A boggy temporal fossa is also a useful sign. In the emergency room one may have to place burr holes in this clinical setting. The death in the epidural hematoma is due to an expanding clot forcing the temporal lobe against the brainstem causing secondary brain stem injury. These patients

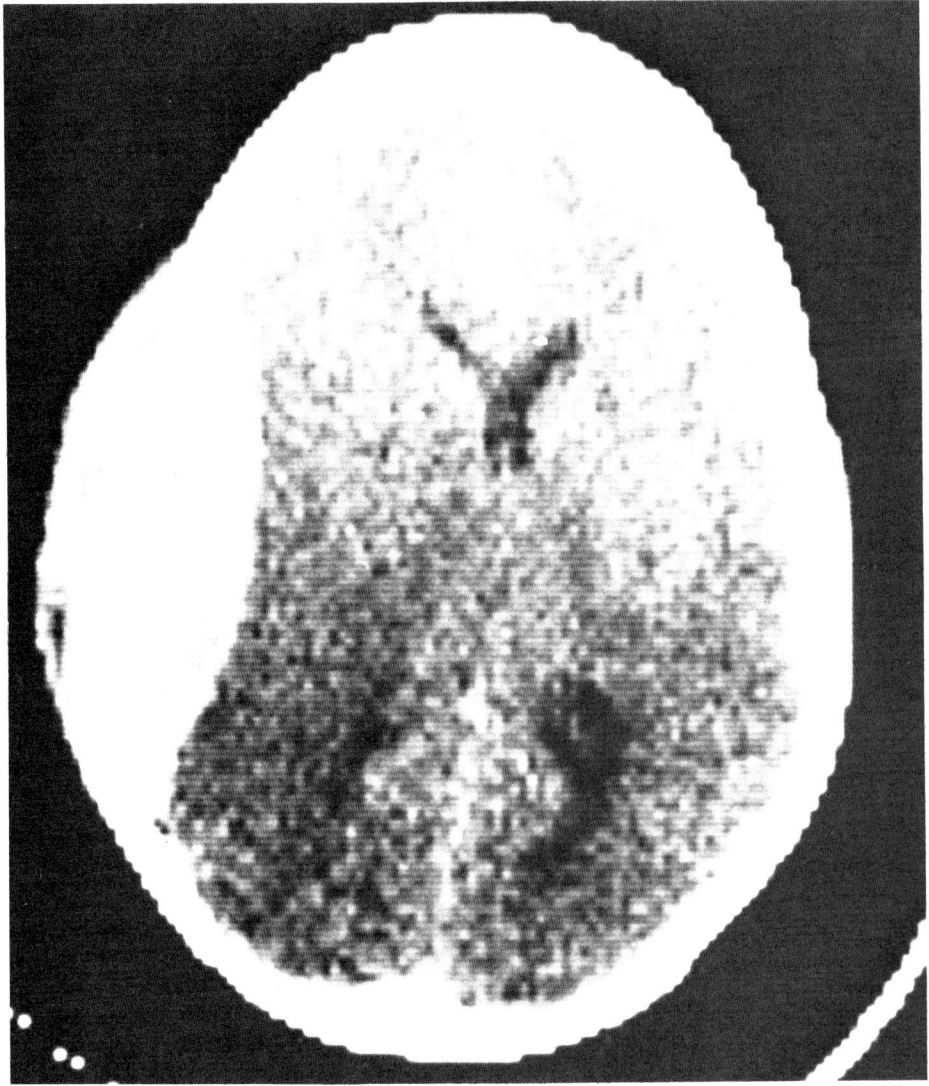

Figure 43.3. The epidural hematoma is lenticular shaped. The acute blood clot is radio dense on CT scan.

should be decompressed prior to herniation. Definitive surgical therapy or CT scanning should follow the burr hole.

Surgical management can best be achieved via a linear incision and frontotemporal craniectomy. The hematoma is removed, and bleeding of the middle meningeal or other vessels is controlled. The dura is tented to the bone edges and the skull defect repaired with a stainless steel cranioplasty or by replacement of the bone flap if one has been turned. If there is any question of an associated subdural, the dura should be opened for inspection.

Rarely, an occipital fracture causes a posterior fossa epidural hematoma by tearing a dipolic vein, the sagittal sinus, the torcula, the lateral sinus, or the sigmoid sinus. These patients may have a depressed mental status with an occipital headache. Ataxia, nystagmus, and gaze palsies are common features of posterior fossa epidural hematomas. Immediate decompression is necessary due to the little time and space for compensation before death from brainstem compression.

Acute Subdural Hematomas (Fig. 43.4)

The therapy of acute subdural hematomas, i.e., those requiring surgery within the first 24–36 hr after injury, carries with it a gloomy prognostic outlook. The poor results following surgical drainage relate to the underlying brain edema and extensive tissue disruption resulting in contusion and laceration of the brain secondary to the forces transmitted at the time of injury. In the past, large craniectomies with dural decompressions have been carried out in an effort to improve the mortality rate associated with these lesions, with ranges from 70 to 90%. It has become evident, however, following review of our own cases that these large flaps and dural decompressions have not significantly altered the outcome. Current therapy for acute subdural hematoma consists, therefore, of making a sufficiently generous flap or craniectomy to provide for definitive clot removal and adequate hemostasis. A wide dural opening should be carried out to provide for inspection of the underlying brain, and grossly contused and lacerated brain tissue should be

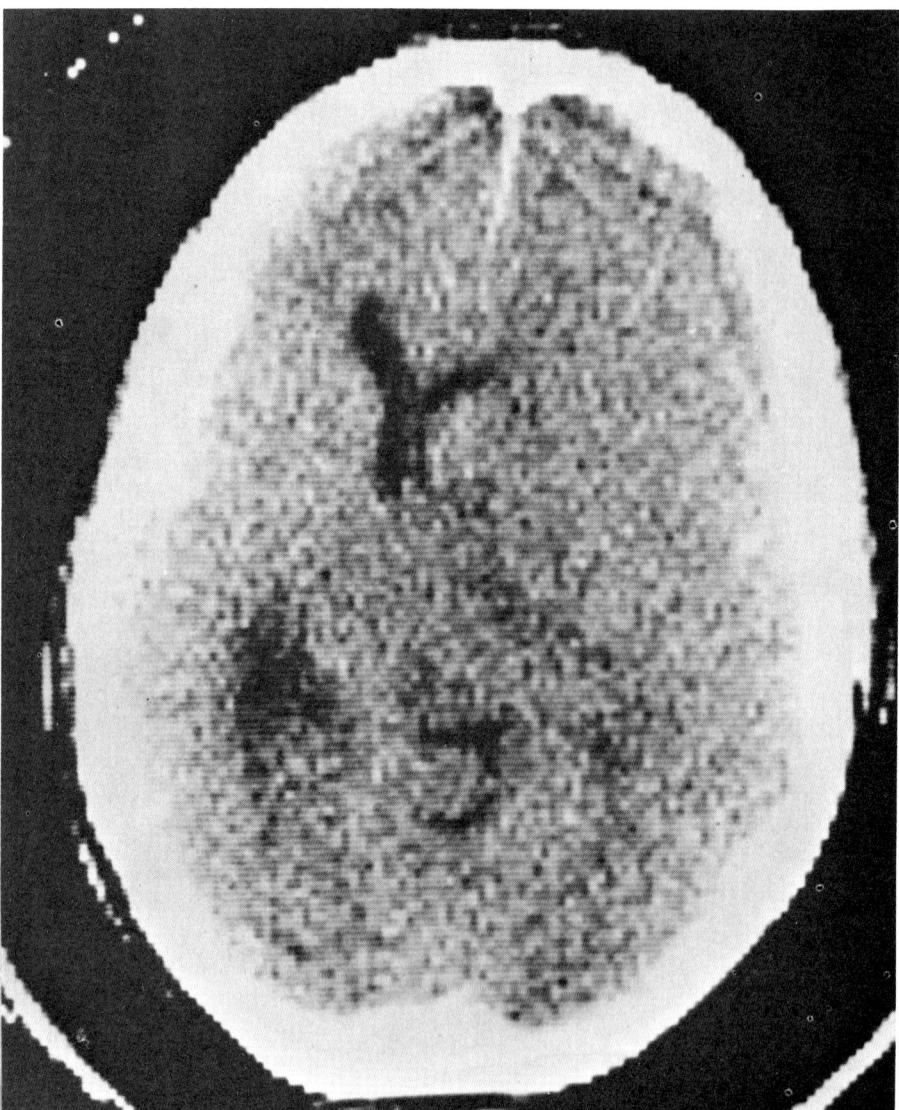

Figure. 43.4. The acute holohemispheric subdural hematoma compresses the ventricular system and shifts the entire brain to the opposite side. The extra-axial collection extends from the frontal to the occipital pole.

removed at the same time, especially the temporal lobe. The bone flap should be replaced. Intracranial pressure should be monitored and vigorous treatment provided for the associated brain edema, including high dose corticosteroids, osmotic and loop diuretics and, if intracranial pressure cannot be controlled, the use of barbiturate hibernation. It seems clear that the management of acute posttraumatic brain edema is not a surgical issue but one which must be resolved by improved medical therapies.

Intracerebral Hematomas (Fig. 43.5)

With the increased usage of CT scanning in the evaluation of patients with head trauma, the recognition of acute intracerebral hematomas and delayed intracerebral hematomas (those occurring 12–48 hr after injury), as distinguished from diffuse brain swelling, is now easily established. By and large, with the exception of very large intracerebral hematomas, these are best initially managed by medical means unless the patient is in a life-threatening situation as a result of uncal herniation and/or uncontrolled increased intracranial pressure. Early drainage of intracerebral hematomas is often followed by reaccumulation of the clot, whereas delayed drainage, if necessary, can be carried out through a small cortical plug with minimum brain damage and a minimum risk of reaccumulation. Intracerebral hematomas often can be treated conservatively and may be resorbed without the need for surgical intervention.

Skull Fractures

The simple fracture is not of serious consequence unless associated with underlying pathology. In the basal skull fracture with spinal fluid leak, patients are placed at bedrest, and the leak resolves within several days. Should the spinal fluid leakage not clear, several lumbar punctures removing 40–50 cc may be carried out. Should this not be successful, the patient is placed on spinal drainage with the removal of up to 300 cc of spinal fluid in 24 hr over several days. This most often will close the leak. We do not recommend prophylactic antibiotics but rather prefer to obtain serial cultures of the nasopharynx or the external auditory meatus every few days. It is only occasionally that operative means must be used to close the fistula.

In depressed fractures, the choice of therapy is dictated by whether the fracture is compound, or whether the fracture results in small depressions over the midline sagittal sinus or at the extreme frontal and occipital poles of the skull, which need not be elevated. Frontoparietal and temporal fractures should be elevated. If the fracture is compound, a wide exposure and removal of devitalized tissue is indicated. If the bone fragments are macerated and obviously contaminated, they may be carefully cleaned with Beta-dine and replaced, particularly in the frontal region, in order to preserve the contour of the face. Other than in the frontal region, the skull defect may be repaired after debridement by an immediate stainless steel wire mesh cranioplasty or, at a later date, by a wire mesh acrylic cranioplasty if contamination is severe or surgery delayed for over 6 hr. Dural lacerations underlying depressed fractures should be closed in a water-tight manner, utilizing facial or pericranial grafting if necessary. Cultures are always taken at surgery, and broad spectrum antibiotics given in meningitic doses may be used. In compound-depressed fractures over 12 hr old in the neurologically intact patient, the scalp laceration is repaired primarily, and the depressed fracture is raised electively when wound healing is assured. Simple depressed skull fractures are generally repaired electively within 48 hr.

Gunshot Wounds

Civilian gunshot wounds to the head, even with small caliber missiles, are usually devastating once they penetrate the skull, and the survival of these patients can be closely correlated to their level of consciousness upon admission. In patients admitted in extremis with evidence of the bullet track crossing the midline, surgical therapy is usually not indicated. One can be aggressive in these cases where the injury appears to be involving only one hemisphere. Following CT scan, ventriculography, and angiography, these patients should be brought to the operating room where debridement of the

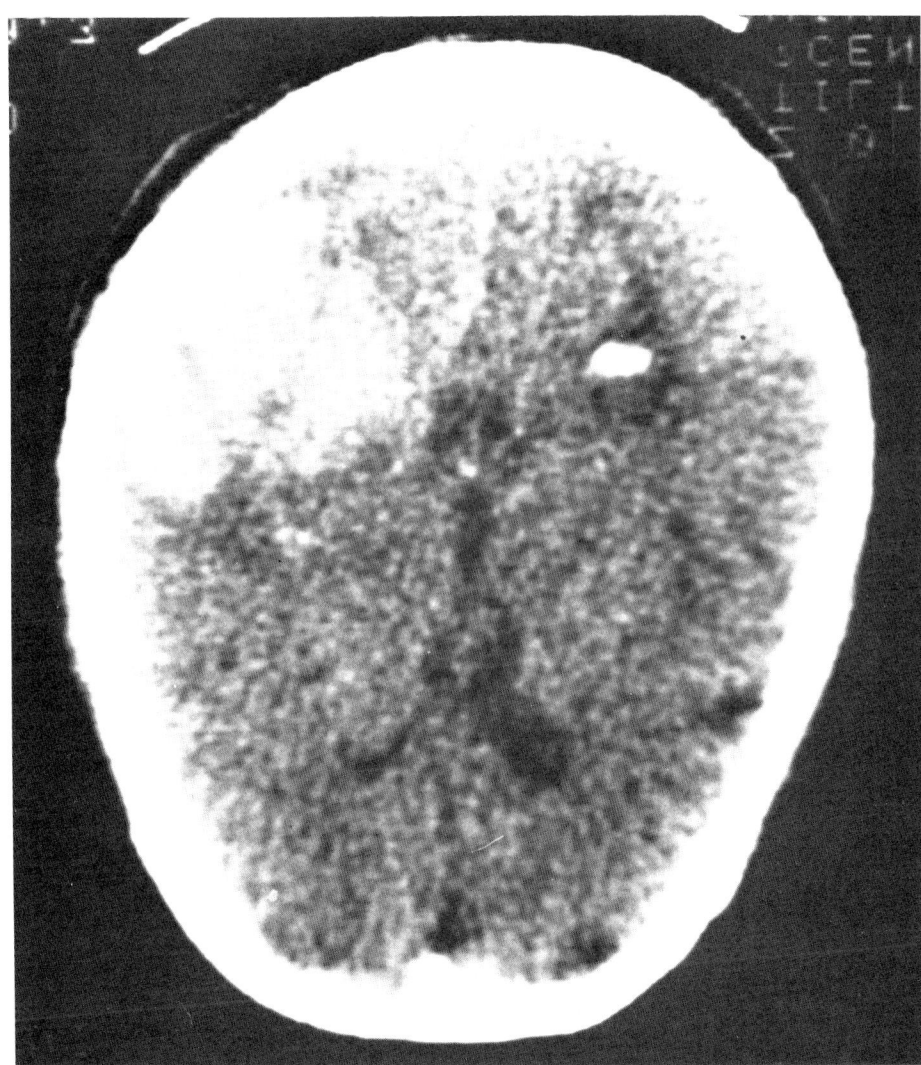

Figure 43.5. The traumatic intracranial hematoma is a mixture of clot and contused brain.

entry and exit wounds can be carried out, with the removal of bone fragments and devitalized tissue including brain. Large metallic fragments should be removed if easily located in the bullet track. Extensive exploration for these fragments, however, is not justified.

POSTHEAD INJURY PROBLEMS

Post-traumatic Seizures

The incidence of post-traumatic seizures varies from less than 5% in the minor closed head injury to 50-60% in those with cerebral laceration or penetrating wounds. Seizures may begin at any time, the majority being seen in the first few months up to 18 months. Recent experimental studies have suggested that prophylactic anticonvulsants started acutely decrease the chance of formation of an epileptogenic focus. The drugs themselves are of low toxicity with few side effects and may be of considerable help in keeping some patients functioning in an automobile-oriented society, where the loss of a driving license can be a social and economic disaster. One occasionally finds the post-traumatic epileptic who is refractory to drug treatment. These patients should be completely re-evaluated by specialists in the field of epilepsy.

Postconcussion State

The postconcussion syndrome is a many faceted syndrome seen following head injury. It consists of headaches, fatigability, muscle spasm, transient visual loss, benign positional vertiginous attacks, and emotional lability with or without coincident depression. It generally starts in the hospital and, if not treated aggressively in the beginning, may with the passage of time progress to an incapacitating syndrome. The symptoms should be treated empirically, and professional psychiatric help should be used early in the management if necessary.

Post-Traumatic Hydrocephalus (Fig. 43.6)

This condition is occasionally noted in surgical and nonsurgical head-injured patients who remain in an akinetic, mute state or who are apparently improving and then regress after several weeks of steady improvement. Their difficulties may be attributable to communicating hydrocephalus due to basal arachnoid block. The literature is replete with cases in which dramatic improvement in the level of functioning has occurred following shunting procedures, although this response to treatment is by no means standard. It is best diagnosed by a CT scan.

Persistent or Late CSF Leakage

Whereas most patients in the period following head trauma associated with basal skull fractures may have transient CSF otorrhea or rhinorrhea as mentioned above, this problem is usually self-limiting. The appearance of late spinal fluid leakage or its persistence for a number of weeks requires surgical intervention. Successful surgical management is dependent upon an accurate anatomical identification of the site of the intracranial defect. Skull films and, in particular, careful polytomography are the initial steps in the preoperative evaluation. RISA cisternography with serial scans can be helpful in identifying the route of CSF egress. More recently, the fluorescein examination of the nasopharynx and paranasal sinuses following the injection of this material into the cerebrospinal fluid pathways via the lumbar route has also proven to be helpful. Finally, serial CT scanning following the lumbar injection of the newer water soluble contrast agent (metrizamide) has also proven to be helpful in identifying the site of leakage.

The surgical approach to repair of spinal fluid fistulae can be either intracranial, extracranial, or a combination of these avenues. If the site of drainage can be identified as occurring in the sphenoid or ethmoid sinuses, an extracranial approach and repair of the fistula with the use of fat, methylmethacrolate, and split thickness skin grafting can often be extremely successful. A similar approach can be utilized if leakage occurs through the mastoid air cells. If a large skull dehiscence exists at the base, then the combination of an intracranial and extracranial approach during the same operative procedure carries with it a higher chance of success than does either by itself. In general, the institution of lumbar CSF drainage and its maintenance for a period of 3-7 days following repair is also advisable. In recurrent fistulae following initial surgical failures, the institution of permanent lumbar peritoneal shunting in association with reoperation should be considered.

Late Skull Defects

Significant skull defects that persist following craniotomy for acute brain injury should be repaired with appropriate materials to afford protection of the underlying brain. Whereas improvement in neurological function and decreased severity of post-traumatic seizure can occur following repair of large skull defects, these significant benefits should not be considered as indications for cranioplasty. They definitely do occur but, unfortunately, all too infrequently. It is generally believed advisable to delay repair of a secondary nature for a period of 6-12 months following the initial injury in order to avoid the potential of secondary wound infection. A heavy gauge stainless steel screen is probably the best material for this purpose.

Management of Chronic Subdural Hematoma (Fig. 43.7)

Chronic subdural hematoma, which can occur at any time from weeks to months following a relatively mild head trauma or which can become symptomatic at varying intervals after the injury, is a problem which has led to many controversies concerning the optimum management technique. In younger individuals with normal sized ventricular systems and no cortical atrophy, drainage through a small, strategically placed craniectomy is clearly the surgical procedure of choice. In older individuals with atrophic brains, these lesions may be found

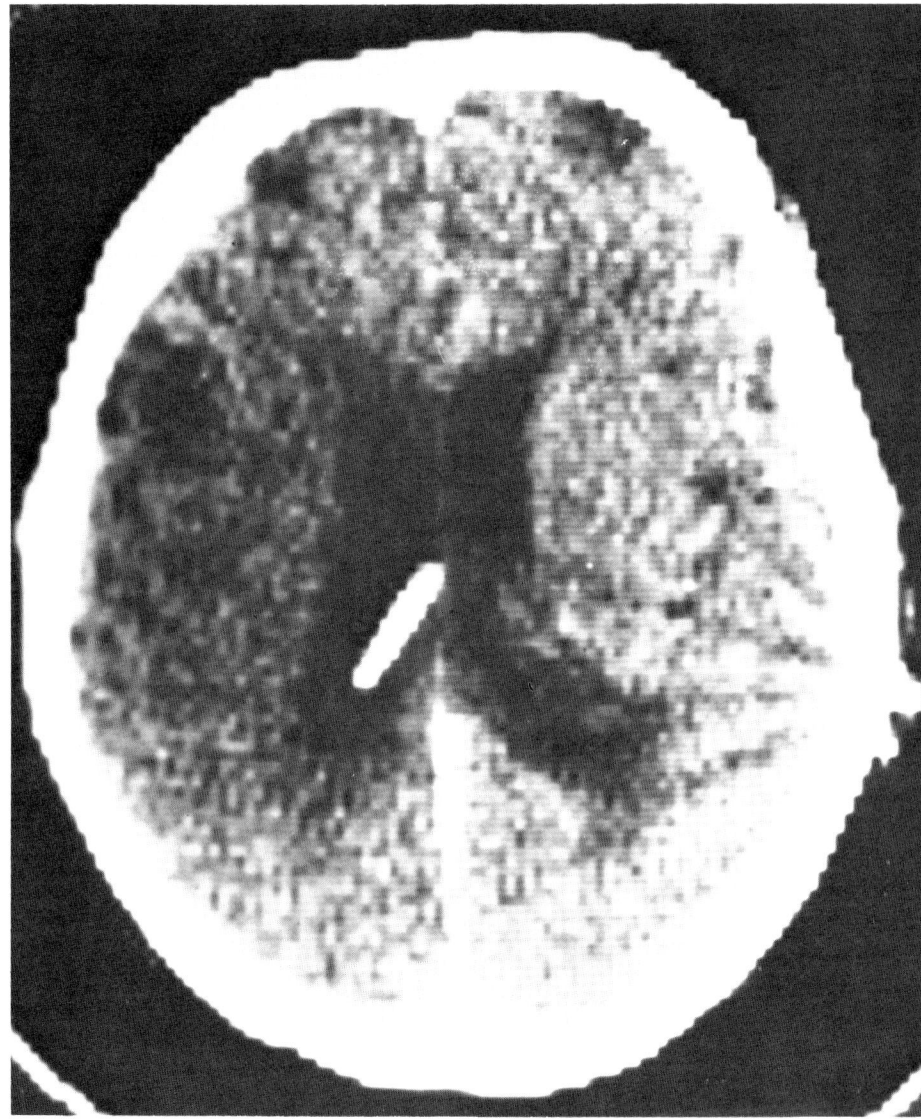

Figure 43.6. Post-traumatic hydrocephalus.

almost incidental to evaluation for diffuse cerebral dysfunction on CT scanning. These collections may often be an admixture of blood and cerebral spinal fluid, so called subdural hygromas. Although it is tempting to attribute the patient's mental dysfunction to these lesions, one often finds that they reaccumulate after drainage and that little benefit accrues from surgical intervention. Chronic subdural collections of this type can be drained through a small twist wire drill hole with the insertion of a sterile external drainage system which can be maintained for several days when surgery is indicated.

It is clear that between these two extremes—i.e., the patient with a normal brain and an enlarging chronic subdural associated with headaches, papilledema, and at times, hemiparesis and the older individual with a relatively asymptomatic lesion—there are a number of patients for whom the choice between drainage versus conservative management may represent a difficult clinical decision. When in doubt, serial CT scanning without and with contrast can be helpful in reaching a final opinion in this matter. An interval of a month to 6 weeks is sufficient to demonstrate the increased size of the mass versus the spontaneous regression.

MANAGEMENT OF CNS TRAUMA IN ASSOCIATION WITH SYSTEMIC TRAUMA

The recognition of the presence of CNS injury in the patient with various systemic trauma, long bone, abdominal, or thoracic, is the first step in the decision-making process leading to the correct management of these patients. This statement may seem obvious; however, a developing subdural in a patient who is in shock from blood loss and who is somewhat confused may be difficult to recognize. Similarly, a low thoracic spinal cord injury may be easily overlooked in the patient with serious abdominal trauma. It is particularly easy to miss the gunshot or stab wound that passes through the head

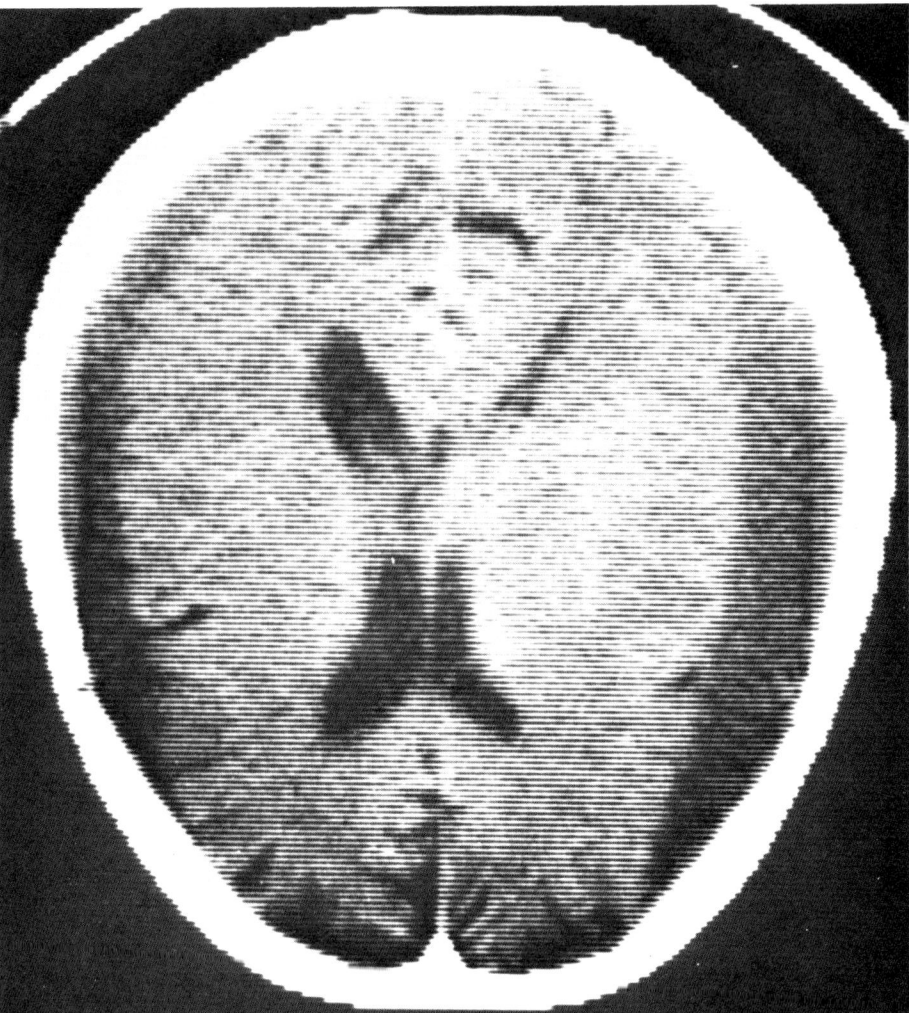

Figure 43.7. The subacute subdural hematoma is the same density as the brain on CT scan, but the large shift of the ventricular system with the ipsolateral frontal horn also shifted posteriorly helps to diagnose the extra-axial collection.

or spinal cord. The combinations of CNS and systemic injuries are legion and require alertness on the part of the emergency room physicians.

Shock does not occur from CNS trauma, with the exception of very high cervical cord injury and in small children with massive scalp lacerations and blood loss. Hypotension, on the other hand, with poor tissue perfusion can produce irreversible damage to already compromised CNS tissue and must be treated with great energy in patients with combined injuries.

Specific recommendations are difficult to make. Patients with a history of loss of consciousness should be examined by a neuroconsultant prior to anesthetic induction. With the increasing availability of CT scanning, this will be the obvious preoperative study unless surgery is mandated on an immediate basis. Air metrizamide ventriculography can be done on a patient in shock during resuscitation if there is evidence of serious head trauma.

If these patients are operated on without neuroevaluation, they should be watched very carefully in the immediate postoperative period. All too often, the patient who fails to awake from anesthesia is not suspected of harboring an intracranial clot until irreversible brain damage has occurred.

Patients complaining of neck or back pain should be evaluated for signs of spinal cord dysfunction, including motor, sensory, and sphincteric difficulties. X-rays of the cervical and/or thoracolumbar spine should be obtained, particularly in patients in whom palpation of the spine reveals areas of tenderness and/or malalignment.

The final decision as to the method and order of operative procedures to be carried out in patients with CNS and systemic injuries must be made by the physicians on the spot. The simultaneous approach, for example, to a subdural hematoma and a ruptured viscus can be considered, but it is usually wiser to manage the more serious life-threatening condition first with the second following immediately. Once again, it must be stressed that hypotension to shock levels may convert a reversible CNS injury to a complete lesion with permanent paralysis or coma and death.

References

Becker, D.P., Miller, J.D., Ward, J.D., Greenberg, R.P., Young, H.F., and Sakalasas, R.: The outcome from severe head injury with early diagnosis and intensive management. J. Neurosurg. *47:*491–502, 1977.

Bender, M.B., and Christoff, N.: Neurosurgical treatment of subdural hematomas. Arch. Neurol. *31:*73, 1974.

Coates, C., and Mierowsky, A. (Eds.): *Neurological Surgery of Trauma.* Office of the Surgeon General, Department of the Army, Washington, DC, 1965.

Cooper, P.: Treatment of head injuries, In: *The Treatment of Neurological Diseases,* edited by Rosenberg. Spectrum, New York, 1979.

Fisher, R.G., Kim, J.K., and Sachs, E.: Complications in posterior fossa due to occipital trauma: their operability. J.A.M.A. *167:*176, 1958.

Flamm, E.S., Demopoulous, H.B., Seligman, M.D., Tomasula, J.J., and Ransohoff, J.: Ethanol potentiation of central nervous system trauma. J. Neurosurg. *46:*328, 1977.

French, B.N., and Dublin, A.B.: The value of computerized tomography in the management of 1000 consecutive head injuries. Surg. Neurol. *7:*171, 1977.

Hammon, W.M.: Analysis of 2187 consecutive penetrating wounds of the brain from Vietnam. J. Neurosurg. *34:*121, 1971.

Lundberg, N., Kjallquist, A., Kullberg, G., Ponten, U., and Sundbarg, G.: Non-operative management of intracranial hypertension. In *Advances and Technical Standards of Neurosurgery,* edited by H. Krayenbuhl. Springer-Verlag, Berlin, 1974.

Marshall, L.F., Smith, R.W., and Shapiro, H.M.: The outcome with aggressive treatment in severe head injuries: acute and chronic barbiturate administration in the management of head injury. J. Neurosurg. *50:*26, 1979.

Matson, D.D.: Neurosurgery of Infancy and Childhood, ed. 2. Charles C Thomas, Springfield, IL, 1969.

McLaurin, R. (Ed.): Head injuries. *Proceedings of the Second Chicago Symposium on Neural Trauma.* Grune & Stratton, New York, 1976.

Miller, J.D., Leech, P.J., and Pickard, J.D.: Volume-pressure response in various experimental and clinical conditions. In: *Intracranial Pressure II,* edited by N. Lundberg, U. Ponten, and M. Brock. Springer-Verlag, Berlin, 1975.

Miller, J.D., Becker, D.P., Ward, J.D., Sullivan, H.G., Adams, W.E., and Rosner, M.J.: Significance of intracranial hypertension in severe head injury. J. Neurosurg. *47:*503, 1977.

Plum, F., and Posner, J.B.: *Diagnosis of Stupor and Coma,* ed. 2. F. A. Davis, Philadelphia, 1972.

Raimondi, S.J., and Samuelson, G.H.: Craniocerebral gunshot wounds in civilian practice. J. Neurosurg. *32:*647, 1970.

Reulen, H.J., and Schurmann, K. (Eds.): *Steroids and Brain Edema.* Springer-Verlag, Berlin, 1972.

Teasdale, G., and Jenett, B.: Assessment of comma and impaired consciousness: A practical scale. Lancet *2:*81, 1974.

Walker, A.E., Caveness, W.E., and Critchley, M. (Eds.): *The Late Effects of Head Injury.* Charles C Thomas, Springfield, IL, 1969.

Youmans, J.R. (Ed.): *Neurological Surgery.* W.B. Saunders, Philadelphia, 1973.

CHAPTER 44

Spinal Cord Injury

HAROLD F. YOUNG
DONALD P. BECKER

It is widely recognized that major spinal cord trauma usually does not produce complete anatomical transection of the spinal cord, but usually there is complete and permanent loss of motor and sensory function below the level of the lesion (Rivlin and Tator, 1979) (Fig. 44.1). This loss of function may be due to microscopic physical interruption of all axons at the lesion site, even though the cord is grossly intact, or to progressive hemorrhage and spreading edema, or to ischemia and subsequent infarction. Neurological deficit may not be fixed at the time of spinal cord injury, but may become ultimately permanent from ongoing pathophysiological events occurring minutes to hours after the injury. A "secondary injury" may thus be a factor contributing to long-term post-traumatic spinal cord dysfunction. Progression of the lesion from gray to white matter seen in experimental spinal cord injury correlates with neurological deficit and reversibility of paraparesis seen in the clinical state.

The above concepts imply that continued intensive investigation of spinal cord injury mechanisms is war-

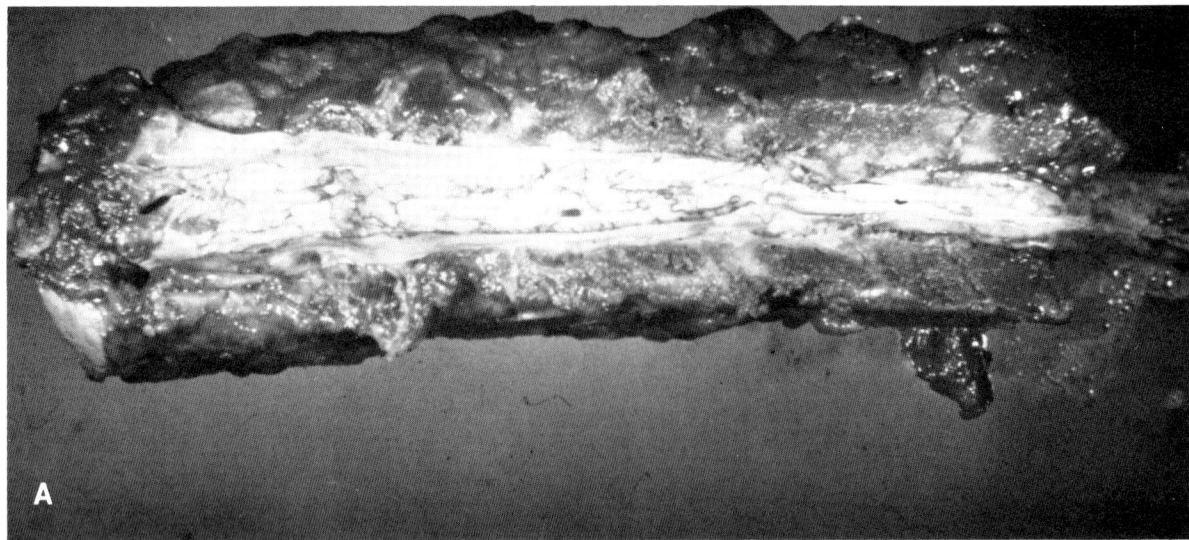
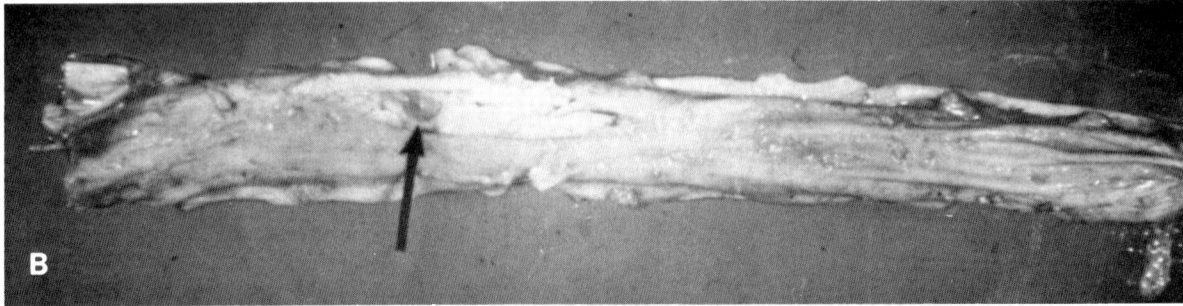

Figure 44.1. *A*, spinal cord from patient with cervical 4–5 dislocation and immediate quadriplegia. Patient expired 4 weeks after injury. The dura is intact and there is anatomical continuity of the spinal cord. The dura may protect cord from severance. *B*, lesion (*arrow*) seen grossly at C4 level of spinal cord.

ranted. The spinal cord must not be considered as an independent organ separated from the brain by the foramen magnum of the skull, but rather as an extension of the brain, undergoing pathophysiological reactions as does the brain. Both the brain and spinal cord respond to severe injury by initial changes in blood flow and by eventual cavitation. In the small diameter spinal cord, cavitation must be prevented.

BACKGROUND

The Edwin Smith papyrus lists among ailments not to be treated six cases of injury to the spine. Generally, this was the pessimistic viewpoint on spinal injury through the subsequent centuries, although Ambrose Paré advocated the care of spinal dislocations by traction. During this time interval vertebral body injury was well recognized and described, but it was not until the observations of Allen (1908) that the spinal cord impact injury lesion itself was well described. Allen (1911, 1914) performed experiments where specific gram-calibrated weights were dropped via a vented tube onto the exposed spinal cord of dogs. The central hemorrhagic lesion described by him in the gray matter of the spinal cord has withstood the test of time as the classic early lesion of experimental impact injury to the spinal cord. The reported series of pathology of human spinal cord injuries (Wolman, 1964, 1965) are remarkably similar to the experimental lesion initially described by Allen. Research in spinal cord injury, except for advances in spinal traction, decubitus ulcer treatment, and bowel and bladder care of paraplegics, remained dormant for the next 60 yr.

Albin and White (1968) presented evidence that spinal cord injury might well be a treatable condition; this initiated a renewed intense interest in spinal cord injury. The remainder of this chapter describes work done during the past decade.

THE ANIMAL MODEL OF IMPACT INJURY TO THE SPINAL CORD

Most of the recent and current spinal cord injury research is based on the impact spinal cord injury model as originally described by Allen (1914). This consists of dropping a specific gram-calibrated weight (g) through a vented guide tube (cm) to strike the surgically exposed spinal cord. The magnitude of each injury is by convention expressed in gram-centimeters (g-cm force), which represents the product of weight of mass and distance of fall. In this chapter, force will be defined as energy exerted per unit area. In actuality a proper description of the impact should include the measure of impulse (momentum transfer), velocity, deceleration, mass, contour, and surface area of the striker. Mechanical alterations in structures supporting the spinal cord, as well as mass of the weight, are significant when attempting to quantitate the force of experimental spinal cord trauma (Dohrmann et al., 1978; Molt et al., 1979). In general, less than a 300 g-cm force to the lower cervical or thoracic cord will cause a moderate spinal cord injury with transient paraparesis compatible with recovery in most animals. A 400 g-cm force or greater is considered severe trauma, producing irreversible paraplegia in the cat, dog, and monkey. Rabbits and rats require only a 50 g-cm force for severe wounding. Throughout this chapter, both the g-cm force and animal species will be identified, since these two considerations are often identified as sources of crucial variability in spinal cord injury experiments. The diameter of the cord and its viscoelectric properties vary from species to species.

An inflatable balloon cuff compression model has been used by some investigators. Circumferential cuff compression to a specified pressure can be used to perform both acute and chronic spinal cord injury.

THE LESION OF IMPACT INJURY TO THE SPINAL CORD

The following is now known to be true in spinal cord impact injury. Even though the impact injury is to the surface of the spinal cord, the early lesion includes a central hemorrhagic necrosis of the central gray matter and is definitely related to impact force (Fig. 44.2). There is a linear relationship between impact force and the extent of the spinal cord lesion. The changes in the spinal cord shortly after a traumatic injury that cause paresis or paralysis have been studied extensively experimentally in a wide species of animals as postmortem reports are rare for the early period after injury. The hemorrhagic spinal cord lesion has been well described by many investigators both at the light and electron microscopic level. In primates, a 300 g-cm force to the spinal cord will result in an initial complete motor and sensory paralysis with some recovery by 12 hr and a return to

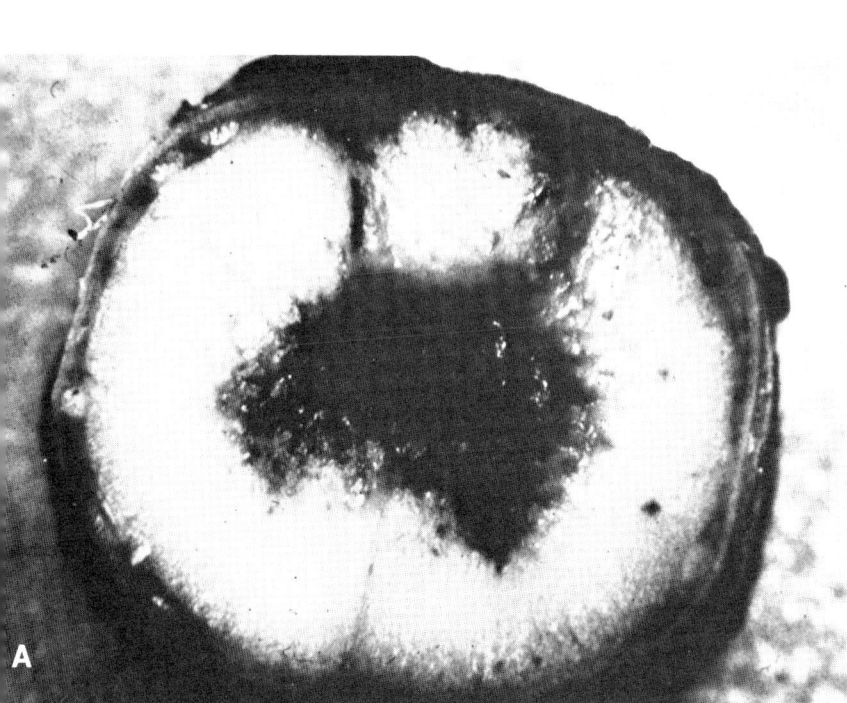
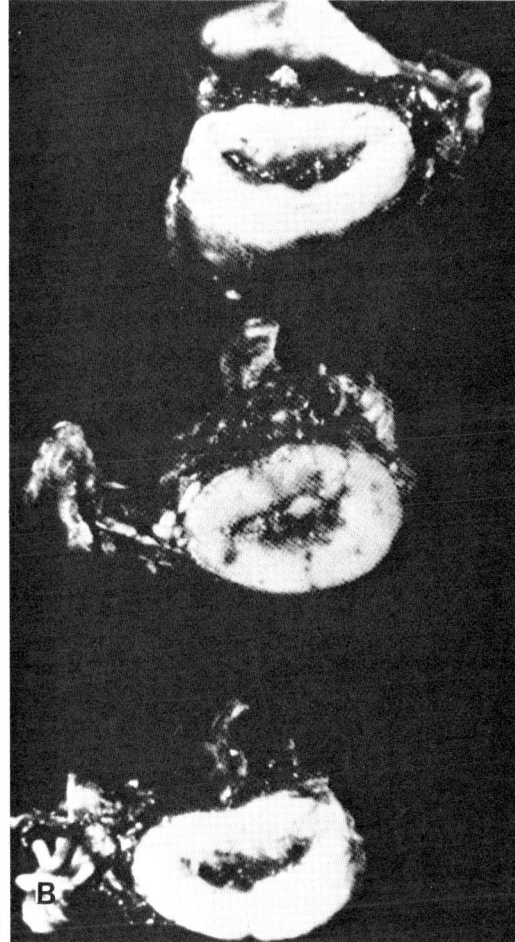

Figure 44.2. *A*, acute spinal cord injury showing central gray and dorsal epidural and subdural hemorrhage. *B*, the acute injury demonstrating central gray hemorrhage over several segments. (Reprinted with permission from D. Yashon: *Spinal Injury*, ch. 7, pp. 71–103. Appleton-Century-Crofts, New York, 1979.)

normal neurological function by 6 months (Wagner et al., 1971). In those monkeys sacrificed 5 min following a 300 g-cm force, the appearance of the cord is similar to normal cord, revealing only distention of the less muscular vessels surrounding the central canal. Light microscopic examination at 15 min reveals isolated, thin walled vessels with leakage of erythrocytes into the perivascular spaces of the gray matter. At 30 min erythrocytes and serous fluid can be found in the central canal area perivascular spaces (Fig. 44.3). By 4 hr the perivascular hemorrhages coalesce and spread throughout the gray matter. Chromatolysis, vacuolization, and alterations in cytoplasmic density and stainability are observed in the neurons. With this force, edema of the white matter is minimal and probably explains why the paraplegia is transient.

Wagner and coworkers (1978) performed long-term studies (4 hr to 4 months) on spinal cords of cats subjected to increasing amounts of trauma (100–700 g-cm force). At 4 hr in animals with the trauma of 500–700 g-cm, the hemorrhages were more extensive and widespread in the gray matter then when lesser forces were used. At 4 weeks, the spinal cord receiving a 100–300 g-cm impact revealed mainly an increase in cellularity of the gray matter, whereas those spinal cords receiving the 500–700 g-cm impact revealed compound granular cells in areas of cystic necrosis (Fig. 44.4). Communication often existed between the central canal and larger cysts and at times even with the subarachnoid space. Thinned, enlarged myelin sheaths and an increase in glial fibers were observed in the white matter as the impact force increased.

At 4 months, cavitation exists in the central gray matter at the site of the early hemorrhage, and in the 700 g-cm impact marked alteration also occurs in the dura mater and leptomeninges, with the latter often adherent to the spinal cord. Only small amounts of white matter remain in those spinal cords subjected to severe trauma. The remainder of the white matter is replaced by an astrocytic gliosis and fibrosis from the leptomeninges. This replacement of spinal cord by cystic spaces has been described by Wolman (1964) as a late change in the traumatized human spinal cord. The dense fibrosis and adherence of the leptomeninges to the cord with obliteration of the subarachnoid space seen experimentally and clinically following trauma are thought due to hemorrhage in the subarachnoid space. Ducker—who has categorized human spinal cord pathology into an "initial phase," an "ischemic phase," and a "repair phase"—also reported graded, progressively severe spinal cord injuries in primates in 1971 (Ducker et al., 1971a). He found stepwise sequential changes, with the center of the cord most vulnerable. He also stressed the difference in the anatomy of the gray and white matter of the spinal cord. The gray matter consists of neurons with mostly short axonal and dendritic processes and mostly supportive glial structures easily separated by blood or fluid. The white matter is made up of long,

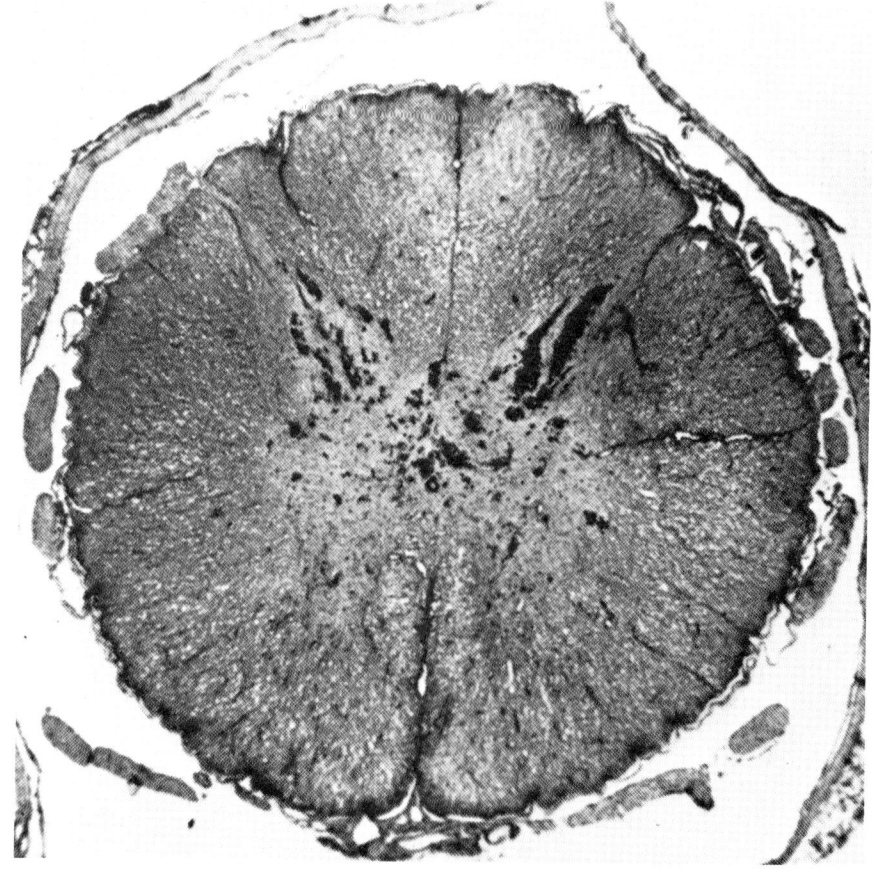

Figure 44.3. Impact spinal cord injury sufficient to cause transitory paraparesis. Photomicrograph showing hemorrhages in the pericentral area and dorsal horns of the gray matter 30 min postcontusion. (Hematoxylin and eosin × 20.) (Reprinted with permission from F. C. Wagner, G. J. Dohrmann, and P. C. Bucy: Journal of Neurosurgery 35:272–276, 1971.)

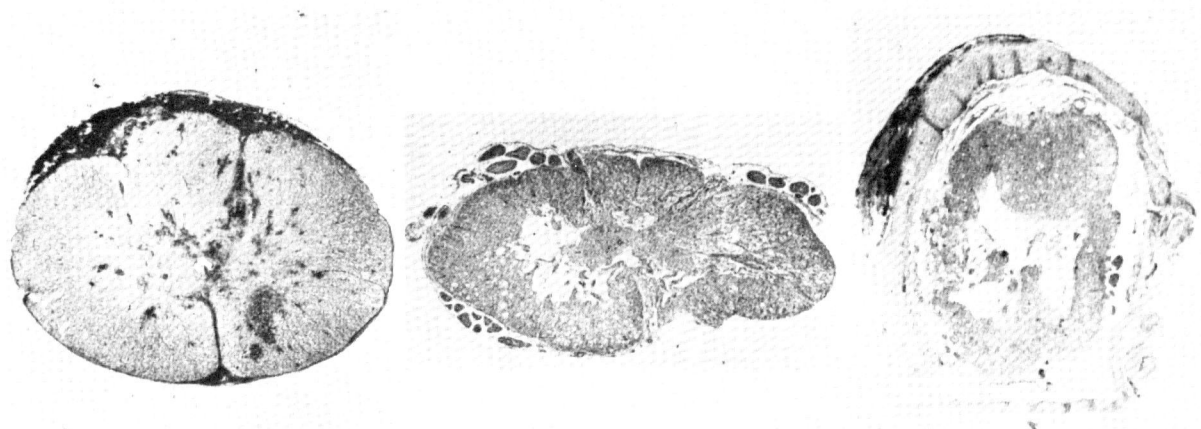

Figure 44.4. Sections of spinal cord from cats receiving 500 g-cm force, showing central and subarachnoid hemorrhages at 4 hr (*left*), cystic necrosis at 4 weeks (*center*), and cavitation and arachnoiditis at 4 months (*right*). Hematoxylin and eosin × 2.5. (Reprinted with permission from F. C. Wagner, J. C. Van Gilder, and G. J. Dohrmann: Journal of Neurosurgery 48:92–98, 1978.)

tightly packed fiber tracts, not easily separated. He demonstrated central necrosis and increasing white matter pathology in severe spinal cord injury by 5–6 days posttrauma. In less severe injury to the spinal cord (200–400 g-cm force), Ducker showed that clinical improvement could occur even while the pathological changes were progressing over the first week.

ULTRASTRUCTURAL OBSERVATIONS

Electron microscopic studies on acute spinal cord injury in the primate have been reported by Dohrmann et al. (1971) and Goodman et al. (1979). By employing a 300 g-cm force, Goodman et al. observed gaps in the endothelial lining as early as 1½ min following the trauma. There is separation of endothelial junctions with exposure of the underlying basic lamina, which tends to remain intact and preserve the continuity of the vessel wall. Platelets occur singly with fibrin strands, or as complex thrombi covering small or large areas of basement membrane. These platelet thrombi may totally occlude small vessels in and adjacent to the hemorrhagic region and, therefore, may contribute to decreased blood flow in the gray matter of the spinal cord following injury. Dohrmann observed the muscular venules of the central gray matter to be distended with erythrocytes at 5 min postinjury. Erythrocytes were in the perivascular spaces of the postcapillary venules and muscular venules 15–30 min postinjury, and gray matter hemorrhage was observed at 1 hr postinjury. There was vacuolation and endothelial swelling at 4 hr, and Dohrmann concluded that, in transitory paraplegia, the principle changes were early perivascular and parenchymal hemorrhages followed by later evidence of ischemic endothelial injury in the microvasculature. These findings have important relationships to post-traumatic spinal cord blood flow (SCBF) studies (to be discussed later).

METABOLIC CHANGES IN SPINAL CORD INJURY

Vascular damage appears important histologically in spinal cord injury. This injury can lead to ischemia, which in the brain is known to induce alterations in cerebral mitochondria (Ginsberg et al., 1977; Schutz et al., 1973). The possibility of similar changes has been investigated in experimental spinal cord trauma. Ito and coworkers (1978) analyzed cytochrome oxidase, since it is the terminal and rate-limiting enzyme of the electron transport series and since its location on the inner membrane might make it vulnerable to the mitochondrial injury. A drop in cytochrome oxidase activities to approximately 50% of normal occurred 15 min following a 400 g-cm impact force. The greatest decrease was at the trauma center; it correlated with histological estimates of gray matter and neuronal damage but was partially independent of these processes. Ito et al. suggested that the mitochondrial injury in impact spinal cord injury may be similar to that which occurs in brain ischemia with involvement of inner membrane or cristae of the mitochondria. These changes in spinal cord mitochondria occur early, possibly within 2 min of injury, unlike cerebral ischemia, in which the defects in mitochondrial function occur relatively late.

Locke et al. (1971) demonstrated increased lactate accumulation in monkey spinal cord tissue following trauma, supporting the concept that ischemia plays a role early in spinal cord injury. CSF lactate levels have been shown to be elevated for up to 9 days following spinal cord compression injury in cats (Anderson et al., 1976). In the same study Ca^{2+} ions were significantly elevated on days 3, 9, 11, 13, and 15; K^+ concentration was elevated on days 9 and 11 postinjury. Chloride levels were significantly reduced during the first 24 hr following the injury. The significant elevation of CSF K^+ concentrations probably represent K^+ loss from necrotic edematous cord where Lewin found a net loss of K^+ from injured and adjacent spinal cord segments 7 and 9 days following impact injury (Lewin et al., 1974).

The findings of early tissue and late CSF lactate accumulation following injury suggest that the spinal cord edema, which was evident from 5 min to 15 days following trauma in the studies of Yashon et al. (1973), may well be related to hypoxia or ischemia. Goodman et al. (1976) demonstrated both cellular swelling and extracellular space enlargement in spinal cord edema. Leakage of Evans blue albumin into the gray matter spreading into the dorsolateral white matter has been demonstrated in acute compression experiments in the dog spinal cord, consistent with the presence of vasogenic edema. In these experiments by Griffiths (1975a), protein leak was observed after the removal of chronic compression but not during chronic compression, suggesting a reactive hyperemia. Traumatically induced hypoxia with associated edema may be extremely important, as the spinal cord is contained in a relatively inelastic pia arachnoid. Edema of the cord encased by pia mater may lead to increased interstitial pressure with further vascular collapse. As will be discussed later, this may alter SCBF and cause further ischemia, resulting in infarction and subsequent late repair by cavitation.

Also, edema may have damaging effects on the activity of the membrane-bound enzyme $(Na^+ + K^+)$-activated adenosine triphosphatase (ATPase). Clendenon et al. (1978) reported a prompt and significant fall in ATPase activity within 5 min of injury, and activity remained below control for the 1 hr time period studied. Others have observed free radical damage to lipids in severe trauma to the cat spinal cord (Milvy et al., 1973). These findings may play an important role in platelet aggregation, which depends on regulated production of prostaglands from polyunsaturated lipids within the platelet membrane. Abnormal free radical reactions due to trauma at the membrane level may alter this process.

SPINAL CORD BLOOD FLOW

Spinal cord injury is clearly associated with vascular changes that are either the primary or secondary cause of spinal cord dysfunction. Extensive light and electron microscopic studies as well as microangiographic studies have documented these changes. The vascular injury in the gray matter must be distinguished from the injury in the white matter, since the latter appears to be the main determinant of eventual neurological dysfuntion. It is necessary to know the normal gray and white matter blood flow in the spinal cord.

Attempts to quantitate normal and abnormal SCBF have produced significantly different results, and only recently has the resolution been obtained to differentiate gray and white matter SCBF (Table 44.1). Landau et al. (1955) used the gas trifluoro-iodomethane ^{131}I uptake and autoradiography to measure regional cerebral blood flow and regional cervical SCBF simultaneously in the cat. Blood flow in the cord white matter was 14.0 ml/100 g/min and in the cord gray matter 63.0 ml/100 g/

Table 44.1
Quantitative Measurements of Normal Spinal Cord Blood Flow

Author	Method	Species	Spinal Cord Blood Flow	
			Gray Matter	White Matter
			ml/100 g/min	
Landau et al. (1955)	ICCF$_3$ ^{131}I	Cat	63	14
Griffiths (1973)	^{133}Xe washout	Dog	48.4	15.7
Griffiths et al. (1975)	H$_2$ clearance	Dog	10.8	11.5
	H$_2$ clearance	Baboon	16.5	13.7
Kobrine et al. (1974, 1975)	H$_2$ clearance	Monkey	14.0	17.5
Sandler and Tator (1976a)	^{14}C-antipyrine autoradiograph	Monkey	57.6	10.30
Sentor and Venes (1979)	H$_2$ clearance	Cat		10.99
Boggan et al. (1977)	H$_2$ clearance	Rat	49.4	
Rivlin and Tator (1979)	C-antipyrine autoradiograph	Rat	61.4	15.2
Takaoka et al. (1977)	Microsphere	Monkey	28.5	14.0
Smith et al. (1978b)	Microsphere	Dog	26.3	7.1
			White and Gray	
Ducker and Perot (1972)	^{133}Xe washout	Dog	16.2	

min. Griffiths (1973) employed the xenon^{133} washout technique in which xenon-saturated saline was injected into the dog spinal cord and SCBF was estimated from its subsequent washout into the systemic circulation. He found that the white matter flow was 15.7 ml/100 g/min and the gray matter flow was 48.4 ml/100 g/min. Kobrine et al. (1974) used the hydrogen clearance method to measure SCBF in primates. The rate at which inhaled hydrogen was washed out of the cord was measured by changes in potential in electrodes inserted into the cord substance. This method measures small discrete areas; allows measurement of spinal cord blood flow by the Fick principle; allows multiple determinations to be made over long periods of time; and, although invasive, seems not to injure tissue significantly. The technique has been criticized for its inability to truly differentiate gray from white matter SCBF. The white matter flow was 17.5 ml/100 g/min, while the "central" cord flow was 14 ml/100 g/min. Griffiths et al. (1975) used the hydrogen clearance method to measure SCBF in dogs and found the value for white matter to be 11.5 ml/100 g/min and only 10.8 ml/100 g/min in the gray matter. In baboons the white matter flow was 13.7/100 g/min and the gray matter flow only 16.5 ml/100 g/min. Sandler and Tator (1976a) measured SCBF in the primate spinal cord using the ^{14}C-antipyrine autoradiographic technique and found white matter flow to be 10.3 ml/100 g/min while gray matter flow was more variable at a mean value of 57.6 ml/100 g/min. These results for spinal cord white matter agree closely with the recent values for cat spinal cord white matter, 10.99 ml/100 g/min, reported by Senter and Venes (1978), who used an extensive modification of the hydrogen clearance method. Smith et al. (1978b) and Takaoka et al. (1977) using the microsphere method reported values of 7.1 and 14.0 ml/100 g/min, respectively, for white matter. In several of the above mentioned studies, the SCBF ratio between gray and white matter is about 5:1, as is the gray-white flow rate for the brain. The normal studies cited here suggest that white matter SCBF in the spinal cord may have little, if any, reserve and function may be compromised by very slight changes in blood flow. This compromise may occur by direct vascular injury, vasogenic edema, release of vasogenic amines, or constant pressure, as by a displaced vertebral fracture.

Spinal cord injury quantitative SCBF studies have been done by a number of investigators during the past decade. Ducker and Perot (1971) measured SCBF in spinal cord impact injury in dogs by the Xe^{133} washout method after microintramedullary xenon injection into the cord. Although gray and white matter cannot be differentiated and some trauma is caused by needle insertion, sequential measurements are possible in each animal. Following trauma, SCBF in the center of the cord fell from a pretrauma level of 15.2 ml/100 g/min to 9.3 at 1 hr, 6.1 at 2 hr, and finally 6.1 ml/100 g/min at 3 hr. Ducker (1976) also measured SCBF in primates by the argon washout technique, which requires insertion of a 1-mm probe into a 5-mm diameter cord. In the completely paraplegic group, SCBF was significantly reduced during the post-traumatic period ranging from 1 hr to 1 week. In the group of animals rendered paraparetic, SCBF values did not differ significantly from normal, leading Ducker to conclude that progressive, persistent decrease in SCBF was a factor in loss of function in the paraplegic primates. Although the investigations of both Bingham et al. (1975a) and Kobrine et al. (1975) showed loss of SCBF in gray matter following impact injury, they showed increased SCBF in the white matter. Bingham used the indicator fractionation technique of flow measurement, while Kobrine, as mentioned above, used the hydrogen washout technique. The finding of hyperemia in spinal cord white matter, surrounding a necrotic central lesion, would be analogous to the so-called "luxury perfusion syndrome" surrounding a cerebral infarct or traumatized cerebral tissue (Lassen, 1966; Overgard and Tweed, 1974). Griffiths (1975b) also has used the hydrogen clearance method to measure SCBF in moderate to severe impact injury of the dog spinal cord. He found similar pretrauma levels for gray matter of 12.5 and central white matter of 14.4 ml/100 g/min. With moderate injury, gray and white matter flow decreased progressively over 5 hr. Also the normal physiological responses of SCBF to CO_2 and hypoxia were lost after trauma. He concluded that the central area of the spinal cord demonstrated a rapid, progressive decrease in flow, whereas the white matter retained a "reasonably normal flow" depending on severity of injury. Also the spinal cord vasculature lost the ability to respond to normal physiological stimuli after trauma. Thus, in these later experiments there is a suggestion of a loss of SCBF autoregulation following impact trauma.

Sandler and Tator (1976b) used the ^{14}C-antipyrine autoradiographic technique to measure SCBF in primates after an inflatable circumferential cuff technique to produce injury. After severe cord injury, which produced paraplegia in almost all animals, SCBF in gray and white matter was reduced to extremely low levels for 24 hr after trauma, but in moderate injury there was return of normal flow to the white matter at 6 hr and occurrence of hyperemia by 24 hr. This is another demonstration that the vasculature in the white matter is capable of perfusing tissue after these time periods.

Recently, Senter and Venes (1978) have reported a refinement of the hydrogen clearance technique to study SCBF. They stabilized the spinal column and dampened the negative intrathoracic pressure of the cats in their experiments. Furthermore, they used a relatively atraumatic and stereotaxic technique for placement of electrolytically etched platinum microelectrodes, modified the amplifier circuitry, and standardized the electrode resistance, impedance, and current from site to site over time. These facts, plus the fact that their reported normal values for SCBF of 10.99 ml/100 g/min in the dorsolateral funiculus of the cat spinal cord correlate so well with the 10.30 ml/100 g/min reported by the noninvasive technique of Sandler and Tator, lend strong credibility to the data and the conclusions of Senter and Venes. The white matter study of the latter investigators on spinal cords undergoing severe trauma (500 g-cm force) demonstrated ischemia both at the level of the injury and 1 cm below the level of the injury. At the level of trauma, ischemia was delayed in onset for 1 hr, and a 2-hr delay occurred 1 cm below the level of the lesion. They concluded that, in their model, spinal cord ischemia occurs in the white matter during the post-traumatic period and could possibly constitute a "secondary injury" contributing to neurological dysfunction. The delay in onset of ischemia 1 cm below the lesion is highly suggestive of a vasoactive substance diffusing away from the trauma site. Likewise, in their studies, while the onset of ischemia was uniform, the return of blood flow 7 hr post-trauma was variable. Blood pressure, pretrauma SCBF, PCO_2, and/or the degree of histological damage had no correlation with return of blood flow. Their finding of a return of flow to the white matter at 7 hr would fit well with the findings of Fairholm and Turnbull (1971) seen on microangiographs of vessels in rabbit spinal cords following trauma. Vessels in the white matter were able to be perfused 7 days after injury, when the tissue of the central cord was disrupted and vessels did not fill (Fig. 44.5). Unfortunately, after 7 hr of ischemia it is doubtful that axonal or neuronal function would be restored.

Normally, there is autoregulation of SCBF in a normal and constant range when the mean arterial blood pressure (MAP) is in a range of 50–135 mm Hg in the monkey (Kobrine et al., 1976). When α-adrenergic receptors are blocked by intravenous administration of phenoxybenzamine, autoregulation is abolished. This suggests a role of the sympathetic nervous system in control of spinal circulation, since intact autoregulation after cervical cord section has been demonstrated (Ko-

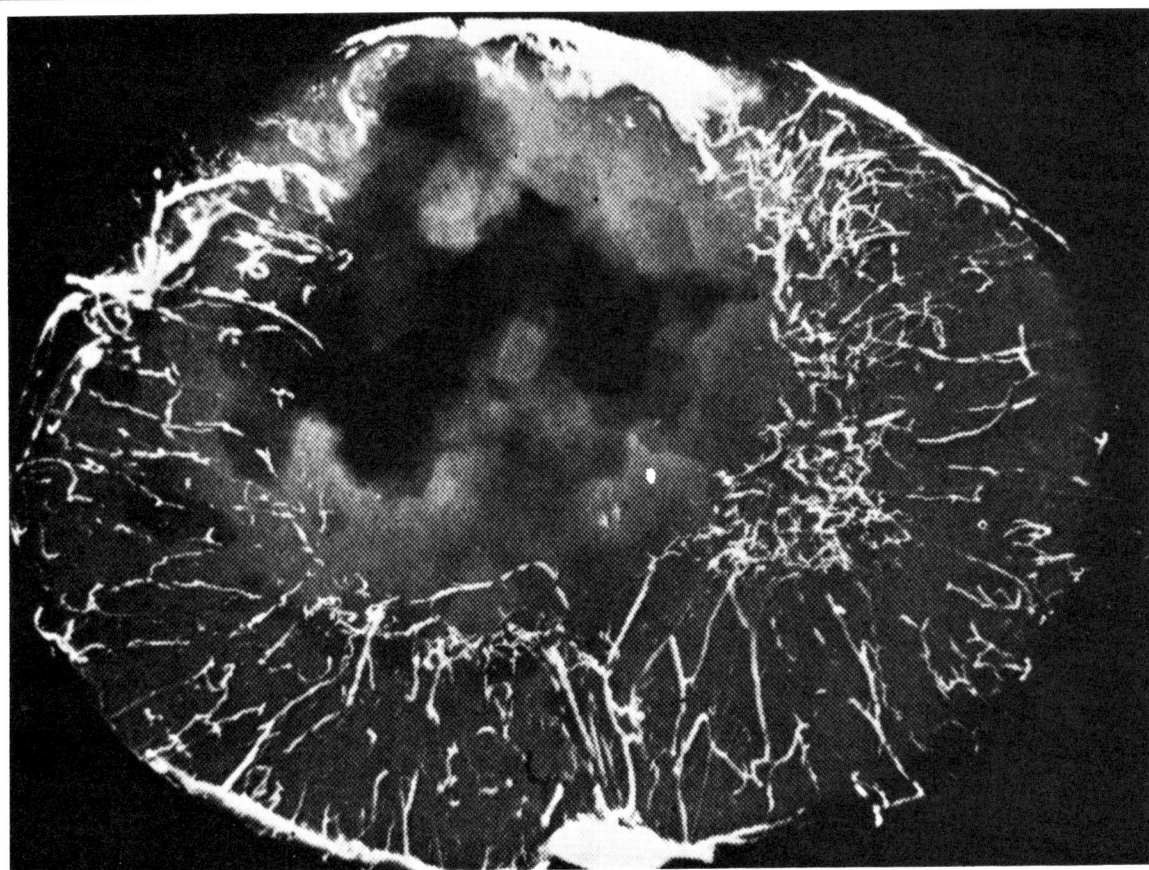

Figure 44.5. Microangiographic study of rabbit cord 7 days after injury. Tissue is disrupted and vessels do not fill in central part of cord. (Reprinted with permission from D. J. Fairholm and I. M. Turnbull: Journal of Neurosurgery 35:277–286, 1971).

brine et al., 1977a). α-Adrenergic receptors must be intact for control of vessel tone and, therefore, for autoregulation of blood flow in the spinal cord. Kobine et al. (1977b) also demonstrated that at high MAP levels, the β-adrenergic component is involved in initiating a significant vasodilatation and an increase in SCBF. The primary importance of the sympathetic nervous system in control of SCBF is further emphasized by the fact that SCBF is less sensitive than cerebral blood flow to changes in $PaCO_2$ (chemical control). Further studies by Senter and Venes (1979) on impact injury of the cat spinal cord, again using the modified hydrogen ion technique, have shown intact autoregulation of SCBF for the initial 60–90 min after injury. However autoregulation is lost with the onset of ischemia. Even though mean systemic arterial pressure (mSAP) fell 30–40 mm Hg within 10 min after trauma, SCBF was maintained over 1 hr. Not only was autoregulation of SCBF intact at the zone of trauma during the first hour, but it remained intact for nearly 2 hr 1 cm below the lesion site. If blood pressure was elevated with Aramine, SCBF increased dramatically at the site of the lesion and 1 cm below. Nitroprusside-induced hypotension at 4 hr post-injury reproduced severe ischemia. Their data suggested that the ischemic response to spinal cord injury is mediated both by the loss of autoregulation and by relative vasoconstriction of the resistant vessels.

In a chronic study of impact spinal cord injury in the same species, Smith et al. (1978a) have shown hyperemia of white matter at 2 weeks following the injury, as did Bingham et al. (1975a) and Kobrine et al. (1975) in acute experiments. The possible existence of early hyperemia was not studied by Smith, but, in addition to late hyperemia, he also demonstrated loss of autoregulation that appeared limited to the injury site. Although the loss of autoregulation of blood flow seems to be under local control, the delay in onset is difficult to explain. It is interesting to note that the loss of autoregulation of SCBF corresponds in time with appearance of gray matter hemorrhages as described by Dohrman et al. (1971). The delayed loss of autoregulation of SCBF may possibly be explained on the basis of release of certain vasoactive substances, such as norepinephrine, serotonin, dopamine, or histamine. Each has been implicated as a mediator of spinal cord post-traumatic ischemia, and they will be reviewed next.

BIOGENIC AMINES

Since a vascular lesion is evident in spinal cord injury and appears time-based, it is important to further consider other metabolic changes that could mediate progressive ischemia. There are naturally occurring cord neurotransmitter substances with recognized vasospastic properties. Trauma may induce an excessive neuronal discharge, leading to release of transmitter substances. These substances in toxic concentrations would have access to spinal cord vascular smooth muscle sites and could potentially cause vasospasm, hypoxia, and subsequent tissue necrosis. Osterholm and Mathews (1972a) found a four-fold increase in norepinephrine (NE) concentrations and a four-fold decrease in dopamine (DA) concentration at cat spinal cord injury sites within 1 hr after a 500 g-cm injury (Table 44.2). Trauma not only increased NE fluorescence in its normal gray matter location but introduced NE into the white matter, where it is not found normally. Vise, in dogs, using a fluorescent microscopy technique, found increased NE in traumatized spinal cord 1–2 hr after wounding. He proposed that the NE came from intravascular sources (Vise et al., 1974). Using a controlled microinjection technique, Osterholm and Mathews (1972a) injected NE (Levophed) into the spinal cord and produced areas of hemorrhage and necrosis not seen in saline control injection sites. One of the most intriguing aspects of the early NE experiments in spinal cord injury performed by Osterholm and Mathews (1972b) was the treatment of acute and spinal cord injury in animals with α-methyltyrosine (AMT), which blocks tyrosine hydroxylase and, therefore, NE synthesis. When given 15 min after injury, AMT reduced the size of the hemorrhagic necrotic area by a factor of eight (23.3% of cross sectional area reduced to 2.9%). This suggested that the development of acute hemorrhagic necrosis required the continued synthesis of a catecholamine neurotramsitter. Other drugs shown by the same investigators to be effective in decreasing the size of acute experimental hemorrhagic necrosis were reserpine, levodopa, α-methyldopa, phenoxybenzamine, disulfiram, 6-hydroxydopamine, fusaric acid, guanethidine, and Bretylium.

Unfortunately, this finding of elevated NE levels at spinal cord injury sites has not been substantiated by other investigators. Hedeman et al. (1974) using the dog spinal cord found a significant elevation of dopamine especially above but also at the level of the injury 15–45 min after the injury, and they demonstrated a significant reduction of NE above and at the injury site. Pretreatment with α-methyltyrosine depleted cord catecholamines and prevented dopamine elevation, but posttreatment did not prevent this elevation. Thus, their study, although unable to substantiate the findings of Osterholm and Mathews, did confirm an adrenergic component in response to spinal cord trauma.

Naftchi et al. (1974) also measured biogenic amines in the spinal cord of cats and found no increase in NE or serotonin at, above, or below the injury site. This group of investigators found a significant increase in DA and histamine at all three levels 1 hr after impact. Pre- and postinjury treatment with ε-aminocaproic acid (EACA) decreased the concentrations of both NE and histamine below control spinal cord values. EACA has antiproteolytic activity and may preserve membrane integrity by neutralizing lysosomal enzymes. Thus, the rise in dopamine seen in the studies of Hedeman and Naftchi may be explained on continued biosynthesis of DA, since dopa decarboxylase is not membrane-bound, whereas dopamine β-hydroxylase (DBH), the enzyme responsible for the conversion of dopamine to norepinephrine, exerts its synthetic effect in the central nervous system only when membrane-bound. This normal state is probably altered by trauma and DBH activity is reduced, decreasing the conversion of DA to NE.

Naftchi's finding of elevated histamine values and Kobrine's observation of hyperemia in the lateral funiculus of spinal cord after trauma prompted Kobrine and Doyle (1976) to study the effect of pretreatment of animals with antihistamines. Using chlorpheneramine and metiamide to block both H_1 and H_2 receptor sites, neither hyperemia nor ischemia was demonstrated in monkeys. They concluded that the hyperemia is a histamine-related phenomenon.

Bingham et al. (1975a), in a 300 g-cm impact injury to the monkey spinal cord, showed a progressive decrease in NE activity at the trauma site over a 4-hr span and no change in DA activity using a spectrophotofluorometric measurement technique. This group of investigators could not prove that catecholamines played a significant role in spinal cord injury due to blunt trauma, although they observed the fall in NE activity to occur during the gradual expansion of the central necrosis. Thus, loss of NE content appeared related to tissue destruction and not deamination by monoamine oxidase. de la Torre et al. (1974) found no increase in NE, DA, and serotonin in spinal cord injuries in cats and dogs. Albin and Bunegin (1974) found no increase in intrinsic spinal fiber NE synthesis rates 1 hr after trauma in dogs and monkeys, while Zivin et al. (1976) found that NE decreases

Table 44.2
Determination of Biogenic Amines in Spinal Cord Trauma

Author	Species	Norepinephrine	Dopamine	Serotonin	Histamine	Prostaglandin
Osterholm and Mathews (1972a and b)	Cat	↑	↓			
Vise et al. (1974)	Dog	↑				
Hedeman et al. (1974)	Dog	↓	↑			
Naftchi et al. (1974)	Cat	↔	↑	↔	↑	
Bingham et al. (1975b)	Monkey	↓	↔			
Rawe et al. (1977a)	Cat	↔				
de la Torre et al. (1974)	Dog, Cat	↔	↔	↔		
Albin and Bunegin (1974)	Dog, Monkey	↔				
Zivin et al. (1976)	Rabbit	↓	↔			
Jonsson and Daniell (1976)	Cat					↑

considerably at the lesion center in traumatized rabbit spinal cords. Jonsson and Daniell (1976) found an increase in prostaglandin in spinal cord injury in cats.

Inasmuch as it seems that SCBF is an important factor in spinal cord trauma, it is necessary to know what effect NE may have on SCBF. The blood-cord barrier, similar to the blood-brain barrier, has been shown to be disrupted in spinal cord trauma. Goodman has shown loss of integrity of the endothelial pentalaminar junctions in the central gray matter within 90 sec following injury (Goodman et al., 1976). In the brain after disruption of the blood-brain barrier, there is a 4-fold increase in NE permeability. If in spinal cord trauma there may be excessive release of NE into the extracellular space, as suggested by Osterholm and Mathews (1972a), and if NE is not removed normally in the hypoxic or ischemic situation, these small or normal amounts of NE may alter SCBF. Crawford et al. (1977) found no overall effect of intra-arterial infusion of NE (12 μg/min and 30 μg/min) on SCBF unless the blood-cord barrier was disrupted, and then these amounts of NE resulted in large reductions in SCBF. If pretreatment was carried out with phenoxybenzamine, there were no reductions in SCBF, suggesting that flow reductions are mediated via α-adrenergic mechanisms. Without treatment, though, there was reduction in SCBF. After barrier disruption, there was no histological evidence of NE-induced hemorrhagic necrosis.

Rawe et al. (1977b, 1978) could not find a significant tissue increase in NE measured sequentially over a 4-hr period following impact injury to the cat spinal cord. Pretreatment with AMT or reserpine did not reduce the hemorrhagic involvement of gray or white matter at 1 hr or improve the long-term recovery of four animals over controls. In another study by Rawe and Perot (1979), phenoxybenzamine pretreatment caused a 32% reduction in systemic blood pressure before trauma with a marked reduction in hemorrhages 1 hr post-trauma, leading this group of investigators to conclude that blood pressure was of greater etiological significance in the pathogenesis of experimental spinal cord hemorrhages than tissue levels of NE. They demonstrated the ability to retard or enhance not only the hemorrhagic lesion but the formation of edema as well by lowering or raising post-traumatic blood pressure while injury was kept constant. This ability was related directly to vascular damage in gray and white matter and to the loss of autoregulation of SCBF (Rawe et al., 1978; Rawe and Perot, 1979).

Currently, the weight of the evidence is that NE is not increased at the spinal cord injury site, but, nevertheless, Osterholm and Mathews' (1972a) ability to produce hemorrhagic necrosis by direct NE injection into the spinal cord has not been refuted. Tibbs et al. (1978, 1979) have shown a brief but dramatic 276% increase over baseline in circulating plasma NE after acute cervical cord transection associated with a transient phase of hypertension. Therefore, it is possible that NE may enter the spinal trauma site during the first hour after disruption of the blood-cord barrier and may contribute to the ischemic process that occurs in the injured spinal cord.

SUMMARY

Impact injury to the spinal cord initially results in a central gray matter ischemic hemorrhagic necrosis. The magnitude of the necrosis and the degree of involvement of spinal cord white matter are proportional to the force of the injury. Shearing forces, possibly compressive forces, initially disrupt vessels, but neurons are involved as well. In transient pareses the lesion may progress while clinical improvement occurs, whereas in permanent paraplegia, the initial lesion is a complete transection or certainly progresses to involve spinal cord white matter. After a decade of intensive investigation, the interaction of biogenic amines, systemic blood pressure, and SCBF has not been clarified. For instance, as of this writing, free and bound NE in the traumatized spinal cord has yet to be measured. The presence of hyperemia versus ischemia of the white matter must be convincingly determined and correlated with electrical studies and quality of survival. The fact remains that the spinal cord often is not transected by trauma and that a delayed detrimental pathophysiological event occurs that can be reversed. It is possible that a secondary injury of the spinal cord may be prevented by proper immobilization, manipulation of blood pressure, and alteration of biogenic amines or other metabolites at the trauma site.

References

Albin, M.S., and Bunegin, L.: Catecholamine synthesis rates in traumatized spinal cord (abstract). Anat. Rec. *178*:296–297, 1974.

Albin, M.S., White, R.J., Acosta-Rua, G., et al.: Study of functional recovery produced by delayed localized cooling after spinal cord injury in primates. J. Neurosurg. *29*:113–120, 1968.

Allen, A.R.: Injuries of the spinal cord with the study of nine cases with necropsy. J.A.M.A. *50*:941–952, 1908.

Allen, A.R.: Surgery of experimental lesion of spinal cord equivalent to crush injury of fracture dislocation of spinal column: A preliminary report. J.A.M.A. *57*:878–880, 1911.

Allen, A.R.: Remarks on the histopathological changes in the spinal cord due to impact: An experimental study. J. Nerv. Ment. Dis. *41*:141–147, 1914.

Anderson, D.K., Prockop, L.D., Means, E.D., and Hartley, L.E.: Cerebrospinal fluid lactate and electrolyte levels following experimental spinal cord injury. J. Neurosurg. *44*:715–722, 1976.

Bingham, W.G., Goldman, H., Friedman, S.J., et al.: Blood flow in normal and injured monkey spinal cord. J. Neurosurg. *43*:162–171, 1975a.

Bingham, W.G., Ruffolo, R., and Friedman, S.J.: Catecholamine levels in the injured spinal cords of monkeys. J. Neurosurg. *42*:174–178, 1975b.

Boggan, J.E., de la Torre, J., and Mullan, S.: A rat model for the investigation of spinal cord injury (abstract). In *Approaches to the Cell Biology of Neurons*, edited by W.M. Cowan, vol. 2, p. 961. Society for Neuroscience, Bethesda MD, 1977.

Clendenon, N.R., Allen, N., Gordon, W.A., and Bingham, W.G., Jr.: Inhibition of Na^+-K^+-activated ATPase activity following experimental spinal cord trauma. J. Neurosurg. *49*:563–568, 1978.

Crawford, R.A., Griffiths, I.R., and McCulloch, J.: The effect of norepinephrine on the spinal cord circulation and its possible implications in the pathogenesis of acute spinal trauma. J. Neurosurg. 47:567–576, 1977.

de la Torre, J.C., Johnson, C.M., Harris, L.A., Kijihara, K., and Mullan, S.: Monoamine changes in experimental head and spinal cord trauma: Failure to confirm previous observations. Surg. Neurol. 2:5–11, 1974.

Dohrmann, G.J., Wagner, F.C., and Bucy, P.C.: The microvasculature in transitory traumatic paraplegia: An electron microscopic study in the monkey. J. Neurosurg. 35:263–271, 1971.

Dohrmann, G.J., Manohar, M.M., and Banks, D.: Biomechanics of experimental spinal cord trauma. J. Neurosurg. 48:993–1001, 1978.

Ducker, T.B.: Experimental injury of the spinal cord. In *Handbook of Clinical Neurology*, edited by P. Vinken and G.W. Bruyn, vol. 25, p. 926. North-Holland, Amsterdam, 1976.

Ducker, T.B., Kindt, G.W., and Kempe, L.G.: The pathological findings in acute experimental spinal cord trauma. J. Neurosurg. 35:700–708, 1971a.

Ducker, T.B., and Perot, P.L., Jr.: Spinal cord oxygen and blood flow in trauma. Surg. Forum 22:413–415, 1971b.

Fairholm, D.J., and Turnbull, I.M.: Microangiographic study of experimental spinal cord injuries. J. Neurosurg. 35:277–286, 1971.

Ginsberg, M.D., Mela, L., Wrobel-Kuhl, K., et al.: Mitochondrial metabolism following bilateral cerebral ischemia in the gerbil. Ann. Neurol. 1:519–527, 1977.

Goodman, J.H., Bingham, W.G., and Hunt, W.E.: Ultrastructural blood-brain barrier alterations and edema formation in acute spinal cord trauma. J. Neurosurg. 44:418–423, 1976.

Goodman, J.H., Bingham, G., Jr., and Hunt, W.E.: Platelet aggregation in experimental spinal cord injury: Ultrastructural observations. Arch. Neurol. 36:197–201, 1979.

Griffiths, I.R.: Spinal cord blood flow in dogs. I. The "normal flow." J. Neurol. Neurosurg. Psychiatr. 36:34–41, 1973.

Griffiths, I.R.: Vasogenic edema following acute and chronic spinal cord compression in the dog. J. Neurosurg. 42:155–165, 1975a.

Griffiths, I.R.: Spinal cord blood flow after impact injury. In *Blood Flow and Metabolism in the Brain*, edited by A.M. Harper, W.B. Jennett, and J.D. Miller, ch. 4, pp. 27–29. Churchill, Edinburgh, 1975b.

Griffiths, I.R., Rowan, J.O., and Crawford, R.A.: Spinal cord blood flow measured by a hydrogen clearance technique. J. Neurol. Sci. 26:529–544, 1975.

Hedeman, L.S., Shellenberger, M.K., and Gordon, J.H.: Studies in experimental spinal cord trauma. Part I. Alterations in catecholamine levels. J. Neurosurg. 40:37–43, 1974.

Ito, T., Allen, N., and Yashon, D.: A mitochondrial lesion in experimental spinal cord trauma. J. Neurosurg. 48:434–442, 1978.

Jonsson, H.T., Jr., and Daniell, H.B.: Altered levels of PGF in cat spinal cord tissue following traumatic injury. Prostaglandins 11:51–62, 1976.

Kobrine, A.I., and Doyle, T.F.: Role of histamine in post-traumatic spinal cord hyperemia and the luxury perfusion syndrome. J. Neurosurg. 44:16–20, 1976.

Kobrine, A.I., Doyle, T.F., and Martins, A.N.: Spinal cord blood flow in the rhesus monkey by the hydrogen clearance method. Surg. Neurol. 2:197–200, 1974.

Kobrine, A.I., Doyle, T.F., and Martins, A.N.: Local spinal cord blood flow in experimental traumatic myelopathy. J. Neurosurg. 42:144–149, 1975.

Kobrine, A.I., Doyle, T.F., and Rizzoli, H.V.: Spinal cord blood flow as affected by changes in systemic blood pressure. J. Neurosurg. 44:12–15, 1976.

Kobrine, A.I., Evans, D.E., and Rizzoli, H.V.: The effect of alpha adrenergic blockade on spinal cord autoregulation in the monkey. J. Neurosurg. 46:336–341, 1977a.

Kobrine, A.I., Evans, D.E., and Rizzoli, H.V.: The effect of beta adrenergic blockade on spinal cord autoregulation in the monkey. J. Neurosurg. 47:57–63, 1977b.

Landau, W.M., Freygang, W.H., Jr., Roland, L.P., et al.: The local circulation of the living brain: Values in the unanesthetized and anesthetized cat. Trans. Am. Neurol. Assoc. 80:125–129, 1955.

Lassen, N.A.: The luxury-perfusion syndrome and its possible relation to acute metabolic acidosis localized within the brain. Lancet 2:1113–1115, 1966.

Lewin, M.G., Hansebout, R.R., and Pappius, H.M.: Chemical characteristics of traumatic spinal cord edema in cats: Effect of steroids on potassium depletion. J. Neurosurg. 40:65–75, 1974.

Locke, G.E., Yashon, D., Feldman, R., and Hunt, W.M.: Ischemia in primate spinal cord injury. J. Neurosurg. 34:614–617, 1971.

Milvy, P., Kakari, S., Campbell, J.B., et al.: Paramagnetic species and radical products in cat spinal cord. Ann. N.Y. Acad. Sci. 222:1102–1111, 1973.

Molt, J.T., Nelson, L.R., Poulos, D.A., and Bourke, R.S.: Analysis and measurement of some sources of variability in experimental spinal cord trauma. J. Neurosurg. 50:784–791, 1979.

Naftchi, N.E., Demeny, M., DeCrescito, V., et al.: Biogenic amine concentrations in traumatized spinal cord of cats: Effect of drug therapy. J. Neurosurg. 40:52–57, 1974.

Osterholm, J.L., and Mathews, G.J.: Altered norepinephrine metabolism following experimental spinal cord injury. Part I. Relationship to hemorrhagic necrosis and post-wounding neurological deficits. J. Neurosurg. 36:386–394, 1972a.

Osterholm, J.L., and Mathews, G.J.: Altered norepinephrine metabolism following experimental spinal cord injury. Part 2. Protection against traumatic spinal cord hemorrhagic necrosis by norepinephrine synthesis blockade with alpha methyl tyrosine. J. Neurosurg. 36:395–401, 1972b.

Overgard, J., and Tweed, W.A.: Cerebral circulation after head injury. Part I. J. Neurosurg. 41:531–541, 1974.

Rawe, S.E., and Perot, P.L., Jr.: Pressor response resulting from experimental contusion injury to the spinal cord. J. Neurosurg. 50:58–63, 1979.

Rawe, S.E., Roth, R.H., Boadle-Biber, M., and Collins, W.F.: Norepinephrine levels in experimental spinal cord trauma. Part I. Biochemical study of hemorrhagic necrosis. J. Neurosurg. 46:342–349, 1977a.

Rawe, S.E., Roth, R.H., and Collins, W.F.: Norepinephrine levels in experimental spinal cord trauma. Part 2. Histopathological study of hemorrhagic necrosis. J. Neurosurg. 46:350–357, 1977b.

Rawe, S.E., Lee, W.A., and Perot, P.L., Jr.: The histopathology of experimental spinal cord trauma: The effect of systemic blood pressure. J. Neurosurg. 48:1002–1007, 1978.

Rivlin, A.S., and Tator, C.H.: Regional spinal cord blood flow in rats after severe cord trauma. J. Neurosurg. 49:844–853, 1978.

Rivlin, A.S., and Tator, C.H.: Effect of vasodilators and myelotomy on recovery after acute spinal cord injury in rats. J. Neurosurg. 50:349–352, 1979.

Sandler, A.N., and Tator, C.H.: Regional spinal cord flow in primates. J. Neurosurg. 45:647–659, 1976a.

Sandler, A.N., and Tator, C.H.: Effect of acute spinal cord

compression injury on regional cord blood flow in primates. J. Neurosurg. 45:660–676, 1976b.

Schutz, H., Silverstein, P.R., Vapalahti, M., et al.: Brain mitochondrial function after ischemia and hypoxia. I. Ischemia induced by increased intracranial pressure. Arch. Neurol. 29:408–416, 1973.

Senter, H.J., and Venes, J.L.: Altered blood flow and secondary injury in experimental spinal cord trauma. J. Neurosurg. 49:569–578, 1978.

Senter, H.J., and Venes, J.L.: Loss of autoregulation and posttraumatic ischemia following experimental spinal cord trauma. J. Neurosurg. 50:198–206, 1979.

Smith, A.J.K., McCreery, D.B., Bloedel, J.R., and Chou, S.N.: Hyperemia, CO_2 responsiveness, and autoregulation in the white matter following experimental spinal cord injury. J. Neurosurg. 48:239–251, 1978a.

Smith, D.R., Smith, H.I., and Rajjoub, R.K.: Measurement of spinal cord blood flow by the microsphere technique. Neurosurgery 2:27–30, 1978b.

Takaoka, Y., Billiar, R.B., White, R.J., and Little, B.A.: Microsphere determination of regional spinal cord blood flow in the primate. Presented at the 45th Annual Meeting of the American Association of Neurological Surgeons, Toronto, Ontario, April 28, 1977.

Tibbs, P.A., Young, B., McAllister, R.G., Jr., Brooks, W.H., and Tackett, L.: Studies of experimental cervical spinal cord transection. Part I. Hemodynamic changes after acute cervical spinal cord transection. J. Neurosurg. 49:558–562, 1978.

Tibbs, P.A., Young, B., Ziegler, M.G., and McAllister, R.G., Jr.: Studies of experimental cervical spinal cord transection. Part II. Plasma norepinephrine levels after acute cervical spinal cord transection. J. Neurosurg. 50:629–632, 1979.

Vise, W.M., Yashon, D., and Hunt, W.E.: Mechanisms of norepinephrine accumulation within sites of spinal cord injury. J. Neurosurg. 40:76–82, 1974.

Wagner, F.C., Dohrmann, G.J., and Bucy, P.C.: Histopathology of transitory traumatic paraplegia in the monkey. J. Neurosurg. 35:272–276, 1971.

Wagner, F.C., Jr., VanGilder, J.C., and Dohrmann, G.J.: Pathological changes from acute to chronic in experimental spinal cord trauma. J. Neurosurg. 48:92–98, 1978.

Wolman, L.: The neuropathology of traumatic paraplegia: A critical historical review. Paraplegia 1:233–251, 1964.

Wolman, L.: The disturbance of circulation in traumatic paraplegia in acute and late stages: A pathological study. Paraplegia 2:213–226, 1965.

Yashon, D., Bingham, W.G., Faddoul, E.M., and Hunt, W.E.: Edema of the spinal cord following experimental impact trauma. J. Neurosurg. 38:693–697, 1973.

Zivin, J.A., Doppman, J.L., Reed, J.L., et al.: Biochemical and histochemical studies of biogenic amines in spinal cord trauma. Neurology 26:99–107, 1976.

CHAPTER 45

Treatment of Spinal Cord Injury

THOMAS G. SAUL
THOMAS B. DUCKER

The human spinal cord is an amazing structure in several respects. Anatomically, the cylinder-shaped spinal cord measures 8–9 mm and 10–14 mm in the sagittal and transverse diameters, respectively (Truex and Carpenter, 1970). This approximates the size of a dime. In spite of this small size, the internal structure is remarkably complex. It consists of literally millions of neurons, dendrites, myelinated and unmyelinated axon fiber tracts, and synaptic connections. The organization and circuitry of this structure are unmatched by any computer. It mediates every movement, perceives external stimuli, assimilates and transmits all of this information to higher centers in the neuroaxis, and receives information from these centers. It controls musculoskeletal as well as visceral activities. It is not surprising, then, that injury to the spinal cord can result immediately in some of the most devastating disabilities involving all body systems. Furthermore, this same complexity makes the treatment of spinal cord injury a difficult and frustrating endeavor on the part of neurotraumatologists. This chapter will deal with the treatment of cord injuries based on current concepts of the tissue and cellular changes that result from such injuries. In particular, we will discuss the consequences and treatment of: 1) me-

Treatment of Spinal Cord Injury

chanical insults, 2) hemodynamic changes, 3) biochemical derangements, and 4) ancillary problems that account for the neurological deficits in cord injuries.

MECHANICAL INSULTS

The mechanical insults that accompany spinal cord injury are of three types: 1) direct tissue disruption due to the injury impact, 2) movement of an unstable spine in the acute phase of injury, and 3) compression of neural tissue secondary to bone or soft tissue material (intervertebral disc and/or ligament). Each of these insults has specific consequences and modes of treatment.

Tissue Disruption

The central nervous system (CNS), including the spinal cord, is unique in that there is no inherent regenerative process that will aid in a functional recovery of anatomically disrupted tissue. The regenerative efforts of the CNS produce only meager sprouts and no new distal growth that would appear to be of any use to humans and/or primates. After cord injury, the pathological events that lead to the irreversible damage begin in the central gray. Electron microscopic studies in the monkey have shown that the muscular venules in the gray substance distend within 5 min of impact. Red cells appear in the perivascular space of the capillaries and venules within 15–30 min. Small hemorrhages occur in the gray matter within 1 hr. Progressive vacuolation and swelling of the endothelium of the capillaries are marked within the first few hours (Dohrmann et al., 1971). The central ischemic and hemorrhagic lesions become present in routine histological sections 4 hr after trauma. Thereafter, there is progressive gray matter necrosis, but the white matter changes do not begin until 3 or 4 hr after injury. The periphery of the cord is initially spared except for the occasional flame-shaped hemorrhage that occurs with the original impact (Assenmacher and Ducker, 1971). The white matter pathology follows the changes in the gray matter. Initially, there is edema; the edema leads to distorted perfusion, and the white matter undergoes destruction over the next few days. The total amount of destruction is generally related to the amount of trauma inflicted (Ducker, 1976). Figure 45.1 illustrates the pathological picture as it relates to the severity of trauma and passage of time. This is a schematic summary of the cross sectional appearance of the injured cords. Figures 44.2–44.5 are the actual microscopic sections of the monkey spinal cords documenting these pathological changes and their time course.

Humans can withstand the initial gray matter injury. This alone represents a segmental, affordable loss of only a small proportion of the total gray matter neuronal pool. If this were the limit of injury, neurologic deficit

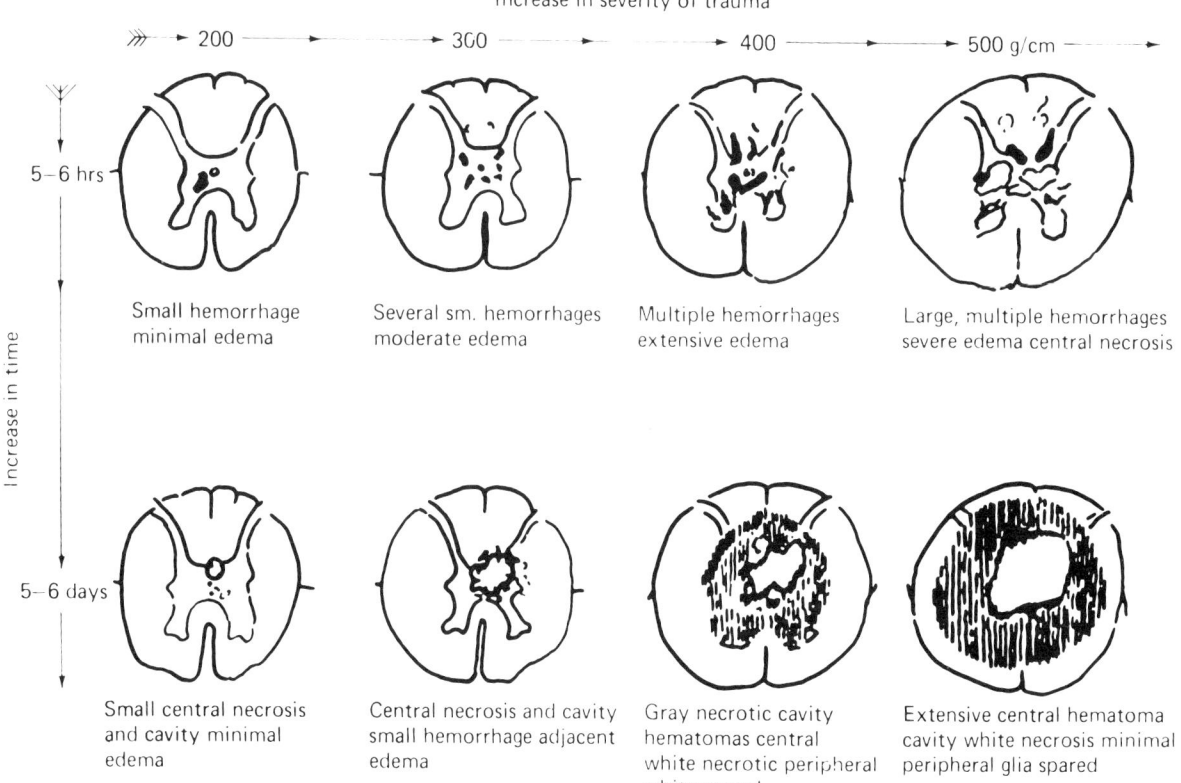

Figure 45.1. The pathological picture as it relates to trauma and time. (Reprinted with permission from T.B. Ducker: In *Handbook of Clinical Neurology*, edited by P.I. Vinken and G.W. Bruyn, vol. 25, ch. 2, pp. 9–26. American Elsevier, New York, 1976.)

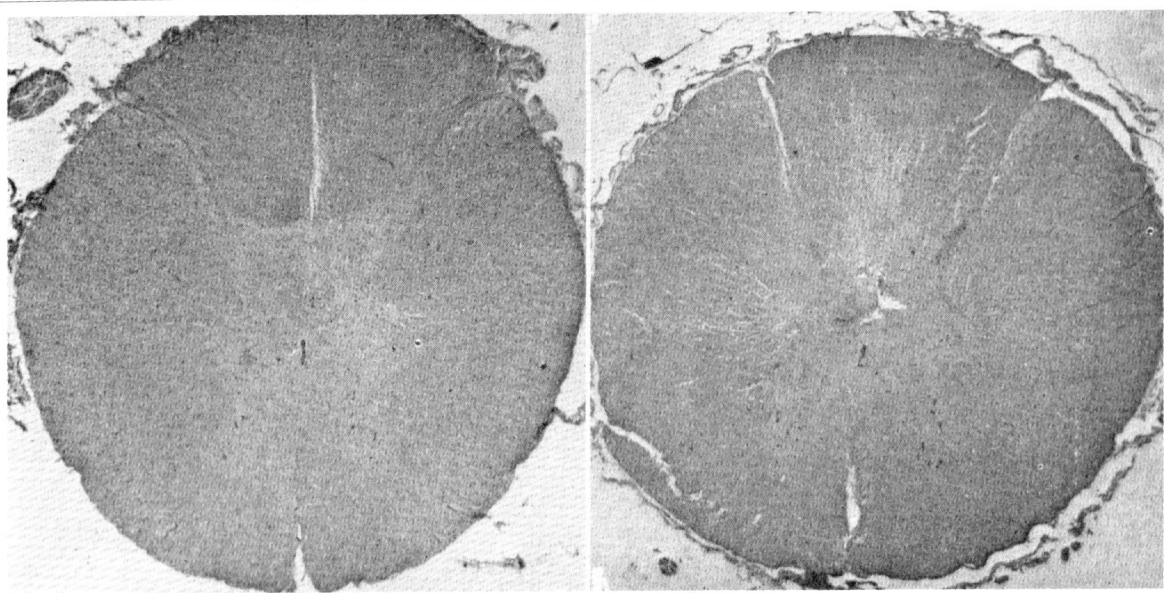

Figure 45.2. Spinal cord sections taken from monkeys 5–6 hr after trauma. *Left,* a spinal cord that sustained a 200 g-cm force. *Right,* a spinal cord that sustained a 300 g-cm force. (Reprinted with permission from T.B. Ducker, G.W. Kindt, and L.G. Kempe: Journal of Neurosurgery 35:700–708, 1971.)

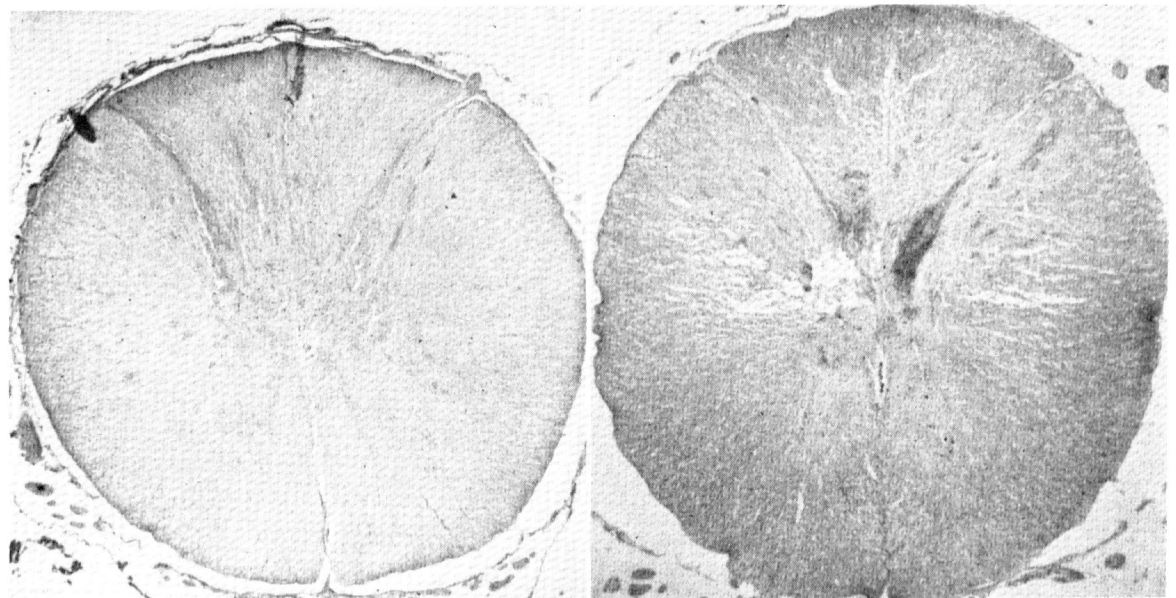

Figure 45.3. Spinal cord sections 5–6 hr after trauma. *Left,* after 400-g-cm force. *Right,* after 500-g-cm force. Note the stepwise increase in gray matter hemorrhages from one to multiple, the increase in edema from minimal to severe, and the development of central necrosis with the heavier blows. (Reprinted with permission from T.B. Ducker, G.W. Kindt, and L.G. Kempe: Journal of Neurosurgery 35:700–708, 1971.)

would be minor. Humans cannot tolerate segmental loss of the peripheral white matter. This disrupts ascending and descending fiber tracts and results in loss of distal functioning of those tracts. Neurons are rendered useless, and cord function is lost in varying degrees.

The problem of regeneration of the spinal cord after traumatic disruption has been investigated extensively for many years (Guttman, 1973; Guth, 1975). Phyloge- netically this is known to occur (i.e., reptiles, amphibians, fish, etc.). However, for species of higher phylogenetic rank, the question remains ambiguous and certainly unanswered. Wolman (1966) demonstrated at autopsy well developed axon regeneration in and around the damaged cord segments in 12 patients who died with traumatic paraplegia. These were small axon bundles found above and below the level of maximum cord

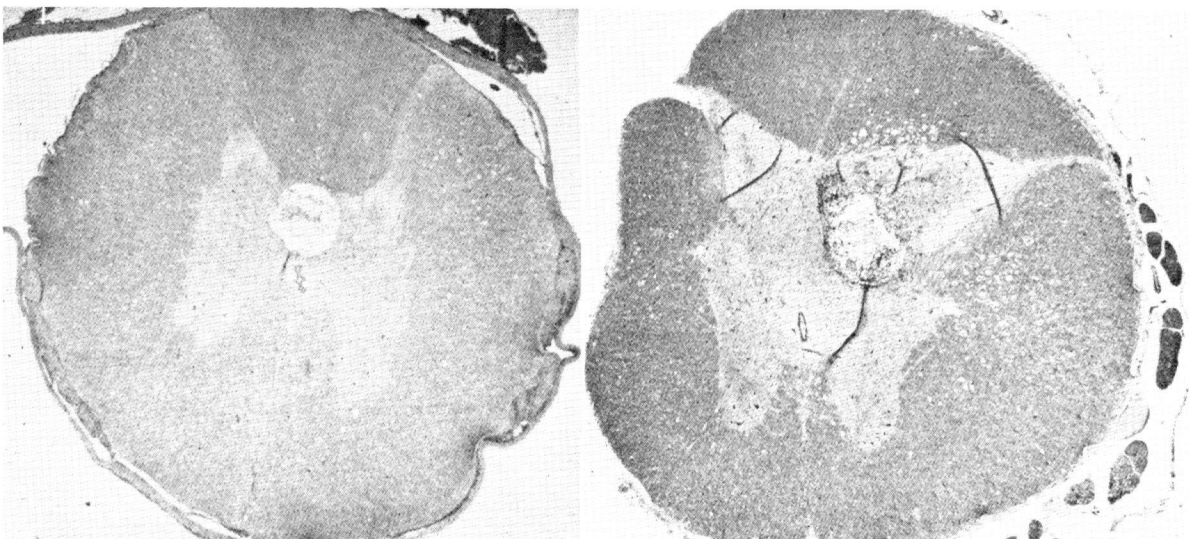

Figure 45.4. Sections of monkey cords from the area of maximum damage 5–6 days after trauma. *Left,* after 200-g-cm force. *Right,* after 300-g-cm force. (Reprinted with permission from T.B. Ducker, G.W. Kindt, and L.G. Kempe: Journal of Neurosurgery *35:*700–708, 1971.)

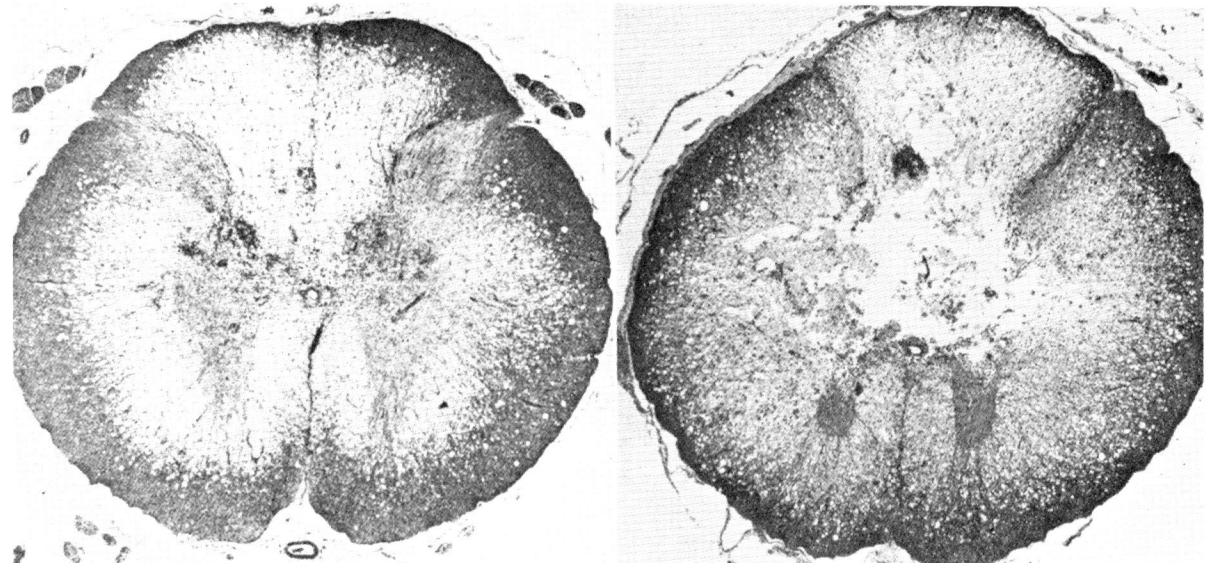

Figure 45.5. Cord sections in the area of maximum damage 5–6 days after injury. *Left,* after 400-g-cm force. *Right,* after 500-g-cm force. Note the progressive development in the size of the central necrosis and the increase in white matter pathology as the amount of trauma is advanced. (Reprinted with permission from T.B. Ducker, G.W. Kindt, and L.G. Kempe: Journal of Neurosurgery *35:*700–708, 1971.)

damage. However, the origins of these nerve fibers were the posterior nerve roots and ganglia.

Investigative efforts have been made to induce a regenerative process in damaged spinal cords. Windle et al. (1952, 1956) demonstrated that the brief phase of active regeneration that normally takes place after cord transections may be extended by the administration of Piromen, a polysaccharide that reduces connective tissue and glial scar formation. This work was done in cats. This work stimulated experimental attempts to diminish scar tissue formation in spine-injured dogs and rats by administering trypsin intrathecally (Freeman et al., 1960). These works demonstrated no functional value in their findings. In 1973, a Russian monograph by Matinian and Andreasian was published and subsequently translated into English in 1976; it reported enzyme therapy to be efficacious in the treatment of experimental paraplegia in rats. The substances employed were trypsin, hyaluronidase, elastase, and Piromen. This study documented a 27–47% functional recovery in the treated group compared to controls who remained paraplegic. Moreover, these authors presented histological evidence of nerve fiber regeneration and electrophysiological evidence of conduction between sciatic nerve and cerebral cortex. Needless to say, such a report caused considerable clamor in this investigative field, not to mention the effect on the cord-injured population of the world. As would be expected, attempts were made to reproduce the Russian findings by a number of different investigators. Guth et al. (1978, 1979), at the University of Maryland, replicated these experiments in 92 rats and demonstrated 1) no recovery from paraplegia; 2) no impulse conduction across the injury site; 3) no histological evidence of nerve fiber regeneration. Subsequent reports from other investigators documented the failure of trypsin and hyaluronidase to effect regeneration in CNS lesion (Pettegrew, 1976; Knowles and Berry, 1978; Feringa et al., 1979).

In spite of the work being done in the area of cord regeneration, there is to date no effective intrinsic spinal cord regenerative process, nor is there any treatment available to induce such a process that could result in effectively reversing direct tissue disruption (Jackson, 1979). Therefore, the only effective way to combat this aspect of cord insult is through primary prevention of these injuries. The incidence of spinal cord injury is three to four per 100,000 population. Easily, 10,000 new injuries occur each year. The majority of these are caused by vehicular accidents and falls. They are also due to recreational, agricultural, and industrial accidents. Physicians in all medical disciplines and other medical personnel need to encourage and promote public and personal safety standards whenever possible. This is the only form of treatment for the irreversible tissue disruption of spinal cord injury.

The other forms of mechanical insults (mobility and compression) can cause additional irreversible damage that can worsen a given neurologic deficit or prevent the recovery of a marginal deficit. Unlike direct tissue disruption, these phenomenon can be altered by therapeutic intervention on the part of the neurotraumatologist.

Mobility of an Injured Spinal Cord

The principle of vertebral immobilization following trauma to the spine has been an undisputed dictum closely observed for many years. It is one that dates back to Hippocrates, who stressed the importance of vertebral alignment and reduction of the fracture. It is this principle that led to the development of the modern day forms of skeletal traction (i.e., Crutchfield, Gardner-Wells, and Halo tongs). The obvious purpose of vertebral immobilization is to prevent movement of an unstable vertebral column with consequent damage to the enclosed spinal cord. All current textbooks and articles stress the importance of this treatment modality, but seldom is the pathophysiological evidence presented. The fact is that physical movement at the site of a spinal cord injury can accentuate the pathology and have a detrimental effect on the clinical course. Ducker et al. (1978a) demonstrated this experimentally by subjecting monkeys to variable degrees of spinal cord contusion at the T11-T12 level. The control group consisted of animals whose injury was inflicted with up to 500 g-cm but without vertebral immobilization. The experimental group received injuries from forces in the 500–800 g-cm range, and rigid vertebral immobilization immediately followed in every case. Clinical neurological evaluation of the animals was made at 6 hr and on each day for 7 days. The system for motor assessment was as follows: no voluntary movement (grade 0); trace movement (grade 1); definite movement of joints but could not run (grade 3); the animals walked and ran normally (grade 4). The results of this experiment revealed that rigid immobilization of the vertebrae surrounding an injured spinal cord altered the clinical course of that lesion. A 500-g-cm injury consistently produced paraplegia in the nonimmobilized animal (Fig. 45.6). However, injuries of 750–800 g-cm are required to consistently produce paralysis when the animal is treated with vertebral immobilization (Fig. 45.7). Figure 45.8 is a composite of Figures 45.6 and 45.7, emphasizing the difference in the biological response curves of the two groups. The mechanisms that account for this improved response curve associated with immobilization are unknown. It is possible that further stretch injury is prevented, thus maintaining the integrity of surviving fiber tracts, glia, and neurons. In addition, the immobilization may optimize the vascular supply to the cord, preserving marginally injured regions.

Therefore, the proper management of a cord-injured patient should include immediate immobilization of the spine. In the early phase of management, this can be accomplished with a spine board with straps, sandbags, or a rigid collar for a cervical injury. A thoracolumbar

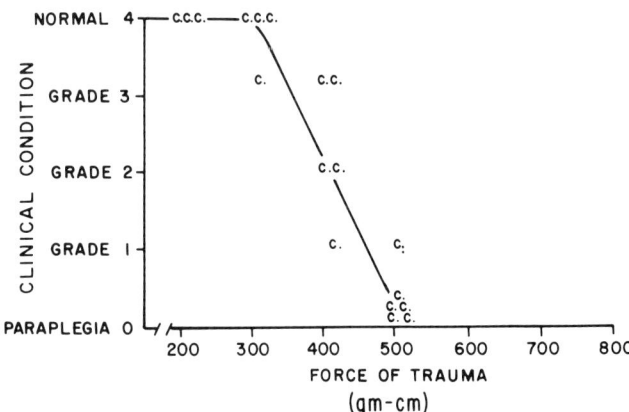

Figure 45.6. Clinical response of monkeys subjected to experimental spinal cord injury. This graph is the biological response curve of control monkeys in the first phase of the study. Clinical outcomes by grades are plotted against the trauma force in g-cm. Most animals subjected to 500 g-cm become paraplegic (grade 0), whereas forces less than 300 g-cm leave them normal or nearly so (grades 3 and 4). None of these animals was immobilized. Each monkey is represented by a *C*. (Reprinted with permission from T.B. Ducker, M. Saleman, and H.B. Daniell: Surgical Neurology *10:*71–76, 1978.)

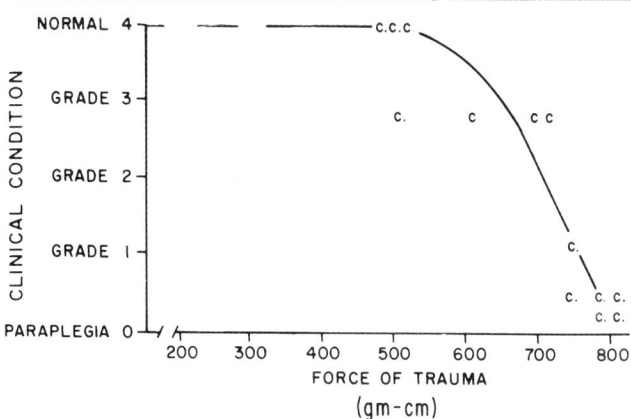

Figure 45.7. Clinical response of immobilized monkeys subjected to experimental spinal cord injury. This graph is the response curve of experimental monkeys in the first phase of the study. Clinical outcomes by grade are plotted against the trauma force in g-cm. Most animals are not rendered paraplegic (grade 0) unless a force of 800 g-cm is employed. At 500 g-cm the monkeys remain normal or nearly so (grades 3 and 4). Each of these animals was immobilized immediately following injury. Each monkey is represented by a *C*. (Reprinted with permission from T.B. Ducker, M. Salcman, and H.B. Daniell: Surgical Neurology *10:*71–76, 1978.)

injury can be immobilized by keeping the patient supine on a firm backboard. After the exact nature of the spine injury has been delineated by radiographic studies, more definitive immobilization and reduction of the fracture should be done. For cervical injuries, one of the various types of skeletal traction can be used to align and immobilize most cervical fractures. After the tongs are inserted, weights are applied for traction force. Except for the rare craniocervical junction injury, the initial poundage is around 2–3 lb (1 kg) per vertebra. The weight is rapidly increased with image fluoroscopy or serial roentgenograms in 5-, 10-, or 20-lb increments, depending on the age and weight of the patient. As traction is being increased, the patient, in certain injuries, can be appropriately positioned—mild hyperextension or flexion—in order to adequately align the bones. Frequent x-rays must be obtained during this time to assess the consequences of each maneuver. If adequate realignment cannot be achieved by this method, open surgical reduction should follow. This is particularly true with dislocated, locked facet joints. Thoracolumbar fractures are treated according to the same principle. These injuries can be realigned and reduced by postural traction, body casts, or jackets or by open surgical reduction and immobilization with Harrington rods.

After this initial immobilization is accomplished, then time can be taken to plan out the more definitive, long term stabilization of the spine. This can be achieved by either elective surgical stabilization or by prolonged skeletal traction. The advantages of an early surgical procedure are early mobilization of the patient and quick entry into a rehabilitation program. This helps prevent the complications associated with prolonged bed rest, especially when kept prone or supine. However, nonsurgical stabilization can be just as effective. If the patient has marked neurological deficit he may be maintained in skeletal traction on a frame or regular bed for approximately 6–8 weeks. After that time, he may be placed in an external cervical brace and the process of mobilization begun. If there is no or incomplete neurological deficit, the patient may be put into traction with a Halo vest apparatus. This will give immobilization and allow the patient to be ambulatory. The patient should remain in this device for 3–6 months to effect proper stabilization (Saul and Ducker, 1981a).

Compression of Neural Tissue

Extra-axial compression of neural tissue, whether it be brain or spinal cord, causes anatomical and physiological changes that result in dysfunction or total loss of function. In spinal cord injuries, there is commonly an initial acute compression of the cord secondary to the abnormal movement of the spine. This results in cord contusion, which leads to the pathological changes described in the earlier section of this chapter on tissue disruption. However, it is also possible that bone and/or soft tissue (intervertebral disc, ligament, hematoma, etc.) may remain in the spinal canal and cause focal compression. During such compression, the blood vessels are often the first to be partially or completely occluded, and this observation has led to some debate as to whether the subsequent dysfunction is the result of the ischemic changes or mechanical distortion. This discussion remains unanswered, which probably indicates that it is a

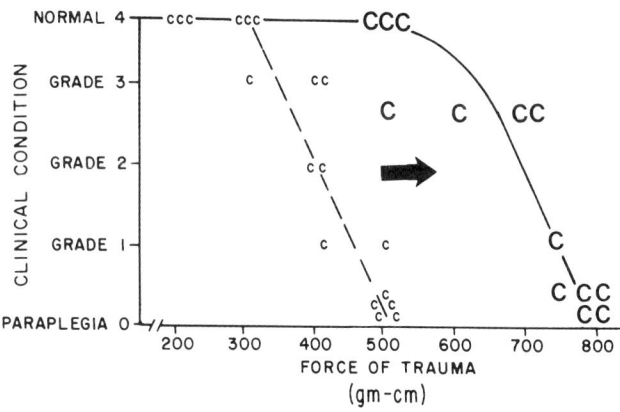

Figure 45.8. Clinical response of control monkeys versus immobilized monkeys. The biological response curve of Figure 45.1 is plotted as a *dashed line* and the experimental response curve of Figure 45.3 as a *solid line*. Each c represents a control monkey and each *C* an immobilized monkey. The net effect of immobilization is to shift the response curve far to the right. (Reprinted with permission from T.B. Ducker, M. Salcman, and H.B. Daniell: Surgical Neurology *10:* 71–76, 1978.)

combination of the two processes. When a compressed cord is examined grossly, one finds it to be edematous, soft, mushy, sometimes grayish-red, and constricted. The meningeal vessels are collapsed and often have undergone hyalization. The white matter demonstrates varying degrees of demyelination. The myelin sheath and axon cylinders are often fragmented, resulting in decreased axoplasmic flow (Davison, 1960).

Some recent experimental studies have been conducted to document the changes that accompany cord compression. Griffiths (1975), using ventrally placed intradural balloon catheters in dogs, examined the effects that acute and chronic compression had on the electrical conductivity and vascular permeability of the cord. He found that evoked potentials through the dorsal column stopped abruptly with acute compression. If the compression was released, these potentials reappeared within 5–15 min. The same was true for chronically applied compression, except the cessation of the evoked potential was delayed. There was marked leakage of Evans blue albumin from the intermediate gray matter in the acute compression. Chronic compression did not increase vascular permeability until after the compression was released, at which time it resembled that of the acute compression. Histologically, all of the animals demonstrated perivascular hemorrhages in the gray matter. Disruption of the gray matter neurophil was also seen. Neuronal degeneration characterized by pallor of staining and loss of the Nissl substances was noted. The white matter changes consisted of separation of the myelinated fibers and disruption of normal architecture. Other investigators have noted similar neurophysiological and anatomical changes (Brodkey et al., 1972) and showed that compression, in association with ischemia, produced an additive effect in cord pathology (Gooding et al., 1975). More recently, Kobrine et al. (1979) have presented further descriptions of the pathophysiology of cord compression. They conducted experiments with acute balloon compression of varying duration on monkey spinal cords. The disappearance and return of spinal cord evoked responses, as well as the spinal cord blood flow (SCBF) were measured. Figures 45.9–45.11 illustrate the varying patterns of these two parameters seen with different durations of compression. They concluded that the major pathological cause for the neural dysfunction seen with compression is physical injury of the neural membrane, irrespective of blood flow changes. They concluded further that the ability of that membrane to recover seems to be related to rapidity and length of time of compression and that focal blood flow changes may not be significant in this mechanism.

Consequently, treatment of spinal cord injuries should include diagnostic tests to demonstrate whether there exists any surgically amenable compression of the cord which, if treated, may result in a better recovery for that patient. This is especially true with incomplete cord lesions (i.e., sparing of some cord function), which have a better prognosis for return of neurologic function (Lucas and Ducker, 1979). The judicious use of plain x-rays, tomography, and myelography is how one identifies bone or soft tissue causing cord compression. If such compression is present, the appropriate surgical decompression can be performed. It should be noted that decompression does not necessarily mean laminectomy. If in a cervical fracture, bone and disc material are impinging ventrally on cord or nerve roots, then an anterior discectomy and/or corpectomy with fusion may be required. If the compression is located posteriorly, secondary to depressed fracture laminae and ligamentum flavum, a laminectomy may be called for. Finally, in thoracolumbar fractures, the insertion of Harrington rods may realign the spine and reduce fractured vertebrae, thus reducing compression. In other words, the decompressive procedure is specifically chosen on the basis of the nature and location of the compressive phenomenon (Saul and Ducker, 1981a).

How aggressive one should be in the use of myelography in acute cord injuries is not clear. The yield of improving the neurological outcome by various types of myelography and subsequent surgery is low. In selected causes, however, recovery is improved. Saul and Ducker (1981b) have reported 90 acute cervical cord-injured patients who underwent Pantopaque myelography; 23 of the patients had abnormal myelograms (seven complete blocks and 16 anterior filling defects); 12 of the 23 patients were operated upon; three of the patients showed greater neurological improvement (greater than 2 SD) based on predicted recovery rates (motor indices) of 500 previously studied patients (Lucas and Ducker, 1979). This represented 3.3% of the total patients studied. Although this is a small proportion, it may indicate that the aggressive approach is appropriate for certain cord injuries.

HEMODYNAMIC CHANGES

When the spinal cord is injured, hemodynamic changes take place that have a profound effect as to the pathological outcome of that lesion. These hemodynamic alterations involve the microscopic vasculature of the cord, as well as the microcirculation. Moreover, systemic hemodynamics may, in turn, effect the intrinsic cord alterations.

Grossly, when injury occurs, there are changes in the vascularity on the surface of the spinal cord. Sludging and stasis occur immediately but soon clear. There is transient disruption of the microscopic flow within vessels on the surface. Any rupture in the vascularity of the surface usually occurs where the capillaries join the veins. This junction forms a right angle as the capillary or small venule comes out of the cord to join this vein. Consequently, flame-shaped hemorrhages can be observed in this area. Surface vessels maintain their flow patterns for at least 12–24 hr. Thereafter, there is progressive traumatic dilation, especially of the veins. They can actually be observed increasing to two to four times their normal size. these observations may persist for several weeks (Assenmacher and Ducker, 1971).

On a more microscopic level, marked changes take place in spinal cord vasomotor responses, blood flow,

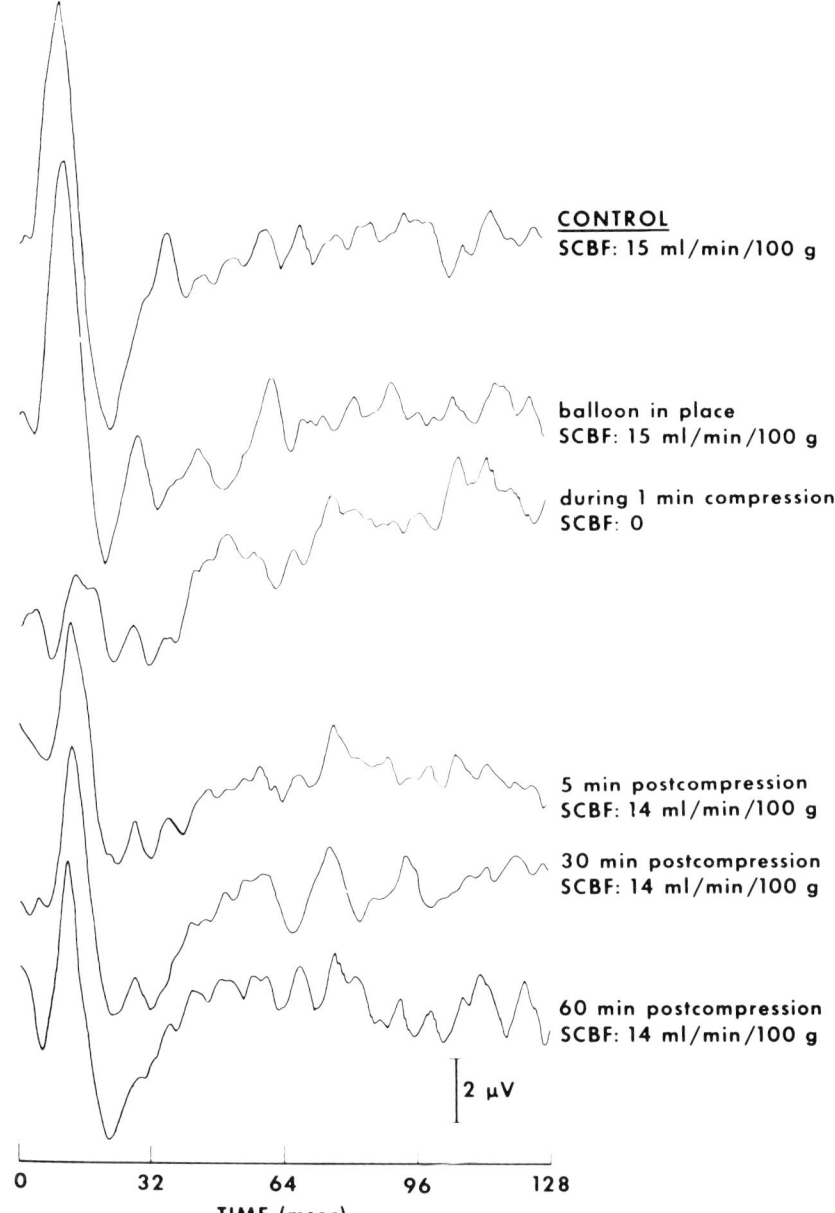

Figure 45.9. Multiple spinal evoked responses (SER) from an animal of the 1-min acute compression group. Note absence of the SER during compression and return of the SER at 5 min postcompression. Note absence of postcompression hyperemia. (Reprinted with permission from A.I. Kobrine, D.E. Evans, and H.V. Rizzoli: Journal of Neurosurgery 51:841–845, 1979.)

oxygen tension, and autoregulation. The vasomotor reactivity of the segment of injured cord is lost almost immediately after injury (Ducker and Kindt, 1971; Smith et al., 1978). As in the brain, increases in the partial pressure of carbon dioxide in arterial blood cause vasodilatation of the spinal cord vascularity and result in increased blood flow (Smith et al., 1969; Kindt et al., 1971). However, when the cord is injured, this response is impaired. In addition, Wagner et al. (1969) have demonstrated by fluorescent studies that circulation time is prolonged in the injured cord segment. The most marked increase is seen in the capillary and venous phases. This correlates with the direct observations of vessels noted by Ducker and Assenmacher (1969).

By using xenon saturation techniques to determine blood flow in the spinal cord, Ducker et al. (1978c) demonstrated a quantitative decrease in flow 2–3 hr after injury. Animals whose baseline spinal cord blood flow was reproducibly 10–20 ml/min/100 g of tissue had their cords traumatized by dropping a 50-g weight through a 10-cm tube. In the animals rendered paraplegic (clinical grade 0), the mean SCBF was initially 15 ml/min/100 g of tissue. Subsequent determinations showed that SCBF was 13 at 30 min postinjury, 9 at 1 hr, and 6 at 2 hr. When the animals were studied at 1 week, the SCBF was 4–5 ml/min/100 g of tissue (Table 45.1). The animals who were paraparetic (clinical grades 1 and 2) showed no significant difference in SCBF from the preinjury baseline measurements. Those animals that were clinically normal (clinical grades 3 and 4) after the cord injury demonstrated *increased* flow rates within 1 hr of the trauma (Table 45.1). In other words, graded clinical motor deficits seemed to parallel alterations in spinal cord blood flow (Fig. 45.12). A similar relationship was

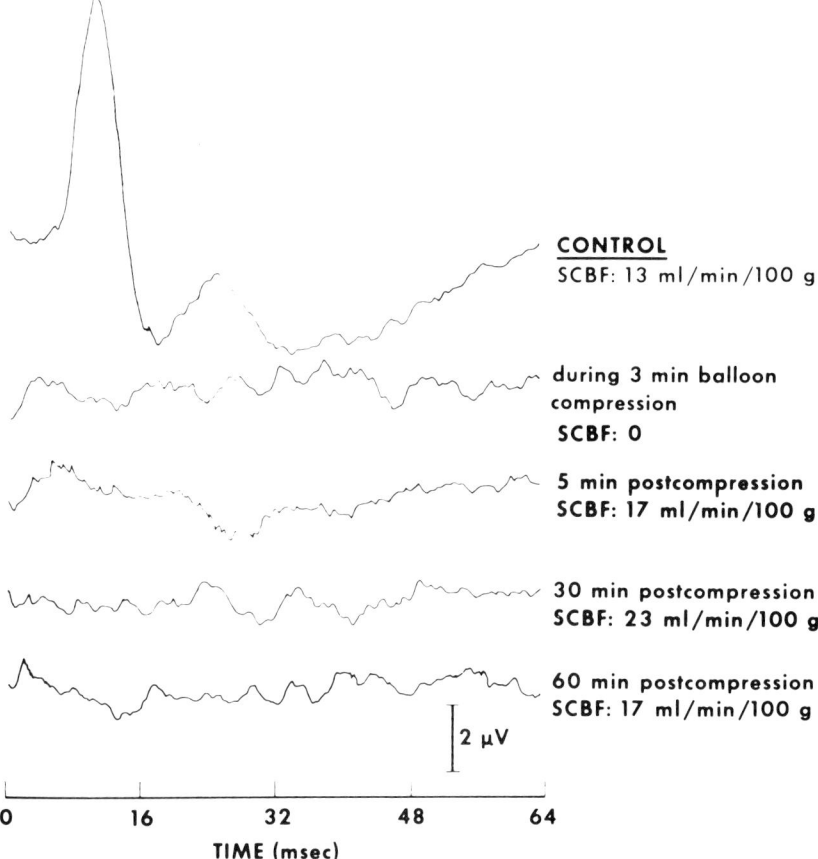

Figure 45.10. Multiple spinal evoked responses (SER) from an animal of the 3-min acute compression group. Note absence of the SER during compression, failure of the SER to return, and a postcompression hyperemia. (Reprinted with permission from A.I. Kobrine, D.E. Evans, and H.V. Rizzoli: Journal of Neurosurgery 21:841–845, 1979.)

found when spinal cord tissue oxygen was measured. The paraplegic animals demonstrated a general depression of tissue oxygen (Fig. 45.13). In the paraparetic animals, no clear pattern emerged. However, in the animals that recovered and moved normally, the tissue oxygen was high, and these vessels persisted for the week of study (Fig. 45.13).

The microangiographic studies of injured spinal cord blood vessels performed by Fairholm and Turnbull (1971) and Dohrman et al. (1973) complement the work by Ducker et al. Both of these studies indicate that there may be an initial ischemic phase for 5–15 min that involves both gray and white matter of the cord. Soon there are hemorrhagic areas within the gray matter. The vascularity there and in the white matter appears normal. Subsequently, peripheral white matter vessels are larger in size and numbers. As the pathophysiology evolves, there seems to be complete cessation of all flow within the central cord and a concomitant increase in vascularity in the periphery. The combination of central ischemia and peripheral hyperemia has also been demonstrated by other blood flow studies of Bingham et al. (1975a) and Kobrine et al. (1975).

The presence of autoregulation in the intact spinal cord has been demonstrated by several investigators (Kobrine et al., 1976; Griffiths, 1973). More recently, Smith et al. (1978) have demonstrated the loss of cord autoregulation. They have also observed these hyperemic states. They offered the theory, however, that the hyperemic may be a consequence of the vasomotor paralysis produced by a direct injury of the cord and vasculature. If hyperemia is associated with a breakdown in the blood-brain barrier, it may cause edema formation and secondary cord injury rather than being associated with better recovery, as Ducker suggested. Furthermore, Rawe et al. (1977b) demonstrated a direct relationship between the post-traumatic systemic blood pressure and cord pathology. Traumatic cord hemorrhages in cats were enhanced or retarded by raising or lowering the systemic blood pressure. They concluded that this further supported the post-traumatic loss of autoregulation and the deletrious effects abnormal blood pressure ranges could have on cord pathology. In 1979, Senter and Venes confirmed these findings when they demonstrated that in experimental cord injury, autoregulation is intact during the initial post-traumatic period and is then lost coincident with the onset of ischemia. They suggested that "maintenance of normal blood pressure during the post-traumatic period of 'spinal sympathetic shock' may be indicated in selective cases."

As one can see, the studies of the effect of trauma on spinal cord blood flow and its relationship to the resulting pathology and neurological deficit remain confusing. Some of the discrepancies of the various experimental reports are related to the difficulty in accurately recording SCBF. In fact, recently Senter and Venes (1978), through a modification of the hydrogen clearance techniques, demonstrated post-traumatic ischemia in the lat-

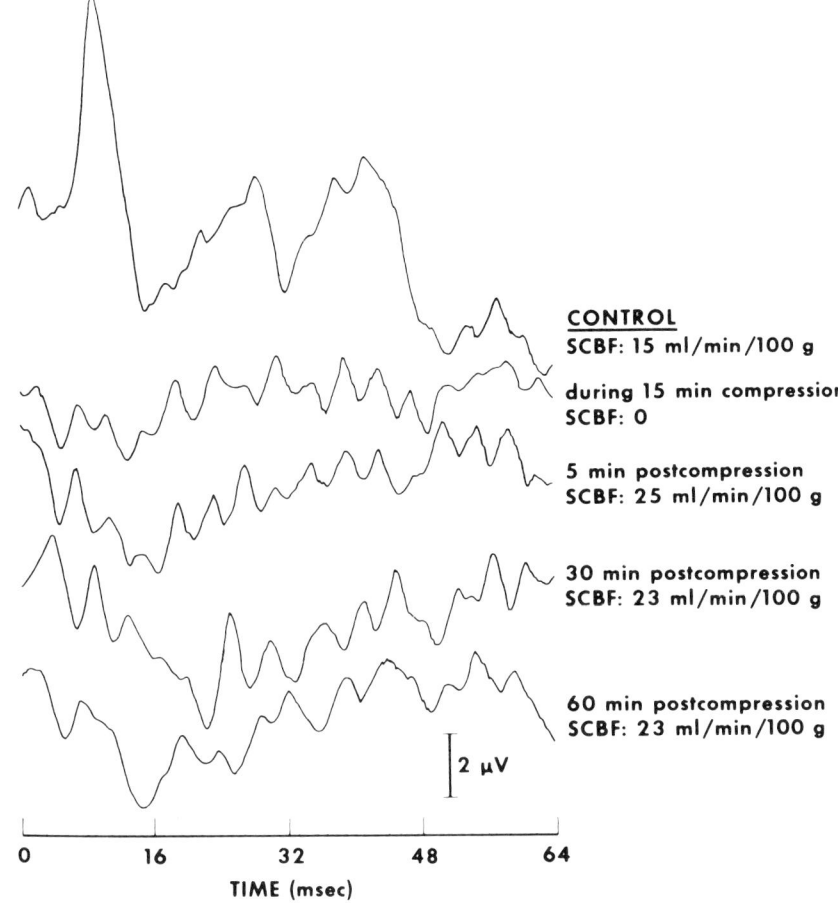

Figure 45.11. Multiple spinal evoked responses (SER) from an animal of the 15-min acute compression group. Notice absence of SER during compression, no return of the SER, and a postcompression hyperemia. (Reprinted with permission from A.I. Kobrine, D.E. Evans, and H.V. Rizzoli: Journal of Neurosurgery 51:841–845, 1979.)

eral white matter—something that has not been well established. They confirmed, however, that there is always a delay in the onset of these ischemic changes. It is probably safe to summarize by stating: 1) Following acute cord injury, there is a short delay before spinal cord blood flow diminishes to dangerous ischemic level. 2) The reduction of SCBF is more marked in the central gray cord than the peripheral white. 3) The loss of vasomotor responsiveness and autoregulation has a profound effect on the development of the pathological lesion. 4) Because of these losses, alterations of blood pressure can dramatically affect the evolution of the lesion. 5) Concomitant with these SCBF changes there are parallel changes in the tissue oxygen tension that will ultimately affect cord metabolic function.

These pathophysiological changes—although they are not completely delineated or understood—have important implications regarding the treatment of acute spinal cord injuries. Since all of these studies show a delay in the onset of the deleterious circulatory changes, strict attention should be paid immediately to assuring adequate spinal cord perfusion and oxygenation. This begins at the scene of the injury with the paramedic personnel. Intravenous lines should be inserted at the first convenient opportunity for vascular volume expansion in the event of hypotension. This may be necessary because of actual blood loss due to associated injuries or to vaso-

Table 45.1
Spinal Cord Blood Flow after Experimental Trauma and Its Relationship to Time and Clinical Grade of Animal[a]

Clinical Grade	No.	Mean Spinal Cord Blood Flow (ml/min/100 gm tissue) before and at Various Times after Spinal Cord Injury				
		Baseline	30 min	1 hr	2 hr	1 week
0 (paraplegic)	4	15	13	9	6	4–5
1 & 2 (paraparetic)	6	14	14	17	17	15–16
3 & 4 (normal or near normal)	4	15	16	26	27	25–26

[a] From Ducker et al., 1978b.

motor paralysis from the cord injury itself. Disruption of descending sympathetic pathways results in loss of vasomotor tone and subsequent hypertension. Concomitantly, the unopposed parasympathetic activity causes a bradycardia in face of hypotension (Table 45.2). Cervical cord injuries cause paralysis of intercostal respiration. Under these conditions, the patient is prone to respiratory distress and hypoxia on the basis of: 1) inability to clear secretions; 2) inability to cough or sigh; 3) development of apnea, secondary to loss of diaphragmatic

Figure 45.12. Spinal cord blood flow versus time in monkeys with graded clinical deficits. Mean spinal cord blood flows pre- and postinjury have been plotted in cc/min/100 g of tissue for three groups of animals: paraplegics (grade 0), paraparetics (grades 1 and 2), and normal or walking animals (grades 3 and 4). An initial increase in blood flow is seen, and this is maintained at 168 hr. (Reprinted with permission from T.B. Ducker, M. Salcman, J.T. Lucas et al.: Surgical Neurology 10:64–70, 1978.)

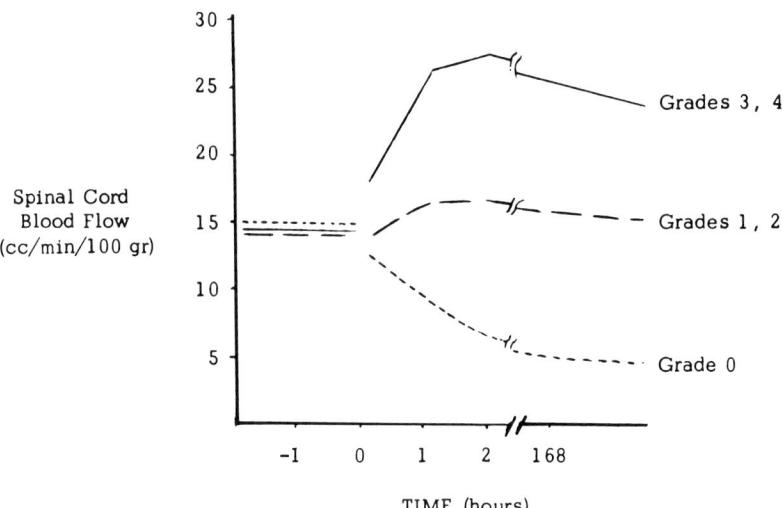

Figure 45.13. Spinal cord tissue oxygen versus time in monkeys with graded clinical deficits. Mean tissue oxygens (PO_2) pre- and postinjury are plotted in mm Hg for three groups of animals: paraplegic or severely paraparetic (grades 0 to 1), moderately paraparetic (grade 2), and animals able to walk (grade 3). Those in the best and worst groups showed a respective increase or decrease in tissue oxygen, and this was maintained at 168 hr. (Reprinted with permission from T.B. Ducker, M. Salcman, J.T. Lucas et al.: Surgical Neurology 10: 64–70, 1978.)

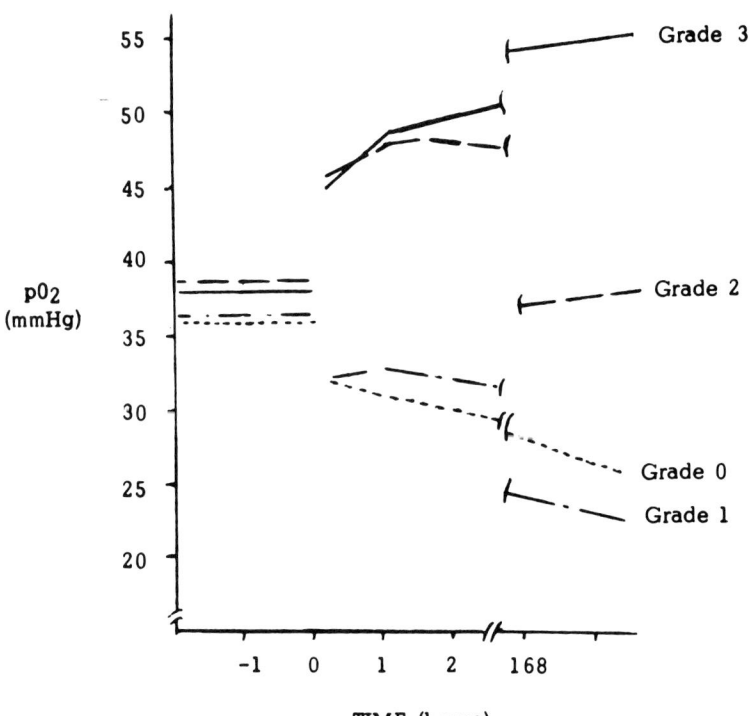

Table 45.2
Frequently Observed Vital Signs in Central Nervous System Trauma

Head injury	BP[a]	P
Increased intracranial pressure	BP	P
Hypovolemic shock	BP	P
Spinal cord injury	BP	P

[a] *BP*, blood pressure; *P*, pulse.

innervation if spinal cord edema involves the upper cervical segments (C3–C5). Therefore, in the treatment of these patients, the protocol should call for meticulous pulmonary therapy, including frequent suctioning, chest physiotherapy, and oxygen administration to maintain normal arterial blood gases. Careful nasotracheal intubation should be performed if the measures above do not effectively support the patient. A nasogastric tube should be inserted to prevent abdominal distension secondary to a paralytic ileus. If untreated, this can result in unwanted vomiting and aspiration; also, respiratory embarrassment can occur due to upward displacement of the diaphragm. It should be noted that all of these initial therapeutic interventions are aimed at optimizing spinal cord oxygenation and perfusion.

From a pharmacological point of view, there is at present no drug that is known to effectively alter this aspect of the pathophysiology of cord injury. Ducker et al. (1978a) could demonstrate no significant beneficial effect on experimental cord injury by using dextran, phenobarbital, methyldopa, phenoxybenzamine, or vasopressors. Killen et al. (1965) also did not find dextran to be helpful in cord injury, even though theoretically—by decreasing sludging and blood viscosity—there should be an increase in arterial bed perfusion. Antifibrinolytic agents such as ε-aminocaproic acid (Amicar) have also been studied (Brodner et al., 1977; Campbell et al., 1974). The rationale for these agents is that they interfere with the proteolytic enzymes that lead to spread of hemorrhagic necrosis. However, these studies do not demonstrate any significant efficacy.

The antiedema and diuretic agents have been associated with a higher degree of efficacy than other drugs. Theoretically, these agents break up the chain of events described as follows: injury leads to ischemia, which leads to necrosis, which leads to edema, which leads to more injury, etc. Mannitol as an osmotic diuretic decreases spinal cord edema rapidly (Yashon, 1978; Parker et al., 1973). Corticosteroids are probably the most widely accepted agents in use. Ducker and Hamit (1969) showed statistically significant improvement and recovery of neurological function associated with dexamethasone in experimental canine studies of incomplete cord injury. The exact mechanisms by which steroids reduce cord edema or improve cord functions remain debated. Moreover, whether steroids are beneficial in the real clinical setting is not settled. Nonetheless, most centers employ steroids in the treatment of acute cord injuries. The dosage used varies from center to center and, at the present time, there is a national randomized study being conducted by the National Institute of Health to compare the response to high dose verses low dose steroids in a large number of cord-injured patients. The present authors recommend the following scheme: dexamethasone, 1 mg/kg/day, or methylprednisolone, 5 mg/kg/day, in divided doses. It is our opinion that, if a cord injury is complete and remains so for 2–3 days, the steroid therapy should be stopped because the risks of continuous steroid treatment (i.e., gastrointestinal bleeding, hyperglycemia, interference with wound healing) may outweigh possible benefits, which are unlikely if not improvement is seen within 3 days. However, in patients with incomplete cord lesions or who are showing neurological improvement, steroid treatment is continued for 1 week and then the dose is tapered quickly.

Dimethyl sulfoxide (DMSO) is a solvent that has been studied and found to have some properties that may be beneficial in treating spinal cord injuries. DMSO appears to diminish adhesiveness and aggregation of platelets and thrombus formation in blood vessels; there is a diuretic effect, as well as an anti-inflammatory effect associated with DMSO. It is also possible that one of the effects is to increase oxygen diffusion in injured tissue (Jacob and Herschler, 1974). Experimental paralysis in dogs injured by a 500 g-cm force has been reversed with DMSO administration (de la Torre et al., 1975). Some clinical trials are presently being conducted to determine the efficacy of this agent.

In 1969, Hartzog et al. reported recovery from experimentally induced paraplegia in baboons treated with hyperbaric oxygen therapy. Kelly et al. (1972) also reported that tissue PO_2 in traumatized spinal cords of dogs was significantly increased by hyperbaric oxygen treatments and that neurological recovery in the animals was greater than control groups. Hyperbaric oxygen therapy increases the tissue oxygen and decreases the tissue edema. Both of these effects would theoretically be advantageous during the early phase after spinal cord injury. Yeo (1976) confirmed this therapeutic effect of hyperbaric oxygen in paraplegic sheep. To date, there are no human trials reported regarding the efficacy of this modality. These are being conducted. At the present time, a randomized double-blind study employing this therapy on cord injuries is being conducted at the Shock Trauma Unit at the University of Maryland.

Albin et al. (1963, 1967, 1968, 1969) introduced early operative localized cooling (hypothermia) of the injured spinal cord. The temperature reduction theoretically decreases metabolic activity, increases ischemic and hypoxic tolerance and possibly reduces inflammation and edema. Ducker and Hamit (1969) confirmed Albin's studies but pointed out that the good results with hypothermia did not differ significantly from those obtained using steroids. Theinprasit et al. (1975) demonstrated an impressive functional recovery rate in cats whose cords were traumatized, resulting in paraplegia and loss of cortical evoked response for more than 6 hr postinjury. The animals treated with laminectomy and cooling recovered enough to be able to walk, compared with inability to walk in both the control animals and those treated with laminectomy alone. The literature contains only small numbers of human trials of local hypothermia (Bricolo et al., 1976; Blume, 1973; White et al., 1972). Many questions remain unanswered regarding this form of treatment. In particular, are the cases of reported beneficial effects truly complete spinal cord lesions? If not, spontaneous and gradual improvement is possible regardless of treatment (Schneider et al., 1973). The fact is that although local hypothermia has theoretical validity, experimental efficacy, and a number of strong advocates, it has not found wide acceptance and implementation among most neurosurgeons. The reasons are mainly that the technique requires a large expenditure of time, personnel, and equipment, and the results are not significantly better than with other forms of therapy. Normothermic perfusion of experimentally injured animal cords has been shown to be as effective as hypothermic perfusion (Tator and Deeke, 1973).

BIOCHEMICAL DERANGEMENTS

In 1972, Osterholm and Matthews (1972a and b) demonstrated a multifold increase in norepinephrine (NE) concentrations within injured spinal cords. They theorized that these substances gain access to spinal cord smooth muscle vascular receptor site and produce vasospasm, ischemia, hypoxia, and subsequent tissue necrosis. These reports excited much interest in the biochemistry of spinal cord injury. Since then, much has been delineated regarding the cellular and ultrastructural changes in cord injuries; however, no effective therapeutic interventions have resulted.

Prior to Osterholm's work, Locke et al. (1971) demonstrated increased lactate levels in injured spinal cord tissue. This was consistent with the known ischemic changes and increase in anaerobic metabolism. Prompted by Osterholm's findings, other investigators began looking at these processes. Hedeman et al. (1974) were unable to confirm the elevation of NE within injured cord tissue. Neither did Naftchi et al. (1974) or Bingham et al. (1975b). Rawe et al. (1977a) also were unable to find elevated levels in injured cords. Furthermore, animals treated with α-methyltyrosine (which interferes with NE synthesis) showed no improvement. Rawe et al. (1978) felt that systemic blood pressure changes mediated by α-adrenergic activity immediately post-trauma had more etiological significance than tissue NE levels. At present, there remains controversy over the role of catecholamine in the production of the pathology seen with spinal cord injury.

The blood-brain barrier (BBB) is the central nervous system's device for keeping itself clean and free of toxic substances. Normally, it allows only oxygen, sugar, and a few select amino acids to cross over into CNS tissue. However, Vise et al. (1974) demonstrated injury to the BBB in spinal cord trauma. They used Evans blue as a fluorescent tracer and demonstrated neuronal staining and extravasation of this tracer into the neuropil of injured canine spinal cords. When the BBB is defective, as they demonstrated, blood-borne substances have access to cord tissue. The significance of this was implied by Tator and Deeke (1973) in their study on normothermic perfusion of the injured spinal cord. They showed that normothermic perfusion of injured monkey spinal cord had a beneficial effect on recovery rates. They theorized that one of the mechanisms could be a "dialysis of noxious substances from the injured cord." What these toxic substances might be was not discussed except for mentioning the proposed catecholamine theory and possibly lactate and other ischemic metabolic products.

Prompted by this attention to the biochemistry of spinal cord injury, some investigators began to examine the changes at the cellular and organelle level. Kao and Chang (1977) demonstrated massive accumulation of lysosomes and release of lysosomal hydrolases in canine spinal cords completely transected by a subpial microscopic technique. They demonstrated that the lysosomal activity peaks for 3-7 days and is associated with autolysis and subsequent cavitation of the cord stumps. Ito et al. (1978) demonstrated mitochondrial alterations as an early manifestation of experimental spinal cord injury. They showed a drop in cytochrome oxidase activities in the center of the traumatic site. Cytochrome oxidase is the terminal and rate-limiting enzyme of the electron transport series and is located on the inner membrane of the mitochondria. Furthermore, Clendendon et al. (1978) showed prompt and significant decrease at the center of the site of experimental cord trauma of $(Na^- + K^+)$-activated ATPase. This enzyme is thought to be localized to the plasma membrane of cells. These studies support the idea that irreversible spinal cord injury may be related to damage to the cell membranes and subsequent metabolic derangements. The etiology of the membrane damage remains an enigma. Some hypotheses include: 1) altered platelet function via abnormal free radical productions (Brody et al., 1974); 2) disruption of long chain fatty acid moieties of membrane phospholipids due to free radical reactions (Kimelberg and Papahadjopoulos, 1974; Milvy et al., 1973).

These investigations into the biochemical derangements accompanying spinal cord injury have not produced any well accepted therapeutic panacea. What they have accomplished is to direct our thinking toward metabolic and biochemical manipulations as possible therapies.

Strict attention should be directed to maintaining the patient in good homeostatic balance. Avoiding high energy consumption states such as fever, infection, and extreme agitation may be appropriate. Endogenous or exogenous toxins should be minimized. This is important since the BBB is known to be defective. Therefore, infection with subsequent sepsis should be warded off. The use of pharmacological agents that may have an adverse effect on cord functions should be avoided. Attempts have been made to reduce the metabolic requirements and activity in the injured cord. This is one of the principles of local hypothermia as discussed previously. Barbiturate therapy has been shown to decrease metabolic rate in CNS tissue (Crane et al., 1978; Pierce et al., 1962). Moreover, barbiturates also are believed to have a membrane stabilization effect by inhibiting the deleterious free radical reactions (Flamm et al., 1979). This has also been shown experimentally with DMSO (Jacob and Herschler, 1974). Steroids are also thought to have some membrane protective effect, thus reducing edema formation. More recently, Senter et al. (1979) have demonstrated alteration of post-traumatic cord ischemia by γ-hydroxybutyrate (GHB), or central nervous system depressant. It is hypothesized that the GHB may interfere with the release of vasoactive substances through depressed central nervous system activity. It has also been shown that GHB can normalize tissue levels of high energy phosphates in hypoxic rat brains (MacMillan, 1978).

ANCILLARY SYSTEMIC CHANGES

This chapter would not be complete if some mention was not made of the changes in other organ systems that are caused by cord injury, which, in turn, can affect the function of that injured cord. These will be discussed according to systems.

Pulmonary

As mentioned earlier, in cervical and high thoracic cord injuries, the patient's respiratory pattern is altered and at risk to such things as developing apnea, atelectasis, pneumonia, etc. Furthermore, pulmonary embolus is a very real danger to cord-injured patients during their hospitalization. Active physical therapy with frequent range of motion of all extremities is an important aid in preventing this. The use of anticoagulants is advocated by some (Guttman, 1973; Silver and Moulton, 1976); others feel it is not warranted (Watson, 1974). Whatever course is chosen, a high index of suspicion is required, and aggressive diagnostic evaluation should be employed if the clinical situation is compatible with this potentially fatal complication. In the patient's acute phase, pulmonary edema is a not uncommon finding. This can result from autonomic changes within the pulmonary system itself as a result of cord transection. It can also be caused by large amounts of fluid replacement in treating hypotension that may be on the basis of peripheral vasomotor paralysis, also secondary to cord transection. It should be emphasized that all of these pulmonary changes can result in hypoxia, sepsis, fever, etc., which can have adverse effects on the already compromised cord function.

Genitourinary

After the acute phase of injury, the patient should be started on a program of intermittent bladder catheterization to prevent bladder dysfunction secondary to overdistension and also to prevent infection that could lead to sepsis and primary renal diseases. Early urological consultation will provide a proper regimen and antibiotic coverage.

Gastrointestinal

Patients should be started on a reasonable bowel regimen of stool softeners and laxatives to maintain good bowel function. When steroids are used, antacids and/or Cimetedine should also be used. Gastrointestinal hemorrhage can be a fatal complication in the cord-injured patient. However, it should also be remembered that the hypotension and debilitation resulting from this complication can hinder cord healing. Abdominal disease accounts for 10% of all fatalities in cord-injured patients (Yashon, 1978). A perforated viscus with peritonitis is most common. The sensory deficit makes the routine abdominal examination virtually useless. Certain clinical signs should draw one's attention to the possibility of this impending disaster. Persistent nausea and vomiting, tachycardia or bradycardia when the pulse has been normal, and pain in the shoulder or clavicular regions referred from subdiaphragmatic irritation may all be signs of intra-abdominal problems. If any of these occur, one should perform the appropriate diagnostic tests.

Skin Care

Special measures for meticulous skin care should be instituted when the patient arrives. Infection and subsequent sepsis from decubitis that form may impede a patient's progress. Paralyzed, anesthetic body parts should be moved and repositioned at least every 2 hr. Specialized foam or rubber mattresses or horizontally rotating frames should be employed. Skin should be washed, massaged, and powdered at least once a day. Bedding should always be dry. Meticulous perineal and sacral skin care is obligatory.

Table 45.3

Spinal Cord Insult	Therapeutic Intervention
Mechanical insults	
Direct tissue disruption	Prevention only; regeneration techniques remain experimental.
Movement of injured spine and cord	Immediate immobilization followed by surgical stabilization or long term (3–6 months) skeletal traction.
Persistent extradural cord compression	Diagnostic myelography in selected cases. If compression is demonstrated, appropriate surgical decompression may be indicated. This should be accompanied by a pretreatment stabilization procedure if required. (The overall efficacy of immediate myelography has not yet been clearly established.)
Hemodynamic changes	
Deminished spinal cord blood flow, loss of autoregulation, and systemic vasomotor paralysis	Maintain normotensive systemic blood pressure for optimum cord perfusion.
Diminished tissue oxygen	Maintain excellent oxygenation: administer O_2; active pulmonary therapy to avoid pneumonia atelectasis; mechanical ventilation if necessary; avoid pulmonary complications: pulmonary embolus, pneumothorax, infection, etc.; reduce cord edema: steroids (generally accepted); DMSO, local hypothermia, hyperbaric O_2 therapy (experimental).
Biochemical derangements	
Accumulation of norepinephrine at site of injury (controversial)	No well accepted therapy; experimental work includes: barbiturates, DMSO, GHB, steroids, local hypothermia, hyperbaric O_2, adrenergic blockers. Also, avoid high energy consumption states: fever, sepsis, agitation.
Defective blood-brain barrier	
Membrane and organelle injury	
Ancillary systemic insults	
Pulmonary complications	Meticulous, aggressive nursing care.
Urinary complications	
Skin complications	

SUMMARY

The treatment of acute spinal cord injury should be directed toward the various types of insults that are known to be part of the pathophysiology creating the neurological deficit. Table 45.3 summarizes what we have presented. At the present time, preventing the cord injury is the only treatment for the initial irreversible tissue disruption that occurs at the time of injury. The remainder of any current treatment protocol consists of minimizing secondary injuries to spinal cord tissue that occur as a result of inadequate immobilization, continued spinal cord compression, and poor oxygenation and blood flow. The goal is to optimize the environment in order to allow the spinal cord to recover as much as possible, depending on the severity of the initial injury.

The experimental work that is being conducted in the areas of biochemical and cellular manipulations as well as regenerative studies are to be encouraged in hopes that in the future a protocol may be adopted that is directed to reversing some of the neurological deficits.

Finally, physicians and researchers in all medical disciplines should encourage and promote public and personal safety standards whenever possible. If we do not, we will continue to experience the high incidence of needless death and disability secondary to spinal injuries.

References

Albin, M.S., White, R.J., and MacCarty, C.S.: Effects of sustained perfusion cooling of the subarachnoid space. Anesthesiology 24:72–80, 1963.

Albin, M.S., White, R.J., Locke, G.S., et al.: Localized spinal cord hypothermia. J. Int. Anesth. Res. Soc. 46:8–16, 1967.

Albin, M.S., White, R.J., Acosta-Rua, G.J., et al.: Study of functional recovery produced by delayed localized cooling after spinal cord injury in primates. J. Neurosurg. 24:113–130, 1968.

Albin, M.S., White, R.J., Yashon, D., et al.: Effects of localized cooling on spinal cord trauma. J. Trauma 9:1000–1008, 1969.

Assenmacher, D.R., and Ducker, T.B.: Experimental traumatic paraplegia: The vascular and pathologic changes seen in reversible and irreversible spinal cord lesions. J. Bone Joint Surg. 53:671–680, 1971.

Bingham, W.C., Goldman, H., Friedman, S.J., et al.: Blood flow in normal and injured monkey spinal cord. J. Neurosurg. 43:162–171, 1975a.

Bingham, W.R., Ruffulo, and Friedman, S.: Catecholamine levels in the injured spinal cord of monkeys. J. Neurosurg. 42:174, 1975b.

Blume, H.: Management of acute spinal cord injuries with local hypothermia and decompression. Presented at the Fifth International Congress of Neurological Surgeons, Tokyo, 1973. Excerpta Med. Int. Congr. Ser. 293:194, 1973.

Bricolo, A., Alle Ore, G., DaPian, R., et al.: Local cooling in spinal cord injury. Surg. Neurol. 6:101–106, 1976.

Broadkey, J.S., Richards, D.E., Blasingame, J.P., et al.: Reversible spinal cord trauma in cats: Additive effects of direct pressure and ischemia. J. Neurosurg. 37:591–593, 1972.

Brodner, R.A., Vangilder, J.C., and Collins, W.F.: The effect of antifibrinolytic therapy in experimental spinal cord trauma. J. Trauma 17:48–54, 1977.

Brody, T.M., Akera, T., Baskin, S.I., et al.: Interaction of Na-K ATPase with chlorpromazine for radical and related compounds. Ann. N.Y. Acad. Sci. 242:527–542, 1974.

Campbell, J.B., DeCrescito, V., Tomasula, J.J., et al.: Effects of antifibrinolytic and steroid therapy on the contused spinal cord of cats. J. Neurosurg. 40:726–733, 1974.

Clendenon, N.R., Allen, N., Gordon, W.A., et al.: Inhibition of Na^+-K^+ activated ATPase activity following experimental spinal cord trauma. J. Neurosurg. 49:563–568, 1978.

Crane, P.D., Braun, L.D., Cornford, E.M., et al.: Dose dependent reduction of glucose utilization by phenobarbital in rat brain. Stroke 9:12–18, 1978.

Davison, C.: General pathological considerations in injuries of the spinal cord. In *Injuries of the Brain and Spinal Cord and Their Covering*, edited by S. Brock, ch. 17, pp. 515–517. Springer, New York, 1960.

de la Torre, J.C., Kawanga, H.M., Rowed, D.W., et al.: Dimethyl sulfoxide in central nervous system trauma. Ann. N.Y. Acad. Sci. 243:362–389, 1975.

Dohrmann, G.T., Wagner, F.C., and Bucy, P.C.: The microvasculature in transitory traumatic paraplegia: An electron microscopic study in the monkey. J. Neurosurg. 35:263–271, 1971.

Dohrmann, G.J., Wick, K.M., and Bucy, P.C.: Spinal cord blood flow patterns in experimental traumatic paraplegia. J. Neurosurg. 38:52–58, 1973.

Ducker, T.B.: Experimental injury of the spinal cord. In *Handbook of Clinical Neurology*, vol. 25, edited by P. J. Vinken and G. W. Bruyn, ch. 2, pp. 9–26. Elsevier, New York, 1976.

Ducker, T.B., and Assenmacher, D.: The microvascular response in experimental spinal cord trauma. Surg. Forum 20:428–430, 1969.

Ducker, T.B., and Hamit, H.F.: Experimental treatments of acute spinal cord injury. J. Neurosurg. 30:693–697, 1969.

Ducker, T.B., and Kindt, G.W.: The effect of trauma on the vasomotor control of spinal cord blood flow. Curr. Top. Surg. Res. 3:163–171, 1971.

Ducker, T.B., Kindt, G.W., and Kempe, L.G.: Pathological findings in acute experimental spinal cord trauma. J. Neurosurg 35:700–708, 1971.

Ducker, T.B., Salcman, M., and Daniell, H.B.: Experimental cord trauma. III. Therapeutic effect of immobilization and pharmacologic agents. Surg. Neurol. 10:71–76, 1978a.

Ducker, T.B., Salcman, M., Lucas, J.T., et al.: Experimental spinal cord trauma. II. Blood flow, tissue oxygen, evoked potentials in both paretic and plegic monkeys. Surg. Neurol. 10:64–70, 1978b.

Ducker, T.B., Salcman, M., Perot, P.L., et al.: Experimental spinal cord trauma. I. Correlation of blood flow, tissue oxygen and neurologic status in the dog. Surg. Neurol. 10:60–63, 1978c.

Fairholm, D. J., and Turnbull, I.M.: Microangiographic study and experimental spinal cord injuries. J. Neurosurg. 35:277–286, 1971.

Feringa, E.R., Kowalski, T.F., Vahlsing, H.L., et al.: Enzyme treatment of spinal cord transected rats. Ann. Neurol. 5:203–206, 1979.

Flamm, E.S., Demopoulos, H.B., Seligman, M.L., et al.: Barbiturates and free radicals. In *Neural Trauma*, edited by A. J. Papp, R. S. Bourke, L. R. Nelson, et al., pp. 289–296. Raven Press, New York, 1979.

Freeman, L.W., MacDougall, J., Turbes, C.C., and Bowman, D.E.: The treatment of experimental lesion of the spinal cord of dogs with trypsin. J. Neurosurg. 17:259–265, 1960.

Gooding, M.R., Wilson, C.B., and Hoff, J.T.: Experimental cervical myelopathy: Effects of ischemic and compression of the canine cervical spinal cord. J. Neurosurg. 43:9–17, 1975.

Griffiths, I.R.: Spinal cord blood flow in dogs: The effect of blood pressure. J. Neurol. Neurosurg. Psychiatry 36:914–920, 1973.

Griffiths, I.R.: Vasogenic edema following acute and chronic spinal cord compression in the dog. J. Neurosurg. 42:155–165, 1975.

Guth, L.: History of CNS regeneration research. Exp. Neurol. 48:3–15, 1975.

Guth, L., Bright, D., and Donati, E.J.: Functional deficits and anatomical alterations after high cervical spinal hemisection in the rat. Exp. Neurol. 58:511–520, 1978.

Guth, L., Albuquerque, E.X., Deshpande, S.S., et al.: Enzyme therapy does not promote regeneration in the transected spinal cord of the rat. In press, 1979.

Guttman, L.: *Spinal Cord Injuries: Comprehensive Management and Research*, ch. 9, pp. 86–88. Blackwell Scientific Publications, London, 1973.

Hartzog, J.T., Fischer, R.G., and Snow, C.: Spinal cord trauma: Effect of hyperbaric oxygen treatment. Proc. Annu. Clin. Spinal Cord Injury Conf. 17:70, 1969.

Hedeman, L.S., and Sil, R.: Studies in experimental spinal cord trauma. part II. Comparison of treatment with steroid, low molecular weight dextran and catecholamine blockade. J. Neurosurg. 40:44–52, 1974.

Hedeman, L.S., Shellenberger, M.K., and Gordon, J.H.: Studies in experimental spinal cord trauma. Part I. Alterations in catecholamine levels. J. Neurosurg. 40:37–44, 1974.

Ito, T., Allen, M., and Yashon, D.: A mitochondrial lesion in experimental spinal cord trauma. J. Neurosurg. 48:434–442, 1978.

Jackson, R.R.: The Russian experience. Spinal Cord Injury Digest 1:3–4, 1979.

Jacob, S.W., and Herschler, R.: Biological actions of dimethyl sulfoxide. In *Conference on the Biological Action of Dimethyl Sulfoxide*. New York Academy of Science, New York, 1974.

Kao, C.C., and Chang, L.W.: The mechanisms of spinal cord cavitation following spinal cord transection. Part I. A correlated histochemical study. J. Neurosurg. 46:197–209, 1977.

Kelly, D.L., Lassiter, K.Z.L., Von Svivut, A., et al.: Effects of hyperbaric oxygenation and tissue oxygen studies in experimental paraplegia. J. Neurosurg. 36:425–429, 1972.

Killen, D.A., Edwards, R.H., Tinsley, E.A., et al.: Effects of low molecular weight dextran, heparin CSF drainage, and hypothermia on ischemic injury of the spinal cord, secondary to mobilization of the thoracic aorta from the posterior parietec. J. Thorac. Cardiovasc. Surg. 50:882–886, 1965.

Kimelberg, H.K., and Papahadjopoulos, D.: Effects of phospholipid-acyl chain fluidity phase transections, and cholesterol on Na^+-K^+-stimulated adenosine triphosphatase. J. Biol. Chem. 449:1071–1080, 1974.

Kindt, G.W., Ducker, T.B., and Huddlestone, J.: Regulation of spinal cord blood flow. In *Brain and Blood Flow*, edited by R. W. Ross Russell, pp. 401–405. Pitman Medical and Scientific Publishing, New York, 1971.

Knowles, J.F., and Berry, M.E.: Effect of enzyme treatment of CNS lesions in rats. Exp. Neurol. 59:450–454, 1978.

Kobrine, A.I., Doyle, T.F., and Martins, A.N.: Local spinal cord blood flow in experimental traumatic myelopathy. J. Neurosurg. 42:144–149, 1975.

Kobrine, A.I., Doyle, T.F., and Rizzoli, H.V.: Spinal cord blood flow as affected by changes in systemic arterial blood pressure. J. Neurosurg. 44:12–15, 1976.

Kobrine, A.I., Evans, D.E., Rizzoli, H.V.: Experimental acute balloon compression of the spinal cord: Factors affecting disappearance and return of the spinal evoked response. J. Neurosurg. 51:841–845, 1979.

Locke, G.E., Yashon, D., Feldman, A., et al.: Ischemia in primate spinal cord injury. J. Neurosurg. 34:614–617, 1971.

Lucas, J.T., and Ducker, T.B.: Motor classification of spinal cord injuries with mobility, morbidity and recovery indices. Am. Surg. 45:151–158, 1979.

MacMillan, V.: The effects of gamma-hydroxybutyrate and gamma-butycolactone upon energy metabolism of the normoxic and hypoxic rat brain. Brain Res. 146:177–180, 1978.

Matinian, L.A., and Andreasian, A.S.: Enzyme therapy in organic lesions of the spinal cord. Akademia Nauk American SSr, p. 94, 1973. (English translation: Brain Information Service, University of California, Los Angeles, p. 156, 1976.)

Milvy, P., Kakari, S., Campbell, J.B., et al.: Paramagnetic species and radical products in cat spinal cord. Ann. N.Y. Acad. Sci. 222:1102–1111, 1973.

Naftchi, N.E., Demeny, M., DeCrescito, V., et al.: Biogenic amine concentrations in traumatized spinal cords of cats: Effect of drug therapy. J. Neurosurg. 40:52–58, 1974.

Osterholm, J.L., and Matthews, G.J.: Altered norepinephrine metabolism following experimental spinal cord injury. Part I. Relationship to hemorrhagic necrosis. J. Neurosurg. 36:386–394, 1972a.

Osterholm, J.L., and Matthews, G.J.: Altered norepinephrine metabolism following experimental spinal cord injury. Part II. Protection against traumatic spinal cord hemorrhagic necrosis by norepinephrine synthesis blockage with alpha-methyl tyrosine. J. Neurosurg. 36:395–401, 1972b.

Parker, A.J., Park, R.D., and Stowater, J.L.: Reduction of trauma-induced edema of spinal cord in dogs given mannitol. Am. J. Vet. Res. 34:1355–1357, 1973.

Pettegrew, R.K.: Trypsin inhibition of scar formation in cordotomized rats. Anat. Res. 184:501, 1976.

Pierce, E.C., Lambertsen, C.J., Duetsch, S., et al.: Cerebral circulation and metabolism during thicopental anesthesia and hyperventilation in mean. J. Clin. Invest. 41:1664–1671, 1962.

Rawe, S.E., Roth, R.H., Boadle-Biber, M., et al.: Norepinephrine levels in experimental spinal cord trauma. Part I. Biochemical study of hemorrhagic necrosis. J. Neurosurg. 46:342–349, 1977a.

Rawe, S.E., Roth, R.H., and Collins, W.F.: Norepinephrine levels in experimental spinal cord trauma. Part II. Histopathological study of hemorrhagic necrosis. J. Neurosurg. 46:350–356, 1977b.

Rawe, S.E., Lee, W.A., and Perot, P.L.: The histopathology of experimental spinal cord trauma: The effect of systemic blood pressure. J. Neurosurg. 48:1002–1007, 1978.

Saul, T.G., and Ducker, T.B.: The spine and spinal cord. In *Early Care of the Injured Patients*, ed. 3. W. B. Saunders Philadelphia, in press, 1981a.

Saul, T.G., Carol, M., and Ducker, T.B.: Immediate minimyelogram in acute cervical cord injury (abstract). Am. Surg., in press, 1981b.

Schneider, R., Crosby, E., Russo, H., et al.: Traumatic spinal cord syndromes and their management. Clin. Neurosurg. 20:424–492, 1973.

Senter, H.J., and Venes, J.L.: Altered blood flow and secondary injury in experimental spinal cord trauma. J. Neurosurg. 49:569–578, 1978.

Senter, H.J., and Venes, J.L.: Loss of autoregulation and posttraumatic ischemia following experimental spinal cord trauma. J. Neurosurg. 50:198–200, 1979.

Senter, H.J., Venes, J.L., and Kauer, J.S.: Alteration of posttraumatic ischemia in experimental spinal cord trauma by a central nervous system depressant. J. Neurosurg. 50:207–216, 1979.

Silver, J.Z., and Moulton, A.: Prophylactic anticoagulant therapy against pulmonary embolus in acute paraplegia. Br. Med. J. *2:*338–340, 1976.

Smith, A.L., Pender, J.W., and Alexander, S.C.: Effects of PCO_2 on spinal cord blood flow. Am. J. Physiol. *216:*1158–1163, 1969.

Smith, A.J., McCreery, D.B., Bloedel, J.R., et al.: Hyperemia, CO_2 responsiveness and autoregulation in the white matter following experimental spinal cord injury. J. Neurosurg. *48:*239–251, 1978.

Tator, C.H., and Deeke, L.: Value of normothermic perfusion, hypothermic perfusion, and decotomy in the treatment of experimental acute spinal cord trauma. J. Neurosurg. *39:*52–64, 1973.

Thienprasit, P., Bantli, H., Bloedel, J.R., et al.: Effect of delayed local cooling on experimental spinal cord injury. J. Neurosurg. *42:*150–154, 1975.

Truex, R.C., and Carpenter, M.B.: *Human Neuroanatomy.* Williams & Wilkins, Baltimore, 1970.

Vise, W.M., Yashon, D., and Hunt, W.E.: Mechanisms of norepinephrine accumulations within sites of spinal cord injuries. J. Neurosurg. *40:*76–82, 1974.

Wagner, F.C., Taslitz, N., White, R.J., et al.: Vascular phenomena in the normal and traumatized spinal cord. Anat. Rec., 163–281, 1969.

Watson, N.: Anticoagulant therapy in the treatment of venous thrombosis and pulmonary embolism in acute spinal injury. Paraplegia *12:*197–201, 1974.

White, R.J., Yashon, D., Albin, M.S., et al.: The acute management of cervical cord trauma with quadriplegia. Presented at the Annual Meeting of the American Association of Neurological Surgeons. Boston, 1972.

Windle, W.F.: Regeneration of axons in the vertebrate CNS. Physiol. Res. *36:*427–440, 1956.

Windle, W.F., Clemente, C.D., and Chambers, W.W.: Inhibition of formation of a glial barrier as a means of permitting a peripheral nerve to grow into the brain. J. Comp. Neurol. *96:*359–370, 1952.

Wolman, L.: Axon regeneration after spinal cord injury. Paraplegia, *4:*175–188, 1966.

Yashon, D.: *Spinal Injury.* Appleton-Century-Crofts, New York, 1978.

Yeo, J.D.: Treatment of paraplegic sheep with hyperbaric oxygen. Med. J. Aust. *1:*538–540, 1976.

Section 4

Vascular Insufficiency

EDITORS' SUMMARY

In their chapter, Garcia and Conger discuss the subcellular pathophysiology of cerebral ischemia syndromes, collectively known under the epidemiologic designation of "stroke." Much has been learned in recent years concerning this pathophysiology; perhaps most importantly, as a result of Garcia's work, is the knowledge that changes in the central nervous system parallel those in other organs, with some important differences, such as the difference in response between the astrocyte and the neuron. One of the central problems in understanding the pathophysiology and probably in designing treatments is the importance of the "no reflow" effect. We would obviously stress a role for calcium in this regard, perhaps through action on the cytoskeletal elements.

Another point that has been made repeatedly through this volume is that there is a very great difference between total and partial or temporary ischemia in the brain. Perhaps this is more important in the brain than in other organs. Most strokes are the result of regional or localized brain ischemia in contrast to global ischemia, which is not occlusive, e.g., after cardiac arrest.

The chapter by Mergner and Schaper reviews the cell and organelle aspects of reaction to injury in the myocardium during infarction. The authors critically review the relevant literature and place particular emphasis on a synthetic analysis of changes during the early phase and at the "point-of-no-return." They emphasize that myocardial infarction induces cell alterations in three different systems: the microvasculature; the Purkinje fibers and conduction system; and the myocardial muscle cells proper.

The review thoroughly analyzes the wealth of literature on the subject as well as the difficulty in answering several pivotal questions related to the precise pathophysiology. Among the central issues discussed by the authors is the potential role of calcium-activated phospholipases which, according to several lines of evidence in the heart as well as in other ischemic cells, play a key role in the loss of reversibility. Even if such is the case, the precise role and location of the important phospholipases in these events remain uncertain. Candidates include those within the mitochondria (possibly outer membrane), those associated with the endoplasmic reticulum and the plasma membrane, and those within the lysosomes. The question of lysosomal leakage of enzymes and their potentially harmful effects has been explored for many years in many tissues, but the relationship of this to cell injury remains uncertain.

Although many different models of myocardial anoxia and ischemia are available for study, none of them has proven to be perfect and the authors attempt to utilize the best features of each to develop an integrated analysis. One of the key questions, for example, is the reason for the difference between global and regional ischemia in the myocardium (see also Ch. 46). The more seemingly relevant model to human acute myocardial infarction is the regional occlusion model, but many complications with regard to border zones, presence and absence of collaterals, and differences in reflow still elude exact description. Additionally, this area needs much better interspecies comparisons. Another key question, which is also discussed in the chapter by Reimer and Jennings (Ch. 9), is the issue of whether cell membrane leakage, which could rapidly accentuate universal injury, occurs prior to or after irreversible mitochondrial damage. Many of the arguments relevant to this dilemma are discussed. Among the many problems is the possible reactivation of the plasmalemma sodium-potassium ATPase following ischemia. Although fatty acid oxidation is deficient and lipid accumulates in some regions of myocardial infarctions, the organelle responsible for this is not known, though it is clear that lipid accumulation is a reversible cellular change. However, based on current data concerning the role of peroxisomes in oxidation of lipids, the relationship of these organelles to this change should be more thoroughly investigated.

A review of attempts to assemble these principles and observations into plans for successful therapeutic interventions constitute the last part of the author's paper. Most of the presently available interventions for reducing the size of myocardial infarction have not really addressed the question of how to inhibit progression of subcellular change—whether or not alternate substrates, membrane protective agents or high energy compounds including ATP could be delivered to an ischemic area and if so would they have an effect remain as further questions for the future.

In his chapter, Roberts reviews the extent of coronary artery narrowing in fatal acute myocardial ischemia. This subject has long been studied in a totally qualitative or semiquantitative fashion, but the present authors, for the first time, performed quantitative studies. These studies reveal the percentage of the internal lengths that are narrowed greater than 75% and percentage of lengths narrowed to lesser degrees. The paper summarizes autopsy in sudden coronary death, clinically isolated unstable angina pectoris, and acute myocardial infarction. Patients with clinically isolated unstable angina had the most extensive coronary narrowing with 48% of the 5 mm long segments 76–100% narrowed, while those with acute myocardial infarction and sudden cardiac deaths had similar but less coronary narrowing. Among the patients studied, those with the least amount of myocardial damage, i.e., angina pectoris, had the most severe degree of coronary narrowing, while those with the severest degree of myocardial damage had less severe coronary narrowing. Findings such as these could explain problems in demonstrating improved survival with coronary bypass procedures in severe angina patients, since less severe coronary narrowing is associated more with myocardial infarction than with angina. Clearly many more studies of this type are needed with better functional correlations if we are to devise more rational interventions.

Muller reviews the current state-of-the-art of myocardial infarction treatment. This is a thorough and thoughtful review which includes all steps from prehospital coronary care to the clinical aspects of diagnosis and treatment in each stage and the complications of each stage.

Considerable data are presented concerning new approaches to the prevention and treatment of myocardial infarction, including efforts designed to prevent the fixed and variable obstructions which result in myocardial ischemia as well as efforts directed toward limitations of the size of the infarct. Among the newer considerations producing variable as opposed to fixed coronary obstruction are platelet aggregations, vascular spasm, and vascular thrombosis. Each of these has received considerable attention.

Platelet aggregation either through direct occlusion or through release of powerful vasoconstrictors including thromboxane A2 may represent important initiating events. Some data using sulfinpyrazone, an inhibitor of platelet function, suggest that we may obtain reduced mortality from sudden death in patients with myocardial infarction. Data are still accumulating on the value of putative antiplatelet therapy with aspirin. Spasm of a coronary artery may be responsible for myocardial infarction. This may be related to the efficacy of nitroglycerin intervention and to that of a new class of potent coronary vasodilators including nifedipine, which interferes with the slow calcium channels essential for contraction of smooth muscle cells. Nifedipine is extremely effective, for example, in Prinzmetal's angina. A multicenter study is underway to look at its long-term effects.

The role of coronary thrombosis still is debated because it is very difficult to determine in any particular case if thrombus was primary or secondary to occurrence of platelet aggregates. In any case, surgical as well as nonsurgical interventions designed to minimize thrombosis including fibrinolytic agents may be useful in the future.

Finally, a variety of methods have been shown to reduce infarct size in experimental animals and some are now under study in patients. These include hyaluronidase, corticosteriods, nonsteroidal antiinflammatory agents such as Ibuprofen, and agents such as isoproterenol which increase infarct size by increasing oxygen demand and others, such as verapamil, which decrease infarct size by decreasing demand. One of the problems in studying interventions in humans is current limitations on precise, early assessment of infarct size, and the difficulties of following the future course. Much more work is needed both on enzymatic methods and on scanning techniques.

At the present time, most of these interventions are still regarded as experimental, though certain principles are recommended by Muller. These include minimizing oxygen demand, avoiding tachycardia, avoiding vasodepressors such as dopamine which cause large increases in myocardial oxygen demand, and, as noted, avoiding isoproterenol. Oxygen still seems to be valuable, since even in the absence of hypoxemia, studies indicate the increased oxygen concentrations limit infarct size even without a significant increase in arterial oxygen content.

CHAPTER 46

Pathology and Pathophysiology of Cerebral Ischemia

JULIO H. GARCIA
KARL A. CONGER

The condition of insufficient blood supply to the central nervous system and, more specifically, to the brain may have the clinical expression of an abrupt, unexpected neurologic deficit, e.g., tingling sensation in the fingers of one hand. This sudden complaint could be secondary to either localized or regional circulatory disturbances, which are known under the epidemiologic designation of *stroke*. The retrospective analysis of a large number of these occurrences has revealed that the vast majority (80%) of strokes are due to localized ischemic injuries, caused by the occlusion of arterial vessels.

Nonischemic strokes develop on the basis of bleeding into either the brain parenchyma (10%) or hemorrhages into the subarachnoid space (3%).

A second variety of circulatory injury to the brain and spinal cord has a diffuse (multifocal) distribution; because of this, a designation of "global circulatory disturbance" has been proposed (Garcia et al., 1975). Some of the causes of global ischemia include: hypotension, shock, cardiac arrest, pulmonary embolism, seizures, and probably blunt head trauma. With the exception of the seizure and trauma cases, the clinical expression of global brain ischemia may be generally designated as *syncope*. In addition to establishing the nature of the mechanism as being either *regional* ischemia, which can be induced by either arterial or venous occlusions, or *global* ischemia, it is important to establish whether the circulatory impairment is either permanent or temporary. Irreversible global ischemia is synonymous with somatic death and is characterized, in its early stages, by relatively moderate and homogeneous cellular changes. Temporary global ischemia, as it exists after episodic cardiac arrest of a few minutes' duration, is reflected in heterogeneous and extensive structural abnormalities, most of which probably develop during the reperfusion period.

The consequences of regional ischemia on the organ architecture are traditionally called *infarction*, particularly once the ischemic injury has become irreversible and the lesion is apparent either to naked eye inspection or to examination by palpation. There is no appropriate noun to designate the wide variety of tissue changes that are seen after temporary global ischemic injuries; the designation of "laminar necrosis" applies only to late occurring cortical changes, which may be absent in some cases, while it ignores structural abnormalities in basal ganglia, cerebellum, and brainstem. Since one of the earliest consequences of any type of brain ischemia is the development of softening (possibly as a consequence of increased water content), it is suggested that the term acute *malacia* be used to designate the anatomical consequences of all types of ischemia. The localized or regional type of encephalomalacia would be the result of a vascular occlusion, whereas diffuse, multifocal encephalomalacia is almost always the result of systemic circulatory disorders. Occlusive arterial factors—such as multiple, simultaneous emboli—could cause bilateral, diffuse, focal areas of softening. However, in contrast to the lesions of global ischemia, brain softenings of embolic origin are asymmetrical in both their size and topographic distribution.

From the above it can be deduced that the pattern of organ injury can vary significantly, depending upon the type of ischemia affecting the brain. No attempt is made in this chapter to cover a large variety of other systemic injuries, which are caused by lowered arterial oxygen tension and known under the designation of hypoxemia. *Ischemia* is defined as a condition in which blood flow is insufficient to support tissue metabolic demands, and this insufficiency is expressed in failure of organ function. The ensuing discussion will analyze the events that take place in various forms of ischemia and stroke; particular emphasis will be given to factor(s) that may determine the various cellular responses observed under several types of ischemia.

Table 46.1 has been modified from a previous publication (Garcia, 1975) and represents a classification of diverse forms of ischemic injury.

Single arterial or venous occlusions induce ischemia,

which is incomplete in almost any organ, but particularly in the brain, because of the abundance of collateral connections that exist in normal human and animal brains (Kamijyo and Garcia, 1975). Thus, it is common to demonstrate, in either humans or animals, that complete interruption of anterograde flow in an occluded artery is followed by prompt retrograde filling of the vessel through the end-to-end anastomoses that connect collateral vessels.

Evidence of the incomplete nature of the ischemia is also derived from cerebral blood flow (CBF) measurements (Morawetz et al., 1978), as well as from the observation that massive increases in wet weight occur after arterial and venous occlusions (Bremer et al., 1978).

Nonocclusive ischemia, e.g., after cardiac arrest, is incomplete in the sense that it is transient or temporary. In this form of injury, tissue swelling may also play an important role in the progression of the lesion, particularly when such swelling affects large portions of the brain. Swelling induces brain volume increases that raise the intracranial pressure and interfere with blood supply, thereby inducing further ischemia.

REGIONAL OR LOCALIZED BRAIN ISCHEMIA

This is one of the most common types of ischemic injury encountered in humans. Ischemic strokes are, in most patients, but a manifestation of a diseased cardiovascular system. Therefore, ischemic strokes are more frequent in persons afflicted with cardiac disease of any kind (congenital defects excluded) and in patients with congenital or acquired vascular disease, e.g., saccular aneurysms and atherosclerosis.

The single most important risk factor for both cerebral

Table 46.1
Causes of Cerebral Ischemia

Vascular occlusions
  Arterial
  Venous
  Simultaneous occlusion of arteries and veins
Nonocclusive circulatory disorders
  Hypotension, shock, temporary cardiac arrest, blunt trauma to the head, status epilepticus

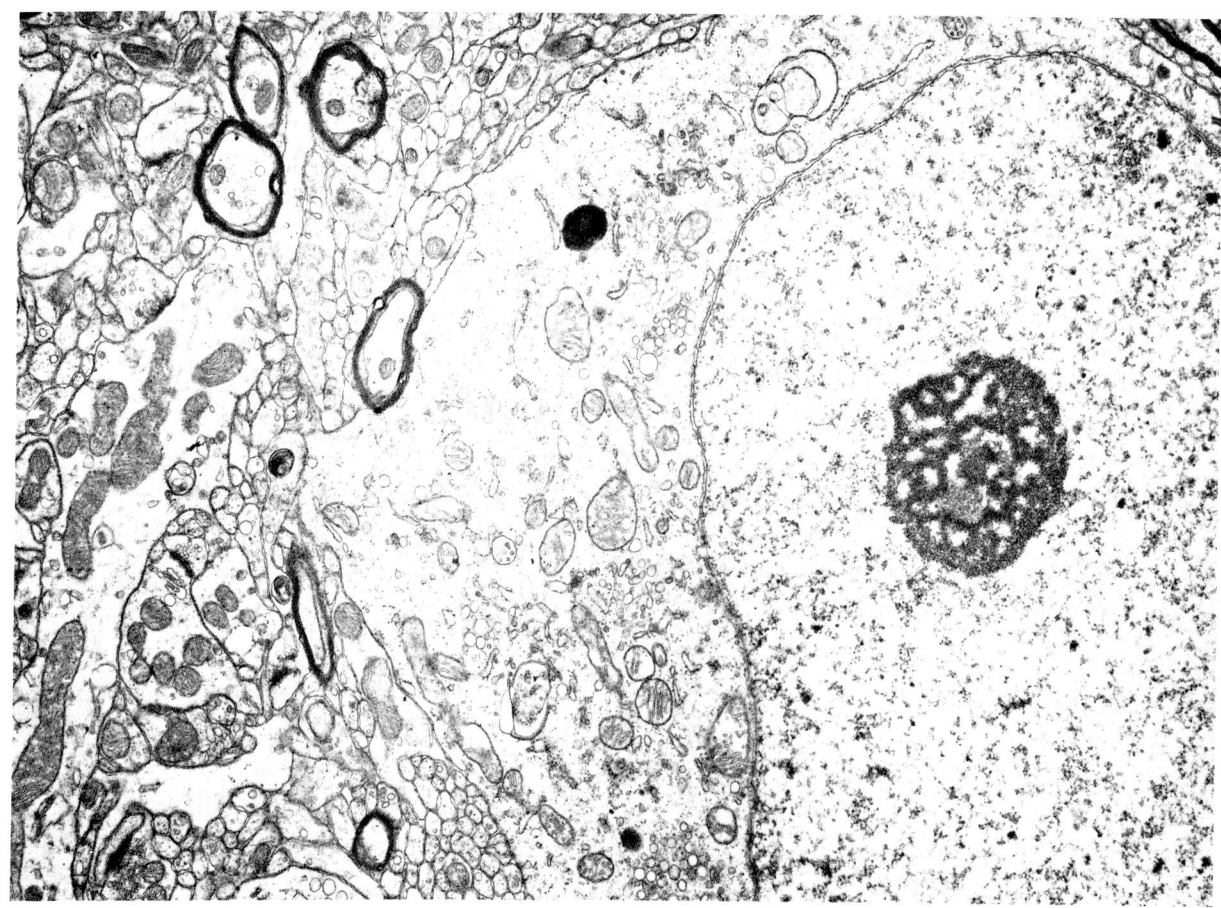

Figure 46.1. Caudate nucleus from rhesus monkey with 6-hr-old occlusion of the middle cerebral artery. This neuronal perikaryon, identified by its large nucleolus and synaptic contacts (not shown in the picture) shows minimal alterations consisting of clearing of cytosol and enlarged volume of nucleus and cytoplasm. Note the increased number of astrocytic mitochondria at extreme *left*. (Original magnification ×5000.)

infarction and brain hemorrhage is systemic hypertensive disease.

Ischemic stroke becomes clinically apparent in one of three ways: 1) transient neurologic deficits, also called TIA, that usually last less than a few hours; 2) progressively worsening neurologic deficit; and 3) completed or nonprogressive stroke. The occurrence of the first clinical variety, i.e., TIA, is a clear indication that some types of cell injury, secondary to focal decreases in CBF, are completely reversible. Although these transient episodes are generally attributed to temporary embolic phenomena, absolute proof of their etiologic mechanism is lacking at present. Fisher (1976) is of the opinion that several features of some TIAs are incompatible with the postulated embolic etiology.

A study of the natural course of ischemic stroke in 180 hospitalized patients showed: 1) no change in the initial neurologic deficit (39%), 2) gradual improvement (35%), and 3) either worsening or remitting-relapsing course in 26% of the cases. Decreased level of consciousness and hemiplegia were associated with a fatal outcome in higher numbers than in patients without these deficits (Jones and Millikan, 1976).

There is no laboratory or contrast study that reflects accurately the evolution of ischemic stroke; the most sensitive and accurate method to appraise the progression of the syndrome is the periodic clinical evaluation of the neurologic deficit (Halsey, 1976).

The analysis of the biological phenomena that ultimately lead to an infarction, that is, to an irreversible lesion, requires the use of an experimental model in which a reproducible lesion can be induced in a predictable area. This is necessary in order to complete prospective analysis of the abnormalities that ultimately lead to an infarction.

On the basis of its relevance to the human condition of ischemic stroke, the experimental model of middle cerebral artery (MCA) occlusion in subhuman primates has been adopted by numerous investigators (Moossy, 1979). Two methods for occluding this vessel have been described: 1) transorbital clipping, a technique that has the advantage of allowing occlusion of the vessel in a reversible manner (Hudgins and Garcia, 1970); and 2) embolization with either silastic material or autologous blood clots (Molinari, 1979).

The common observation that MCA occlusion in

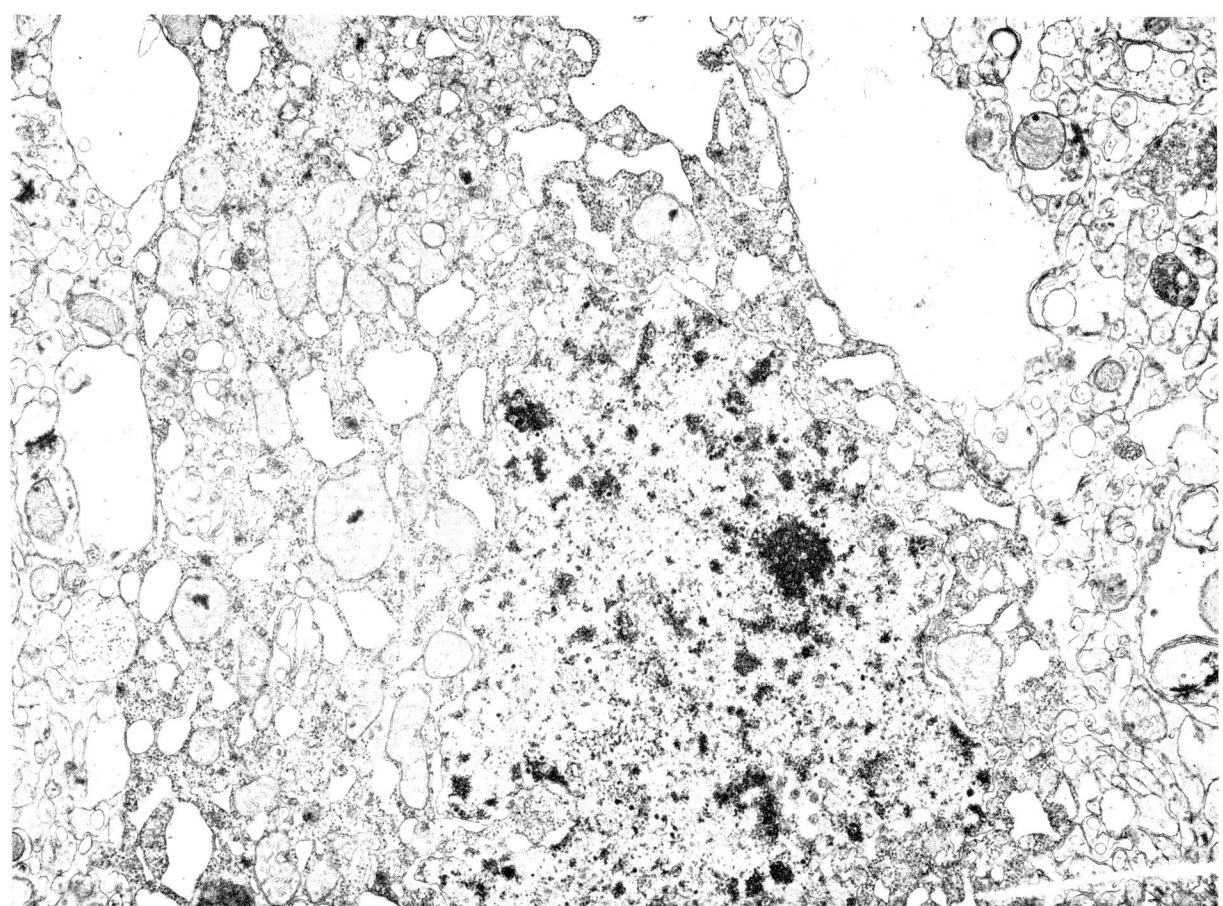

Figure 46.2. Insular cortex from same rhesus monkey as in Fig. 46.1. The type of neuronal abnormality illustrated here is entirely different. Nucleoplasm and cytosol show marked increases in electron density, except for the cisternal endoplasmic reticulum. Note the densities in the inner matrix of the neuronal mitochondria and the swollen astroytic processes around the neuronal perikaryon. (Original magnification ×6,000.)

awake animals leads to instantaneous contralateral deficit, which may or may not disappear spontaneously, has been explained by the fact that the circulatory deficit is promptly compensated by the collateral circulation (Morawetz et al., 1978). Perhaps more intriguing are the observations that brain tissues made ischemic for periods of several minutes recover previously lost functions when circulation is re-established by reopening the vessel (Astrup et al., 1977; Morawetz et al., 1978).

Thus, several questions may be raised by these observations: 1) What are the tolerable limits of occlusive arterial ischemia in humans or animals? 2) What is the nature of the abnormalities responsible for the initial loss of function, and which of these are fully reversible by reperfusion? 3) What determines the irreversibility of the lesion?

The answer to the first question is probably modified by a number of diverse factors, such as age of the animal, body temperature at the time of occlusion, vascular anatomy of the brain, and general cardiovascular condition of the subject. However, it is significant that most healthy subhuman primates subjected to up to 2 hrs of arterial occlusion recover completely, after a 3-hr reperfusion time, in terms of both regional CBF values and disappearance of the neurologic deficit induced by the arterial occlusion (Morawetz et al., 1978).

The nature of the abnormalities developing acutely, i.e., during the immediate postocclusive state, has been analyzed by structural and dynamic means and may be artificially separated into changes affecting: 1) neuronal perikaryon, 2) axis cylinders and myelin sheaths, 3) astrocytes and other glial elements, and 4) capillaries and intraparenchymal vessels.

Some *neuronal perikarya* show marked alterations in mitochondrial volume with massive swelling of inner matrix and rupture of cristae; other neuronal perikarya exhibit profound shrinkage and increased electron density (Garcia et al., 1977; Little et al., 1974). In addition, otherwise intact neurons may be "disconnected" from their afferent input through various mechanisms that include perineuronal astrocytic swelling and swelling of synaptic terminals (Garcia et al., 1979). Several observations confirm that the responses of individual neurons are highly variable even when they are adjacent to one

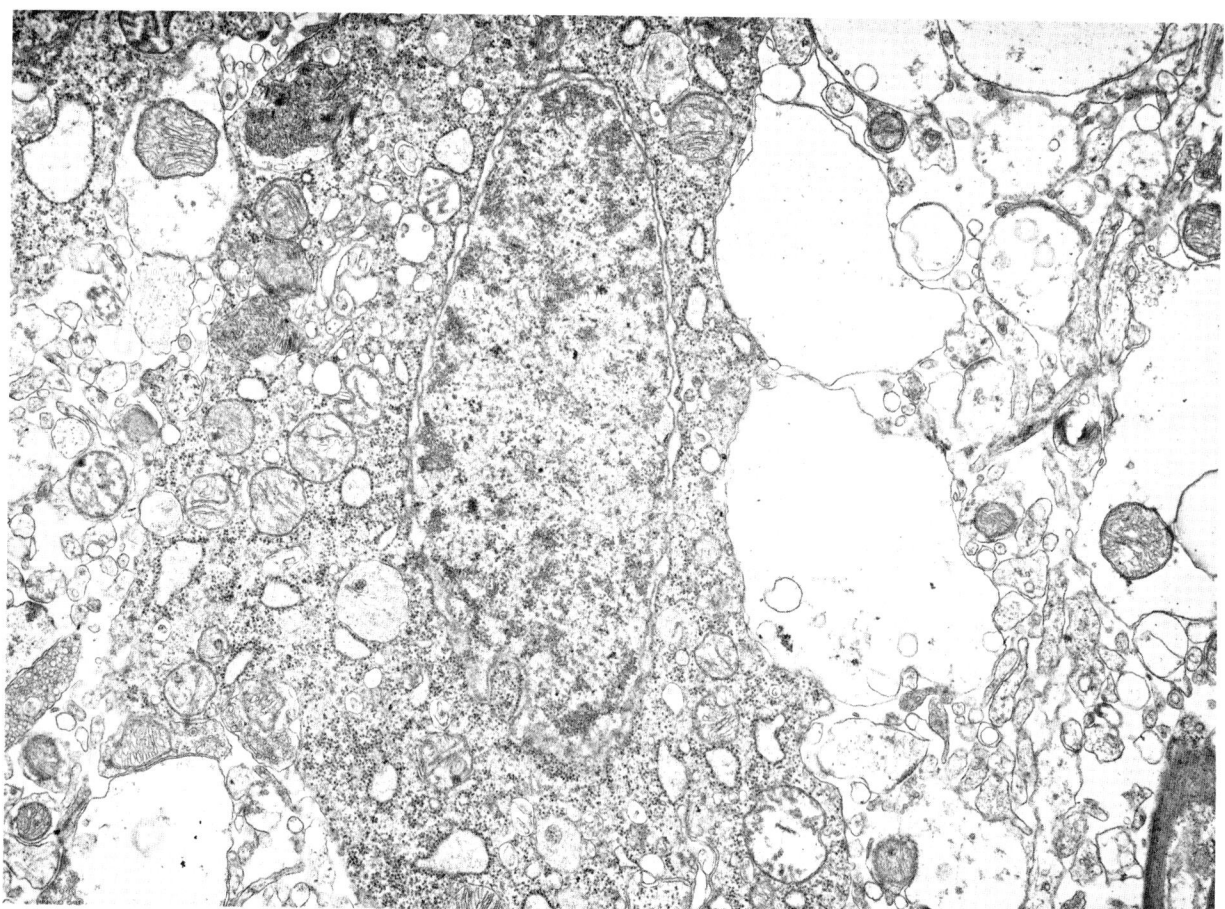

Figure 46.3. Insular cortex from rhesus monkey whose middle cerebral artery remained occluded for 5 hr. The nature of the structural abnormalities visible in this cell is different from that seen in several other neurons injured by the same method. However, it is not possible to decide whether the degree of injury is more or less advanced. (Original magnification ×6,000.)

another, and some have suggested that these individual responses may be determined by the intrinsic metabolic state of each cell (Garcia et. al., 1978) (Figs. 46.1–46.4).

Axis cylinders located in certain areas, e.g., internal capsule, show massive swelling during the acute stage of regional ischemia, at a time when the myelin sheaths are intact (Garcia et al., 1979). These axonal increases in volume develop in the absence of mitochondrial alterations, and it is possible that efferent impulses may be inhibited by this abnormality. Whether there exists a physical connection between the shrunken, "dark" neuronal perikarya and the swollen, lucent axis cylinders remains to be determined. Other changes in axonal ultrastructure, occurring as a consequence of focal ischemia, include increases in neurofilaments and, eventually, fragmentation of plasma membranes (Garcia et al., 1980) (Figs. 46.5–46.8).

In response to acute and incomplete ischemia, *astrocytes* develop massive increases in volume and marked electrolucency that affect both the nucleus and perikaryon; in contrast to neuronal mitochondria, there is no swelling of astrocytic mitochondria in response to ischemia (Garcia et al., 1977) (Figs. 46.9 and 46.10). Although necrosis of some astrocytes becomes apparent after sufficiently prolonged forms of incomplete ischemia, the majority of astroglial elements seemingly thrive under ischemic conditions. Increased numbers of astrocytic nuclei, sometimes in close apposition to one another, are interpreted as signs of cell division. *Oligodendrocytes*, as well as *myelin sheaths*, remain ultrastructurally unchanged after prolonged, incomplete forms of ischemia (Garcia et. al., 1977). The number of microglial nuclei in areas of temporary ischemia continues to increase several days after the episode of ischemia (Neuwelt et al., 1978), suggesting that division of these cells is also stimulated by incomplete blood perfusion.

Capillaries and other components of the microcirculation have been implicated in the pathogenesis of progressive tissue injury after a short episode of ischemia. The initial postulate that the earliest ischemic damage affected mostly capillary endothelium has been proven incorrect by ultrastructural studies (Garcia et al., 1971). The possibility that there may be mechanical obstruction of capillary lumina has also been eliminated by experi-

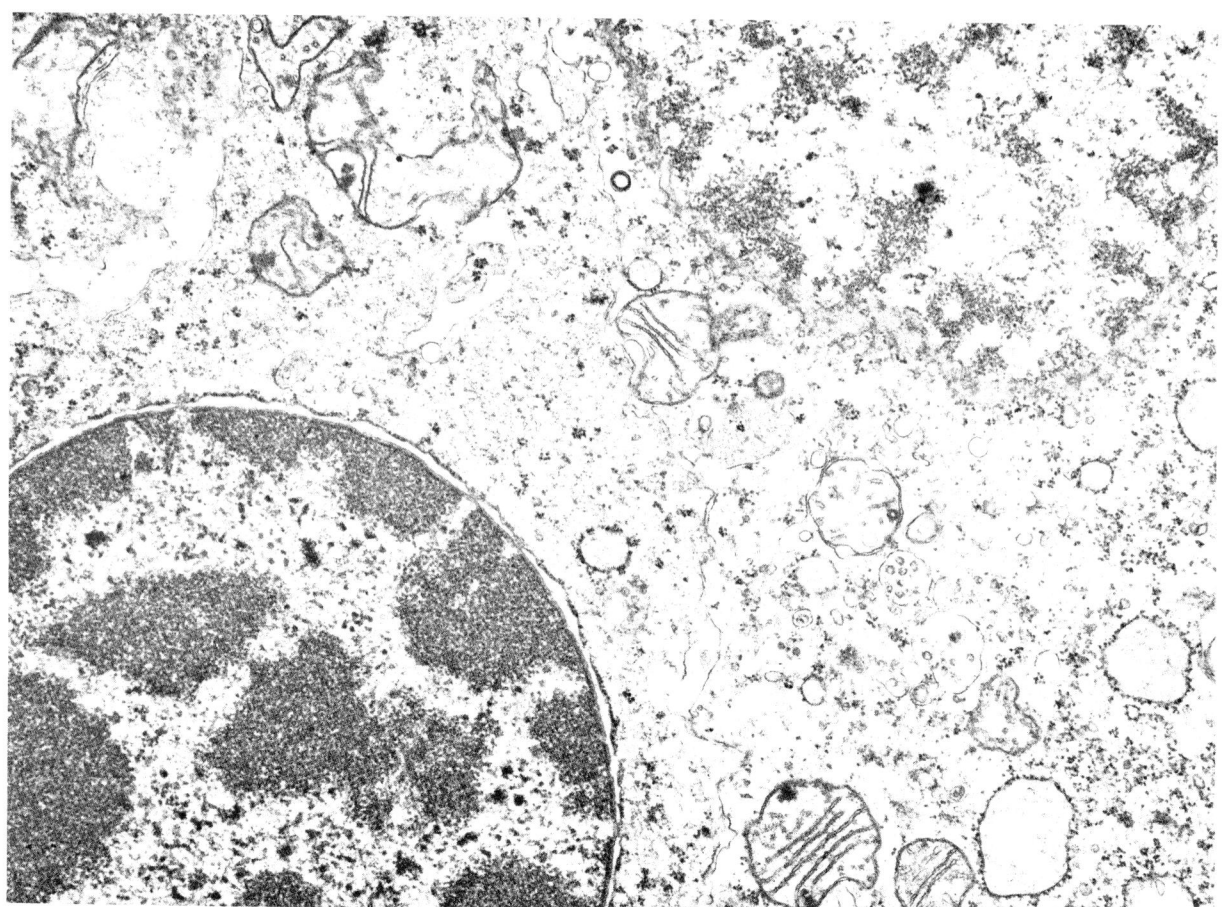

Figure 46.4. Putamen from same animal as in Fig. 46.3. These cells (probably neurons) are considered irreversibly injured on the basis of the inner matrical densities visible in most mitochondria. Following occlusion of the MCA, the putamen is one of the areas where the lowest CBF values are recorded (Morawetz et al., 1978). (Original magnification ×8,000.)

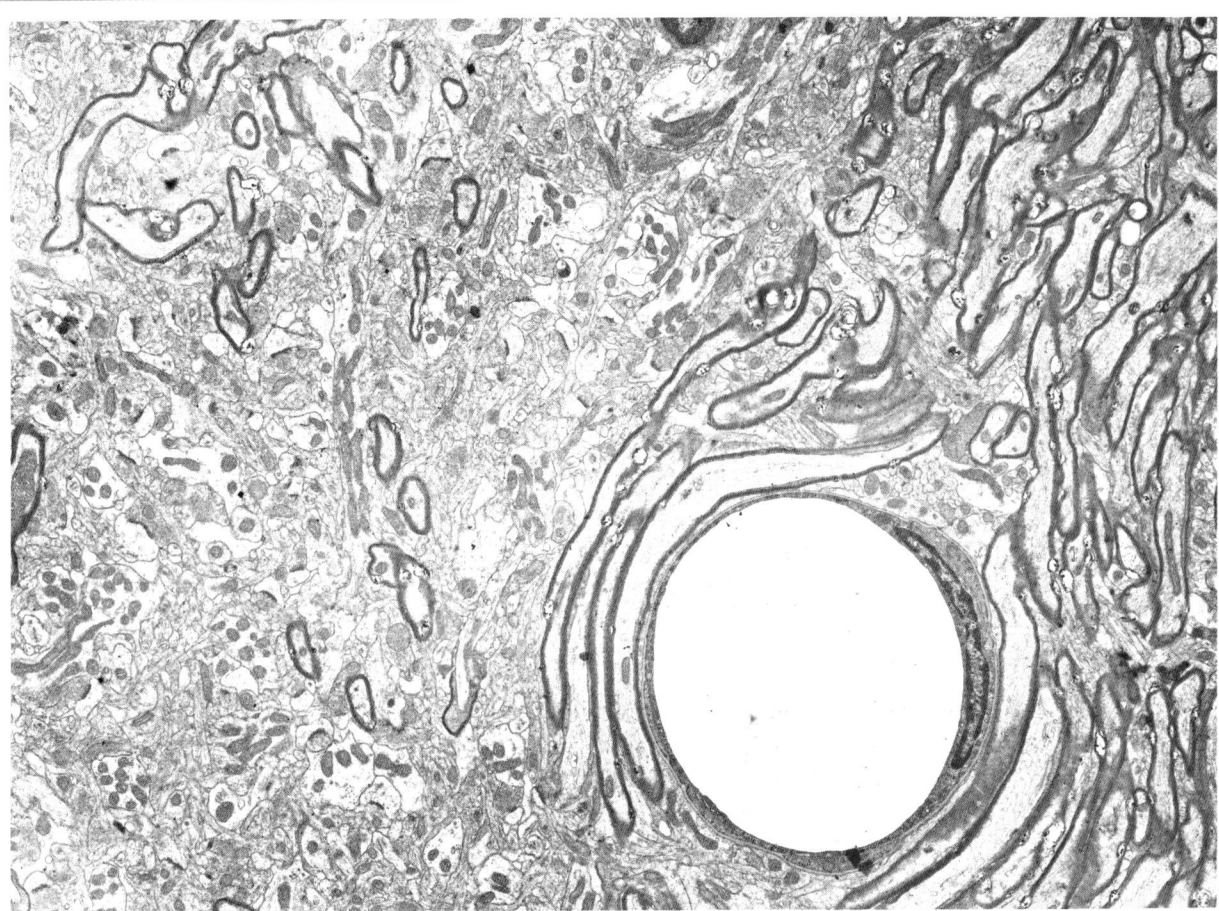

Figure 46.5. Caudate nucleus from rhesus monkey subjected to a sham occlusion of the middle cerebral artery 5 hr before death. This animal and all others reported in this and similar studies were killed, under anesthesia, by cardiovascular perfusion with aldehydes administered at a pressure comparable to the animal's systolic blood pressure (Garcia et al., 1978). A wide open capillary is seen at the right lower corner. Note features of myelinated axons and of intervening neuropil, which are identical to those reported in normal laboratory animals. (Original magnification ×3,000.)

mental tests in which carbon black particles were injected in the circulation after variable periods of ischemia (Fischer et al., 1977). There is, however, significant evidence of functional changes in capillary endothelium in terms of the capability to transport several metabolites (Nishimoto et al., 1978); also there exist data showing profound alterations in water transport, which vary as a function of the region studied and the duration of the ischemic event (Watanabe et al., 1977). Brain water content increases in direct proportion to decreases in CBF and, seemingly, the tissue accumulation of water precedes the development of failure in synaptic transmission and failure in ionic pumps (Symon et al., 1979). A large number of studies have shown that a marked increase in capillary permeability to proteins is a common consequence of ischemia (Klatzo, 1979); however, there is no temporal correlation between water accumulation and increases in protein transport across endothelial cells (Klatzo, 1979; Kamijyo et al., 1977). The relationship between changes in endothelial permeability and the progression of brain ischemic injury remains to be determined. In regional ischemia of short duration, the areas of neuronal injury are not the same areas where abnormally high protein leakage is first demonstrated (Kamijyo et al., 1977; Little et al., 1974).

The phenomenon of "no reflow"—which occurs after temporary ischemia and which originally was attributed to mechanical obstructions in the microcirculation—is currently ascribed to circulating plasma fractions, probably prostaglandins, that may exert either a vasoconstrictive or a hemostatic effect at the level of the microcirculation (Furlow and Hallenbeck, 1978). It seems as if the conditions created by brain ischemia alter platelet aggregation, a condition that may worsen the initial decrease in blood flow by inducing the formation of microthrombi (Dougherty et al., 1979). In terms of changes in regional blood flow after occlusion of a single intracranial artery, e.g., middle cerebral artery, considerable heterogeneity has been noted in various brain areas of the same animal, although the areas of earliest

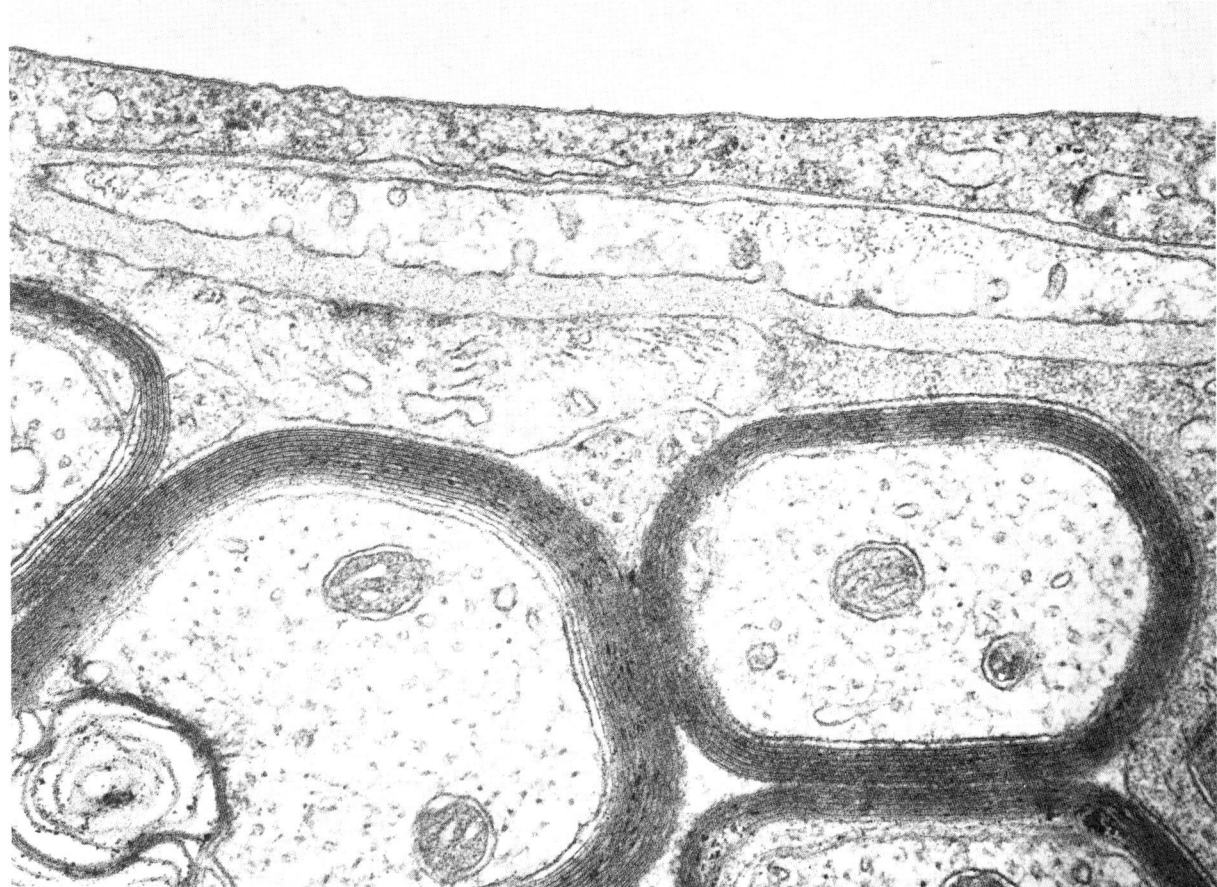

Figure 46.6. Caudate nucleus (rhesus monkey); same animal as in Fig. 46.5. The capillary lumen at the *top* of the picture is separated from the brain parenchyma by the cytoplasm of endothelial cell, pericyte, and a basement membrane. Note detail of myelin sheaths around individual axis cylinders that contain microtubules, filaments, mitochondria, and occasional fragments of endoplasmic reticulum. (Original magnification ×25,000.)

"infarction" or irreversible changes are those where CBF values are the lowest (Symon, 1974). Whenever local blood flow values fall below 12 ml/100 g/min for 2 hr or longer, the regional blood flow remains low even after reopening the artery (Morawetz et. al., 1978). It remains to be determined whether this phenomenon is a reflection of 1) failure of microcirculation, 2) irreversible tissue injury, or 3) a combination of these and other unknown factors.

From the preceding discussion it seems that, in the case of a transient arterial occlusion, the initial loss of hemispheric function, i.e., development of hemiparesis, is not due to irreversible nerve cell injury. Various ultrastructural studies have shown that accelerated phospholipid degradation is related to irreversible ischemic injury (Farber et al., 1978), and it has been suggested that the resultant membrane dysfunctions are first reflected in collections of calcium phosphate in the mitochondria (Hagler et al., 1979). It is noteworthy that such precipitates are not seen in many neuronal mitochondria until at least 2 hr of MCA occlusion (Garcia et al., 1977). Therefore, it is suggested that the electrical silence and the loss of motor function observed after MCA occlusion are initially a reflection of synaptic and, possibly, axonal abnormalities (Garcia et al., 1980) that possibly are a direct consequence of decreased energy supplies.

A new experimental model has been developed for the purpose of determining whether regional drops in CBF correspond to a predictable pattern of cellular abnormalities. In this model of focal ischemia, regional CBF is calculated from the rate of hydrogen clearance, measured through several intracerebrally implanted electrodes. Values obtained before and during occlusion of a middle cerebral artery are correlated with the degree of tissue injury, estimated by both ultrastructural and biochemical methods (Garcia et al., 1980).

DIFFUSE BRAIN ISCHEMIC INJURY

Global ischemic injury to organs such as liver and kidney is a common consequence of episodic cardiac arrest, hypotension, and shock. In the case of the brain, the pattern of global ischemia observed after these injuries can also be seen following blunt trauma to the head

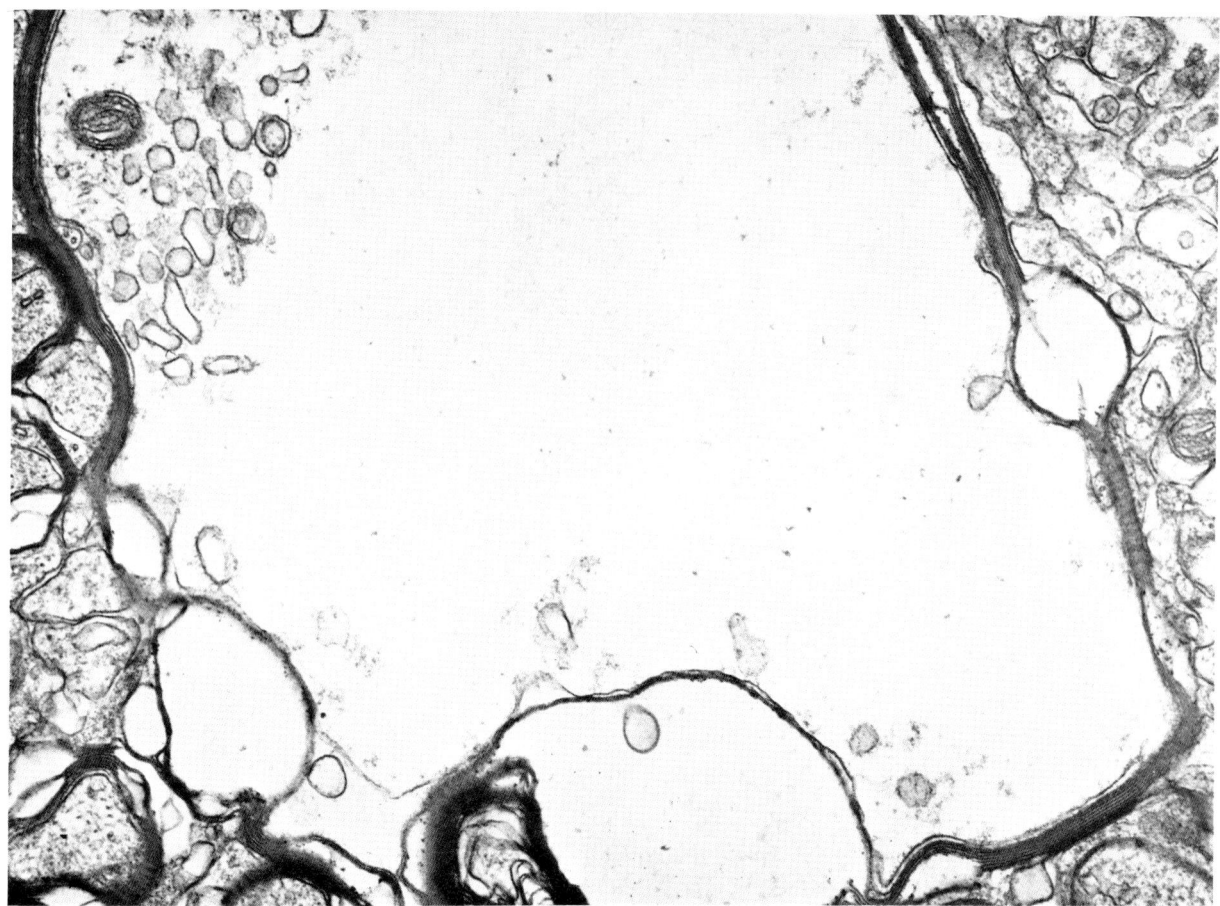

Figure 46.7. Globus pallidus from rhesus monkey whose middle cerebral artery had been occluded by a silastic embolus 24 hr before fixation. Note massive enlargement of the axon; some of its organelles are still recognizable at the *left upper corner*. The orginal myelin sheath is comparatively well preserved. (Original magnification ×20,000.)

and after sustained epileptic seizures. It is traditionally thought that brain global ischemia of a few minutes' duration results in a pattern of cell injury that affects primarily areas of "selective vulnerability," such as the pyramidal cell layer of the hippocampus, the Purkinje cell layer of the cerebellum, and layers three and four of the neocortex (Grenell, 1946). Experimental studies of hypotension in subhuman primates have confirmed the multifocal nature of the injury and emphasized the distribution of the injury along the lines of the arterial border zones (Brierley et al., 1969). Global ischemic injury to cat brains lasting as long as 60 min need not be fatal to *all* cellular elements, as indicated by the recovery of the previously isoelectric electroencephalogram and the evidence of protein synthesis by the ischemic brain tissues (Kleihues et al., 1974). Gamache and Myers (1975) have concluded that the neuropathologic sequelae of global ischemia are probably related to local hypoxemic and acidotic conditions that develop during the recirculation period. Further evidence for the validity of this postulate may be inferred from the result of studying, by electron microscopy, totally ischemic brains. In that study, as late as 60 min after exsanguination, relatively few cells showed evidence of irreversible injury (Kalimo et al., 1977). However, when brain made ischemic in such manner was reperfused, a highly heterogeneous and multifocal pattern of neuronal injury was noted (Jenkins et al., 1979). During global ischemia, extracellular potassium increased from 3.3 to 5.6 mEq/liter, while subarachnoid sodium decreased from 133 to 53 mEq/liter. These abnormalities were promptly reversed by re-establishing brain circulation (Hossmann et al., 1977). It may be concluded that the prompt and pronounced changes in ionic content caused by ischemia are a reflection of dysfunction of ionic pumps in diverse plasma membranes. Such alteration seemingly is irreversible only to a limited number of cells, at any given moment. However, as long as the ischemic condition persists and for reasons unknown at present, there is a progressive increase in the number of individually affected cells. Myocardium made ischemic by coronary occlusion does not contain a significantly large number of necrotic cells until 20–30 min after the vascular occlusion (Jennings et al., 1975). Our structural observations in diverse types of

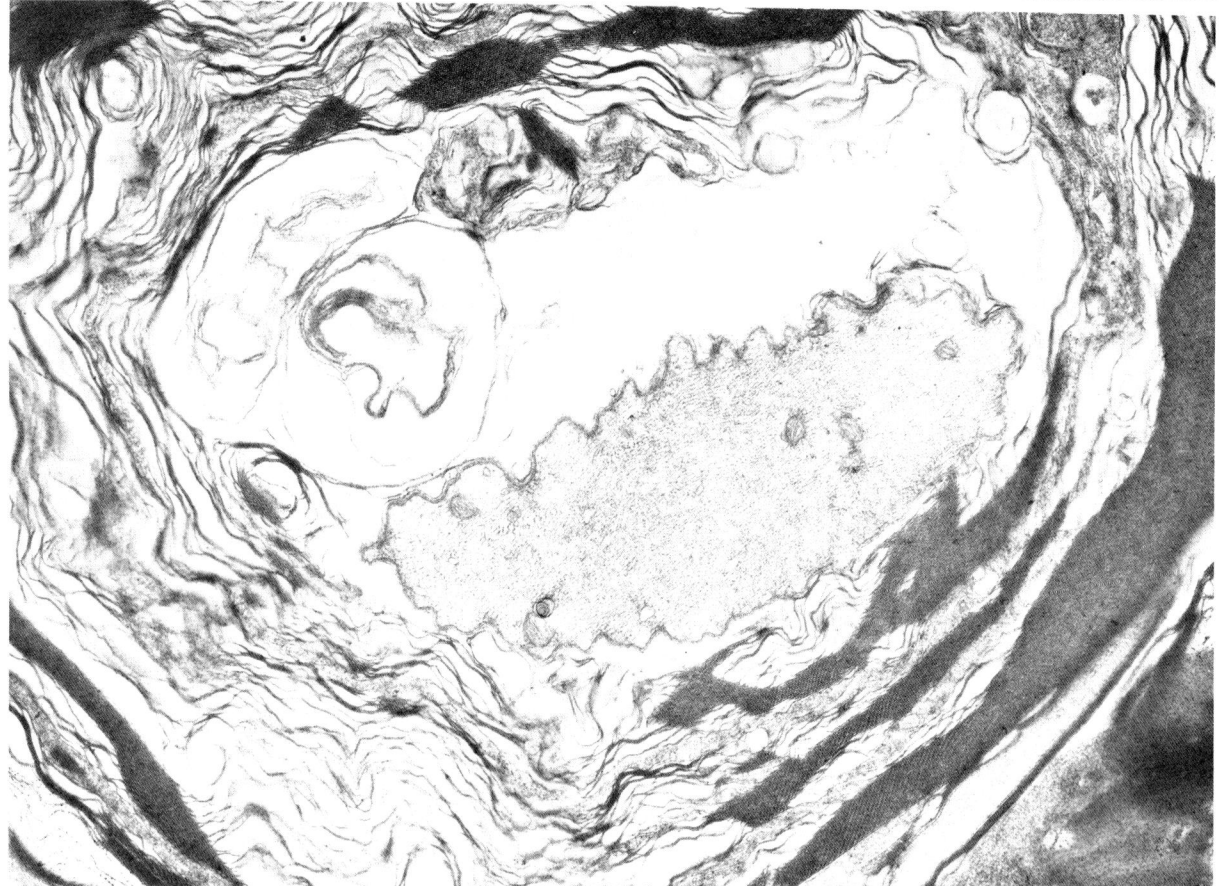

Figure 46.8. Corona radiata from rhesus monkey. The corresponding middle cerebral artery was occluded 7 hr before fixation. In this area, there is beginning of disintegration of the myelin sheaths and marked increase in the number of microfilaments contained in this axon. (Original magnification ×16,000.)

brain ischemic injury are strongly suggestive of a similar evolution, i.e., despite the one time nature of the injury, either arterial occlusion or hypotensive episode, there seems to be, over a period of minutes or hours, a progressive increase in the number of lethally injured units or cells. Corroboration of this postulate requires a reproducible method to quantitate the number of necrotic or irreversibly injured cells. In the past, cell viability has been evaluated by measuring high energy phosphate concentrations and oxidation-reduction states. However, studies of recirculation periods following ischemia have shown that intermediates of energy metabolism return to normal values under conditions that are not compatible with functional recovery (Mrsulja et al., 1976; Levy and Duffy, 1977; Conger et al., 1980). Consequently, concentrations of high energy phosphate metabolites cannot be used as indicators of survival during recirculation. Other classical biochemical approaches that might be used to evaluate tissue viability include measurement of ischemia sensitive enzyme function (Quayle et al., 1976), protein synthesis rates (Cooper et al., 1977; Yanagihara, 1976), and mitochondrial function (Rosenthal et al., 1976). All of the above biochemical determinations have a common limitation, namely, they require either quick frozen or fresh brain homogenates. Although such techniques are appropriate for most biochemical analyses, they are incompatible with most microscopic analyses of acute cell injury.

It has been held that traditional methods used in preparing tissues for light and electron microscopy are inadequate for the measurement of biochemical constituents; however, the heterogeneity of the structural damage encountered following MCA occlusion requires simultaneous application of both biochemical and morphological evaluations.

In studies of the effects of transient ischemia and hypoxia, we noted that derangements in amino acid concentrations persist long after recovery of high energy metabolites (Folbergrova et al., 1974; Ljunggren et al., 1974; Mrsulja et al., 1976; Duffy et al., 1972; Nordstrom et al., 1978). Some amino acids remain constant during global ischemia, while others, particularly alanine, change in proportion with the length of the ischemic episode (Conger et al., 1978). These studies suggested that, if amino acid concentrations could be quantitated in tissue prepared for electron microscopy, their concen-

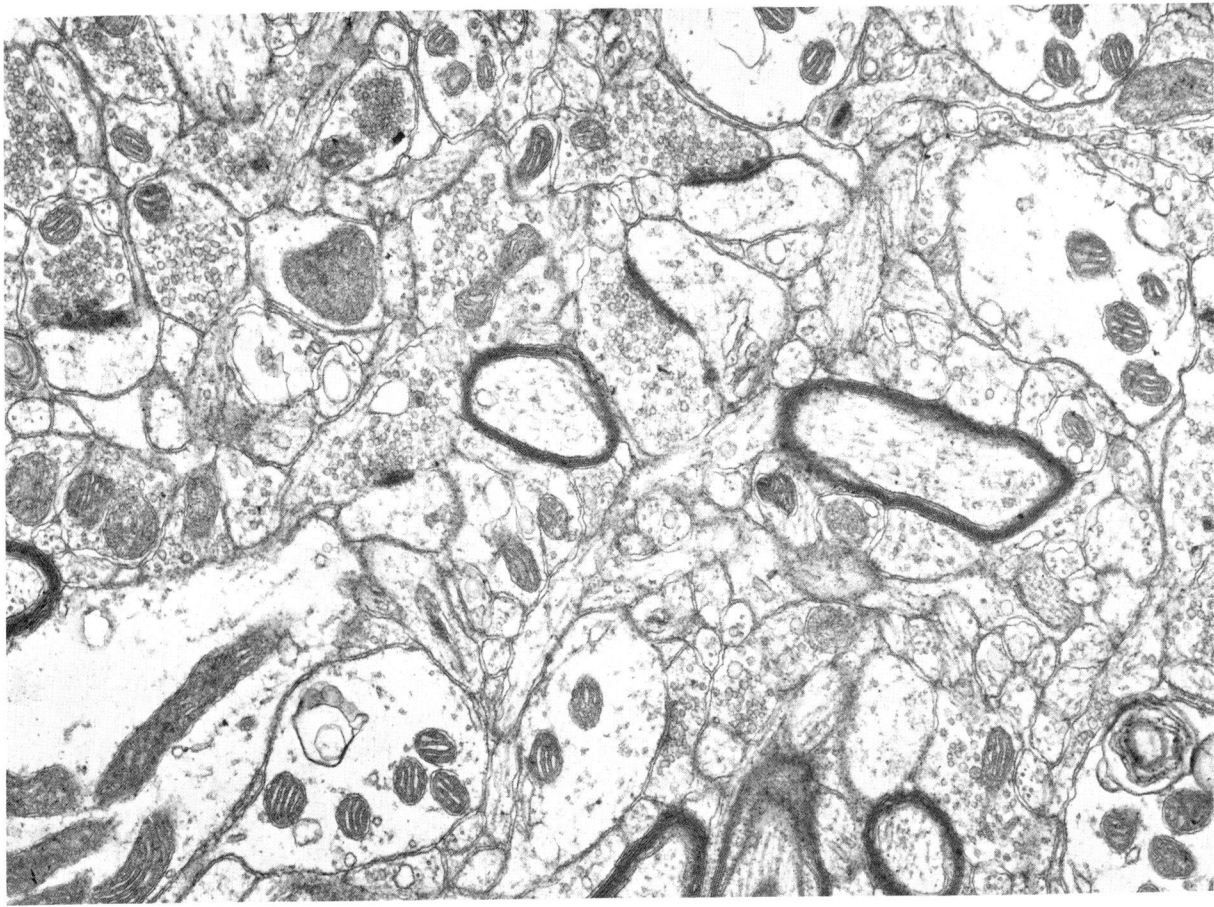

Figure 46.9

Figure 46.9 and **Figure 46.10.** Both samples are from the caudate nucleus of two rhesus monkeys—one subjected to a sham operation (Fig. 46.9) and a second one with an arterial occlusion of 7-hr duration (Fig. 46.10). In contrast to the alterations visible in other areas, the only abnormality consists of increased volume and increased electron lucency of selected compartments, i.e., astrocytic processes and presynaptic terminals (Garcia et al., 1979). (Original magnifications ×5,000 and ×6,000, respectively.)

trations might reflect the severity of structural damage better than the more labile carbohydrate pool.

Therefore, we investigated the feasibility of measuring amino acids in aldehyde-fixed tissue. This study showed that, as expected, glutaraldehyde perfusion of mouse brain causes a rapid decline in high energy phosphate intermediates, which is accompanied by an increase in lactate. Amino acids, however, are considerably more stable during periods of fixation than the intermediates of energy metabolism. For example, concentrations of glutamate and aspartate remained essentially unchanged in mouse forebrain over a 90-min period of complete ischemia. During the same period marked increases in alanine occurred in this tissue. The increase in alanine was dependent upon the time at which perfusion of glutaraldehyde fixatives were started. That is, the longer perfusion was delayed, the higher alanine rose in the tissue. It was postulated that the increase in alanine occurs because the pyruvate glutamate transaminase reaction is widely displaced from equilibrium (Krebs, 1975; Conger et al., 1978). Alanine accumulates due to the high levels of glutamate and pyruvate in ischemic cerebral tissue. The increase in alanine continues until the catalyst, glutamate pyruvate transaminase, is inhibited by the glutaraldehyde fixative. Since glutamate concentrations do not change over prolonged periods, this amino acid can be used as a reference to which changes in alanine can be compared. Measurements of alanine/glutamate (A/G) ratios are more useful than measurements of alanine alone because absolute concentrations of amino acids vary from one brain region to the next (Berger et al., 1977). Furthermore, the ensuing edema of ischemia would dilute all amino acids, including glutamate and alanine. Subsequent measurement of amino acids in aldehyde-fixed primate brain revealed a striking correlation between the degree of ischemic damage, i.e., morphological changes at both the light and electron microscopic level, and values of the A/G ratio (Kauffman et al., 1978).

Concentrations of amino acids in aldehyde-fixed pri-

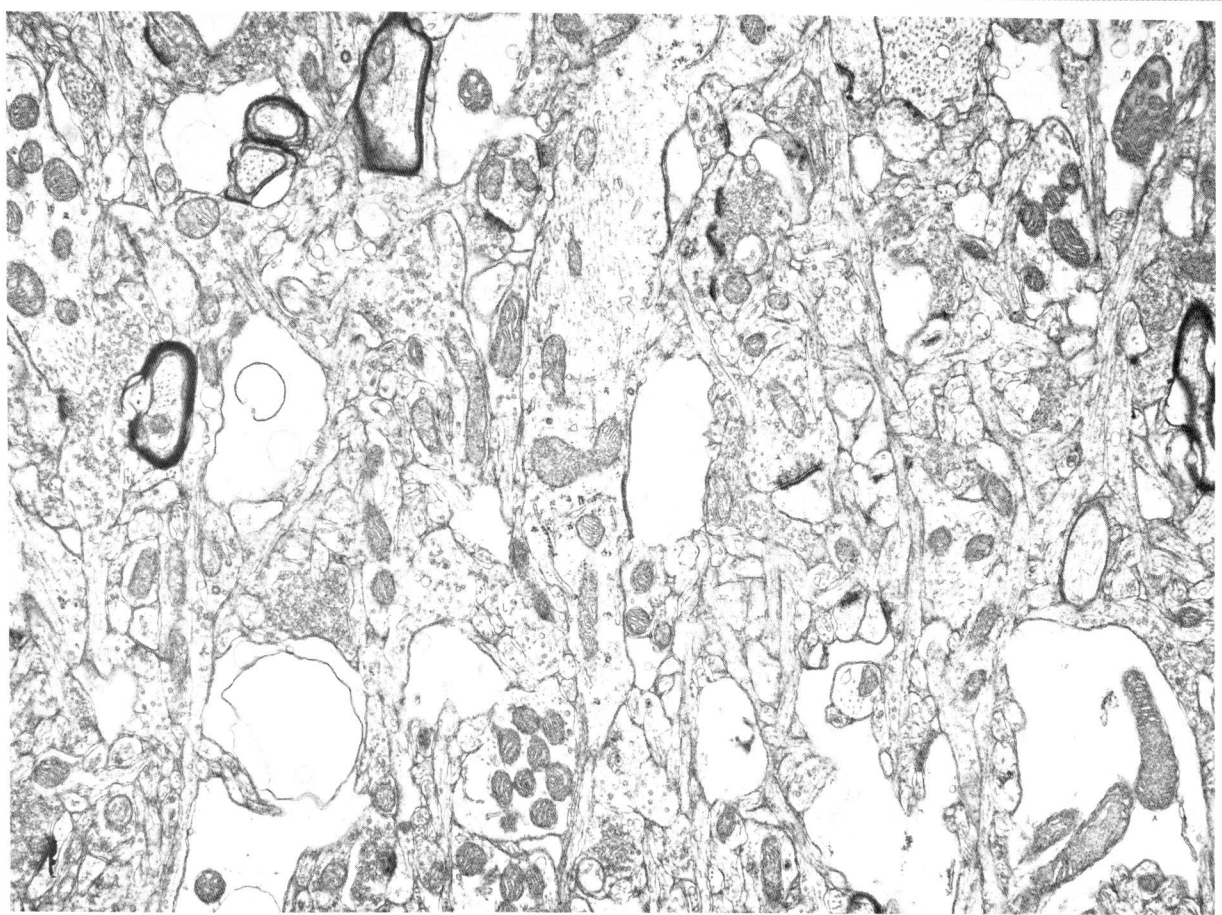

Figure 46.10

mate brain compare very favorably with values obtained in quick frozen mouse brain. For example, quick frozen mouse forebrain concentrations of alanine, aspartate, and glutamate were 0.50, 3.02, and 10.81 mmoles/kg of wet tissue, respectively (Conger et al., 1978), whereas concentrations of these amino acids in aldehyde-fixed samples of superior temporal gyrus of rhesus monkey brain were 0.29, 2.81, and 9.89 mmoles/kg of wet tissue, respectively. Thus, the technique for measuring amino acids in aldehyde-fixed brain is applicable to both rodents and subhuman primates. In addition, this study showed that after an MCA occlusion the changes in amino acid ratios reflect the severity of tissue injury (Kauffman et al., 1978). The severity of acute cell injury can be judged by specific alterations in the ultrastructural appearance of mitochondria and other cell organelles (Hagler et al., 1979). Since biochemical analyses were done on relatively large samples (30–50 mg of wet tissue weight), the results represent averages of values obtained from areas of some heterogeneity. As this study was necessarily of limited scope due to the use of an expensive primate model, we designed a more rigorous study to evaluate the efficacy of the A/G ratio as an indicator of ischemic damage.

A close correlation between the degree of ischemia, recovery from ischemia, and A/G ratios has been observed in a comprehensive study in gerbils involving 95 animals. After unilateral occlusion of the carotid artery, half of the animals displayed mild to severe neurologic symptoms. Animals with mild neurologic symptoms had slight but significant increases in the A/G ratio. Animals with severe neurologic deficits displayed high A/G ratios, particularly marked in the hemisphere ipsilateral to the occluded artery (Kauffman et al., 1978). In addition, a strong correlation was found between lactate levels and A/G ratios. A second study in gerbils explored the effect of short-term bilateral carotid occlusion and reperfusion on A/G ratios and a wide variety of metabolic intermediates. Gerbils' carotid arteries were occluded bilaterally for 1, 5, and 20 min, respectively, after which A/G ratios and other metabolic intermediates were measured. All occlusions, including the 1- and 5-min period, resulted in significant increases in alanine and marked decreases in high energy phosphate intermediates. After reperfusing over a 1 hr period, alanine continued to increase briefly but then returned normal in the 1-min-occluded gerbils. Interestingly, the A/G ratio remained high in the 20 min-occluded animals, which did not survive despite return or even overshoot of concentrations of high energy phosphate intermediates (Conger and Garcia, 1979).

BRAIN HEMORRHAGES AS A TYPE OF STROKE

Two types of spontaneous or nontraumatic intracranial bleedings may become manifest in the form of a stroke: 1) brain hemorrhages and 2) subarachnoid hemorrhage.

Massive spontaneous bleeding into the brain parenchyma is a relatively rare but well known condition that is associated with various diseases that include systemic hypertension, coagulopathies, congenital defects in blood vessels, brain tumors, and systemic bacterial infections (McCormick and Rosenfield, 1973).

The structural abnormalities that hypertensive disease induces in arteriolar walls, such as hyalinization and microaneurysms, have been traditionally incriminated for the brain hemorrhages noted in hypertensive subjects (Cole and Yates, 1967). However, the exact mechanism responsible for the vascular rupture is unknown, and the demonstration of the initial bleeding site in individual cases of brain hemorrhage is extremely difficult to achieve.

Among the causes of death of patients with brain hemorrhage are massive increases in intracranial pressure and flooding of the ventricular cavities by blood.

Primary or nontraumatic subarachnoid hemorrhage is demonstrated in about 3% of stroke patients. Bleeding in the subarachnoid space originates either in congenitally defective intracranial vessels or represents an extension from small, superficially located brain parenchymal hemorrhages. The presence of blood in the subarachnoid space interferes with the circulation of spinal fluid, a condition that may raise the intracranial pressure. Additionally, several vasoactive compounds (probably prostaglandins) that are present in blood cells, e.g., platelets, may be released in sufficiently large amounts so that vasoconstriction and brain ischemia are relatively common consequences of subarachnoid bleeding (Zervas, 1979). As indicated before, ischemia causes brain edema that, because of the closed nature of the skull, may induce further ischemia by exerting extrinsic constriction of the brain blood vessels.

Thus, it can be appreciated that ischemic injury to the brain occurs under a wide variety of circumstances that range from heart disease to blunt head injury. Although considerable progress has been attained in the past decade, the explanation for the progressive nature of the ischemic injury in most cases remains unknown.

Acknowledgment. This work was supported by United States Public Health Service Grant NS 08802.

References

Astrup, J., Symon, L., Branston, N.M., and Lassen, N.A.: Cortical evoked potential and extracellular K+ and H+ at critical levels of brain ischemia. Stroke *8:*51, 1977.

Berger, S.J., Carter, J.G., and Lowry, O.H.: The distribution of glycine, GABA, glutamate and aspartate in rabbit spinal cord, cerebellum and hippocampus. J. Neurochem. *28:*149, 1977.

Bremer, A.M., Yamada, K., and West, C.R.: Experimental regional cerebral ischemia in the middle cerebral artery territory in primates. Part 3. Effects on brain water and electrolytes in the late phase of acute MCA stroke. Stroke *9:* 387, 1978.

Brierley, J.B., Brown, A.W., Excell, B.J., and Meldrum, B.S.: Brain damage in the rhesus monkey resulting from profound arterial hypotension. I. Its nature, distribution and general physiological correlates. Brain Res. *13:*68, 1969.

Cole, F.M., and Yates, P.O.: The occurrence and significance of intracerebral microaneurysms. J. Pathol. Bacteriol. *93:* 393, 1967.

Conger, K.A., and Garcia, J.H.: Alanine and glutamate concentrations as indicators of post-ischemic survival. J. Neuropathol. Exp. Neurol. *38:*308, 1979.

Conger, K.A., Garcia, J.H., Lossinsky, A.S., and Kauffman, F.C.: The effect of aldehyde fixation on selected substrates for energy metabolism and amino acids in mouse brain. J. Histochem. Cytochem. *26:*423, 1978.

Conger, K.A., Garcia, J.H., Kauffman, F.C., Lust, W.D., and Passonneau, J.V.: Alanine to glutamate ratios as an index of reversibility of cerebral ischemia in gerbils. Exp. Neurol. *71:* 370–382, 1981.

Cooper, H.K., Zalewska, T., Kawakami, S., Hossman, K.-A., and Kleihues, P.: The effect of ischemia and recirculation on protein synthesis in the rat brain. J. Neurochem. *28:*929, 1977.

Dougherty, J.H., Jr., Levy, D.E., and Weksler, B.B.: Experimental cerebral ischemia produces platelet aggregates. Neurology *29:*1460, 1979.

Duffy, T.E., Nelson, S.R., and Lowry, O.H.: Cerebral carbohydrate metabolism during acute hypoxia and recovery. J. Neurochem. *19:*959, 1972.

Farber, J.L., Martin, J.T., and Chien, K.R.: Irreversible ischemic cell injury. Am. J. Pathol. *92:*713, 1978.

Fischer, E.G., Ames, A., III, Hedley-Whyte, E.T., and O'Gorman, S.: Reassessment of cerebral capillary changes in acute global ischemia and their relationship to the "no-reflow phenomenon." Stroke *8:*36, 1977.

Fisher, C.M.: Discussion of frequency and symptom analysis of transient ischemic attacks. In *Cerebrovascular Diseases* (Tenth Princeton Conference), edited by P. Scheinberg, pp. 50–53. Raven Press, New York, 1976.

Folbergrova, J., Ljunggren, B., Norberg, K., and Siesjo, B.K.: Influence of complete ischemia on glycolytic metabolites, citric acid cycle intermediates, and associated amino acids in the rat cerebral cortex. Brain Res. *80:*265, 1974.

Furlow, T., Jr., and Hallenbeck, J.M.: Indomethacin prevents impaired perfusion of the dog's brain after global ischemia. Stroke *9:*591, 1978.

Gamache, F.W., and Myers, R.F.: Effects of hypotension on rhesus monkeys. Arch. Neurol. *32:*374, 1975.

Garcia, J.H.: The neuropathology of stroke. Hum. Pathol. *6:* 593, 1975.

Garcia, J.H., Cox, J.V., and Hudgins, W.R.: Ultrastructure of the microvasculature in experimental cerebral infarction. Acta Neuropathol. *18:*273, 1971.

Garcia, J.H., Kalimo, H., Kamijyo, Y., and Trump, B.F.: Cellular events during early cerebral ischemia. I. Electron microscopy of feline cerebral cortex after middle-cerebral-artery occlusion. Virchows Arch. [Cell Pathol.] *25:*191, 1977.

Garcia, J.H., Kamijyo, Y., Kalimo, H., Tanaka, J., Viloria, J.E., and Trump, B.F.: Cerebral ischemia: The early structural changes and correlations of these with known metabolic and dynamic abnormalities. In *Cerebral Vascular Diseases*, edited by J.P. Whisnant and B. Sandok, pp. 313–323. Grune & Stratton, New York, 1975.

Garcia, J.H., Lossinsky, A.S., Kauffman, F.C., and Conger, K.A.: Neuronal ischemic injury: Light microscopy, ultrastructure and biochemistry. Acta Neuropathol. (Berlin) *43:* 85, 1978.

Garcia, J.H., Lossinsky, A.S., Kauffman, F.C., Conger, K.A., and Mena, H.: Fine structure and biochemistry of brain edema in regional cerebral ischemia. In *Cerebrovascular Diseases* (Eleventh Conference), edited by T.R. Price and E. Nelson, pp. 169–189. Raven Press, New York, 1979.

Garcia, J.H., Conger, K.A., Morawetz, R., and Halsey, J.H.: Post-ischemic brain edema: Quantitation and evolution. Adv. Neurol. *28:*147–169, 1980.

Grenell, R.G.: Central nervous system resistance. I. The effects of temporary arrest of cerebral circulation for periods of two to ten minutes. J. Neuropathol. Exp. Neurol. *5:*131, 1946.

Hagler, H.K., Sherwin, L., and Buja, L.M.: Effect of different methods of tissue preparation on mitochondrial inclusions of ischemic and infarcted canine myocardium: Transmission and analytic electron microscopy study. Lab. Invest. *40:*528, 1979.

Halsey, J.H., Jr.: Monitoring the cerebral circulation in progressing stroke. In *Current Concepts of Cerebrovascular Disease (Stroke)*, edited A.G. Waltz, vol. 11, no. 6, pp. 27–32. American Heart Association, Dallas, 1976.

Hossmann, K.A., Sakaki, S., and Zimmerman, V.: Cation activities in reversible ischemia of the cat brain. Stroke *8:*77, 1977.

Hudgins, W.R., and Garcia, J.H.: Transorbital approach to the middle cerebral artery of the squirrel monkey: A technique for experimental cerebral infarction applicable to ultrastructural studies. Stroke *1:*107, 1970.

Jenkins, L.W., Povlishock, J.T., Becker, D.P., Miller, J.D., and Sullivan, H.G.: Complete cerebral ischemia: an ultrastructural study. Acta Neuropathol. (Berlin) *48:*113–125, 1979.

Jennings, R.B., Ganote, C.E., and Reimer, K.A.: Ischemic tissue injury. Am. J. Pathol. *80:*179, 1975.

Jones, H.R., and Millikan, C.H.: Temporal profile (clinical course) of acute carotid system cerebral infarction. Stroke *7:*64, 1976.

Kalimo, H., Garcia, J.H., Kamijyo, Y., Tanaka, J., and Trump, B.F.: The ultrastructure of "brain death." II. Electron microscopy of feline cortex after complete ischemia. Virchows Arch. [Cell Pathol.] *25:*207, 1977.

Kamijyo, Y., and Garcia, J.H.: Carotid arterial supply of the feline brain: Applications to the study of regional cerebral ischemia. Stroke *6:*361, 1975.

Kamijyo, Y., Garcia, J.H., and Cooper, J.: Temporary middle cerebral artery occlusion: A model of hemorrhagic and subcortical infarction. J. Neuropathol. Exp. Neurol. *36:*338, 1977.

Kauffman, F.C., Conger, K., and Garcia, J.H.: Alanine and glutamate concentrations as an index of ischemic brain damage. J. Neuropathol. Exp. Neurol. *37:*640, 1978.

Klatzo, I.: Cerebral edema and ischemia. In *Recent Advances in Neuropathology*, edited by W.T. Smith and J.B. Cavanagh, no. 1, pp. 27–40. Churchill Livingston, Edinburgh, 1979.

Kleihues, P., Kobayashi, K., and Hossman, K.A.: Purine nucleotide metabolism in the cat brain after one hour of complete ischemia. J. Neurochem. *23:*417, 1974.

Krebs, H.A.: The role of chemical equilibria in organ function. Adv. Enzyme Regul. *13:*449, 1975.

Levy, D.E., and Duffy, T.E.: Cerebral energy metabolism during transient ischemia and recovery in the gerbil. J. Neurochem. *28:*63, 1977.

Little, J.R., Kerr, F.W., and Sundt, T.M., Jr.: Significance of neuronal alterations in developing cortical infarction. Mayo Clin. Proc. *49:*827, 1974.

Ljunggren, B., Ratcheson, R.A., and Siesjo, B.K.: Cerebral metabolic state following complete compression ischemia. Brain Res. *73:*291, 1974.

McCormick, W.F., and Rosenfield, D.B.: Massive brain hemorrhage: A review of 144 cases and examination of their causes. Stroke *4:*946, 1973.

Molinari, G.F.: Clinical relevance of experimental stroke models. In *Cerebrovascular Diseases* (Eleventh Princeton Conference), edited by T.R. Price and E. Nelson, pp. 19–34. Raven Press, New York, 1979.

Moossy, J.: Validation of ischemic stroke models. In *Cerebrovascular Diseases* (Eleventh Princeton Conference), edited by T.R. Price and E. Nelson, pp. 3–10. Raven Press, New York, 1979.

Morawetz, R.B., DeGirolami, V., Ojemann, R.G., Marcoux, F.W., and Crowell, R.M.: Cerebral blood flow determined by hydrogen clearance during middle cerebral artery occlusion in unanesthetized monkeys. Stroke *9:*143, 1978.

Mrsulja, B.B., Lust, W.D., Mrsulja, B.J., Passonneau, J.V., and Klatzo, I.: Post-ischemic changes in certain metabolites following prolonged ischemia in gerbil cerebral cortex. J. Neurochem. *26:*1099, 1976.

Neuwelt, E.A., Garcia, J.H., and Mena, H.: Diffuse microglial proliferation after global ischemia in a patient with aplastic bone marrow. Acta Neuropathol. *43:*259, 1978.

Nishimoto, K., Wolman, M., Spatz, M., and Klatzo, I.: Pathophysiologic correlations in the blood-brain barrier damage due to air embolism. Adv. Neurol. *20:*237, 1978.

Nordstrom, C., Rehncrona, S., and Siesjo, B.K.: Effects of phenobarbital in cerebral ischemia. Part II. Restitution of cerebral energy state, as well as of glycolytic metabolites, citric acid cycle intermediates and associated amino acids after pronounced incomplete ischemia. Stroke *9:*335, 1978.

Quayle, E.S., Christian, S.T., and Halsey, J.H.: Effects of ischemia on the Mg^{++} requiring adenosine triphosphatase associated with neuronal synaptic vesicles in gerbil brain. Stroke *7:*36, 1976.

Rosenthal, M., Martel, D., La Manna, J.C., and Jobsis, F.F.: In situ studies of oxidative energy metabolism during transient cortical ischemia in cats. Exp. Neurol. *50:*477, 1976.

Symon, L.: Physiological studies of blood flow in the middle-cerebral-artery territory. In *Current Concepts of Cerebrovascular Disease, (Stroke)*, vol. 9, no. 2, pp. 5–8. American Heart Association, Dallas, 1974.

Symon, L., Branston, N.M., and Chikovani, O.: Ischemic brain edema following middle cerebral artery occlusion in baboons: Relationship between regional cerebral water content and blood flow at 1 to 2 hours. Stroke *10:*184, 1979.

Watanabe, O., West, C.R., and Brewer, A.: Experimental regional cerebral ischemia in the middle cerebral artery territory in primates. Part 2. Effects on brain water and electrolytes in the early phase of MCA. Stroke *8:*71, 1977.

Yanagihara, T.: Cerebral ischemia in gerbils: Differential vulnerability of protein, RNA and lipid synthesis. Stroke *7:*260, 1976.

Zervas, N.T.: Cerebral vasospasm: Introduction. In *Cerebral Vascular Diseases* (Eleventh Princeton Conference), edited by T.R. Price and E. Nelson, p. 269. Raven Press, New York, 1979.

CHAPTER 47

Cellular and Subcellular Changes in Myocardial Infarction

WOLFGANG J. MERGNER
JUTTA SCHAPER

CELL INJURY AND THE HEART

Myocardial infarction induces cellular alteration in three different systems: 1) the microvasculature (Armiger and Gavin, 1975; Borgers et al., 1971; Chimosky et al., 1967; Hearse, 1977; Hearse et al., 1978; Kloner et al., 1974a, 1975a and b; MeNeely, 1974; W. Schaper and J. Schaper, 1976, 1977); 2) the Purkinje fibers and the conduction system and conduction process (Baba et al., 1970; Coraboeuf, 1978; Coraboeuf et al., 1976; Carmeliet, 1978; Corr and Gillis, 1974, 1975, 1978; El-Sherif et al., 1977; Kohlhardt et al., 1977; Podzuweit et al., 1978a–c; Scherlag et al., 1969, 1970, 1974); and 3) the working myocardium. Although progression of cell injury, if it passes the "point-of-no-return," might be similar, vulnerability and time course of cellular reactions in these systems are certainly different (Jennings et al., 1963, 1964, 1978a; Jennings, 1976a; W. Schaper and Pasyk, 1976; Friedman et al., 1973; Lazzera et al., 1973, 1974). The working myocardial cells appear as the most sensitive member of the heart tissue (Lochner et al., 1975, 1976, 1978; Opie, 1976; Shrago, 1976; Shug et al., 1975; Whalen et al., 1974; Kloner et al., 1974b).

Reversible and Irreversible Cell Injury in the Heart

Ischemic cell injury passes from a reversible phase to an irreversible phase if permitted to progress. These phases have been characterized in morphological terms (Trump and Mergner, 1974; Trump et al., 1976a and b; J. Schaper, 1978b, 1980; J. Schaper et al., 1979a). However, much uncertainty exists in identifying the functional events that occur during each phase. Equally, the key event(s) or organelle failure(s) that lead(s) the cell to cell death has been sought in a wide variety of systems (Table 47.1). For example, *decreased cellular energy levels*, based on either inhibited anaerobic flux or mitochondrial failure, have been a hypothetical choice by a number of investigators because critical levels of ATP and creatine phosphate (CP) concentration in the heart seem to correlate with cell survival (Bretschneider, 1964; Bretschneider et al., 1975; Levitzky and Feinberg, 1975; Kammermeier, 1964; Kübler and Spieckermann, 1970; Jennings, 1976a and b). This is not true for other systems. In the kidney, for example, low ATP concentrations are reached early and are tolerated during the reversible phase for some time (Kahng et al., 1978). The relationship between ATP levels and cell survival is always difficult to assess because it is difficult to define the time course of the reversible phase or the advent of cell death.

A *breakdown of the barrier function of the plasma membrane* could also be a cause of irreversibility if it can be shown that a protective function remained during the reversible phase. The plasma membrane should be considered if influx of such ions as calcium could be controlled until irreversibility is reached through some destructive process, such as activated phospholipases (Chien and Farber, 1977; Chien et al., 1977, 1978; Coleman et al., 1976; Ashraf and Halverson, 1977, 1978; Farber et al., 1978; Whalen et al., 1974; Ganote et al., 1976; Franson et al., 1978; Hearse et al., 1978; Hawkins et al., 1977; Lamers and Hülsmann, 1977).

Similarly, it has been proposed that the event of ischemia induces *accumulation of protons* by interrupting oxygen supply, substrate delivery, and perfusion, which, when exceeding local tissue buffering capacity, reach critical levels and permanently alter cellular viability. However, the target of such "acidic destruction" at a pH of 6.0 has not yet been identified, nor has the mechanism by which such a process changes cellular organelle function (J. Schaper, 1978a; Garlick, 1978; Williamson et al., 1976, 1978; Armiger et al., 1975; Jennische et al., 1978).

Loss and failure of resynthesis of important intermediaries of metabolism comprise another mechanism being proposed, for example, by Gerlach et al. (1971). This scheme would permit one to think that at the time of cell death, organelle function such as mitochondria or plasma membrane remains intact, yet substrate of ATP production such as adenine nucleotides cannot be delivered at a satisfactory concentration and speed. Therefore, this deficiency leaves the bioenergetic systems retarded

Table 47.1
Pathogenesis of Irreversibility[a]

A. Decrease of cellular energy levels
   1. Glycolysis inhibited
      a. Substrate depletion
      b. Intermediate excess
      c. Acidosis
      d. Co-factor loss
   2. Mitochondrial failure
      a. Inhibition, acyl-Co-A, ATP-ADP exchange
      b. Loss of adenine nucleotide substrate
      c. Alterations of proteins (DNP-ATPase)
      d. Alteration of phospholipid by mitochondrial phospholipases, Ca^{2+}-activated
B. Loss of cell volume regulation
   1. Na^+-K^+ pump decreased
   2. Permeability increased and membrane defects
      a. Exogenous peroxidation products
      b. Endogenous calcium-activated phospholipases
      c. Exogenous enzymes of leucocyte lysosomes
      d. Activated complement
   3. Calcium-paradox
C. Intracellular acidity
   1. Protein denaturation
   2. Stoppage of glycolysis
D. Failure of resynthesis
   1. Adenine nucleotides
E. Internally released lysosomal enzymes
   1. Lysosomal rupture
   2. Lysosomal phospholipases

[a] Modified from Jennings, 1976a.

in ATP production beyond the level of proper maintenance (Buhl, 1976; Chiong and Parker, 1975).

Another mechanism of cellular destruction could be either the gradual or the sudden *release of lytic enzymes* from cellular stores (proteases, phospholipases), which, under proper conditions, such as low pH or absence of internal inhibitors, destroy certain key functions in cells (Williamson et al., 1976; Welman et al., 1978; Decker and Wildenthal, 1978a and b; Decker et al., 1977, 1979; DeDuve and Beaufay, 1959; Duncan, 1966; Gottwik et al., 1975, 1978; Malbica and Hart, 1971; Mego et al., 1972; Hoffstein et al., 1976; Weglicki et al., 1972, 1975; Welman and Peters, 1976, 1977). The question remains whether or not such conditions exist in ischemia and if they exist at the time of cell death (Hawkins et al., 1972; Wildenthal, 1978).

It is also not clear what type of cell change represents irreversibility: a membrane alteration of phospholipids? an alteration of proteins and enzymes? or substrate exhaustion? Furthermore, the time limits of the reversible phase are uncertain as well, because of the absence of undisputed markers of cell death.

Many of the above mentioned problems have been studied in various other models (single cells, kidney, liver, skeletal muscle), where at least a preliminary answer appeared forthcoming. Therefore, the question we have to consider in comparison to such models is whether the heart—that is, the working myocardium—is similar to or different from other systems and, finally, if the answer put forward is dependent on characteristics of the model studied. We will discuss the ischemic injury as it has been studied in various model systems and as ischemia affects the structural elements of the heart. Subsequently, we will ask for the evidence from current studies implicating one system or the other of key importance in leading the path through the point-of-no-return.

Irreversibility will remain the big puzzle until we have resolved the detailed changes in each organelle system as a function of ischemic time or as a function of the point-of-no-return. Each model utilized has to demonstrate its relevance to the in vivo infarction.

Models of Study

The model selected (Table 47.2) sets the limits of a study, but within the constraint of the experimental system the model should permit a higher precision of the obtained data than the raw natural system. It is particularly difficult to relate data of various model systems to each other in the heart because of the interrelated functions of various structural elements under different conditions, such as microvasculature and Purkinje-fibers. Ideally one would search to study a single cell system first and then transfer data to the higher order of organization step by step back to the in vivo system. In the heart, the single cell systems of adult cells have only recently been developed. Although cultures of fetal and newborn hearts have been used for some time (Glick et al., 1974; Harary et al., 1976; Roeske, 1978; Harary and Farley, 1960; Pretlow et al., 1972; Ingwall et al., 1975), adult heart cell preparations are not generally available as a study object (Vahouny et al., 1970, 1979). The applicability of the single cell system has yet to be demonstrated. Organelle preparations of prior injured tissue also have considerable inherent difficulties both in being representative of the damaged organelles and not being additionally altered during the isolation procedure. Therefore, research in myocardial infarction has obtained the bulk of hemodynamic and cell physiological data from two model systems: 1) regional ischemia with and without reflow and 2) global ischemia with and without reoxygenation. These data have been supplemented by the anoxic perfused heart preparation and by isolated systems such as the papillary muscle preparation, the perfused septum, and free hand slices of myocardial tissue. There still exists a great deal of confusion about the exact definition of the terms ischemia, anoxia, anoxic perfusion, etc. The consequences for cellular metabolism and possible survival may not be the same (Neely et al., 1970, 1973, 1975a and b, 1976a and b;

Table 47.2
Model Systems

Isolated mitochondria, endoplasmic reticulum, lysosomes
Adult heart cell preparation
Regional ischemia
Global ischemial
Anoxic perfusion, beating heart
Cardioplegia
Isolated papillary muscle, septum, tissue slices

Neely and Morgan, 1974; Opie et al., 1971, 1975; Opie, 1976). Therefore, we would like to refer to a paper by Neely and Morgan (1974), where they made this definition very clear: "Availability of oxygen to the heart can be restricted either by lowering or reducing to zero the oxygen tension of the perfusate, thereby inducing hypoxia or anoxia or by restricting the flow of the perfusate containing high oxygen tensions to induce ischemia."

REGIONAL ISCHEMIA, IN VIVO WITH AND WITHOUT REFLOW

The experimental system closest to the situation of myocardial infarction is the regional ischemia system. It does involve the regional microvasculature and arteriolar collaterals and it is also influenced by the occurrence of ventricular arrhythmias and other hemodynamic factors, such as changes of blood pressure and contractility. Furthermore a number of recent studies have demonstrated that the surrounding nonischemic myocardium is affected (Mathes, 1976; Lowe et al., 1978). The model system of the regional ischemia has in the past been a rather imprecise instrument for studying infarction until recently, when this model was developed to fairly high precision (see Table 47.3) by 1) measuring the perfusion bed in relation to infarct size; 2) measuring the microperfusion of the ischemic tissue at various points during ischemia and/or reperfusion; 3) utilizing each animal as its own control; 4) subdividing the tissue in subendocardial, mid- and epicardial regions for which viability, perfusion, etc., were separately determined, 5) standardizing anesthesia and animal maintenance (W. Schaper, 1978; W. Schaper et al., 1979a and b). Still, there are a number of major limitations: *a*) The only sign of irreversible alteration of cellular viability is the p *NTB stain*. This stain identifies the activity of certain dehydrogenases (lactate, dehydroxybutyrate, pyruvate, malate, succinate) using the respective substrate. Recent tests on dehydrogenase concentration in ischemic tissue have demonstrated that the enzymes remain intact for a considerable period of time (Klein et al., 1979). Therefore, it is uncertain what inactivation shown by a negative stain means in regard to remaining cell function. It has been shown, however, that there exists a similar demarcation of myocardial infarction by means of the p NTB stain and conventional light microscopic histological examination (W. Schaper et al., 1979a). Furthermore, it takes a considerable period of time before the stain becomes negative, which excluded this stain for identifying abnormal or irreversible altered cells during early periods of infarction. In spite of those limitations the system has yielded considerable insight into the hemodynamics of regional infarction. Such results include the following:

1. Regional perfusion is reduced to approximately 10% of normal in the subendocardial region following occlusion of a major or medium sized coronary artery.
2. Resistance to collateral circulation is rather high (W. Schaper et al., 1976) during early periods of obstruction of an extramural coronary vessel but will decline within 24 hr, mainly due to passive distension of the

Table 47.3
System to Study Infarcts—Hemodynamics

Identification of perfusion area	Barium injection into coronary vessels
Identification of infarct area and cell viability	pNTB stain using malate as substrate
Perfusion area/infarct size	Computer calculation and display
Identification of regional perfusion before, during early and late period of infarction and reflow	Microsphere injection and estimation of coronary flow against a reference organ
Reversible or irreversible injury	Needle biopsy at various time intervals
Changes in ion influxes	Radioactive ion tracer studies and third compartment calculations, ion selective electrodes in coronary artery and coronary sinus, freezing gun and microprobe measurements on untreated frozen sections

collateral vessels. After 24 hr an active growth process within the collateral wall will further reduce resistance (W. Schaper and Pasyk, 1976; J. Schaper et al., 1976).

3. Resistance to reflow will increase in the infarcted region within 2 hr, mainly in the subendocardium.
4. Early periods of reflow will show a reactive hyperemia, (W. Schaper and Pasyk, 1976), a response that is either of temporary duration, indicating reversible injury, or is prolonged and most likely a phenomenon related to irreversible alteration. Ischemic injury may also be a function of the oxygen requirement of the tissue (Bretschneider et al., 1970).
5. Morphological examination will show during even quite early intervals (45 min) of ischemia extravasation of red blood cells and increased interstitial edema. Polymorphonuclear leucocytes evade into the paravascular space at 60 min of ischemia. With reperfusion, the hemorrhage into the paravascular space increases, but hemorrhagic infarction does not occur in all hearts. Myocardial cells develop fat droplets of neutral lipids prior to the point-of-no-return which, however, are inhomogeneously distributed, probably because of the inhomogeneity of the remaining collateral circulation. With reflow at later intervals, contraction bands develop which can or cannot be associated with simultaneous development of flocculent densities in mitochondria (J. Schaper et al., 1979a).

GLOBAL ISCHEMIA, WITH AND WITHOUT REOXYGENATION

Global ischemia is a "cleaner" model than regional ischemia because the ischemia can be total, unaffected by remaining collateral circulation. The model has relationship to clinical situations such as might occur during cardiac surgery. This system was utilized to describe the morphological changes through which the myocardial cells pass from normal to irreversible injury (J. Schaper, 1978b, 1980; J. Schaper et al., 1979a and b).

Cellular and Subcellular Changes

Stage 1b is reached quite rapidly in the heart and is characterized by early elongation of Z-bands and a transient contraction of the mitochondrial matrix space.

Stage 2 of global ischemia shows loss of mitochondrial granules and early swelling of mitochondria (Fig. 47.1).

Stage 3 shows swelling of mitochondria and some blebbing of peripheral portions of the sarcomere (Fig. 47.2).

At *stage 4* there is generalized swelling of all mitochondria and cristae alteration. Consumption of cristae by the swollen mitochondria occurs in part (Fig. 47.3).

At *stage 5* (Fig. 47.4) there are flocculent densities seen in mitochondrial matrix space, the generally accepted sign of cell death (Trump et al., 1971; Trump and Mergner, 1974; Jennings et al., 1964; J. Schaper et al., 1979a; Buja et al., 1976). The meaning is irreversible injury. Slight fluffy densities have been observed in the matrix space at stage 4 and seem to resolve (Glaumann et al., 1975). A recent study by Jennings et al. (1978b) attempting isolation of intramitochondrial densities differentiated three findings: 1) large flocculent densities consisting of proteins and phospholipids; 2) smaller ring-shaped densities consisting of calcium phosphate; and 3) large spheric densities consisting of calcium, phospholipids, and phosphorous. This agrees well with studies by Collan et al. (unpublished data, 1979), who digested flocculent densities with proteases on frozen sections of renal tissue and subsequently stained those sections for identification of morphology. By disappearance of the flocculent densities it could be shown that they largely consist of protein coagula. This notion was also suggested by their rapid development following exposure to organic mercurials (Sahaphong and Trump, 1972). It is unclear at present what mitochondrial functional changes correspond to the development of flocculent densities. Logically one would expect a deficiency in matrix-located enzymes such as the various nonmembrane-bound dehydrogenases and the Krebs cycle enzymes. Such alteration in ischemic heart mitochondria was determined by Jennings et al. (1969) using pyruvate metabolism; however, when isolated mitochondria from ischemic tissue were tested, no such deficiencies could be shown and activities or levels of mitochondrial Krebs cycle enzymes do not decline until late following ischemic injury. It is obvious that this question requires further studies in order to gain a deeper understanding. Data on isolated mitochondria should be taken with some caution because of the above mentioned limitations (Lochner et al., 1975).

Global ischemia preparations with reoxygenation with perfusion either by whole blood or with oxygenated salt solution represent an important supplement to ischemic studies because such studies assist in determining remaining cell viability and in studying cellular and subcellular systems in response to reoxygenation. By morphological criteria, significant differences exist between regional and global ischemia (J. Schaper, 1978b). These differences are listed in Table 47.4. In regional ischemia, persistence of mechanical work leading to stretching and compression of the ischemic regions and the presence of a low flow perfusion condition due to collateral vessels cause morphological alterations different from those in global ischemia. There the heart is quiet and not perfused at all.

ANOXIC PERFUSION, BEATING HEART

The model of anoxic perfusion of the beating heart

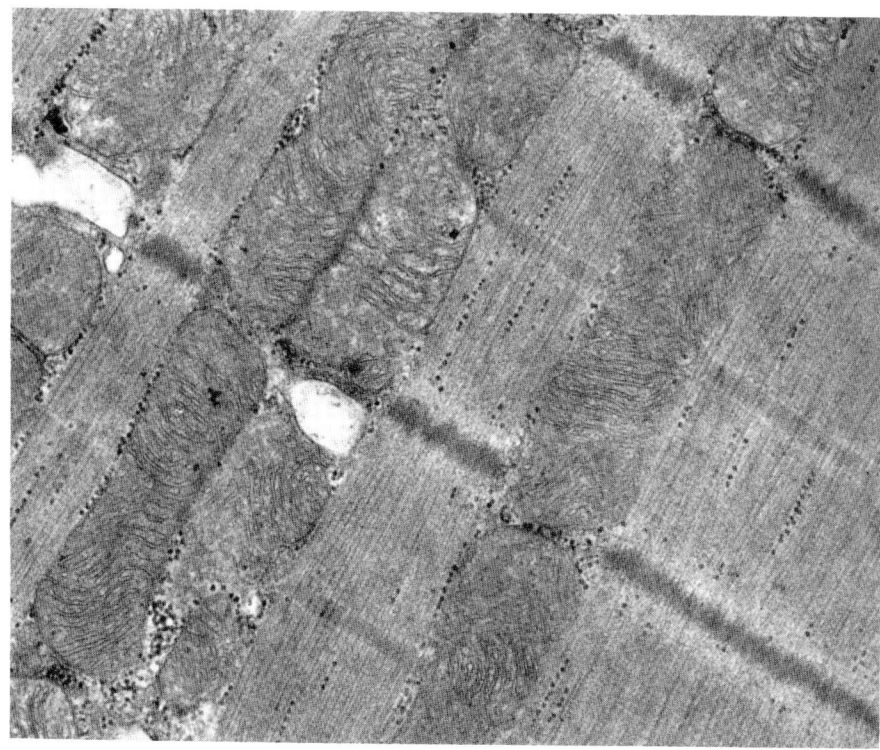

Figure 47.1. Myocardium, early ischemic injury, stage 1b, global ischemia (see text for details). Magnification ×30,000.

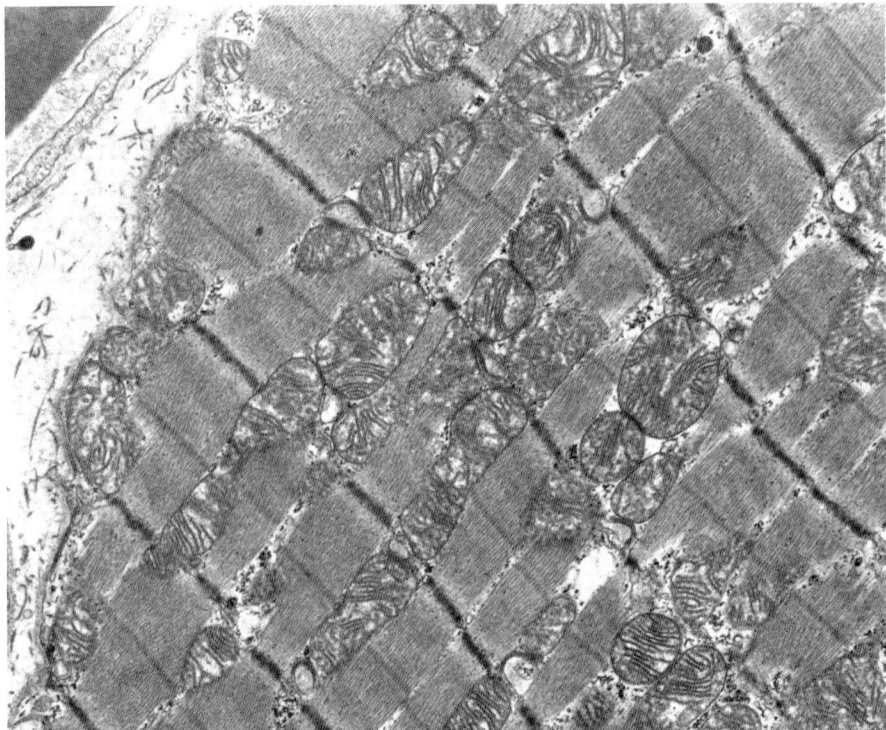

Figure 47.2. Myocardium, global ischemia, reversible ischemic injury, stage 2 (see text for details). ×17,000.

represents a certain situation of hypoxia (or anoxia) while the rate of perfusion is undisturbed. The model can be supplemented by withdrawing substrates, or the selective administration of certain substrates can shed light on specific metabolic functions in hypoxia. This model offers a great latitude in experimental variation. This model, like the globally ischemic heart, may be used like an "in vivo model" or as an isolated heart preparation. Inflow and effluent solutions can be examined for metabolic components, oxygen extraction, etc. A modification of the latter system is the "satellite-heart-model," by which a supply dog does deliver oxygenated blood for perfusion of the coronary system, for the reflow system, and for zero-values (W. Schaper et al., 1976). This is of some importance because the oxygen-carrying capacity, the buffering capacity or the oncotic pressure of oxygen-bubbled solution might significantly differ and vary compared to whole blood preparations. The model of the anoxic (or hypoxic) perfused beating heart has yielded numerous data on anaerobic glycolytic flux as a function of ischemic time and reduced flow. Particularly important data that have been obtained are as follows:

1. Competition between fatty acid and glucose metabolism in normal and hypoxic hearts (Neely and Morgan, 1974; Opie, 1976).

2. The initial rapid acceleration of anaerobic glycolysis in hypoxia which lasts less than 1 min only to return to low levels as a function of internal inhibition probably due to cytoplasmic lactate accumulation. Lactate supposedly inhibits the phosphofructokinase and the 3-P-glyceraldehyde dehydrogenase as does elevated proton concentration (Neely et al., 1976b; Kohn and Garfinkel, 1978; Opie, 1976).

3. The inactivation of anaerobic glycolysis being dependent on the coronary flow is markedly reduced at values lower than 60% flow while above that value there is active flux through this pathway (Neely et al., 1975b; Opie, 1976).

4. Glucose transport is not limiting in ischemia but glucose delivery is (Kohn and Garfinkel, 1978).

5. Glycogen is readily utilized until the branching point of the polysaccharide chains are reached. Limited utilization occurs subsequently (Kohn and Garfinkel, 1978).

6. Fatty acid metabolism is inhibited at the level of β-oxidation in mitochondria and therefore is of no auxiliary function in ischemia. As a matter of fact resynthesis of fatty acid has to be neutralized by formation of cytoplasmic triglycerides, mentioned above (Neely et al., 1976b).

7. There is indeed a rapid washout of adenine nucleotides which, after breakdown from 5'-AMP as adenosine and other metabolites, appear readily in the interstitial space where they possibly execute some effect on microcirculatory function until they are reabsorbed by myocardial parenchymal cells prior to being further metabolized (Kohn and Garfinkel, 1977a and b, 1978; Kohn et al., 1977). 5'-AMPase is cytochemically demonstrated within interstitial parenchymal cells (Borgers et al., 1971). Breakdown of AMP to adenosine that is vasoactive (Schrader et al., 1977) has been shown to occur outside the myocardial cells (Schrader et al., 1977).

CARDIOPLEGIC MODELS

Perfusion of cardioplegic solutions into the coronary circulation produces cardiac arrest. This model is of considerable importance since it represents a means to

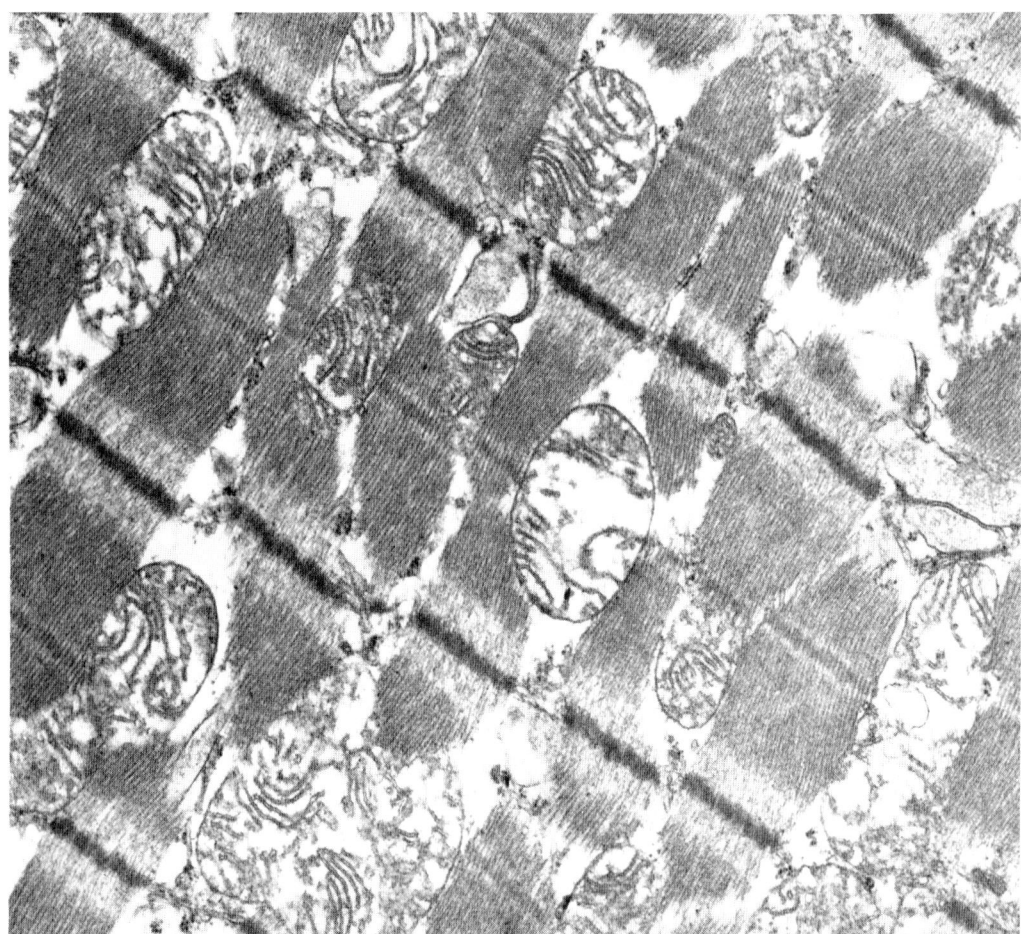

Figure 47.3. Myocardium, global ischemia, severe reversible ischemic injury, stage 4 (see text for details). ×19,400.

maintain myocardial cellular integrity during cardiac surgery. In fact, cardioplegia induced by chemical substances is able to postpone autolytic breakdown of cardiac tissue during the "no-reflow-situation" because of aortic cross clamping. Experiments with the cardioplegic arrested heart are of interest because they permit the study of cardiac metabolism in the nonbeating unperfused heart. Results of these studies are currently applied to increase the safety in human cardiac surgery (Kirsch et al., 1972; Bretschneider et al., 1975; Gay, 1975; Hearse et al., 1976).

SINGLE CELL MODELS

Recent progress in the study of isolated adult heart cells has permitted the exploration of cellular functions under various hypoxic and substrate deficient conditions (Harary et al., 1976). Functional assessment of transport functions, ion and volume control, respiration, and other synthetic or catabolic functions has been made possible by this model as well as by functional and structural correlation, etc., since this model permits study of cell function independent of the vascular and interstitial components (Gerards and Kammermeier, 1978). The same advantages, however, also present disadvantages of this model. Since these isolated adult heart cells are obtained without basement membrane, they remain sensitive to the calcium paradox (see 2.11) and can only be maintained for any length of time without addition of calcium to the medium (Grosso et al., 1977; Dani et al., 1977; Moses and Kasten, 1979). Further studies are needed. These cells are said to have been maintained for 24 hr at room temperature and for 1 week at 0–4°C (Vahouny et al., 1979).

ISOLATED PAPILLARY MUSCLE, PERFUSED SEPTUM AND SLICES

The study of physiological functions of heart tissue in regard to work performance, ion transport, or volume control has lead to the development of models of isolated segments of heart tissue either with blood supply attached (septal preparations) or as isolated tissue preparations, such as papillary muscle. Free hand slices have been used for metabolic and morphological studies (Jennings et al., 1978a; Hawkins et al., 1977).

These models have the advantage of sequestering small pieces of tissue; however, perfusion and nutrition might present a problem if a homogeneous tissue response is to be obtained. A great number of modifications

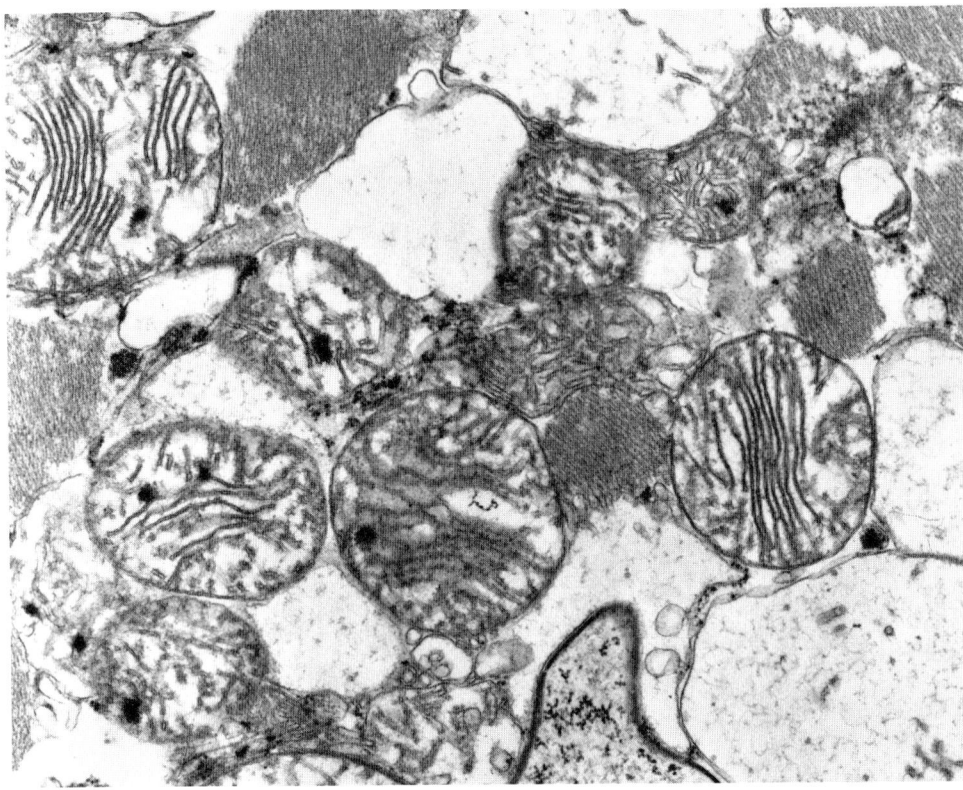

Figure 47.4. Myocardium, global ischemia, irreversible cell injury, stage 5 (see text for details). ×36,000.

of the environment such as acidosis, however, have been studied in these systems (Bing et al., 1973; Pentillä and Trump, 1974a and b, 1975).

REPERFUSION

Remaining viability following a phase of reperfusion and reoxygenation has been accepted as the general test for reversible and irreversible cell injury. Reperfusion itself, however, might prove injurious or be only partially possible because of rising resistance in the vascular bed. In regional ischemia the no-reflow phenomenon occurs, in global ischemia the stone heart.

The observed explosive changes in cells following reperfusion have been thought to represent an unmasking of a prior occurring membrane or cell defect or to lead to an introduction of destructive phenomena such as the calcium paradox. Critical evaluation, however, has shown that the infarct size did not increase following reperfusion; i.e., cell death occurred plus or minus reperfusion. Whether or not changes in the microvascular bed contribute to the no-reflow phenomenon (Kloner et al., 1974a and b, 1976; Reimer et al., 1977) and to an extension of the original infarction needs further investigation. According to studies by Schaper and Pasyk (1976), it appears that the resistance in ischemic perfusion bed rises only after prolonged periods of ischemia.

AWAKE DOG MODELS

Infarctions induced by ligation or clamping of a coronary vessel are usually carried out under anaesthesia. It could be shown that hemodynamic parameters such as pressure, heart rate, PCO_2, and PO_2 are important physiological elements which require good control. It has been argued that such anaesthetized animals do not correspond to the natural infarction and therefore infarction models have been proposed usually in the awake chronically instrumented dog. Chronic instrumentation, however, requires careful observation of the animal; larger series of experiments can, therefore, not be carried out—data can only be obtained from single animals. Furthermore, coronary occlusion by ligation or clamping *is* an artificial condition which again does not permit the study of the true in vivo situation.

Structural Components of the Heart in Ischemia

Ischemic cell injury does affect all structural components of the heart at different rates and to a varying extent. The most striking difference exists between the conduction system, particularly Purkinje fibers and working myocardium, the latter being the very sensitive components. Those differences depend probably on different cellular dependencies on oxidative phosphorylation. Some structures are also affected by external forces such as compression of microvasculature through edema of interstitial space (Ono et al., 1979) and myocardial cells, because loss of cellular volume control leads to cell swelling, a possible factor in increasing resistance in the ischemic vascular region.

THE MYOCARDIAL CELL

An infarction is the result of interrupted blood supply and describes an area of necrotic myocardial cells, i.e.,

Cellular and Subcellular Changes

Table 47.4

Regional Ischemia	versus	Global Ischemia
Heterogeneity of severity of cellular injury		Homogeneous cellular injury
Lipid accumulation		No lipid
Extravasation of blood constituents during ischemia		No blood constituents
Early occurrence of irreversible injury		Late occurrence of irreversible injury
Further cellular deterioration upon reperfusion		Cellular recovery upon reperfusion
Hemorrhagic necrosis after reperfusion		Hemorrhagic necrosis is absent (present only after coronary underperfusion = partial ischemia)

cells which are in a stage of irreversible cell injury. The early response of myocardial cells to ischemic injury is paralysis. The average life span of a myocardial cell in regional ischemia at 37°C varies between 10 and 60 min; i.e., different authors indicate different time intervals. This may be due to different experimental conditions, such as $M\dot{V}O_2$ (myocardial oxygen consumption), etc., as mentioned above (Müller et al., 1979; see 1.21). According to our experience, the first morphological signs of irreversible injury occur between 45 and 60 min after occlusion of a large coronary artery at an $M\dot{V}O_2$ of 6–8 ml/min/100 g. An early functional sign of myocardial ischemia is regional paralysis; i.e., the affected cardiac region ceases to contract. Morphologically this phenomenon is characterized by relaxation of many sarcomeres. Contracted sarcomeres and hypercontractures, however, may also be present. Loss of contractile function may affect the ischemic area locally (passive stretching and compressing by the forcefully contracting surrounding myocardial tissue), and it may also affect the entire heart, causing functional overload on the nonischemic cardiac tissue; the surrounding nonischemic myocardial cells are also altered morphologically, an alteration which requires considerable time for recovery and adjustment even in regions distant from the infarction. Such changes are: edema of myocardial cells, mainly the periphery of the cell and at the perinuclear region; irregularities of sarcomeric arrangement; and occasional extravasation of plasma proteins.

MICROVASCULATURE AND BLOOD COMPONENTS

The microvasculature (capillaries, arterioles, venuoles) can play a role in ischemia as follows:

1. Within the infarcted region, alteration of capillary endothelial cells such as swelling and the occurrence of endothelial blebs could represent mechanical obstruction to proper reperfusion. Abnormal response of arterioles could be responsible for the prolonged reactive hyperemia response following prolonged ischemia; venous compression could interfere with proper efflux from the ischemic region (Kloner et al., 1975a and b; W. Schaper and Pasyk, 1976; W. Schaper, 1978).

2. The components of the blood could propagate vascular damage and/or interfere with perfusion: stiffness of ischemic red blood cells could increase blood viscosity (Weed et al., 1969) reaction of platelets and leucocytes, for example, in response to stimuli from injured cells, could propagate vascular functional and structural changes (J. Schaper, 1978a).

3. Increasing myocardial perfusion by dilatation and regrowth of collateral vessels (W. Schaper et al., 1971) could both contribute to washout of K^+ or adenine nucleotides and metabolic waste products from ischemic tissue and also improve the O_2 supply if sufficient collateral flow were re-established. At that time through regrowth of collaterals (W. Schaper et al., 1971), Purkinje cells, for example, regain access to perfusion. This was shown in an elegant experiment by Dangman et al. (1979), who induced inhibition of spontaneous electrical activity by injecting a pulse of K^+ into the nonoccluded coronary vessels after 24 hr of ischemia. Late increasing collateral flow is not sufficient for working myocardial cells, but Purkinje fibers can benefit from increased flow at that late interval. Many aspects of the microvasculature are still the subject of intense investigation (see Bassingthwaighte et al., 1974; Feigl, 1975a and b; Feldstein et al., 1978; Fitzpatrick et al., 1978; Flameng et al., 1977; Hoffman and Buckberg, 1976; W. Schaper and J. Schaper, 1976, 1977; W. Schaper et al., 1976, 1979a and b; Sherf et al., 1977; Tillmans et al., 1974).

EXTRAMURAL CORONARY ARTERIES AND VEINS AND TRANSMURAL VESSELS

Myocardial infarction commonly occurs in patients who have severe coronary artery disease. Recently a vasospastic mechanism has been observed and postulated to be the major factor in a distinct subgroup of patients (Maseri et al., 1975). Since the atherosclerotic obstruction is impressive, a static concept has been accepted by most investigators (Baroldi, 1978; Cook et al., 1977), but even if the obstruction is unchangeably established, its hemodynamic effect depends entirely on the microvascular flow and the energy demand of the heart muscle. At rest, a 95% obstruction can correlate with satisfactory flow, while with increased energy demand already, 65% obstruction can mean ischemic conditions (Kirkeeide, 1978; Kirkeeide et al., 1979). In what way an active vasoconstrictive component has to be considered is totally unknown at the present time. Studies on the metabolic requirements of extramural arteries revealed that the normal coronary artery can tolerate considerably reduced oxygen tension because it depends on a powerful anaerobic glycolysis, in contrast to intramural arteries and arterioles which require oxidative phosphorylation for proper function (Takenaka et al., 1978; Weiss and Shina, 1978).

CONDUCTION SYSTEM

With the advent of ischemia, the elements of the conduction system do demonstrate electrophysiological abnormalities (Kohlhardt et al., 1977). If ischemic, the sinus node and A-V node may fall silent, resulting in atrial fibrillation (Baba et al., 1970), while conduction time in Purkinje fibers might first be prolonged. Following this phase it might become erratic. Conduction time in Purkinje fibers may also be disturbed in the presence of undisturbed nodal activity (Bailey et al., 1972; Coraboeuf, 1978; Coraboeuf et al., 1976; Corr and Gillis, 1978; Elharrar and Zipes, 1977; El-Sherif et al., 1977; Fenoglio et al., 1979; McGee et al., 1978). The elements of the conduction system, however, are less vulnerable than the working myocardium. Subendocardial Purkinje fibers have been found to be viable at least 24 hr following the infarction, when, in response to lowered collateral resistance, they gain access to re-established collateral circulation as mentioned above (Dangman et al., 1979; El-Sherif et al., 1977; Scherlag et al., 1969, 1970, 1974; Lazzera et al., 1973, 1974).

Yet, functionally the conduction system as a whole appears greatly disturbed, causing three distinct episodes of arrhythmias, ventricular tachycardia, or fibrillation, one at the first few minutes—frequently lethal—one at 18–30 min—also dangerous—and one at 6–18 hr—commonly benign (Gettes, 1974; Gettes and Reuter, 1974; Harris and Rojas, 1943). The mechanism of those episodes is not quite clear at present. The following possibilities have been proposed:

1. Increased and/or altered autonomic nervous activity induces a situation liable to develop an arrhythmic response (Jones et al., 1978; Kolata et al., 1967; Corr and Gillis, 1974, 1975, 1978; Lown and Verrier, 1976; Recordati et al., 1971).

2. Conduction fibers isolated from central excitation develop circus movements of conduction and establish multiple foci responsible for ventricular tachycardia and fibrillation (Wit and Bigger, 1975; Wit and Cranfield, 1978).

3. Alteration of increased cAMP, free fatty acids, and increased extracellular potassium interfere with orderly conduction (Podzuweit et al., 1978a–c).

4. Altered myocardial cells might serve as focal initiators of electrical stimulation (Carmeliet, 1978; Yamazaki et al., 1978).

5. Release of catecholamines secondary to ischemia might disturb myocardial conduction or alter cell metabolism with release of fatty acids (Lammerant et al., 1966; Thoren, 1972; Yamazaki et al., 1978).

Arrhythmia and ventricular tachycardia and fibrillation acutely lower cardiac output, change the hemodynamic support of coronary circulation, and are frequently lethal. Therefore, an understanding of their pathogenesis is of greatest importance. Acidosis has been reported to depress velocity in conduction of Purkinje fibers, which could be partly relieved by organic anions.

PROGRESS AND PATHOGENIC MECHANISM OF ISCHEMIC INJURY

In the study of the pathogenetic mechanism leading to cell death, certain assumptions are being made which have to be verified: 1) cell death is under all circumstances due to the same chain of cellular reactions. It seems as if cells go down an identical path to irreversibility (Trump et al., 1971, 1976b; Trump and Mergner, 1974) after having been disturbed or injured with various events such as interruption of oxygen-substrate supply and perfusion (equals ischemia) or any single element of the ischemic event such as anoxia or lack of substrate alone (Dhalla et al., 1972). Cell injury affecting plasma membrane alone (complement injury, for example) (Hawkins et al., 1972; Shin et al., 1977, 1978), poisoning of plasma membrane with mercurial compounds (Sahaphong and Trump, 1971, 1972), or inhibitors of energy metabolism affecting all cell functions would also produce the same chain of interrelated reactions and finally cell death. 2) There are key changes of organelle functions (Trump and Mergner, 1974; Trump et al., 1971, 1976a and b). Without those, the life of a cell cannot be sustained. If altered by the mechanisms of cell injury, the cell will be destined to die. 3) Interference with those destructive mechanisms means salvage of cells and sustaining of life temporarily until reflow takes place. 4) If able to define the point of attack such as plasma membrane, key proteins, and enzymes, interrelated enzyme systems such as oxidative phosphorylation may put us in a position to identify cell salvaging procedures (Maroko and Braunwald, 1976; Braunwald, 1976).

It follows that the time course of changes in key organelle systems is one possible approach of study.

Cell Organelles

The cell is more than the sum of organelle functions yet, organelles can be considered as single subunits of integrated functions (Kohn and Garfinkel, 1978). Of course, we should realize that some controls and directions depend on the interplay of these functional subunits (Achs and Garfinkel, 1977a and b). Isolated organelles behave differently from those inside the cellular system. This interrelated control becomes apparent if we consider the interwoven relationship of plasma membrane and the bioenergetic system (Trump and Mergner, 1974; Bulkley et al., 1978; Jennings, 1969; Jennings et al., 1963). All the complex reactions of parenchymal cells certainly cannot be understood as being induced by one and only one defective organelle system. Rather there is a network of interrelated alterations which in progression promote cellular alterations; yet it could well be that one organelle system holds the key to irreversibility. Our experimental models are designed to identify this system (Mergner and Mergner, 1981).

PLASMA MEMBRANE

Ischemic cell injury has been described as cell reactions determined by ion and watershifts or loss of volume control (Trump et al., 1971). These are changes which are determined by an altered barrier function of the plasma membrane, a paralysis—so to speak—of the mechanism that establishes the directional gradient which guarantees the internal environment (Rona et al., 1975). There are differences in the resulting ion shifts which depend on the external pool of ions. Although a detailed analysis of the minute to minute changes has not been established in all cell systems, it appears that an efflux of K^+ occurs at an earlier phase (Rau and Langer, 1978) than an influx of Na^+ (Kline and Morrad, 1978; Laiho and Trump, 1975a and b; Hoffman et al., 1978; Mergner et al., 1976), although beginning at the earliest point one can observe, at least in anoxic perfusion experiments, that the sodium space expands at the earliest moment of anoxia and recovers even at points of time which are beyond repair (Winkler et al., 1979; see also "Ionshifts and Ionsequestration").

On the other hand, it was observed by Jennings (1976b), Kloner et al. (1974b), and Whalen et al. (1974) in regional ischemia that there was following reflow an explosive expansion of the inulin accessible space at critical time intervals (Jennings, 1976b). This was interpreted as a nonrepairable opening of the plasma membrane to admit such large molecules as inulin in a large number of cells, because not all parts become equally ischemic in regional ischemia. At the same time the water increases in the ischemic tissue, the water shifts being identical to the increase of the inulin space. There are some questions which can be addressed to this system: Is the analytical technique sensitive enough to show ion shifts between cells and interstitial space and between cell organelles and cytosol? Taken at face value these data indicate that at the time of reflow a distinct change occurs at the level of the plasma membrane. Whether this change has occurred before and is detected at the time of reflow, as suggested by the authors (Whalen et al., 1974; Jennings et al., 1964; Jennings, 1976a and b), or whether reflow itself induces some changes (Bulkley et al., 1978) has to be determined. The difference between Purkinje cells and myocytes in the same ischemic region has to be explained as well; these cells differ in their energy metabolism and most likely not in plasma membrane response to cell injury in ischemia.

Sodium-Potassium-ATPase

Reactivation of sodium potassium-ATPase following ischemia can be shown in a great number of systems, from simple (e.g., squid axons) to complex [e.g., skeletal muscle (Komaha et al., 1971), heart (Winkler et al., 1979; Shine et al., 1977), and renal cortex]. Recent data, however, have been presented by Dhalla (personal communication) that Na^+-K^+-activated ATPase declines at critical times (60 min) of ischemia and does not recover upon reflow (Nagatomo et al., 1978).

Glucose Transport and Fatty Acid Transport

If ischemic cell injury would interfere with orderly glucose transport, cells might starve (Elbrink and Bihler, 1975). A number of studies, however, have shown that glucose transport is enhanced rather than limited during or following periods of ischemia (Garfinkel, 1976; Kohn and Garfinkel, 1978). Vascular glucose delivery, however, is a limiting factor, a fact which is included in the definition of ischemia. Since many parenchymal organs including the heart depend in their normal metabolism on fatty acids, transport, and cellular metabolism during or following limited periods of ischemia is of considerable interest. Yet there are no good studies of fatty acid transport. As will be shown, fatty acid metabolism is inhibited during ischemia (Neely et al., 1976a and b; Hochachka et al., 1977; Randle et al., 1970). If and when it can be activated following transient ischemia has not been studied sufficiently, although models have been worked out (Rose and Goresky, 1977).

Lactate Transport

Lactate in heart muscle cells is transported in two directions: into and out of myocytes. This translocation is the function of a hypothetical lactate permease (Spencer and Lehninger, 1976) which has been shown to exist in Ehrlich ascites tumor cells and which is also suggested to exist in myocytes because of its inhibition in ischemia (Garfinkel, 1976). During very early phases of ischemia there appears to be a parallel increase in lactate production and in lactate transport. Soon, however, that is, within minutes, lactate translocation is reduced and accumulation of lactate occurs only intracellularly in the cytosol compartment (Kohn and Garfinkel, 1978). Response to reflow of this sequestered lactate pool, however, seems to exist, although exact studies related to time of ischemia have not been conducted. The cytosolic accumulation of lactate might have metabolic consequences, as will be shown below (Rovetto et al., 1973, 1975).

Calcium Translocation

In normal myocytes, active calcium translocation during resting condition goes into the extracellular phase. From this extracellular pool controlled by binding to basement membrane sialic acids residues, a small amount enters the cell during each excitation through the slow channels (Langer, 1978; Coraboeuf, 1978), possibly triggering calcium release from intracellular binding or sequestration sites. Therefore, three processes are controlling calcium influx into the intracellular phase: passive calcium leaks; calcium influx through slow channels; and sodium calcium exchange.

In partial (or total) ischemia this inward current persists during early periods of ischemia, while the leakage rate of extracellular calcium into the intracellular compartment increases as a function of ischemic time. Whether or not during ischemia there is a sudden severe alteration of the carrier function towards calcium signaling irreversibility or whether this is a gradual erosion process is unknown (Shen and Jennings, 1972a and b; Lee and Dhalla, 1976).

An exact description of intra- and extracellular calcium shifts is most desirable for formulation of concepts of calcium in ischemic cell injury. A disturbance of calcium can:

1. alter the flux of glycogenolysis and glycolysis (Elbrink and Bihler, 1975);
2. activate plasma membrane bound phospholipases and lead to membrane alteration (Farber et al., 1978; Franson et al, 1978; Chien et al., 1977; Geissler et al., 1976; Newkirk and Waite, 1971, 1973; Nachbaur et al., 1972);
3. activate mitochondrial phospholipases and lead to

membrane disturbances interfering with oxidative phosphorylation (Mergner and McDonnell, 1978; Mergner et al., 1977b, French et al., 1972)

4. activate SR-bound phospholipases and contribute to the release of fatty acids in ischemia (Chien and Farber, 1977);
5. activate lysosomal phospholipases and affect general membrane alteration (Franson et al., 1971; Waite et al., 1976; Weglicki et al., 1972); and
6. interfere with energy conservation and affect the ability of cellular maintenance.

Calcium Paradox

Myocytes exposed to short periods of calcium-free perfusion at 37°C and with energy metabolism uninhibited (Ruigrok et al., 1978) are subject to an unlimited influx of calcium if calcium-free perfusion is followed by calcium-containing solutions (Zimmerman et al., 1967; Zimmerman and Hülsman, 1966). Cell functions subsequently decline due to excessive accumulation of calcium by mitochondria, with a decline in CP and ATP and explosive cell swelling. Whether or not the calcium paradox plays a role in ischemia, as suggested by Bulkley et al. (1978), is unknown. It may, however, play a role in cardioplegia induced by various cardioplegic solutions. The calcium paradox seems to be an energy-dependent process (Ruigrok et al., 1978). It has been suggested that calcium-free perfusion affects the relationship between plasma membrane and the surrounding basal lamina, which might have a controlling function on the extracellular calcium pool (Hearse et al., 1978).

Recovery of cells from the calcium paradox has been attempted (Nayler, personal communication) but not successfully obtained yet. The functional equivalent of calcium accumulation after calcium-free perfusion is increased is "stiffness of the ventricles," resulting in the stone heart phenomenon. This represents an irreversible injury of myocardial cells.

Calcium-Activated Phospholipases

Recently through the work of Chien et al. (1977, 1978) on liver cells and Weglicki et al. (1975) on heart cells the proposal has been made that phospholipases located in the plasma membrane could be activated in ischemia. This activation leads to a hormone-sensitive response of membranes (Franson et al., 1978) or to a self-destruction of membranes such as plasma membrane (Farber et al., 1978). Inhibition by chlorpromazine of this process (Chien et al., 1977) has been reported. This concept is of key importance if it can be shown that the activation of membrane-located phospholipases is fast enough and extensive enough to explain permanent or temporary membrane alteration. Of course, it would also be essential to obtain an exact idea of the type of interaction (complement type, ion carrier type, etc.) and the resulting functional alteration. These questions, however, have yet to be studied (Seeman, 1974).

LYSOSOMES

The concept that lysosomes as bags of lytic enzymes contribute to cell destruction prior to cell death (suicidal bag hypothesis), to autolysis of cells after cell death, or to cell repair if cells should survive is old, proposed almost as early as lysosomes were discovered (DeDuve and Beaufay, 1959). Whether or not lysosomes indeed cause irreversibility, however, has not sufficiently been proven. Their role in reversible and irreversible cell injury is unclear. For example, loading of lysosomes with protein markers (ferritin) (Hawkins et al., 1972) did show that with immune injury (plasma membrane) or ischemic injury there was no release of ferritin even when cells were severely destroyed.

Release of Lytic Enzymes and Their Activation

In the heart, lytic enzymes were found in part of the endoplasmic reticulum, the Golgi complex, and secondary lysosomes—a system thought to be functionally in continuity (cytocavitary network) (Trump, 1975). Ischemia then could be related to early release of lytic enzymes, interestingly, though, clear evidence of release could only be achieved with cathepsin (Decker and Wildenthal, 1978a and b; Lesch, 1977), while acid phosphatase could not be demonstrated to be released. This data differed from Hoffstein et al., (1976), Gottwik et al. (1975, 1978), and Welman et al. (1976, 1977, 1978). Therefore, one has to include release *and* activation of lytic enzymes from lysosomes in theoretical consideration of the pathogenesis of irreversible ischemic injury. Whether there are also inhibitors of lysosomal enzymes in the cytosol or organelles is unknown at present.

Changes in Lysosomal Functional Parameters in Ischemia

Ischemia does involve changes in lysosomal membranes, which most likely can be observed during early intervals when the ATP concentration noticeably falls. At that time, it can be shown that the pH gradient across the inner membrane falls, leaving the content of lysosomes less acidic and moving the pH in such a way that the acid optimum for lytic function does not exist anymore. Ischemia most likely also affects the various transport functions across the membrane and the volume control based on cation and anion gradients (Mego et al., 1972; Malbica and Hart, 1971); lysosomes swell (Trump and Mergner, 1974).

Permeability Towards Lytic Enzymes as a Function of Ischemic Time

Of critical importance, however, for including lysosomes into consideration, is the determination of their permeability towards bigger substances such as proteins (Riciutti, 1972a and b; Majno et al., 1960).

The following points should be considered:
1. Is there a point of rupture?
2. Is the change in permeability gradual?
3. Can it be shown that enzymes thus released are active?
4. Are there cytosolic inhibitors of lytic enzymes and if so are they active at ischemic conditions?
5. If there is lysis of lysosomal integrity and activation

of enzymes, what is the point of attack: general digestion, proteinolysis, lipo- and phospholipolysis (Wildenthal, 1978; Kennett and Weglicki, 1978a and b)?

SARCOPLASMIC RETICULUM (SR) AND PEROXISOMES

Inactivation of functions such as inhibition of the calcium transport mechanism and SR-ATPase are early findings related to declining ATP concentration. These indeed may be significant findings since they contribute to the cytosolic increase of calcium. Whether or not there are any other mechanisms, such as self-destruction of membranes due to activation of lytic enzymes, is currently unknown. Evidence of peroxisomes function in ischemia has been presented by Herzog and Fahimi (1974).

CYTOSOL

The cytosol can contribute to cellular reactions to ischemia through its control over glycogenolysis, anaerobic glycolysis, and anabolic functions as well as ATP-consuming functions related to cytosol filaments such as myofilaments. Furthermore, the cytosolic calcium concentration contributes to an altered regulation, as do other ions such as inorganic phosphate and magnesium (Achs and Garfinkel, 1977a and b; Elbrink and Bihler, 1975; Jacobus, 1978; Kübler and Katz, 1977; Neely et al., 1973, 1975a and b, 1976a and b; Rovetto et al., 1973, 1975).

Anaerobic Glycolysis

Anaerobic glycolysis in the heart is stimulated within several seconds (Neely et al., 1973; Opie, 1976; Achs and Garfinkel, 1977a and b). Therefore, a number of investigators assume that increased energy production through this pathway represents a normal auxiliary energy system to heart cells. During the same interval the outer branches of glycogen are quickly lysed, a reaction which stops at the outer branching points of the glycogen molecule (Achs and Garfinkel, 1977a and b; Kohn and Garfinkel, 1978).

After this initial burst, glycolytic flux is very much reduced, being inhibited at several critical control sites such as phosphofructokinase or 3-P-glyceraldehyde dehydrogenase (Neely et al., 1975a, 1976b; Kohn and Garfinkel, 1978).The inhibition at these critical points may be partially a function of metabolic interactions with ATP/ADP/P_i concentrations at these controlling enzyme steps and partially a function of the decreasing intracellular pH (Opie, 1975). Particularly experimentally well defined is the inhibition of anaerobic glycolysis at the level of 2/3-P-glyceraldehyde dehydrogenase by increased levels of lactate which could be linked to the cytosolic lactate accumulation secondary to partial inhibition of plasma membrane lactate permease (Kohn and Garfinkel, 1978). The key question is, how irreversible is such inhibition? Preliminary studies by Holsinger et al. (1978) seem to indicate that anaerobic glycolysis can recover during reflow while oxidative phosphorylation (see "mitochondria") may not (Opie et al., 1971, 1975).

Filaments

The prominent feature of the reflow phase is the development of prominent contraction bands. There are numerous questions related to this morphological phenomenon which, if answered, might provide more insight into the cytosol phenomena during reflow. Some of these questions are:

1. Are contraction bands a sign of irreversible cell alteration or are they transient?
2. Are contraction bands due to increased cytosol concentrations of calcium or are ATP-deficiency or other phenomena contributing factors? Lack of ATP is an established cause of contraction band formation in skeletal muscle. The role of calcium there is questioned.
3. Since there are different types of contraction bands, the question remains as to which ones are correlated to what cellular metabolic status?
4. Does the process which causes contraction band formation also signal or even contribute to the advance of destructive processes such as increase of free cytosolic calcium inhibition of myosin ATPase and excess consumptions of myosin ATP or rupture of plasma membrane (Ganote et al., 1976)?

The development of blebs at the surface of ischemic heart cells can be observed. These blebs possibly are related to an alteration of the gel fiber consistency of these superficial sites secondary to the influx of calcium, possibly related to the process of altered calcium permeability of the plasma membrane (Trump et al., 1978b).

Fat Droplet

Glycogen synthesis is inhibited during periods of partial or complete regional ischemia; however, regional ischemia having some degree of remaining perfusion shows a significant amount of accumulation of triglycerides. These are seen as cytosolic fat globules (J. Schaper, 1978b, 1980). This phenomenon is more frequently seen in models of chronic cell injury in liver and kidney cells. Its rapid appearance in heart cells might be related to the high dependency on fatty acid metabolism and its inhibition of β-oxidation in mitochondria (Neely et al., 1976a) in ischemia as an emergency depoisoning and storage measure. Cells containing fat droplets have been observed to function and survive. Therefore, it may be concluded that accumulation of lipids in heart cells by itself may be consistent with viability.

MITOCHONDRIA

Organelle changes in mitochondria leading to a defective organelle function such as oxidative phosphorylation are an essential part in all schemes of irreversibility. The sequence being constructed and the importance of events as it is being designed might differ in detail. Mitochondria are numerous in working myocardial cells and the surface of the inner membrane alone makes them the major provider of ATP and the major sequestration site of calcium (Carafoli and Crompton, 1976). Studies on isolated organelles, however, are particularly difficult in heart tissue due to mechanical and chemical factors of the isolation process, including factors of the isolation medium (Lochner et al., 1975; Nayler et al., 1976; Nayler, personal communication). Therefore, schemes have to be worked out by which the time course of observed organelle changes have to be traced back to the intact tissue or parts of the tissue for proper timing of the ischemic change. This can be done by examining oxidative phosphorylation and related functions in whole tissue, tissue slices, isolated mitochondria, and submitochondrial preparations (Mergner et al., 1977a, 1979b).

Substrate-Transport, Krebs Cycle and Respiration

A number of mitochondrial transport processes are altered in ischemic tissue, as demonstrated for metabolite-dependent shuttle mechanisms (Achs and Garfinkel, 1977a and b; Klingenberg, 1970). In reconstituted systems (isolated mitochondria) or under reflow conditions, a number of these inhibitions do recover during early periods of ischemia, that is, during the reversible phase. Therefore, one may assume that translocation across the inner membrane is not a limiting reaction in ischemic cell injury (Mergner et al., 1977a, 1977d). The same is true for Krebs cycle metabolisms and dehydrogenation steps including respiration (state IV, substrate supported). The persistence of respiration and substrate metabolism can be found until the early phase of *irreversible cell injury*, when NAD-requiring substrates (NADH dehydrogenase) may not continue to support respiration (Mergner et al., 1977a). One may conclude, therefore, that until irreversibility is reached there is no evidence of proteolytic destruction of transport proteins and proteins of the respiratory chain (Mergner et al., 1977e).

Oxidative Phosphorylation

Oxidative phosphorylation is affected fairly early and shows functional defects in a reconstituted system. Such functional defects are: 1) early: a reduced state III respiration (ADP + substrate), b) uncoupling of mitochondria, and c) declining ATPase activity (DNP-stimulated); and 2) later: a) reduced P/O ratio which occurs approximately when the time of irreversibility is reached.

Functional changes in the later phase of ischemic injury in oxidative phosphorylation appear to be related to a decline in the proton gradient (Mitchell, 1961) across the inner membrane of mitochondria (Mergner et al., 1977a). In the presence of a persistent electron transport (state IV respiration) (Chance and Williams, 1955), the declining proton gradient could indicate either reduced translocation of protons or reduced gradient of protons, considering that charge separation still occurs (that is, protons and electrons are being produced) (Blondin and Green, 1975). This change occurs at the same time when the P/O ratio declines. We postulate, therefore, a relationship between these declining functions (Mergner et al., 1972a and b, 1977a, 1977c, 1977d, 1979a; Laiho and Trump 1975a; Lochner et al., 1975, 1976, 1978, 1979; Trump et al., 1976a and b).

Calcium Sequestration

The ability to accumulate or sequester calcium declines as an early phenomenon of ischemia (Göring and Spieckermann, 1978; Mergner et al., 1977b). When mitochondria are examined in a reconstituted system it becomes apparent that the rate of calcium accumulation declines. However, there is still calcium translocation (Lee and Dhalla, 1976) and precipitation in paramembranous punctate densities in ischemic mitochondria. This calcium appears as calcium phosphate (Buja et al., 1976; Jennings et al. 1978a; Ashraf and Bloor, 1976). The exact relationships still have to be worked out. It appears that the presence of punctate densities in paramembranous sites of isolates ischemic mitochondria or within fixed tissue or even frozen sections is an indication of injured membranes. The calcium may be rather immobile (Mergner et al., 1976, 1977b, 1977e; Dhalla et al., 1972, 1978).

Göring and Spieckermann (1978) determined that ischemia affects calcium uptake and the calcium release reactions of mitochondria (Crompton et al., 1976a and b; Lehninger et al., 1978). The decline of mitochondrial function that occurs during the critical transitional phase affects certain key functions of mitochondrial inner membranes involved in calcium accumulation, proton gradient, and oxidative phosphorylation, while other functions such as respiration remain intact. Therefore, we wanted to define the ischemic impact causing irreversibility as a destructive process which affects the integrity of the machinery of oxidative phosphorylation. In our hypothesis the key of reversible injury rests with calcium-activated destruction and alteration of the phospholipid layer of the inner membrane of mitochondria, as will be pointed out in detail below (Mergner and McDonnell, 1978).

Nucleus and Anabolic Processes During Ischemia and Reflow

Ischemia interferes with some anabolic processes directed by nuclear synthetic functions and mitochondrial synthetic functions (Albin et al., 1970; Aschenbrenner et al., 1970; Kao et al., 1976; Peterson and Lesch, 1975; Rabinowitz, 1971; Wollenberger and Krause, 1968). It could be that failure of synthesis of substrates of oxidative metabolism such as adenine nucleotides (Atkinson, 1968; DeJong et al., 1977; Gerlach et al., 1971) limits survival because of an inability of cells to transfer the energy of a reactivated oxidative phosphorylation machinery in reflow situations (Gerlach et al., 1971). The potential contribution could be visualized in situations with relatively high remaining flow causing a washout effect, and it could be a factor if resynthesis of adenine nucleotides is only a staggering and slow process, that is, at borderline reversibility. Therefore, hypoxia and hypoxic perfusion could differ from complete ischemia in the relative washout of substrate and also of ions, for example, K^+ and Mg^{2+}, known to be important for energy delivery and synthetic processes (Höfer and Pressman, 1966; Gomez-Pyou et al., 1970, 1972).

Although nuclei of myocytes are morphologically altered quite early following ischemic cell injury, there is no evidence that their ability to recover declines prior to the point-of-no-return. Isolated nuclei (Kleitke et al.,

1973) taken from ischemic rat kidney demonstrate synthetic activity in a reconstituted system, and there is evidence that a certain key synthetic activity of proteins can recover following short periods of ischemia, providing ATP is generated and control over the inner environment is re-established. An example for accelerated synthesis has been reported for cytochromes (Kao, 1976). On the other hand, it could be shown that stopped protein synthesis by itself does not cause cell death (Shelburne and Trump, 1968). Therefore, it may be concluded that nuclear synthetic function is not directly related to irreversible changes in subcellular changes of myocardial infarction.

Mechanism of Irreversibility

Among the numerous proposed possibilities which have been related to the event of irreversibility, we have shown that irreversibility rests with nonretrievable loss of functions which represent the expression of the life of a cell. Key functions to be considered in such a discussion are:

1. The ability to maintain an homeostatic inner environment. Homeostasis represents control over water in- or efflux, ion in- and efflux as well as production of an ion gradient and the distinct topographic control of ions such as calcium within cellular compartments (cytosol, SR, mitochondria).

2. New generation of certain substrates such as adenine nucleotides for transfer of metabolic energy. The generation itself of energized products by the cellular machinery of mitochondria is an essential characteristic of viability.

3. The confinement and/or inhibition of lytic enzymes such as reside in lysosomes or such as are a part of all organelles (phospholipases).

Since all these functions rest within cellular membranes, viability may be defined as a state of cellular maintenance, where these membrane functions are unaffected.

IONSHIFTS AND IONSEQUESTRATION

The idea that ion shifts could be a critical step in the sequence leading to irreversibility is based on two assumptions. 1) A number of ions which represent the internal environment are essential to the normal function of key enzymes such as Mg^{2+} for DNP-ATPase and K^+ for P_i-ATP exchange, etc. (Chefurka, 1966; Höfer and Pressman, 1966; Gomez-Pyou et al., 1970, 1972). It has been proposed that certain biological functions can only be carried out under ideal concentration of key ions. Therefore, leakage and loss of these ions should interfere with resuming proper functions, a fact which still has to be tested. 2) Other ions which penetrate cells should reach uncontrolled concentration—ischemia interfering with normal sequestration and release functions—and lead to activation of other enzymatic functions. An example for this relationship may be seen in cellular accumulation of P_i and Ca^{2+} during early phases of ischemia (Mergner et al., 1979b; Dhalla et al., 1972, 1978; Göring and Spieckermann, 1978; Kübler and Katz, 1977; Lee and Dhalla, 1976; Hoffman et al., 1978; Nayler et al., 1976; Nayler, personal communication; Shen and Jennings, 1972a and b).

Potassium in Ischemia and Reflow

Microprobe analysis of frozen sections of canine myocardium in regional ischemia shows a rapid loss (within 15–30 min) of potassium from mitochondria and cytosol (Mergner et al., 1976; Hoffman et al., 1978; Trump et al., 1978a). This loss is not immediately discovered by tissue extraction (Jennings 1976b, Jennings et al., 1978a; Kloner et al., 1974a; Whalen et al., 1974). Therefore, it may be that such loss occurs into the interstitium with an enlargement of this space (Ono et al., 1979). Short-term reflow after ischemia of longer duration does not immediately correct this change, although studies on isolated heart preparations with isotopes have shown an immediate activation of Na^+, K^+-ATPase (Winkler et al., 1979). In single cell preparations the K gradient is reversed if cells are viable, offering this ion shift as an indicator of reversibility of cell injury in that system (Laiho and Trump, 1974a and b).

Mg^{2+} in Ischemia, Isolated Mitochondria and Ascites Tumor Cells

Elemental Mg^{2+} levels are not clearly seen in microprobe analysis studies unless instruments are used with high resolution. Therefore, intracellular data from this source are insufficient. Isolated cell preparations indicate an early loss of magnesium (Laiho et al., 1971; Laiho and Trump, 1975a and b), while mitochondria isolated from ischemic kidney reveal loss of Mg^{2+} only after 60 min of ischemia (Collan, unpublished data). This change, if confirmed, could be of interest because it would indicate a membrane-related release of a structurally important ion.

Elemental Shifts of Phosphorous

According to the hypothesis by Kübler and Katz (1977) one finds a striking elevation of inorganic phosphate during early phases of ischemia, and indeed microprobe analysis does reveal an elevation of phosphorous over cells, mainly over mitochondria (Mergner et al., 1976, 1979b). This change is not accompanied by a similar calcium elevation during the early phase of ischemia. Increase of calcium is only seen during the later phase of ischemia where precipitates form between calcium and phosphate, when the so called "paramembranous punctate" or "amorphous densities" are present (Buja et al., 1976; Jennings et al., 1978b; Mergner et al., 1977b and d). It is unknown if and how phosphorous contributes to cellular degeneration in ischemia. The role of phosphate translocation into mitochondria under ischemic condition requires further studies.

CALCIUM

The most critical ion shift, however, appears to be the uncontrolled elevation of cytosolic calcium. Very recent evidence by microprobe analysis has shown that such cytosolic elevation indeed does take place during early phases of ischemia in the heart (Trump et al., 1979; Mergner et al., 1979b)—prior to the point-of-no-return—

so that such elevation could be related to an activation of calcium-dependent phospholipases (see "Phospholipases"). The first question which has to be considered is, What is the source of the cytosolic calcium? The following possibilities exist: (1) plasma membrane (see "Plasma Membrane"), calcium leakage from the outside through passive or activated exchange processes; (2) SR; and (3) mitochondria secondary to a shifted balance due to energy deficiency.

Poole-Wilson (personal communication) in recent studies showed by repeated pulses of radioactive calcium that the plasma membrane barrier became gradually more leaky as a function of ischemic time during anoxic perfusion.

Mitochondrial calcium translocation and its precipitation of calcium as calcium phosphate during certain phases of ischemia and ischemia with reflow requires further study (Buja et al., 1976; Jennings et al., 1978b; Ashraf and Bloor, 1976; Mergner et al., 1977b).

The energized mitochondrial calcium translocation may be assumed to be stopped, while at the same time during ischemia the mitochondrial ability of accumulation is paralyzed and on reflow the rate of calcium accumulation is slowed down (Mergner et al., 1977b).

It has been proposed that these calcium phosphate densities are signs of an altered inner membrane in ischemia. They are seen frequently accompanying reflow (Kloner et al., 1974a) when cells have also other severe changes such as blebs, interruption of the continuity of the plasma membrane, contraction bands, and flocculent densities in the matrix of mitochondria. Studies attempting to differentiate calcium binding and calcium translocation show no significant change in membrane binding or the rate of binding to the inner membrane of mitochondria. We believe, therefore, that calcium plays an essential role in the progression of the ischemic cell injury. The processes leading to an uncontrolled cytosolic calcium are 1) loss of sequestration power, mitochondria, SR, and 2) increased leaks, either from within cells or from outside the cells. There is no evidence that a sudden change of permeability with increased permeability towards calcium leads to cell death, but there is no doubt that prolonged elevation of calcium in the cytosol could be instrumental in activation of destructive processes.

PHOSPHOLIPIDS, PHOSPHOLIPASES, AND BREAKDOWN PRODUCTS

Recent studies to determine the level and rate of activity of a large series of enzymes in ischemia have shown that most enzyme systems retain high levels and activity, *even* during time periods, which are distinctly beyond the point-of-no-return (Klein et al., 1979). This has been shown to be true for respiratory enzymes, lactate dehydrogenase, DNP-ATPase, Na^+, K^+ ATPase, etc. (Komaha et al., 1971). It is not clear at all if the earlier and reversible periods of ischemia include degradation of proteins. In studies by Majno et al. (1960), liberation of amino acids was a late phenomenon accompanied by a change of tissue pH. We see evidence that ischemic damage which leads to irreversibility represents an alteration of phospholipids or of a change of phospholipid-protein interaction (Mergner and McDonnell, 1978). Alterations of the intactness of membrane functions of biologically essential membranes such as mitochondria could represent an irreversible loss of viability.

Ischemic Dysfunction

Membranes of ischemic tissue, organelles, and cellular membranes show early dysfunction (Boime et al., 1970; Chien et al., 1978; Coleman et al., 1976; Ashraf and Halverson, 1977, 1978; Nayler, personal communication; Farber et al., 1978). Part of this dysfunction is certainly due to inhibition because of an energized substrate deficiency; part of this dysfunction, however, is due to membrane changes themselves or changes of distinct barrier functions.

There is increased leakage from and into the cytosol through the plasma membrane, even while the pumps show increased activation in reflow (Winkler et al., 1979; Jennings, 1976b; Jennings et al., 1978a; Chiong and Parker, 1975; Van Rossum, 1972; Rau and Langer, 1978). Mitochondrial membranes lose their ability to maintain volume in a potassium chloride solution and swell in tissue sections after passing a contracted state (Armiger et al., 1975; Mergner et al., 1976, 1977f); microsomal ribosomes dissociate from the membrane, and transfer of ions through channels changes as a function of ischemia (Carmeliet, 1978; Coraboeuf, 1978). Finally, massive leaks occur through plasma membrane with expansion of the inulin and water spaces (Jennings, 1976b; Jennings et al., 1978a; Rona et al., 1975), the proton gradient of mitochondria disappears (Mergner et al., 1977a) and lysosomes loose cathepsin D (Decker et al., 1977; Decker and Wildenthal, 1978a and b; Kennett and Weglicki, 1978a and b; Lesch, 1977).

Phospholipids

There have been a few studies of isolated membranes and their content of phospholipids following ischemia. Chien et al. (1978) and Chien and Farber (1977) examined isolated plasma membrane of liver cells and showed changes in phospholipid content after ischemic injury. Changes in phospholipid content by isolated mitochondria were shown by Smith et al. (1980), Trump et al. (1976b) and Mergner et al. (1977e). The latter studies revealed a loss of cardiolipin and phosphatidylethanolamine as a function of ischemic time. Boime et al. (1970) showed increased fatty acid release from ischemic rat liver microsomes. The ischemic process therefore appears to induce destructive changes of phospholipids which, if prevented, can prolong viability (Farber et al., 1978).

Phospholipases

Studies on all organelle membranes have shown that all membranes contain phospholipases. This is true for plasma membrane of liver (Chien et al., 1977), heart (Franson et al., 1978; Waite et al., 1976), lysosomes (Weglicki et al., 1972; Waite et al., 1976), mitochondria (French et al., 1972; Mergner and McDonnell, 1978;

Parce et al., 1978), etc. These phospholipases are frequently or in most cases activated by elevated levels of calcium, whereby a distinct level of calcium concentration is needed above which inhibition occurs (Franson et al., 1978; Mergner and McDonnell, 1978). It has not been demonstrated yet by what mechanism of membrane alteration such phospholipases are being instrumental in causing significant membrane changes and if the rate at ischemic conditions of 37°C, pH 6.0–6.7 is sufficient. Possibly there exist auxiliary phenomena such as peroxidation (Yasuda and Fujita, 1977).

Mechanism of Membrane Alteration

One crucial target of such membrane alteration may be mitochondrial inner membranes. This alteration determines viability. The mechanism of such a proposed membrane alteration is speculative. At present one could visualize several possibilities of such ischemic membrane alteration (Mergner and Mergner, 1981): 1) a change in membrane properties through insertion of alien substances such as fatty acids and lysophosphatides; and 2) a change in membranes through introduction of structural disorder (altered arrangement of phospholipids, altered protein phospholipid interaction, loss of phospholipids).

Fatty Acids. Mitochondria change their membrane properties through insertion of free fatty acids into the inner membrane. These free fatty acids could act as proton carriers (Hinkle and McCarthy, 1978) and induce uncoupling in in vitro systems. Whether or not such mechanism is active in ischemia as proposed by Boime et al. (1970) for rat liver system is unclear.

Lysophosphatides. Recent studies on the role of lysophosphatides have shown that these substances are fairly toxic to membranes. All membrane systems therefore contain lysophospholipases for further breakdown of these intermediary metabolic substances. It is possible that these substances are formed in ischemia with increased numbers and that they remain in the membrane. Recent studies have shown that externally added lysophosphatides could simulate the permeability disorders seen in ischemia.

Altered Arrangement of Phospholipids. Altered arrangement and/or mobility of phospholipids has its distinct possibility in certain membrane changes such as it is seen in the complement injury of the plasma membrane where channels are being formed for ionic leakage (Shin et lal., 1977, 1978; Seeman, 1974).

Altered Protein Phospholipid Interaction. Altered protein to protein or protein phospholipid interaction (Van Deenen, 1975) could exist in the inner membrane ATPase system with dissociation of the inner membrane ATPase unit from the membranous unit. The base pieces located within the inner membrane could act as proton channels (Hinkle and McCarthy, 1978).

Not only do those degradative processes have to be proved to be active in ischemica, but it also has to be established in what sequence, rate, and direction they are being activated. There is some evidence through comparison of studies of mitochondria being altered by externally added phospholipase (Burstein et al., 1971a and b).

In these studies it was shown that the sequence of functional degradation was identical to the ischemic alteration if phospholipase was incubated with intact mitochondria in increasing concentration. When external phospholipases acted on intact mitochondria, the above described pattern of ischemic changes occurred, such as loss of rate of calcium accumulation, loss of phosphorylation, and preservation of respiration.

If, however, inside out submitochondrial particles were exposed to phospholipase (Burstein et al., 1971b), respiration was eliminated. Therefore, the following sequence of events could be postulated: cytosolic elevation of calcium leads to external activation of phospholipases which induce irreversible inner membrane degradation and therefore loss of ATP-producing power of mitochondria.

Changes in the plasma membrane which have been proposed by Farber et al. (1978) and Jennings et al., (1978a) seem to be repairable if a source of ATP is available.

FAILURE DURING REGENERATION AND WASHOUT PROCESSES

As cells approach the point-of-no-return, however, they may loose more and more regenerative power. It could then be that the morphological state 4 (Trump and Mergner, 1974) represents a certain gray zone, where addition of further events such as loss of adenine nucleotides or lack of regeneration of adenine nucleotides and loss of potassium and magnesium slow down or prohibit recovery. This has to be considered for two reasons:

1. Our only test system for remaining viable are studies on reconstituted systems and reflow studies. Could such reflow be instrumental in further destruction by washout or washin of substances, for example, exposure to excess calcium?

2. Therapy will be aimed at restoring normal conditions. Shouldn't such therapy be programmed according to the phasic recovery of cells?

CONCLUSION

Is ischemic cell injury to myocardial cells identical to ischemic cell injury to cells of other organs?

We have attempted to describe ischemic cell injury to myocytes as identical to other parenchymal cells where irreversibility represents an event of exhaustion of regenerative functions. Life as a process is based on the constant energy-requiring, actively maintained balance of multiple integrated systems. If such energy supply is not forthcoming degradative processes ensue. In our presentation we have proposed the possibility that such degradative processes are activated during the reversible phase through increasing influx of calcium into cytosol, and that this uncontrolled cytosolic elevation of calcium is instrumental in altering phospholipids of numerous membranes. The key membrane in such degradative processes, it seems, is the mitochondrial membrane. If an alternative energy source would be forthcoming, cells would be able to maintain viability and repair ischemia-induced alterations, and so stay alive.

Irreversible cell injury, therefore, seems to be due to a number of different cellular events that involve all components of the myocardium. The inability to reverse the above described degradative changes upon withdrawal of the noxious stimulus (i.e., ischemia) produces lack of contractile function and action potential, destruction of the morphological integrity of the tissue, and various subcellular functional defects. Irreversibility may be defined as the permanent loss of the energy-producing functions, but we have to bear in mind that this definition may yet simplify too much the complexity of events as we have described them. There is no doubt, however, that ischemia resulting in irreversible progression of destructive cellular events produces myocardial infarction and necrosis.

Acknowledgment. This work was supported by National Institutes of Health Grant No. 1-R01-7222281-01, National Blood, Heart and Lung Institute. Written during tenure as visiting professor at Max-Planck Institut, Bad Navheim (WJM).

References

Achs, M.J., and Garfinkel, D.: Computer simulation of energy metabolism in anoxic perfused rat heart. Am. J. Physiol. *232:*164–174, 1977a.

Achs, M.J., and Garfinkel, D.: Computer simulation of rat heart metabolism after adding glucose to the perfusate. Am. J. Physiol. *232:*175–184, 1977b.

Albin, R., Aschenbrenner, V., and Rabinowitz, M.: Increased turnover of mitochondrial constituents in cardiac hypertrophy and acute hypoxia in the rat. J. Clin. Invest. *29:*2A, 1970.

Armiger, K.C., and Gavin, J.B.: Changes in the microvasculature of ischemic and infarcted myocardium. Lab. Invest. *33:*51, 1975.

Armiger, K.C., Herdson, P.B., and Gavin, J.B.: Mitochondrial changes in dog myocardium induced by lowered pH in vitro. Lab. Invest. *32:*223–226, 1975.

Aschenbrenner, V., Druyan, R., Albin, R., Rabinowitz, M., and Haue, A.: Cytochrome C and total protein turnover in mitochondria from rat heart and liver. Biochemistry *9:*157–160, 1970.

Ashraf, M., and Bloor, C.M.: X-ray microanalysis of mitochondrial deposits in ischemic myocardium. Virchows Arch. [Cell. Pathol.] *22:*287–297, 1976.

Ashraf, M., and Halverson, C.: Structural changes in the freeze-fractured sarcolemma of myocardium. Am. J. Pathol. *88:* 583–594, 1977.

Ashraf, M., and Halverson, C.: Ultrastructural modifications of nexuses (gap junctions) during early myocardial ischemia. J. Mol. Cell. Cardiol. *10:*263–269, 1978.

Atkinson, D.E.: The energy charge of the adenylate pool as regulatory parameter: Interaction with feedback modifiers. Biochemistry *7:*4030–4040, 1968.

Baba, N., Leighton, R.F., and Wissler, A.M.: Experimental cardiac ischemic observation of the sinoatrial and atrioventricular nodes. Lab. Invest. *23:*168–177, 1970.

Bailey, J.C., Greenspan, K., Elizari, M.V., Anderson, G.J., and Fisch, C.: Effects of acetylcholine on automaticity and conduction in the proximal portion of the His-Purkinje specialized conduction system of the dog. Circ. Res. *30:*210–216, 1972.

Baroldi, G.: Coronary stenosis: Ischemic or non-ischemic factor. Am. Heart J. *96:*139–143, 1978.

Bassingthwaighte, J.B., Yipintsoi, T., and Harvey, R.B.: Microvasculature of the dog left ventricular myocardium. Microvasc. Res. *7:*229–249, 1974.

Bing, O.H.L., Brooks, W.W., and Messer, T.V.: Heart muscle viability following hypoxia: Protective effect of acidosis. Science *80:*1297–1298, 1973.

Blondin, G.A., and Green, D.E.: A unifying model of bioenergetics. Chem. Eng. News *10:*26–42, 1975.

Boime, F., Smith, E.E. and Hunter, F.E.: The role of fatty acids in mitochondrial change during liver ischemia. Arch. Biochem. Biophys. *139:*425–443, 1970.

Borgers, M., Schaper, J., and Schaper, W.: Adenosine-producing sites in the mammalian heart: A cytochemical study. J. Mol. Cell. Cardiol. *3:*287–296, 1971.

Braunwald, E. (Ed.): *Protection of the Ischemic Myocardium.* American Heart Association, Dallas, 1976.

Bretschneider, H.J.: Überlebenszeit und Wiederbelebungszeit bei Normo-und Hypothermie. Verh. Dtsch. Ges. Kreislaufforsch. *30:*11–34, 1964.

Bretschneider, H.J., Cott, L.A., Hensel, I., Kettler, P., and Martel, J.: Ein neuer komplexer haemodynamischer Parameter aus 5 additiven Gliedern zur Bestimmung des O_2-Bedarfs des linken Ventrikels. Pfluegers Arch. Ges. Physiol. *319:*14–28, 1970.

Bretschneider, H.J., Hübner, G., Knoll, D., Lohr, B., Notbeck, H., and Spieckermann, P.G.: Myocardial resistance and tolerance to ischemia: Physiological and biochemical basis. J. Cardiovasc. Surg. *16:*241–260, 1975.

Buhl, M.R.: The postanoxic regeneration of 5′-adenine nucleotides in rabbit kidney tissue during in vitro perfusion. Scand. J. Clin. Lab. Invest. *36:*175–181, 1976.

Buja, L.M., Dees, J.H., Harling, D.F., and Willerson, J.T.: Analytical electron microscopic studies of mitochondrial inclusions in canine myocardial infarcts. J. Histochem. Cytochem. *24:*508–516, 1976.

Bulkley, B., Nunnally, R.L., and Hollis, D.P.: "Calcium paradox" and the effect of varied temperature on its development: A phosphorous nuclear magnetic resonance and morphological study. Lab. Invest. *39:*133–140, 1978.

Burstein, C., Loyter, A., and Racker, E.: Effects of phospholipases on structure and function of mitochondria. J. Biol. Chem. *246:*4075–4082, 1971a.

Burstein, C., Kandrach, A., and Racker, E.: Effects of phospholipases and lipases on submitochondrial particles. J. Biol. Chem. *246:*4083–4089, 1971b.

Carafoli, E., and Crompton, M.: Calcium ions and mitochondria. In *Calcium in Biological Systems,* edited by C.J. Duncan, pp. 89–116. Cambridge University Press, Oxford, 1976.

Carmeliet, E.: Cardiac transmembrane potentials and metabolism. Circ. Res. *42:*577–587, 1978.

Chance, B., and Williams, G.R.: Respiratory enzymes in oxidative phosphorylation in the steady state. J. Biol. Chem. *217:*407–427, 1955.

Chefurka, W.: Oxidative phosphorylation of in vitro aged mitochondria. I. Factors controlling loss of dinitrophenol stimulated adenosine triphosphatase activity and respiratory control in mouse liver mitochondria. Biochemistry *5:*3887–3903, 1966.

Chien, K.R., and Farber, J.L.: Microsomal membrane dysfunction in ischemic rat liver cells. Arch. Biochem. Biophys. *180:*181–198, 1977.

Chien, K.R., Abrams, J., Pfau, R.G., and Farber, J.L.: Prevention by chlorpromazine of ischemic liver cell death. Am. J. Pathol. *88:*539–558, 1977.

Chien, K.R., Abrams, J., Serroni, A., Martin, J.T., and Farber,

J.L.: Accelerated phospholipid degradation and associated membrane dysfunction in irreversible ischemic liver cell injury. J. Biol. Chem. *253:*4804–4817, 1978.

Chiong, M.A., and Parker, J.O.: Metabolic indicators of myocardial ischemia in man. Recent Adv. Stud. Cardiac Struct. Metab. *10:*141–157, 1975.

Coleman, S.E., Duggan, T., and Hackett, R.L.: Plasma membrane changes in freeze fractured rat kidney cortex following renal ischemia. Lab. Invest. *35:*63–70, 1976.

Cook, B.H., Granger, H.J., and Taylor, A.E.: Metabolism of coronary arteries and arterioles: A histochemical study. Microvasc. Res. *14:*145–159, 1977.

Coraboeuf, E.: Ionic basis of electrical activity in cardiac tissue. Am. J. Physiol. *234:*H101–H116, 1978.

Coraboeuf, E., Deronbaix, E., and Hoerter, J.: Control of ionic permeabilities in normal and ischemic heart. Circ. Res. (Suppl. I) *38:*92–98, 1976.

Corr, P.B., and Gillis, R.A.: Role of the vagus nerves in the cardiovascular changes induced by coronary occlusion. Circulation *49:*86–97, 1974.

Corr, P.B., and Gillis, R.A.: Effect of autonomic neural influences on cardiovascular changes induced by coronary occlusion. Am. Heart J. *89:*766–774, 1975.

Corr, P.B., and Gillis, R.A.: Autonomic neural influences on the dysrhythmias resulting from myocardial infarction. Circ. Res. *43:*1–9, 1978.

Crompton, M., Capano, M., and Carafoli, E.: The sodium-induced efflux of calcium from heart mitochondria. Eur. J. Biochem. *69:*453–462, 1976a.

Crompton, M., Sige, E., Salzmann, M., and Carafoli, E.: A kinetic study of the energy-linked influx of Ca^{2+} into heart mitochondria. Eur. J. Biochem. *69:*429–434, 1976b.

Dangman, K.H., Wang, H.H., and Wit, A.L.: Effects of intracoronary potassium chloride on electrograms of canine Purkinje fibers in six hours to four week old myocardial infarction: An indication of time dependent changes in collateral blood flow. Circ. Res. *44:*392–405, 1979.

Dani, A.M., Cittadini, A., Flamini, G., Festuccia, G., and Terranora, T.: Preparation and some properties of isolated beating myocytes from adult rabbit heart. J. Mol. Cell. Cytol. *9:*777–784, 1977.

Decker, R.S., and Wildenthal, K.: Influence of methylprednisolone on ultrastructure and cytochemical changes during myocardial ischemia: Selective effects on various cell inclusions and organelles including lysosomes. Am. J. Pathol. *92:*1–22, 1978a.

Decker, R.S., and Wildenthal, K.: Sequential lysosomal alterations during cardiac ischemia. II. Ultrastructural and cytochemical changes. Lab. Invest. *38:*662–673, 1978b.

Decker, R.S., Poole, A.R., Griffin, E.E., Dingle, J.T., and Wildenthal, K.: Altered distribution of lysosomal cathepsin D in ischemic myocardium. J. Clin. Invest. *59:*911–921, 1977.

Decker, R.S., Poole, A.R., Dingle, J.T., and Wildenthal, K.: Lysosomal alterations in autolysing rabbit heart. J. Mol. Cell. Cardiol. *11:*189–196, 1979.

DeDuve, C.H., and Beaufay, H.: Tissue fractionation studies. 10. Influences of ischemia on the state of some bound enzymes in rat liver. Biochem. J. *73:*610–616, 1959.

De Jong, J.W., Verdouw, P.D., and Ramme, W.J.: Myocardial nucleoside and carbohydrate metabolism and hemodynamics during partial occlusion and reperfusion of pig coronary artery. J. Mol. Cell. Cardiol. *9:*297–312, 1977.

Dhalla, N.S., Yates, J.C., Watz, D.A., McDonald, V.A., and Olsson, R.E.: Correlation between changes in the endogenous energy stores and myocardial function due to hypoxia in the isolated perfused rat heart. Can. J. Physiol. Pharmacol. *50:*333–345, 1972.

Dhalla, N.S., Das, P., and Sharma, G.P.: Subcellular basis of contractile failure. J. Mol. Cell. Cardiol. *10:*363–385, 1978.

Duncan, C.J.: Properties and stabilization of the lysosomal membrane. Nature *210:*1229–1230, 1966.

Elbrink, J., and Bihler, I.: Membrane transport: Its relation to cellular metabolism rates. Science *188:*1179–1184, 1975.

Elharrar, V., and Zipes, D.P.: Cardiac electrophysiological alterations during myocardial ischemia. Am. J. Physiol. *233:*H329–345, 1977.

El-Sherif, N., Hope, R.R., Scherlag, J., and Lazzera, R.: Reentrant ventricular arrhythmias in late myocardial infarction period. I. Conduction characteristics in the infarction zone. Circulation *55:*686–702, 1977.

Farber, J.L., Martin, T.J., and Chien, K.R.: Irreversible ischemic cell injury. Am. J. Pathol. *92:*713–732, 1978.

Feigl, E.O.: Reflex parasympathetic coronary vasodilatation elicited from cardiac receptors in the dog. Circ. Res. *37:*175–182, 1975a.

Feigl, E.O.: Control of myocardial oxygen tension by sympathetic coronary vasoconstriction in the dog. Circ. Res. *37:*88–95, 1975b.

Feldstein, M.L., Henquell, L., and Honig, C.R.: Frequency analysis of coronary intercapillary distances: Site of capillary control. Am. J. Physiol. *253:*H321–H325, 1978.

Fenoglio, J.J., Karaguenzian, H.S., Friedman, P., Albala, A., and Wit, A.: The course of infarct growth toward the endocardium after coronary occlusion. Am. J. Physiol. *236:*H356–H370, 1979.

Fitzpatrick, T.M., Alter, I., Corey, E.J., Ramwell, P.W., Rose, J.C., and Kol, P.A.: Cardiovascular responses to PG_2 (prostacyclin) in dog. Circ. Res. *42:*192–198, 1978.

Flameng, W., Winkler, B., Wüsten, B., and Schaper, W.: Minimum requirements for the measurement of regional myocardial flow using tracer microspheres. Bibl. Anat. *15:*24–29, 1977.

Franson, R.C., Waite, M., and LaVia, M.: Identification of phospholipase A_1 and A_2 in the soluble fraction of rat liver lysosomes. Biochemistry *10:*1942–1946, 1971.

Franson, R.C., Pang, D.C., Towle, D.W., and Weglicki, W.B.: Phospholipase A activity of highly enriched preparations of cardiac sarcolemma from hamster and dog. J. Mol. Cell. Cardiol. *10:*921–930, 1978.

French, S.W., Todoroff, T., Norum, M.L., and Ihrig, T.J.: Effects of lipid hydrolysis and phosphate swelling on the structural and functional integrity of mitochondria. Exp. Mol. Pathol. *16:*16–33, 1972.

Friedman, P.L., Stewart, J.R., Fenoglio, J.J., Jr., and Wit, A.L.: Survival of subendocardial Purkinje fibers after extensive myocardial infarction in dogs: In vitro and in vivo correlations. Circ. Res. *33:*517–611, 1973.

Ganote, C.E., Warstell, J., and Kaltenbach, J.P.: Oxygen induced enzyme release after irreversible myocardial injury: Effects of cyanide on perfused hearts. Am. J. Pathol. *84:*327–350, 1976.

Garfinkel, D.: Lactate permeation. Circ. Res. (Suppl. I) *38:*I-13–I-14, 1976.

Garlick, P.: The measurement of intracellular pH with NMR in ischemia. In *Acidosis and the Heart.* Cardiac Muscle Research Group, Autumn Meeting, London, 1978.

Gay, W.: Potassium-induced cardioplegia. Ann. Thorac. Surg. *20:*95–99, 1975.

Geissler, D., Mentz, P., Bayer, B.L., and Forster, W.: Action of phospholipase A on isolated heart preparations. Acta Biol. Med. Ger. *35:*1171–1172, 1976.

Gerards, P., and Kammermeier, H.: Isolated myocardial cells of adult rats: Interrelationship of shape, energy metabolism and enzyme release. Pfluegers Arch. (Suppl.) *373:*R18, 1978.

Gerlach, E., Maroko, P., Zimmerman, H.G., Peterson, I., and Trendelenberg, C.H.: Different response to adenine nucleotide synthesis de novo in kidney and brain during aerobic recovery from anoxia and ischemia. Experientia 27:876–878, 1971.

Gettes, L.S.: Electrophysiologic basis of arrhythmias in acute myocardial ischemia. In *Modern Trends in Cardiology*, edited by M.F. Oliver, pp. 219–246. Butterworth, London, 1974.

Gettes, L.S., and Reuter, H.: Slow recovery from inactivation of inward currents in mammalian myocardial fibers. J. Physiol. (Lond.) 240:703–724, 1974.

Glaumann, B., Glaumann, H., Berezesky, I.K., and Trump, B.F.: Studies on the pathogenesis of ischemic cell injury. II. Morphological changes of the pars convoluta ($P_1 \pm P_+$) of the proximal tubule of the rat kidney made ischemic in vivo. Virchows Arch. [Cell. Pathol.]19:281–302, 1975.

Glick, M.R., Burns, A.H., and Reddy, W.J.: Dispersion and isolation of beating cells from adult rat heart. Anal. Biochem. 61:32–42, 1974.

Gomez-Pyou, A., Sandoval, F., Chavez, E., and Tuena, M.: On the role of potassium on oxidative phosphorylation. J. Biol. Chem. 245:5239–5247, 1970.

Gomez-Pyou, A., Sandoval, F., Chavez, E., Freites, D., and de Gomez-Pyou, M.: Dependency of the ATPase and ^{32}P-ATP exchange reaction on mitochondrial K^+ and electron transport. Arch. Biochem. Biophys. 153:215–225, 1972.

Göring, G.G., and Spieckermann, P.G.: Ca^{2+}-uptake and -release phenomena from cardiac mitochondria under normal and ischemic conditions. Basic Res. Cardiol. 73:126–132, 1978.

Gottwik, M.G., Kirk, E.S., Hoffstein, S., and Weglicki, W.B.: Effect of collateral flow on epicardial and endocardial lysosomal hydrolases in acute myocardial ischemia. J. Clin. Invest. 56:914–923, 1975.

Gottwik, M.G., Kirk, E.S., Kennett, F.F., and Weglicki, W.B.: Release of lysosomal enzymes during ischemic injury of canine myocardium. Recent Adv. Stud. Cardiac Struct. Metab. 12:431–443, 1978.

Grosso, D.S., Frangakis, C.J., and Carlson, E.C.: Isolation and characterisation of myocytes from adult rat heart. Prep. Biochem. 7:383–401, 1977.

Harary, J., and Farley, B.: In vitro studies of single isolated beating heart cells. Science 131:1674–1675, 1960.

Harary, J. Hoover, F., and Farley, B.: The isolation and cultivation of rat heart cells. Methods Enzymol. 32:740–744, 1976.

Harris, A.S., and Rojas, A.G.: Initiation of ventricular fibrillation due to coronary occlusion. Exp. Med. Surg. 1:105–133, 1943.

Hawkins, H.K., Ericsson, J.L.E., Biberfeld, P., and Trump, B.F.: Lysosome and phagosome stability in lethal cell injury. Am. J. Pathol. 68:255–287, 1972.

Hawkins, H.K., Lowe, J.E., Hill, M.L., and Jennings, R.B.: Loss of cell volume and electrolyte control in slices of ischemic myocardium. Am. J. Pathol. 86:449, 1977.

Hearse, D.J.: Reperfusion of the ischemic myocardium. J. Mol. Cell. Cardiol. 9:605–615, 1977.

Hearse, D.J., Stewart, D.A., and Brainbridge, M.V.: Myocardial protection during bypass and arrest. J. Thorac. Cardiovasc. Surg. 72:880–884, 1976.

Hearse, D.J., Humpfrey, S.M., and Bullock, R.R.: The oxygen paradox and the calcium paradox: Two facets of the same problem? J. Mol. Cell. Cardiol. 10:641–668, 1978.

Herzog, V., and Fahimi, D.: Microbodies (peroxisomes) containing catalase in myocardium: Morphological and biochemical evidence. Science 185:271–273, 1974.

Hinkle, P.C., and McCarthy, R.E.: How cells make ATP. Sci. Am. 238:104–107, 1978.

Hirche, H.J., Franz, C., Bös, L., Bissig, R., Lang, R., and Schramm, M. Myocardial extracellular K^+ and H^+ increase and noradrenaline release as possible cause of early arrhythmia following acute coronary artery occlusion in pigs. J. Mol. Cell. Cardiol. 12:579, 1980.

Hochachka, P.W., Neely, J.R., and Driedzic, W.R.: Integration of lipid utilisation with Krebs cycle activity in muscle. Fed. Proc. 36:2009–2015, 1977.

Höfer, M., and Pressman, B.F.: Stimulation of oxidative phosphorylation in mitochondria by potassium in the presence of oligomycin. Biochemistry 5:319–329, 1966.

Hoffman, J.I.E., and Buckberg, G.D.: Transmural variation in myocardial perfusion. In *Progress in Cardiology*, edited by J.F. Joachim, pp. 321–330. Lea & Febiger, Philadelphia, 1976.

Hoffman, M., Mergner, W.J., Hickey, J., and Mergner, G.W.: Electrolyte shifts following permanent coronary artery occlusion. Fed. Proc. 37:495, 1978.

Hoffstein, S., Weissmann, G., and Fox, A.C.: Lysosomes in myocardial infarction: Means of cytochemistry, subcellular fractionation, with observations on the effect of methylprednisolone. Circulation (Suppl. I) 53:I-34–I-40, 1976.

Holsinger, J.W., Ramey, C.A., and Allison, T.B.: Transmural gradients in ischemic canine left ventricle: Effects of blood reflow and glycolytic intermediates. Recent Adv. Stud. Cardiac Struct. Metab. 12:579–583, 1978.

Ingwall, J.S., DeLuca, M., Sybers, H.D., and Wildenthal, K.: Fetal mouse hearts—a model for studying ischemia. Proc. Natl. Acad. Sci. U.S.A. 72:2809–2813, 1975.

Jacobus, W.E.: Alteration of heart mitochondrial energy transport by Pi. J. Mol. Cell. Cardiol. (Suppl. I) 10:38, 1978.

Jennings, R.B.: Early phase of myocardial ischemic injury and infarction. Am. J. Cardiol. 24:753–765, 1969.

Jennings, R.B.: Relationship of acute ischemia to functional defects and irreversibility. Circulation (Suppl. 1) 53:I-26–I-29, 1976a.

Jennings, R.B.: Cell volume regulation. Acta Med. Scand. 587:83–93, 1976b.

Jennings, R.B., Kaltenbach, J.P., Sommers, H., Bahr, G.F., and Wartman, W.B.: Studies of the dying myocardial cell. In *Etiology of the Myocardial Infarction*, edited by T.N. James and J.W. Keyes, pp. 189–204. Little, Brown, Boston, 1963.

Jennings, R.B., Sommers, H.M., Herdson, P.B., and Kaltenbach, J.P.: Ischemic injury of myocardium. Ann. N.Y. Acad. Sci. 156:61–68, 1964.

Jennings, R.B., Herdson, P.B., and Hill, M.L.: Pyruvate metabolism in mitochondria isolated from dog myocardium. Lab. Invest. 20:548–557, 1969.

Jennings, R.B., Hawkins, H.K., Lowe, J.E., Hill, M.L., Klotman, S., and Reimer, K.A.: Relation between high energy phosphate and lethal injury in myocardial ischemia in the dog. Am. J. Pathol. 92:187–214, 1978a.

Jennings, R.B., Shen, A.C., Hill, M.L., Ganote, C.E., and Herdson, P.B.: Mitochondrial matrix densities in myocardial ischemia and autolysis. Exp. Mol. Pathol. 29:55–67, 1978b.

Jennische, E., Enger, E., Medegård, A., Applegren, L., and Haljamae, H.: Correlation between tissue pH, transmembrane potentials, cellular energy metabolism during shock and during ischemia. Circ. Shock 5:251–260, 1978.

Jones, C.E., Beck, L.Y., DuPont, E., and Barnes, G.E.: Effects of coronary ligation on the chronically sympathectomized dog ventricle. Am. Physiol. Soc. 235:H429–434, 1978.

Kahng, M.W., Berezesky, I.K., and Trump, B.F.: Metabolic and ultrastructural response of rat kidney cortex to in-vitro ischemia. Exp. Mol. Pathol. 29:183–198, 1978.

Kammermeier, H.: Verhalten von Adenin-Nukleotiden und Kreatinphosphat im Herzmuskel bei funktioneller Erholung nach länger dauernder Asphyxie. Verh. Dtsch. Ges. Kreislaufforsch. 30:206, 1964.

Kao, R., Rannels, D.E., and Morgan, H.E.: Effects of anoxia and severe ischemia on the turnover of myocardial proteins. Acta Med. Scand. 587:117–123, 1976.

Kennett, F.F., and Weglicki, W.B.: Lack of effect of methylprednisolone on lysosomal and microsomal enzymes after two hours of well-defined canine myocardial ischemia. Circ. Res. 43:759–768, 1978a.

Kennett, F.F., and Weglicki, W.B.: Effects of well-defined ischemia on lysosomal and microsomal enzymes in a canine model. Circ. Res. 43:750–758, 1978b.

Kirkeeide, R.L.: Mechanism of normal and stenotic coronary blood flow. Ph.D. Thesis, Iowa State University, Ames, Iowa, 1978.

Kirkeeide, R.L., Young, D.F., and Cholvin, N.R.: Mechanics of stenotic coronary blood flow. Ger. J. Cardiol. 68:263, 1979.

Kirsch, V., Rodewald, G., and Kalmar, P.: Induced ischemic arrest, clinical experience with cardioplegia in open heart surgery. J. Thorac. Cardiovasc. Surg. 63:121–130, 1972.

Klein, H.H., Puschmann, S., Wissler, J.H., Winkler, B., and Schaper, W.: Studies on limiting metabolic features controlling heart muscle tissue integrity. Hoppe Seyler's Z. Physiol. Chem., 360:1169, 1979.

Kleitke, B., Hinterberger, V., Ohnen, K., Rabitsch, G., and Wollenberger, A.: Einfluss von totaler Ischemie auf die Ribonucleinsäure und Eiweißsynthese im Herzmuskel der Ratte, untersucht in Schnitten und zellfreien Systemen. Acta Biol. Med. Ger. 30:33–55, 1973.

Kline, R., and Morrad, M.: Potassium efflux and accumulation in heart muscle: Evidence from K^+ electrode experiments. Biophys. J. 16:367–372, 1978.

Klingenberg, M.: Metabolite transport in mitochondria: An example of intracellular membrane functions in essays. In *Biochemistry*, edited by P.N. Campbell and F. Dickens, vol. 6, pp. 146–150. Academic Press, New York, 1970.

Kloner, R.A., Ganote, C.E., and Jennings, R.B.: The "noreflow" phenomenon after temporary coronary occlusion in the dog. J. Clin. Invest. 34:1496–1508, 1974a.

Kloner, R.A., Ganote, C.E., Whalen, D., and Jennings, R.B.: Effect of a transient period of ischemia on myocardial cells. II. Fine structure during the first few minutes of reflow. Am. J. Pathol. 74:399–422, 1974b.

Kloner, R.A., Ganote, C.E., Jennings, R.B., and Reimer, K.A.: Demonstration of the "no-reflow" phenomenon in the dog heart after temporary ischemia. Recent Adv. Stud. Cardiac Struct. Metab. 10:463–474, 1975a.

Kloner, R.A., Ganote, C.E., Reimer, K., and Jennings, R.B.: Distribution of coronary arterial flow in acute myocardial ischemia. Arch. Pathol. 99:86–94, 1975b.

Kloner, R.A., Reimer, K.A., Wilkerson, J.T., and Jennings, R.B.: Reduction of experimental myocardial infarct size with hyperosmolar mannitol. Proc. Soc. Exp. Biol. Med. 151:677–683, 1976.

Kohlhardt, M., Münich, Z., and Maier, G.: Alterations of the excitation process of the sinoatrial pacemaker cell in the presence of anoxia and metabolic inhibitors. J. Mol. Cell. Cardiol. 9:477–488, 1977.

Kohn, M.C., and Garfinkel, D.: Computer simulation of ischemic rat heart purine metabolism. I. Model construction. Am. J. Physiol. 232:H386–H393, 1977a.

Kohn, M.C., and Garfinkel, D.: Computer simulation of ischemic rat heart purine metabolism. II. Model behavior. Am. J. Physiol. 232:H394–H399, 1977b.

Kohn, M.C., and Garfinkel, D.: Computer simulation of entry into glycolysis and lactate output in the ischemic heart. J. Mol. Cell. Cardiol. 10:779–796, 1978.

Kohn, M.C., Achs, M.J., and Garfinkel, D.: Distribution of adenine nucleotides in the perfused rat heart. Am. J. Physiol. 232:R158–R163, 1977.

Kolata, T., Ascanio, G., Tallarida, R.J., and Openheimer, M.J.: Action-potentials in the sensory vagus at the time of coronary occlusion. Am. J. Physiol. 213:71–78, 1967.

Komaha, A., Boyd, W.A., Ballinger, L.M., and Ueda, I.: Adenosine in phosphatase activity of subcellular fractions of normal and ischemic muscle. J. Surg. Res. 11:297–302, 1971.

Kübler, W., and Katz, A.M.: Mechanism of early pump failure of the ischemic heart: Possible role of adenosine triphosphate depletion and inorganic phosphate accumulation. Am. J. Cardiol. 40:467–482, 1977.

Kübler, W., and Spieckermann, P.G.: Regulation of glycolysis in the ischemic and the anoxic myocardium. J. Mol. Cell. Cardiol. 1:351–377, 1970.

Laiho, K.U., and Trump, B.F.: Relationship of ionic, water and cell volume changes in cellular injury of Ehrlich ascites tumor cells. Lab. Invest. 31:207–215, 1974a.

Laiho, K.U., and Trump, B.F.: The relationship between cell viability and changes in mitochondrial ultrastructure, cellular ATP, ion and water content following injury of Ehrlich ascites tumor cells. Virchows Arch. [Zellpathol.] 5:267–277, 1974b.

Laiho, K.U., and Trump, B.F.: Mitochondrial changes and ion and water shifts in the cellular injury of Ehrlich ascites tumor cells. Beitr. Pathol. 155:237–247, 1975a.

Laiho, K.U., and Trump, B.F.: Studies on the pathogenesis of cell injury: Effects of inhibitors of metabolism and membrane function on the mitochondria of Ehrlich ascites tumor cells. Lab. Invest. 32:163–182, 1975b.

Laiho, K.U., Shelburne, J.D., and Trump, B.F.: Observations on cell volume, ultrastructure, mitochondrial conformation and vital-dye uptake in Ehrlich ascites tumor cells: Effects of inhibiting energy production and function of the plasma membrane. Am. J. Pathol. 65:203–230, 1971.

Lamers, J.M.J., and Hülsmann, W.C.: Inhibition of ($Na^+ + K^+$)-stimulated ATPase of heart by fatty acids. J. Mol. Cell. Cardiol. 9:343–346, 1977.

Lammerant, J., De Herdt, P., and de Schryner, C.: Direct release of myocardial catecholamines into the left heart chambers: The enhancing effect of acute coronary occlusion. Arch. Int. Pharmacodyn. Ther. 163:219–226, 1966.

Langer, G.A.: The structure and function of myocardial cell surface. Am. J. Physiol. 235:H461–468, 1978.

Lazzera, R., El-Sherif, N., and Scherlag, B.J.: Electrophysiological properties of canine Purkinje cells in one-day-old myocardial infarction. Circ. Res. 33:722–734, 1973.

Lazzera, R., El-Sherif, N., and Scherlag, B.J.: Early and late effects of coronary artery occlusion on canine Purkinje fibers. Circ. Res. 35:391–399, 1974.

Lee, S.L., and Dhalla, N.S.: Subcellular calcium transport in failing hearts due to calcium deficiency and overload. Am. J. Physiol. 231:1159–1165, 1976.

Lehninger, A., Vercesi, A., and Bababummi, E.A.: Regulation of Ca^{2+} release from mitochondria by oxidation-reduction state of pyridine nucleotides. Proc. Natl. Acad. Sci. U.S.A. 75:1690–1694, 1978.

Lesch, M.: Kinetics of solubilisation of cathepsin D in autolyzing rabbit myocardium. Circulation 56:111–209, 1977.

Levitzky, S., and Feinberg, H.: Biochemical changes in ischemia. Ann. Thorac. Surg. 20:21–29, 1975.

Lochner, A., Opie, L.H., Owen, P., Kotzé, J.C.N., Bruyneel, K., and Gevers, W.: Oxidative phosphorylation in infarcting baboon and dog myocardium: Effects of mitochondrial isolation and incubation media. J. Mol. Cell. Cardiol. 7:203–217, 1975.

Lochner, A., Kotzé, J.C.N., and Gevers, W.: Mitochondrial oxidative phosphorylation in myocardial anoxia: Effects of albumin. J. Mol. Cell. Cardiol. 8:465–480, 1976.

Lochner, A., Kotzé, J.C.N., Benade, A.J.S., and Gevers, W.: Mitochondrial oxidative phosphorylation in low-flow hypoxia: Role of free fatty acids. J. Mol. Cell. Cardiol. 10:857–875, 1978.

Lochner, A., Kotzé, J.C.N., Gevers, W., and Benade, A.J.S.: Substrate effect on mitochondrial function and tissue lipid in low flow hypoxia of isolated perfused rat hearts. Basic Res. Cardiol. 74:303–312, 1979.

Lowe, J.E., Reimer, K.A., and Jennings, R.B.: Experimental infarct size as a function of the amount of myocardium at risk. Am. J. Pathol. 90:363–380, 1978.

Lown, B., and Verrier, R.L.: Neural activity and ventricular fibrillation. N. Engl. J. Med. 294:1165–1170, 1976.

Majno, G., Laguttata, M., and Thompson, T.E.: Cellular death and necrosis: Chemical, physical and morphological changes in rat liver. Virchows Arch. [Pathol.] 333:421–465, 1960.

Malbica, J.O., and Hart, L.G.: Effect of ATP and some inflammatory agents on a purified lysosomal fraction having high acid phosphatase and labile β-glucuronidase activity. Biochem. Pharmacol. 20:2017–2026, 1971.

Maroko, P.R., and Braunwald, E.: Effects of metabolic and pharmacologic interventions on infarct size following coronary occlusion. Circulation (Suppl. I) 53:I-162–I-168, 1976.

Maseri, A., Mimmo, R., Chierdia, S., Pezola, A., and L'Abbate, A.: Coronary artery spasms—a cause of acute ischemia in patients, hemodynamic and angiographic documentation. Clin. Res. 23:195A, 1975.

Mathes, P., Ronnig, D., Sack, D., and Erhardt, W.: Experimental myocardial infarct in the cat. I. Reversible decline in contractility of noninfarcted tissue. Circ. Res. 38:540–546, 1976.

McGee, J., Singer, D.H., TenEick, R.E., Kloner, R., Belic, N., Reimer, R., and Elson, J.: Cellular electrophysiologic marker of irreversible ischemic myocardial injury. Am. J. Physiol. 235:H559–H568, 1978.

MeNeely, G.R.: The capillary factor in myocardial infarction. Am. J. Cardiol. 34:583–587, 1974.

Mego, J.L., Farb, R.M., and Barnes, J.: An adenosine triphosphate dependent stabilisation of proteolytic activity of heterolysosomes, evidence of a proton pump. Biochem. J. 128:763–769, 1972.

Mergner, W.J., and McDonnell, M.: Phospholipase activity of normal, aged and ischemic mitochondria. Lab. Invest. 38:357, 1978.

Mergner, W.J., and Mergner, G.: Subcellular aspects of ischemic heart disease: Studies on acute myocardial infarction. In *Pathobiology of Human Disease*, edited by B.F. Trump, R.T. Jones, and A. Laufer. Fischer Verlag, Stuttgart, in press, 1981.

Mergner, W.J., Garbus, J., Dees, J.H., Valigorsky, J.M., and Trump, B.F.: Structural and functional changes in human kidney and liver mitochondria after shock and trauma. Am. J. Physiol. 66:36, 1972a.

Mergner, W.J., Smith, M.A., and Trump, B.F.: Mitochondrial coupling factor and permeability in the early phase of ischemia. Lab. Invest. 26:485, 1972b.

Mergner, W.J., Hickey, J.M., Chang, S.H., Berezesky, I.K., Weissman, H.I., and Trump, B.F.: Studies on ischemia of the myocardium: Stereometry and microprobe analysis. In *Proceedings of the International Association of Pathologists XIth International Congress*, p. 180. Washington, DC, 1976.

Mergner, W.J., Marzella, L., Mergner, C., Kahng, M.W., Smith, M.W., and Trump, B.F.: Studies on the pathogenesis of ischemic injury. VII. Proton gradient and respiration of renal tissue cubes, renal mitochondria and submitochondrial particles following ischemic cell injury. Beitr. Pathol. 161:230–243, 1977a.

Mergner, W.J., Smith, M.W., Sahaphong, S., and Trump, B.F.: Studies on pathogenesis of ischemic cell injury. VI. Accumulation of calcium by isolated mitochondria of ischemic rat kidney cortex. Virchows Arch. [Cell Pathol.] 26:1–16, 1977b.

Mergner, W.J., Smith, M.W., and Trump, B.F.: Studies on the pathogenesis of ischemic cell injury. XI. P/O ratio and acceptor control. Virchows Arch. [Cell. Pathol.] 26:17–26, 1977c.

Mergner, W.J., Chang, S.H., Jones, R.T., and Trump, B.F.: Microprobe analysis and fine structure of mitochondrial granules in ultrathin frozen sections of rat pancreas. Exp. Cell. Res. 108:429–432, 1977d.

Mergner, W.J., Collan, Y., Kahng, M.W., and Trump, B.F.: Pathophysiology of acute renal failure: Mitochondrial changes in pars convoluta following temporary ischemia. Am. J. Pathol. 86:47a–48a, 1977e.

Mergner, W.J., Smith, M.W., and Trump, B.F.: Studies on pathogenesis of ischemic cell injury. IV. Alteration of ionic permeability of mitochondria from ischemic rat kidney. Exp. Mol. Pathol. 26:34–46, 1977f.

Mergner, W.J., Chang, S.H., Marzella, L., Kahng, M.W., and Trump, B.F.: Studies on pathogenesis of ischemic cell injury. XIII. ATPase of rat kidney mitochondria. Lab. Invest. 40:686–694, 1979a.

Mergner, W.J., Mergner, G., Yim, S., Chang, S.H., and Trump, B.F.: Subcellular ionshifts in ischemia: Microprobe analysis. Ger. J. Cardiol. 68:265, 1979b.

Mitchell, P.: Coupling of phosphorylation to electron and hydrogen transfer by a chemi-osmotic type of mechanism. Nature 191:144–148, 1961.

Moses, R.L., and Kasten, H.: Ultrastructure of dissociated adult mammalian myocytes. J. Mol. Cell. Cardiol. 11:161–172, 1979.

Müller, K.D., Klein, H., Naujocks, S., and Schaper, W.: Manipulation der Infarktgröße durch drastische Änderung des kardialen Sauerstoffverbrauchs nach 45' Koronarokklusion. Ger. J. Cardiol. 68:266, 1979.

Nachbaur, J., Colbeau, A., and Vignais, P.M.: Distribution of membrane-confined phospholipase A in the rat hepatocyte. Biochim. Biophys. Acta 274:426–446, 1972.

Nagatomo, T., Jarmakani, J.M., Philipson, K., and Nakazawa, M.: The effect of anoxia on membrane bound ATPase and K^+-p nitrophenyl phosphatase activities in the rabbit heart. J. Mol. Cell. Cardiol. 10:981–989, 1978.

Nayler, W.G., Grau, A., and Scade, A.: A protective effect of verapamil on hypoxic heart muscle. Cardiovasc. Res. 10:650–662, 1976.

Neely, J.R., and Morgan, H.E.: Relationship between carbohydrate and lipid metabolism and the energy balance of heart muscle. Annu. Rev. Physiol. 36:413–459, 1974.

Neely, J.R., Whitefield, C.T., and Morgan, H.E.: Regulation of glycogenolysis in hearts: Effect of pressure development glucose and FFA. Am. J. Physiol. 219:1083–1088, 1970.

Neely, J.R., Rovetto, M.J., Whitmer, J.T., Morgan, H.E.: Effects of ischemia on function and metabolism of the isolated working heart. Am. J. Physiol. 225:651–658, 1973.

Neely, J.R., Whitmer, J.T., and Rovetto, M.J.: Inhibition of glycolysis in hearts during ischemic perfusions. Recent Adv.

Neely, J.R., Whitmer, J.T., and Rovetto, M.J.: Effect of coronary blood flow on glycolytic flux and intracellular pH in isolated rat hearts. Circ. Res. *37*:733–741, 1975b.

Neely, J.R., Rovetto, M.J., and Whitmer, J.T.: Rate limiting steps of carbohydrate and fatty acid metabolism in ischemic hearts. Acta Med. Scand. Suppl. *587*:9–15, 1976a.

Neely, J.R., Whitmer, K.M., and Mochizuki, S.: Effects of mechanical activity and hormones on myocardial glucose and FFA utilisation. Circ. Res. (Suppl. I) *38*:I-22–I-30, 1976b.

Newkirk, J.D., and Waite, M.: Identification of phospholipase A_1 in plasma membrane of rat liver. Biochim. Biophys. Acta *225*:224–233, 1971.

Newkirk, J.D., and Waite, M.: Phospholipid hydrolysis by phospholipases A_1 and A_2 in plasma membranes and microsomes of rat liver. Biochim. Biophys. Acta *298*:562–576, 1973.

Ono, Y., Schraven, E., Gruber, C., and Schaper, J.: Extracellular edema and homogeneity of tissue perfusion in the isolated working rat heart. J. Mol. Cell. Cardiol., (Suppl. 2)*11*:43, 1979.

Opie, L.H.: Effect of extracellular pH on formation and metabolism of isolated perfused rat heart. Am. J. Physiol. *209*:1075–1080, 1975.

Opie, L.H.: Effects of regional ischemia on metabolism of glucose and fatty acids: Relative rates of aerobic and anaerobic energy production during myocardial infarction and comparison with effects of anoxia. Circ. Res. (Suppl. I) *38*:I-52–I-74, 1976.

Opie, L.H., Mansford, K.R.L., and Owen, P.: Effect of increased heart work on glycolysis and adenine nucleotides in the perfused heart of normal and diabetic rats. Biochem. J. *124*:475–490, 1971.

Opie, L.H., Owen, P., and Lubbe, W.: Estimated glycolytic flux in the infarcting heart. Recent Adv. Stud. Cardiac. Struct. Metab. *7*:249–255, 1975.

Parce, W.J., Cunningham, C.C., and Waite, M.: Mitochondrial phospholipase A_2 activity and mitochondrial aging. Biochemistry *17*:1634–1639, 1978.

Penttilä, A., and Trump, B.F.: Extracellular acidosis protects Ehrlich ascites tumor cells and rat renal cortex against anoxic injury. Science *185*:277–278, 1974a.

Penttilä, A., and Trump, B.F.: Protective effect of acidosis on viability of Ehrlich ascites tumor cells (EATC) exposed to anoxia. Am. J. Pathol. *74*:60a, 1974b.

Penttilä, A., and Trump, B.F.: Studies on modification of the cellular response to injury. I. Protective effect of acidosis on p-chloromercuribenzenesulfonic acid-induced injury of Ehrlich ascites tumor cells. Lab. Invest. *32*:690–695, 1975.

Peterson, M.B., and Lesch, M.: Studies on the reversibility of anoxic damage to the myocardial protein synthetic mechanism. J. Mol. Cell. Cardiol. *7*:175–190, 1975.

Podzuweit, T., Dalby, A.J., Cherry, G.W., and Opie, L.H.: Cyclic AMP levels in ischaemic and non-ischaemic myocardium following coronary artery ligation: Relation to ventricular fibrillation. J. Mol. Cell. Cardiol. *10*:81–94, 1978a.

Podzuweit, T., Els, D.J., and Shanley, B.C.: Catecholamine-cAMP induces arrhythmias in the infarcting pig heart. J. Mol. Cell. Cardiol. (Suppl. I) *10*:77, 1978b.

Podzuweit, T., Louw, G.C.J., and Shanley, B.C.: Catecholamine-cAMP-Ca^{2+} induces arrhythmias in the healthy pig heart. J. Mol. Cell. Cardiol. (Suppl. I) *10*:78, 1978c.

Pretlow, T.G., Glick, M.R., and Reddy, W.J.: Separation of beating cardiac myocytes from suspensions of heart cells. Am. J. Pathol. *67*:215–226, 1972.

Rabinowitz, M.: Control of metabolism and synthesis of macromolecules in normal and ischemic myocardium. J. Mol. Cell. Cardiol. *2*:277–292, 1971.

Randle, P.J., England, P.J., and Denbon, R.M.: Control of the tricarboxylate cycle and its interaction with glycolysis during acetate utilisation in rat heart. Biochem. J. *117*:677–695, 1970.

Rau, E.E., and Langer, G.E.: Dissociation of energetic state and potassium loss from anoxic myocardium. Am. J. Physiol. *235*:H537–543, 1978.

Recordati, G., Schwartz, P.J., Pagani, M., Malliani, A., and Brown, A.M.: Activation of cardiac vagal receptors during myocardial ischemia. Experientia *27*:1423–1424, 1971.

Reimer, K.A., Lowe, J.E., Rasmussen, M.M., and Jennings, R.B.: The wavefront phenomenon of ischemic cell death. I. Myocardial infarct size as duration of coronary occlusion in dogs. Circulation *56*:786–794, 1977.

Riciutti, M.: Myocardial lysosomes stability in the early stages of acute ischemic injury. Am. J. Cardiol. *30*:492–498, 1972a.

Riciutti, M.: Lysosomes and myocardial cellular injury. Am. J. Cardiol. *30*:499–502, 1972b.

Roeske, W.R., Deluca, M., and Ingwall, J.: Factors influencing enzyme release from cultured fetal mouse hearts deprived of oxygen and glucose. J. Mol. Cell. Cardiol. *10*:907–919, 1978.

Rona, G., Bentet, M., and Hüttner, I.: Membrane permeability alterations as manifestation of early cardiac muscle cell injury. Recent Adv. Stud. Cardiac Struct. Metab. *6*:445–455, 1975.

Rose, C.P., and Goresky, C.A.: Constraints on uptake of labeled palmitate by the heart: The barrier at the capillary and sarcolemmal surfaces and the control of intracellular sequestration. Circ. Res. *41*:534–545, 1977.

Rovetto, M.J., Whitmer, J.T., and Neely, J.R.: Comparison of the effects of anoxia and whole heart ischemia on carbohydrate utilisation in isolated working rat hearts. Circ. Res. *32*:699–711, 1973.

Rovetto, M.J., Laberton, W.F., and Neely, J.R.: Mechanism of glycolytic inhibition in ischemic rat heart. Circ. Res. *37*:742–751, 1975.

Ruigrok, T.J.C., Boink, A.B.T.J., Spies, F., Block, F.Y., Maas, A.H.J., and Zimmerman, A.N.: Energy dependence of calcium paradox. J. Mol. Cell. Cardiol. *10*:991–1002, 1978.

Sahaphong, S., and Trump, B.F.: Studies of cellular injury in isolated kidney tubules of the flounder. V. Effects of inhibiting sulfhydryl groups of plasma membrane with the organic mercurials PCMB (parachloromercuribenzoate) and PCMBS (parachloromercuribenzenesulfonate). Am. J. Pathol. *63*:277–298, 1971.

Sahaphong, S., and Trump, B.F.: Mitochondrial matrix densities in cell injury. Am. J. Pathol. *66*:34a, 1972.

Schaper, J.: Ultrastructure and pH of isolated human papillary muscle. In *Acidosis and the Heart*. Cardiac Research Group, Autumn Meeting, London, 1978a.

Schaper, J.: Ultrastructural characteristics in regional versus global myocardial ischemia. J. Mol. Cell. Cardiol. (Suppl. I) *10*:I-95, 1978b.

Schaper, J.: Ultrastructure of the myocardium in acute ischemia. In *Pathophysiology of Myocardial Perfusion*, edited by W. Schaper, ch. 19, pp. 581–673. Elsevier, Amsterdam, 1980.

Schaper, J., König, R., Franz, D., and Schaper, W.: The endothelial surface of growing coronary collateral arteries: Intimal margination and differentiation of monocytes: A combined SEM and TEM study. Virchows Arch. [Pathol. Anat.] *370*:193–205, 1976.

Schaper, J., Pasyk, S., Hofmann, M., and Schaper, W.: Early ultrastructural changes in myocardial ischemia and infarction. In *Ischemic Myocardium and Antianginal Drugs*, edited by M. Winbury. Raven Press, New York, 1979a.

Schaper, J., Mulch, J., Winkler, B., and Schaper, W.: Ultrastructural, functional and biochemical criteria for estimation of reversibility of ischemic injury: A study on the effect of global ischemia of the isolated dog heart. J. Mol. Cardiol. *11:* 521–541, 1979b.

Schaper, W.: Experimental coronary artery occlusion. III. The determinants of collateral blood flow in acute coronary occlusion. Basic Res. Cardiol. *73:*584–594, 1978.

Schaper, W., and Pasyk, S.: Influence of collateral flow on the ischemic tolerance of the heart. Circulation (Suppl. I) *53:*I-57–I-62, 1976.

Schaper, W., and Schaper, J.: Pathophysiology of myocardial perfusion. Pathobiol. Annu. *6:*317–363, 1976.

Schaper, W., and Schaper, J.: The coronary microcirculation. Am. J. Cardiol. *40:*1008–1012, 1977.

Schaper, W., deBrabander, M., and Lewi, P.: DNA-synthesis and mitoses in the coronary collateral vessels of the dog. Circ. Res. *28:*671–679, 1971.

Schaper, W., Frenzel, H., and Hort, W.: Experimental coronary artery occlusion. I. Measurement of infarct size. Basic Res. Cardiol. *74:*46–53, 1979a.

Schaper, W., Frenzel, H., Hort, W., and Winkler, B.: Experimental coronary artery occlusion. II. Spatial and temporal evolution of infarction in the dog heart. Basic Res. Cardiol. *74:*233–239, 1979b.

Scherlag, B.J., Werman, B., and Lazzera, R.: The effect of hypoxia on automaticity and contractility in canine Purkinje fibers. J. Physiol. *200:*255–265, 1969.

Scherlag, B.J., Helfant, R.H., Haft, J.C., and Damato, A.N.: Electrophysiology underlying ventricular arrhythmias due to coronary ligation. Am. J. Physiol. *219:*1665–1671, 1970.

Scherlag, B.J., El-Sherif, N., Hope, R., and Lazzera, R.: Characterization and localization of ventricular arrhythmias resulting from myocardial ischemia and infarction. Circ. Res. *35:*372–383, 1974.

Schrader, J., Nees, J., and Gerlach, E.: Evidence of cell surface adenosine receptors on coronary myocytes and atrial muscle cells: Studies with an adenosine derivative of high molecular weight. Pfluegers Arch. *369:*251–257, 1977.

Seeman, P.: Ultrastructure of membrane lesions in immune lysis, osmoticlysis and drug induced lysis. Fed. Proc. *33:*2116–2124, 1974.

Shelburne, J.D., and Trump, B.F.: Inhibition of protein synthesis in flounder kidney tubules. Fed. Proc. *27:*419, 1968.

Shen, A.C., and Jennings, R.B.: Myocardial calcium and magnesium in acute ischemic injury. Am. J. Pathol. *67:*417–440, 1972a.

Shen, A.C., and Jennings, R.B.: Kinetics of calcium accumulation in acute myocardial ischemic injury. Am. J. Pathol. *67:*441–452, 1972b.

Sherf, L., Ben Shaul, Y., and Lieberman, Y.: The human coronary microcirculation: An electron microscopic study. Am. J. Cardiol. *39:*599–605, 1977.

Shin, M.L., Paznekas, W.A., Abramovitz, A.S., and Mayer, M.M.: On the mechanism of membrane damage by C: Exposure of hydrophosphates on activated C proteins. J. Immunol. *119:*1358–1364, 1977.

Shin, M.L., Paznekas, W.A., and Mayer, M.M.: On the mechanism of membrane damage by complement. The effect of length and unsaturation of the acyl chains in liposomal bilayers and the effect of cholesterol concentration in sheep erythrocytes and liposomal membrane. J. Immunol. *120:*1996–2002, 1978.

Shine, K.I., Douglas, A.M., and Ricchuti, N.: ^{42}K exchange during myocardial ischemia. Am. J. Physiol. *232:*H564–570, 1977.

Shrago, E.: Myocardial adenine nucleotide translocase. J. Mol. Cell. Cardiol. *8:*498–500, 1976.

Shug, A.L., Koke, J.R., Folts, J.D., and Bittar, N.: Role of adenine nucleotide translocase in metabolic change caused by ischemia. Recent. Adv. Stud. Cardiac Struct. Metab. *10:*365–378, 1975.

Smith, M.W., Collan, Y., Kahng, M.W., and Trump, B.F.: Changes in mitochondrial lipids of rat kidney during ischemia. Biochem. Biophys. Acta. *618:*192–201, 1980.

Spencer, T.L., and Lehninger, A.L.: L-lactate transport in Ehrlich ascites tumor cells. Biochem. J. *154:*405–414, 1976.

Takenaka, F., Sakanashi, M., and Higuchi, M.: High-energy phosphate metabolism of isolated coronary arteries in the dog. Blood Vessels *15:*190–197, 1978.

Thoren, P.: Left ventricular receptors activated by severe asphyxia and by coronary artery occlusion. Act. Physiol. Scand. *85:*455–463, 1972.

Tillmans, H., Ideda, S., Hansen, H., Sarma, J.S.M., Fauvel, J.M., and Bing, R.: Microcirculation in the ventricle of the dog and turtle. Circ. Res. *34:*561–569, 1974.

Trump, B.F.: The network of intracellular membranes. In *Cell Membranes, Biochemistry, Cell Biology and Pathology*, edited by G. Weissmann and R. Claibone, pp. 123–135. Hospital Practice Text, New York, 1975.

Trump, B.F., and Mergner, W.J.: *Cell Injury in the Inflammatory Process*, edited by B.W. Zwiefach, L. Grant, and R.T. McClusky, vol. 1, pp. 115–257. Academic Press, New York, 1974.

Trump, B.F., Croker, B.P.J., and Mergner, W.J.: The role of energy metabolism, ion and water shifts in the pathogenesis of ischemic cell injury. In *Cell Membranes: Biological and Pathological Aspects*, edited by G.W. Richter and D.G. Scarpelli, pp. 84–128. Williams & Wilkins, Baltimore, 1971.

Trump, B.F., Mergner, W.J., Kahng, M.W., and Saladino, A.J.: Studies on subcellular pathophysiology of ischemia. Circulation (Suppl. I) *53:*I-17–I-26, 1976a.

Trump, B.F., Berezesky, I.K., Collan, Y., Kahng, M.W., and Mergner, W.J.: Recent studies on the pathophysiology of ischemic cell injury. Beitr. Pathol. *158:*353–388, 1976b.

Trump, B.F., Berezesky, I.K., Pendergrass, R.E., Chang, S.H., Bulger, R.E., and Mergner, W.J.: X-ray microanalysis of diffusible elements in scanning electron microscopy of biological thin sections: Studies of pathologically altered cells. Scan. Electron Microsc. *2:*1027–1039, 1978a.

Trump, B.F., Jones, R.T., Berezesky, I.K., Phelps, P.O., and Laiho, K.U.: Role of calcium in cell injury. Fed. Proc. *37:*403, 1978b.

Trump, B.F., Berezesky, I.K., Chang, S.H., Pendergrass, R.E., and Mergner, W.J.: The role of ion shifts in cell injury. Scan. Electron Microsc. *3:*1–14, 1979.

Vahouny, G.V., Wei, R.W., Starkweather, R., and Davis, C.: Preparation of beating heart cells from adult rats. Science *167:*1616–1618, 1970.

Vahouny, G.V., Wei, R.W., Tamboli, A., and Albert, E.N.: Adult canine myocytes: Isolation, morphology and biochemical characteristics. J. Mol. Cell. Cardiol. *11:*339–357, 1979.

van Deenen, L.L.M.: Lipid-protein interaction in model systems and biomembranes. In *Biomembranes: Structure and Function*, edited by G. Gardos and I. Szasz, Proc. FEBS, vol. 35, pp. 3–16. Elsevier, New York, 1975.

van Rossum, G.D.V.: The relation of sodium and potassium transport to the respiration and adenine nucleotide content

Stud. Cardiac Struct. Metab. 7:243–248, 1975a.
of liver series marked with inhibitors of respiration. Biochem. J. 129:427–438, 1972.

Waite, M., Griffin, H., and Franson, R.: The phospholipases A of lysosomes. Front. Biol. 45:257–305, 1976.

Weed, R.I., La Celle, P.L., and Merrill, E.W.: Metabolic dependence of red cell deformability. J. Clin. Invest. 48:793–809, 1969.

Weglicki, W.B., Owens, K., Urschel, C.W., Serur, J.R., and Sonnenblick, E.H.: Hydrolysis of myocardial lipids during acidosis and ischemia. Recent Adv. Stud. Cardiac Struct. Metab. 3:781–793, 1972.

Weglicki, W.B., Ruth, R.C., Gottwik, M.G., McNamara, D.B., and Owens, K.: Lysosomes of cardiac and skeletal muscle: Resolution by zonal centrifugation. Recent Adv. Stud. Cardiac Struct. Metab. 8:503–517, 1975.

Weiss, H.R., and Shina, A.K.: Regional oxygen saturation of small arteries and veins in the canine myocardium. Circ. Res. 42:119–126, 1978.

Welman, E., and Peters, T.J.: Properties of lysosomes in guinea pig hearts: Subcellular distribution and in vitro stability. J. Mol. Cell. Cardiol. 8:443–464, 1976.

Welman, E., and Peters, T.J.: Enhanced lysosome fragility in the anoxic perfused guinea pig heart: Effect of glucose and mannitol. J. Mol. Cell. Cardiol. 9:101–120, 1977.

Welman, E., Selwyn, A.P., Peters, T.J., Colbeck, J.F., and Fox, K.M.: Plasma lysosomal enzyme activity in acute myocardial infarction. Cardiovasc. Res. 12:99–105, 1978.

Whalen, D.A., Hamilton, D.G., Ganote, C.E., and Jennings, R.B.: Effect of a transient period of ischemia on myocardial cells. Am. J. Pathol. 74:381–398, 1974.

Wildenthal, K.: Lysosomal alteration in ischemic myocardium: Result or cause of myocellular damage. J. Mol. Cell. Cardiol. 10:595–604, 1978.

Williamson, J.R., Schaffer, S.W., Ford, C., and Safer, B.: Contribution of tissue acidosis to ischemic injury in the perfused rat heart. Circ. Res. (Suppl. I) 53:I-13–I-14, 1976.

Williamson, J.R., Steenberger, C., and DeLeeuw, G.: Nature of flow and oxygen border zones in hypoxic and ischemic myocardium. J. Mol. Cell. Cardiol. (Suppl. I) 10:134, 1978.

Winkler, B., Hofmann, M., Naujocks, S., Puschmann, S., Stämmler, G., and Schaper, W.: Rapid Recovery of the Membrane Ion Pumps in Irreversible Ischemic Injury. American Heart Association, Dallas, 1979.

Wit, A.L., and Bigger, J.T., Jr.: Possible electrophysiological mechanisms for lethal arrhythmias accompanying myocardial ischemia and infarction. Circulation (Suppl. III) 52:96–115, 1975.

Wit, A.L., and Cranfield, P.F.: Reentrant excitation as a cause of cardiac arrhythmias. Am. J. Physiol. 235:H1–17, 1978.

Wollenberger, A., and Krause, E.G.: Metabolic control characteristics of the acutely ischemic myocardium. Am. J. Cardiol. 22:349–359, 1968.

Yamazaki, N., Suzuki, Y., Kamikawa, T., Ogawa, K., Mizutani, K., Kakizawa, N., and Yamamoto, M.: Arrhythmogenic effects of acute free fatty acid mobilization on ischemic heart. Recent. Adv. Stud. Cardiac Struct. Metab. 12:271–277, 1978.

Yasuda, M., and Fujita, T.: Effect of lipid peroxidation on phospholipase A$_2$ activity of rat liver mitochondria. J. n. J. Pharmacol. 27:429–435, 1977.

Zimmerman, A.N.E., and Hülsman, W.C.: Paradoxical influence of calcium ions on the permeability of the cell membranes in isolated rat heart. Nature 211:646–647, 1966.

Zimmerman, A.N.E., Daenes, W., Hülsman, W.C., Snyder, J., Wisse, E., and Durrer, D.: Morphological changes of heart muscle caused by successive perfusion with calcium-free and calcium-containing solution (calcium paradox). Cardiovasc. Res. 1:201–209, 1967.

CHAPTER 48

Fatal Acute Myocardial Ischemia: An Analysis of the Extent of Coronary Narrowing at Necropsy

WILLIAM C. ROBERTS

Postmortem angiographic studies by Blumgart and associates (1940) 40 yr ago disclosed severe narrowing of the lumens usually in two of the three major coronary arteries (right, left anterior descending, and left circumflex) in patients with fatal acute myocardial infarction. Roberts and Buja (1972), by histologic study of cross sections of 5-mm long segments of the three major coronary arteries, also found among patients with either fatal acute myocardial infarction or sudden coronary death that usually two of the three major coronary arteries were greater than 75% occluded by atherosclerotic plaques. Of patients with clinically isolated, unstable angina pectoris studied by Roberts in 1976, even severer degrees of coronary narrowing were found.

The above quoted studies were of a *qualitative* nature in that they sought to determine only the number of major coronary arteries narrowed greater than 75% in cross sectional area by atherosclerotic plaque per patient. The present study is of a *quantitative* nature in that it asks not only whether a coronary artery is 76–100% narrowed at some point along its course but what percentage of its entire length is greater than 75% narrowed by atherosclerotic plaques and what percentages of its entire length is narrowed to lesser degrees (51–75%, 26–50%, and 0–25% in cross sectional area). The present study summarizes necropsy observations in patients with *sudden coronary death* (Roberts and Jones, 1979), clinically isolated *unstable angina pectoris* (Roberts and Virmani, 1979) and *acute myocardial infarction* (Roberts and Jones, 1980).

PATIENTS STUDIED AND METHODS

A total of 80 necropsy patients, each of whom had had an acute coronary event, were studied. They included 27 patients with transmural (involving greater than the inner half of the left ventricular wall) *acute myocardial infarcts* that by history and by histologic examination were between 24 hr and 30 days old; 31 patients with *sudden coronary death*, i.e., death within 6 hr after onset of chest pain, which if present began outside the hospital, who never had evidence of congestive cardiac failure, who at necropsy had >75% cross sectional area narrowing by atherosclerotic plaque of at least one of the four major coronary arteries and no ventricular wall myocardial coagulation necrosis; and 22 patients with clinically isolated, *unstable angina pectoris* (without historical evidence at any time of acute myocardial infarction or congestive heart failure) and death within 3 days of an aortocoronary bypass operation. Patients with associated valvular, congenital, or pericardial heart diseases, patients with hypertrophic cardiomyopathy and other myocardial diseases not secondary to coronary disease, and patients who had had a cardiac operation (other than the angina group) were excluded.

The coronary arteries in all 80 patients were studied in similar fashion. The hearts were fixed for at least 1 day in formalin. The four major epicardial coronary arteries were then excised intact, x-rayed, and fixed for at least 1 more day. Following decalcification (if necessary), each of the four major coronary arteries was cut transversely to its longitudinal axis into approximately 5-mm long segments; each segment was labeled sequentially from either its aortic ostium or from its origin from the left main. Of the coronary arteries, the average length of the right was 11 cm; left main, 1 cm; left anterior descending, 10 cm; and left circumflex, 6 cm. The 5-mm segments were labeled, processed in alcohol and xylene, dehydrated, and embedded in paraffin. Two histologic sections were cut and stained from each paraffin block. The Movat stain was used on one histologic section, and all determinations of luminal narrowing were based on examination of the Movat-stained sections. The degrees of narrowing were based on histologic examination of each cross section magnified 25–50 times. The judgment regarding the degree of luminal narrowing of each 5-mm segment was based on the degree of luminal obliteration within the luminal circle bordered by the internal elastic membrane. The circle was visually subdivided into four equal sized quadrants. The degree of narrowing in each 5-mm segment was determined as follows: 0–25%, 26–50%, 51–75%, and 76–100%. A total of 4016 5-mm long segments of coronary artery were examined in the 80 patients. The observations in the patients with fatal acute myocardial ischemia were compared to those of age and sex-matched controls for each of the three groups of coronary patients. The control subjects all died from noncardiac causes (mainly acute leukemia), none had evidence of cardiac dysfunction during life, all had had normal (<140/90 mm Hg) systemic arterial pressures, and all had normal sized (<351 g in women and <401 g in men) hearts at necropsy.

RESULTS

The results are summarized in Table 48.1. Of the 4016 5-mm long segments of major coronary artery examined in the 80 patients, 1538 segments (38%) were 76–100% narrowed in cross sectional area by atherosclerotic plaque, 1368 (34%) were 51–75% narrowed, 808 (20%)

Table 48.1
Quantification of Coronary Narrowing in Acute Myocardial Ischemia[a]

Group	No. Patients	Total 5-mm Segments of CA	No. (%) of 5-mm Segments with Extent of Cross Sectional Area Narrowing by Atherosclerotic Plaques			
			0–25%	26–50%	51–75%	76–100%
AMI	27	1403	72 (5)	319 (23)	528 (38)	484 (34)[b]
C	22	1003	285 (28)	437 (44)	250 (25)	31 (3)
SCD	31	1564	111 (7)	360 (23)	536 (34)	557 (36)[b]
C	25	1100	363 (33)	470 (42)	237 (22)	30 (3)
AP	22	1049	119 (11)	129 (12)	304 (29)	497 (48)[c]
C	20	955	214 (22)	454 (48)	274 (29)	13 (1)
Totals						
Patients	80	4016	302 (8)	808 (20)	1368 (34)	1538 (38)
Controls	40	1858	588 (31)	812 (44)	404 (22)	54 (3)

[a] *AMI*, transmural acute myocardial infarction <31 days old; *AP*, clinically isolated *unstable* angina pectoris with death within 3 days of aortocoronary bypass operation or cardiac catheterization; *C*, controls, i.e., death from a noncardiac condition (usually acute leukemia), no evidence of cardiac dysfunction during life, normotension, normal heart weight at necropsy; *SCD*, sudden coronary death, i.e., that occurring within 6 hr of onset of chest pain associated with >75% cross-sectional area luminal narrowing (by atherosclerotic plaque) of at least one of the four major (right, left main, left anterior descending, and left circumflex) coronary arteries and unassociated with foci of myocardial necrosis or other types of heart disease; *CA*, coronary artery.
[b] $p < 0.05 =$ [b] to [c].

were 26–50% narrowed, and 302 (8%) were 0–25% narrowed. The percentages of 5-mm long segments 76–100% narrowed in cross sectional area by atherosclerotic plaques were similar in the patients with acute myocardial infarction and sudden coronary death (about 35%); the patients with clinically isolated unstable angina had the highest percentage of 5-mm long segments 76–100% narrowed (48%), and this difference between the other two groups of coronary patients was significant ($p < .05$). In contrast, the percentage of 5-mm long segments of major coronary artery narrowed 76–100% in the control subjects ranged from 1 to 3%, and this difference between study patients and control subjects was highly significant ($p < .001$). The percentage of 5-mm segments narrowed 51–75% in cross sectional area also was significantly greater in the study patients than in the control subjects (34% versus 22%). Thus, 72% of the 5-mm long segments of major coronary artery in the study patients were >50% narrowed in cross sectional area, whereas only 25% of the segments in the control patients were narrowed to this degree ($p < .05$). In contrast, 28% of the 5-mm segments in the study patients and 75% in the control subjects were equal to or less than 50% narrowed in cross sectional area ($p < 0.05$).

COMMENTS

This study describes in *quantitative* detail the degree and extent of luminal narrowing by atherosclerotic plaque in each of the four major epicardial coronary arteries in patients with fatal acute myocardial ischemia. Among the 80 patients studied, 38% of the major coronary tree was 76–100% narrowed in cross sectional area by atherosclerotic plaque, and another 34% was 51–75% narrowed—for a total of 72% >50% narrowed. Only 3% of the 5-mm long segments in the control subjects were narrowed 76–100% in cross sectional area, and only 25% were >50% narrowed. Only 8% of the 5-mm long segments in the study patients were 0–25% narrowed in cross sectional area, and few were entirely normal. Thus, coronary atherosclerosis among necropsy patients with fatal acute myocardial ischemia is a *diffuse* process.

The present study also shows differences in the extent of severe narrowing in the three acute coronary event groups. The patients with clinically isolated unstable angina pectoris had the most extensive coronary narrowing, with 48% of the 5-mm long segments 76–100% narrowed in cross sectional area by atherosclerotic plaque. The patients with acute myocardial infarction (34%) and those with sudden coronary death (36%) had similar but less coronary narrowing. The patients with unstable angina pectoris, i.e., those with the severest degrees of coronary narrowing, paradoxically had the least amount of myocardial damage (Roberts, 1976), usually normal sized hearts, and normal cardiac outputs; in contrast, the patients with acute myocardial infarcts had less severe coronary narrowing but the most myocardial damage.

SUMMARY

Each of the four major epicardial coronary arteries in 80 patients with fatal acute coronary events was divided into 5-mm long segments, and a Movat-stained histologic section was prepared and examined from each segment. An average of 56 5-mm long segments were examined from each of the 80 patients. Of the 4016 5-mm segments of coronary artery examined, 1538 (38%) were 76–100% narrowed in cross sectional area by atherosclerotic plaque (controls = 3%), another 34% of the segments were 51–75% narrowed (controls = 22%), 20% were 26–50% narrowed (controls = 44%), and only 8% were 0–25% narrowed (controls = 31%). Thus, coronary atherosclerosis among patients with fatal acute coronary events is diffuse and severe.

The 22 patients with clinically isolated *unstable angina pectoris* had the highest percentage of 5-mm long segments 76–100% narrowed in cross sectional area by atherosclerotic plaque, namely 48%; the 27 patients with *acute myocardial infarction* and the 31 patients with *sudden cardiac death* had a similar percentage (about 35%) of coronary segments narrowed 76–100%. Among the 80 necropsy patients studied, those with the least amount of myocardial damage, i.e., angina pectoris, had the severest degree of coronary narrowing, and those with the severest degree of myocardial damage, i.e., acute myocardial infarction, had less severe coronary narrowing.

References

Blumgart, H.L., Schlesinger, M.J., and Davis, D.: Studies on the relation of the clinical manifestations of angina pectoris, coronary thrombosis, and myocardial infarction to the pathologic findings with particular reference to the significance of the collateral circulation. Am. Heart J. *19:*1, 1940.

Roberts, W.C.: The coronary arteries and left ventricle in clinically isolated angina pectoris. Circulation *54:*388–390, 1976.

Roberts, W.C., and Buja, L.M.: The frequency and significance of coronary arterial thrombi and other observations in fatal acute myocardial infarction: A study of 107 necropsy patients. Am. J. Med. *52:*425–443, 1972.

Roberts, W.C., and Jones, A.A.: Quantitation of coronary arterial narrowing at necropsy in sudden coronary death: Analysis of 31 patients and comparison with 25 control subjects. Am. J. Cardiol. *44:*39–45, 1979.

Roberts, W.C., and Jones, A.A.: Quantitation of coronary arterial narrowing at necropsy in acute transmural myocardial infarction: Analysis and comparison of findings in 27 patients to those in 22 control. Circulation *61:*786–790, 1980.

Roberts, W.C., and Virmani, R.: Quantification of coronary arterial narrowing in clinically-isolated unstable angina pectoris: An analysis of 22 necropsy patients. Am. J. Med. *67:* 792–799, 1979.

CHAPTER 49

Treatment of Myocardial Infarction

JAMES E. MULLER

Myocardial infarction (MI) is a serious and widespread disorder that accounts for hundreds of thousands of deaths each year in the United States. The clinical presentation of this disorder was first described in 1910 by Obraztsov and Strazhesko in Russia and by Herrick in 1912 in the United States (Herrick, 1912; Muller, 1977). Since these early descriptions, knowledge about MI has greatly expanded. The improved treatment that physicians now offer to patients with this condition may well be contributing to the declining mortality from cardiovascular disease (Chartbook, 1978).

PREHOSPITAL CORONARY CARE

Unfortunately the majority of deaths from MI occur before the patient reaches the hospital (Fulton et al., 1969). In order to decrease the time interval from the onset of pain to the initiation of medical care, extensive efforts have been made both in the community—to alert the public to the signs and symptoms of a myocardial infarction so that they might seek medical care more rapidly—and by hospitals—to extend coronary care outward to the community (Moiseev, 1962; Pantridge, 1970; Pantridge et al., 1974).

Over the past 10 years a large number of emergency medical technicians have been trained to provide acute care for victims of MI. These technicians often reach the patient at the scene of the MI within minutes after notification of the health care system. They are trained to identify the signs and symptoms of an acute MI, interpret electrocardiographic findings, provide emergency cardiopulmonary resuscitation (CPR), and treat arrhythmias. The primary purpose of this prehospital care is to stabilize the patient in a normal rhythm with an adequate blood pressure for transport to the hospital. If this is not possible, CPR is continued while the patient is transported to the hospital.

The function of the technician varies depending upon the level of training and the licensure specifications of the particular area. The type of prehospital coronary care administered in the city of Baltimore is an example of a highly developed system. These personnel, called Cardiac Rescue Technicians (CRTs), work as part of a statewide emergency care program coordinated by the Maryland Institute for Emergency Medical Services. When a pair of CRTs reaches a patient presumed to have had an MI and cardiopulmonary arrest, one initiates CPR and the other calls for assistance and special equipment. When a defibrillator is available, the paddles are placed on the patient's chest and the heart rhythm is determined from an oscilloscopic recording. If ventricular fibrillation is present, a single shock of 400 W-sec can be administered without the need for prior consultation with a physician. If asystole is present, CPR is carried out while the patient is being transported as rapidly as possible to the hospital.

Additional care at the scene of the cardiac arrest can be coordinated by means of telemetric communication with a physician at a referral facility. A secure intravenous line should be established to allow the administration of drug therapy; EKGs are transmitted to the physician, who may then direct repeat defibrillation or the injection of lidocaine, epinephrine, sodium bicarbonate, or atropine. Such emergency measures should be continued during rapid transport of the patient to a hospital emergency room. In some areas of the country, inhalation of nitrous oxide is employed to reduce the pain of infarction (McLaughlin et al., 1977).

EMERGENCY ROOM CARE

Once the patient reaches the hospital emergency room, morphine should be given intravenously in doses of 2–4 mg every 5 min if moderate or severe pain is present. If respiratory depression and hypotension do not ensue, 40 mg or more may be given. Sudden hypotension may occur as a result of vasodilatation, but this complication will usually respond to elevation of the patient's legs and infusion of a volume expander.

After pain has been controlled, the decision about whether or not to admit the patient to the hospital must be made rapidly. Generally, a brief history of the event and a complete 12-lead EKG are sufficient to determine whether an MI is definitely present. In many cases it is useful to compare the present electrocardiogram with a previous tracing, if this is available. It is generally accepted that patients with a definite acute MI should be hospitalized and, if possible, treated in a specialized unit in which EKG monitoring, defibrillation, and hemodynamic monitoring are available (Day, 1963; Sobel, 1974). Several studies from England have suggested that for *selected* patients, home care might yield equally good results (Hill et al., 1978). These studies suffer from the "beta error," i.e., a significant detrimental effect of home care may have gone undetected because of the relatively small size of the sample. Hence, for the present, it remains reasonable to admit all such patients to a coronary care unit (CCU).

Patients with suspected, but not proven, MI may present a major dilemma to the physician responsible for CCU admission. In some instances, the availability of CCU beds is limited, and the physician must balance the needs of the new patient requiring emergency care against those of patients previously admitted who require continued care. The difficulty of this choice is diminished when a patient area that provides intermediate EKG monitoring capabilities is available (Resnekov, 1977).

Once the decision for CCU admission has been made, the patient should be moved as soon as possible from the emergency room to the CCU and should be accompanied by a physician and a nurse or trained technician. A portable EKG monitor should be attached to the patient; a syringe with 100 mg of lidocaine and a syringe with 2 mg of atropine should be available. A secure intravenous line should also be present.

ADMISSION TO THE CORONARY CARE UNIT

During the initial contact with a patient admitted to the CCU, the physician should be highly sensitive to the difficult events the patient has just experienced. In many instances the onset of an acute MI rapidly transforms a perfectly healthy individual into a patient who has experienced great pain and knows that he or she has a disease that may have been responsible for the death of a close friend or relative. If possible the patient should be assured immediately that the most dangerous phase of the heart attack has passed and that the CCU will provide increased safety during the recovery period.

Prior to a complete history and physical examination the physician should determine the following:

1. Is the patient comfortable and free of moderate or severe pain?
2. Are heart rate, respiratory rate and blood pressure within acceptable limits?
3. Is the patient free of significant conduction disturbances and ventricular ectopic activity?

If none of these difficulties is present, the situation is uncomplicated and no immediate special action need be taken. (The recognition and treatment of complications of infarction are discussed later in this chapter.) The physician should then obtain a detailed history and perform a complete physical examination. The new EKG, previous EKGs (if available), chest x-ray, electrolytes, and possibly an early creatine kinase (CK) determination should be reviewed. The details of this evaluation are described below.

CLINICAL FINDINGS

History

Identification of patients in whom an MI is likely to occur aids in the diagnosis. Individuals with risk factors such as advanced age, a history of heavy cigarette smoking, elevated serum cholesterol, hypertension, diabetes mellitus, or a family history of severe atherosclerosis are more likely to have significant coronary atherosclerosis and MI than those without such conditions. Infarction is also more common in those with known ischemic heart disease, as indicated by prior angina pectoris or MI.

The patient with acute MI frequently experiences premonitory symptoms. Patients with stable angina may note a change in their anginal pattern. Previously healthy individuals may suffer an infarction a short time after the onset of stable angina.

The pain of infarction is generally described by patients as extremely severe, crushing, substernal chest pain or pressure and is often associated with marked anxiety, diaphoresis, nausea, and vomiting. Occasionally the pain may be localized in the abdomen, arm, or head and mistaken for another disorder. Patients who have experienced angina may note that the pain is similar to anginal pain but more intense, of longer duration, and not relieved by nitroglycerin. Many patients will describe it as the worst pain they have ever experienced.

Although the typical patient has severe pain, in some the discomfort is mild. In perhaps 20% of cases, MI occurs in the absence of chest pain. A MI may also present as an otherwise unexplained increase in congestive heart failure. In rare cases, systemic arterial embolism from a left ventricular mural thrombus may be the first sign of MI.

Physical Findings

When the patient is first seen, the primary physical findings will be those associated with the severe pain. Patients are generally extremely agitated and may show pallor and diaphoresis. Hypertension is frequently present during the acute stage, before the pain is relieved, but generally resolves spontaneously. After the pain of infarction has ceased or has been relieved by analgesics, the physical examination is of relatively limited value for diagnosis of the condition. Low blood pressure in association with peripheral signs of vasoconstriction may be a warning that cardiogenic shock is present or imminent. Tachycardia that persists after the pain is relieved may be an ominous sign that an increased heart rate is required to compensate for a stroke volume that has been seriously decreased by MI. The temperature is generally normal at the onset of infarction, but it frequently rises several days postinfarction as the inflammatory process peaks in the sterile necrotic myocardium. Examination of the eyes may reveal xanthelasma, indicative of hyperlipidemia. Fundoscopic examination may show changes of hypertension or diabetes mellitus. Examination of the neck may reveal increased jugular venous pressure, an indication of right heart failure. Auscultation may reveal the presence of pulmonary rales, which could result from left ventricular failure or intrinsic lung disease from smoking. Examination of the heart may reveal cardiomegaly or a dyskinetic precordial bulge. An S3 gallop may be heard, and a murmur indicative of papillary muscle dysfunction may be present at the apex. The second heart sound may be paradoxically split. The presence of a thrill in association with a holosystolic murmur suggests a ventricular septal defect. When the thrill is absent, a holosystolic murmur may indicate mitral regurgitation. The peripheral pulses may reveal signs of diffuse atherosclerosis or may in some instances be absent because of arterial embolism.

Laboratory Findings

ELECTROCARDIOGRAM

The EKG is of great value since it often provides instantaneous information about the presence and location of acute MI (Marriott, 1972). Electrocardiographic signs differ in transmural and subendocardial MIs.

In *transmural myocardial infarction* the following sequence of events occurs: the earliest change of acute transmural ischemia is marked ST segment elevation with an increase in R wave height. Three to 6 hr after the onset of ischemia the ST segment elevation begins to decline as Q waves develop. By 12–24 hr after the onset of ischemia, the EKG may show development of a large Q wave with partial or complete loss of R wave voltage and further diminution of ST segment elevation. T waves are generally inverted by this time.

A *subendocardial myocardial infarction* is defined electrocardiographically as an infarction in which pathologic Q waves do not develop. In such infarcts the primary finding is ST segment depression that persists for longer than 12 hr. In most cases subendocardial infarction is also accompanied by T wave inversions that also persist for longer than 12 hr. There may also be loss of R wave voltage without the development of Q waves.

Several pitfalls attend the use of the EKG in identifying the presence of acute ischemia and MI. Early repolarization with ST segment elevation of several millimeters is a normal variant that may simulate infarction. It can be differentiated from acute ischemia by the absence of chest pain in the patient with early repolarization. Left bundle branch block, which radically alters the spread of electrical activity through the heart, completely obscures the normal electrocardiographic findings of acute infarction. The Wolff-Parkinson-White syndrome, in which depolarization travels through an abnormal pathway, can also simulate the QRS findings of MI. In patients who have had previous infarction, a new infarction may occur in the opposite side of the heart and cancel the electrocardiographic signs of both infarctions.

In extreme cases, it is possible for an MI to occur without any changes in the QRS complex, ST segment, or T wave. This could occur with a subendocardial infarction in the posterior portion of the heart, an area not well represented on the surface EKG. Thus, the absence of EKG changes does not exclude the diagnosis of MI.

The EKG is most useful in the diagnosis of infarction when a careful search is made for *serial changes*. Comparison between an EKG taken during an attack of pain and an EKG recorded several weeks or months prior to the event is often of great value. Likewise, when a patient is hospitalized for several days in a coronary care unit and the electrocardiographic diagnosis of infarction remains in doubt, it is useful to compare the first and last EKGs obtained in the CCU to detect minor changes that might not be noted in comparisons of sequential EKGs.

The strong correlation between the EKG leads in which the signs of infarction are observed and the location of the infarction at autopsy (Myers et al., 1948a and b, 1949) has led to the use of anatomic terms such as "inferior" and "anteroseptal" to describe infarctions, although their meanings remain imprecise. Table 49.1 presents a proposed usage of terms that is inclusive and nonoverlapping.

SERUM ENZYME MEASUREMENTS

An abnormal elevation in the serum of enzymes from cardiac tissue provides support for the diagnosis of acute MI. This method first utilized the determination of serum glutamic-oxaloacetic transaminase (SGOT), which, although present in heart tissue, is also present in many other tissues. In recent years attempts have been made to study enzymes that are more specific to the myocardium. Creatine kinase, or CK (formerly called creatine phosphokinase, or CPK), is now the serum enzyme most widely used to diagnose MI. However, since CK is contained in brain and skeletal muscle as well as myocardium, tests have been developed to determine the MB isoenzyme of CK, which is found in appreciable quantities only in cardiac muscle (Roberts et al., 1975a). The only limitations of the use of the MB isoenzyme are the cost of its determination and its more rapid disappearance from serum than total CK. Determination of CK-MB is of greatest value when the total CK is elevated but the clinician suspects that a MI is not present and that the CK elevation is produced by some other source, such as skeletal muscle. A practical method for use of the CK-MB determination is to obtain routinely a single sample from each patient drawn approximately 18 hr after the onset of the most severe pain, when the isoenzyme is most likely to be elevated. The time of appearance of the common enzymes utilized to diagnose MI is shown in Figure 49.1. It is apparent that if the patient is seen several days after the suspected infarction, determination of the lactate dehydrogenase (LDH) enzyme would be of greatest utility.

OTHER TESTS

Arterial Blood Gases

These need not be determined routinely on every patient. However, when the patient's pulmonary status is uncertain, determination of an arterial PO_2 may be of value. In many patients with MI, arterial PO_2 is de-

Table 49.1
The Electrocardiogram and Location of a Myocardial Infarction

Location of EKG Changes	Anatomic Term
II, III, aVF	Inferior
V1–V2	Septal
V3–V4	Apical
V5–V6	Lateral
I, aVL	High lateral

This is a proposed system of nomenclature for infarct locations. The advantage of this system is that all the portions of the heart that produce direct EKG changes are named, and, at the same time, none of the terms are overlapping. Infarcts that include more than one location can be described with combined terms, e.g., inferolateral, lateral-high lateral.

pressed because of shunting in the pulmonary circulation (Fillmore et al., 1971).

Chest X-ray

In most patients with acute MI, only a portable chest x-ray is obtained. This technique generally exaggerates the width of the mediastinum and the size of the cardiac silhouette. The x-ray is of some value in detecting the presence or absence of pulmonary edema and pulmonary vascular redistribution, but there are only weak correlations between radiographic findings and pulmonary capillary wedge pressures as determined by means of the Swan-Ganz catheter (Montero et al., 1979).

Technetium-99m (^{99m}Tc) Pyrophosphate Scintigraphy

After intravenous injection, pyrophosphate accumulates in ischemic and infarcted myocardium. When the pyrophosphate is linked to the radionuclide ^{99m}Tc, an image of the area of accumulation can be obtained with a bedside gamma scintillation camera (Parkey et al., 1974). Since pyrophosphate accumulates in ischemic as well as infarcted tissue, the test cannot be used to confirm the presence or absence of infarction in borderline cases. Hence, its value is limited to situations in which CK determination and the EKG would not be helpful, such as several days after the onset of pain or when left bundle branch block is present. The technique may also be useful for detecting the extension of the infarct and for the sizing of infarcts for research purposes.

Radionuclide Ventriculography

Red blood cells labeled with ^{99m}Tc can be utilized to obtain an image of the motion of the cardiac chambers (Strauss et al., 1974). With this technique a noninvasive measurement of ejection fraction and ventricular wall motion can be obtained. If cardiac output appears low clinically, the technique can be used to distinguish mitral regurgitation with a high regurgitant fraction from low output due to diminished myocardial contractility.

Differential Diagnosis

When the patient is first seen, numerous potential causes for the chest pain should be explored. In most

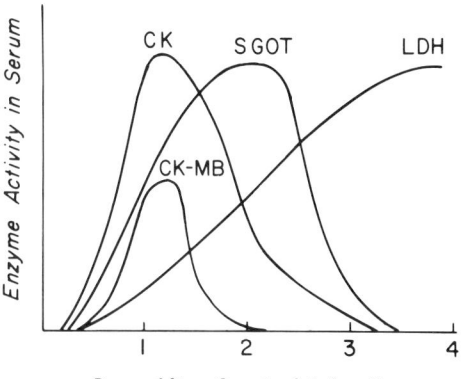

Figure 49.1. The dynamics of serum enzyme changes during acute MI. Several features are of importance. First, if a sample is drawn too early (less than 4 hr after the onset of pain), it may fail to demonstrate an enzyme elevation despite the presence of an infarction. Second, since the rise in CK-MB is of shorter duration than the rise in CK total, an improperly timed sample might fail to show CK-MB elevation in the presence of infarction. Third, the LDH is of greater value than CK when the patient is first seen more than 48 hr after the presumed infarction because it remains elevated for 8–14 days.

instances the EKG provides immediate assistance in determining whether or not the pain is produced by myocardial ischemia. In some cases, however, there are no obvious signs of myocardial ischemia on the EKG, and it is necessary to conduct a careful search for the various cardiovascular, gastrointestinal, musculoskeletal, pulmonary, and neurologic disturbances listed in Table 49.2 that can mimic the pain of MI (Becker et al., 1957; Bennett and Atkinson, 1966; Inouye et al., 1967; Sasahara, 1974; Dale and Lewis, 1975). In most cases a satisfactory explanation for the pain can be found.

Classically, the diagnosis of MI is confirmed retrospectively by the presence of two or more of the following features: a typical history, characteristic EKG changes, and a rise in myocardial enzyme levels in the serum. With the development of the isoenzyme method, a rise in CK-MB can be considered to be the gold standard for the presence or absence of infarction, if appropriately timed samples are available. It is understood that an extremely small infarction may occur that can be detected pathologically but causes no detectable alteration in serum CK-MB. Failure to diagnose such small infarctions does not present a major difficulty, since these are unlikely to be attended by serious electrical or hemodynamic consequences.

TREATMENT OF UNCOMPLICATED MYOCARDIAL INFARCTION

With the information obtained from the admission history, physical examination, and laboratory data, the

Table 49.2
Conditions That Can Mimic the Pain of Myocardial Infarction

Cardiovascular
Prolonged angina
Pericarditis
Myocarditis
Dissecting aneurysm
Gastrointestinal
Esophageal spasm
Esophageal rupture
Peptic ulcer
Cholecystitis
Pancreatitis
Musculoskeletal
Costochondritis
Myositis
Pulmonary
Pulmonary embolism
Spontaneous pneumothorax
Pleurodynia
Pulmonary hypertension
Neurologic
Herpes zoster
Nerve root compression
Thoracic outlet compression

physician should have an adequate understanding of the patient's condition. If the patient is free of significant chest pain, hemodynamic abnormalities, ventricular ectopic activity, and conduction disturbances, the infarction is considered uncomplicated. Treatment of uncomplicated infarction is straightforward and the diagnosis is good.

Routine Admission Orders

For most patients a standard set of admission orders can be used. These should include orders for frequent monitoring of vital signs and for routine CK sampling. Initially, activity should be limited to bed rest and the patient should be kept NPO (nothing by mouth). If needed, medications should be prescribed for the relief of pain and anxiety. There remain a number of other medications whose use in uncomplicated infarction remains controversial.

Specific Medications

LIDOCAINE

There is general agreement that lidocaine should be given to suppress frequent ventricular premature beats (VPBs), multifocal VPBs, couplets, or ventricular tachycardia (VT). If hepatic function is normal, the recommended dose is an intravenous bolus of 1.5 mg/kg followed by a continuous intravenous infusion of 2–4 mg/min.

Controversy surrounds the prophylatic use of lidocaine to prevent ventricular tachycardia-ventricular fibrillation (VF) in the absence of VPBs (Lie et al., 1974). Studies indicate that lidocaine not only suppresses VPBs that cause VT but that it also raises the fibrillation threshold. It is argued that since the agent is generally well tolerated, it should be given to all patients with acute myocardial infarction even in the absence of VPBs.

For most patients it is our practice to await the appearance of VPBs for the initiation of lidocaine. However, young patients seen within several hours of the onset of pain are generally given prophylactic lidocaine because of the high incidence of VF in this setting. Lidocaine should also be administered prophylactically if continuous EKG monitoring is not available.

ANTICOAGULANTS

Despite numerous clinical trials designed to evaluate the role of anticoagulants in the therapy of acute MI, the issue remains controversial (Gifford and Feinstein, 1969). It is our practice to fully anticoagulate patients at high risk for thromboembolic events (i.e., patients with a history of thromboembolism, low cardiac output, or ventricular aneurysm). Others are given low dose heparin unless a contraindication to anticoagulation is present (Wessler, 1976).

PREINFARCTION β-BLOCKADE

With the widespread use of β-adrenergic receptor blockade for patients with angina pectoris and previous MI, it is increasingly common to encounter patients with acute MI in whom a decision must be made to continue or discontinue β-blockade. At the present time there is no clear indication as to the proper course. Discontinuation could lead to worsening of the infarct because of the propranolol rebound effect (Alderman et al., 1974). Continuation of β-blockade represents an attempt to limit infarct size, which is currently an experimental maneuver with unknown long term consequences. Hence, at the present time, the physician must make the decision on the basis of incomplete data. It is our practice to continue β-blockade unless such contraindications as bradycardia, congestive heart failure, atrioventricular (AV) block, or asthma are present.

Ambulation and Recovery

Several days postinfarction, if no complications have occurred, attention should be directed to the patient's gradual return to full activity. Coronary care unit nurses, who generally spend extensive time with each patient, should take an active role in this process. Efforts should be made to diminish the patients psychologic dependence on monitoring and the CCU environment, in preparation for transfer from the CCU (Hackett et al., 1968).

The rate of resumption of physical activity must be decided individually for each patient. Early ambulation and discharge decrease the risk of pulmonary embolism, diminish the psychologic effect of the infarct upon the patient, and decrease the amount of costly resources that must be expended for each patient (Levine and Lown, 1951; Hutter et al., 1973; Thornley and Turner, 1977). However, patients with large infarcts should probably have a period of at least 2 weeks of limited activity so that the tensile strength of the infarcted area can increase. This rest may diminish postinfarction aneurysm and expansion of the infarcted zone.

During the recovery period patients frequently experience depression (Cassem and Hackett, 1973). This should be accepted as part of the process of recovery, while at the same time efforts should be made by the physician to emphasize the positive features of the long term outlook. This process can be aided by a specialized cardiovascular nurse who assists with the instruction of the patient during the post-MI period.

Discharge

By the time of hospital discharge, the complications of infarction should be controlled or absent and the patient should have resumed the activity level that will be required at home. In particular, the patient should walk a flight of stairs with a physician or nurse in the hospital, if this will be required at home.

The physician should make specific recommendations regarding the level of activity that should be undertaken at home. The physician should state whether driving is permitted, stairs may be climbed, or sexual activity resumed. It is often useful to ask the patient to engage in only limited activity during the 1st week at home until a follow-up examination has been completed.

The time of hospitalization varies for each patient. It is our practice to hospitalize patients with a small, uncomplicated infarction for 7–10 days; others with large transmural infarction are hospitalized for 18–21 days. Laboratory tests prior to discharge should include a standard chest x-ray, electrolytes, and a 24-hr Holter monitor if ventricular ectopic activity (VEA) has been a significant problem. It should be emphasized to the patient that hospital care was only one phase of the help he will receive in his return to health.

RECOGNITION AND TREATMENT OF COMPLICATIONS OF ACUTE MYOCARDIAL INFARCTION

Arrhythmias

Myocardial ischemia and necrosis cause major instabilities in the electrical activity of the heart (Fig. 49.2). Cell disruption produces local changes in refractoriness, conductance, and automaticity that lead to a wide range of arrhythmias. These individual arrhythmias may be harmful in themselves or may be harbingers of more serious arrhythmias. The approach by the physician to these arrhythmias may have a decisive influence on the final outcome of the infarction.

The first task in managing an arrhythmia is to search for a readily treatable cause, such as systemic hypokalemia, hypoxia, acidosis, or alkalosis. It is also worthwhile to recall that a central venous catheter may be the cause of an arrhythmia if it is in contact with the heart. In most cases, treatable causes are not found and the physician must then decide whether attempts should be made to terminate or suppress the arrhythmia.

ATRIAL ARRHYTHMIAS

Sinus Bradycardia (Sinus Rhythm with Heart Rate Less Than 60 Beats/min)

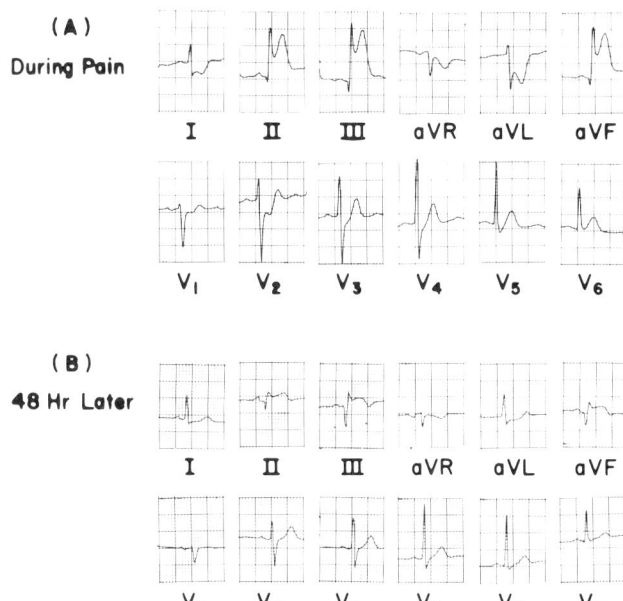

Figure 49.2. EKG changes of a transmural inferior MI. *A*, marked ST segment elevation in II, III, and aVF during the early stages of myocardial ischemia. ST segment depression in I and aVL could be the reciprocal of ST segment elevation in the inferior leads or could result from primary subendocardial ischemia in the high lateral myocardium. *B*, 24 hr later the infarction has evolved with an increase in Q wave depth and a decrease in ST segment elevation in II, III, and aVF. Although its height has decreased, the R wave is still present, indicating persistence of some viable myocardium in that area.

Vagal tone, with or without ischemia and edema of the sinatrial node, may produce heart rates so low (less than 40 beats/min) that cardiac output and arterial pressure are seriously compromised. Sinus bradycardia is more common with inferior than with anterior infarction. Some contend that extreme bradycardia may also allow VEA to occur, but others claim bradycardia is protective against arrhythmias (Rotman et al., 1972). It is our practice to treat bradycardia with atropine only when the rate is so slow that systemic arterial pressure is compromised.

Sinus Tachycardia

When a ventricular rate above 100 is encountered, the physician should first determine if sinus rhythm is present. Atrial flutter with 2:1 AV block is frequently mistaken for sinus tachycardia. Carotid sinus massage will often produce higher grade AV block that will clearly reveal the flutter waves. Sinus tachycardia might be harmful since the increased oxygen demand of the rapid rate might enlarge the infarct by increasing oxygen demand in marginally perfused tissue. Hence, such treatable causes of sinus tachycardia as fever, hypovolemia, and excessive anxiety should be sought and corrected if possible. The ominous finding of a sinus tachycardia, which reflects pump failure, has been mentioned previously.

Atrial Fibrillation, Atrial Flutter (Liberthson et al., 1971)

These atrial arrhythmias do not have the same potential as the ventricular arrhythmias for rapid deterioration to lethal conditions. However, they may be harmful by increasing O_2 demand and thus enlarging the infarction. Also the loss of the atrial contribution to ventricular filling may cause a significant fall in cardiac output in patients with compromised ventricular function.

The vigor of attempts to terminate, control, or prevent an atrial arrhythmia should be based on the amount of difficulty the arrhythmia is causing. Rapid electrical cardioversion should be used in a case in which the atrial arrhythmia is accompanied by ischemic chest pain, pulmonary edema, or significant hypotension (Lown, 1967). If these complications are not present, digoxin—0.25 mg every 3 hr intravenously until the ventricular rate is less than 100—may be given and quinidine—200-400 mg every 6 hr orally—may be given to terminate the rhythm and prevent its recurrence.

VENTRICULAR ARRHYTHMIAS

Ventricular Premature Beats

VPBs occur in almost all patients with infarction. They are of concern only because of their potential to lead to ventricular tachycardia (VT) and ventricular fibrillation (VF) (El-Sherif et al., 1976). Multifocal VPBs and VPBs that occur in couplets are considered more likely to lead to VT/VF than unifocal, single VPBs. It is important to identify VPBs caused by parasystole (varying coupling interval, interectopic intervals that are multiples of a basic interval). These VPBs are most resistant to therapy and less in need of therapy than regular VPBs since they rarely degenerate into VT/VF.

Most VPBs respond to treatment with intravenous lidocaine (Morgensen, 1970). If this is ineffective, intravenous procaine amide (100 mg intravenously slowly every 5 min up to 1 g followed by 2-4 mg/min continuous infusion) is the usual drug of second choice (Giardina et al., 1973).

The goal of therapy is suppression of dangerous VPBs without development of side effects from this medication. In some patients chronic VEA may persist despite vigorous antiarrhythmic therapy, and the physician must accept the level of ectopy that had been present prior to the MI.

Ventricular Tachycardia

VT is defined as a sequence of three or more VPBs occurring at a rate greater than 100 beats/min. With VT the systemic arterial pressure may be adequate or it may be so low that the rhythm itself is lethal. Even with an adequate arterial pressure VT is dangerous because of its tendency to degenerate into ventricular fibrillation. If the arterial pressure is adequate, VT can be treated with an intravenous bolus of 50 mg of lidocaine, which may terminate the arrhythmia. If the arterial pressure is not adequate, immediate cardioversion should be performed. Intravenous lidocaine, oral quinidine, and oral procainamide are the medications most commonly given to prevent VT.

Ventricular Fibrillation

With VF there is a total loss of synchronous contraction of the ventricles. Cardiac output falls drastically, and death will occur within minutes. VF should be treated with a transthoracic shock of 400 W-sec as soon as possible. CPR should be initiated when VF occurs and continued while the defibrillator is being readied.

Accelerated Idioventricular Rhythm (AIVR)

AIVR is a rhythm similar to VT in that it arises in the ventricle; it differs from VT in that it occurs at a rate of less than 100 beats/min. It is generally accompanied by an adequate cardiac output and does not progress to VT or VF. Hence it need not be treated. It is important, however, to recognize that AIVR frequently occurs in patients who develop VT at some time during their infarction (deSoyza et al., 1974).

Conduction Disturbances

During infarction the specialized conducting pathways of the heart suffer the same dysfunction and destruction as do the contractile tissues. Disturbances of conduction are of importance only to the degree that they presage the occurrence of complete heart block (CHB) with an adequate escape focus. Although CHB is less frequent than ventricular fibrillation, it occurs with the same lightning speed and is more difficult to treat unless a temporary pacemaker has been inserted prophylactically.

Conduction disturbances are more likely to be progressive with anterior than with inferior infarction since with anterior infarction the disturbances more often result from actual necrosis of the conducting system. In addition, the disturbance is generally further below the AV junction than with inferior MI; hence the block is below most pacemakers that could rescue the ventricle with an adequate rate. With inferior infarction the conduction disturbance is more likely to result from an increase in vagal tone than from myocardial necrosis.

FIRST DEGREE AV BLOCK

In this type of block, the P-R interval exceeds 0.2 sec, but all P waves are conducted to the ventricle. With this, and with the other conduction disturbances, it is important to review previous EKGs to determine whether the delay is new or old. New first degree AV block may result from an increase in vagal tone or from ischemia or necrosis in the vicinity of the AV node. It is not harmful in itself and generally does not lead directly to CHB.

SECOND DEGREE AV BLOCK

In this condition, some but not all P waves are conducted to the ventricle. Two forms exist: 1) Mobitz type I, in which the P-R interval gradually lengthens until a

Treatment of Myocardial Infarction

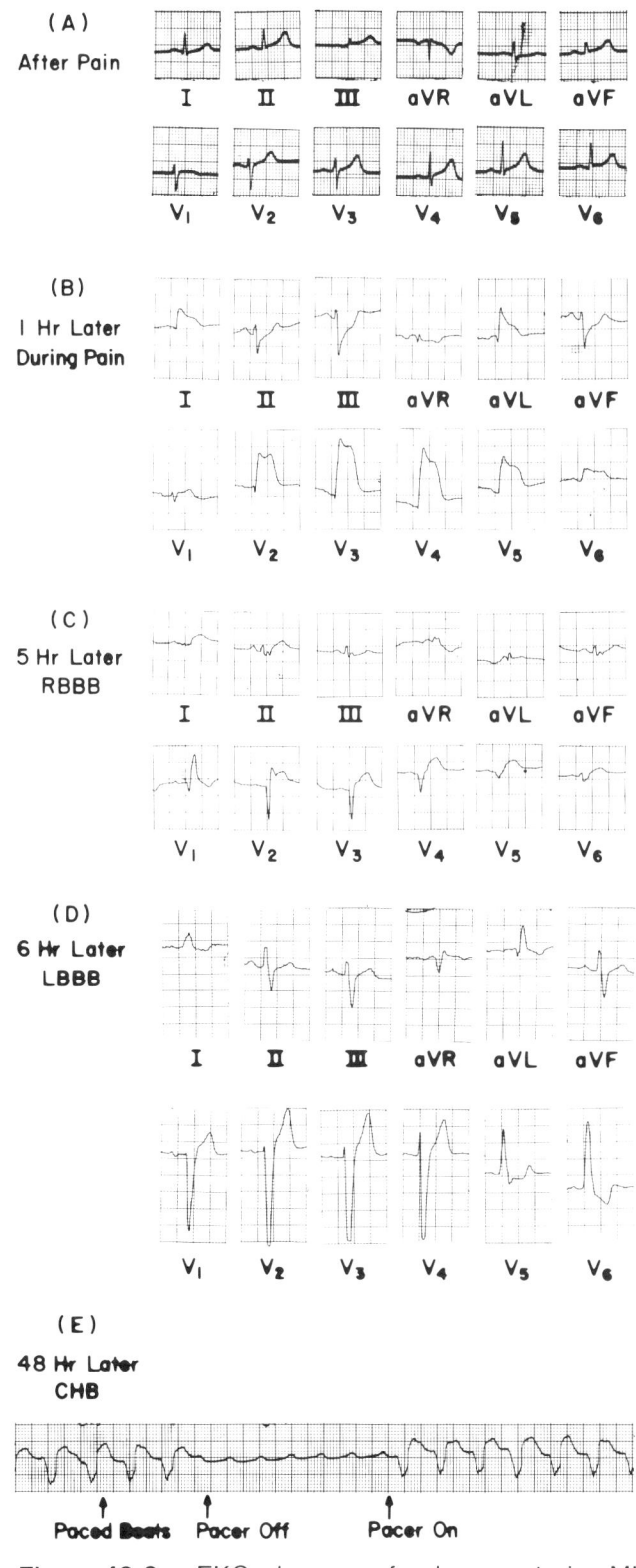

Figure 49.3. EKG changes of a large anterior MI complicated by conduction disturbances. A, EKG taken in the emergency room after an episode of chest pain shows minor ST segment elevation in II, III, and aVF, suggesting inferior transmural ischemia. B, 1 hr later severe chest pain developed with massive ST segment elevation in anteroseptal, apical, lateral, and high lateral leads. In addition, the first sign of conduction difficulty is present with the appearance of left anterior hemiblock. C, 5 hr after admission complete RBBB is present but does not obscure the anterior Q waves or ST segment elevation of the ongoing infarction. D, 6 hr after admission RBBB resolved but complete LBBB developed, altering all previous signs of the infarction. E, 48 hr after admission complete heart block developed. The rhythm strip shows QRS complexes produced by a temporary transvenous pacemaker. When the pacemaker is turned off, only P waves are present. Although AV conduction returned on the following day, a permanent pacer was placed because of the probability that CHB would eventually recur.

P wave is not conducted, is generally associated with inferior infarction and does not progress directly to CHB. 2) Mobitz type II, in which the P-R interval is constant for conducted P waves but some P waves are not conducted to the ventricle, generally occurs with anterior infarction and represents necrosis of the conducting system distal to the bundle of His. It may suddenly progress to CHB.

If only 2:1 AV block is present (50% of all P waves are not conducted), it is impossible to distinguish Mobitz type I from type II.

THIRD DEGREE AV BLOCK

In this type, known as complete heart block, the P waves have no fixed relationship to the QRS complexes. The condition of the patient is entirely dependent on the rate of the fastest ventricular pacemaker below the block. During infarction these lower ventricular pacemakers may be damaged by ischemia or suppressed by lidocaine that had been required to treat VPBs. Hence a dangerous emergency situation may rapidly develop unless a pacemaker was inserted prophylactically. In such an emergency, atropine may be given to decrease AV block and isoproterenol may be used to increase the rate of a ventricular pacemaker while a temporary transvenous pacemaker is inserted.

BUNDLE BRANCH AND FASCICULAR BLOCK

During infarction right bundle branch block (RBBB), left bundle branch block (LBBB), or blockage of the anterior fascicle [left anterior hemiblock (LAH)] or posterior fascicle [left posterior hemiblock (LPH)] of the left bundle may occur (Atkins et al., 1973). Again the primary importance of these disorders is the degree to which they signal the occurrence of CHB and indicate the need for pacemaker insertion.

PROPHYLACTIC PACEMAKER INSERTION

This aspect of the care of patients with acute MI remains extremely controversial since the probabilities for progression to CHB of each of the numerous combinations of conduction disturbances remain poorly defined (Resnekov and Lipp, 1972). In addition, the ease of insertion and complication rate of prophylactic pacemakers vary with the equipment and experience of each CCU. Several situations in which it is generally agreed that a pacemaker should be inserted are (Alpert and Francis, 1977): 1) Mobitz type II AV block, 2) new LBBB, 3) new RBBB with anterior infarction, 4) RBBB plus LAH or LPH, and 5) CHB with a slow ventricular rate and a wide QRS complex.

A more detailed consideration of this problem is contained in the report of a multicenter study on indications for pacing in acute MI (Hindman et al., 1978). A major conclusion of this study is that patients who demonstrate a high degree of AV block during infarction have a high risk of sudden death or recurrent block postinfarction and thus should receive permanent pacing.

Hemodynamic Disturbances

With the successful control of arrhythmias and conduction disturbances in CCUs, impairment of pumping function of the heart has emerged as a major problem. In many cases only congestive heart failure is present, but in others cardiogenic shock occurs.

CONGESTIVE HEART FAILURE (CHF)

During infarction CHF may occur in the absence of cardiomegaly by physical examination or chest x-ray because there is no time for ventricular dilatation to occur. The other distinctive feature of CHF during MI is that an increased compliance of the left ventricle may make a major contribution to elevation of left atrial pressure and the production of rales.

Diuretics and afterload reduction are used to treat CHF during MI. Digoxin is used with caution since it may potentially increase VEA and AV block. It is also possible that administration of digoxin to a patient without cardiomegaly might increase oxygen demand and extend myocardial injury.

CARDIOGENIC SHOCK

The mortality of this unfortunate consequence of MI is over 90%. Cardiogenic shock is caused by destruction of over 40% of the left ventricular myocardium (Page et al., 1971). A patient is considered to be in shock by clinical criteria if the systolic arterial pressure is less than 80 mm Hg and urine output is less than 20 cc/hr in the absence of hypovolemia. The skin is generally cool and diaphoretic, and mentation may be impaired. Since the clinical signs of shock may originate from several different mechanisms, patients thought to be in cardiogenic shock should be instrumented with an arterial catheter and a Swan-Ganz pulmonary artery catheter to determine their true intra-arterial pressure, left ventricular filling pressure, and cardiac output (Ratshin et al., 1972; Russell and Rackley, 1974). During infarction the jugular venous pressure, which reflects right sided filling pressure, is a poor index of left sided filling pressure.

When these measurements are completed, patients will be found to be in one of the four hemodynamic categories proposed by Forrester et al. The short-term mortality rate increases from 3% in class I to 51% in class IV, which includes patients with cardiogenic shock (Forrester et al., 1976).

Class I: Hemodynamically Uncomplicated Cardiac index (CI) >2.2 liters/min/m^2

Pulmonary capillary wedge pressure (PCW) ≤18 mm Hg

Most patients in this category need no specific therapy. Occasionally a patient will demonstrate hypotension resulting from inappropriate peripheral vasodilation (a Bezold-Jarisch reflex). In such a case methoxamine, a peripheral vasoconstrictor, may be used to maintain arterial pressure.

Class II: Pulmonary Congestion without Peripheral Hypoperfusion

$$CI > 2.2 \text{ liters/min/m}^2$$
$$PCW > 18 \text{ mm Hg}$$

In these patients diuretics should be the initial therapy followed by vasodilator therapy if the systemic vascular resistance is elevated. Digoxin may also be utilized.

Class III: Peripheral Hypoperfusion without Pulmonary Congestion

$$CI \leq 2.2 \text{ liters/min/m}^2$$
$$PCW \leq 18 \text{ mm Hg}$$

These patients suffer from intravascular *volume depletion*. Fortunately this treatable condition is rather commonly encountered. The causes are multiple: nausea and NPO orders may decrease fluid intake, pressors may force fluid out of the vascular space, and diuretics may cause excessive urine output. These patients, in whom cardiogenic shock was suspected, respond extremely well to intravenous volume expansion (Crexells et al., 1973). Volume replacement should be continued until the PCW reaches the range of 18–20 mm Hg.

Class IV: Combined Pulmonary Congestion and Peripheral Hypoperfusion

$$CI \leq 2.2 \text{ liters/min/m}^2$$
$$PCW \geq 18 \text{ mm Hg}$$

This category includes patients with cardiogenic shock, in whom therapy is most difficult. If systemic vascular resistance is elevated, a peripheral vasodilator, such as nitroprusside, may increase the CI without causing an unacceptable fall in systemic arterial pressure (Armstrong et al., 1975). If arterial pressure is below 90 mm Hg systolic, a pressor with inotropic activity, such as dopamine, may be needed. Occasionally a combination of dopamine with a vasodilator may be useful (Miller et al., 1977). Intra-aortic balloon counterpulsation can be used to stabilize these patients, but the long-term outlook remains bleak unless a specific mechanical defect is present that can be corrected surgically (Buckley et al., 1971; Scheidt et al., 1973).

Mechanical Defects

Infarction, particularly if extensive, may cause major alterations in the geometry of the ventricle, with potentially serious clinical consequences. If recognized, these defects can in some cases be repaired surgically.

MITRAL REGURGITATION

In many patients a murmur of mitral regurgitation may occur unaccompanied by significant hemodynamic changes. This generally results from papillary muscle dysfunction produced by changes in the supporting myocardium (Burch et al., 1968). In a few patients with infarction the papillary muscle may rupture, causing severe mitral regurgitation and shock (Morrow et al., 1968). An apical holosystolic murmur radiating to the axilla is generally present, although in some cases the defect may be so severe that no murmur is produced. Differentiation of a rupture of a papillary muscle from perforation of the ventricular septum, its closest imitator, can be made with the Swan-Ganz catheter. A ruptured papillary muscle will produce large "V" waves in the PCW tracing, whereas a septal perforation will produce an oxygen step-up between blood samples taken from the right atrium and the pulmonary artery. Immediate treatment for a ruptured papillary muscle consists of afterload reduction with vasodilators or intra-aortic balloon counterpulsation to increase the proportion of cardiac output that goes through the aortic, as opposed to the mitral, valve. The goal of immediate therapy is to stabilize the patient until the myocardium has sufficient strength to permit definitive surgical repair.

RUPTURE OF THE VENTRICULAR SEPTUM

As discussed above, this complication is best diagnosed with the use of a Swan-Ganz catheter. It may be suspected clinically when shock, a holosystolic murmur, and a precordial thrill suddenly develop. The immediate therapy for a ventricular septal defect (VSD) is the same as that for a ruptured papillary muscle (Longo and Cohen, 1976). Surgery is also delayed, if possible, until the septum has sufficient strength to permit suturing.

RUPTURE OF THE FREE WALL OF THE VENTRICLE

This is an unfortunate complication that is almost always immediately fatal unless the pericardium restricts the loss of blood and emergency surgery is performed (VanTassel and Edwards, 1972).

LEFT VENTRICULAR ANEURYSM

With large infarcts the myocardial wall may have such low tensile strength during the healing process that it bulges outward. An aneurysm may be formed that may decrease cardiac output (by absorbing some of the motion of the blood during systole), produce arrhythmias, and serve as a location for formation of a mural thrombus (Loop et al., 1973). Clinically an aneurysm may be suspected when ST segment elevation persists beyond the 1st week postinfarction. If no contraindications are present, anticoagulation is advisable to prevent thromboembolism. If severe CHF or shock is present, surgical resection of an aneurysm, after tensile strength of the margins has returned (2-3 weeks post-MI), can result in improved ventricular function.

Causes of Continued Chest Pain Postinfarction

The most common causes of chest pain after the initial infarction are pericarditis, postinfarction angina, and infarct extension. Since each requires different therapy, proper identification of the cause of the pain is essential.

PERICARDITIS

Pericarditis may occur at any time after the 1st day of infarction. Pericarditis that occurs during the 1st week or two postinfarction results from the normal inflammatory response that accompanies transmural myocardial necrosis. Pericarditis occurring several weeks or months postinfarction is termed Dressler's syndrome and occurs on an autoimmune basis (Dressler, 1956).

Clinical recognition of pericarditis is based on the presence of pain that varies with position or with respiration and, in some cases, a pericardial friction rub (Spodick, 1976). The pain generally responds well to therapy with salicylates or indomethacin. It is important to emphasize that the pains of pericarditis in the postinfarction setting are often attributed to continuing myocardial ischemia and are inappropriately treated with nitrates, β-blockade, and morphine.

POSTINFARCTION ANGINA

Since infarctions occur at different rates it is impossible to identify an exact time that separates the pain of the infarction from postinfarction angina for all patients. In most patients, however, transient pain occurring more than 24 hr after the onset of infarction represents a different process. If the pain is similar to the original ischemic pain but is of shorter duration and not associated with a re-elevation of serum CK, the diagnosis of postinfarction angina can be made. Reversible EKG changes that appear with the pain strengthen the diagnosis but are not essential. The pain should be treated with routine antianginal therapy, if no contraindications are present.

INFARCT EXTENSION

In a number of patients additional myocardial necrosis occurs after the initial event. Extension is suspected when a postinfarction patient develops prolonged pain with persistent evidence of ischemia or new evidence of necrosis on the EKG. Confirmation of extension is based on a re-elevation of myocardial enzymes in the serum. At the present time, extension of infarction is treated in the same manner as the original infarction with primary reliance on morphine for the relief of pain. On-going studies of protection of ischemic myocardium may alter the therapy for extension, since extension is a situation in which pretreatment, or very early treatment, of ischemia is possible.

Thromboembolism

The use of prophylactic anticoagulation to prevent thromboembolism has been discussed previously. In the absence of anticoagulation, and sometimes despite prophylactic anticoagulation, thromboembolism may occur in either the pulmonic or systemic circulation (Thompson, 1974; Sasahara et al., 1975).

Pulmonary embolism should be suspected if episodic tachypnea occurs, particularly in an obese, immobile patient with diminished cardiac output. If available, a portable lung scan is often useful to support or exclude the diagnosis. Full anticoagulation with intravenous heparin should be instituted when the diagnosis is certain.

Arterial embolism may produce a wide variety of signs and symptoms, depending upon the location of the embolus. The most frequent presentations are pain and pallor of an extremity or a cerebrovascular accident (CVA). Surgical removal of an embolus from an extremity is often successful. For an embolic CVA, anticoagulation should be delayed until it is certain that cerebral hemorrhage has not occurred.

Right Ventricular Infarction

In recent years the techniques of Swan-Ganz catheterization and radionuclide ventriculography have revealed a surprisingly high incidence of right ventricular (RV) infarction. Clinical identification of right ventricular infarction is of great importance to the selection of proper therapy (Lorell et al., 1979). The proper treatment of RV infarction with reduced cardiac output is administration of fluid to passively assist the flow of blood through the lungs. If the RV infarction is not recognized, the physician may mistakenly administer a diuretic since the distended neck vein might be interpreted to represent fluid overload.

With RV infarction the Swan-Ganz study reveals elevated right atrial and right ventricular end diastolic pressures with a reduced RV systolic pressure. The radionuclide ventriculogram shows decreased motion of the right ventricle. Autopsy studies have confirmed the high incidence of RV infarction and have also revealed that it is most commonly associated with inferior infarction.

PROGNOSIS

Short and long-term survival following MI vary greatly for different types of patients. At one extreme a patient with a single, complete coronary occlusion producing a small infarct uncomplicated by congestive heart failure or ventricular ectopy may have a life expectancy near that of the general population. At the other extreme a patient with a large infarct, with congestive heart failure and significant ectopy may have a shorter life expectancy than a patient with a malignant neoplasm. Several prognostic indices have been developed that relate certain features of a patient's presentation to prognosis (Peel et al., 1962; Norris et al., 1969).

REHABILITATION

Recovery from a MI presents a difficult task that requires determination on the part of the patient and skill in evaluation and recommendation on the part of the physician.

Three to four weeks after the patient is discharged from the hospital, it is useful to perform a submaximal exercise tolerance test (ETT) limited by a heart rate of 120 beats/min. This test will provide information on the patient's ability to exercise and the occurrence of arrhythmias or ischemic ST segment changes during exertior. It can serve as an invaluable aid to the physician in recommending additional activity for the patient. A Holter monitor should also be obtained at this time if the patient had experienced persistent ventricular ectopic activity during hospitalization (The Coronary Drug Project Research Group, 1973).

Indications for cardiac catheterization post-MI are not well defined. In some institutions cardiac catheterization is recommended for all patients who have suffered a MI, unless contraindications exist. It is our practice to recommend catheterization to patients in the following categories: 1) moderate to severe angina pectoris requiring therapy with propranolol and long acting nitrates; 2) a positive ETT with the development of ST segment elevation at sites that do not have Q waves; 3) a positive ETT with ST segment depression greater than or equal to 2 mm in any lead.

In some instances catheterization may be recommended for a young patient who is asymptomatic with an equivocal ETT and who wishes to know his prognosis with greater certainty (Humphries et al., 1974). Other factors that should be evaluated several months postinfarction are the patient's cholesterol and triglyceride levels and the status of modifiable risk factors. The patient should be instructed in a low cholesterol diet and encouraged to discontinue smoking.

Drug therapy after infarction should be tailored to the complications that are present (angina, CHF, VEA). Many patients need only be given sublingual nitroglycerin for use if ischemic pain returns. There is evidence that prophylactic β-blockade after infarction might substantially reduce subsequent mortality (Multicentre Study, 1975; Anderson et al., 1979). Definitive recommendations on this practice must await the results of a large national study that is currently in progress.

Finally, the physician must make every effort to counteract the fear and self-doubt that may afflict a patient after an infarction. If appropriate, it may be emphasized to the patient that, although some of the heart muscle has been permanently damaged, the remaining muscle is more than adequate for continued function. In many patients a fixed routine of exercises and walking may be extremely helpful to overcome the psychologic reluctance to exercise and the deconditioning that may follow an infarction. With this management many patients return to normal activity following their infarction.

NEW APPROACHES TO THE PREVENTION AND TREATMENT OF MYOCARDIAL INFARCTION

Although care for the patient with necrotic myocardium has vastly improved in the past decade, it remains imperative to seek methods to prevent such an event. Therefore, intensive efforts are in progress to prevent the fixed and variable coronary obstructions that produce the myocardial ischemia that leads to infarction. In addition, other efforts have been directed toward limitation of the size of infarction that results from a given coronary occlusion.

Fixed Coronary Obstruction (Coronary Atherosclerosis)

From the preceding chapter it is readily apparent that coronary atherosclerosis is the underlying cause of most cases of MI. Prevention of atherosclerosis would be the optimal method to prevent MI.

There are currently major investigative efforts under way to understand the manner in which the atherosclerotic plaque develops. It is apparent that elevated serum cholesterol has a major role in plaque formation, and many attempts are in progress to lower serum cholesterol through dietary and pharmacologic measures. The role of platelets and the clotting system in the genesis of plaques is also being investigated. However, at the present time there are no proven medical means by which coronary atherosclerosis can be controlled. Surgical therapy, with coronary artery bypass grafting, is only a partial solution to the problem of coronary atherosclerosis, and its efficacy in preventing MI is not yet proven.

Although the complete prevention of coronary atherosclerosis remains an elusive goal, the falling cardiovascular mortality in the United States may be due in part to a decline in atherosclerosis caused by alterations in risk factors. In the United States the average serum cholesterol has fallen, control of hypertension has improved, and middle aged men, who are at greatest risk for coronary events, have decreased their use of cigarettes. These gains are encouraging, but the causal link between risk factor modification and declining cardiovascular mortality has yet to be proven. The Multiple Risk Factor Intervention Trial (MRFIT) currently in progress could provide such proof.

Variable Coronary Obstruction

Over the past 5 years there has been growing awareness among cardiologists that variable coronary obstruction may have an important role in the pathogenesis of MI. Interest in the role of variable obstruction is heightened by the availability of numerous drugs that might be of immediate value in the effort to prevent or reverse such obstruction and prevent MI.

Evidence for the role of variable obstruction in infarction has been provided by the angiographic studies of Drs. Maseri (Maseri et al., 1978) and Oliva (Oliva and Breckinridge, 1977). These investigators have proven that at least some cases of MI are caused by a variable obstruction. In some the variable obstruction occurs at a location in which a coronary artery is partially blocked by a fixed obstruction. In a few cases variable obstruction may cause infarction even in the absence of obstructive coronary atherosclerosis. The onset of variable obstruction would explain the unusual circumstances that often surround the onset of MI. It is well known that the pain of MI may begin while the patient is sleeping or at rest and myocardial oxygen consumption is unlikely to be increased. One or a combination of the following three processes might produce sudden obstruction to coronary flow sufficient to cause MI.

PLATELET AGGREGATION

Platelets may be stimulated by intimal injury to aggregate in a coronary artery. Such an aggregation could cause occlusion itself or could liberate quantities of thromboxane A2, an extremely powerful coronary vasoconstrictor, which could in turn cause complete coronary occlusion. Suspicion that platelets may initiate the obstruction leading to MI has been heightened by the report that sulfinpyrazone (Anturane), an inhibitor of platelet function, reduced mortality from sudden death in patients who had suffered a myocardial infarction (Sulfinpyrazone, 1978). A large national multicenter study of the value of antiplatelet therapy with aspirin in patients with coronary artery disease is now in progress.

SPASM

In certain patients spasm of a coronary artery is clearly responsible for the complete occlusion that produces MI. It was demonstrated that in 6 of 15 patients with acute MI, intracoronary nitroglycerin could restore patency of the vessel when given soon after the onset of infarction (Oliva and Breckinridge, 1977).

If spasm causes MI, it is possible that some infarctions could be prevented by a new class of potent coronary vasodilators. These agents act by blocking the slow calcium channel responsible for the contraction of smooth muscle cells in the walls of the coronary arteries.

Nifedipine is a calcium antagonist with which considerable experience has accumulated (Muller and Gunther, 1978). It is extremely effective for the control of spasm in cases of Prinzmetal's angina refractory to conventional medical therapy (Antman et al., 1979). A multicenter study is now under way to determine whether the administration of nifedipine soon after the onset of chest pain to patients with threatened MI could prevent infarction from occurring by eliminating coronary spasm. The study is being conducted at the Georgetown University School of Medicine; North Shore Hospital in Manhasset, New York, an affiliate of Cornell University School of Medicine; and the Waltham Hospital in Waltham, Massachusetts. The coordinating center is located at the Peter Bent Brigham Hospital and Harvard Medical School. The study, which will include over 200 patients, will be completed in 1982.

THROMBOSIS

More than 50 years ago the presence of thrombosis in the coronary arteries of patients with MI was so well recognized that the disease was called "coronary thrombosis." There was, however, a persistent concern over the time at which these clots occurred; their late appearance led many to consider them insignificant secondary events. A recent surgical study reveals that clots are frequently present in the early stages of infarction (Phillips et al., 1979). Coronary artery bypass grafting was performed a mean of 6.5 hr after the onset of chest pain in 75 patients with MI. A fresh thrombosis was present in most cases. Even from this experience it remains impossible to determine whether the thrombosis is a primary event or a secondary event resulting from platelet aggregation and spasm. Nevertheless, thrombosis occurs early and attempts to reverse spasm should perhaps include measures to lyse a secondary thrombus.

As with platelet aggregation and spasm, the role of thrombosis is important therapeutically. Potent fibrinolytic preparations are available that can be injected directly into a coronary artery or can be infused systemically for a less direct and less invasive approach. The favorable results from a large cooperative European study of fibrinolytic therapy for acute infarction indicate that this may be a useful therapeutic approach (European Cooperative Study Group, 1979).

Limitation of Infarct Size

Even in the presence of complete, fixed coronary occlusion, it may be possible to prevent a certain amount of ischemic myocardium from becoming necrotic.

Studies in experimental animals 10 years ago by Dr. Eugene Braunwald and Dr. Peter Maroko demonstrated that the quantity of myocardium that becomes necrotic following coronary occlusion is not predetermined by the anatomy of the coronary vasculature (Maroko et al., 1971). It was shown that numerous interventions could be applied that either increased or decreased the amount of ischemic myocardium that finally became necrotic.

Over the past 10 years these findings have been confirmed in numerous laboratories. Quantitative studies have now been performed that have shown that 30% or more of the ischemic area can be prevented from infarcting (Redwood et al., 1972; Reimer et al., 1973; Kjekshus and Mjos, 1973; Kloner et al., 1978). It has also been shown in animals that interventions can be beneficial even when given 6 hr following occlusion (Hillis et al., 1977).

The interventions act through several different mechanisms. Some, such as isoproterenol, increase infarct size by increasing oxygen demand. Others, such as propranolol, decrease infarct size by decreasing oxygen demand. Interventions such as nitroglycerin act in part by increasing the supply of blood to the ischemic area through collateral vessels. Other interventions, such as ibuprofen, presumably act by decreasing the inflammatory response and limiting the nonspecific injury of myocardial cells that such inflammation produces. Table 49.3 indicates the broad range of interventions that have been found to be useful.

STUDIES IN PATIENTS

Methods of Measurements

The major impediment to clinical assessment of agents designed to limit infarct size has been the absence of a totally satisfactory method to measure salvage of ischemic myocardium. A number of methods have been developed, each with its own advantages and limitations.

CREATINE KINASE. Measurement of serum creatine kinase (CK) may be used to quantitate the size of an infarction as well as to determine its presence (Roberts et al., 1975). Infarct size determined from CK curves has been shown to correlate closely with infarct size measured at autopsy in a group of patients dying with acute MI (Bleifeld et al., 1977).

A difficulty with the method is the possibility that an intervention being measured can alter the relationship between cell death and the amount of CK released. However, the presence of such an interaction can be excluded by animal experimentation with the agent to be tested in patients. The major disadvantage of this method is that the extreme variability in size of infarcts in a control group necessitates the use of an extremely large patient population to achieve sufficient power to detect a beneficial effect.

QRS MAPPING. There is a close correlation between the amount of necrosis produced by ischemia in myocardial biopsy specimens and changes in the local epicardial QRS complex (Hillis et al., 1976). Specimens that show a moderate amount of necrosis show moderate development of Q waves and a moderate loss of R wave voltage. Specimens that show 100% necrosis show a complete loss of R wave voltage. There is also a close relationship between changes in the epicardial EKG and changes in the precordial EKG (Muller et al., 1975). These relationships form the basis for the use of the precordial EKG to assess effectiveness of interventions to limit infarct size (Muller et al., 1978). The method can be used only in patients with acute anterior or lateral transmural MI who do not develop conduction disturbances. In these patients the electrical signs of ischemia are directly reflected in the precordial EKG. The method is used in the following manner. 1) The height of the precordial R waves at sites with ST segment elevation is measured. 2) The patient is randomly assigned to treated or control group. 3) An EKG is recorded 1 week later from the same sites. 4) The percentage loss of R wave voltage from prerandomization to 1 week later is calculated for treated and control groups.

This method may be used with the standard six precordial leads, but its sensitivity is greater with multiple precordial leads. The advantage of the method is that it provides the opportunity for each patient to serve as his own control for the amount of R wave voltage present initially. The disadvantages of the method are that it is not quantitative and that, at the present time, it can be applied only to relatively few patients. It is possible that the use of the vectorcardiogram can extend the applicability of the method to a larger number of patients (Cowan et al., 1979).

TECHNETIUM-99M PYROPHOSPHATE SCINTIGRAMS. The area of uptake of technetium-99m-labeled pyrophosphate during acute MI is correlated with infarct size. The limitations of this method are similar to those of the CK method.

First, there is a wide variation in size of infarcts and each patient does not serve as his or her own control since the measurement is taken after the intervention is given and the infarction has occurred.

Second, the intervention may alter the relationship between the scintigram and the actual extent of infarction.

RADIONUCLIDE VENTRICULOGRAPHY. The radionuclide ventriculogram (RVG) is a noninvasive technique that can be used to measure ejection fraction and local wall motion during acute MI. The RVG measures the effect of the infarct on ventricular function, an end point of greater clinical significance than the size of the infarct itself. The ejection fraction can be measured prior to randomization to treatment or control groups and at some time after therapy. In this manner each patient serves as his or her own control, and the number of patients required to detect a beneficial effect of therapy upon ventricular function is greatly reduced.

Clinically Important Interventions

Pilot studies in patients have been completed which indicate that a number of interventions may limit infarct size. The following studies have yielded encouraging results, but none is sufficient to warrant a change in therapy at the present time.

β-ADRENERGIC BLOCKADE. In a small group of patients it has been shown that acute ST segment elevation during the infarction was reduced when intravenous propranolol was administered (Gold et al., 1976). A large study is currently in progress in Sweden in which metoprolol is being given to patients with acute MI. In patients without prerandomization LDH elevation, the

Table 49.3
Interventions that Modify Myocardial Injury Following Coronary Occlusion[a]

I. Interventions that reduce myocardial injury
  A. By decreasing myocardial oxygen demand
    1. β-adrenergic blockade[b]
    2. Pranolium
    3. Reserpine
    4. Cardiac glycosides in the failing heart[b]
    5. Counterpulsation
      a. Intra-aortic balloon[b]
      b. External counterpulsation[b]
    6. By decreasing afterload in hypertensive individuals—trimethaphan camsylate[b]
    7. By inhibition of lipolysis—β-pyridylcarbinol, lipid-free albumin, glucose-insulin-potassium
    8. Calcium antagonists—verapamil,[b] nifedipine
    9. Pentobarbital
  B. By increasing myocardial oxygen supply
    1. Directly
      a. Coronary artery reperfusion
      b. Elevating arterial PO_2[b]
      c. Thrombolytic agents
      d. Heparin
    2. Through collateral vessels
      a. Elevation of coronary perfusion pressure by methoxamine, neosynephrine, or norepinephrine.
      b. Intra-aortic balloon counterpulsation[b]
      c. External counterpulsation[b]
      d. Nitroglycerin[b]
      e. "Reverse coronary steal," or favorable redistribution of regional myocardial blood flow—methoxamine, oxygen[b]
    3. By increasing plasma osmolality
      a. Mannitol
      b. Hypertonic glucose
  C. By augmenting glycolysis (presumed)
    1. Glucose-insulin-potassium[b]
    2. Hypertonic glucose
    3. Pyruvate
    4. Carnitine
    5. Sodium dicloroacetate
  D. By enhancing transport to the ischemic zone of substrate utilized in energy production (presumed)—hyaluronidase[b]
  E. By protecting against autolytic and heterolytic processes (presumed)
    1. Cobra-venom factor
    2. Aprotinin
II. Interventions that increase myocardial injury
  A. By increasing myocardial oxygen requirements
    1. Isoproterenol
    2. Glucagon
    3. Ouabain
    4. Bretylium tasylate
    5. Tachycardia
  B. By decreasing myocardial oxygen supply
    1. Directly
      a. Hypoxemia
      b. Anemia
    2. Through collateral vessels
      a. By reducing coronary perfusion pressure (hemorrhage)
      b. By "coronary steal," or unfavorable redistribution of regional myocardial blood flow, dipyridamole, nitroprusside[b]
  C. By decreasing substrate availability—hypoglycemia

[a] Reprinted with permission from J.E. Muller, P.R. Maroko, and E. Braunwald: *Preservation of the Ischemic Myocardium*; Upjohn Company, Kalamazoo, MI, 1977.
[b] Denotes intervention that has received some clinical application.

infarct size is reduced as calculated by an LDH method similar to the CK method (Hjalmarson et al., 1979). The study is continuing to determine whether metoprolol has a beneficial effect on mortality. Alprenolol, another β-blocker, has recently been shown to reduce mortality by 50% when given soon after infarction (Anderson et al., 1979).

NITROGLYCERIN. It has been shown that intravenous nitroglycerin limits infarct size as judged by the EKG (Borer et al., 1975; Come et al., 1975). A recent study from Chiche et al. (1979) in France again demonstrated beneficial changes in the EKG following intravenous nitroglycerin; in addition mortality was lower in the treated group. Intravenous nitroglycerin seems to be most effective in limiting infarct size in patients with left ventricular failure.

HYALURONIDASE. Hyaluronidase is an enzyme that depolymerizes hyaluronic acid in the myocardium and presumably improves diffusion of substrates to, and waste products from, ischemic myocardium. In a clinical study 91 patients with acute anterior transmural MI were randomized to control or hyaluronidase treatment less than 8 hr after the onset of pain. The control group lost 70.9 ± 3.6% of their R wave voltage from pretreatment to 10 days postinfarction. The hyaluronidase-treated group, however, lost only 54.2 ± 5.0% of their R wave voltage. Ventricular function was not measured in this study, and the clinical significance of this difference in R wave loss is unknown (Maroko et al., 1977).

GLUCOSE-INSULIN-POTASSIUM (GIK). There has been great controversy over the value of GIK therapy for acute MI. Recently a randomized study by Rogers et al. (1979) demonstrated improved ventricular function in GIK-treated patients compared to controls.

THROMBOLYTIC THERAPY. A large multicenter trial of the use of streptokinase for patients with acute MI has recently been completed in Europe. The mortality rate 6 months after infarction was one-half as high in the patients who received streptokinase as in the control group. There was no direct evidence indicating the mechanism through which the beneficial effect occurred. Infarct size was not measured, but it was postulated that a beneficial effect upon infarct size could have occurred (European Cooperative Study Group, 1979).

Studies in Progress

At the present time there are several major studies in progress that will clarify the role of various interventions to limit infarct size in the treatment of patients with acute MI. The studies of GIK and of metoprolol mentioned above are currently continuing. In addition, the National Heart, Lung and Blood Institute has launched a major study to determine whether propranolol or hyaluronidase is of value to patients with infarction. This study is named the Multicenter Investigation of the Limitation of Infarct Size (MILIS). More than 1000 patients will be randomized to control, propranolol, or hyaluronidase treatment during acute infarction. End points will include CK infarct size, QRS mapping, technetium-99m pyrophosphate scintigrams, and changes in ejection fraction as determined by the RVG. In addition, the study will include Holter monitoring and exercise test performance 6 months postinfarction to determine whether possible harmful effects of successful limitation of infarct size are present. For example, it is possible that limitation of infarct size may leave the patient with an area of poorly perfused myocardium that causes ventricular ectopy or angina pectoris. The possibility that such harmful effects may occur is one of the primary reasons that major interventions to limit infarct size are not yet recommended as standard therapy.

Therapy at the Present Time

Although major interventions are not yet recommended, there is sufficient evidence that infarct size can be modified to warrant several changes in the routine care of patients with myocardial infarction. Oxygen demand should be minimized during the early stages of infarction. This can be accomplished by careful attention to relief of pain, with its attendant sympathetic hyperactivity, and to control of fever. Tachycardia should be avoided if possible since this is a major determinant of myocardial oxygen consumption. Therefore, atropine should be used for bradycardia only when required to maintain blood pressure. Pressors, such as dopamine, should be avoided if possible because they cause large increases in myocardial oxygen demand. However, pressors must sometimes be used to maintain blood pressure despite the likelihood that they will enlarge the infarct. Isoproterenol should be avoided if possible since it increases myocardial oxygen demand through its inotropic and chronotropic properties and decreases oxygen supply by causing peripheral vasodilation that decreases coronary perfusion pressure.

The optimal level of systemic arterial pressure during infarction is unknown. A high systemic arterial pressure increases myocardial oxygen demand but also increases oxygen supply through improved coronary perfusion. A low systemic arterial pressure decreases myocardial oxygen demand but also decreases supply. The proper balance between these two opposite tendencies will probably vary for each patient.

Finally, it would appear valuable to administer oxygen to patients with MI even in the absence of arterial hypoxemia since studies have indicated that an increase in PO_2 may also limit infarct size even without a significant increase in arterial oxygen content (Maroko et al., 1975; Madias and Hood, 1975).

SUMMARY

Myocardial infarction continues to be a major health problem. Patients who survive the dangerous prehospital period generally received specialized care in a CCU. In this setting arrhythmias can be prevented or rapidly treated. The hemodynamic disturbances associated with MI can often be corrected with invasive pressure monitoring and the proper use of volume expansion, afterload reduction, and inotropic agents. With proper evaluation and encouragement by the physician, many patients can return to full activity after their infarction.

Eventually, it is likely that control of atherosclerosis will prevent almost all cases of MI. Since such a goal remains elusive, attention has also been directed to several other approaches that offer somewhat less but could be implemented in the near future. Reversal of variable coronary occlusion by antiplatelet drugs, calcium antagonists, or fibrinolytic agents or limitation of infarct size by numerous agents are two approaches that are now under intense investigation.

Acknowledgments. I am grateful to Drs. Elliott Antman, John Rutherford, and Peter Stone for review of the manuscript and to Ms. Deidre Bernard for its preparation.

References

Alderman, E.L., Coltart, D.J., Wettach, G.E., et al.: Coronary artery syndromes after sudden propranolol withdrawal. Ann. Intern. Med. *81:*625, 1974.

Alpert, G.S., and Francis, G.S.: *Manual of Coronary Care.* Little, Brown, Boston, 1977.

Andersen, M.P., Becksgaard, P., Frederiksen, J., et al.: Effect of alprenolol on mortality among patients with definite or suspected acute myocardial infarction. Lancet *2:*865, 1979.

Antman, E., Muller, J., Goldberg, S., et al.: Nifedipine therapy for coronary spasm: Clinical experience in the United States. Circulation (Suppl. II)*60:*II–76, 1979.

Armstrong, P.W., Walker, D.C., Burton, J.R., et al.: Vasodilator therapy in acute myocardial infarction: A comparison of sodium nitroprusside and nitroglycerin. Circulation *52:*1118, 1975.

Atkins, J.M., Leshin, S.J., Bloomqvist, G., et al.: Ventricular conduction blocks and sudden death in acute myocardial infarction. N. Engl. J. Med. *288:*281, 1973.

Becker, W.F., Powell, J.L., and Turner, R.J.: A clinical study of 1,060 patients with acute cholecystitis. Surg. Gynecol. Obstet. *104:*491, 1957.

Bennett, J.R., and Atkinson, M.: The differentiation between oesphageal and cardiac pain. Lancet *2:*1123, 1966.

Bleifeld, W., Mathey, D., Hanrath, P., et al.: Infarct size estimated from serial creatine phosphokinase in relation to left ventricular hemodynamics. Circulation *55:*303, 1977.

Borer, J.S., Redwood, D.R., Levitt, B., et al.: Myocardial ischemia treated with nitroglycerin plus phenylephrine. N. Engl. J. Med. *293:*10008, 1975.

Buckley, M.J., Mundth, E.D., Daggett, W.M., et al.: Surgical therapy for early complications of myocardial infarction. Surgery *70:*814, 1971.

Burch, G.E., DePasquale, N.P., and Phillips, J.H.: The syndrome of papillary muscle dysfunction. Am. Heart J. *75:*399, 1968.

Cassem, N.H., and Hackett, T.P. Psychological rehabilitation of myocardial infarction patients in the acute phase. Heart Lung *2:*328, 1973.

Chartbook for the Conference on the Decline in Coronary Heart Disease Mortality. National Center for Health Statistics, Hyattsville, MD, 1978.

Chiche, P., Baligadoo, S.J., and Derrida, J.P.: A randomized trial of prolonged nitroglycerin infusion in acute myocardial infarction. Circulation (Suppl. II)*60:*II–165, 1979.

Come, P.C., Flaherty, J.T., Baird, M.G., et al.: Reversal by phenylephrine of the beneficial effects of intravenous nitroglycerin in patients with acute myocardial infarction. N. Engl. J. Med. *293:*1003, 1975.

The Coronary Drug Project Research Group: Prognostic importance of premature beats following myocardial infarction: Experience in the Coronary Drug Project. J.A.M.A. *223:*1116, 1973.

Cowan, M.J., Reichenbach, D.D., and Bruce, R.A.: Quantification of infarct size in humans by spatial vectorcardiography. Circulation (Suppl. II)*60:*I–71, 1979.

Crexells, C., Chatterjee, K., Forrester, J.S., et al.: Optimal level of filling pressure in the left side of the heart in acute myocardial infarction. N. Engl. J. Med. *289:*1263, 1973.

Dale, W.A., and Lewis, M.R.: Management of thoracic outlet syndrome. Ann. Surg. *181:*575, 1975.

Day, H.W.: Preliminary studies of an acute coronary care area. Lancet *83:*53, 1963.

deSoyza, N., Bissett, J.K., Kane, J.J., et al.: Association of accelerated idioventricular rhythm and paroxysmal ventricular tachycardia in acute myocardial infarction. Am. J. Cardiol. *34:*667, 1974.

Dressler, W.: A post-myocardial infarction syndrome. J.A.M.A. *160:*1379, 1956.

El-Sherif, N., Myerburg, R.J., Scherlag, B.J., et al.: Electrocardiographic antecedents of primary ventricular fibrillation: Value of the R-on-T phenomenon in myocardial infarction. Br. Heart J. *38:*415, 1976.

European Cooperative Study Group for streptokinase treatment in acute myocardial infarction. N. Engl. J. Med. *301:*797, 1979.

Fillmore, S.J., Guimaraes, A.C., Scheidt, S.S., et al.: Blood-gas changes and pulmonary hemodynamics following acute myocardial infarction. Circulation *45:*583, 1971.

Forrester, J.S., Diamond, G., Chatterjee, K., et al.: Medical therapy of acute myocardial infarction by application of hemodynamic subsets. N. Engl. J. Med. *295:*1356, 1404, 1976.

Fulton, M., Julian, D.G., and Oliver, M.F.: Sudden death and myocardial infarction. Circulation (Suppl IV)*40:*182, 1969.

Giardina, E.G., Heissenbuttel, R.H., and Bigger, J.T., Jr.: Intermittent intravenous procaine amide to treat ventricular arrhythmias. Ann. Intern. Med. *78:*183, 1973.

Gifford, R.H., and Feinstein, A.R.: A critique of methodology in studies of anticoagulant therapy for acute myocardial infarction. N. Engl. J. Med. *280:*351, 1969.

Gold, H.K., Leinbach, R.C., and Maroko, P.R.: Propranolol-induced reduction of signs of ischemic injury during acute myocardial infarction. Am. J. Cardiol. *38:*689, 1976.

Hackett, T.P., Cassem, N.H., and Wishnie, H.A.: The coronary care unit: Appraisal of its psychological hazards. N. Engl. J. Med. *279:*1365, 1968.

Herrick, J.B.: Clinical features of sudden obstruction of the coronary arteries. J.A.M.A. *59:*2015, 1912.

Hill, J.B., Hampton, J.R., and Mitchell, J.R.: A randomized trial of home-versus-hospital management for patients with suspected myocardial infarction. Lancet *1:*837, 1978.

Hillis, L.D., Askenazi, J., Braunwald, E., et al.: Use of changes in the epicardial QRS complex to assess interventions which modify the extent of myocardial necrosis following coronary artery occlusion. Circulation *54:*591, 1976.

Hillis, L.D., Fishbein, M.C., Braunwald, E., et al.: The influence of the time interval between coronary artery occlusion and the administration of hyaluronidase on salvage of ischemic myocardium in dogs. Circ. Res. *41:*26, 1977.

Hindman, M.C., Wanger, G.S., JaRo, M., et al.: The clinical significance of bundle branch block complicating acute myocardial infarction. 2. Indications for temporary and permanent pacemaker insertion. Circulation 58:689, 1978.

Hjalmarson, A., Ariniego, R., Herlitz, J., et al.: Limitation of infarct size in man by beta-blocker metoprolol. Circulation (Suppl. II)60:II-164, 1979.

Humphries, J.O., Kuller, L., Ross, R.S., et al.: Natural history of ischemic heart disease in relation to arteriographic findings: A twelve-year study of 224 patients. Circulation 49:489, 1974.

Hutter, A.M., Sidel, V.W., Shine, K.I., et al.: Early hospital discharge after myocardial infarction. N. Engl. J. Med. 228:1141, 1973.

Inouye, W.Y., Berggren, R.B., and Johnson, J.: Spontaneous pneumothorax: Treatment and mortality. Dis. Chest 51:67, 1967.

Kjekshus, J.K., and Mjos, O.D.: Effect of inhibition of lipolysis on infarct size after experimental coronary artery occlusion. J. Clin. Invest. 52:1770, 1973.

Kloner, R.A., Braunwald, E., and Maroko, P.R.: Long term preservation of ischemic myocardium in the dog by hyaluronidase. Circulation 58:220, 1978.

Levine, S.A., and Lown, B.: The "chair" treatment of coronary thrombosis. Trans. Assoc. Am. Physicians, 64:316, 1951.

Liberthson, R.R., Salisbury, K.W., Hutter, A.M., et al.: Atrial tachyarrhythmias in acute myocardial infarction. Am. J. Med. 60:956, 1976.

Lie, K.I., Wellens, H.J., van Capelle, F.J., et al.: Lidocaine in the prevention of primary ventricular fibrillation. N. Engl. J. Med. 291:324, 1974.

Longo, E.A., and Cohen, L.S.: Rupture of interventricular septum in acute myocardial infarction. Am. Heart J. 92:81, 1976.

Loop, F.D., Effler, D.B., Navia, J.A., et al.: Aneurysms of the left ventricle: Survival and results of a ten-year surgical experience. Ann. Surg. 178:399, 1973.

Lorell, B., Leinbach, R.C., Pohost, G.M., et al.: Right ventricular infarction: Clinical diagnosis and differentiation from cardiac tamponade and pericardial constriction. Am. J. Cardiol. 43:465, 1979.

Lown, B.: Electrical reversion of cardiac arrhythmias. Br. Heart J. 29:469, 1967.

Madias, J.E., and Hood, W.B.: Acute myocardial infarction: ST-segment elevation maps and O_2 breathing (abstract). Clin. Res. 23:194A, 1975.

Maroko, P.R., Kjekshus, J.K., Sobel, B.E., et al.: Factors influencing infarct size following experimental coronary artery occlusions. Circulation 43:67, 1971.

Maroko, P.R., Radvany, P., Braunwald, E., et al.: Reduction of infarct size by oxygen inhalation following acute coronary occlusion. Circulation 52:360, 1975.

Maroko, P.R., Hillis, L.D., Muller, J.E., et al.: Favorable effects of hyaluronidase on electrocardiographic evidence of necrosis in patients with acute myocardial infarction. N. Engl. J. Med. 296:898, 1977.

Marriott, H.J.L.: *Practical Electrocardiography*, ed. 5. Williams & Wilkins, Baltimore, 1972.

Maseri, A., L'Abbate, A., Baroldi, G., et al.: Coronary vasospasm as a possible cause of myocardial infarction. N. Engl. J. Med. 299:1271, 1978.

McLaughlin, P.R., Doherty, P.W., Martin, R.P., et al.: Myocardial imaging in a patient with reproducible variant angina. Am. J. Cardiol. 39:126, 1977.

Miller, R.R., Awan, N.A., Joye, J.A., et al.: Combined dopamine and nitroprusside therapy in congestive heart failure: Greater augmentation of cardiac performance by addition of inotropic stimulation to afterload reduction. Circulation 55:881, 1977.

Moiseev, S.G.: The experience of rendering first aid to myocardial infarction patients in Moscow. Sov. Med. 26:30, 1962.

Montero, A.C., Archibald, D., Franciosa, J.A., et al.: Value and safety of pulmonary artery catheterization in a multihospital study of acute myocardial infarction. Circulation (Suppl. II)60:165, 1979.

Morgensen, L.: Ventricular tachyarrhythmias and lignocaine prophylaxis in acute myocardial infarction. Acta Med. Scand. 168(Suppl. 513):30, 1970.

Morrow, A., Cohen, L., Roberts, W., et al.: Severe mitral regurgitation following acute myocardial infarction and ruptured papillary muscle. Circulation (Suppl. II)37 and 38:124, 1968.

Muller, J.E.: Diagnosis of myocardial infarction: Historical notes from the Soviet Union and the United States. Am. J. Cardiol. 40:269, 1977.

Muller, J.E., and Gunther, S.J.: Nifedipine therapy for Prinzmetal's angina. Circulation 57:137, 1978.

Muller, J.E., Maroko, P.R., and Braunwald, E.: Evaluation of precordial electrocardiographic mapping as a means of assessing changes in myocardial ischemic injury. Circulation 52:16, 1975.

Muller, J.E., Maroko, P.R., and Braunwald, E.: Precordial electrocardiographic mapping: A technique to assess the efficacy of interventions designed to limit infarct size. Circulation 57:1, 1978.

Multicentre Study: Improvement in prognosis of myocardial infarction by long-term β-adrenoceptor blockade using practolol. Br. Med. J. 3:735, 1975.

Myers, G.B., Klein, H.A., and Kiratzke, T.: 2. Correlation of electrocardiographic and pathologic findings in large anterolateral infarcts. Am. Heart J. 36:838, 1948a.

Myers, G.B., Klein, H.A., and Stofer, B.E.: 1. Correlation of electrocardiographic and pathologic findings in anteroseptal infarction. Am. Heart J. 36:535, 1948b.

Myers, G.B., Klein, H.A., and Stofer, B.E.: Correlation of electrocardiographic and pathologic findings in lateral infarction. Am. Heart J. 37:374, 1949.

Norris, R.N., Brandt, P.W.T., Caughey, D.E., et al.: A new coronary prognostic index. Lancet 1:274, 1969.

Oliva, P.B., and Breckinridge, J.C.: Arteriographic evidence of coronary arterial spasm in acute myocardial infarction. Circulation 56:366, 1977.

Page, D.L., Caulfield, J.B., Kastor, J.A., et al.: Myocardial changes associated with cardiogenic shock. N. Engl. J. Med. 285:133, 1971.

Pantridge, J.F.: Mobile coronary care. Chest 58:229, 1970.

Pantridge, J.F., Webb, S.W., Adgey, A.A.J., et al.: The first hour after the onset of acute myocardial infarction. In *Progress in Cardiology*, vol. 3. Lea & Febiger, Philadelphia, 1974.

Parkey, R.W., Bonte, F.J., Myer, S.L., et al.: A new method of radionuclide imaging of acute myocardial infarction in humans. Circulation 50:540, 1974.

Peel, A.A.F., Semple, T., Wang, I., et al.: A coronary prognostic index for grading the severity of infarction. Br. Heart J. 24:745, 1962.

Phillips, S.J., Kongtahworn, C., Zeff, R.H., et al.: Emergency coronary artery revascularization: A possible therapy for acute myocardial infarction. Circulation 60:241, 1979.

Ratshin, R.A., Rackley, C.E., and Russell, R.O., Jr.: Hemodynamic evaluation of left ventricular function in shock

complicating myocardial infarction. Circulation 45:127, 1972.
Redwood, D.R., Smith, E.R., and Epstein, S.E.: Coronary artery occlusion in the conscious dog: Effects of alterations in heart rate and arterial pressure of the degree of myocardial ischemia. Circulation 46:323, 1972.
Reimer, K.A., Rasmussen, M.M., and Jennings, R.B.: Reduction by propranolol of myocardial necrosis following temporary coronary artery occlusion in dogs. Circ. Res. 33:353, 1973.
Resnekov, L.: Invited article: The intermediate coronary care unit: A stage in continued coronary care. Br. Heart J. 39:357, 1977.
Resnekov, L., and Lipp, H.: Pacemaking and acute myocardial infarction. Prog. Cardiovasc. Dis. 14:475, 1972.
Roberts, R., Gowda, K.S., Ludbrook, P.A., et al.: Specificity of elevated serum MB creatine phosphokinase activity in the diagnosis of acute myocardial infarction. Am. J. Cardiol. 36:433, 1975a.
Roberts, R., Henry, P.D., and Sobel, B.E.: An improved basis for enzymatic estimation of infarct size. Circulation 52:743, 1975b.
Rogers, W.J., Mantle, J.A., McDaniel, H.G., et al.: Prospective randomized trial of glucose-insulin-potassium in acute myocardial infarction. Circulation (Suppl. II)60:165, 1979.
Rotman, M., Wagner, G.S., and Wallace, A.G.P.: Bradyarrhythmias in acute myocardial infarction. Circulation 45:703, 1972.
Russell, R.O., Jr., and Rackley, C.E.: *Hemodynamic Monitoring in a Coronary Intensive Care Unit*. Futura, Mount Kisko, NY, 1974.
Sasahara, A.A.: Current problems in pulmonary embolism: Introduction. Prog. Cardiovasc. Dis. 17:161, 1974.
Sasahara, A.A., Sonnenblick, E.H., and Lesch, M.: *Pulmonary Emboli*. Grune & Stratton, New York, 1975.
Scheidt, S., et al.: Intra-aortic balloon counterpulsation in cardiogenic shock: Report of a cooperative clinical trial. N. Engl. J. Med. 288:979, 1973.
Sobel, B.E.: The cardiac care unit: 1974. In *The Myocardium: Failure and Infarction*, edited by E. Braunwald. H.P. Publishing Co., New York, 1974.
Spodick, D.H.: *Pericardial Diseases*. F.A. Davis, Philadelphia, 1976.
Strauss, H.W., Pitt, B., and Everette, J.A., Jr. (Eds.): *Cardiovascular Nuclear Medicine*. C.V. Mosby, St. Louis, 1974.
Sulfinpyrazone in the prevention of cardiac death after myocardial infarction: The anturane reinfarction trial. N. Engl. J. Med. 298:289, 1978.
Thompson, J.E.: Acute peripheral arterial occlusion. N. Engl. J. Med. 290:950, 1974.
Thornley, P.E., and Turner, R.W.D.: Rapid mobilization after acute myocardial infarction: First step in rehabilitation and secondary prevention. Br. Heart J. 39:471, 1977.
VanTassel, R.A., and Edwards, J.E.: Rupture of heart complicating myocardial infarction: Analysis of 40 cases including nine examples of left ventricular false aneurysm. Chest 61:104, 1972.
Wessler, S. Prevention of venous thromboembolism by low-dose heparin. Mod. Concepts Cardiovasc. Dis. 45:105, 1976.

EPILOGUE

Cultivating a Climate of Research. The Wangensteen* System, 1930–1967

RICHARD C. LILLEHEI

Long years ago I resolved that as an after dinner speaker I would not show slides to a group which had already suffered a surfeit of the same during the immediately preceding hours and I would also be brief.

But what to add to that which this distinguished group has already provided? The program is already overflowing with new data and ideas; this area, I believe, is best left to the younger investigators who have usually done the work. Moreover, my long time friend and colleague from the University of Minnesota of 25 years ago, Max

---

* Dr. Wangensteen died suddenly on January 13, 1981. He was in his 83rd year. Characteristically, on January 12th, he spent a full day correcting galley proofs of a new book. Thus ended a grand life.

Harry Weil, has already given you an "overview" of shock studies.

What was the common denominator at the University of Minnesota in the 1950s when C. W. Lillehei, F. John Lewis, Norman Shumway, Alan Thal, Lloyd MacClean, Hal Weil, Lerner Hinshaw and others were drawn together? It was, I believe, a climate where the spirit of inquiry and a love of learning reigned supreme; a climate established by Owen Wangensteen in Surgery, Maurice Visscher in Physiology, and Wesley Spink in Internal Medicine.

I have noted in the past decade or so that interest in research has declined while the primary emphasis has been on more adequate distribution of medical care with accentuation of the need for a large increase in medical graduates. With this, I believe has come a decline in new advances which medicine, and the study of shock in particular, greatly needs. This decline is due as much to a decrease in the quality of our teachers as to the paucity of research money.

The history of the advance in any discipline is the story of individuals of imagination and accomplishment who left their mark upon its development. In the hope that a brief description of Dr. Wangensteen's imagination and accomplishments might be an inspiration for some of you or your students, vicariously, as it was for me directly, I will recount some of the highlights of the Wangensteen years.

When we recognize someone as unusually good in a profession or skill, we look for ways to repeat this experience or tradition. What is tradition, if not the handing down of statements, beliefs, legends, and customs from generation to generation by word of mouth or by practice?

To define the Wangensteen tradition, we have to define more than the man and include the time and place as well. When Dr. Wangensteen took over as Chief of the Department of Surgery at the University of Minnesota in 1930, there were no full-time men. The department was run by part-timers who, for the most part, donated their time from busy downtown practices. The School of Medicine's part-timers were largely an undistinguished lot. The only scholars of note were mostly in the basic sciences and these could probably be counted on one hand. Before Dr. Wangensteen was offered the chair, a number of well known surgeons, mainly from the East, had looked at the position and had expressed, in one way or another, the feeling of Dr. Mont Reid, a Halsted-trained man: "There is nothing here and there never will be."

So much for the place, let's look at the time. The Mayo brothers in Rochester reigned supreme as surgical technicians, and the Mayo Clinic was the mecca for surgeons from the world around. In the East, the influence of Halsted was still paramount, although he had died 8 years previously. The surgical principles advanced by the Mayos, Halsted, and various distinguished European surgeons had greatly decreased the mortality from most abdominal surgical procedures, and, except for the availability of antibiotics, we have not greatly improved on these results since that time. But something was lacking and clinical surgery seemed to be "stalled." The reason for this was largely due to a preoccupation with surgical technique, to the virtual exclusion of *experimental surgery*. New concepts and new approaches to the surgical treatment of disease would come only very slowly, if at all, without the use of the experimental method. A modern day counterpart might be the specialties of cardiology and neurosurgery. They have only recently discovered the experimental laboratory, which probably explains why progress has been so slow in these areas.

Now to the man, Owen Wangensteen. In 1930 he was 31 when he became the Chairman of the Department of Surgery. Raised on a farm in the northwest corner of Minnesota, he had an early experience in caring for farm animals, which he believed was the beginning of his interest in medicine. All of his undergraduate education and most of his medical training took place at the University of Minnesota. He did spend a year at the Mayo Clinic after graduation and later, after his surgical training at Minnesota, a brief period in Europe; but these interludes only sharpened his desire to return to the University of Minnesota.

Dr. Wangensteen came to this post with unusual intellectual abilities, untainted by tradition, unspoiled by background, unsophisticated, a relative greenhorn who had no connection with the reigning surgical schools which were centered almost exclusively east of the Mississippi. He had an almost abnormal singlemindedness; an ability to neglect everything for that "greatest of paymaster," opportunity, and he knew that work is still the best way to get the better of life.

The growing number of residents and young staff members over the ensuing years became his family. He was our surrogate father, and we his children. A father figure with enough fallibilities to keep him human, but never enough to address him by any other term but Dr. Wangensteen, Sir, or "The Chief." Even now in private conversation most of us have never used any other terms.

He liked to describe himself as a type of Gunga Din, the regimental water carrier, administering to the needs of his staff, but I think my colleague Aldo Castenada, now chief of cardiovascular surgery at the Children's Hospital in Boston, has a better description. He called him a "player-coach." His methods would seem, in retrospect, rather simple. Perhaps this is why they worked so well.

There was certain naiveté that he instilled in all of us—a feeling that every facet of surgery could be challenged—and the fact that the authorities had said something couldn't be done often had little more factual basis than a statement of Galen. A favorite phrase occurred over and over in his conversations: "We should not genuflect to the authorities." He combined this naiveté with a tolerance for a wide variety of personalities and ideas. No idea was too far afield to test in the experimental laboratory. Like Thomas Edison, he knew that there was always a better way, if we could just find it.

The department was never comfortable nor complacent. In most areas, two, three, and sometimes four different individuals were working on the same subject, each sure that he had Dr. Wangensteen's full support, and each did. This resulted in intense competition and is best illustrated in the development of cardiac surgery at the University of Minnesota and in the study of shock.

I should not neglect the great influence of others in the medical school on the Department of Surgery. Foremost was Maurice Visscher, who came to the University of Minnesota as Professor of Physiology in 1936. For nearly 30 years Dr. Wangensteen and Dr. Visscher cooperated in joint studies and in training of the surgical residents. Almost without exception those members of the Department of Surgery who made significant contributions have the mark and influence of Dr. Visscher.

At this same time, Dr. Wesley Spink in the Department of Internal Medicine was carrying on an active research program which also attracted many of our best surgical residents and physiologists, for example, Drs. MacClean, Hinshaw, Waisbren, and Weil.

I should say something about the various personalities that we had in the department. Performance and consecutiveness were Dr. Wangensteen's measure of the man. He cared little about background or appearance, or whether one was a good old boy or a regular fellow—probably because he wasn't one himself. Compatibility was not a prerequisite for success in this department. Perhaps just the opposite was true, for Dr. Wangensteen was always an outsider himself. Not a bad position to be in since it is often easier to get perspective from the periphery than from the center of a group.

His peers in surgery only reluctantly recognized him initially because he wasn't one of them. He kept talking about dog cages instead of hospital beds. Eventually, however, he won the approval of almost all of them. Perhaps the best example of this was his election to the Presidency of the American College of Surgeons—a post which usually involved thousands of tedious hours on committees and boards as a prerequisite. These were tasks that Dr. Wangensteen rarely did, having spent his time in other ways to improve the art and science of surgery.

I must emphasize that during these golden years, it was not just his own performance but that of his whole department which shone like a beacon out of Minneapolis. He had the type of ego which grew in proportion to the triumphs of his surgical family. This is really the essence of his success; his ability to keep good men around him, a characteristic of only a few in medicine, or in any other field.

A number of contemporaries of Dr. Wangensteen's have retired in recent years who exemplify just the opposite. I won't mention names, but you could travel to numerous university surgical centers in recent years and find that when the *man* retired, there was nothing left, no tradition, no school, and no "surgical descendants" of any stature. Gifted young men in these departments had long since been encouraged to go elsewhere so the spotlight would shine on the chairman without pause. But with the retirement of such chairmen, "the name died before the man";[†] not so with Dr. Wangensteen.

[†] From "To an Athlete Dying Young," by A. E. Housman.

One of the criticisms of the Wangensteen program was the wide range of qualities of its graduates. Dr. Wangensteen was responsible for more of the best than any other surgeon in this country. There were also a few at the other end of the scale. This was the result of a program which was never the same for any resident. It might take less than 3 years or nearly 10, depending on the man. Flexibility was the cornerstone of the program. Such a program would never satisfy most department heads in this or any other country. Uniformity is too often their cornerstone. Rigidity may ensure a uniform end product, but it will never give the best! In such an environment, it is no accident that open heart surgery or the use of vasodilators and steroids for treating shock began in Minneapolis, rather than in Boston, New York, Philadelphia, Chicago, or Rochester.

Some of our most imaginative surgeons weren't always the most skillful in the operating room. Technical skills can be learned but an inquiring mind is developed at the mother's knee and is not easily taught. Such a mind can only be carefully nurtured and given opportunity for expansion. Dr. Wangensteen provided this opportunity in abundance. In this respect, no country has a surplus of such minds. Hence, the new rule that foreign medical graduates can now come for only two years of training is a harbinger of eventual decline. A department like Dr. Wangensteen's, a United Nations in microcosm, is now no longer possible.

The characteristics of the Wangensteen tradition would seem to be *tolerance* and *flexibility*—would unorthodoxy cover both? In modern surgery, there are few who can match Dr. Wangensteen and his school. Drs. John Hunter, Theodore Billroth, and probably Halsted most readily come to mind, but in my opinion, Hunter is his peer.

I have defined the tradition as I see it, but what can we do to perpetuate it? Shall we use the vehicle of societies? Do these perpetuate the tradition? Do they encourage new ideas? Can we recreate a Wangensteen type of surgical department? Can we recreate the age of Pericles, the age of Enlightment of the 18th century in Europe with its Beethoven, Mozart, and Goethe or in the United States with Franklin, Jefferson, Hamilton, and Washington? Can we recreate a Vienna of the 1880s or a Rochester, Minnesota in the early 20th century? These ages can no more be reproduced than we can create another Hunter, Billroth, or Wangensteen. The time, the place, the man will never again combine in the identical chemistry. Lightening may strike twice in the same place but these eras do not!

If we can't recreate the situation or the man, what can we perpetuate? Obviously, the ideas that made the era. The feeling that no area of medicine is immune to change. The ability of the old to give way graciously to the young. The knowledge that immortality is gained only by passing our ideas and knowledge on to others.

If we can do this, then at some other time, at some other place, and under the guidance of someone like Dr. Wangensteen, another era of great progress will occur. Yet, the ideas behind this new era will be the same as they have been since the beginning of time, the encouragement of young minds to develop to their ultimate in an environment of encouragement and tolerance.

It may seem that I have delivered an eulogy to this great man—but let me hasten to tell you that he is alive and well. In his 80s, he is the embodiment of one of the teachings of Leroy, Robert "Satchel" Page who asked, "How old would you be if you didn't know how old you were?"

Dr. Wangensteen truly does not know how old he is. The best example I can cite is the publication of the book, *The Rise of Surgery—From Empiric Craft to Scientific Disciple*, by Dr. Wangensteen and his wife, Sally Wangensteen. It is the testament of a way of life of this great teacher; we are desparately in need of such men and women at this time as in all times. Perhaps this brief account of the life of a man who imparted so much to others will be of aid to some readers of this book; I hope so!

Ecclesiastes said, "A good life has its number of days, but a good name can triumph forever."

Index

Acid-base balance, correction, future treatment of shock, 504
Adenosine and creatine phosphate, treatment of shock, 211
Adenosine monophosphate, cyclic
  levels during shock, 207
  treatment of shock, 211
Adenosine triphosphatase, sodium-potassium, 120
Adenosine triphosphate
  cellular transport, shock, liver, 129
  transfusion therapy, 447
  treatment of shock, 201, 211
Adrenal cortical steroids, hemorrhagic shock and, 466
β-Adrenergic blockade, myocardial infarction and, 697
Adrenocorticotropic hormone, hemorrhagic shock and, 467–470
Afferent arteriolar vasoconstriction, acute renal failure and, 330
Ageing, cellular, 23
Airway
  control, 409
  head injury and, 603
  obstruction, control during resuscitation, 414
Alveolar wall, pathobiology of, shock, lung, 358–370
Alveoli, integrity, lung, 389
Amino acids
  plasma level, multiple systems organ failure, 202
  sepsis, 201
Aminoglycosides, septic shock treatment, 488
Ammonia, liver, shock, 290
Anaerobiosis, 3, 66
Angina, postinfarction, 693
Angiotensin I, 166
Angiotensin II, 155, 167
Angiotensin III, 155, 168
Angiotensins
  cardiovascular actions, 166
  formation, 166
  shock-inducing actions, 169
Anoxia
  cardiac output, 156
  microcirculation and, 155
Anoxic perfusion, beating heart, 661
Antibiotics, septic shock treatment, 410, 485–490
Anticoagulants, myocardial infarction, 688
Arterioles, microcirculation in shock, 181
Astrocytes, ischemia, 649
Atalactasis, lung, 156
Atrial arrhythmias, myocardial infarction, 689
Atrial fibrillation, myocardial infarction, 690
Axis cylinders, ischemia, 649
Azotemia, acute renal failure and, 326

Bacteremia
  bacterial flora in, 483
  prognostic factors, 484
  sources of infection, 484
Biogenic amines, spinal cord injury and, 620
Bleeding
  intracranial extracerebral, 558
  treatment of underlying process, 449, 502
Blood
  artificial, 430

components, ischemia, 665
oxygen content, hyperbaric therapy, 523
oxygen transport, 509
plasma substitutes and, 429
preservative solutions, hemorrhagic shock transfusion therapy, 448
rheology, 410
  hypovolemic shock, 454
stored
  acid base, 449
  adenine, 450
  ammonia, 449
  chemical changes in, 448
  citrate toxicity, 449
  coagulation, 448
  hemorrhagic shock and, 447
  hypothermia, 449
  microaggregates, 450
  potassium, 449
synthetic, future treatment of shock, 507
urea nitrogen, liver, shock, 290
volume, hemorrhagic shock, 203
Blood-brain barrier, normal and abnormal, 555, 570
Blood flow
  cerebral, 578
    changes, 583
    regulation, 579
  optimal
    characteristics, 158
    factors jeopardizing, 160
  redistribution of, ischemia and shock, 155, 165
  shock, 201
  spinal cord injury, 556, 618
Blood gas
  arterial
    myocardial infarction, 686
    treatment of shock, 501
  liver, shock, 287
Blood pressure, shock and, lung, 359
Blood vessels, gastric, toxic rupture of, shock, 307
Bradykinin, lung injury and, 402
Brain
  contusions, 559, 562
  displacement, ischemia, 592
  generalized swelling, 555, 565
  gray matter, necroses, 566
  hemorrhage, type of stroke, 656
  ischemic injury, 651
  wound or laceration, 558, 561
Bundle branch, block, infarction, 691
Burns, lung injury and, 396

Calcium
  acute cell injury and, 30
  calmodulin and, 104
  cell, regulation, 4
  concentration
    acute renal failure, 349
    during shock, 208
  damaging effects of, 28
  dependent reactions, 96
  efflux, plasma membrane, 99
  endoplasmic reticulum transport, 100
  influx, plasma membrane, 98
  ionized, control, 155
  ion shift, ischemia, 671
  metabolism, 3

mitochondrial transport, 101
paradox, ischemia, 667
sarcoplasmic reticulum transport, 100
sodium-induced release, 103
translocation, ischemia, 667
transport and regulation, cell membrane, 95–104
Calcium-activated phospholipases, ischemia, 668
Calmodulin, calcium, 104
Capacitance system, cardiac output and, 156
Capillaries
  cardiac output and, 156
  deficient flow, shock, 186
  endothelial/epithelial cell swelling, acute renal failure and, 329
  factors controlling fluid flux, 184
  increased permeability, 155
  ischemia, 649
  leakage, 156
  microcirculation in shock, 182
  permeability, ischemia and shock, 165
Carbenicillin, septic shock treatment, 489
Carbohydrate metabolism, shock, 207
Carbon monoxide
  fire casualties, 202
  laboratory diagnosis, 273
  pathology and pathophysiology, 202, 270
  poisoning
    central nervous system, 202
    hyperbaric oxygenation in, 525
    myocardium, 202
  toxicity, 271
  treatment, 273
Cardiac arrest
  exsanguination, 422
  resuscitation, 411
Cardiac output
  determination, 502
  low, shock, 439
Cardiogenic shock
  infarction and, 692
  treatment, 499, 503
Cardioplegic models
  awake dog, 664
  papillary muscle, perfused septum and slices, 663
  reperfusion, 664
  single cell, 663
Cardiopulmonary-cerebral resuscitation, 413
Cardiopulmonary failure, multiple systems organ failure, 202
Cardiopulmonary resuscitation, 409
  closed chest, 419
  open chest, 420
Cardioscopes, treatment of shock, 501
Cardiovascular decompensation, mediators and, 156
Catabolic hormones, future treatment of shock, 505
Catecholamine, stress phase, 3, 60, 62
Catheter
  central venous insertion, 425
  peripheral venous insertion, 425
  pulmonary artery, 410, 425
  systemic artery, 425
Cell
  death, multiple systems organ failure, 202
  energy metabolism, shock, 208
  flow distribution, shock, 455

705

Cell—*continued*
  function, shock, 209
  metabolism, regulation, 121
  organelles, ischemia, 666
  regeneration, failure during, 673
  response, qualitative dynamics, 47
  washout process, failure during, 673
Cell-mediated immunity, endotoxic shock, 228
Cell volume
  defective regulation, cell injury and, 138
  regulation, 121, 135
    ion transport and, 133
    shock, liver, 128, 129
Cellular injury
  acute lethal, 6
    direct attack on membrane, 16
    irreversible phase, 6
    ischemia, 6
    point-of-no-return, 6
    recovery, 16
    reversible phase, 6
  behavior of cells following, 3
  calcium, 6, 25
  chronic, 17
    ageing, 23
    atrophy, 22
    fatty metamorphosis, 17
    hypertrophy, 21
    lysosome formation, 19
    neoplastic transformation, 23
  dynamics of cell response to, 3, 47
  heart
    models, 658
    reversible and irreversible, 658
  hypothesis of changes, 40
  ion shifts, 23
  lytic enzymes and, 659
  metabolic responses, 3
  no-reflow phenomenon, 143
  organelle changes, 30
    cell junctions, 33
    cell membrane, 30
    endoplasmic reticulum, 35
    lysosomes, 36
    membrane constituents, 32
    mitochondria, 38
    nucleus, 38
    peroxisomes, 38
    secretory granules, 36
  origin of disease, 6
  stability aspects, 52
  stages of change, 3, 8
  swelling and volume regulation, 132, 138
  system aspects, 48
  therapeutic interventions and, 4, 5
  vascular mediators and, 155
Central nervous system
  ischemia, 555
  responses, after head injury, 603
  resuscitation, 409
  tissue insults, 625
  trauma, management of, 611
Central venous pressure
  treatment of flow-directed pulmonary artery catheter, 502
  treatment of shock, 501
Cephalosporins, septic shock treatment, 490
Cerebral metabolism
  blood flow and, 578
  depression, 582
  energy, 578
  hypoxemia effects on, 578

Cerebrospinal fluid
  changes, ischemia, 591
  leakage, 610
Cerebrovascular reactivity
  dysautoregulation, 581
  impaired chemical regulation, 582
  intracerebral steals, 582
Circulatory shock, 454
Clotting factors, shock, 189
Coagulation, 188
  defect, 189
  future treatment of shock, 505
  liver, shock, 287
Colitis, pseudomembranous, septic shock, 304
Colloid
  concentration levels, shock, 410, 460
  future treatment of shock, 504
  plasma substitutes, 427
Colloid osmotic pressure, hypovolemic shock, 455
Coma, resuscitation, 411
Congestive heart failure, myocardial infarction and, 692
Contractile filaments, 155
Coronary arteries
  ischemia, 665
  narrowing, ischemia, 643, 681–683
  spasm, myocardial infarction and, 695
Coronary atherosclerosis, myocardial infarction and, 695
Coronary care unit, myocardial infarction, 685
Coronary obstruction, 695
Coronary veins, ischemia, 665
Corticosteroids
  adrenal, future treatment of shock, 505
  drug treatment with, shock, 431
  hemorrhagic shock, 155, 410
    pharmacologic dosages, 468–470
    treatment, 465–477
Creatine kinase, myocardial infarction measurement, 696
Crystalloids, future treatment of shock, 504
Cyanide
  fire casualties, 202
  laboratory diagnosis, 276
  metabolism and treatment, 274
  pathology and pathophysiology, 202, 270, 275
  poisoning, 202
    hyperbaric oxygenation in, 525
  toxicity, 274
Cytoplasm, ionized calcium in, 98
Cytoskeleton, microcirculation and, 155
Cytosol, ischemia, 669

Desoxycorticosterone, hemorrhagic shock and, 466
Dexamethasone, hemorrhagic shock and, 469
Dextran, plasma substitute, 428
Dextrose, plasma substitute, 426
Dialysis, acute renal failure treatment, 353
2,3-Diphosphoglycerate, hemorrhagic shock and, 450
Disseminated intravascular coagulation, 156, 480
  factors promoting, 186
  microinfarction of tissues, 190
  syndromes of
    diagnosis, 193
    treatment, 194
Diuretics, acute renal failure treatment, 342
Duodenum, shock and, 304

Edema
  biochemical aspects of formation, 575
  cerebral, 555, 570
  fluid
    composition of, 572
    spread of, 575
  hydrostatic, 374
  ischemia effects, 586
  localized, 566
  mechanisms of resolution, 576
  morphological aspects of formation, 574
  physiological aspects of formation, 573
  pulmonary, 283, 358, 368, 382, 384
  vasogenic, 571, 576
Edematous swelling, 566
Efferent arteriolar dilatation, acute renal failure and, 330
Electrocardiogram, myocardial infarction, 686
Electrolytes, liver, shock, 289
Electrolyte solution, plasma substitute, 426
Electron microscopy
  liver, shock, 294
  pancreas, 310
Endoplasmic reticulum, 35
  calcium transport, 100
Endothelium
  anoxia effects, 155
  lung, shock and, 359
  septic and endotoxic shock effects, 155
Endotoxemia
  gluconeogenesis and, 410
  lung injury and, 396
  mitochondrial function, 89
Endotoxic shock
  endothelium and, 155
  hemodynamic responses, 222
  history, 219
  septic shock and, 220
Endotoxin
  DIC and, 156
  energy charge changes, 75
Energy charge, endotoxin and, 75
Energy metabolism
  cell, shock, 208
  comparative, tissues, 66
  hemorrhagic shock and, 4
  septic shock and, 4
  shock and, 74–82
Energy pathway, shocked cells, 74
Enzymes, liver, shock, 291
Epinephrine, chemical effects on stress, 61
Epithelium, lung, necrosis, 362
Esotropy, 19
Exotropy, 19
Exsanguination, cardiac arrest, 422
Extracellular space, normal and abnormal, 555, 572

Fat metabolism, shock, 207
Fatty acid, transport, ischemia, 667
F emulsion, 509, 510
Fever, multiple systems organ failure, 202
Fibrinolysis
  diffuse gastric hemorrhage, 307
  lung, shock, 359
Fibrosis, shock-induced, lung, 364
Fick equation, rationale for transfusion, 447
Flow-directed pulmonary artery catheter, 410
Fluid
  balance, acute renal failure, 346
  exchange, lung, 373

Index

Fluorocarbons
  emulsions
    oxygen transport, 508
    treatment of shock, 499, 504, 520
Fluosol-DA, composition of, 514

Gas, solubility of, 508
Gastric hemorrhage
  shock and, 307
  toxic rupture of blood vessels, 307
Gastrointestinal systemic changes, spinal cord injury and, 637
Gastrointestinal tract, shock, ischemia and hypoxemia, 301
Genitourinary systemic changes, spinal cord injury and, 637
Glomerular capillary hydrostatic pressure, acute renal failure and, 329
Glomerular filtration, renal failure and, 282, 326, 327
Glomerular permeability, acute renal failure and, 329
Glucocorticoids
  cell survival uses, 4
  hemorrhagic shock and, 468–470, 474–476
Gluconeogenesis
  endotoxemia and, 410
  sepsis, 201
Glucose
  plasma level, multiple systems organ failure, 202
  transport, ischemia, 667
  treatment of shock, 211
Glucose-insulin-potassium
  myocardial infarction and, 698
  treatment of shock, 211
Golgi apparatus, 35
Granulocytes
  sticking, shock, lung, 359
  transfusion
    septic shock and, 491
    shock, 410

Head injury
  circulatory alterations, 565
  cutaneous, 558
  diagnostic studies, 604
  evaluation, 556, 602
  fluid management, 604
  gunshot wound, 609
  hyperbaric oxygenation in, 524
  indirect circulatory necroses, 559, 565
  intracranial extracerebral bleeding, 558
  intracranial primary lesions, 559
  medical therapy, 605
  neurological examination, 603, 604
  pathology of, 555, 558–568
  pathophysiology, 555
  post-traumatic, 570
  post-traumatic internal hydrocephalus, 568
  pretraumatic alterations, 558
  primary traumatic lesions, 558
  problems after, 610
  surgical therapy, 606
  treatment, 601–612
  vital signs and associated injuries, 603
Heart
  cellular injury and, 658
  ischemia, structural components, 664
  monitoring in septic shock, 481
Hematology, liver, shock, 287

Hematoma
  epidural, acute, 606
  extradural, 559
  intracerebral, 608
  intraventricular, 561
  subarachnoid hemorrhage and, 561
  subdural, 560
    acute, 607
    chronic, 610
Hemoblood, future treatment of shock, 507
Hemodilution, treatment, hypovolemic shock, 454–463
Hemoglobin, future treatment of shock, 504
Hemorrhage
  control, 409
    external, 423
    internal, 423
  DIC and, 156
  subarachnoid, brain, 561
Hemorrhagic shock, 4, 409
  cardiorespiratory pattern during early period, 440–442
  corticosteroid treatment, 465–477
  definition, 203
  energy metabolism and, 80
  factors, 201
  gastrointestinal tract disorders and, 301
  glucocorticoid effects, 476
  hyperbaric oxygenation in, 524
  liver, model, 299
  lung injury and, 395
  pancreas, 322, 323
  pathophysiology and therapy, 201, 439–446
  resuscitation, 411
  transfusion therapy, 409, 447–452
  treatment, 211
Histamine
  lung injury and, 399
  shock and, 155
Hormonal alterations, shock, 206
Hormonal manipulation, future treatment of shock, 505
Hormones, stress and, 60
Hyaluronidase, myocardial infarction and, 698
Hydrocephalus, post-traumatic, 568, 610, 611
Hydrocortisone, hemorrhagic shock and, 467
Hydrostatic edema, 374
Hyperbaric oxygen therapy, 499, 522–526
  applications, 523
  barometric pressure, 522
  carbon monoxide poisoning, 525
  cyanide poisoning, 525
  head injury, 524
  myocardial infarction, 525
  pressure unit comparison, 523
  spinal cord injury, 524
  stroke, 525
Hyperbilirubinemia, multiple systems organ failure, 202
Hypercoagulability, 188
Hyperemia, cerebral, 585
Hyperemic swelling, 565
Hyperparic oxygen therapy
  carbon monoxide poisoning, 202
  cyanide poisoning, 202
Hypertension, intracranial, consequences of, 591
Hypertrophy, 21
Hypoalbuminemia, multiple systems organ failure, 202
Hypoperfusion, liver, 286

Hypothermia, future treatment of shock, 505
Hypovolemia
  compensations, 205
  treatment, 502
Hypovolemic infarction, shock syndromes and, 439
Hypovolemic shock
  energy metabolism and, 80
  mathematical modeling, 536, 540
  pancreas, 322, 323
  plasma expanders and hemodilution as treatment, 454–463
  plasma lipase levels, pancreas, 319
Hypoxemia
  effect on cerebral metabolism, 578
  gastrointestinal tract and, 301
Hypoxia
  acute, mitochondrial adaptation, 91
  cardiac output and, 156
  cell, blood flow in, 201
  cell volume regulation and, 135
  chronic, mitochondrial adaptation, 91
  sublethal tissue, 90

Infection, septic shock, 482–493
Infusion strategies
  central venous catheter insertion, 425
  deliberate hemodilution, 426
  peripheral venous catheter insertion, 425
  pulmonary artery catheterization, 410, 425
  systemic artery catheterization, 425
Inotropic drugs, shock, 431
Insulin
  effects on stress, 60, 62
  future treatment of shock, 505
Intestines, shock and, 303
Intracranial pressure
  changes, 587
  Cushing reflex, 556
  Glasgow coma scale, 556
  increased, 590
Intracranial volume, changes, 587
Ions
  altered movements, relationship to cellular injury, 3
  cell volume regulation and transport, 133
  defective regulation, 155
  gradients, resting potential and, 112
  membrane, transport alterations, 122
  shifts, 23, 201
    cellular, 132
  sodium and potassium, regulation of transport, 115
Ischemia, 6
  blood flow in, 201
  brain, 651
  cardiac output, 156
  causes, 646
  cell volume regulation and, 135
  central nervous system, 555
  cerebral, 643, 645
  complete, mitochondrial function, 84
  gastrointestinal tract and, 301
  global, cellular injury, 660
  incomplete, mitochondrial function, 84
  microcirculation and, 155
  microvasculature and blood components, 665
  mitochondrial metabolic response reversibility, 86
  myocardial, acute fatal, 643, 681–683
  myocardial cell, 664

Ischemia—continued
  other effects, 586
  progress and pathogenic mechanism, 666
  progressive cell deterioration, 210
  regional, cellular injury, 660
  regional or localized, 646
  renal failure and, 282
  reversibility mechanism, 671
  vascular mediators and, 155, 165

Ketone body, formation, sepsis, 201
Kidney, monitoring, septic shock, 481
Kidney failure
  acute
    fluid and electrolyte management, 346
    initial phase, 341
    maintenance phase, 346
    prevention, 341
    recovery phase, 354
    treatment, 341–354
  adenosine triphosphate and magnesium treatment, 201
  experimental theories, 325
  passive backleak, 326
  pathology of, 324–334
  shock and, 282
Kidney tubules
  acute renal failure and, 334
  proximal, reabsorption defect, 331
Krebs cycle intermediates, treatment of shock, 211

Lactate
  liver, shock, 290
  transport, ischemia, 667
Lidocaine, myocardial infarction, 688
Light microscopy
  liver, shock, 294
  pancreas, 310
Lipid, plasma level, multiple systems organ failure, 202
Lipolysis, lung, shock, 359
Liver
  cellular adenosine triphosphate and sodium-potassium, shock, 129
  cell volume regulation, shock, 128
  electrogenic sodium-potassium pump, 118
  hematology and coagulation, shock, 287
  hemodynamics, shock, 287
  membrane permeability, 118
  monitoring in septic shock, 481
  pathology, 285–299
  shock, morphology of, 294
  sodium-potassium ATPase, shock, 128
  sodium-potassium transport, 123
Lung
  alveolar integrity maintenance, 389
  atelectasis, 156
  expansion, positive end-expiratory pressure, 390
  fluid and solute exchange, shock, 373
  injury
    hemorrhagic shock and, 395
    mediators and modulators of, 396
  monitoring in septic shock, 481
  shock, 155, 156, 358–370
    pathology, 283
    reversibility, 365
Lysosomal enzymes
  lung injury and, 397

shock, 208, 283
Lysosomal hydrolase-myocardial depressant factor system, pharmacological modulation, 173, 176
Lysosomal hydrolases, 155
Lysosomes
  formation, 19
  ischemia, 668
Lytic enzymes
  ischemia, 668
  release, cellular destruction, 659

Macula densa, sodium-chloride concentration, 332
Magnesium, hemorrhagic shock treatment, 201
Mallory-Weiss syndrome
  microthrombosis and, 306
  shock, 305
Mannitol, acute renal failure treatment, 344
Mathematical models, 528–544
  construction of, 528
  hypovolemic shock, 536, 540
  respiratory, 530, 544
  variables and components, 538, 539
Medical registries
  data base definition, 546
  data input, 550
  data retrieval, 551
  design and principles for, 545–552
  errors, 548
  man-computer interaction, 550
  prototype example, 549
  purpose, 546
  user modifications, 551
Membrane
  biological, calcium interaction with, 96, 97
  calcium transport and regulation, 95–104
  damage, 5
  intracellular, calcium transport, 104
  lipid peroxidation, ischemia effects, 586
  permeability
    shock and, 201
    sodium and potassium, liver, 118
  plasma, calcium transport across, 98, 104
  transport system, sodium-potassium, 4, 112
Metabolic alterations, during shock, 208, 287
Metabolic control mechanisms, 155
Metabolic fuel-energy deficit, 247
Metabolic inhibition, cell volume regulation and, 135
Metabolic tissue acidosis, drug treatment, 430
Metabolism
  see also specific subject and site
  during shock, ischemia, anoxia, 67
    degradation of adenine nucleotides, 68
    gluconeogenesis, 70
    glycolysis, 70
    lipid, 71
    regulation, 67
  intermediary, 3, 66
  response to cellular injury, 3
Metabolites, liver, shock, 290
Metamorphosis, fatty, 17
Methylprednisolone, hemorrhagic shock and, 470, 475
Microcirculation
  alterations, 155
  biochemical techniques, 155
  microscopic techniques, 155
  principles of regulation, 185

safety factors, 184
shock, 181, 206
terminology, 155, 156
Microthrombi, lung, shock, 360
Microthrombosis, Mallory-Weiss syndrome, gastrointestinal tract, 306
Microtubules, 155
Microvasculature, ischemia, 665
Mitochondria
  adaptive response mechanism, 92
  calcium
    release, 103
    transport, 101
    uptake, 102
  damage, cell recovery and, 3, 4
  endotoxemia effects, 89
  ischemia, 86, 669
  phosphorylative activity, endotoxin and, 75
  shock effects, 84, 87
    protection against damage, 89
  swelling, multiple systems organ failure, 202
Mitral valve, regulation, infarction and, 693
Multiple systems organ failure, 202
  clinical syndrome, 254
  etiologic considerations, 266
  metabolic time course, 257
  physiologic time course, 255
  therapeutic considerations, 268
  time course correlations, 265
Myelin sheaths, ischemia, 649
Myocardial cells, ischemia, 664
Myocardial depressant factor, 155
  biological actions, 175
  cardiovascular actions, 175
  corticosteroids and, 473
  formation, 173
  pharmacologic prevention of antagonism, 175
Myocardial infarction
  acute, recognition and treatment, 689
  ambulation and recovery, 688
  cellular and subcellular changes, 658–674
  conditions mimicking, 688
  continued chest pain, 693
  coronary care unit, 685
  differential diagnosis, 687
  emergency room care, 684
  extension, 693
  hemodynamics, 660, 692
  hospital discharge, 689
  hyperbaric oxygenation in, 525
  laboratory findings, 686
  mechanical effects, 693
  methods of measurement, 696
  other tests, 686
  prehospital coronary case, 684
  prevention and treatment, new approaches, 695
  prognosis, 694
  rehabilitation, 694
  shock syndromes and, 439
  specific medications, 688
  therapy, 698
  treatment, 684–699
Myocardium, contractility, MDF effects, 156
Myoendothelial cell junctions, 155
Myogenic control mechanisms, 155
Myo-myo cell junctions, 155

Neoplastic transformation, 23

Index

Neurologic deficit, progressive or worsening, 647
Neuronal perikarya, ischemia and, 648
Neutropenic patient, prevention of infection, 493
Nicotinamide, treatment of shock, 211
Nitroglycerin, myocardial infarction and, 698

Nonelectrolytes, liver, shock, 289
No-reflow phenomenon, 143, 155
Nucleotide
  cyclic, role of, 5
  reduction, 3
Nutrition
  acute renal failure, 349
  future treatment of shock, 505

Oligemic swelling, 565
Oligodendrocytes, ischemia, 649
Oliguria, acute renal failure and, 326
Organ
  dysfunction, shock, 282
  function, shock, 209
Organelle, changes, 30
Oxidative metabolism, sepsis, 201
Oxygen
  availability, shock, liver, 287
  carriers, 430
    future treatment of shock, 504
  consumption
    plasma expanders and, 459
    survival and, 460
  solubility, 512
  toxicity, 526
Oxygenation, resuscitation and, 417

Pacemaker, prophylactic insertion, 691
Pancreas
  cell injury, 282
  shock effects, 309
  structure and function, 310
Peptides, 156
Peptide-steroid
  stress phase, 3, 60, 62
  hormonal effects, 63
Pericarditis, myocardial infarction, 693
Peripheral perfusion, monitoring in septic shock, 481
Peroxisomes, ischemia, 669
Phagocytic cells, endotoxic shock, 227
Phosphate, concentration, acute renal failure, 349
Phospholipases, 3
  ischemia, 671
Phospholipids, ischemia, 671
Plasma
  expanders
    hypovolemic shock treatment, 454–463
    metabolic responses to infusion, 459
    oxygen consumption after, 459
    rheologic and microcirculatory effects, 458
  lipase, hypovolemic shock effects, pancreas, 319
  membrane, ischemia, 666
  parenteral, substitutes for, 426
  substitutes, evaluation of, 462
  volume expansion, shock, 456
Platelet aggregation
  ischemia and shock, 165

myocardial infarction, 695
thromboxane-induced, 155, 156
Point-of-no-return, 5
Portal system, circulation, shock, 285
Positive end-expiratory pressure
  hemodynamic effects of, 391
  lung expansion, 390
Positive pressure ventilation, clinical use, 392
Potassium
  active, fluxes, 114
  balance, acute renal failure, 348
  intracellular, diffusibility of, 118
  ion regulation of transport, 115
Preinfarction β-blockade, myocardial infarction, 688
Pressure-volume relations, brain, 587
Prostacyclin, formation, 170
Prostacyclin-thromboxane system, 155, 169
Prostanoids, lung injury and, 402
Protein, intravascular loss, shock, 455
Protein metabolism, shock, 207
Pulmonary edema
  common causes, 384
  fibrosis and, shock, 368
  septic, 382
  shock, 283, 358
Pulmonary fibrosis
  pulmonary edema and, shock, 368
  shock-induced, 367
Pulmonary resistance, microcirculation in shock, 182
Pulmonary systemic changes, spinal cord injury and, 636

QRS mapping, myocardial infarction measurement, 696

Radionuclide ventriculography, myocardial infarction, 687, 697
Renin-angiotensin system, 155, 166
  axis, acute renal failure mediator, 331, 333
  cardiovascular effects, 170
  shock, 168
Resistance, high peripheral, shock, 439
Respiratory distress syndrome
  adult, 480
  permeability effect, 383
  sepsis, 283
  septic, pulmonary alveolarcapillary permeability and, 372–385
  treatment, 387–394, 393
Respiratory insufficiency, shock, 363
Respiratory therapy, shock and, lung, 156
Resting potential
  ion gradients and, 112
  sodium-potassium pump, 117
Restitutio ad integrum, in shock-induced pulmonary fibrosis, 367
Resuscitation
  cerebral, 432
  fluid, 423
  hemorrhagic shock, coma and cardiac arrest, 411–434
  shock-trauma victims, steps, 416
Reticuloendothelial function, mediators and, 156
Reticuloendothelial system, shock, 208

Sarcoplasmic reticulum
  calcium transport, 100

ischemia, 669
Schwartz-Mann phenomenon, 156
Secretory process, pancreatic, shock effects, 312
Seizures, post-traumatic, 610
Sepsis
  DIC and, 156
  lung injury and, 396
  pneumococcal, splenectomized patient, 493
Septic pulmonary edema, 382
Septic shock
  antibiotic treatment, 485
  as a cause of death, 201
  bacterial flora in, 483
  cardiorespiratory pattern during early period, 442
  cardiovascular adaptive response, 236
  clotting factors, 189
  diagnosis, 480
  endothelium and, 155
  endotoxic shock and, 220
  energy metabolism and, 80
  gastrointestinal tract disorders and, 301
  general treatment, 410, 479–481
  granulocyte transfusion, 491
  hemodynamic responses, 222
  human response to, 201, 235
  hyperbaric oxygenation in, 524
  infection, 482–493
  liver, model, 299
  mitochondrial function, 4, 87, 88
  monitoring, 481
  prognostic factors, 484
  renal failure and, 282
  sources of infection, 484
  stages, 4
  steroids and, 491, 492
Serotonin
  lung injury and, 401
  shock and, 155
Serum enzyme, measurements, myocardial infarction, 686
Shock
  see also specific type
  adenosine triphosphate and sodium-potassium, liver, 129
  cardiorespiratory variables, 440
  cell and organ function during, 122, 209
  cell volume regulation, liver, 128
  circulatory, membrane sodium-potassium transport, 112
  clinical examination, 501
  colloid concentration levels and, 460
  diagnosis, 501
  disseminated intravascular coagulation and, 189
  drug treatment, 409, 430
  duodenum, 304
  energy metabolism and, 74–82
  extravascular water accumulation, 458
  gastrointestinal tract and, 301
  hemodynamic disturbances, 204
  hepatic perfusion and function, 285
  hormonal alterations during, 206
  intestine, effect on, 303
  intravascular protein loss, 456
  laboratory procedures for diagnosis, 501
  lung, 155, 156, 358–370
    pathology, 283
    reversibility, 365
  mediators and, 156
  metabolic alterations, 208

Shock—*continued*
  microcirculation in, 181
  mitochondrial function, 84
  organ dysfunction and, 282
  oxygenation, 281
  physiologic defects of, 442
  plasma volume expansion, 456
  respiratory insufficiency, 363
  resuscitation, 409
  sequential stages, 439
  socioeconomic problems, 505
  sodium-potassium ATPase, liver, 128
  sodium-potassium transport, liver, 123
  stomach, 304
  strategies for future treatment, 499, 500
  systemic blood pressure and, 281
  therapeutic goals, 442
  therapy principles, 440, 444, 445
  tissue perfusion, 281
  treatment response, 501
  ultrastructural changes, 208
  vascular mediators in, 155, 165
  vasoactive agents in, 205
  vasoconstrictor effects, 166
Sinus tachycardia, myocardial infarction, 689
Skin, spinal cord injury and, 637
Skull
  defects, 610
  fracture, 558, 608
Sodium
  active, fluxes, 114
  balance, acute renal failure, 347
  intracellular, diffusibility of, 118
  ion regulation of transport, 115
Sodium bicarbonate, drug treatment with, shock, 431
Sodium-chloride, macula densa, 332
Sodium-potassium
  cellular, shock, liver, 129
  transport
    energetics, 118
    functional aspects of, 121
    membrane, circulatory shock, 112
    shock, liver, 123
Sodium-potassium ATPase, 120
  ischemia, 667
  shock, liver, 128
Sodium-potassium pump
  liver, 118
  resting potential and, 117
Solute exchange, lung, 373
Spinal cord injury, 613–622
  ancillary systemic changes, 556, 636
  biochemical derangements, 635
  biogenic amines, 620
  blood flow, 556, 618
  hemodynamic changes, 630
  hyperbaric oxygenation in, 524
  impact
    animal model of, 614
    lesions, 615
  mechanical insults, 625
  medical therapy, 555
  metabolic changes, 617
  mobility, 628
  neural tissue compression, 629
  surgical therapy, 555
  treatment, 555, 624–638
  ultrastructural observations, 617
Splenectomy, pneumococcal sepsis, prevention of, 493
Steroids, septic shock treatment, 491, 492
Stomach, shock and, 304
Stress
  hormonal nature of
    biphasic, 60
    chemical response to, 60
  hormonal phases
    catecholamine, 3, 60, 62
    peptide-steroid, 3, 60, 62, 63
Stroke
  brain hemorrhage, 656
  completed or nonprogressive, 647
  hyperbaric oxygenation in, 525
  pathophysiology, 643
Substrates, sources, 3
Suicide bag hypothesis, 37
Swelling, generalized, brain, 565

Technetium-99M pyrophosphate scintigrams, myocardial infarction measurement, 697
Thromboembolism, myocardial infarction and, 694
Thrombolytic therapy, myocardial infarction and, 698
Thrombosis, myocardial infarction and, 696
Thromboxane A_2, 155
Thromboxanes, formation, 170
Thrombus, formation, 155
Ticarcillin, septic shock treatment, 489
Tissues, microinfarction, disseminated intravascular coagulation and, 190
Transfusion, hemorrhagic shock treatment, 447
Transient neurologic defects, 647
Transmural vessels, 665
Transpiration, 514–516
Traumatic shock, 409
  cardiorespiratory pattern during early period, 442
  clotting factors, 189
  pathophysiology and therapy, 439–446
Tuboglomerular feedback mechanism, acute renal failure, 331

Urine, hourly testing, treatment of shock, 501

Vacuoles, autophagic, multiple systems organ failure, 202
Vascular mediators
  microcirculation and, 155
  shock and ischemia, 165
Vascular occlusion, 3
Vascular permeability, cell junction permeability, 155
Vascular resistance, reduction, 156
Vascular response, endotoxic shock, 228
Vascular volume, increase, 156
Vascular wall, 188
Vasculotoxins, shock and, 165
Vasoactive agents, shock, 205
Vasoconstriction, 155
  ischemia, 165
Vasoconstrictors
  drug treatment with, shock, 431
  shock and, 166
Vasodilators
  drug treatment with, shock, 431
  future treatment of shock, 505
Vasopressors, future treatment of shock, 505
Vasospasm, 155
Veins
  cardiac output and, 156
  microcirculation in shock, 181
Venous gases, mixed, shock, 502
Ventilation
  resuscitation and, 417
  resuscitation for shock, 503
Ventilation-oxygenation, 409
Ventricle, free wall rupture, infarction and, 693
Ventricular aneurysm, left, infarction and, 693
Ventricular arrhythmias, myocardial infarction, 690
Ventricular fibrillation, myocardial infarction, 690
Ventricular septum, rupture, myocardial infarction and, 693
Venules, cardiac output and, 156
Viability, transfusion therapy, hemorrhagic shock, 448

Wangensteen System, 701–704
Washout process, failure during, 673
Water
  extravascular accumulation, shock, 458
  shifts, cellular, 132